**Educational Principles and
Practice in Veterinary Medicine**

Educational Principles and Practice in Veterinary Medicine

Edited by

Katherine Fogelberg, *DVM, PhD (Science Education), MA (Educational Leadership)*
Virginia-Maryland College of Veterinary Medicine
Blacksburg, Virginia, USA

WILEY Blackwell

Library of Congress Cataloging-in-Publication Data
Names: Fogelberg, Katherine, editor.
Title: Educational principles and practice in veterinary medicine / edited
  by Katherine Fogelberg.
Description: Hoboken, New Jersey : Wiley-Blackwell, [2024] | Includes
  bibliographical references and index.
Identifiers: LCCN 2023023538 (print) | LCCN 2023023539 (ebook) | ISBN
  9781119852759 (hardback) | ISBN 9781119852766 (adobe pdf) | ISBN
  9781119852773 (epub)
Subjects: MESH: Education, Veterinary
Classification: LCC SF756.3 (print) | LCC SF756.3 (ebook) | NLM SF 756.3
  | DDC 636.0890711–dc23/eng/20231002
LC record available at https://lccn.loc.gov/2023023538
LC ebook record available at https://lccn.loc.gov/2023023539

Cover Design: Wiley
Cover Images: Courtesy of Melissa Stiles; Courtesy of Cassandra Cartmill

Set in 9.5/12.5pt STIXTwoText by Straive, Pondicherry, India

SKY10063514_122923

This book is dedicated to all my past and future students, and my fellow education nerd colleagues/friends.
It is also dedicated to my husband, John, who has always believed in me more than
I believed in myself and encouraged me to follow my dreams.

Contents

List of Contributors

Stacy L. Anderson
Lincoln Memorial University College of Veterinary
Medicine, Harrogate, TN
USA

Misty R. Bailey
College of Veterinary Medicine
University of Tennessee
Knoxville, TN
USA

Sarah Baillie
Bristol Veterinary School
Bristol, UK

Sarah A. Bell
University of Florida College of Veterinary Medicine
Gainesville, FL
USA

Freyca Calderon
Pennsylvania State University-Altoona
Altoona, PA
USA

Patricia Butterbrodt
Richard A. Gillespie College of Veterinary Medicine
Lincoln Memorial University
Harrogate, TN
USA

Meghan Byrnes
Virginia-Maryland College of Veterinary Medicine
Blacksburg, VA
USA

Sherry A. Clouser
University of Georgia College of Veterinary Medicine
Athens, GA
USA

Bobbi J. Conner
Virginia-Maryland College of Veterinary Medicine
Blacksburg, VA
USA

Kimberly S. Cook
Texas Christian University
Fort Worth, TX
USA

Peter Doolittle
Virginia Tech University, School of Education
Blacksburg, VA, USA

Ryane E. Englar
University of Arizona College of Veterinary Medicine
Oro Valley, AZ
USA

Katherine Fogelberg
Virginia-Maryland College of Veterinary Medicine
Blacksburg, VA
USA

Lawrence Garcia
University of Florida College of Veterinary Medicine
Gainesville, FL
USA

Philippa Gibbons
Texas Tech School of Veterinary Medicine
Amarillo, TX
USA

Lisa M. Greenhill
American Association of Veterinary Medical Colleges
Washington, DC
USA

Erik H. Hofmeister
College of Veterinary Medicine, Auburn University
Auburn, AL
USA

Gabriel Huddleston
Texas Christian University
Fort Worth, TX
USA

Julie A. Hunt
Richard A. Gillespie College of Veterinary Medicine
Lincoln Memorial University
Harrogate, TN
USA

Katrina Jolley
Richard A. Gillespie College of Veterinary Medicine
Lincoln Memorial University
Harrogate, TN
USA

Jill R. D. MacKay
The Royal (Dick) School of Veterinary Sciences
University of Edinburgh
Midlothian, Scotland
UK

Susan M. Matthew
Washington State University College of Veterinary
Medicine, Pullman, WA
USA

Lynda M.J. Miller
Richard A. Gillespie College of Veterinary Medicine,
Lincoln Memorial University
Harrogate, TN
USA

Donald B. Mills
Texas Christian University
Fort Worth, TX
USA

Karla O'Donald
Texas Christian University
Fort Worth, TX
USA

Sraavya M. Polisetti
American Association of Veterinary Medical Colleges
Washington, DC
USA

Malathi Raghavan
Purdue University College of Veterinary Medicine
West Lafayette, IN
USA

Shane M. Ryan
Medical University of South Carolina College of
Pharmacy
Charleston, SC
USA

Micha C. Simons
Virginia-Maryland College of Veterinary Medicine
Blacksburg, VA
USA

Matthew Schexnayder
IDEXX Laboratories, Inc.
Baton Rouge, LA
USA

Stephanie L. Shaver
University of Arizona College of Veterinary Medicine
Oro Valley, AZ
USA

Jo R. Smith
University of Georgia College of Veterinary Medicine
Athens, GA
USA

Dawn M. Spangler
Richard A. Gillespie College of Veterinary Medicine
Lincoln Memorial University
Harrogate, TN
USA

Myrah Stockdale
Campbell University College of Pharmacy and
Health Sciences
Lillington, NC
USA

Stephanie Thomovsky
Purdue College of Veterinary Medicine
West Lafayette, IN
USA

Ying Wang
Plano East Senior High School
Plano, TX
USA

Jesse Watson
North Carolina State University College of Veterinary
Medicine, Raleigh, NC
USA

Shelly Wu
Peter O'Donnell Jr. School of Public Health, University of
Texas Southwestern Medical Center, TX, USA

Kendall P. Young
American Association of Veterinary Medical Colleges
Washington, DC
USA

Preface

When you leave your soul to a teacher, it demands confidence – Svein Loeng, 2017
There is a wide gulf between what we want in education and what we do in education – Benjamin Bloom, 1972

I have fought long and hard to get the profession of veterinary medicine to recognize the value of learning about and understanding the discipline of education. I entered veterinary school at age 31, almost 10 years older than most of my classmates and far more seasoned in life than many of them, as well. I came into the program off active duty with the Army, with whom I had spent the previous decade after growing up in difficult circumstances. Also, both my parents were lifelong educators, and I rebelled against the idea that I would follow in their footsteps, mostly because I had loftier goals and a strong desire to be more financially stable than either of them!

However, my stint in the Army helped me realize that curriculum design was super cool and fun. It tapped into my creative brain while also challenging my logical brain, and it allowed me to dabble across a variety of content and ways of knowing. I figured this out during my last duty assignment, where I was provided the opportunity to update a 20-year-old curriculum and ensure our military medical providers fully understood how to care for themselves and their patients on the battlefield – the *current* battlefield, as at the time, terrorism was becoming the more prevalent form of warfare and the battlefield lines were increasingly blurring – there was no longer a "front line;" the child down the street or the woman coming toward you might just as well have a hand grenade or machine gun as the man wearing camouflage. This is how and where I earned my educational wings, so to speak, and I loved it.

Having been rejected from veterinary school twice prior to landing back on active duty as a commissioned officer (I had previously enlisted as a flute player, then was awarded a scholarship to complete my undergraduate degree and earn my commission), I was lucky to find education as another career option. I completed my Master's in Educational Leadership while on active duty, fully intending to go into education – likely teaching high school – when I left the military. But, as usual, life had other plans for me. My last boss in the Army convinced me to try for vet school again and, after agonizing through a correspondence course (yes – the preview to online learning was snail mail correspondence courses!) to complete the required second semester of physics, I found myself heading out of the Army and into veterinary school.

It was clear really quickly that veterinary school was going to be the biggest academic challenge I had faced to that point; the pace was fast and the content was variably challenging. But mostly it was the sheer volume of information being thrown at me and my classmates, starting on the first day. I was older and a step or two slower mentally than my classmates, too, which did not help things. But mostly I was frustrated by the less-than-ideal educational practices we experienced regularly in the classroom. Day after day we sat in lectures where faculty stood up and read – literally *read* – their PowerPoint slides to us. To be clear, I fully understood many were doing their best; that they probably had no training in how to teach. And I like to think I would have been just as frustrated had I not already earned a graduate degree in education, but it doesn't matter in the end. My graduate training certainly gave me specific reasons, rooted in theory and philosophy, for pointing out how inadequate the teaching was, but we have all experienced that poor teaching at the university level – and it is the majority of the time rather than the exception. My vet school experience was certainly *good enough*, but I felt strongly I could make things better. As I always say, veterinary school is hard. It should be hard and it will always be hard. It does not have to be made harder by crappy teaching.

I say all this to remind you that I came to veterinary education – and therefore this textbook – for a reason. From the beginning of my nontraditional career, I wanted to help veterinary educators be *better* – and perhaps more than better, maybe even exceptional. There are a few out there who are already exceptional, of course – I had a few myself and I do believe the group is growing. But those who are exceptional have had to work really hard to get there; they have learned by trial and error, through self-reflection and absorbing the good and bad of their own learning experiences. They have embraced the idea that education – of which teaching is a part – is a discipline in and of itself and come to understand that content knowledge and expertise is helpful, but it is not everything when it comes to educating. Educating, I often say, is the second hardest job in the world.

I have practiced in small animal general practice as a paid veterinarian for over 10 years – some full time, some as a locum. I have worked in some of the most prestigious zoos and wildlife conservation centers as a student and volunteer veterinarian, and I have been lucky to interact with and work on some of the most amazing animals known to humankind. I have mentored a number of new veterinarians and taught hundreds – perhaps thousands – of public health and human medical students. My career has been varied and vast and not what I ever could have anticipated, but it has surely provided me a strong foundation for doing what I do now as I get back to what I love – education. Not just the teaching part, which is one of the best bits, but the rest of it – theory, philosophy, research, curriculum, assessment, classroom management, and on and on. . .so many I have spoken with in veterinary education who are considering advanced training in the field are surprised that there are specialties, just as in veterinary medicine. I certainly don't know everything about every piece of the education pie, but I do know quite a bit about some of it.

What I do know I have written about in this textbook. What I know not quite enough about I have either found someone who does or taken up the Herculean task of immersing myself in it enough to make a passable attempt at conveying it to you (see: Chapters 1 and 2). For those sections I had no knowledge of, I asked a slew of contributing authors to cover; authors who come from a variety of backgrounds in both education and veterinary medicine; who have experience in K-12 classrooms, undergraduate, graduate, and professional classrooms. I have authors who have written numerous chapters for numerous books, and authors who are contributing to a textbook for the very first time. I have worked hard to provide comprehensive and inclusive content with a focus on veterinary education but with broad enough implications to be useful to those in other health professions and, potentially, even those in higher education programs. From theory to leadership, clinical teaching to technology in the classroom, and philosophy to the structure and function of higher education institutions in the United States, I suspect you will find something useful to you if you are in academia at all.

This is my first attempt at editing a textbook and I am so excited to have it completed and published. If I had known then what I know now, it might not ever have happened. But what I find, sometimes, is that diving into the deep end can be the best way to go. Living a life of fear is never going to be a productive one; live boldly and, while there are always risks of failure, there are also opportunities for huge rewards. In this textbook, I find huge reward – not only for the end product, which you hold in your hands, but also in the experience I have gained, the knowledge I have absorbed, and the relationships I have built during the process. You may not find this book as satisfying as I do, but I do hope you will find it useful and a great addition to your library all the same.

Happy reading!
Katherine

1

Educational Philosophy and Philosophers

Katherine Fogelberg, DVM, PhD (Science Education), MA (Educational Leadership)
Virginia-Maryland College of Veterinary Medicine, Blacksburg, VA, USA

Ying Wang, PhD (Curriculum studies)
Plano East Senior High School, Plano, TX, USA

Section 1: Introduction and Overview

Katherine Fogelberg and Ying Wang

What is philosophy? Merriam-Webster online defines philosophy in numerous ways, with several of the definitions relating specifically to teaching and learning, including "all learning exclusive of technical precepts and practical arts; the sciences and liberal arts exclusive of medicine, law, and theology (i.e., a doctor of philosophy); the 4-year college course of a major seminary; a discipline comprising as its core logic, aesthetics, ethics, metaphysics, and epistemology; pursuit of wisdom; a search for a general understanding of values and reality by chiefly speculative rather than observational means; the most basic beliefs, concepts, and attitudes of an individual or group" (accessed 8 March 2022). It appears the scholarly definition of philosophy is most likely a combination of the *pursuit of wisdom* and *a search for a general understanding of values and reality by chiefly speculative rather than observational means*. Philosophy, in general, is certainly a thinking person's discipline.

Philosophy is also, as you have read, far-reaching and broad in its aims. It asks the great questions of the universe, whether it is in relation to supreme deities or if particles exist that affect us daily even though we cannot see them. Philosophers ask questions that we often cannot answer; or that we can answer based only on our current knowledge and experiences, knowing that those answers will change and evolve alongside any expansion of knowledge and amassing of new experiences. And, as with anything that becomes too large, pieces have broken off over the ages to form new areas of philosophical thought and inquiry. One of those pieces is the philosophy of education.

Though mostly ignored in preservice teacher preparation programs and largely nonexistent within in-service teacher professional development, educational philosophies are foundational to educational policies and practices; put differently, we can always trace any decisions and practices in education to some philosophical roots. Unlike most educational courses that exemplify specific skills and what to do in concrete educational scenarios, educational philosophies offer answers to the question of why we do certain things and justify why we forgo other ones in education. This is one reason it is important and helpful for teachers to have a written or otherwise clearly articulated teaching philosophy; it is an opportunity for them to contemplate their beliefs about curriculum, their responsibilities and expectations of students, and how learning takes place in the classroom (Moss and Lee 2010). It is through developing a teaching philosophy that a teacher can better understand why they teach the way they do and how their practice is or is not reflective of their contemporaries. It can also illuminate for other readers the educator's understanding of knowledge, reality, pedagogy, curriculum, ethics, goals of teaching, and so on.

Different educational philosophies have come to prominence and then declined throughout history, sometimes overlapping each other. They have influenced educational policy-making processes and curriculum components across time and space and continue to do so today. Though not necessarily in opposition to each other, the demise of one educational philosophy is usually accompanied by the rise of another, one that criticizes the current educational philosophy and claims to mitigate, if not fully resolve, certain shortcomings of the one it looks to replace.

What drives these ebbs and flows of different philosophical stances? Most often it is moments in history where significant societal changes occurred; this will be further explored later in the chapter as discussions of the varying educational philosophies are presented in more depth.

Part 1: Philosophy of Education Defined

The word "philosophy" consists of two ancient Greek word roots, namely "philo" (love) and "sophia" (wisdom); accordingly, when put together, the word "philosophy" means "love of wisdom." Thus, philosophy explores worldviews that explain phenomena in usually coherent but abstract terms and provides guiding principles for people in reality. Likewise, educational philosophies reference philosophies that consider practices in education. Educational philosophies underlie educational components ranging from creating curricula to determining classroom instruction, from understanding learning processes to selecting assessments, from writing learning objectives to setting the overall goals of education, and so forth.

The discipline of philosophy generally consists of three branches: metaphysics, epistemology, and axiology. Metaphysics delves into the study of ontology, rendering questions of what reality is, how we know what is real, and by extension, what is/are truth(s) in our universe. Closely related to ontology, epistemology outlines questions of what knowledge is, what is worth knowing, and how we know. And axiology explores questions of value, or aesthetics and ethics, asking about what is good, beautiful, or valuable. Correspondingly, when these three branches are applied in educational theories, people ponder what curriculum is; question what the nature of knowledge is, and, therefore, what is worth teaching and learning; and ask what the goals or aims of education are. In answering such questions systematically, and based on the major philosophical movements (idealism, realism, pragmatism, and existentialism) four primary schools of educational philosophy emerged – essentialism, perennialism, progressivism, and reconstructivism/resconstructionism (Harmon and Jones 2005; Sandovnik et al. 2018). A fifth has more recently come to prominence: humanism. Humanism is driven by some of the more contemporary educational philosophers – primarily Abraham Maslow, of Maslow's hierarchy fame, created in 1943. However, humanism's roots are ancient, as with most philosophies, and it will also be explored more deeply later in this chapter.

In defining philosophy writ large, however, it is necessary to define any subplots within the larger plot of philosophy as a discipline. Philosophy of education is a subplot, if you will, of philosophy as a whole, and is defined by Siegel (2009) as "that branch of philosophy that addresses philosophical questions concerning the nature, aims, and problems of education" (p. 3). Although central to the evolution and practice of education, it is rarely taught in traditional philosophy courses; rather, if it is taught, it is generally delivered within departments or programs of education (Noddings 2016). While this may seem odd, philosophy as a whole is often too large to tackle in a single course of study, thus some of its branches are often left to be taught by the discipline under which its title falls, e.g., philosophy of education, philosophy of science, philosophy of goodness or value, philosophy of logic, and others. While these offshoots are seemingly discipline-specific, it is important to keep in mind that each branch has a common starting place, at least in the Western world: ancient Greece.

Socrates, Plato, and Aristotle laid the foundations of Western philosophy through the ages; a philosophy that allowed discipline-specific philosophies to emerge and, in some cases, burgeon into a full-blown area of study. Nel Noddings (2016) acknowledges this explicitly in the introduction to her fourth edition of *Philosophy of Education*, where one section in her first chapter is dedicated to Socrates and Plato; another to Aristotle. In fact, Noddings briefly discusses some of the most impactful historical philosophers of education, from Rousseau (1700s) through Pestalozzi, Herbart, and Froebel (mid-1800s). Randall Curren (2007) also covers some of the ancient philosophers; both will be referred to extensively in the next section, covering a brief history of educational philosophy.

Before moving into its history, however, let us be sure that we understand what it is that philosophers of education actually *do*. While philosophers traditionally analyze and work to clarify anything with ambiguity within a content or topic, philosophers of education specifically reflect upon, consider, discuss, and explore "concepts, arguments, theories, and language" (Noddings 2016, p. xiii) related to education as a discipline and as a practice. For example, Noddings (2016) reminds us that questions asked in ancient times about education are still relevant today: "What should be the aims or purposes of education? Who should be educated? Should education differ according to natural interests and abilities? What role should the state play in education?" (p. 1). As you can clearly see, she is not mistaken; these questions are still played out every day in the United States, as we continue to question educational equity and how to attain it; how to best encourage and support students in their efforts to achieve the skills and knowledge needed to both contribute to society and earn a decent living; the extent to which each school is beholden to state policies, procedures, and politics (as I write this there are numerous efforts to ban certain teachings and books across the country, as well as lawsuits from students and parents against schools who have forced religious beliefs and gatherings onto them on school grounds during school hours); and what the real purpose of an education is. Are students required to get a high school education because it is deemed necessary for them to survive and thrive, or because it is necessary for parents to have a place to deposit their children during the workday? Should everyone obtain a university degree? What is the purpose of a university degree, especially if such a degree does not guarantee work in the area studied? So many questions about education. All of these and more are considered by educational philosophers; all of these and more are pieces to the puzzle that is education.

With this in mind, let us dive into a brief history of educational philosophy – both Western and Eastern, after which you will dig into some of the more influential ancient (Eastern) and contemporary (Western) philosophers of education as we lay the foundation for upcoming chapters in this text. The third section begins to group the types of educational philosophies that have evolved over time, beginning with teacher-centered educational philosophies, moving to learner-centered educational philosophies in Section 4, and concluding with socially centered educational philosophies in Section 5. You will notice they progress historically from early to present day; however, keep in mind that just because one set of philosophies has fallen out of favor does not mean that it is completely off the radar. It is highly likely that any educator you speak to has beliefs in and approaches to education that are rooted in several of these -*isms*, as I call them; perhaps they would not explicitly recognize them as such, but all have heavily influenced education and educational practices over the centuries.

Section 2: A Brief History of Western Educational Philosophy

Katherine Fogelberg

The Classical Era (600 BCE–476 CE) is widely acknowledged as the birth of Western philosophy as a discipline. It is also where we find the foundations of educational philosophy as we know it established. It is important to acknowledge that the term "classical" should also encompass those rooted in Chinese, Indian, and Arab classical texts; the Chinese roots of educational philosophy are covered later in this chapter. The Indian and Arab roots are not included only because of the editor's lack of connections to scholars with this knowledge; should those emerge and a second edition of this text be warranted, they would be happily incorporated.

From the Western perspective, Socrates (469–399 BCE) is well-established as the originator of the philosophy of education. It should be noted that Socrates did not use his time to address questions he considered inconsequential; he chose to pursue conversations about big questions – those he felt were meaningful in the larger picture of society and life. You will note, too, that throughout the discussion of Socrates the term "conversation" is more often applied than the term "teaching"; this is because Socrates was never a formal teacher. He never charged for his services; he met his students in their homes and in various public gathering places, and those students were always free to leave or join at their will, answer or not answer as they chose. Thus, it seems fitting to refer to his discussions with students as conversations rather than as lessons or teachings, as the latter terms imply a more formal atmosphere and the compelled presence of students.

Although Socrates did no writing himself, preferring to engage in verbal sparring to make his points, we are familiar with his work through his best-known student, Plato. Plato's writings were voluminous and are broken into evolutionary units by Classicists that span the early, or Socratic, dialogues, the transitional dialogues, the middle dialogues, and the late dialogues (Curren 2007).

The early dialogues present Socrates as he truly was; constantly questioning and using questions to lead those interested in his conversations into deeper thought about a given topic. His use of constant questioning may be familiar to you as the Socratic method, although not all who use it are as adept at doing so as he was. While many view the Socratic method as merely answering every question with a question, there are finer points to this method that are often overlooked. Noddings (2016) notes that Socrates always started his conversations – that led to learning – with a seemingly simple question, such as "What is truth? or What does it mean to be just?" (p. 3). As the student responded, Socrates would ask a follow-up question, prompting her or him to think more deeply and come up with a new response. This process – also known as *elenchus*, or destructive cross-examination – continued until the teacher, the student, or both believed the analysis had been taken as far as possible in the moment (Noddings 2016). Based on examples of such Socratic conversations, it is apparent that logic, *logos*, is at the heart of many – perhaps most – of Socrates teachings; he is leading the student into understanding the logic – or lack thereof – behind their original answers when the conversation concludes.

Plato's transitional dialogues depicted Socrates as his true self but begin to interject Plato's attempts at identifying and overcoming issues he sees with Socrates' thinking, while the late dialogues leave Socrates largely out of the writings and are where Plato largely abandons some of the important ideas characteristic of the middle dialogues (Curren 2007). It is the middle dialogues, however, that continue to resonate with today's educational philosophers, as it is here where Plato's utopian state and greatest work, *Republic*, appears (Curren 2007; Noddings 2016).

Republic is about the equivalent of 10 modern-day chapters (called books in the translation) and much of its content is focused on the problems of education (Noddings 2016; Curren 2007). In its introduction, Plato provides a cast list, with Socrates being identified as the narrator throughout. As the writing unfolds, the reader witnesses Plato, through Socrates, opine that citizens should have education suited to their capacities, dividing students into three categories: those destined to be artisans and workers; those he called guardians (soldiers), to whom the safety and security of the state were entrusted; and those who would lead (rulers and those in the upper echelons of the guardian class). According to Benjamin Jowett's 2012 translation with introduction, the work reaches its apex in Books V, VI, and VII, where "philosophy reaches the highest point…to which ancient thinkers ever attained" (Jowett 2012, p. 1). This thought is echoed in Curren's text, although in slightly less hyperbolic terms.

As Curren (2007) highlights, there were others who also provided blocks to build the foundation of the philosophy of education upon; more often referred to as sophists and orators, such individuals developed and defended their own approaches to higher education. One of the more prominent orators of his time, Isocrates was a contemporary of Plato who established a school of rhetoric just a few years after Plato opened his Academy. A staunch defender and practitioner of rhetoric as philosophy in the service of politics, Isocrates also believed that "practical wisdom" was gained through education grounded in the study of speech (*logos*), or the ability to speak well and persuasively (Curren 2007). This is in contrast to Plato's ideas about how practical wisdom was gained; he believed that such wisdom was grounded in systemic knowledge (*episteme*) – something Isocrates did not believe was attainable by humans (Curren 2007).

However, "*The Republic* of Plato is also the first treatise upon education, of which the writings of Milton and Locke, Rousseau, Jean Paul, and Goethe are the legitimate descendants" (Jowett 2012, p. 1). Truly, Plato's tome is a foundational writing in educational philosophy; though his ideas started with interactions with Socrates, he would go on to make his mark in the field as the first true philosopher of education. Socrates was his narrator, but it is Plato who historically persists as the primary "influencer" of educational philosophy in ancient times. Although Plato's model of education may be viewed as elitist because he believed that education was primarily to educate the few who were "capable of attaining understanding of the highest forms of knowledge" so they could exercise political power responsibly (Peters et al. 2015, p. 6), it is still his philosophical foundations upon which current Western educational philosophy stands.

The Western philosophers, orators, and sophists persisted until the fall of the Roman Empire, which led to the Dark Ages – the early part of what is collectively known as the Middle, Medieval, or Postclassical era. Spanning from 476 to 1450 ADE, the Middle Ages saw significant strife with the collapse of the Roman Empire and rebuilding efforts during the Dark Ages, an oppressive and often violent Catholic church reaching the height of its power, and the Black Death sweeping through Europe. It is also this era, however, that produced the printing press, an invention that would influence the entire world as it hastened the distribution of the written word to a pace previously unattainable. While not the sole reason for the return to the Classical Era values and philosophies, the printing press certainly aided humanity as it strove to emerge from a difficult social time and helped define the Age of Enlightenment as a pivotal time in human history – as well as educational philosophy.

It would not be until the Early Modern Era that we would see the emergence of additional philosophers who can be viewed as moving educational philosophy forward. During this era, we see philosophy speaking to "eternal truths about rational man as the fount of knowledge" (Peters et al. 2015, p. 6), with Immanuel Kant separating experience from a priori forms of knowledge (a moralist approach). However, John Locke viewed education as an imperative for maintaining and sustaining the social contract (realism), while Jean-Jacques Rousseau (a naturalist) viewed the power of knowledge as being polluted by society (Peters et al. 2015).

Contemporaries Locke and Rousseau had similar ideas about the importance of education through practical and sensorial experiences, though both protested the likeness of their thought (Peters et al. 2015). Locke is widely acknowledged as the father of liberalism, and his primary aim for education was the production of individuals able to make rational decisions as a citizen within society (Peters et al. 2015). As with Locke, "Kant believed in the importance of inculcating through education a cultivated and ethical sensibility" (Peters et al. 2015, p. 6). However, Kant split from Locke's belief that education was to teach children the adult characteristics required to be part of a civil society. Instead, Kant's view was that children should be viewed as distinct from the adult (Peters et al. 2015). Rousseau also celebrated the notion of childhood, as demonstrated in his well-known text *Emile*; he also lauded the natural morality of the child and blamed society for all its deficiencies (Rousseau 1957, as cited in Peters et al. 2015).

Plato (Classical), Kant, Locke, and Rousseau (each from the Enlightenment) are the four foundational masters of Western philosophy; each made contributions to conceptions of what education "ought" to be that were "both pivotal articulations and emblematic of their wider theoretical perspectives on knowledge and the conditions of existence" (Peters et al. 2015, p. 6).

Although in reading the works of each of these philosophers, one might not view education as being overly prominent, all did explicitly recognize education's importance both for achieving some of their societal and theoretical aims and belief that education was the primary site for such aims to be developed (Peters et al. 2015). It should be noted that these philosophers were primarily speaking about educating boys and men, a theme that was not uncommon in Western societies and has had far-reaching effects that continue today.

With the movement into the Early Modern Era, the European Renaissance began and the oppressive ideals and actions of the Middle Ages receded. This cultural renaissance saw an embrace and valuation of art, music, literature, and philosophy, paving the path to a society in the West built by Europe's exploration and colonization of numerous continents, including Africa and the Americas. Such expansion – coming from significant violence and repression – ultimately resulted in resistance and loss of power, particularly in areas that were so geographically far away from Europe. This diaspora of Europeans who then became different countries resulted in parallel industrialization, urbanization, technological advances, and regional and global conflicts – all of which have led us to the information age, in which we are now fully entrenched.

As with the rest of the world, in the United States through the late nineteenth and early twentieth centuries, there were social, cultural, intellectual, and historical pressures that affected the creation of the educational discipline known as philosophy of education. However, Kaminsky (1992) argues that such pressures culminated in a specific date of origin for the philosophy of education as a discipline, that being Sunday, 24 February 1935, in Atlantic City, when the John Dewey Society was established by a group of school superintendents and academics. The formalization of a national public school movement in the early twentieth century, the emergence of the belief that education could be studied as "laboratory science," and a burgeoning awareness that education was inextricably intertwined with the nation's social order provided the opportunity for John Dewey and a group of other less known scholars and teachers who ended up forming the

backbone of the progressive movement in education to take the spotlight (Kaminsky 1992).

Peters et al. (2015) reinforce the idea that a variety of influences created opportunities for changing philosophical views of education. Postwar in the twentieth century, for example, we saw the rise of the analytic tradition, "in which a liberal philosophy that drew very heavily on certain aspects of classicism proposed to analyze education through conceptual analyses" (Peters et al. 2015, p. 6). Although public schools (first known as "common schools") had been established for almost a century by the time World War II ended (Kober and Rentner 2020), Dewey's emergence during this postwar era in the United States was a bit of luck. In a time during which the U.S.'s receptivity to education as experience was heightened, Dewey and his educational philosophy found widespread acceptance. His philosophy and theories would ultimately shape the educational landscape in the United States and beyond, particularly with respect to increasing child-centered approaches in the classroom (Peters et al. 2015).

Dewey's – among others – influence cannot be overstated. But his was not the only loud voice in the crowd, as with the establishment of the formal public school system came the inevitable power struggles that accompany any large-scale institution. As Kaminsky summarizes nicely:

> Herbert Spencer and John Dewey made education and educational philosophy an intellectual issue. Populism and progressivism made education a political issue. The muckrakers made education a public issue. And, finally, the social reform movement. . .was central in confirming the discipline's social conscience. The American Social Science Association placed educational philosophy within the aegis of the social sciences. Then, like the various social sciences, educational philosophy found its way into U.S. universities (p. 180).

And while the educational philosophers in the U.S. were having their moment, others in the Western world were also emerging as scholar leaders. In South America, Paulo Freire was publicly exploring the entrenched inequalities in education, while in Austria Ivan Illich was publishing his ideas about a "deschooling approach" (Peters et al. 2015), akin to the current home-schooling movement in the United States. Both Freire and Illich contributed significantly to building the foundations for exploring knowledge, power, and the oppression that often mars the ideals of public education.

While the philosophy of education, as we view it today, may have started with the ancient Greeks, the Eastern world has had its influence as well (and is explored in much greater depth later in this chapter). But regardless of where the discipline began, the questions remain similar. As you hopefully gleaned from your reading thus far, philosophers of education have historically explored the questions of power, ethics, politics, epistemology, and ontology; it is an exploration that continues today and will likely continue as long as education remains a staple of human society. As Peters et al. (2015) write:

> The fundamental question for philosophy of education is that of the nature or possibility of knowledge. What is the criterion for the constitution of knowledge? Who decides what knowledge is important? Who should have access to knowledge? How should knowledge be judged, changed, or modified? Should everyone have access to all knowledge, or should there be limits placed on who can be exposed to certain knowledge and limits on when this exposure should take place? (p. 5).

These are echoes of the questions posed by Noddings, introduced earlier in this chapter. It may seem like educational philosophy continues to ponder the same questions from era to era, and this may very well be true. But the answers to these questions continue to change and, thus, the asking of the same questions continues to be important for ensuring the discipline moves forward thoughtfully; it is only through asking such questions and closely examining the evolution of the thoughts that accompany their answers that we can continually improve our educational approaches and processes.

Section 3: The Eastern Origins of the Philosophy of Education

Ying Wang

Similar to understanding Western educational philosophies, it would be inappropriate to claim it was possible to summarize all the major schools of Asian educational philosophies in several paragraphs or book pages. Given the complexity and richness of Asian culture, this section mainly focuses on Chinese educational philosophies, within which Confucianism and Taoism have been the most influential. This fact has two immediate implications regarding exploring Chinese educational philosophies. On the one hand, it is no exaggeration to say that anyone who tries to understand Chinese culture, and for that matter, Asian cultures, will fail if they do not start with Confucianism and Taoism. On the other hand, while the words and deeds of Confucian and Taoist scholars in ancient China were meant to engage people and guide

social lives during their eras, throughout history, they have been continuously (re)interpreted by people. Some of the interpretations attempt to gauge the original meanings of masters like Confucius, Mencius, Lao-tzu, and Chuang-tzu, yet others interpreted canonical texts of Confucianism and Taoism to serve their own political or cultural agendas.

The following section will discuss Confucianism, major Confucius literature, how Confucianism is embodied in society, how Confucianism is implemented in education, and by extension the consequences of such implementation. In particular, we will also explore the concept of "*junzi* (君子)," an exemplary person with talent and virtue and an ideal personality used to educate students in China. We will also discuss the criticism of Confucianism, especially from the feminist perspective. With that said, the Confucianism defined and discussed in this section references earlier Confucian literature and concepts, and does not include later expansions of Confucian ideas, including but not limited to Neo-Confucianism (*song ming li xue* 宋明理学) and New-Confucianism (*xin ru jia* 新儒家) (Hansen 1999; Ho 2018; Metzger 1986).

Part 1: Confucianism

Confucianism is known as *rujia xuepai* (儒家学派) in China, and it was named after the sage Confucius, who lived around 1700 years ago in China, or what is referred to as the Spring and Autumn historical period (771–476 BCE) in China. Confucianism broadly covers societal, political, and ethical aspects, yet is often considered a civil religion (Bellah 1975), which prescribes the sense of an ideal identity, social rituals, and "common moral understanding at the foundation of a society's central institution" (Berling n.d., n.p.). In other words, Confucianism provides the social rules that bind people's behaviors in society. By the same token, Confucianism highlights what are supposedly proper social interactions between different members based on how two parties are positioned or related in the society. These rules sometimes are also identified as the gist of Confucian role ethics (CRE; Foust and Tan 2016). Confusing as it appears, Confucian teachings intentionally merged ethics, education, and politics, such that rulers could use them to keep the society in order. Especially after the chaotic pre-Qin period, the emperors of the Han dynasty prioritized Confucianism in their political beliefs (*ba chu bai jia, du zun ru shu* 罢黜百家, 独尊儒术). Such integration of different aspects of social lives also led to these individual aspects referencing each other to make standards and evaluations.

Throughout Chinese history, many dynasties adopted Confucianism to govern because rulers believe it delineated people's roles and outlined rules about morality, making it easier to govern and maintain the social hierarchy. Additionally, Confucian literature is required in the imperial examination or civil service examination (*ke ju kao shi* 科举考试), which first originated in kingdoms during the Han dynasty to select candidates to work for the government and was standardized in the Tang dynasty until its abolishment in the Qing dynasty. However, the tradition of selecting proper candidates for civil servants still survives if one compares the imperial examination with the contemporary College Entrance examination (*gaokao* 高考) and the civil service exam (*gong wu yuan kao shi* 公务员考试) in China. The logic of all three examinations is based on the merits of the candidates, but how much each exam stays true to meritocracy remains in question. For instance, in the Han dynasty, the nine-rank system (*jiu pin zhong zheng zhi* 九品中正制) used in combination with the imperial exam signified one's family background and one's political career outlook to a large extent. Though contemporary exam systems in China do not necessarily require student's familiarity with Confucian literature (such as the civil service exam), the exam systems themselves are fraught with alternative "aristocracy," which features people with social capital. It is still common for incumbent government officials to use their power (*guan xi* 关系) to favor their children or their relatives.

The major Confucian literature used in history, and even in contemporary Chinese textbooks, includes the *Four Books* (*Si shu* 《四书》) and *Five Classics* (*Wu jin* 《五经》). *Four Books* consist of *Analects* (*Lun yu* 《论语》), *Great Learning* (*Da xue* 《大学》), the *Doctrine of the Mean* (*Zhong yong* 《中庸》), and *Mencius* (Meng zi 《孟子》). The *Five Classics* refers to *the Book of Poetry* (*Shi jing* 《诗经》), *the Book of History* (*Shang shu* 《尚书》), *the Book of Rites* (*Li ji* 《礼记》), *the Book of Changes* (*Yi jing* 《易经》), and *the Spring and Autumn Annals* (*Chun qiu* 《春秋》). Labeled as Confucian literature, these books were often also the texts required to be well memorized for students in ancient China. Though in contemporary China, memorization of all these books is not required, selected chapters or excerpts in Chinese textbooks are still frequently tested, thus making students recite them is a common practice in K-12 education.

Among these canonical books, *Analects* is the one authored collectively by students of Confucius. Though not written by Confucius, it recorded his most famous and significant quotes. Most of the sayings are dialogues between Confucius and his disciples, like those between Socrates and his students in *The Republic* (Gu 2015; Plato 2021; Sandovnik et al. 2018). Yet notably, in Chinese education, schools and tests not only require the above-mentioned key texts to be memorized, but also ask students to interpret and apply the ideas in their writings (Ho 2018). In contemporary China, though oftentimes K-12 Chinese textbooks do not require students to memorize the whole texts of the *Four Books* and *Five Classics*, textbook presses – usually funded by the government – consistently make sure the most significant sections are included in the textbooks.

As indicated earlier, Confucianism has been widely endorsed by rulers and governments in different historical periods, as it emphasizes rituals and social mores that guide people's behaviors. This explains why it remains the core of education as well. Confucianism features "Three cardinal guidelines and five constant virtues" (*san gang wu chang* 三纲五常) (Li 2019, para. 4). The three cardinal guidelines refer to three fundamental social relationships: father-son, king-subject, and husband-wife. It is said that in these relations, the latter should always obey the former. The five constant virtues are *ren* (benevolence 仁), *yi* (righteousness 义), *li* (rites or propriety 礼), *zhi* (knowledge and/or wisdom 智), and *xin* (integrity or trustworthiness 信) Law 2016a,b; Sun 2014; Waley 2005).

Part 2: *Junzi* as the Core of Person-Making and Citizen-Making in Confucianism

In early Chinese education, education is more than obtaining knowledge; as explained previously, education is closely connected with personal ethics and morality, thus cultivating the young into an ethical and competent person (*shu ren* 树人) (Fraser 2006). Confucian educational philosophy believes cultivating students allows them to connect abstract morality in their daily actions; this belief is also exemplified in his rendition of an ideal Confucian person *junzi* in *Analects*. To some extent, the logic of Confucian educational philosophy agrees with the idealism proposed by Socrates and Plato. In articulating how to teach and implement Confucian ethics like the three cardinal guidelines and five constant virtues, the word *junzi* is mostly quoted in Confucian literature and when people discuss Confucian ethics. It is still prevalent in today's conversations when people try to justify the decency of their behaviors or discipline themselves, but in Confucian literature, there is not an explicit definition of what a *junzi* is, though Confucius has provided many explanations and assumptions of how a *junzi* would behave daily.

Very often, *junzi* is translated into English as "gentleman" in Western cultures, yet it should be noted that though both are considered ideal personalities in their respective cultures and histories, the word "gentleman" implies nobleness, decorum, and knighthood, while *junzi* implies ethics, morality, constant self-discipline, nobility, and knowledge. *Junzi* are cautious in what they say and reflect on a daily basis (Confucius 2010). For instance, in

Analects, Confucius constantly explains with concrete examples how *junzi* would behave in myriad situations. One such example is from his conversation with his disciple Zengzi, who says, "Every day I examine myself many times. Do I do my best when doing things for others? Am I honest and reliable when associating with friends? Whether do I review and practice what my teachers teach me? (曾子曰:"吾日三省吾身。为人谋而不忠乎?与朋友交而不信乎?传不 习乎?") (Confucius 2010, pp. 5–6). More examples are list below:

> ...Not being well understood, but I neither complain nor get angry. Isn't that a gentleman bearing? (人不知，而不愠，不亦君子乎?)... (Confucius 2010, pp. 8–9).
>
> ...Gentlemen don't depart from humanity and virtue just in a short period of time of dinner. Even at the most critical moment, gentlemen must act according to the principle of humanity and virtue. And even destitute and homeless, they can act according to the principle of humanity and virtue. (君子去仁，恶乎成名?君子无终食之间违仁， 造次必于是，颠沛必于是。)(Confucius 2010, pp. 79–80)
>
> ...Confucius (2010) said, "As far as a gentleman is concerned, he cannot become a man of high prestige if he does not behave solemnly" (子曰:"君子不重则不威;学则不固。) (pp. 11–12).

Confucius (2010) also indicates personality and attributes according to how *junzi* would treat others in society:

> If gentlemen sincerely love their kinsfolk, people will uphold love and humanity; if gentlemen truly take care of their old friends, people couldn't be indifferent. (君子笃[4]于亲，则民兴于仁，故旧[5]不遗，则民不偷。) (p. 125).
>
> Gentlemen give relief only to the poor but don't add property to the rich. (君子周急不济富) (pp. 135–136).
>
> Confucius said, "Gentlemen live in harmony with others but don't wallow in the mire with others. Yet vulgarians do exactly the opposite." (子曰:"君子和[1]而不同[2]，小人同而不和。" (p. 292).

Clearly, *Analects* recorded many of Confucius's sayings on what he should or not should do.

Another characteristic we can note by reading *Analects* is that Confucius often compared the behaviors of a *junzi* with those of a vulgarian or villain; the contrast often suggests what we are discouraged from doing, echoing the rationale of rulers adopting Confucianism as a ruling philosophy, since the binary opposition between a *junzi* and a villain (and sometimes the opposite can also be a woman)

offers people a quick reference of laws and regulations. Thus, although there is no clear definition of *junzi*, the concept has helped Confucius' students, past and present, understand how to live as a *junzi* in daily life even if they cannot fully claim to represent the *junzi* personality (Fingarette 1998; Lorraine 2011). Therefore, it should be no surprise that Confucianism as a person-making educational philosophy is mostly taken as a citizen-making philosophy as well (Li and Xue 2020; Xue and Li 2020).

Part 3: Women and Confucianism

While Confucianism has been the most famous and consistently adopted educational, ethical, and political philosophy in China's history, it is also widely criticized. Among the fiercest criticism is that Confucianism is anti-feminist. Women in Confucian literature are peripheral at best, and "subhuman beings" at worst (Gao 2014, p. 114). Since its inception in the Spring and Autumn period, Confucianism has not only codified proper behaviors of citizens in general but also for women (Gao 2014). Though in Confucian literature there does not exist an ideal persona concept about women, relevant works have indicated how women should behave themselves in social contexts, especially in the collection called *Four Books for Women* (*Nv Sishu* 《女四书》). These books include *Lessons for Women* (*nv Jie* 《女诫》), *The Analects for Women* (*nv lun you* 《女论语》), *Teachings for the Inner Court* (*nv xun* 《女训》), and *Short Records of Models for Women* (*nv fan jie lu* 《女范捷录》). Generally speaking, women were not allowed to study publicly historically, let alone be selected to become civil servants; if allowed study, they were taught "Three Obediences and Four Virtues" (*san cong si de* 三从四德). As opposed to the three cardinal guidelines and five constant virtues of a *junzi*, "three obediences" prescribe that women follow their father before marriage, obey their husbands in marriage, and are subjugated to their sons after the husband passed away. The "four virtues" include chastity, modesty (in speech), neatness (of appearance to please men), and capability to do household chores (needlework and cooking). Countless practices are borne out of these four virtues. Most notorious among them is foot binding (*gun jiao* 裹脚), abolished only in the first half of the twentieth century; women were asked to bind their feet from toe to heel when they were little girls so their feet would remain 3 in. long (san can jin lian 三寸金莲), because the androcentric sense of beauty in Confucianism adores short feet. Though it requires more research on how such Confucian concepts on women's education have influenced other Asian countries, as scholarly research demonstrates, similar concepts surely guided numerous women's practices in some Asian countries (Foust and Tan 2016; Herr 2016).

The stark contrast between educational expectations held for girls/women and those for boys/men is analogous to the one between Emile and Sophia in *Emile, Or On Education* (Rousseau (1979), if you will. While Emile in Rousseau's rendering was expected to learn critical thinking, reasoning, and exploring the world, Rousseau (1979) indicated his female counterpart should only learn how to be an eligible wife. If one takes a glimpse of any Chinese ancient literature mentioning women, it is not difficult to reach the conclusion that historical situations for women can be much worse than Sophia's. The power dynamics between males and females in China are often referred to as *yin-yang* (阴阳) and *nei-wai* (内外) (Lin 1935). *Yin* means the shade and usually means complimentary to the *yang* or the male. Similarly, *nei* means inside, and *wai* outside, implying that women should handle things like household chores, while men work outside the home and are often the breadwinners of a family. Both *yin* and *nei* suggest that women are restricted to the home, their existence is supplementary to men, and what they do should be helpful but secondary to men's deeds. By extension, the historical labor division between men and women has enduring impacts on how both genders are treated in society. In the book *Hanfeizi*:

> If a boy is born, the parents congratulate each other, if a girl is born, they kill her. [Both boys and girls] all come from the same parents, yet boys are celebrated, and girls are killed; this is because they [i.e., the parents] consider the benefits (of having a boy) in the long run (as cited in Rosenlee 2006, p. 122).

The quote above shows that girls are taken as almost useless to the family. Sadly, this ancient practice has been reflected in contemporary Chinese culture. Still today, women were discouraged from obtaining too much education, especially if such pursuit might take away their brothers' opportunities. And they are taught that too much education (usually suggested by a master's or doctoral degree) will intimidate potential bachelors who might date or marry them otherwise. Women have also been considered as "water is thrown out of the maiden family once she is married (*po chu qu de shui* 泼出去的水)," since once married, they are not likely to contribute financially to the maiden family. In the backward waters of China, girls sometimes are addressed as "goods that lose money" (*pei qian huo* 赔钱货). In the early twentieth century, the May Fourth movement fought against Confucianism. When people engaged in such iconoclasm, one of the major arguments they upheld was to set women free from the three tyrannies in Confucianism, as "the way of Confucius" was at odds with modern life (Chen 1916/2000, p. 353).

Though the gender preference sounds out of date, and women were touted as equally important as men ("half of the sky" *ban bian tian* 半边天) after the People's Republic of China was founded, girls and women are still somewhat inferior and shunned when families and society are pushed to make gender choices. When the Chinese government implemented the brutal One Child Policy in the 1980s, women often aborted girls. Similarly, abandoning girl babies and girl infanticide was most people's lived experiences if some girl babies were actually born. One such example is the newly released Netflix documentary *Found* (Gou et al. 2021), where three Chinese American girls adopted from Canton, China, embarked on the journey to find their biological parents and understand their own identities. All three girls were abandoned around the marketplace in their biological hometowns due to their gender.

Scholars (Foust and Tan 2016; Herr 2016) note that the labor division was necessary in most cultures throughout history, and the labor division stipulated by Confucian scholars like Confucius and Mencius also resulted from social and historical limitations; as such, feminist criticisms should refrain from blaming them for the adversity experienced by women in Confucian cultures. Yet, the point here is not how justified Confucian educational philosophies and social expectations for women were in ancient Chinese feudalism, but instead, what malicious and enduring consequences have come into being due to relevant Confucian philosophies and expectations toward women in the first place that presuppose people to think and interact with the society they lived in. It appears that gender equality has largely been realized in China. For instance, women are allowed to go to college and work; and statistically, the number of women going to college has surpassed that of male students (National Bureau of Statistics of China 2021).

However, there are still rampant social abuses of gender inequality if one examines individual social issues closely. One example is "gender segregation" that indicates more women take social sciences as their major than men, and opposite patterns can be found when it comes to science majors (Yuan 2019, p. 2). Another example is the flamboyant sexist practice that job advertisements prescribe the job applicants' gender for job positions, which obviously would immediately cause legal issues if it were applied in the United States. Likewise, on the job market, employers include questions about dating, marriage, and children in their initial interviews, because they automatically connect women job applicants' situations with how long they will work, or how consistent and intensively they can work (especially how much overtime they can work), etc. Meanwhile, when the impacts of feudal Confucian thoughts are studied, we should also be aware of the differences among geographical locations (Jacka 2006). For instance, in urban areas where educational resources are more available than those in rural or much less developed areas, the remanence of feudal Confucian thoughts is much less than the rural or less developed areas.

Some scholars (Li 2000; Rosenlee 2006; Duncan and Brasovan 2016; Batista 2017; Yuan 2019) hold that there are parallel thoughts between feminism and Confucianism, and therefore feminists can take a leaf from Confucian philosophy to suit their own agendas against patriarchy. One similarity is the caring ethics and Confucian role ethics, in the sense that both believe one person lives in relation to others in the society and rendering feminist caring relations with others becomes critical to rearticulate women's identity politics in society (Cahill and Li 2001; Yuan 2019). While Confucian role ethics centers on the submission of one to a superior/senior other (wife to husband, son to father, and subject to the king), care ethics begins with the affirmation of interdependency and equality among people such that the care should be mutual. We should also be aware that the care concept in Confucian role ethics often requires the inferior party to care for the superior party. In the case of women, women are usually portrayed as the caregiver and in most texts and traditions they are there only to serve the androcentric culture.

Part 4: Taoism

Taoism, also known as Daoism (*dao iia xue pai* 道家学派), became popular during the Spring and Autumn period when multiple schools were vying for dominance in kingdoms in this historical period, including, but not limited to, Mohism (*mo jia xue pai* 墨家学派), Confucianism (*ru jia xue pai* 儒家学派), and Legalism (*fa jia xue pai* 法家学派), etc. Daoism is often considered as important as, if not more significant than, Confucianism in Chinese culture and history. Having already learned that Confucianism was adopted in Chinese dynasties for ruling people and keeping society in order, we see that while Taoism is somewhat eclipsed by Confucianism, rulers also adopted Taoist political ideology when necessary to supplement the shortcomings of Confucianism.

The most famous Taoist scholars/founders include Lao-tzu (*lao zi* 老子) and Chuang-tzu (*zhuang zi* 庄子); both were Confucius contemporaries. As a matter of fact, Lao-tzu was slightly senior to Confucius, as historical records show that Confucius used to ask Lao-tzu the question about the way (*dao* 道). Major Taoist texts include *Tao Te Ching* (*Dao De Jing* 《道德经》) and *Zhuangzi* (《庄子》), both of which are widely referenced in different disciplines and daily life when people address Taoism. Additionally, these two scholars and works are also most frequently studied by Western scholars who study Chinese ancient philosophy or compare western and eastern philosophies.

Notably, keywords like *dao/tao* (the way), *de/te* (virtue), *wu* (non-being), *wu-wei* (inaction, or non-action), *qi* (force), *yin*, and *yang* are most referenced, and scholars usually engage in their interpretations of these key words/ideas of Taoism, as there was no agreed-upon interpretation from Lao-tzu and Chuang-tzu. One example is that for politicians and emperors, *wu-wei* from Lao-tzu's perspective indicates nonaction as a best way to govern people; a contemporary western concept similar to *wu-wei* is laissez-faire. Whereas, from the perspective of Chuang-tzu, *wu-wei* indicates wisdom to pursue the ultimate happiness.

Similar to Confucianism, Taoism has been widely accepted in Chinese culture and history, such that it is impossible to wrap Taoism in any single discipline or facet of societal life. For instance, Taoist ideas, such as living with nature, *wu-wei*, and the dialectic relationship between power and weakness are taught through Chinese ancient texts such as *Laotzu* (《老子》) and *Wandering at Ease* (*xiao yao you* 《逍遥游》) in Chinese K-12 education. Similarly, the government engages with the philosophy of *wu-wei*, often translated as effortless action or inaction, in making certain policies. Taoism is also another major civil religion, in addition to Buddhism and Confucianism, and as a religion, it is practiced widely. Some people who claim to be Taoist may engage in daily religious rites, or simply adopt Taoist life philosophy but have nothing to do with any religious rites.

In Weijin and the Northern and Southern period (AD 220–420), *xuanxue* (玄学), or what is often translated as "neo-daoism" (D'Ambrosio 2016, p. 261), became popular among intellectuals, especially those who were demoted or marginalized by the government due to the power conflicts between them and the rulers. Weijin *Xuanxue* is also argued as an intellectual reaction to the hypocrisy and corruption in the government. It features the priority of *wu* (non-being) as the start of the universe, living with nature, and indifference to politics. In its development, *xuanxue* also merges with Confucianism and Buddhism, given that intellectuals were mainly Confucian scholars who tried to reconcile their frustrations with their political careers with life itself. Though not discussed in detail here, *xuanxue* can be understood as one example where educational philosophies, Confucianism and Taoism in particular, supplement each other in Chinese history not only when rulers need different political ideologies to rule the society, but also when individuals need consolation to explain their predicaments.

Part 5: Taoism Versus Confucianism

Despite the disparity between Taoism and Confucianism, these two predominant schools of thought are constantly compared (D'Ambrosio 2016, 2020; Defoot 2007; Hue 2007;

Zhang 1993; Zhou 2006, 2019). For instance, D'Ambrosio (2020) notes that the Confucian comprehensive notion of person-making centers on the person in relation to "a family and ancestry, a community and state, and the world and cosmos" (p. 8). In other words, the Confucian standard of being a successful person in society, or *junzi*, entails pragmatically practicing ethics based on one's socially assigned roles. In contrast, Taoist self-cultivation stipulates that people should be perceived according to their relationship with nature or their places in the cosmos. An example is from different interpretations of *dao* (the way) in Confucianism and Taoism. Confucianism holds that *dao*, the way to success, is characterized by constant learning of texts and emulating models like *junzi*, yet the taoist way means one living with the force that permeates around the cosmos, without being fixated on the success or failures in the human world. According to Chuang-tzu, the idea of *you* (游/遊), often translated as roaming, wondering, or playing, is significant in achieving *dao*. Perhaps due to the emphasis on cosmos and nature in its philosophy, while the other aspect of *wu-wei* as a political concept is employed to encourage people to submit themselves to their born places at times, other scholars also put Taoist *wu-wei* as a gesture toward anarchism posed against Confucianism endorsing monarchism and social hierarchy (Yu 2008; Zhang 1993; Lenehan 2020).

Part 6: Coda on Asian Educational Philosophies

As a major educational philosophy, Confucianism has overshadowed other educational philosophies both in Chinese culture in general and in school curricula. Like any other word ending with "ism," Confucianism also entails contested ideas, especially when Confucianism is coupled with politics throughout history and taken up by scholars for different research agendas. But at the core of Confucianism is the cultivation of the pupil. The ideal personalities exhibited by *junzi* can channel many values embraced by American cultures. To a large extent, Confucianism can be complementary to the existing curriculums in American public education (Chan et al. 2017). Despite numerous negative impacts of Confucianism on Chinese women, Confucian role ethics does stipulate care as essential to individual identities and one's relationship with people in their social circles. Another value of Confucianism to preservice teachers in the United States is teaching the increasing Asian student population. The knowledge of Confucianism allows a teacher to understand the work ethics and cultural backgrounds of most students who have Asian cultural roots, especially those that were impacted by Confucianism. The knowledge of eastern educational philosophies does not only echo culturally responsive teaching but also makes teachers to better engage and motivate students to learn in the classrooms.

By the same token, though Taoism appears to advocate inaction, it advocates for a dialectical interpretation of what we oftentimes take as negativity in classroom teaching. Such dialectical stance often expands into numerous concepts we are taught to connect with negative connotations. For instance, Smythe (2019) has suggested "emptiness" from the Taoist perspective can be utilized to ease anxiety experienced in American classrooms. Similarly, *wu wei*, or the passivity toward the power in Taoism also can be applied to transitioning traditional classroom instructional strategies to student-centered curriculums and instructional approaches (Jeffrey and Clark 2019). The change from teachers as instructors to teachers as facilitators often comes with challenges and questions about loss of teachers' authoritative power in the classroom. Yet, Taoist *wu wei* can help teachers understand sharing the power in the classroom through learner-centered teaching leads to more students' participation and realization of responsibilities in learning and assessments. In other words, giving away traditional instructional power and sharing power in the classroom results in maximizing students' learning potential.

Section 4: Ethics and Aims of Education

Ying Wang

In this section, the notion of axiology is introduced, the connections between axiology/philosophy and education are made, and how the aims of education are intertwined with ethics is explored. Attentive to this book's intended readership, we will also discuss what it means for classroom teachers and administrators to reflect on the ethics and aims of education.

Part 1: Axiology and Education

In general, philosophy consists of three branches: ontology, epistemology, and axiology. Ontology asks the question of being and reality, and epistemology deals with the question of knowledge and how to learn. The last branch of philosophy, axiology, deals with the question of what the good is and the question of what beauty is. As has been made clear earlier in this chapter, philosophy remains pertinent in education, and, thus, so is axiology. Within education, if we are pondering what to teach with ontology and how to teach with epistemology, ethics compels us to ask the question of why we teach at all.

As a Foundations instructor during my graduate program, I often heard preservice teachers complain in the hallway that philosophy was too abstract to understand

and that my course was intimidating. One primary reason for these complaints might be that we often think philosophy is isolated from the daily jobs we do. This is demonstrated in teacher preparation programs that generally focus on classroom management and lesson prep skills, with efforts to train preservice teachers such skills overshadowing reflections on educational practice and the understanding that the moral richness of everyday teaching refuses to provide quick and easy answers to teachers' dilemmas. By extension, this trend includes neglect in preparing them to reflect on why they need these skills and what they are trying to achieve in the long run.

However, when we ponder educational components such as curriculum, pedagogy, and educational goals, we are, in fact, tackling philosophy of education. Similar to the corresponding relationship between ontology and curriculum, and that between epistemology and pedagogy, ethics is often considered significant in understanding and/or stipulating the aims of education on different levels. In multiple educational theories, the goals or aims of education are the starting point for creating curricula. For example, critical inquiries prioritize forming social justice, undoing inequality, and challenging oppression (Counts 1969), while postmodern educational ethics focuses on attentiveness to difference and intertextuality (Slattery 2006), and feminist educational ethics pays attention to women's bodily experiences, critiques of patriarchy, and proposes that alliances with other marginalized groups is essential. By articulating these major aims of education, educators upholding the axiological aspects of educational philosophy make questioning the status quo, understanding across contexts, and awareness of differences and heterogeneity essential in their curricula and pedagogies.

The aims of education must also include disparities among different stakeholders. What the parents hold dear in terms of the aims of education for their children may not be the same aims from the government's perspective. Similarly, the best education in parents' or educators' eyes does not necessarily meet the job market's expectations. In some cultures, this disagreement often translates into the assumption that we think students with greater intellectual achievements should be financially successful after they become part of the workforce. Furthermore, aims at different educational levels, namely the K-12 educational institutions and higher educational institutions, often do not align with each other (Sandovnik et al. 2018; White 2010).

Part 2: Morality Versus Ethics

According to poststructuralist scholarship (Mazzei 2013; Wallin and Sandlin 2018), language is merely one object of the world rather than being a mirror of the world. In other words, using language to represent the world and reality is impossible, let alone using a language with consensus. In a similar vein, the usages of the two words "morality" and "ethics" in philosophy, and for that matter, educational philosophies, are unruly edges. Hence, we want to define what we mean by morality and ethics specifically in this section. According to the Stanford Encyclopedia of Philosophy website, the two denotations of the word "morality" are (i) "descriptively to refer to certain codes of conduct put forward by a society or a group (such as a religion), or accepted by an individual for her own behavior, or (ii) normatively to refer to a code of conduct that, given specified conditions, would be put forward by all rational people" (SEP website 2020).

Despite the fact that the word "morality" is hard to define, people tend to connect the word with moral judgment in general (Binkley 1961; Copp 2005). When discussing whether moral judgments are objective or subjective, Binkley (1961) holds that some people think moral judgments are objective, since such judgments are made based on "the accepted standards of human society, or on the accepted standards of a particular civilization" (p. 190). By contrast, others argue that moral judgments are subjective because they recognize the patterns of propaganda and are thus inclined to search for their own evaluations. These two stances on whether moral judgments are objective can also be read as what we define as the difference between "morality" and "ethics" in this section. According to Deleuze (1997),

> The difference is that morality presents us with a set of constraining rules of a special sort, ones that judge actions and intentions by considering them in relation to transcendent values (that is good, that's bad. . .); ethics is a set of optional rules that assess what we do, what we say, in relation to the ways of existing involved (p. 100).

In other words, though both words underline codes of conduct and principles that define what is good and bad in society, morality prescribes the rules and principles agreed upon by the society; whereas ethics suggests more autonomy on the part of individuals to render moral principles, given daily actions and responses constantly become the site of praxis. Additionally, morality often uses the question of whether someone is hurt as the standard to judge if one's actions are moral, yet the question of whether one's behaviors are ethical often hinges on the individuals who decide if they ought to do or ought not to do something on a daily basis (Gardner et al. 2003; Haynes et al. 2013). Put differently, ethics requires one to live an examined life constantly. It is in this sense we are discussing the relationship between ethics and the aims of education.

Ethics often entails criteria for the right action, and this begs the question: what are some major theories regarding ethics? This question is then followed by another: what is the right action? Based on different answers to this question, ethical theories are categorized into deontology, consequentialism, virtual ethics, ethics of care, etc. (Carr and Steutel 2005; Copp 2005). According to Brink (2005), "consequentialism identifies right action as action that promotes value" (p. 382). This is to say that what results from the action determines if the action is a correct one and thus ethical. By contrast, deontology takes correct action as having intrinsic value, and, thus, it is independent of what is caused by such action. Sans the question of what consequences are from one's action, deontology also indicates that the person taking action has a moral duty and is able to engage in rational thinking. In a yet different school of thought, virtue ethics emphasizes virtue as moral character (Annas 2005). Last, but hardly least, the ethics of care highlights that caring for others and caring relations as the starting point of ethics; this stance on ethics is built on caring relations and meeting people's needs rather than putting the burden of care solely on a socially inferior party (Yuan 2019).

Though addressing ethics differently, all four notions of ethics are relevant to classroom teachers' identities and teaching practices in the classroom. Also, worth mentioning here is that these four notions can coexist in individual teachers' and school administrators' philosophies. For instance, when a student suffers from anxiety and depression, a teacher may choose to prioritize accommodating the student's needs so that they are not stressed by their academic performance. The teacher's choice signifies that they view academic success as secondary to the student's health. This choice is thus based on deontology and ethics of care since the teacher makes the decision based on the individual student's mental health and their moral judgment involves a caring relationship with the student. To illustrate further, instructional decisions in classrooms are often based on consequentialism, since teachers often need to ask questions in the decision-making process such as: what are the results of the choices they make? What are the effects if they take these actions rather than those actions?

Part 3: Why Ethics Is Important for Classroom Teachers

The question regarding ethics can surface at places where teachers and school leaders wrestle with dilemmas and daily scenarios that resist easy answers (Ayers 2004; Infantino 2009). As teachers prepare for daily lessons, they face numerous decisions, from how to teach lessons to how to engage students in class, to whether to give students certain options in doing assignments or taking tests, and whether to make exceptions in class based on extenuating circumstances, to name a few. Some decisions are trivial and have few moral impacts, while others have significant bearing on ethics and what the teacher takes as the aims of education.

For example, studying the cultural stories of student teachers, Britzman and Greene (2003) found student teachers find the student teaching process is a constantly uncanny and uneasy one due to "clashes between authoritative and internally persuasive discourses" (p. 73). As indicated earlier, such conflicts are mostly due to how institutions and stakeholders define the aims of education differently. What preservice teachers have absorbed from their teacher preparation programs is often at odds with what the actual schools have stipulated as teaching. On the other hand, teacher preparation programs cannot fully predict all classroom hiccups, so such programs guide education students to make decisions that appear right for teachers that often conflict with the student teaching element in their preparation program (Noddings 2008). It is during student teaching that they find dilemmas not always covered in their own classroom learning, and these dilemmas force student teachers to reflect on practices and engage in moral reasoning before reaching a decision or conclusion (Sellman 2012).

Another great example in today's education is that we often hear how important it is to "hold teachers accountable" in professional development workshops and other attacks on public education. The word "accountability" has, to a large extent, been substituted for the word "responsibility" in our evaluation of teachers (Biesta 2010; Noddings 1992). Standards and accountability often entail a rhetorical gimmick used to manipulate curricula taught in schools, and most teachers are thus not teaching lessons of their own making because they are instructed to teach toward the goal of having students pass standardized testing as much as they can (Pinar 2004). When justifying teachers' ratings, school administrators will use a form with itemized lists that suggest criteria for exemplary teaching. Thus, the number of times teachers use teaching strategies highly approved by administrators becomes key if they are teaching lessons with fidelity. However, if we allow ourselves to raise Biesta's question of the difference between good education and measurable education in reflection upon our own teaching, it will help us understand why accountability is problematic. While good education and measurable education overlap with each other in making sure students grasp lessons and demonstrate their learning in classes, measurable education can engender sacrificing learning experiences and unmeasurable outcomes of good education. As Biesta (2010) notes, managerial accountability in measurable education "has shifted from questions of aims and ends of educational practices to questions about the smoothness and effectiveness of educational processes" (p. 6). I would surely be remiss to assume one cannot easily understand the difference between the word "measurable" and the word "good," yet knowing the difference is insufficient, and such knowledge only predisposes a teacher to wrestle daily with when to teach toward accountability for the sake of job security and when to teach based on what they deem to be good education. On a larger scale, knowing the difference also presses them to ask how much they should teach toward accountability and how much they can teach toward what they see as good education against the stipulated curriculums.

As Levinson and Fay (2019) contend, questions and policies are usually considered as places where the right decisions are easy to reach, but because educators and policymakers are obliged to take moral values and principles into consideration, there are very few occasions where one can easily find "the right decision." Hence, ethical dilemmas in teaching and other educational policymaking scenarios must be deliberated by individuals concerning "practices, cultures, personalities, rules, politics, and even legal requirements" (Levinson and Fay 2019, p. 7).

Wrapping up this section, we can think of practicing ethics in classrooms with the word *phronesis*, or what the Aristotelian philosophy has defined as "practical wisdom" (Kinsella and Pitman 2012, p. 1). *Phronesis* recognizes that abstract knowledge, training in teacher preparation programs, and actual teaching life work in silos. *Phronesis* is not meant to underestimate the importance of abstract moral principles, but it does indicate that daily practices and decisions need to be informed by abstract moral principles, though they are not an answer key to teachers' dilemmas. As practical wisdom, *phronesis* bridges abstract knowledge and daily practices in the sense that it involves individuals' ethical deliberations, judgment, and reflection (Kinsella and Pitman 2012; Wakeham 2019). When certainty is missing from the daily events in schools, *phronesis* values teachers' agency to develop their ethics and put their ethics to use in making instructional decisions (Higgs 2012).

Section 5: Educational Philosophers of Note

Katherine Fogelberg

Before diving into the different views of educational philosophy, it is important to provide a foundation in some educational philosophers of note, some of whom you have already been indirectly introduced to via citations within this chapter (e.g., Noddings and Dewey), and one who is recognized as bringing an important perspective to educational philosophy but is not always the first person to come to mind when the topic arises (hooks). This section is a very brief overview of some of the recognized titans within the philosophy of education – at least those within the US's view. Those with more in-depth learning and backgrounds in this specific area of education may disagree, but for this audience, Noddings, Dewey, and hooks are those who standout as foundational educational philosophers. They are introduced here but will be, along with a variety of others, further profiled in later chapters covering their theories of education more deeply.

Part 1: John Dewey

John Dewey (1859–1952) is perhaps the most recognized and vaunted person in the realm of educational philosophy; there is an entire society named for him and as a white male educator in the wake of the Second Great War in the United States, he was uniquely situated to influence the field to which he committed his professional life: education. Born in 1859 and living until 1952, he was also the first in the line of the contemporary educational philosophers in the United States who had significant impact on the discipline. Dewey is an outsized figure within the field, as his influence was felt early and continues to resonate with educators today; very few discussions about education as a discipline occur without some direct or indirect reference to John Dewey. Although his theories and philosophies primarily focused on K-12 teaching, much of his work is easily transferable to higher education, including professional education.

Dewey is the educational theorist and philosopher who you may be most familiar with; he is indeed a towering figure within the world of education. A prolific writer, Dewey's collected works can be found in David Reed's e-book published by PergamonMedia. In these works, Dewey philosophizes about education as a whole and about individual components of education, as demonstrated by his titles, which include *Studies in Logical Theory* (1903), *Psychology and Social Practice* (1900), *Moral Principles in Education* (1909), *How We Think* (1910), and *Democracy and Education: An Introduction to the Philosophy of Education* (1916); it is this last title that is viewed as his most impactful and enduring work. In *Democracy and Education*, Dewey philosophizes upon the issues faced in the attempt to provide high-quality education for the public in a democratic society, ultimately calling for a full revision of public education and emphasizing the need for universal education to advance both individuals and the society within which they serve. The text continues to be relevant over 100 years after its original debut and is widely lauded as the foundational work in public education in the United States.

Part 2: Nel Noddings

Nel Noddings (1929–2022) was born a decade after Dewey's foundational work in education was first published; a work that cracked open the door for her to explore care ethics in the classroom. While less discussed and potentially less heavily emphasized on a regular basis in his work, Dewey's writings on ethics permeated his writings, in some cases directly but in most less so (Hildebrand 2023). But this discussion of ethics in relation to education provided an opportunity for others to build on the idea, and Noddings took full advantage of this with her philosophical approach to education from a caring perspective, which she called care ethics. Within this philosophical approach to education, Noddings incorporated the idea that caring was the foundation of morality, and that only through the development of a caring relationship between teacher and student could morality be achieved.

Sadly, Noddings passed in 2022. But her work in educational philosophy will continue to influence teachers and students alike; her legacy coming from her gender, her grace, and her intellectual impact on the field of education writ large. She is referenced often in this textbook, and there is a more in-depth exploration of the Noddings' care ethic in Chapter 6 – Roles of the Professional Program Instructor.

Part 3: bell hooks

Born almost 25 years after Noddings, bell hooks (1952–2021), nee Gloria Jean Watkins, was a Black, queer woman feminist, scholar, and educational philosopher. "That shift from beloved, all-black schools to white schools where Black students were always seen as interlopers, as not really belonging, taught me the difference between education as the practice of freedom and education that merely strives to reinforce domination" (hooks 1994, p. 4). Educational philosopher is something she might not have called herself, nor did anyone necessarily recognize her explicitly as such. However, among her prodigious number of books and publications, two that addressed education specifically provided insights into hooks' personal experiences as a teacher and as a student, and lay the groundwork for overcoming the racial, sexual, and class boundaries imposed upon those in the classroom to achieve what she viewed as the teacher's most important goal: freedom.

In *Teaching to Transgress: Education as a Practice of Freedom* (1994), hooks demonstrated her educational philosopher's hat: "education was about the practice of freedom" she says, in her introduction (hooks, p. 4). Through education, hooks (1994) goes on to explain, she was able to grow beyond the boundaries society placed on her, which made it possible for her to create and implement teaching practices that directly addressed ways to interrogate curricular biases that reinforced the systems of domination, including racism and sexism while at the same time figuring out new ways to teach diverse groups of college students.

> The classroom remains the most radical space of possibility in the academy. For years, it has been a place where education has been undermined by teachers and students alike who seek to use it as a platform for opportunistic concerns rather than as a place to learn. With these essays, I add my voice to the collective call for renewal and rejuvenation in our teaching practices. Urging all of us to open our minds and hearts so that we can know beyond the boundaries of what is acceptable, so that we can think and rethink, so that we can create new visions, I celebrate teaching that enables transgressions – a movement against and beyond boundaries. It is that movement which makes education the practice of freedom (hooks 1994, p. 12).

hooks's approach to teaching was situated within her educational philosophy – that learning should be engaging and fun; that learning was a partnership between student and teacher; and that education was, above all, about providing students the tools they needed to effect social change that challenged and overcame oppression. Philosophically she was strongly influenced by Paulo Freire and aligned, perhaps unwittingly, with W.E.B. DuBois, all of whom, along with hooks, are profiled in Chapter 2.

Part 4: The -isms

Mostly based on four major philosophies, namely, idealism, realism, pragmatism, and existentialism, five corresponding schools of educational philosophies emerged: perennialism, essentialism, progressivism, social reconstructionism or reconstructivism (Harmon and Jones 2005; Sandovnik et al. 2018), and humanism or humanistic education. Before we go too much further, a little note on "-isms." There are, as you likely know, many nouns that can be "ism'ed" (e.g., fanaticism, liberalism or conservatism, and mysticism), although Google's Oxford Languages dictionary defines ism as a standalone noun; one that identifies a "distinctive practice, system, or philosophy, typically a political ideology or an artistic movement" (n.d., n.p.). It does also identify -ism as a suffix, and of the examples provided, the addition of -ism to words "denoting a system, principle, or ideological movement" (Oxford Language Dictionary online n.d., n.p.) is directly related to philosophy. Much like the scientific "-ologies," (biology, physiology, toxicology, and so on), education also has its own unique and sometimes confounding language. Acquiring the words is important and relatively easy; truly understanding them is always the challenge, particularly when dealing with concepts as abstract and often seemingly esoteric as philosophy (and theory!). Sometimes breaking words into their constituent parts can help with the understanding, which is why this interlude has been provided before diving into the -isms of education.

The emergence of educational philosophies corresponding to major philosophical movements in society should not be especially surprising; societal pressures continue to shape how education is imagined and delivered, something you will see clearly in Chapter 2 and may have some experience with in your own teaching practice. We are currently, for example, entrenching ourselves in a firmly constructivist approach to learning in veterinary (and other medical professional) education programs. This has happened before and will likely happen again after the current trends give way to other trends; society right now has created a generation of learners who have been raised in an educational system that tells them they are customers rather than students – an approach to education that is very business-centered and, in such an approach, also very student-oriented (though not always for reasons that educational philosophies argue we should be student-oriented). In short, it should not be terribly difficult to understand how the philosophies driving society (even if you may not be aware of it) also drive the philosophical stances of educators.

Section 6: Teacher-Centered Educational Philosophies: Perennialism and Essentialism

Ying Wang and Katherine Fogelberg

Part 1: Introduction

There are, as you can imagine, a lot of intricacies involved with each of the many extant philosophies, so the most pertinent of each has been extracted in its appropriate place to provide you with the basic information needed to understand how the corresponding educational philosophies were built upon them. For this section, we will lightly explore idealism and realism, as the educational philosophies of perennialism and essentialism are mainly built upon these two overarching philosophies.

Idealism as a movement was most prominent in the eighteenth and nineteenth centuries, although there are some allusions to it in the seventeenth century and some who clung to it even through the twentieth century (Guyer and Horstmann 2021). There are a number of divisions within idealism, including (but not limited to), metaphysical, epistemological, aesthetic, moral, ethical, subjective, objective,

and absolute idealism (Guyer and Horstmann 2021). In modern philosophy, idealism is generally divided into ontological idealism, or the idea that the ultimate foundation of reality is something mentally internal to humans, and epistemological idealism, or the idea that existence independent of the mind does exist, but everything we know about the reality independent of the mind is so fully permeated by the mind's constructive activities that all claims to knowledge are, in reality, a form of self-knowledge (Guyer and Horstmann 2021). In other words, idealists currently believe either that reality only exists in our individual minds or there are aspects of reality independent of our minds but we have created them and, thus, reality is still created by humans' mental machinations.

Realism, on the other hand, approaches reality through claims of *existence* and claims of *independence* (Miller 2019). The claim of existence states that objects exist and those objects can be factually described: paper, doors, plants, and so on; in addition, facts about these items also exist: paper is thin; doors are rectangular; plants have roots. The claim on independence states that regardless of what anyone says or thinks, existing items have those properties – saying or thinking that plants do not have roots does not make it so (Miller 2019). In other words, a person's beliefs, language, ideas, or conceptions of reality *do not alter reality*; you can probably see how this is very different from the idealist's view of the world. Miller (2019) succinctly states that idealists concede the existence of objects but reject that their existence is independent of our minds – this is where the true difference lies between these two philosophies.

Despite the fact that perennialism, which emerged primarily from idealism, and essentialism, which emerged primarily from realism, disagree on multiple curriculum components, such as curriculum emphases, major classroom instruction methods, teachers' specific roles, goals of education, and assessments, they both stress the importance of the teacher's roles in teaching and learning. This is why, in addition to being labeled as knowledge-centered and subject-centered educational philosophies, perennialism and essentialism are also sometimes referred to as teacher-centered educational philosophies, versus student-centered educational philosophies (e.g., progressivism; Sadker and Zittleman 2016; Kooli et al. 2019).

As an exemplar of perennialism, the *Paideia Proposal* (Adler 1982) contends that teachers should be placed at the center of instruction; as the experts of content area knowledge they teach, they co-learn with students through lecturing and dialectic dialogues with students, so that the students come to their own knowledge in the process. In the essentialist philosophy, teachers are also considered the authority in the classroom, and thus, lecturing is the main method to transmit knowledge. The difference between the teacher authority in the perennialism philosophy and that in the essentialism philosophy lies in the question of how much autonomy students are allowed to have to reach and produce knowledge.

Part 2: Perennialism

Though rarely referenced nowadays when capitalism and the logic of efficiency predetermine most educational decisions, perennialism was the most predominant educational philosophy in US history through the 1990s, when significant public education reform occurred. When perennialism is referenced, people often perceive it as the most traditional and conservative school of educational philosophy. As part of the word perennialism, "perennial" means lasting forever or coming back year after year. Similarly, the name perennialism suggests that reality is absolute, enduring, and independent of worldly matter; only great ideas and traditional disciplines should be taught in education since great ideas transcend time and space (Adler 1982; Ellis 2003).

Scholars agree that perennialism found its root in idealism (Ornstein and Hunkins 2018). Tracing back to ancient Greek philosophers like Socrates and Plato, idealism upholds that the mind is the most important, and worldly matter secondary in education. As they think reality is spiritual and unchanging, philosophers of idealism, such as Socrates and Plato, also posit that truth is absolute and external (Harmon and Jones 2005). Modern representative philosophers of idealism include Rene Déscartes, Immanuel Kant, George W.F. Hegel, Ralph Waldo Emerson, and Henry David Thoreau. For idealists, to educate means to raise student awareness and help them appreciate enduring truths and values through dialectic dialogue and studying great ideas from the past; translated, this means studying male- and Euro-centric ideas that were considered great. Moral education and the question of "what is a good life" are at the core of idealism, and according to idealists, as soon as you find your own understanding of this question through education, you should easily navigate other aspects of life.

Although primarily influenced by idealism, some scholars contend that realism also contributed to perennialism in education (Tan 2006; Ornstein and Hunkins 2018). This contention is supported by the fact that the curriculum of perennialism proposes that elementary education should put its emphasis on the three Rs: reading, writing, and arithmetic – topics that are viewed to concretely exist and students need to be able to do and understand – before students are introduced to great ideas and critical thinking at the secondary level.

Goal of Education

Perennialists pushed the idea that good education and meritocracy should be the focus of education; they believed the nature of man was most important, and, thus, demanding academic standards were necessary to ensure both the quality of educators and the quality of students. This idea that knowledge should and did transcend time is reflected in the idealist's approach to the world: reality is only constructed by our minds, and, thus, education for endurance makes sense. The increasing pace of industrialization and urbanization in the Western world spurred the movement toward perennialism as an urgent need to teach students basic skills they could apply to living in an ever-evolving society and rapidly shifted the social and political landscape.

Perennialism stipulates that the goal of education is to teach morality, critical thinking, and what a good life is. With this educational philosophy in mind and understanding that educational philosophy informs educational elements such as curriculum, classroom instruction, learning, and assessments, a typical perennialist curriculum consists of great ideas and classical literature in Western and European history and culture. As previously referenced, one widely cited example in the United States was the *Paideia Proposal* (*paideia* originates from Greek, meaning "the upbringing of a child") by Mortimer Adler (1982, 1984). Adler also participated in editing the *Great Books of the Western World* series, featuring (male and Euro-centric) scholars including Plato, Aristotle, Kant, Shakespeare, and Homer, among others.

Paideia Proposal supporters believed that schooling should prepare students to "earn a decent livelihood," "to be a good citizen of the nation and the world," and "to make a good life for one's self" (Roberts and Billing, as cited in Ellis 2003, p. 132). Though advocates of the *Paideia Proposal* listed preparing students to make a living as one of the goals of education, they also insisted that a solid education on morality and citizenship through great ideas in an organized sequence would naturally lead to students obtaining skills to make a living (Adler 1982, 1984; Roberts and Billings 1999).

Curriculum

According to the *Paideia Proposal*, the same curriculum should be taught to all students and all students should learn in the same way. There should be no elective or vocational courses because, even if provided with elective courses, young students are too intellectually immature to make good choices by themselves. Vocation-related training should be postponed until students go to college.

Hutchins (1936), a significant proponent of the perennialist philosophy who also participated in editing the *Great Books of the Western World Series*, argued that "education implies teaching. Teaching implies knowledge. Knowledge is truth. Truth is everywhere the same. Hence, education should be everywhere the same" (p. 66). Hutchins's quote epitomizes the essence of perennialism, that is, education is about teaching enduring ideas and absolute truths, and that education should be the same for everyone, regardless of the individual student's interests or social contexts.

Perennialist scholars insist that studying permanent truths and great ideas from the past offers a liberal education that enables individuals to ponder on morality and contemplate what a good life is. Through this process, they become intellectually mature and will become adept at using critical thinking skills. Perennialists also believe that the curriculum should be subject/knowledge-centered (Ellis 2003; Ornstein and Hunkins 2018); academic disciplines emphasized in the perennialist approach are language, literature, the arts, science, mathematics, history, geography, and social studies (Adler 1982, 1984). From a moral education perspective, it is acceptable to perennialists that moral teaching and moral beliefs based on religions sometimes overlap with each other in classroom instruction (Bloom 1987; Ellis 2003; Murray 2012; Ornstein and Hunkins 2018).

To some extent, we can argue that perennialism is contrary to the idea that education should cater to the job market or any other worldly matter. Especially at the elementary and secondary level, proponents of perennialism note that we should have rigorous academic standards and offer few elective courses or vocational training because putting students on the vocational tracks would deny them the chance for equal and liberal education. Besides Robert M. Hutchins and Mortimer J. Adler, other scholars of perennialism include Allan Bloom and Charles Murray. Both Bloom (1987) and Murray (2012) contend that eclipsing liberal education and foundational values in American public education leads to indifference to morality and major societal problems.

Teacher's Role and Classroom Instruction

In line with the principles in the *Paideia Proposal*, the teacher in a perennialist classroom has absolute intellectual authority. Yet, in spite of being the authority in the classroom, unlike essentialists, the perennialist teacher presents lesson topics without hammering knowledge into the students' minds; instead, the perennialist teacher encourages students to develop their own knowledge through inquiries and critical thinking. With that said, perennialism in education does require teachers to be the role model in terms of

living a moral life, modeling logical reasoning, and critical thinking in inquiries (Adler 1984; Tan 2006; Kooli et al. 2019). Additionally, given the curricular emphasis on the classics and great literature, a teacher in the perennialist classroom should also be familiar with factual information in textbooks and be capable of engaging students in deep discussions and dialectic dialogues. Since perennialism in education finds most of its philosophical root in idealism, it takes lecture-based instruction, coaching, and the Socratic method as its main instructional methods in the classroom (Adler 1982, 1984; Ellis 2003). Although teachers are the experts in the content area and have the intellectual authority in the classroom, they serve more as a facilitator in the classroom, posing open-ended questions and offering feedback to push the discussions on subject topics further such that students raise their awareness and develop morally through discussion (Adler 1982, 1984).

Part 3: Essentialism: Roots in Realism

The slogan of essentialist educational philosophers was "back to basics" (Ellis 2003; Harmon and Jones 2005; Ornstein and Hunkins 2018), which was widely endorsed in education during the height of this educational movement. Essentialism came to prominence at a time when public education became the norm and was accessible to all populations. It was built on the idea that students should progress through a series of increasingly difficult tasks and topics that, once mastered, indicated their readiness to be promoted to the next level; it is not unlike many of the systems we see even today in educational systems throughout the world. This educational philosophy is somewhat aligned with realism in that it is an objective and structured approach to learning – just as realism is an objective and structured approach to reality.

Realism is believed to date back to Aristotle in ancient Greece, the most famous student of Plato. Unlike Plato and Socrates who believe the mind endures, comes before worldly matter, and thus, is of the utmost importance to gain knowledge about a good life and understand morality, Aristotle believed that people learned from empirical activities. His reasoning was that enduring truths or laws should be observable from the material world. Similarly, realists like Aristotle believed that reality was independent of the mind; knowledge should be obtained through making scientific queries about the world. Other well-known realists are Thomas Aquinas, Francis Bacon, John Locke, and Bertrand Russell.

Modern realism mainly stresses scientific reasoning as the core of education. Though some scholars (Tan 2006; Ornstein and Hunkins 2018) posit that parts of essentialism also originated from idealism because essentialists also believe in the value of transmitting cultures and history to younger generations. However, the main argument of essentialism is that we learn the facts and concepts of cultures and history to function in society rather, and this is more important, than cultivating the young student's mind or developing their critical thinking skills. Compared with perennialist educators, who stress moral and intellectual development, and accordingly educate students to become intellectual elites in society, essentialist educators are more concerned about educating students – including through traditional education and through vocational training – so that they can function in the physical world. Ellis (2003) suggests that the Committee of Ten, led by Charles Eliot, and the Committee of Ten Report in the 1890s served as the landmark transition from perennialism to essentialism in the curriculum of American public schools. It is also true that essentialism was a response to the progressive education movement that swept education in the United States in the 1920s and 1930s (Arslan 2018).

Goal of Education

In essentialists' eyes, education is not so much to incite change as it is to instill the most essential skills and facts in Western history to younger generations that meet the accepted standards of society. Unlike perennialism, which focused on moral and intellectual development through learning "great ideas" in the past, essentialists called for curricular emphasis on teaching students reading, writing, and arithmetic skills so that students could survive in society (Bagley 1938; Ellis 2003). Facts, basic concepts, and essential skills are the center of the essentialist curriculum; typical subjects in its curriculum are English, foreign languages, mathematics, writing, physics, arts, music, and the like.

Similar to perennialism, however, essentialism also does not consider students' social needs, emotional needs, or academic interests under consideration in its educational scope. Though such skills are also hinted at in the perennialist approach, essentialist scholars deem the mastery of essential skills indispensable to survival in society. What are the implications for educational policies? A glimpse of *A Nation at Risk, No Child Left Behind* (NCLB), and "Race to the Top" helps elucidate how education has witnessed the return of essentialist philosophy in education in the United States. It is clearly the rationale for the return to teaching basics in education; one that is anchored in the perception that this will resume the US's educational standing internationally in the post-sputnik era. Essentialism continues to be the prevalent educational philosophy in today's public education system, with most classes being taught to ensure student success on standardized testing that are focused on standards explicitly prescribed by state and federal educational agencies.

Curriculum

As a teacher-centered/subject-centered educational philosophy, essentialism also shares the perennialists' view that students are too immature to choose what to learn, and, thus, curriculum should be handpicked by adults who know and can identify the essential knowledge and necessary skills for students to succeed in society. As a result of the philosophical beliefs and corresponding policies, the curriculum in essentialism focuses on the "essential" part of academic disciplines; the three Rs, the basic skills of what Hirsch et al. (1988) call "core knowledge" are stressed both at the elementary level and the secondary level, because all three are what students need to function in society. As a result, whether students should be promoted to the next higher level should be decided by whether they have mastered the required skills in the corresponding grade level.

The leading proponents of essentialism were William Bagley and E.D. Hirsch, Jr. Both scholars (Bagley 1934; Hirsch et al. 1988) expressed their concerns about the gap between education, needs, and accepted standards in society. Bagley was a professor of education and founder of the Essentialist Education Society, and Hirsch et al. (1988) published *Cultural Literacy: What Every American Needs to Know*. In this book, he argued that schools should return to the basics and teach practical skills like reading, writing, and computing, so students are able to survive and function in society after they graduate.

Worrying that perennialist education was inadequate and progressive education was indifferent to society's needs, essentialists proposed that schools should hold strict standards regarding mastering critical skills and techniques from textbooks. The curriculum should feature memorization of facts rather than rhizomatic inquiries (nonlinear questions that end up connecting to each other) or exploration of the great ideas proposed by perennialism.

Teacher's Role and Classroom Instruction

Like a teacher from the perennialism school, a teacher in the essentialists' eyes should be an expert in their subject area and assume absolute authority in the classroom. Since factual knowledge and essential skills are what essentialists believe to be most significant to master, lecturing is the major and most efficient instructional method. In a typical essentialist's classroom, the teacher lectures from the front of the classroom while students memorize facts and practice skills through assignments. With explicit academic standards prescribed by federal and state-level agencies, the teacher uses standardized tests to diagnose students' weaknesses and gauge their academic competence and achievements. In the essentialist classroom, teaching for accountability is the shortcut to being the "best" teacher. Because whether learning and mastering essential concepts and skills takes place in the classroom depends on the mastery of specific facts and skills, backward mapping of what to teach and how to teach is the characteristic of an essentialist teacher's classroom instruction.

Section 7: Learner-Centered Educational Philosophies: Pragmatism and Existentialism

Katherine Fogelberg

Part 1: Introduction

Learner-centered educational philosophies are rooted in two foundational philosophies, specifically, pragmatism and existentialism. Pragmatism laid the groundwork for progressivism, constructivism, and reconstructionism (the last of which is covered more fully in the section covering socially-centered educational philosophies), while existentialism was the philosophy upon which humanism in education was built.

Pragmatism originated in the United States in the latter third of the nineteenth century and currently presents a growing alternative to the analytic and "Continental" philosophies (Radu 2011; Legg and Hookway 2021). Broadly understood, pragmatism is the idea that agency within the world cannot be separated from knowing the world – translated, that you cannot separate what you know about the world from your ability to live within and affect the world (Legg and Hookway 2021). However, it went through a couple of philosophical generations to get to this broad and somewhat abstract idea. The first iteration started with "classical pragmatism" as put forth by Charles Sanders Peirce and William James and was strongly influenced by evolutionary theory and the scientific revolution this theory spawned (Curren 2009; Legg and Hookway 2021). The focus of the first-generation pragmatists was on "inquiry, meaning and the nature of truth," while the second generation turned "more explicitly towards politics, education and other dimensions of social improvement," and was heavily influenced by the thoughts and ideas of John Dewey (Curren 2009; Chennault 2013; Legg and Hookway 2021, n.p.).

Existentialism as a philosophical movement can be difficult to explain, as it had a broad reach and diverse range of foci in its heyday (Aho 2023). The name itself, first used in 1943 by the French philosopher Gabriel Marcel, does not reference a specific system or philosophical school; in fact, existentialism houses a group of apparently divergent views, many of whom in retrospect fall under this philosophical camp but, during their lives did not necessarily explicitly identify as such (Aho 2023). And while the most prominent proponents of existentialism were Marcel's compatriots, including Jean-Paul Sartre, Simone de Beauvoir, Albert Camus, and Maurice Merleau-Ponty, nineteenth-century philosophers Søren Kierkegaard and Friedrich Nietzsche, along with twentieth-century German philosophers such as Edmund Husserl, Martin Heidegger, and Karl Jaspers, and prominent Spanish intellectuals José Ortega y Gasset and Miguel de Unamuno, were responsible for laying the conceptual groundwork for this movement (Aho 2023).

Part 2: Progressivism: Roots in Pragmatism

As originally perceived by Peirce, the core of pragmatism was his *pragmatic maxim*, a rule that appeared more positivist than progressive, as it essentially stated that "If and only if assertion and denial of a sentence imply a difference capable of observational (experiential, operational, or experimental) test does the sentence have factual meaning" (Feigl, as cited in Curren 2009, p. 490). For both Peirce and James, an essential component of the maxim was clarifying truth as a concept, which produced a broad outlook that ended up splitting the pragmatists into two camps. The first consisted of those who followed Peirce and believed pragmatism should be a scientific philosophy following monism, or the idea truth is a singular entity that can only be supported or disproven. The second camp followed James and, importantly for educators, John Dewey (more on this later), who took an alethic view of truth – one that believed it should be a more broad-based philosophy allowing for multiple interpretations of what was true (Legg and Hookway 2021).

Ultimately, the unifying idea behind pragmatism is that of *experience*, all interactions that occur between subjects and objects, between individual selves and the world (Radu 2011). As such, epistemologically pragmatists view their philosophy as paving the path back to common sense, centered on experience, resulting in the rejection of what they considered a flawed philosophical heritage that had "distorted the work of earlier thinkers" (Legg and Hookway 2021).

Progressivism's roots in pragmatism emerge when considering that experience and common sense are the core tenets of this approach to the classroom. Although Peirce would eventually go a distinctly different direction from

James and Dewey (who would further break from James), Peirce did have some prescience regarding pedagogy, indirectly discussing both inquiry-based learning and evidence-based teaching, though these are not found in a single writing (Legg and Hookway 2021). James also wrote about education early on, though his ideas are certainly more aligned with essentialism and perennialism, as can be seen in his advice to teachers recommending they view children as able and open to learning different ideas at different ages, with younger children needing to first learn "sensible properties of material things" (harkening back to essentialism) so that later in adolescence they are able to understand "the more abstract aspects of experience" (reflecting some perennialist views) – including science and morality (James, as cited in Curren 2009, p. 495).

It is Dewey, however, who is viewed as the main figure in progressivist education and, indeed, in philosophy of education in general (see earlier overview in this chapter; more in-depth discussion of his educational theory in Chapter 2). Within the realm of progressive education (and the pragmatism from which it sprouted), Dewey's three fundamental commitments are the roots of this educational philosophy: "a naturalistic and evolutionary conception of human nature and human affairs; a high regard for the methods and norms of experimental, scientific inquiry; and a conception of democracy as a form of social life consistent with individual growth" (Curren 2009, p. 496). As such, Dewey viewed education as a means for disseminating the tools of inquiry and growth, and believed education to be the "most fundamental vehicle of social reconstruction" (Curren 2009, p. 497).

From this perspective, then, the traditional schools and methods of instruction that placed the teacher at the center of the learning process with students expected to memorize and recite back information were unfavorably looked upon (Legg and Hookway 2021). Instead, Dewey advocated for a more learner-centered approach, where students were provided the opportunity to explore and experience learning with guidance from the teacher; a classroom that developed the skills and attitudes necessary to engage in scientific inquiry that is socially based (Curren 2009). In other words, Dewey wanted students to learn how to *think* rather than how to *know*, a concept that professional programs continue to struggle with even today (Legg and Hookway 2021).

Goal of Education

From Dewey's perspective, then, the traditional schools and methods of instruction that placed the teacher at the center of the learning process with students expected to memorize and recite back information were unfavorably

looked upon (Legg and Hookway 2021). Instead, Dewey advocated for a more learner-centered approach, where students were provided the opportunity to explore and experience learning with guidance from the teacher; a classroom that developed the skills and attitudes necessary to engage in scientific inquiry that is socially based (Curren 2009).

The goals of a progressivist's education are to teach students how to *think* rather than how to *know*, a challenge we experience regularly even today in our classrooms, labs, and clinics. Epistemologically, progressivists wish to encourage students to carry out inquiry in a logical, appropriate, and successful manner (Legg and Hookway 2021). In this, it may appear that progressivism is just a reworked version of essentialism (or positivism, covered in Chapter 2). However, progressivists view the *process* of seeking knowledge and how it can be improved as being the ultimate goal of education (Legg and Hookway 2021). Thus, the main differences between progressivism and essentialism are that in progressivism, the focus is on the student and the process, whereas in essentialism, the focus is on the teacher and the outcome.

Curriculum

As an educational philosophy, progressivism also views students as able and willing to learn if provided the right structure, environment, and opportunities to interact with each other, their teacher(s), and the world. In this way, while the learning environment should be somewhat flexible and loose, the curriculum should still be selected by the teacher while being driven by the interests of students and guided by student questions.

According to Lerner (1962, as cited in Perez 2022a), there are key features that a progressive curriculum incorporates, including being student-centered, emphasizing growth, being action-oriented, focusing on process and change, being centered on equality, and ensuring a community-centric learning environment. In the original spirit of Dewey, who was a strong proponent of co-ed classrooms, vocational, and liberal arts education, progressivist curricula emphasized the three Rs but also included the arts, sciences, and vocational training (Curren 2009).

Clearly, progressivism is very student-centered – which aligns with the pragmatist's view that solving society's issues was the heart of action and value in thinking. Thus, a progressivist's curriculum is structured but still engaging and is focused on having students think about and attempt to solve real-world problems through directed activities that incorporate the scientific method but are also open to multiple "truths" that might emerge from such inquiry.

Teacher's Role and Classroom Instruction

As a student-centered philosophy of education, progressivists believe teachers are facilitators rather than deliverers of education, as might be found in an essentialist or perennialist classroom. This means that progressivist instructors direct students in the classroom but view the instructional time as a conversation – a speaking *with* versus a speaking *at* students. In this process, teachers must help students figure out how to *learn* – or, as you read about Dewey earlier, students needed to be taught how to *think* rather than how to *know* (Perez 2022a; Legg and Hookway 2021).

In progressive classrooms, learning is viewed as a collaborative, social process that places the burden of learning on the learner; they must figure out how to ask the questions to be answered, determine how to answer the questions posed, and, in doing so, learn how to become a fully functioning and contributing member to a democratic society – with the help of a facilitator who is there to support them in their endeavors when needed. The pedagogical practices of a progressivist educator generally include active learning that promotes self-discovery; self-directed learning; cooperative learning strategies; enhancing students' problem-solving skills; and nurturing critical thinking skills that are delivered through group work focused on meaningful, relevant projects that promote experiential learning opportunities in addition to the people skills students acquire through working in peer groups (Perez 2022a). Such projects are to be approached through the application of the scientific method, but not to verify truth, as perennialists and essentialists seek to do; rather, progressivists approach the use of the scientific method as an opportunity to validate student experiences – hence, the alethic view of truth that second-generation pragmatists adhered to, although it should not be forgotten that first generation pragmatists were explicitly interested in inquiry, meaning, and the nature of truth as well (Legg and Hookway 2021).

If you are already familiar with constructivism as an educational theory, you may be finding yourself feeling as if progressivism and constructivism are essentially the same. This is not an unfair thought or observation, though there are some subtle differences between these two schools of educational thought – even while they both emerged from pragmatism. Fortunately, this is a great segue to the next educational philosophy covered in this section, which just happens to be constructivism (the philosophy, not the theory – that is covered in Chapter 2).

Part 3: Constructivism: Roots in Pragmatism

Constructivism is the theory that says learners construct knowledge rather than just passively take in information. In its extreme, constructivism proposes that only when we figure things out by engaging in learning that is followed to a satisfying conclusion do we truly accept anything as knowledge, and, thus, the preexistence of knowledge cannot truly occur because what others may have learned and recorded was not learned by every individual – and only the individual who constructed the knowledge may truly own it (Gruender 1996). Fortunately, most constructivist educators are not willing to go this far, settling instead for the idea that students construct their knowledge within the confines of their experiences, and these experiences encompass their pasts as well as the pasts of others. Couched in philosophical terms, constructivism admits that what we view as knowledge is truly just a claim or group of claims about the world – it is our *construction* of the thing we believe about our lives and our world (Colliver 2002). Thus, knowledge claims are only justified if we collectively agree that they help us reach our practical goals, which is in contrast to the belief that knowledge claims are *verified* when they prove to correspond to reality, as perennialists and essentialists contend (Legg and Hookway 2021; Colliver 2002).

Because construction of knowledge necessarily requires action and experience, it is easy to see how pragmatism provided the basis for constructivism to emerge. It is, perhaps, a more evolved permutation of progressivism, though it can also be traced back to an eighteenth-century philosopher named Giambattista Vico, who admired René Descartes, in spite of the fact that Descartes writings had been banned by the church (Gruender 1996). Vico's philosophy was focused on history, and asked for "rational and historical explanations of the origins of human cultures," a question that was in direct conflict to the doctrine of the time that believed in Divine providence and the idea that societies could only be properly ruled by royalty – and specifically kings – who were beholden only to God (Gruender 1996). To get around this contradiction and get his philosophy published, Vico posed the idea that humans could only construct their own ideas about the world with the understanding that no such ideas would ever reach the heights of God's knowledge, as God had created the world and therefore only He could know all its possibilities (Gruender 1996). Constructivism in the historical sense was born, and though Vico's work would inform the extreme constructivist views, it is pragmatism, the uniquely American philosophy, that is widely accepted as the intellectual movement that inspired constructivism.

Goal of Education

Confucius is famously credited with the quote "I hear and I forget. I see and I remember. I do and I understand," a succinct summary of the constructivist's view of the goals of education. Teaching students from the front of the room without engaging them in conversation effectively creates students whose only goal is to repeat back information using rote memory that quickly becomes lost. Using demonstrations is a step closer to the constructivist's ideal, but still lacks the ability to fully engage students in the learning process. Students taught through demonstration will make a stronger connection to the information, but they will not truly absorb it in a way that an educator might desire. Students are provided the chance to actively engage in learning, however, allows students to hear, see, do, and absorb knowledge, because in doing so students are creating connections to past experiences and information that provide them the basis for true discovery of knowledge and truth (Adom et al. 2016).

Given this background information, then, it should not surprise you that the goals of education for the constructivist teacher include students learning through *experience* and gaining an understanding of the world through connecting new experiences with old experiences. Constructivists aim to shift from the concept of *knowledge as a product* to *knowing as a process* – something that should feel similar to, but not the same as, the progressivist's goal of education (Jones and Brader-Arage 2002). As with progressivism, constructivism is focused on the student and the process. Where these two differ in their approach to knowledge itself: whereas progressivism views knowledge as already existing – something that students need to be taught to seek out, with the *process* of seeking being the focus, constructivism believes that knowledge is actively constructed by each student and is based on their *assimilation* (fitting new information into existing *schemas*) and *accommodation* (revising and creating new schemas that incorporate the old schemas) of new knowledge with prior information and experiences.

Curriculum

The approach to curriculum from the constructivist's perspective is counter to the more traditional classroom in that it begins with the whole and expands to address individual parts. In other words, it emphasizes the big picture first rather than the individual pieces that continue to be delivered in a stepwise fashion, moving students toward understanding how those pieces fit to make the whole, which occurs in more traditional classrooms. The curriculum is structured in a manner that provides teachers with information about what students already know and proceeds to build upon prior knowledge in a way that allows students to actively engage in the learning process. It uses real-life, authentic, and relevant problems to teach students how to connect new information and experiences with their prior learning – in other words, the curriculum is constructed in a way that supports students in learning how to negotiate meaning.

To do this, constructivist curricula contain lessons based on an instructor's understanding of what students have come to their classrooms knowing, and this serves as a basis for determining where the incoming class sits with respect to the expectations of knowledge set by precedent or teacher expectation. From there, the teacher elicits prior knowledge from the students and refines their lessons to meet students where they are; intentionally incorporates exercises or lessons that create cognitive dissonance – meaning, challenges students to reconsider their prior knowledge in light of new information and provides them support as they revise their existing understandings; and asks students to reflect on their learning in a way that demonstrates what they have learned (University at Buffalo n.d.)

Teacher's Role and Classroom Instruction

Similar to progressivism, constructivism views teachers as facilitators rather than deliverers of knowledge. However, the facilitator role in the constructivist classroom is less formalized and structured than in the progressivist's classroom; instructors with this philosophical stance also view instructional time as an opportunity to engage in discourse with students, although in this view, instructors do not drive the conversations, students do. This can be seen in the types of activities constructivists may incorporate in their classrooms, which include peer teaching, and IBL, or inquiry-based learning, approaches (University at Buffalo n.d.).

Inquiry-based learning approaches encompass problem-based learning (PBL), team-based learning (TBL), and case-based learning (CBL), with which some of you may be familiar. In particular, CBL – or some iteration of it – is being increasingly used in professional programs, including veterinary medicine (see Fogelberg et al. 2021; Crowther and Baillie 2016; Pereira et al. 2018). PBL, which originated in human medicine at McMaster University in Canada (Servant-Miklos 2019), was quite popular for some time and has faded in the last few decades. And TBL, the most recent iteration of IBL approaches, is seeing some resurgence now, with the University of Arizona's veterinary program being fully TBL based. It is safe to say that the constructivist philosophy of education is alive and well, if in slightly different forms and functions.

As with progressivist classrooms, constructivist classrooms view learning as a collaborative, social process that places the burden of learning on the learner; they must figure out how to ask the questions to be answered and determine how to answer the questions posed. However, constructivism asks students to do this more autonomously than does progressivism, with some pedagogical practices relying more fully on the students to lean on each other and their prior experiences than on the facilitator to solve the problems posed. The facilitator, in the extreme constructivist classroom, does little more than provide the problem to be solved, leaving students to figure out resources, create the questions they think need to be answered, and answer the questions they have created. In such classrooms, facilitators often do not intervene when students are going down a road that may be viewed as inaccurate or outright incorrect, instead encouraging students to rethink certain aspects of their work without influencing students with regard to the "correctness" of their learning. Most constructivist classrooms are not quite this hands-off, but if such learning environments are encountered, it is important to know that this is certainly in keeping with the scope of this educational philosophy.

Part 4: Humanism: Roots in Existentialism

Existentialism was prominent throughout literature and academia, not unlike other intellectual movements. But what truly sets existentialism apart from other philosophical movements in the West is its long reach - into the movies of Ingmar Bergman, Michelangelo Antonioni, Jean-Luc Goddard, Akira Kurosawa, and Terrence Malick, and in paintings by Edvard Munch, Marcel Duchamp, Pablo Picasso, Paul Cézanne, and Edward Hopper, who captured its moods. It also impacted politics, with Martin Luther King, Jr. and Malcolm X focusing on its underlying principles of "freedom and the struggle for self-creation" to inform what were viewed as their "radical and emancipatory politics," while those same principles influenced a distinguished cadre of Black intellectuals including Ralph Ellison, Richard Wright, and W.E.B. Du Bois (Aho 2023, n.p.). Other aspects of this seemingly disparate philosophy also helped shape theological debates and profoundly impacted the field of psychotherapy (Aho 2023).

If you are wondering why existentialism as a movement was so far-reaching in comparison to other intellectual movements, it is helpful to understand the social context that fertilized the philosophy. Existentialism has been described "as a historically situated event that emerged against the backdrop of the Second World War, the Nazi death camps, and the atomic bombings of Hiroshima and Nagasaki," creating the perfect storm of circumstances and forcing an entire generation to face the human condition, and confront the fact that death was inevitable, freedom was not necessarily reality, and that life could just as easily be meaningless as it could be meaningful (Aho 2023, n.p.). It is likely *nihilism,* or the belief that nothing in life truly exists, that you have heard most commonly couched in the existentialist's modern-day musings. While it is certainly one of the more consistent ideas running through existentialism, it is not the only one, though the others are beyond the scope of this chapter and textbook.

Goal of Education

According to Wichita State University, humanism as a philosophy is rooted in Ancient Greece, as with many of the philosophies presented in this chapter. Although ancient, it did not come to prominence until the Italian Renaissance, when society pushed back on the heavy influence of the church and determined that focusing on the inherent good that existed in humanity was more important (Wichita State University n.d.). However, other scholars have made the case that the humanism to which Wichita State University refers ultimately resulted in the *humanities* as a conceptual group of subjects to be taught, whereas *humanism* as an educational philosophy really emerged from existentialism (Zovko and Dillon 2017).

The teacher who chooses to approach education philosophically as a humanist refutes the essentialist, perennialist, and behaviorist (see text later in this chapter) approaches to education, all of which explicitly recognize authority and focus on the teacher as the center of the classroom and learning experience. In place of the traditional authoritative, hierarchical structure favored, humanists view education as a partnership between students and educators that focuses on the individual student and their inherent goodness simply because they are human. To this end, the goal of education for a humanism-minded teacher is to help students achieve self-actualization (Aung 2020).

Curriculum

For a humanism-oriented educator, the curriculum is fairly wide open and driven more by the student than the educator (Augsburg University n.d.; Huitt 2009). Options for learning are provided by the teacher, but ultimately students are allowed to choose what content they wish to pursue and learn, because the information itself is secondary to developing the student as a human: one who knows themself and is interested in learning throughout their lives – currently referred to as a lifelong learner (Zovko and Dillon 2017; Huitt 2009). This is accomplished through a learner-centric curriculum that engages learners in figuring out how to effectively self-evaluate, addresses the emotional, physical, and intellectual aspects of learning, and teaches students *how* to learn without dictating *what* they learn (Wichita State University n.d.)

However, there are some subjects that are generally favored by those with a humanistic philosophy of education. During the Italian Renaissance, humanists favored grammar and rhetoric, history and poetry, moral philosophy (but not logic), science (in the form of natural philosophy), and physics (Zovko and Dillon 2017). In more contemporary humanistic curricula, music, visual arts, literature, philosophy, mathematics, and physical science are viewed as important – somewhat similar to ancient humanistic education but different enough to warrant making the distinction (Aung 2020).

Teacher's Role and Classroom Instruction

A clearly student-centered philosophy of education, humanist educators view their roles as being facilitators and guides; they are in the classroom to support students on their journey to self-actualization and provide them enough knowledge to enable them to continue on their paths. Teachers are there to question students, probe their thinking, and guide them in acquiring the knowledge and skills needed to morally mature and become whole. Humanistic educators do this through promoting independence and positive self-direction, developing students' ability to take responsibility for their own learning, supporting and developing creativity, encouraging knowledge-seeking and curiosity, and cultivating an interest in the arts (Huitt 2009).

Humanism has been less developed and implemented in the United States, as it is still considered an emerging educational philosophy and, given its divergence in approaches, thoughts, and ideas (much like its parent philosophy of existentialism), is somewhat challenging to qualify (Huitt 2009). Importantly, if you are aware of its historical roots philosophically, recognize it as the most flexible and student-centered of the student-oriented educational philosophies, and understand that its purpose is to nurture and grow the whole student so they become lifelong learners who might eventually become self-actualized beings, you will likely be in better shape than most.

Section 8: Socially-Centered Educational Philosophies: Behaviorism and Reconstructionism

Katherine Fogelberg

Socially-centered educational philosophies consider that learning is a function of societal interactions; those who fall into this camp believe that it is society and/or individual interactions between people that ultimately determines what should be learned and how one should behave. However, the two philosophies discussed in this section put "social" at the center of their approaches in very different ways – hence the seemingly disparate roots of these educational philosophies in realism and pragmatism (see previous sections if you need to refresh your memories on these beyond what is covered here).

Behaviorism is grounded in realism, and more specifically the idea of logical positivism, or the belief that knowledge only truly exists if it is verified through observation and/or experience (empiricism). It is the idea that truth is only real if it is observable and testable; it is the basis for the positivist movement and the push to ensure that everything is "supported" or "proven" through experimentation and observation. Logical positivism, often referred to as simply positivism (covered in slightly more depth in Chapter 2), laid the groundwork for the scientific revolution and continues to significantly impact our educational systems today – particularly through behaviorism, which while considered a socially-centered educational philosophy, comes at it from the perspective of empirical science rather than socially-centered understandings.

On the other end of the socially-centered educational philosophy spectrum, reconstructionism's biggest influence is pragmatism (with a wave to progressivism), covered in the section just previous to this in discussions of student-centered educational philosophies. In some ways this makes sense, as pragmatists, if you recall – particularly the first-generation pragmatists – emerged from the scientific revolution that started with Darwin's theory of evolution. Thus, the groundwork for the value of teaching scientific reasoning and empirical processes was laid. As pragmatism evolved into its second generation of philosophers, however, remember that while they were also interested in the value of inquiry, the quest for meaning, and the desire to figure out the nature of truth, second-generation pragmatists were becoming more interested in the social aspects of philosophy – politics, social improvement, and the role of education in both (Curren 2009; Chennault 2013; Legg and Hookway 2021).

Part 1: Behaviorism: Roots in Realism and Logical Positivism

Recall that realism was the philosophical movement that views reality as claims of *existence* and claims of *independence* (Miller 2019). The claim of existence states that objects exist and those objects can be factually described and those facts are reality, while the claim of independence states that, regardless of what anyone says or thinks, existing items have those properties (Miller 2019). Importantly, in the realist's view of the world, no matter what anyone thinks or believes, what exists is reality and it cannot be altered (Miller 2019).

Logical positivism took realism to the extreme: science, and thus reality, was only valid if it was observed, organized, and systematized through mathematics and logic: "Observation provided the *content,* mathematics and logic the *form* of scientific knowledge" (Hocutt 1997, p. 77). And while philosophically behaviorism is recognized as being traditionally rooted in realism, from a practical standpoint, behaviorism is modeled as much in the vein of positivism as it is in realism.

Like constructivism, behaviorism is varyingly viewed as a philosophy, a theory, and/or both – and has many faces. For our purposes, it is both – philosophically, it is grounded in science – realism and positivism – and underlies the science known as behavior analysis, which is an attempt to "analyze and explain an organism's approach to a science of behavior" (Moore 2022, p. 711). Although John Watson is widely recognized as the founder of behaviorism, it reached its apex with B.F. Skinner (who coined the term and would ultimately be tied to it through the moniker *radical behaviorism* that it would eventually morph into) in the mid-twentieth century (Moore 2022; Samelson 1981). Both Watson and Skinner are further profiled in Chapter 2.

As an educational philosophy, both realism and positivism guide the behaviorist's approach to education: it is teacher-centered and essentially ignores the inner workings of learners, focusing instead on the external expression (in the form of behaviors) of intelligence. Why, then, you may be asking yourself, is it being covered in the socially-centered section? Because although it is a teacher-oriented approach to education, it is the interactions between the teachers and the students – along with, to a lesser extent, the interactions between students – that are the heart of this educational philosophy.

Goal of Education

In behaviorism, there is a belief that free will and autonomous action do not exist; behaviorists additionally view human nature as neutral – behaviors are a product of the individual's environment, which is shaped by society and the human interactions that occur every day. As such, while this is a distinctly teacher-centered educational philosophy (due to its realist and positivist roots), ultimately the learning that occurs in a behaviorist's classroom is about social interaction and the bigger society within which those interactions happen. This means that the goals of education for a behaviorist are *observable* and *measurable* changes in student behaviors that adhere to the norms of society.

It is also, however, important to behaviorists (and specifically radical behaviorists) to "search for relationships between learners' behavior and the variables of which it is a function, and. . .using the knowledge thus discovered to design and demonstrate measurably superior instruction" (Heward and Cooper 1992). In other words, behaviorists are interested in the most effective stimuli to elicit the most appropriate responses (i.e., behavior changes), but they are also interested in using this information to contribute to improving instruction as a whole – something that is often lost in the reductionist description of behaviorism as only a stimulus-response approach to education. Of note, the historical roots of behaviorism when viewed as a theory of education are further explored in Chapter 2, where Pavlov is cited as the primary building block of behaviorism but is (hopefully) more fully explained in a manner that gives you a greater appreciation for his genius, which should transcend (but rarely does) the similarly reductionist description of his experiments with dogs.

Curriculum

For a behaviorist, the curriculum is driven by science that is empirically driven and theory-based. As you might expect for a curriculum arising from realism and positivism, the teacher is responsible for selecting the content and delivering it through primarily lecture-based means. However, in contrast to the true realist or positivist, behaviorists believe the transfer of knowledge to students can only occur through finding the correct stimulus – meaning, the stimulus that will motivate the student to adjust their behavior appropriately (Western Governors University 2020).

Curricula designed by behaviorists emphasize science and reasoning; it is driven by teacher modeling of appropriate responses to specific stimuli to passive students who are to essentially mimic the demonstrated behavior (Western Governors University 2020). Such behaviors are repeatedly displayed by the teacher and, when students achieve the "correct" behavior, they are positively reinforced – consider the earning of "good" grades, an almost ubiquitous carryover of behaviorism in education. On the flip side, students who engage in "incorrect" behaviors are either ignored (negatively reinforced – often used in animals and labeled as operant conditioning) or they are punished, which is punitive and intended to decrease the "incorrect" behavior (but often fails to do so). This speaks to the importance of student motivation in behaviorism: positive reinforcement tends to be viewed as more effective in creating behavior change, while negative reinforcement is a great way to get students, over time, to stop investing time into something that the teacher may not view as important (Western Governors University 2020).

The last piece of the curricular design likely to be incorporated into a behaviorist's classroom is the ability to revisit and repeat information. Repetition, in combination with positive and negative reinforcement, is a key element to student learning in the behaviorist's view. As such, content is created in a manner that provides explicit opportunities to revisit information – both across subjects and within a given topic course. This means that the importance of a physical exam might be introduced in one course and practiced several times over the duration of that course while also being taught in a different, but concurrent, course. Reinforcement occurs in each course, with one assessing the requisite behavior changes through a written exam asking what the steps of a physical exam are, and another assessing the changes through a skills station that asks the student to perform a physical exam while explaining what they are doing. Those students answering correctly and performing the physical exam appropriately might earn verbal praise and/or a good grade. Those students struggling might earn verbal correction, a failing grade, and/or nothing at all – the first two would be punishment, the last negative reinforcement.

You are all likely most familiar with the first two, though you might be surprised by the categorization of the latter as negative reinforcement, though this is a common complaint by students – "I turned in my paper and got a C, but there were no comments to help me understand what I did wrong or how I could improve to earn an A!" Grades and non-comments are all carryovers from the behaviorist movement, so are commonly found in existing curricula in some form or fashion.

Teacher's Role and Classroom Instruction

The types of activities typically used in a behaviorist teacher's classroom include drills, question and answer periods, guided practice, regular reviews, positive and negative reinforcement (see above), and punishment (Western Governors University 2020). As a teacher-centric classroom, the teacher is there to be the provider of knowledge and is viewed as the authority on whatever topic is being delivered. Instruction is planned beforehand, structured, and provides ample opportunity for regular revisiting of previous information to ensure students get the necessary repetition to effect lasting behavior change.

When delivering information, the material increases in difficulty as students respond to and change their behaviors to adapt to new challenges. This is not unlike the *scaffolding* and *spiral curriculum* approaches to education proposed by Bruner, whose *cognitivism* is explored further in Chapter 2. Briefly, however, it is the idea that students need information provided in a way that decreases the distractors from that information, allowing the student to concentrate on the challenging skill they are attempting to learn (Ozdem-Yilmaz and Bilican 2020). As the student gains skill and

confidence, the distractors can be reduced, which increases the cognitive load required. An example is how surgical skills are taught; students are provided the information in lectures and the skills – one at a time and with increasing complexity – for many weeks and months prior to performing the fully integrated task of spaying a dog.

With such scaffolding, information can also be spiraled back to related content, allowing for the repetition behaviorists believe in – though the *spiral curriculum* was also proposed by Jerome Bruner, who was not a behaviorist but created educational theories that certainly had echoes of behaviorism in them. Notably, Bruner was also a proponent of *social learning theory*, which, while very different from behaviorism philosophically, still aligned with it in the sense that he believed learning was a social construct. As such, behaviorism as an educational philosophy may seem somewhat sterile on the surface, but when digging deeper, reveals some connections to other educational philosophies and learning theories that may provide us insights into how many of its features have endured in the classroom for well over a century.

Reconstructionism: Roots in Pragmatism

Pragmatism laid the foundations for both progressivism and reconstructionism (sometimes referred to as social reconstructionism or reconstructivism), though as you will read, the two differ in specific and significant ways. First thought of by Theodore Brameld during the 1940s (though the name was borrowed from I.B. Berkson via John Dewey), he published two books in 1950 outlining this "new" educational philosophy (Brameld 1977). Having studied philosophy at the University of Chicago under George H. Mead, James H. Tufts, and others who were philosophically aligned with Dewey's Chicago School, unsurprisingly created with the pragmatist's philosophy of education in mind, Brameld's reconstructionism is intended to be an amendment to the pragmatist's philosophy (Brameld 1977). Though many would perceive reconstructionism as an attempt to create a utopian society, as Mosier did in 1951, the key features of reconstructionism, as identified by Brameld in 1977, were not meant to create a utopian society or repudiate Dewey's philosophies, though Brameld's many critics were able to obscure the original educational philosophy through selectively attacking individual tenets of the reconstructionist philosophy.

Brameld (1977) outlines the features of reconstructionism he feels are the most often misinterpreted or misshapen in his article reappraising his own philosophy almost three decades after his original reshaping of progressivism was published. In it, he makes clear that he feels we can learn from Marxian theory "not in any orthodox or doctrinaire fashion, but by means of (i) its 'sociological realism' as an expose of the dominant forces of exploitative power, and (ii) its aggressive methodology of class action for social change" (Brameld 1977, p. 69). Building upon this idea, reconstructionism believes in the concept of consensual validation – or the idea that seeking the truth is "an actively social dialogic rather than. . .an individualized process" (Brameld 1977, p. 70). Brameld (1977) viewed this as an important part of education and specifically calls out those interested in forwarding competency-based education as a fad that regresses education back to "social conservation" (though he does not elaborate on this somewhat peculiar phrase).

The last of Brameld's (1977) tenets of reconstructionism that will be covered here is the idea of social-self-realization, which he deliberately double-hyphenated because "it symbolizes the highest value of human life as a fulfilling of people of all classes, races, and nations by the transactional effect of self on society and of society on self" (p. 71). It is this transactional nature of education that has been lost by progressivists, he argues, who have moved too far into the realm of the student-centered school (Brameld 1977). It is his concern for the lost interplay between student and educator that Brameld retrospectively emphasizes, reminding his readers that social-self-realization is not intended to subordinate, but that it is an important part of maintaining a viable, planned democracy through its insistence that "the self is most meaningful and realizable through the rigorous process of consensual validation while warmed by the colorful and subliminal (or, if you prefer, mythological) qualities of human experience" (Brameld 1977, p. 71).

It is the reconstructionist's socially-oriented purpose of education that ultimately breaks with progressivism. Thus, progressivism is presented in the student-centered educational philosophies section because its pedagogical practices focus on the learner and its philosophical stance is that the individual learner's interests and growth are the key goals of education (Sutinen 2014). In contrast, while reconstructionism is student-centered in its delivery, its intent lies in the social aspect of education and its value to society (Sutinen 2014). For the reconstructionist, education produces citizens of society who are capable of shaping social and political policies (Sutinen 2014). Lastly, in direct contrast to the progressivist's view that an individual's self-discipline should be nurtured through education, reconstructionists push for a social discipline, defined as an agreement among the majority about how the program should be ordered so groups can effectively unite in a systematic effort to outline and achieve their goals (Mosier 1951).

Goal of Education

Learning, in the reconstructionist's view, is social-realization (Mosier 1951). Because reconstructionism views philosophies as cultural interpretations and educational philosophies as theories of cultural change, its proponents believe that sufficient social and educational purposes are not provided by societal experiences (Mosier 1951; Sutinen 2014). As a result, learning is both a normative and descriptive process, meaning that the goal of education for a reconstructionist is to create a self-actualized, socially realized human (Mosier 1951; Sutinen 2014). Reconstructionists desire, as do those who follow humanism as an educational philosophy, to educate the whole child. And, in doing so, reconstructionists believe the goal of education is to produce a citizen of society who is "able to evaluate social reality and. . .change social practices as appropriate" (Sutinen 2014, p. 20).

Curriculum

The reconstructionist's curriculum is oriented around activities that enable learners to "act justly and morally in social situations" (Sutinen 2014, p. 19). Thus, educational activities are based on forming projects that are interesting to the learner and are related to community and social activities (Sutinen 2014). As such, the curriculum of reconstructionism cultivates learners' abilities to critically examine culture; commitment to advocate for and pursue social reform; and ability, desire to plan for, implement, and assess programs intended to influence cultural change (Gutek, as cited in Sutinen 2014).

To achieve these goals, learners are taught subjects similar in breadth to the progressivist's curriculum: the basic literacy skills (reading, writing, and mathematics); the arts; science; and vocational skills. However, unlike the progressivist's classroom, these skills are delivered to students through a curriculum that is focused outside of the individual learner, encompassing socially-oriented activities that span disciplines and teach students through experiences. Think PBL – touched on in the constructivism section – with a specific slant toward helping learners critically appraise social issues and work toward implementable solutions to affect change and shift cultural norms.

Teacher's Role and Classroom Instruction

The reconstructionist's role as educator is very similar to that of the teacher who follows one of the student-centered educational philosophies, so there is little reason to repeat the information here (see earlier section for the initial, more in-depth explanation). In brief, this generally means that the teacher in a reconstructionist classroom lectures little and provides a generous amount of time for cooperative group work, functions as a facilitator (rather than giver) of knowledge, and encourages students to form ideas and opinions grounded in their own research rather than relying on the teacher to influence them (Perez 2022b).

Mosier (1951) states it a bit more succinctly, if less descriptively: the reconstructionist teacher's goal is to provide purposeful, goal-seeking activities that motivate and enhance intelligent beings.

Summary

Educational philosophy, for those who are less abstract in their thinking, can certainly be mind-bending – and the theory chapter immediately following is not any less so. But to truly appreciate and understand *what* you do in the classroom, you must also understand the *why*. It is the why, after all, that helps you to continually and critically appraise the practices you engage in when teaching. If you are simply doing what you have seen others do, or mimicking the teaching you experienced as a student, you are essentially performing surgery without having the underlying skills and knowledge to manage the problems that arise during that extremely complex procedure. Perhaps you will get through the surgery unscathed because nothing critical will occur, and perhaps this is the case for the first 100 surgeries you do. But when that 101st surgery presents you with an issue you have not been adequately prepared for, your patient suffers – all because you were not provided the foundational knowledge and skills in physiology, anesthesia, anatomy, pharmacology, and the like.

You may laugh at this analogy, and that is perfectly fine. However, once you are done (and feeling better!), consider this: we ask educators like you to walk into classrooms every day and engage in teaching, one of the most complex and difficult professions in the world, without providing anything other than personal experience as a foundation on a regular basis. This is the norm; it is an accepted and acceptable practice. There are many in higher education who have no idea what an educational philosophy is, have no concept of educational theory, have never read an educational research article, and have never been provided the opportunity to learn more about the discipline of education. Each of these individuals still calls themselves a teacher (or educator, or professor), yet each would balk at someone else calling themselves a veterinarian, physician, engineer, or scientist, if that someone else did not have the proper training and earned credentials to do so. It would be viewed, in fact, as absurd. Why is it then, that education has been relegated to a title that is taken rather than earned?

I leave that soapbox to say, we hope that as you read this chapter you recognized elements of your educational experiences and practices that you perhaps were unable to fully previously articulate. It should be relatively easy to identify the behaviorist approaches you were likely subjected to throughout your own education; it is behaviorism that tends to jump out at us the most in our experience. But you are highly likely, as professional or vocational program educators, to see flashes of perennialism, essentialism, progressivism, and constructivism in your training as well. Humanism and reconstructionism are potentially less prominent, but if you ever took a social studies course, subscribed to the Montessori system of schooling (Maria Montessori is profiled in Chapter 2), or have heard anything about critical theory, these two educational philosophies have touched your lives as well.

In short, we hope you see now that there are reasons for how our educational systems have been set up and the way education is delivered. We hope this chapter has opened your mind to new ideas and approaches to teaching and learning and has provided you with some building blocks to create a solid foundation for your thinking about education moving forward. And, if we have fallen short in that regard, we at least hope that you have been provoked into thinking more carefully about your own ideas when it comes to education, while supplying an accessible and understandable string of philosophical terms that you can use to impress your friends and colleagues.

Keep in mind that this chapter is intended to provide you a solid grounding in what educational philosophy is, the major movements in educational philosophy and from which intellectual movements as a whole they emerged, and why it is important to at least be familiar with this area of education. It is not intended to transform you into an educational philosopher, nor is it a comprehensive view of the discipline – there are a variety of other texts you can refer to if this chapter sparks a desire in you to read further (see: Curren 2007; Siegel 2009; Noddings 2016; Horkheimer 1993; hooks 1994, 2003).

References

Adler, M. (1982). *The Paideia Proposal*. Macmillan.

Adler, M. (1984). *The Paideia Program: An Educational Syllabus*. Macmillan.

Adom, D., Yeboah, A., and Ankrah, A.K. (2016). Constructivism philosophical paradigm: implication for research, teaching, and learning. *Global Journal of Arts Humanities and Social Sciences* 4 (10): 1–9.

Aho, K. (2023). Existentialism. In: *The Stanford Encyclopedia of Philosophy* (ed. E.N. Zalta and U. Nodelman). https://plato.stanford.edu/entries/existentialism (accessed 13 February 2023).

Annas, J. (2005). Virtue ethics. In: *The Oxford Handbook of Ethical Theory* (ed. D. Copp), 515–536. Oxford University Press.

Arslan, H. (ed.) (2018). *An Introduction to Education.* Cambridge Scholars Publishing.

Augsburg University (n.d.). *Educational philosophies definitions and comparison chart.* https://web.augsburg. edu/~erickson/edc490/downloads/comparison_edu_ philo.pdf (accessed 15 February 2023).

Aung, Y.M. (2020). Humanism and education. *International Journal of Advanced Research in Science, Engineering, and Technology* 7 (5): 13555–13561.

Ayers, W. (2004). *Teaching Toward Freedom.* Beacon Press.

Bagley, W.C. (1934). *Education and Emergent Man.* Ronald Press.

Bagley, W.C. (1938). An essentialist's platform for the advancement of American education. *Educational Administration and Supervision* 24: 242–256.

Batista, J. (2017). *The Confucianism-feminism conflict: why a new understanding is necessary.* Schwarzman Scholars (29 August). https://www.schwarzmanscholars.org/ events-and-news/confucianism-feminism-conflict- new-understanding-necessary.

Bellah, R.N. (1975). *The Broken Covenant: American Civil Religion in a Time of Trial.* Seabury Press.

Berling, J.A. (n.d.). *Confucianism.* Asia Society https://asiasociety.org/education/confucianism.

Biesta, G. (2010). *Good Education in an Age of Measurement: Ethics, Politics, and Democracy.* Routledge.

Binkley, L.J. (1961). *Contemporary Ethical Theories.* Philosophical Library, INC.

Bloom, A. (1987). *The Closing of the American Mind.* Simon and Schuter.

Brameld, T. (1977). Reconstructionism as radical philosophy of education: a reappraisal. *The Educational Forum* 42 (1): 67–76. https://doi.org/10.1080/ 00131727709338153.

Brink, D.O. (2005). Some forms and limits of consequentialism. In: *The Oxford Handbook of Ethical Theory* (ed. D. Copp), 380–423. Oxford University Press.

Britzman, D.P. and Greene, M. (2003). *Practice Makes Practice: A Critical Study of Learning to Teach (Revised).* State University of New York Press.

Cahill, S. and Li, C. (2001). Book review: The sage and the second sex: confucianism, ethics, and gender edited by Chenyang Li. Chicago: Open Court, 2000. xiii, 256 pp. $24.95 (paper). *The Journal of Asian Studies* 60 (4): 1160–1163. https://doi.org/10.2307/2700049.

Carr, D. and Steutel, J. (2005). *Virtue Ethics and Moral Education.* Routledge.

Chan, T., Jiang, B., and Xu, M. (2017). U.S. Teachers' perception of Confucian teaching philosophies and methodologies. *New Waves Educational Research & Development* 20 (2): 20–34.

Chen, D. (1916/2000). The way of Confucius and modern life. In: *Sources of Chinese Tradition: From 1600 Through the Twentieth Century*, 2e, vol. 2 (ed. W.T. de Bary and R. Lufrano), 353–356.

Chennault, R.E. (2013). Pragmatism and progressivism in the educational thought and practices of Booker T. Washington. *Philosophical Studies in Education* 44: 121–131.

Colliver, J.A. (2002). Constructivism: the view of knowledge that ended philosophy or a theory of learning and instruction? *Teaching and Learning in Medicine* 14 (1): 49–51.

Confucius (2010). *The Analects of Confucius* (D. Song, Trans.) (《论语》汉英对照). University of International Business and Economics Press.

Copp, D. (2005). *The Oxford Handbook of Ethical Theory.* Oxford University Press.

Counts, G.S. (1969). *Dare the School Builds a New Social Order?* Arno Press.

Crowther, E. and Baillie, S. (2016). A method of developing and introducing case-based learning to a preclinical veterinary curriculum. *Anatomical Sciences Education* 9: 80–89.

Curren, R. (ed.) (2007). *Philosophy of Education: An Anthology.* Malden, MA, USA: Wiley-Blackwell.

Curren, R. (2009). Pragmatist philosophy of education. In: *The Oxford Handbook of Philosophy of Education* (ed. H. Siegel), 489–507. New York, NY: Oxford University Press.

D'Ambrosio, P.J. (2016). Wei-Jin period Xuanxue "Neo-Daoism": re-working the relationship between Confucian and Daoist themes. *Philosophy Compass* 11 (11): 621–631. https://doi.org/10.1111/phc3.12344.

D'Ambrosio, P.J. (2020). Confucianism and Daoism: on the relationship between the Analects, Laozi, and Zhuangzi: part I. *Philosophy Compass* 15 (9): 1–11. https://doi.org/ 10.1111/phc3.12702.

Defoot, C. (2007). Daoism explained: from the dream of the butterfly to the fishnet allegory (review). *China Review International* 14 (1): 179–185.

Deleuze, G. (1997). *Negotiations, 1972–1990* (M. Joughin, Trans.). Columbia University Press.

Duncan, T. and Brasovan, N.S. (2016). Contemporary ecofeminism and confucian cosmology. In: *Feminist Encounters with Confucius* (ed. M.A. Foust and S. Tan), 226–251. Brill https://doi.org/10.1163/9789004332119.

Ellis, A.R. (2003). *Exemplars of Curriculum Theory.* Routledge.

Fingarette, H. (1998). *Confucius: The Secular as Sacred.* Waveland Press.

Fogelberg, K., Hunt, J., and Baillie, S. (2021). Young and evolving: a narrative of veterinary educational research from early leaders. *Education in the Health Professions* 4 (3): 124–133.

Foust, M.A. and Tan, S. (ed.) (2016). *Feminist Encounters with Confucius*. Brill.

Fraser, C. (2006). Zhuangzi, Xunzi, and the paradoxical nature of education. *Journal of Chinese Philosophy* 33 (4): 529–542. https://doi.org/10.1111/j.1540-6253.2006.00380.x.

Gao, X. (2014). Women existing for men: confucianism and social injustice against women in China. *Race, Gender & Class* 10 (3): 114–125.

Gardner, R., Cairns, J., and Lawton, D. (ed.) (2003). *Education for Values: Morals, Ethics and Citizenship in Contemporary Teaching*. Kogan Page.

Gou, A. Lipitz, A., Raskin, J. et al. (2021, October 9). *Found [Motion picture]*. United States: Amanda Lipitz Productions.

Gruender, D. (1996). Constructivism and learning: a philosophical appraisal. *Educational Technology* 36 (3): 21–29.

Gu, N. (2015). *Brief Introduction of the Four Books and the Five Classics* (顾农: 略谈四书五经). Guoxue. http://www.guoxue.com/?p=31166 (accessed 3 July 2022).

Guyer, P. and Horstmann, R.-P. (2021). Idealism. In: *The Stanford Encyclopedia of Philosophy* (ed. E.N. Zalta and U. Nodelman). https://plato.stanford.edu/entries/idealism (accessed 10 February 2023).

Hansen, M. (1999). *Lessons in Being Chinese: Minority Education and Ethnic Identity in Southwest China*. Hong Kong University Press.

Harmon, D. and Jones, T. (2005). *Elementary Education: A Reference Handbook*. ABC-CLIO.

Haynes, J., Gate, K., and Parker, M. (ed.) (2013). *Philosophy and Education: An Introduction to Key Questions and Themes*. Routledge.

Herr, R.S. (2016). Confucian mothering: the origin of tiger mothering? In: *Feminist Encounters with Confucius* (ed. M.A. Foust and S. Tan), 40–68. Brill.

Heward, W.L. and Cooper, J.O. (1992). Radical behaviorism: A productive and needed philosophy for education. *Journal of Behavioral Education* 2 (4): 345–365.

Higgs, J. (2012). Realising practical wisdom from the pursuit of wise practice. In: *Phronesis as Professional Knowledge: Practical Wisdom in Professions* (ed. E.A. Kinsella and A. Pitman), 73–86. Sense Publishers.

Hildebrand, D. (2023). John Dewey. In: *The Stanford Encyclopedia of Philosophy* (ed. E.N. Zalta and U. Nodelman). https://plato.stanford.edu/archives/fall2023/entries/dewey/ (accessed 10 December 2022).

Hirsch, E.D., Kett, J.F., and Trefil, J. (1988). *Cultural Literacy: What Every American Needs to Know*. Vintage Books.

Ho, W. (2018). *Culture, Music Education, and the Chinese Dream in Mainland China*. Springer Singapore.

Hocutt, M. (1997). From logical positivism to scientific realism: A review of Robert Klee's *Introduction to the philosophy of science: cutting nature at its seams*. *Behavior and Philosophy* 25 (1): 77–80.

hooks, b. (1994). *Teaching to Transgress: Education as the Practice of Freedom*. New York, NY: Routledge.

hooks, b. (2003). *Teaching Community: A Pedagogy of Hope*. New York, NY: Routledge.

Horkheimer, M. (1993). *Between Philosophy and Social Science: Selected Early Writings*. Hunter, G.F., Kramer, M.S., and Torpey, J. (translators). Cambridge, MA, USA: MIT Press.

Hue, M.-T. (2007). The influence of classic Chinese philosophy of Confucianism, Taoism and legalism on classroom discipline in Hong Kong junior secondary schools. *Pastoral Care in Education* 25 (2): 38–45. https://doi.org/10.1111/j.1468-0122.2007.00406.x.

Huitt, W. (2009). Humanism and open education. In: *Educational Psychology Interactive*. Valdosta, GA: Valdosta State University http://www.edpsycinteractive.org/topics/affect/humed.html (accessed 14 February 2023).

Hutchins, R.M. (1936). *The Higher Learning in America*. Yale University Press.

Infantino, R. (2009). *Tough Choices for Teachers: Ethical Challenges in Today's Schools and Classrooms*. R & L Education.

Jacka, T. (2006). *Rural Women in Urban China*, 2006. Armonk, NY: M.E. Sharpe.

Jeffrey, D. and Clark, R. (2019). Supplementing western perspectives of learner-centered instruction with a Daoist approach toward authentic power sharing in the classroom. *International Journal of Contemporary Education* 2 (1): 9–16. https://doi.org/10.11114/ijce.v2i1.4016.

Jones, M.G. and Brader-Arage, L. (2002). The impact of constructivism on education: language, discourse, and meaning. *American Communication Journal* 5 (3): 1–10.

Kaminsky, J.S. (1992). A pre-history of educational philosophy in the United States: 1861–1914. *Harvard Educational Review* 62 (2): 179–198.

Kinsella, E.A. and Pitman, A. (ed.) (2012). *Phronesis as Professional Knowledge: Practical Wisdom in the Professions*, 73–86. Sense Publishers.

Kober, N. and Rentner, D.S. (2020). *History and Evolution of pPblic Education in the US*. For the Center on Education Policy at The George Washington University www.cep-dc.org (accessed 8 January 2023).

Kooli, C., Zidi, C., and Jamrah, A. (2019). The philosophy of education in the Sultanate of Oman: between perennialism and progressivism. *American Journal of Education and Learning* 4 (1): 36–49.

Law, W.W. (2016a). Cultivating Chinese citizens: China's search for modernization and national rejuvenation. In: *Re-Envisioning Chinese Education: The Meaning of Person-Making in a New Age* (ed. G. Zhao and Z. Deng), 34–54. Routledge.

Law, W.W. (2016b). Social change, citizenship, and citizenship education in China since the late 1970s. In: *Spotlight on China: Changes in Education under China's Market Economy* (ed. S. Guo and Y. Guo), 35–51. Sense Publishers.

Legg, C. and Hookway, C. (2021). Pragmatism. In: *The Stanford Encyclopedia of Philosophy* (Summer 2021 Edition) (ed. E.N. Zalta). https://plato.stanford.edu/archives/sum2021/entries/pragmatism (accessed 13 February 2023).

Lenehan, K. (2020). Zhuangzi's discourse on "contented acceptance of fate" and its relation to catastrophe. *Educational Philosophy and Theory* 52 (13): 1388–1399. https://doi.org/10.1080/00131857.2020.175.

Levinson, M. and Fay, J. (ed.) (2019). *Dilemmas of Educational Ethics: Cases and Commentaries*. Harvard Education Press.

Li, C. (ed.) (2000). *The Sage and the Second Sex: Confucianism, Ethics, and Gender*. Open Court.

Li, J. (2019). *The thoughts, systematic structure, and contemporary meaning of essential Confucian values. Rujia Website*. (24 May) https://www.rujiazg.com/article/16426 (accessed 9 July 2022).

Li, J. and Xue, E. (2020). Unveiling the "logic" of modern university in China: historical, social and value perspectives. *Educational Philosophy and Theory* 52 (9): 986–998. https://doi.org/10.1080/00131857.2020.171.

Lin, Y. (1935). *My Country and my People*. John Day Company.

Lorraine, T.E. (2011). *Deleuze and Guattari's Immanent Ethics: Theory, Subjectivity, and Duration*. SUNY Press.

Mazzei, L.A. (2013). A voice without organs: interviewing in posthumanist research. *International Journal of Qualitative Studies in Education* 26 (6): 723–740.

Metzger, T. (1986). *Escape from Predicament: Neo-Confucianism and China's Evolving Political Culture*. Columbia University Press.

Miller, A. (2019). Realism. In: *The Stanford Encyclopedia of Philosophy* (ed. E.N. Zalta and U. Nodelman). https://plato.stanford.edu/entries/realism (accessed 10 February 2023).

Moore, J. (2022). Conceptual foundations: teaching the historical development of radical behaviorism as a philosophy of science. *Perspectives on Behavior Science* 45: 711–742.

Mosier, R.D. (1951). The educational philosophy of reconstructionism. *The Journal of Educational Sociology* 25 (2): 86–96.

Moss, G. and Lee, C. (2010). A critical analysis of philosophies of education and INSTASC standards in teacher preparation. *International Journal of Critical Pedagogy* 3 (2): 36–46.

Murray, C. (2012). *Coming Apart: The State of White America, 1960–2000*. Crown Forum.

National Bureau of Statistics of China (2021, December). *Final Statistical Monitoring Report on the Implementation of China National Program for Women's Development (2011–2020)*. National Bureau of Statistics of China. www.stats.gov.cn/enGLISH/PressRelease/202112/t20211231_1825801.html.

Noddings, N. (1992). *The Challenge to Care in Schools: An Alternative Approach to Education*. Teachers College Press.

Noddings, N. (2008). *Critical Lessons: What our Schools Should Teach*. Cambridge University Press.

Noddings, N. (2016). *Philosophy of Education*, 4e. Boulder, CO, USA: Westview Press.

Ornstein, A.C. and Hunkins, F.P. (2018). *Curriculum Foundation, Principles, and Issues*, 7e. Pearson.

Oxford Language Dictionary (n.d.). https://www.oed.com/ (accessed 8 January 2023).

Ozdem-Yilmaz, Y. and Bilican, K. (2020). Discovery learning-Jerome Bruner. In: *Science Education in Theory and Practice: An Introductory Guide to Learning Theory* (ed. B. Apkan and T.J. Kennedy), 177–190. Cham, Switzerland: Springer Texts in Education.

Pereira, M., Artemiou, E., Conan, A. et al. (2018). Case-based studies and clinical reasoning development: teaching opportunities and pitfalls for first year veterinary students. *Medical Science Educator* 28: 175–179. https://doi.org/10.1007/s40670-017-0533-y.

Perez, D. (2022a). Progressivism. In: *Social Foundations of K-12 Education*. https://kstatelibraries.pressbooks.pub/dellaperezproject/chapter/chapter-5-progressivism (accessed 14 February 2023).

Perez, D. (2022b). Social reconstructionism. In: *Social Foundations of K-12 Education*. https://kstatelibraries.pressbooks.pub/dellaperezproject/chapter/chapter-5-progressivism (accessed 14 February 2023).

Peters, M.A., Tesar, M., and Locke, K. (2015). *Oxford bibliographies: philosophy of education*. https://www.researchgate.net/profile/Marek-Tesar/publication/322076772_Philosophy_of_Education/links/5a432df5aca272d294591411/Philosophy-of-Education.pdf (accessed 8 January 2023).

Pinar, W. (2004). *What Is Curriculum Theory?* Lawrence Erlbaum.

Plato. (2012). *Trans. By Jowett. B. The Republic. Free in the public domain*. https://www.amazon.com/Republic-Plato-ebook/dp/B0082SV87G/ref=sr_1_6?crid=1II9FKSYRTHV6&keywords=the+republic+by+plato&qid=1646774367&s=digital-text&sprefix=the+republic+by+plato%2Cdigital-text%2C128&sr=1-6 (accessed 8 March 2022).

Plato (2021). *The Republic*. Maven Books.

Radu, L. (2011). John Dewey and progressivism in American education. *Bulletin of the Transilvania University of Brasov* 4 (53): 85–90.

Roberts, T. and Billings, L. (1999). *The Power of Paideia Schools: Defining Lives through Learning*. ASCD.

Rosenlee, L.L. (2006). *Confucianism and Women: A Philosophical Interpretation*. SUNY.

Rousseau, J. (1979). Emile: Or on Education (A. Bloom, Trans). Basic Books. Tho, N. N. (2016). Confucianism and humane education in contemporary Vietnam. International Communication of Chinese Culture, 3(4), 645–671. https://doi.org/10.1007/s40636-016-0076-8

Sadker, D.M. and Zittleman, K.R. (2016). *Teachers, Schools, and Society: A Brief Introduction to Education*. McGraw-Hill Education.

Samelson, F. (1981). Struggle for the scientific authority: the reception of Watson's behaviorism, 1913–1920. *Journal of the History of the Behavioral Sciences* 17: 399–425.

Sandovnik, A.R., Cookson, P.W., Semel, S.F., and Coughlan, R.W. (2018). *Exploring Education: An Introduction to the Foundations of Education*, 5e. Routledge.

Sellman, D. (2012). Reclaiming competence for professional phronesis. In: *Phronesis as Professional Knowledge: Practical Wisdom in the Professions* (ed. E.A. Kinsella and A. Pitman), 115–130. Sense Publishers.

Servant-Miklos, V.F.C. (2019). Fifty years on: a retrospective on the World's first problem-based learning programme at McMaster University medical school. *Health Professions Education* 5 (1): 3–12.

Siegel, H. (ed.) (2009). *The Oxford Handbook of Philosophy of Education*. New York, NY, USA: Oxford University Press.

Slattery, P. (2006). *Curriculum Development in the Postmodern Era*, 2e. Routledge.

Smythe, J. (2019). Inviting emptiness into a cluttered curriculum: infusing pedagogical practice with Taoist philosophy as a healing balm. *Journal of Curriculum and Pedagogy*. 17: 1–20. https://doi.org/10.1080/15505170.2019.1627618.

Stanford Encyclopedia of Philosophy (2020). *The definition of morality*. https://plato.stanford.edu/entries/morality-definition (accessed 20 September 2022).

Sun, L. (2014). *Shangdong students make posters promoting "socialist core values"*. *Shanghaiist*. http://shanghaiist.com/2014/12/31/shandong- students-make-posters-promoting-socialist-core-values.php (accessed 31 December).

Sutinen, A. (2014). Social reconstructionist philosophy of education and George S. Counts: observations on the ideology of indoctrination in socio-critical educational thinking. *International Journal of Progressive Education* 10 (1): 18–31.

Tan, C. (2006). Philosophical perspectives on education. In: *Critical Perspectives on Education: An Introduction* (ed. C. Tan, B. Wong, J.S.M. Chua, and T. Kang), 21–40. Prentice Hall.

University at Buffalo (n.d.). *Office of curriculum, assessment, and teaching transformation*. https://www.buffalo.edu/catt/develop/theory/constructivism.html (accessed 14 February 2023).

Wakeham, J. (2019). Navigating rocky choices with practical wisdom. In: *Dilemmas of Educational Ethics: Cases and Commentaries* (ed. M. Levinson and J. Fay), 44–48. Harvard Education Press.

Waley, A. (2005). *The Books of Song*. Routledge.

Wallin, J.J. and Sandlin, J.A. (ed.) (2018). *Paranoid Pedagogies: Education, Culture, and Paranoia*. Palgrave Macmillan.

Western Governors University (2020). *What is behavioral learning theory?* https://www.wgu.edu/blog/what-behavioral-learning-theory2005.html (accessed 16 February 2023).

White, J. (ed.) (2010). *The Aims of Education Restated*. Routledge.

Wichita State University (n.d.). https://www.wichita.edu/services/mrc/OIR/Pedagogy/Theories/humanism.php (accessed 16 February 2023).

Xue, E. and Li, J. (2020). What is the ultimate education task in China? Exploring "strengthen moral education for cultivating people" ("Li De Shu Ren"). *Educational Philosophy and Theory* 52 (9): 986–998. https://doi.org/10.1080/00131857.2020.1754539.

Yu, J. (2008). Living with nature: Stoicism and Daoism. *History of Philosophy Quarterly* 25 (1): 1–19.

Yuan, L. (2019). *Confucian Ren and Feminist Ethics of Care: Integrating Relational Self, Power, and Democracy*. Lexington Books.

Zhang, D. (1993). The impact of the thought of the school of Confucianism and the school of Daoism on the culture of China. *Chinese Studies in philosophy* 24 (4): 65–85.

Zhou, Y. (2006). Under Confucian eyes: writings on gender in Chinese history, and: women in Daoism (review). *Philosophy East and West* 56 (4): 684–687. https://doi.org/10.1353/pew.2006.0065.

Zhou, X. (2019). Daoism and dialogism: a dialogue between China and the West. *Culture & Psychology*, 1354067X1984507. https://doi.org/10.1177/1354067x19845072.

Zovko, M.E. and Dillon, J. (2017). Humanism vs competency: traditional and contemporary models of education. *Educational Philosophy and Theory* 50 (6–7): 554–556. https://doi.org/10.1080/00131857.2017.1375757.

2

Educational Theory and Theorists

Katherine Fogelberg, DVM, PhD (Science Education), MA (Educational Leadership)
Virginia-Maryland College of Veterinary Medicine, Blacksburg, VA, USA

Kimberly S. Cook, EdD, MBA
Texas Christian University, Fort Worth, TX, USA

Freyca Calderon, PhD
Pennsylvania State University-Altoona, Altoona, PA, USA

Karla O'Donald, PhD
Texas Christian University, Fort Worth, TX, USA

Section 1: Introduction

Katherine Fogelberg

Philosophy and theory are two terms that we often encounter in the field of education – most often in academia, but certainly in everyday education for those who have been formally trained in the discipline (and even for those who have not, though most often in this case indirectly and/or unwittingly). However, there is sometimes confusion about the differences between the two, which is not surprising given how blurry the lines truly are. As you have learned in the previous chapter, philosophy asks questions about the nature of three big things: knowledge (epistemology), reality or being (ontology), and value or why (axiology).

This chapter dives into educational theory – the premises upon which learning practices are built. By definition, theory is "a supposition or a system of ideas intended to explain something, especially one based on general principles independent of the thing to be explained" (from the Oxford Languages dictionary, Google's lexicon of choice). This, then, is the key difference to keep in mind when considering the separation (however thin) between philosophy and theory: philosophy asks and tentatively answers Big Questions, while theory explains things – or tries to, at least. Thus, educational philosophers ask and ponder ideas about Big Questions and through these ponderings, define important challenges embedded within education, while theories develop ways to move toward solutions for overcoming such challenges. This is a nice line of demarcation to return to as

you wander through the first two chapters of this textbook, as there are some educational philosophies that carry the same name as some of the educational theories covered in this chapter (behaviorism and constructivism, to be exact). Therefore, upon completion of these two chapters, you should be able to disentangle behaviorism and constructivism as philosophies (asking Big Questions and through them, defining the important challenges of education) from behaviorism and constructivism as theories (developing and moving toward solutions for overcoming the challenges).

Most – if not all – of those reading this textbook likely consider themselves "scientists." However, just like there is more than one type of doctor, there is also more than one type of scientist. There are those who are bench scientists (previously known as "hard" scientists, and inclusive of physical, earth, biomedical, environmental, etc. sciences) and those who are social scientists (previously not overtly acknowledged or called "soft" scientists, inclusive of sociologists, psychologists, educators, and the like). There is no hard line between these, of course, but it is important to recognize this distinction because educational philosophy falls in the realm of social science but impacts bench science, too. And because theory is taught very differently to bench scientists than it is to social scientists – as you may be gleaning already.

There is still a commonly taught fallacy in many science disciplines that theories are formed and tested so that they can be proven and then they become laws. Some of you may have learned this yourself; perhaps even passed this along as canonical knowledge. But now, knowing the difference between philosophy and theory, I hope you are comparing this misconception with the struggles many have delineating the differences between philosophy and theory. The connection here is *theory* – ideas that move us toward solutions for overcoming challenges. Bench scientists strive to do this, too – perhaps such challenges do not emerge from philosophy (perhaps they do!), but such challenges are presented in Big Questions and often result in a questioning – or even reimagining – of our world. The discovery of DNA, photons, neutrons, atoms, ions . . . they were all a result of questions and a desire to answer those questions. Theories then were created to provide a possible way forward – the theory of thermodynamics or theories that help us investigate whether quarks really exist are not things to be proven but roads to be explored. The main difference from social science theory is that there tends to be less, if any, empirical data in the theories of social science. But the fundamental concept of social science theory is not really different – it is just different language.

For this chapter – and the rest of this text – you can think of theories as sets of statements, principles, or ideas that guide us in making claims about the world (Hagen 2005). It provides an explanatory construct to help structure action through identification of key relationships that can be used to explain, predict, or change a phenomenon (Jaeger et al. 2013). This chapter will attempt to introduce you to a broad range of foundational theories in education and to some of the more notable theorists in the field of education, just as the previous chapter laid the groundwork for educational philosophy and philosophers of note.

Importance of Educational Theories

According to Biesta (2013), in *The Handbook of Educational Theories*, educational theories are important for these reasons: they help us understand what is not understood and is foreign; they provide new descriptions of educational principles and practices; they give us tools to shift from gathering data to understanding that data and how it applies to our classrooms; and they allow us to conceptualize phenomena that we wish to investigate – in other words, they produce a subject that allows that subject to be studied. There are some who have argued that education is not a discipline in and of itself, but Biesta argues that regardless of whether it is its own discipline or not, educational theories are unique unto themselves. While psychology, for example, may produce ideas about education that evolve into theories, Biesta argues that these are psychology theories that participate in education but they cannot be educational theories because they are unable to generate educational perspectives, ways of seeing, concerns, and ways of questioning. And when we fail to recognize and embrace this, we risk allowing others to guide our discipline without our input.

I agree with Biesta – and see this happening in academia routinely as many who call themselves educators have failed to engage with educational theories in a way that allows them to gain insights into and knowledge of the unique and complex challenges that education poses. I also see the contradictory approaches to education that frustrate those in higher education who are delivering content, especially in veterinary medicine. If you feel that students must actively engage in their learning – whether that be in the form of small group assignments, discussions within small or large groups, working through cases, or seeing cases on the clinical floor – but you find yourself feeling as if the only way to "teach" is to deliver lectures using slides and/or notes packets, an understanding of your theoretical (albeit potentially unknown) stance may help you gain insights into ways you might better align your theory and your practice. This can only make you a better teacher!

To be sure, there are hundreds of educational theories available to you. You need only Google search "educational theories" to verify this. I encourage you to go through this exercise so you can see the dizzying array of educational theories that are out there, then come back to this chapter. Upon your return, you will see some theories that align with what you found and some differences. Know that this is OK. This textbook is not intended to be a comprehensive dive into all the educational theories out there; others have already taken on that task. It is simply intended to introduce you to the theories upon which all other educational theories have been built and provide you with a basic understanding of their histories, impacts, similarities, and differences. If you become enamored with educational theory (and I hope a few of you do), also know that as you do your own research into the theories of learning that interest you the most, they may not be what we have chosen to focus on in this text – and that is also OK. Just as with bench scientific theories, educational theories are varied and mostly unproven, though not necessarily unsupported.

The first part of this chapter will introduce you to "The Big Three" – the overarching "camps" into which most educational theories fall. These three, behaviorism, cognitivism, and constructivism, are evolutions of each other, and the fourth that will be touched on – positivism – is one that gained momentum through the rise of bench science and its emergence as the "gold standard" for all things – even those beyond bench science. While not always discussed in the broader references to educational theory, it is imperative you understand it because of its heavy influence on teaching today, particularly in the sciences, but really across the board. The vast majority of higher education teachers likely start their careers using a positivist approach without even realizing it; another reason it is included in this chapter.

Once the Big Three and their "other sibling" (positivism) have been covered, the chapter will move into specific theorists and their theories. Each theorist will be connected to one of the foundational educational theories, though be forewarned that trying to fully box them in is an exercise in futility and will not be attempted. Instead, each section will attempt to elucidate the ways that positivism, behaviorism, cognitivism, and constructivism have influenced their stances and theories, and help clarify the places where each theory resonates with or contradicts these foundational educational theories.

In the end, you should be well familiar with the Big Three and their other sibling, understand generally where each of the theorists explored in this chapter falls on the spectrum of those foundational theories, and be able to articulate why you do or do not align educationally with each of the foundational theories. You might also find yourself interested in learning more about an individual theory, which would be fantastic, and that is why there is a provided list of resources and references for you to consult as you further explore the theories that should be driving our teaching, no matter where that teaching occurs.

Finally, you will not see some of the more contemporary theorists presented here; some are covered in another chapter (specifically, Malcolm Knowles), and others are occasionally referenced throughout the textbook as appropriate. This chapter is dedicated to the foundational theories of education, upon which the likes of Ericsson, Knowles, Miller, and others built their more contemporary theories. This is not to slight them, nor to insinuate that their work is less important or valuable. It is merely due to the limited amount of time and space available, as well as the purpose of this textbook. Perhaps, if another edition is requested, such theorists will find their way into this text!

Section 2: The Big Three and Their Other Sibling

Katherine Fogelberg

Part 1: Positivism: The Launching Pad for Behaviorism and Other Learning Theories

"Positivism is the view that the only way to obtain knowledge of the world is by means of sense perception and introspection and the methods of the empirical sciences" (Acton 1951, p. 291). As many of you reading are likely bench scientists, this quote may resonate with you. However, given that you are reading *this* text, you also likely consider yourself a teacher – perhaps even an educator. As such, it is imperative to understand how the wave of positivism, which is rooted deeply in the "scientific method" we have all been so indoctrinated into, has impacted the very thing we do regularly: teach.

Auguste Comte [1798–1857] was a French philosopher and is the man credited with starting positivism (and sociology). In what feels a long-ago precursor to Bloom's Taxonomy of learning, Comte proposed the Law of Three Stages: "the theological or fictive stage; the metaphysical or abstract stage; and finally the scientific or positive stage" (Comte 1822, as cited in Acton 1951, p. 292). It is this final stage, explained as the stage where "facts are linked in terms of ideas or general laws of an entirely positive order suggested or confirmed by the facts themselves . . ." (Comte 1822, as cited in Acton 1951, p. 292), that modern positivism grew from. It was this "positive order" that would stick, and thus "positivists" view the world in observable, quantifiable chunks of information. They believe new knowledge is created carefully, through observation, creation of hypotheses, testing of hypotheses, and either retesting hypotheses to provide repeatable support of its truth or adjusting hypotheses to find the truth. It is a fairly linear sequence, starting with an observation and ending with the results of an experiment.

Comte's positivism was initially created for the study of human society – thus birthing the field of sociology – though it ended up having far-reaching impacts, particularly in the social sciences. The impacts were felt in his newly formed sociology and, later, psychology and education. Because he felt that even humans could be objectively quantified, Comte's movement started the quest to bring human behavior out of the realm of the mystical and wondrous and into the realm of science.

This approach to science has had an enormous influence on the way we teach – not only science but all subjects – as it is the epistemological stance that has been taken for decades and was the driving force behind the idea that the teacher knows all and the students are vessels to be filled (Hinchey 2010). If you have heard the phrases "sage on the stage," "sit and get," and the like, you can now recognize that all of these originated from the positivist movement. Thus, while it is perhaps not widely acknowledged as a current learning theory, it is certainly rooted in the idea that knowledge is only achieved through observation and rigorous testing, which led to the idea that only scientists – and then researchers – held knowledge that was then to be passed down to students in our traditional top-down education systems and teaching approaches.

All of you have experienced this epistemological view of teaching and learning throughout your education, beginning in elementary and going up through your veterinary program. As Hinchey (2010) points out, our very school systems are built on this concept of subject-specific instruction that becomes increasingly specialized as we advance through the education system. She additionally reminds us that the further up the ladder you climb educationally, the more expertise is required of the teachers to ensure they have enough knowledge to pass on to the novices; this reaches its heights at the level of the university and, certainly, within the medical professions. Now you have the education-related knowledge and language to recognize and describe this practice, as well as a better understanding of why it is so deeply entrenched in our education system. Fortunately, we are seeing the pendulum swing back toward a somewhat opposing epistemological stance, which we will cover later in this chapter.

Hopefully, you might see more clearly now why positivism is not necessarily considered an educational theory but is important to understand when discussing educational theory. The origins of positivism trace back to the early 1800s and have embedded themselves into our society so thoroughly that it is close to impossible to imagine what things would look like without it. The process and ideas of positivism are certainly useful and have created opportunities for bench scientists around the world to make breakthroughs that have been replicated and confirmed; there is no arguing that. And while the downsides of applying positivism to social sciences are many, its mere existence opened the doors to educational theories being created – first in its likeness and later straying from that likeness while still being rooted in the idea that all unexplained phenomena in the world – human or otherwise – can be explained through careful observation, creation of hypotheses, and conducting of experiments to determine the veracity of such hypotheses.

Part 2: Behaviorism: The Foundations of Outcomes-Based Education

While Biesta may make compelling arguments that psychology and education theories are distinctly different, there is little to no pushback against the idea that education theories owe a lot of their foundations to psychology. Behaviorism, the original of the Big Three educational theories, was created and forwarded by three recognizable psychologists: Edward Thorndike, John Watson, and B.F. Skinner. In coming up with and refining what would ultimately be taught as an educational theory, all three drew on their backgrounds in psychology and the idea of Comte's positivism. None of them predicted their ideas would become so influential in the broader realm of education, though one did end up teaching only because the job market for psychological research was so poor (some things truly never change).

The psychologists turned educators who created and applied this theory were determined to observe, categorize, and measure all aspects of learning, through experiments that we find abhorrent today but were looked upon with significant interest during their day. Ultimately, for example, the experiments performed by Watson were incredibly harmful to those involved, but because such harms failed

to manifest until much later and his theory had already spread like wildfire, an entire generation of children was affected. While potentially less extreme, both Thorndike and Skinner tended toward the extreme in their experiments as well. In the end, while behaviorism still has a heavy influence on today's approaches to education, we have seen its edges somewhat blunted by later and more contemporary theories and theorists.

Born just eight years before Comte died, Ivan Pavlov [1849–1936] is perhaps the world's best-known behaviorist, though he would not have labeled himself as such. A Nobel-prize-winning physiologist, Pavlov's experiments with dogs occurred as a result of his studies directed toward determining the physiology of digestion combined with his earlier work demonstrating the existence of a basic pattern in the reflex regulation of circulatory organ activity (nobelprize. org). After discovering the reflex regulation, he moved on to figuring out the physiological processes involved with digestion. It was here that he developed the surgical method of using chronic fistulas, a monumental breakthrough in research because it allowed continuous observation of *in situ* organs under relatively normal conditions (nobelprize. org). This innovative solution to organ study allowed him to definitively determine and demonstrate that the nervous system was a dominant force in regulating digestive processes, a discovery that is acknowledged as the basis of modern digestive physiology (nobelprize.org).

During his study of digestive gland activity and its reflex regulation, Pavlov was particularly interested in "psychic secretions," which occurred in animals who were stimulated by food, even if that food was some distance from the animal. Through use of fistulated salivary gland ducts, pioneered by a colleague in 1895 but based on Pavlov's own use of fistulas to study other digestive organs, he was able to determine that salivary secretion was not psychic; rather, it was a reflex that could be conditioned. It was this discovery that made it possible to experimentally investigate, rather than subjectively speculate about, "the most complex interrelations between an organism and its external environment" (nobelprize.org, n.p.). While today Pavlov's groundbreaking work has been reduced to the bell-ringing inducement of salivating dogs, it is clear that the experiments were much more sophisticated than this summary indicates. His work also had far-reaching implications for medicine, as well as other disciplines that he likely could never have anticipated – education being one, by way of psychology.

John Watson [1878–1958]

Behaviorism essentially took Pavlov's somewhat revolutionary (at the time) conditioned responses in dogs to a new level by applying his ideas to conditioning people. The groundwork was laid by Darwin, who first "attributed mental processes to lower organisms" (Skinner 1959, p. 197); this caused others to react and point out that Darwin's anecdotal evidence of such claims could be explained in other ways. Ultimately, Pavlov's experiments combined with the initial observations of Darwin resulted in Watson asking, "If there were other explanations of mental processes in lower organisms, why not also in man?" (Skinner 1959, p. 197). It was through his desire to answer this question that behaviorism was born.

John Watson, as Samelson (1981) states, was credited with being the "founder of behaviorism" about 50 years after his reading of a paper at a meeting of the American Psychological Association's New York branch. The first in a series of eight lectures delivered at Columbia University in 1913 covering animal psychology (Samelson 1981), Watson opened with: "Psychology as the behaviorist views it is a purely objective experimental branch of natural science. Its theoretical goal is the prediction and control of behavior" (Watson 1994, p. 248). With this bombshell, Watson questioned the entirety of the newly (approximately 50 years old) formed discipline of psychology, although he apparently did not wish to be viewed as a harsh critic: "I do not wish unduly to criticize psychology" (Watson 1994, p. 249). Later in 1913, Watson would publish his *The Behavioral Learning Theory*, which further moved psychology toward behavior as an "-ism" (Weegar and Pacis 2012).

Watson's (1994) explanation for his statements comes later in his paper when he states that in comparison to other sciences, the esoteric nature of psychology is problematic. "If you fail to reproduce my findings. . . The attack is made upon the observer and not upon the experimental setting. In physics or chemistry the attack is made upon the experimental conditions" (p. 249). In other words, in other sciences, better technique provides better results, whereas in psychology, it is based on feelings – which are never cut and dry. A clear disciple of positivism, this lack of adherence to measurable outcomes and processes was a sticking point for Watson; one he used to make the argument that his discipline's search for answers through consideration of the consciousness was fruitless. It was time, he felt, to create a study of psychology based on observable, measurable responses – this was a mantra he continued to repeat, delivering a speech in 1925 to the Fifty-First Annual Meeting of the American Neurological Association that reiterated his commitment to making psychology a more objective science (Watson 1925). In this address, he stated, "I do not believe there is any such thing as instinct. . . our studies on the conditioned responses, both of animals and of human beings, have shown that we can condition the. . . responses" (Watson 1925, p. 185).

In this same speech, Watson outlined several experiments indicating that babies can be conditioned to "fear every other object in the universe. All one has to do is to show the object and strike the steel bar behind his head and repeat the procedure one or two times" (p. 191). In fact, this conditioning experiment was actually conducted. Dubbed the "Little Albert Experiment," Watson and a graduate student exposed 9-month-old "little Albert" to several White furry objects, including a White rat, noting that he enjoyed playing with them. After a short time, as Albert played with the White rat, Watson made a loud sound behind his head on several occasions – his "conditioning" intervention. After several repetitions of the condition intervention, the White rat – as well as the other objects Albert had enjoyed – became a source of fear even without the scary noise being made (APA.org 2010). The child was never deconditioned and, sadly, died of acquired hydrocephaly at a very young age (APA.org 2010), which may be why the adult impacts of such experiments were never truly seen until it was a bit too late.

Ultimately, Watson would become somewhat extremist in his claims about behaviorism in response to attacks on his work. This resulted in his book, *Psychological Care of the Infant and Child*, which urged parents to show little affection to their children. Although he publicly regretted the book after its production, he had already impacted many families with his parenting theory of cold detachment, and it is often these extreme views for which he is remembered. Fortunately, the year before he died, the American Psychological Association remembered him for the impact made on the field in a citation that read:

> To Dr. John Watson B. Watson, whose work has been one of the vital determinants of the form and substance of modern psychology. He initiated a revolution in psychological thought, and his writing have been the point of departure for continuing lines of fruitful research (Skinner 1959, p. 129).

Regardless of how anyone feels about the later extreme views and human experiments Watson did, it cannot be denied that his work laid the foundation for others in the field. It also cannot be denied that his formalization of a theory of behavior provided the basis of educational theories that we continue to study and use today.

Edward Thorndike [1874–1949]

Edward Thorndike, an American psychologist, had lots of ideas about lots of things, ranging from his thoughts on genetics to his ideas about education, all of which were rooted in his training in – and beliefs about – psychology. While Watson was working diligently to ensure his study of psychology was aligned with the positivist approach to inquiry, Thorndike was explicitly connecting psychology to education. Indeed, he would become known as the father of educational psychology, although he started his work in animals and transitioned to education only when the job market became such that he needed to find some work (Beatty 1998).

As someone who was interested in a lot of little measurements, Thorndike did not believe behaviorism would be a unifying theory of education; he actually did not believe such a thing could – or should – ever exist (Beatty 1998). He was, in his approach, far more bench scientist than theorist, adhering strongly to the idea that facts and the measurability of *all* things (including human behavior, morality, and learning) was possible, but that such measures could only be accomplished through observation of objects.

But Thorndike's prominence was established over a decade earlier – in 1898, with the publication of his doctoral thesis, which called into question and aggressively mocked the state of behavior research in animals. At the time, observation and introspection on the part of the observer were reported anecdotally, and accepted by much of the scientific community as evidence that animals had feelings and behaved in certain ways as a result of those feelings. He, however, strongly believed that behaviors could and should be measured using "A representative sample of subjects. . . examined in a carefully described, standardized situation" (Galef 1998, p. 1130). In other words, Thorndike was the first behaviorist studying animals to actively apply the scientific method – or the approach to psychological research that would be lamented as missing by Watson 15 years later.

As with most innovators, Thorndike's methods were soundly rejected, and even reviled, by many of his contemporaries. Wesley Mills suggested that Thorndike's methods were cruel and thus the animals studied had their baseline intellects "grossly underestimated," while C.L. Morgan went so far as to say that his subjects should be referred to as victims (Galef 1998). However, as the true nature of Thorndike's work became clearer, the outrage cooled and a plethora of laboratories were set up and began studying comparative psychology in the manner of Thorndike's experiments. These laboratories have descendants that remain active today at Harvard University and the University of Chicago (Galef 1998). By 1910, however, the ability to make a living studying animal behavior, particularly as he had created it, had become untenable and he had moved to the realm of education.

In Thorndike's essay titled "The contribution of psychology to education," originally printed in 1910, it is easy to see the connections he makes between psychology and education:

Psychology contributes to a better understanding of the aims of education by defining them, making them clearer; by limiting them, showing us what can be done and what can not; and by suggesting new features that should be made parts of them (Thorndike 1910, p. 1).

He then continues on to support each of the statements he has made with fuller explanations of what he believes to be true. He ends the essay by pointing out that psychology will not do the only heavy lifting: "The science of education can and will itself contribute abundantly to psychology . . . School-room life itself is a vast laboratory in which are made thousands of experiments of the utmost interest to 'pure' psychology" (Thorndike 1910, p. 8). His view, then, was clearly a reciprocal one: psychology would provide structure and process to education, and education would provide a "vast laboratory" from which psychology could draw innumerable experiments. In moving a positivist psychology to the classroom, Thorndike effectively introduced behaviorism, as well. A move from animal to human studies in behavior was not a huge leap, given his views on the classroom as laboratory.

While Thorndike's contributions to education cannot be ignored, they must always be tempered with the knowledge that, as with many early scholars – regardless of field – he was also a classist who was opinionated about who should be educated and why. He did not believe in education for all and felt that a liberal arts education was a waste, essentially trying to squash the idea that good citizens were only produced through a renaissance approach to teaching – in direct contrast to the ideals of the ancient educational philosophers – among others – discussed in Chapter 1. While he did go against the popular idea of his contemporaries that only children could really learn (Beatty 1998), he also believed that a superior human race could and should be created through selective breeding and was, therefore, a self-proclaimed eugenicist. As a recognized educational expert, he played a prominent role in convincing teachers of the value of eugenics and incorporating this ideology into the educational programs of the US at the time (Kurbegovic 2022). But regardless of this somewhat negative history, Thorndike is still viewed as a great thinker and one of the more impactful behaviorists of all time.

B.F. Skinner [1904–1990]

The educational theory that grew from the seeds of Pavlov and his dogs reached its height through BF Skinner – who some of you may know through his semi-fictional novel *Walden Two*, written in 1948. Skinner's novel appeared to be science fiction at the time but was eventually deemed prescient in light of the ensuing behavioral methodologies he employed to "train" humans – beginning with his own children. His successes were widespread enough to influence the way teachers delivered content in school, in spite of the bad press he received about the "air crib" he constructed and raised his second child, a daughter, in until she was two years old.

He was firmly aligned with Watson in his approach to education (Weegar and Pacis 2012), and could even be credited with creating the precursor to our computer adaptive tests that have been implemented in several professional licensing exams, such as the NCLEX – the nursing licensing exam. Because he believed that mental processes are not important to learning, an idea he would have to have had based on his positivist approach to studying learning, his behaviorism would retroactively be renamed radical behaviorism.

The bulk of Skinner's experimental work was done on lab animals and evolved into what you may know as operant conditioning today, a behavioral approach used more explicitly in animals than humans. In classical conditioning, a stimulus was used to obtain a response. This stimulus was continued until an association between an object and a stimulus was ingrained so firmly that, absent the stimulus, the presence of the associated object still induced a response. This is the watered-down version of Pavlov's salivating dogs and was demonstrated clearly by Watson's human Little Albert experiment. However, it was later found that such conditioning was temporary and unpredictable. Thus Skinner, acknowledging the limits of such conditioning, determined that additional stimuli were needed to increase the reliability and durability of the conditioned response. In searching for methods to do this, he introduced positive and negative reinforcement, a concept that is highly nuanced and is often incorrectly interpreted.

In Skinner's version of behaviorism, positive reinforcement consists of providing some type of reward when a desired behavior is exhibited. This is similar to clicker training your favorite animal, with the click first being associated with a treat after performing a certain behavior, and eventually being viewed as the reward in lieu of the treat. It satisfies, albeit in a different manner, just as the treat did. Negative reinforcement, on the other hand, is not punishment, as many often interpret it to be; rather, it is the removal of something unpleasant in response to a stimulus. Thus, if someone reacts positively to a specified stimulus, something causing discomfort or displeasure is removed, and, over time, the desired behavior changes with the expectation that the noxious item will be removed. A sort of positive reinforcement in reverse, if you will. It may be easiest to think of positive reinforcement as the addition of something pleasant and negative reinforcement as the removal of something unpleasant in an attempt to condition the response of a subject. As you can see, while it is a somewhat challenging thing to explain and remember, it is clearly different than a reward and punishment system – at least different than the punishment part. Behaviorism's Evolution The *Stanford Encyclopedia of Philosophy* (https://plato.stanford.edu) defines three types of behaviorism: methodological, psychological, and analytical or logical (Graham 2019). Methodological behaviorism, the realm of Watson, believes that psychology should study only animal and human behavior and not be concerned with their mental states because mental states have no impact on the sources of behavior (Graham 2019). Psychological behaviorism, practiced by Pavlov, Thorndike, Skinner, and a bit of Watson, proposes that animal and human behavior can be explained through conditioning (or learning) by observing and testing responses to external physical stimuli, and, in some cases, positive or negative reinforcements. Analytical or logical behaviorism focuses on the mental state and its effects on behavior but does not explain the mental state, per se (Graham 2019). Rather, when someone is viewed as having a specific belief, for example, it is not to say that person is in a particular mental state but is a prediction of what they might do in a specific situation or within particular environments (Graham 2019). This third type of behaviorism came about around the same time as the other two and had a bit of a resurgence in the early 2000s, but it is Watson, Thorndike, and Skinner who are primarily associated with behaviorism.

A commitment to the positivist epistemology of the time and with the publication of a variety of human experiments that were both sensational and impactful, behaviorism became embedded in society and influenced practices from parenting to teaching. But while Graham (2019) focuses on the current labels within behaviorism on the macro level, it is important to understand the evolution of Watson's behaviorism on the micro level, as well, because it is this form – referred to as methodological by Graham – that continues to influence, often unknowingly, education today.

Within the macro label of methodological behaviorism, Pavlov laid the groundwork and his work and those extensions are referred to as *associationism*. Associationism is the idea that an animal can be conditioned to behave in a certain way through external forces, and early work by Watson and Thorndike affirmed this was also the case in people, giving birth to behaviorism proper (Pavlov 1967). With its strict adherence to a positivist paradigm (in this case, positivist being used in its original form as the scientific approach rather than as a teaching approach), the products of Watson's and Thorndike's experiments were viewed as breakthroughs. Highly impactful, it is important to note that conditioned behaviors were often temporary, especially in people. It is also important to understand that whatever external stimulus was used lost its effectiveness over time and its impact was varied, making the length of the desired behavior unpredictable, rendering the theory imperfect at best.

This idea that mental processes and/or states (referred to as mentalism at the time) had no place in teaching behaviors was pretty radical, given the origination of mentalism with Darwin. Skinner would recognize the radical nature of behaviorism well after Watson had begun his work, first using the term "radical behaviorism" in reference to his own work as early as the 1940s (Schneider and Morris 1987). Interestingly, the term had been used as early as 1920 in reference to Watson's work by others, though the moniker did not stick at the time. Today, the term is generally used to refer only to Skinner's work, in spite of the fact that it was Watson who first coined the term behaviorism and that his views were more similar to Skinner's than different (Schneider and Morris 1987). Whether referred to as behaviorism or radical behaviorism, the roots are essentially the same: behavior can be taught through conditioning, there is no consciousness or need to introspect, because behaviors are merely responses to training.

In the spirit of competitive science, perhaps, it is a fun piece of trivia that in spite of the forward movement Thorndike contributed to behaviorism and its positivist investigations into shaping behavior, Skinner would purport Thorndike to believe in some sort of consciousness in an early 1960s essay:

> Thorndike's experiments, at the end of the 19th century. . . showed that the behavior of a cat in escaping from a puzzle box might seem to show reasoning but could be explained instead as the result of simpler processes. Thorndike remained a mentalist, but he greatly advanced the objective study of behavior which has been attributed to mental processes (Skinner 1963, pp. 951–952).

Thus, while on the micro level behaviorism appears to have evolved into radical behaviorism, in reality, the change is not so easy to parse. It first started with Watson, certainly, but given that Skinner openly viewed Thorndike as a mentalist, it appears there was a very small schism early in the beginnings of behaviorism.

You may be asking yourself, then, did behaviorism ever really exist in the beginning, or was it always radical? Did Skinner merely name it such so that he could distinguish himself from his contemporary Watson, who is still viewed as the originator of behaviorism, even though Skinner was doing concurrent and parallel work? Or is it merely semantics – the realm of the esoteric and somewhat meaningless when all is said and done? Regardless of how it is viewed, behaviorism's "second act" is widely accepted as radical behaviorism, given the back-and-forth noted in the literature at the time between those who were radical behaviorists (Watson, Skinner), and their contemporaries, who were slightly softer (Thorndike, Warren, Culkins), who acknowledged that a consciousness or other mental phenomena might have a role to play in shaping behavior (Schneider and Morris 1987). For purposes of this text, it is important you understand there is a fuzzy line of demarcation between behaviorism and radical behaviorism, though they both started in the same place.

The third and final evolution of behaviorism, social behaviorism, is more clear-cut as an iteration of what was a psychology theory and has morphed over time into an educational one. It takes into account the impact of an individual's environment on modifying behavior and learning and acknowledges the role that internal processes – which cannot be seen or empirically measured – play in learning. While the founders of behaviorism would scoff at this idea, it was a natural evolution given that radical behaviorism could not consistently predict or reproduce its effects in every situation with every learner (even with Skinner's introduction of negative and positive reinforcement). What seemed to work for some did not work for others, and even within a single individual, external stimuli could be the same but vary in their effects from day to day or week to week. Therefore, something else had to be influencing the outcome. While mental processes could not – and still cannot, to our great chagrin – be observed and objectively measured, the environment in which learners are taught most certainly can be. Environment would be defined and redefined as social behaviorists continued to apply and test their work, but it currently encompasses everything in the physical and social environment; from lighting and the color of the walls to the number of students and how they interact in the classroom.

Albert Bandura [1925–2021] was one of the more influential psychologists who believed in social behaviorism; his prodigious theorizing impacted a number of fields, including psychology, education, and social work. Bandura's ideas about behavior and how it could be shaped are epitomized in social learning theory, which is based on behaviorism but recognizes that mediating processes occur between a stimulus and a response, and includes the premise that students learn by observing others in their environments (Bandura 1971).

Eventually, as with all evolutions, there comes a point when something reaches its apex and can no longer be contained within the boundaries created by its origination. Theories are no different, and while behaviorism still influences many facets of human existence and learning, the movement toward social behaviorism supplied the foundations for subsequent educational theorists to begin exploring other causes of learned behavior – responses, changes, and developments. This led to a new era of educational theories built on behaviorism but willing to acknowledge that there had to be something beyond the observable influencing the responses. In coming to this conclusion, the "mentalism" first proposed by Darwin became relevant once again, although it would be more sophisticated and highly influenced by the positivist movement that had become a mainstay in psychology and education.

It is important to note that while this text discusses the evolutions of the Big Three educational theories, there is significant overlap in the theorists who were proponents of each. It is true from an educational perspective that behaviorism seems to come first and constructivism last temporally, but you will see that each of the three main theories came about around the same time – the late 1800s and early 1900s. Had the appetites or intellectual movements of society been slightly different, it is quite possible that we would not be discussing behaviorism today and instead would have built constructivist schools that had potentially endured for over 100 years. In the end, the evolution of educational theories is a bit of a façade. However, it does make it slightly easier to consider them as a chronological series when looking at each historically and how they affected our approaches to education in the US, because their rise and fall correspond with a chronological timeline, even if their initial creation does not.

Behaviorism in Education

Thorndike's influence on education cannot be denied; it started in the US in the early part of the twentieth century and continues even today in some classrooms, as it was Thorndike who popularized the practice and repetition approach (perhaps more currently recognizable as the memorize and regurgitate mantra of today) to teaching (Bruner 2004). Ultimately, educators who follow a behaviorist approach are focused on shaping students' behavior. It is this approach that has been used for many decades, as it imbues the teacher with control and views students as empty vessels to be filled (Wortham 2003). This allows educators to deliver rewards, punishments, and positive and negative reinforcements to get students to behave in the desired manner; while we may not explicitly recognize this to be true, with some reflection it is easy to see that this approach is still in full swing within our current education systems. For example, we reward students who do their homework and answer questions correctly with "good" grades, punishing those who fail to do so with "bad" grades. Likewise, those bad grades are often erased or updated if the student repeats an exam, assignment, or course and responds "correctly" (i.e., the way the educator wishes them to respond).

Given that there was further evolution of this theory as applied to education, why do we continue to use it? As with many things that have become embedded in society, behaviorism was the bedrock upon which many educational

practices were built. It is difficult to eradicate approaches that seem to work, even when we have ample evidence to support that it does not work the way we would like it to all the time. Such is the case with behaviorism; in spite of well over 70 years of research demonstrating that behaviorism does not adequately induce learning, it continues to have strong influence in our educational institutions, because, according to Wortham (2003), it works – at least well enough to provide educators and students a reasonable amount of evidence that reinforcements can shape behavior. However, the lack of attention paid to the mental (cognitive) processes that also contribute to behavior is where this theory as applied to education falls short. Fortunately, recognition that people could learn in the absence of external reinforcements allowed the theory to evolve into one that did focus on mental processes.

Part 3: Cognitivism: Recognition that Mental Processes Matter

Rooted, once again, in psychology, cognitivism as a learning theory emerged as a reaction to behaviorism within the borders of the classroom and within its original discipline. Cognitivism rejects the idea that learning is simply a stimulus–response process, and although the cognitivist movement started just shy of a decade after behaviorism took off, it was alongside the rise of social behaviorism, which believed mental processes were where true learning was happening with behaviors merely being the manifestations of that learning, that this school of thought began to take hold.

Edward Chase Tolman [1886–1959] is considered the pioneer who started cognitivism within psychology (Yilmaz 2011; Bruner 2004). While he is less known and discussed today, having been replaced by more recognizable theorists including Jean Piaget, Lev Vygotsky, and Jerome Bruner, you might have noticed that Bruner himself clearly recognized the impact of Tolman's work on educational psychology in the early 2000s. His thoughts on learning were somewhat overshadowed by the zeal that accompanied the behaviorist movement and had dominated educational practices through the early twentieth century. Nonetheless, Tolman was publishing results about his experiments with rats in mazes that appeared to have mental maps of the different mazes into which they were placed (Yilmaz 2011; Bruner 2004). However, it would not be until the mid-twentieth century that cognitive psychology would truly begin to bloom (Garnham 2019).

Cognitivist theorists center their ideas on the thinking processes, the brain functions, and the ways in which the mind solves complex tasks. To them, the acquisition of knowledge is not based on behavior. Instead, learning occurs by linking new information with previous knowledge and creating mental structures and schemas. The learner is an active participant in the learning process and is perceived as someone who is capable of learning and complex thinking.

However, this is not to be confused with the mentalism that had given rise to the behaviorist movement before. Mentalists believed there were things happening in the mind that could not be fully elucidated but could be interpreted (Watson and Coulter 2008). Cognitivists, on the other hand, viewed the workings of the mind in the way we essentially view computers today: there is an input, that input is processed through an internal symbol system using discrete abstract symbols – in other words, acquisition of knowledge involves something internal that involves coding and structuring of that coding by the learner (Garnham 2019; Yilmaz 2011). As a result, learners are active participants in the learning process for those taking a cognitivist stance, unlike behaviorists who viewed learning as a passive reaction to external stimuli.

In this theoretical view, the idea of *schemes, schemas,* or *schematas* is central (all are synonymous). Schemas are abstract units of knowledge, skill, and understanding that can be woven into complex relationships with other schemas and/or hierarchically categorized (Clark 2018; Flavell 1996). For example, counting is an abstract idea that can be both hierarchically categorized – as in 100 is larger than 50 is larger than 1 – and woven into complex relationships with other schemas – as in counting money, which has different value than counting flowers in a field. It is these individual pieces of information that contribute to larger clumps of information and allows our minds to organize and connect the pieces in ways that make sense to us; it is estimated that adults have hundreds of thousands of these variably sized schemas, and new schemas are created every time new information is received (Clark 2018). Thus, it is when schemas change that learning takes place in the cognitivist's view.

As such, cognitivists attempt to make knowledge meaningful and work to help learners be more organized in ways that allow them to relate new information to their existing stored knowledge. They recognize that thought processes, including "memory, thinking, reflection, abstraction, and metacognition," are inherent to learning (Al-Shammari et al. 2019, p. 410). In this regard, cognitivism focuses on how learners know what they know and how that knowledge has been acquired rather than their behavior. It is this emphasis on the processes and the learning that particularly detaches it from behaviorism.

Distilled into the principle most pertinent to classroom instruction, the idea of organization is what bubbles to the surface. In keeping with the computer analogy, the famous "garbage in, garbage out" euphemism potentially sums up the cognitivist's approach to teaching. Because cognitivists view learning as a process of organizing many bits of information into larger and larger schemas, instruction must be presented in a logically sequenced and organized way that is digestible and relatable for the learner (Ozdem-Yilmaz and Bilican 2020). It is also important to support learners in retaining new information and being able to recall such information within the context of the appropriate existing schemas, which provides them the opportunity to build upon those existing schemas and, therefore, learn.

There are many prominent educational psychologists connected to cognitivism, including Piaget and his theory of individual cognitive development, Vygotsky and his theory of social cognitive growth, including his ideas about the zone of proximal development (ZPD), and Bruner's cognitive constructivist learning theory (Yilmaz 2011). One with whom you may be very familiar on the surface level is Benjamin Bloom [1913–1999], an educational psychologist best known for his taxonomy of learning (Lasley 2022), which is one of the most widely used cognitivist tools in education today. You may also be familiar with Albert Bandura and his social cognitive theory (SCT), which is covered in-depth in Chapter 3. It is, however, generally recognized that Piaget and Vygotsky were two of the most influential theorists in the movement from behaviorism to cognitivism and from cognitivism to constructivism.

Perhaps not surprisingly, there were numerous iterations of cognitivist theory, but in contrast to the evolution from behaviorism to cognitivism, where the lines of demarcation are pretty clear, the differences between cognitivism and constructivism are much blurrier. This makes it difficult to outline the work of any fully committed cognitivists in this section, as most of those who believed in cognitivism (and even started it!) ultimately landed in the constructivist camp. That is not to say that there are no committed cognitivists out there; it is simply to justify the lack of introduction to explicit cognitivists while there are clearly dedicated sections to behaviorists and constructivists. As you become more familiar with these educational theories and the theorists behind them, perhaps you will find cognitivism more to your liking and will choose to explore those theorists on your own. For now, I have left the majority of this work to the authors of Chapter 3, which explores more deeply learning and cognition through the lens of cognitivism.

Part 4: Constructivism: The Student as an Active and Reflective Learner

Likely not surprisingly, there are many versions of constructivism, the most popular of which include cognitive, developmental, critical, radical, and social (Boghossian 2006;

Ozdem-Yilmaz and Bilican 2020). Regardless of the version, all have at their core the belief that learning is an active process that occurs through the creation of meaning and connection with previous experiences; therefore, there is not a "correct" or "incorrect" meaning; instead, meaning is a personal interpretation. These internal representations of knowledge are constantly changing as the learner's experience changes. Thus, the context of learning is central to the constructivist's approach to education because learners construct their own personal interpretations of the world based on their experiences and interactions, meaning that social interactions and cultural context play important roles in the construction of an individual learner's knowledge (Rannikmae et al. 2020). It is constructivism writ large that is explored below, with occasional nods to social constructivism (Vygotsky, Bruner, Piaget), as this is the most well-known "branch" of constructivism. *Note*: radical constructivism, the movement led by Ernst von Glaserfield, has gained some traction in contemporary science and mathematics education. The goal of this text is to provide a deep enough overview of educational theories to help you understand the language and perspectives of the primary educational theorists so that, if you should desire to do so, you may read further on the micro levels of theory with a better understanding of its roots.

It should be easy to see how cognitivism gave way to constructivism; the tenets of constructivism are seen in cognitivism's nod to the internal processes that organize and chunk information into schemas that expand as new information is obtained, as well as in the idea that learning is a primarily internally motivated act. The later evolution of behaviorism into social behaviorism also provides a glimpse into the eventual emergence of constructivism, with Bandura laying the groundwork in his acknowledgment that the environment plays a role in shaping the behavior of children.

Of the learning theories presented here, constructivism is potentially the most abstract; it lends itself to a more philosophical stance – one that emerged from a change in thought from a positivist, objective epistemological belief and evolved into a subjective, postmodernist perspective (Boghossian 2006). In plain language, the subjective turn differed from both the objective (what is known independent of an examiner) and metaphysical (knowledge that is independent of the knower) epistemological stances in that it focused on individual experiences (Boghossian 2006). Alongside postmodernism or the idea "that there are multiple perspectives, interpretations and truths, and that each perspective has its own validity" (Boghossian 2006, p.715), these two philosophical stances provided the basis for constructivism's emergence.

Although in so many ways diametrically opposed to behaviorism, constructivism certainly owes its beginnings to the behaviorist movement. No one plays a game without an opponent; even in solitaire, the player is working against lady luck and/or the card deck, depending on which view is taken. You cannot have an opposite without opposition, and behaviorism was the opponent for which constructivism eventually came into being. It would be a mistake, however, to write that behaviorism was older than constructivism, as the opposite is actually true, with the idea of constructivism originating in 1896 (see *John Dewey* later in this chapter for additional information).

It is possible that the landscape of education in the US might look very different today had Dewey's approach to education taken hold over Thorndike's. We will never know. What we do know is that "one cannot understand the history of education in the United States during the twentieth century unless one realises [sic] that Edward L. Thorndike won and John Dewey lost" (Ellen Condliffe Lagerman, as cited in Tomlinson 1997, p. 367). Perhaps Thorndike "won" because his concepts were more easily digested by society; perhaps he was simply more persuasive than Dewey. No matter the cause, Thorndike, and thus behaviorism, took the educational reins in the early twentieth century and did not let go until cognitivists poked enough holes in the theory to move it to the bench, to use a well-worn sports analogy. The singularity of the behaviorists' focus and their unwillingness to bend was likely a huge contributor to its sidelining. This focus is clear, too, in the sense that behaviorists worked off the premise that there was a single reality.

However, as thinking about learning expanded, Dewey's ideas gained traction and allowed later theorists to create a more abstract educational theory; one in which multiple, individual realities were recognized as existing. These realities are concurrent and potentially parallel, but because each person experiences and interprets situations differently and uses such experiences and interpretations to construct their own reality, no two people can share the same reality. As a bench science analogy, consider Einstein's theory of relativity: two people viewing the same moment at the exact same time from different angles see two different things. Which of these realities is the True reality? A behaviorist would argue that there is only one reality – the one that exists according to an external "other," which super cedes any individual's experience of the moment; a constructivist would argue that there are 2 realities – or 3 or 100, depending upon the number of viewers (i.e., students) present.

Perhaps the easiest way to think of the differences between behaviorism and constructivism is to view the earlier as a belief that knowledge acquisition is externally focused and the latter as a belief that knowledge acquisition is internally focused. With an external focus, objectivity reigns. With an internal focus, subjectivity reigns. But on a simpler, less philosophical level, constructivists (like cognitivists) believe that learners are active participants in their learning and that such learning both requires and relies upon prior knowledge and experience. Hence, the focus of learning is on making connections for learners between new knowledge and prior knowledge while making it relevant to them.

Where constructivism differs from cognitivism is in the way the processing of new information is believed to occur; with the latter, mental processes are viewed as computers, if you recall. With constructivists, it is not just the taking in and organizing of various bits of information that constitutes learning, it is also reflection upon new information and where it fits within the extant knowledge contained within the mind. Therefore, while cognitivists also believe in the active nature of learning and the importance of prior knowledge (schemas), constructivists extend this idea to include reflection upon the active process of learning to inform the construction of new knowledge within the context of prior knowledge and lived experience, a concept emphasized by Dewey in 1910: ". . . the ground or basis for a belief is deliberately sought and its adequacy to support the belief examined. This process is called reflective thought; it alone is truly educative in value. . ." (p. 1). It is a very fine line between cognitivism and constructivism, which may also be why so many educational theorists are not easily categorized as one or the other.

In summary, constructivism as a theory of learning places the learner, instead of the teacher, at the center of the learning process. Constructivists as a general rule believe that learners play an active role in their own learning because they construct their own knowledge based on previous experiences and/or perceptions. Such construction of knowledge requires reflection and interpretation of their experiences and inputs and includes the impact of the social environment, cultural norms, and the like. Because each learner must construct their own knowledge through acquisition of experience and interpretation of those experiences, the learning process is subjective rather than objective, although the subjective experience of learning is an important part of learning objective approaches to information.

The next section of this chapter will cover a variety of educational theorists who generally fall under the constructivist umbrella. It is hoped that the brief overviews of positivism, behaviorism, cognitivism, and constructivism have provided ample enough background to view each as both discrete and foundational educational theories that all began around the same time but ultimately ended up reaching their heights in a somewhat natural appearing succession. We are currently in the educational age of constructivism, though elements of behaviorism and cognitivism still impact our educational institutions and delivery methods on a regular basis and in ways that we may never shed. Each has contributed significantly to our understanding of how people learn, and with the advent of neuroimaging, we are increasingly learning to appreciate the true genius of many of the theorists who have been introduced to this point and are covered in the remainder of this chapter.

This is not an exhaustive list, of course; there are too many educational theories and theorists to count – some with more reach and influence than others. There are many you may be familiar with that are not listed here (Miller, Ericsson, Bloom, and Knowles, for example); it is not because they are not important, but because those listed here are the foundational theorists who provided the original theories on which those "others" built their ideas. With that, let us dive into the constructivist theorists with whom every student of education should be at least somewhat familiar. They are presented in alphabetical order by last name; this seemed to be the simplest way to introduce each theorist given the already outlined overlaps and emergences within their respective fields. Each is explored quite briefly, as the hope is to introduce you to each of them and provide you with enough information to help you understand their contributions while leaving you potentially wanting more. Also, with each of those included in this textbook, keep in mind that they have all written volumes and had volumes written about them – this is the tiniest scratch on the surface of each. Hopefully, the scratches are deep enough to allow you an appreciation of their work.

Jerome Bruner [1915–2016]
Introduction and Early Work
American-born, specifically New York-born, Jerome Bruner is widely viewed as being the leading figure in helping us understand how children learn and what educators can – and should – aspire to be (Gardner 2001). After completing his psychology training at Duke and Harvard Universities, he published his first paper in 1939 covering a more traditional psychology study for the time, involving thymus extract and its effects on the sexual behavior of female rats (Gardner 2001). Shortly after, he began researching public opinion, propaganda, and social attitudes as a social psychologist during World War II (WWII), after the end of which he began focusing on human perception and cognition (Gardner 2001).

After the war, Bruner's studies continued and ultimately led him to become "increasingly concerned with the development of human cognition" (Gardner 2001, p. 91). As a result, he joined his colleagues to form Harvard's Center of

Cognitive Studies, where they turned their work toward children (Gardner 2001). Leaving the US in 1970 for Oxford University, where he studied infant agency and children's language, he returned to the US around 1980, where he demonstrated increasing concerns centered on social and cultural phenomena, and began rejecting the contemporary turn that cognitivism had taken toward the concrete computational analogy (Gardner 2001; Takaya 2008; Rannikmäe et al. 2020).

It is cognitivism that launched Bruner's brand, however. Just five years after WWII ended, an alignment of the beginning of the cognitive revolution led by Bruner and the launching of Sputnik, convinced the US that more resources needed to be poured into education, with a particular emphasis on science, technology, and mathematics (Gardner 2001) – a movement that has not waned as this book is written; science, technology, engineering, and math, or STEM, is still on the tip of everyone's tongues in the US. In response, the National Academy of Sciences and the National Science Foundation invited a number of high-profile scholars, including scientists, psychologists, and educators, to participate in a meeting to discuss how to move forward; Bruner was named chair of this gathering (Gardner 2001).

It could be argued that Bruner's allegiance to cognitivism began its end with the postconference publication of his book, *The Process of Education*, in which he described the main themes that had emerged from the meeting and which directly influenced educational programs developed at the same time (Gardner 2001; Takaya 2008; Ozdem-Yilmaz and Bilican 2020). One of the most important points was that children should be learning the structures of disciplines rather than the facts and procedures associated with each discipline, which was at the time the current approach to teaching (Gardner 2001; Takaya 2008). Instead, the conference attendees had come to the conclusion that if students understood the basic principles in a subject area, they could then think "generatively about new issues" (Gardner 2001, p. 92). Said differently, Bruner helmed the movement that changed "the understanding of knowledge from *gathering* as the correlation of sensory input and behavioral output to *construction* as an active selection and culturally situated meaning-making of experience" (Bruner 1983, p. 103, as quoted in Ozdem-Yilmaz and Bilican 2020, p. 179; emphasis original). Taking inspiration from Piaget and Inhelder, the conferees further rejected the idea that children were little adults who should be assimilating information and determined that children were actually problem-solvers who had their own ways of making sense of the world (Gardner 2001; Ozdem-Yilmaz and Bilican 2020).

In yet another ground-breaking proposal, and in a break from Piaget on this topic, Bruner and his colleagues concluded that children were capable of learning any topic at any age, this time going explicitly against the four stages of learning that Piaget had so carefully laid out (Ozdem-Yilmaz and Bilican 2020). Thus, they argued that school curricula should be spiraled – the idea being that topics should be introduced in appropriate ways beginning early in the school years, then revisited later with increasing depth and complexity (Gardner 2001; Takaya 2008; Ozdem-Yilmaz and Bilican 2020). For those of you familiar with the term "spiral curriculum," you now understand where it came from and why. Such concepts, however, were a clear break with the cognitivist movement to which Bruner had committed earlier in his career; it is here we see the beginning of his evolution into the constructivist he would be until the end of his storied career and life.

Bruner's book – inspired by the meeting that he chaired with eminent scholars from around the US – was immediately and widely embraced. Translated into 19 languages, it remained one of Harvard University Press's best-selling books for many years (Gardner 2001). Apparently, its impact also impacted Bruner, as he chose to remain involved in educational efforts within the US and in Great Britain during his tenure at Oxford University (Gardner 2001). During his heyday in the late 1960s and early 1970s, Bruner led the "Man: A Course of Study" project, which worked to create a full school curriculum based on the behavioral sciences that were emerging around the same time (Gardner 2001). The effort engaged all manner of individuals – from students to full professors in academic institutions – and produced engaging and educative materials that were circulated widely and made openly available throughout the US and overseas (Gardner 2001).

The headiness of the experiment was bound to end at some point, however, and the rise of poverty, racism, and a highly divisive war in the US drained the education reform movement (Gardner 2001). The National Science Foundation eventually pulled its support from the curriculum, as it sustained attacks from conservative social groups who felt it was too elitist and relativistic, claims that Bruner could not deny when asked: "We never quite solved the problem of getting the materials from Widener (library at Harvard University) to Wichita (largest city in Kansas, the heartland of America)" (Gardner 2001, p. 93).

The Basis for a Move Toward Constructivism

While he burst onto the scene in the 1950s, Bruner became increasingly interested in and aligned with Vygotsky's work in the early 1960s, in particular, his ideas about the role of culture in education (Rannikmäe et al. 2020). Bruner became convinced that culture, which in Bruner's view is a complex and layered environment that is a "toolkit for sense-making and communicating" (Bruner 1996, p. 3, as cited in Takaya 2008, p. 2) was an integral part of shaping the mind. It is this idea of culture, which is a product of society, that appears to have led Bruner to the conclusion that the social environment played a large role in child development. It is through "enculturation," Bruner reasoned, that individuals form complex thinking structures that interact with their environment, resulting in a model of the world being individually constructed through their interactions with people, objects, language, and ideas (Ozdem-Yilmaz and Bilican 2020). It is these interactions that allow learners to create appropriate social frameworks, with such frameworks influencing subsequent acquisition of knowledge (Ozdem-Yilmaz and Bilican 2020).

It is this idea that provides us insights into the "cognitive constructivism" that Bruner would eventually come to espouse as an educational theory; his belief in the influence of social interactions combined with language being integral to learning is fully aligned with the constructivist movement. The building of appropriate social frameworks requires conscious or unconscious reflection upon the experiences contributing to such frameworks. Without such reflections, the theorist must revert to the computational model of learning. Clearly, Bruner was not willing to subscribe to such an approach.

In another nod to Vygotsky, specifically the concept of the ZPD, Bruner felt strongly that adults should help children learn through *scaffolding*, which he describes as "the steps taken to reduce the degrees of freedom in carrying out some task so that the child can concentrate on the difficult skill (which) she is in the process of acquiring" (Bruner 1978, p. 19, as quoted in Ozdem-Yilmaz and Bilican 2020, p. 180). It was through the act of the interaction between the instructor and learner, in other words, that enabled the learner to acquire new knowledge and help them grow intellectually, socially, and culturally.

Although it would not be until the 1990s that Bruner would become openly disenchanted with the cognitive revolution he started (Rannikmäe et al. 2020), it could be argued that the seeds of his evolution were sown well before then. His explorations and adaptations of Vygotsky's work certainly resonate more with the idea of constructivism than with the cognitivism he broached in the 1960s and supported through its heights. It is, perhaps, his social constructivism that enabled him to reconcile his original thoughts on learning with his ideas regarding culture, language, and a complex environment and their importance for learning in children.

Contemporary Impact

Cognitivism, cognitive constructivism, social constructivism, active learning, spiral curriculum, scaffolding, and discovery learning – each of these terms or phrases are connected directly or indirectly with Jerome Bruner. His

work provided, and continues to provide, approaches to learning in the classroom that moved the center of education away from the teacher and toward the learner during the cognitivist revolution and beyond. We see echoes of his influence in K-12 classrooms, undergraduate programs, and, perhaps most relevantly for you, in professional training programs around the world. Inquiry-based learning approaches (case-based, problem-based, and team-based learning) have their roots in social constructivism, as do assessment practices such as objective structured clinical examinations (OSCEs) and direct observation of procedures (DOPs).

Bruner's wide-ranging and deep knowledge of psychology was applied relentlessly to diving into the black box of the mind and its learning processes. His storied career continues to be celebrated by psychologists and educators, linguists, and anthropologists alike. His influence in the educator's classroom simply cannot be denied; so many teaching approaches have been shaped by his work, as has the language of education itself. This section has barely touched on the major points of Bruner's work and influence, but it has laid a solid foundation for you to understand his enormous and mostly positive impacts he has had on education today.

Many references to spiral curriculum and scaffolding in professional programs, including veterinary medicine, are made, often without knowing how they came about or who originated them. While some routinely pair Vygotsky with the ZPD and Piaget with the four stages of learning, fewer seem to be able to trace Bruner's concepts back to him. This is somewhat of a travesty, for as a contemporary thinker (or, at least, more contemporary than most educational theorists enshrined as great thinkers), Bruner remains "the Compleat Educator in the flesh" (Gardner 2001, p. 94). His passion for improving our understanding of learning propelled and spanned two full theoretical movements in education, and his willingness to consider and reconsider his colleagues' and his own ideas about learning were unending. It is this excitement for his work that shined throughout his career and is encapsulated beautifully in *The Process of Education* over 60 years ago: "Intellectual activity is anywhere and everywhere, whether at the frontier of knowledge or in a third-grade classroom" (p. 14, as quoted in Gardner 2001).

John Dewey [1859–1952]
Introduction and Early Work

John Dewey is revered as one of the most influential educational theorists of all time. Born around the middle of the nineteenth century in Burlington, Vermont, United States, he cofounded pragmatism, pioneered functional psychology, theorized extensively on democracy (and how education was an integral part of it), and led the progressive education movement in the US (Williams 2017; Gouinlock 2022).

Dewey's undergraduate work was completed in his home state of Vermont, after which he attended Johns Hopkins University, where he completed his PhD in 1884 and then took a position teaching philosophy and psychology at the University of Michigan (Gouinlock 2022). During his years at Michigan, his interests shifted away from philosophy and toward psychology, which evolved into an interest in child psychology and ultimately led him to develop his philosophy of education that he felt would meet the needs of a changing democratic society (Gouinlock 2022). He moved to the University of Chicago in 1894, where he started his university lab schools after developing his progressive pedagogy (Thayer-Bacon 2012; Gouinlock 2022).

It was during his time in Chicago that he would publish an article in the journal *Psychological Review* in 1896 titled "The reflex arc concept in psychology" (about 20 years prior to Thorndike's well-known publication), in which he proposed an organismic ontology, his attempt at replacing the two dualisms of his time: the mind and body dualism of Descartes and the physical stimulus and response dualism pushed by Thorndike (Tomlinson 1997). In ascribing to the need for a naturalistic psychology while rejecting Thorndike's behaviorist approach, Dewey determined that there was purpose behind human behavior and that such purpose combined with complex physiological circuitry was what resulted in change or, in his view, adaptation (Tomlinson 1997).

In this article, Dewey refutes the concept of the arc, referring instead to the reflex circuit – one that is a coordinated circle, some of whose members have come into conflict with each other. It is the temporary disintegration and need of reconstitution which occasions, or afford the genesis of, the conscious distinction into sensory stimulus on one side and motor response on the other (Dewey 1896, p. 370).

In other words, the reflex arc cannot be viewed in isolation as a curve moving back and forth, thoughtlessly and with no input from the mind; it is not a simple response to an external stimulus. Dewey is arguing that the physical movements and physiological responses are not simply the result of an external stimulus, but that something must mediate that response because occasionally the stimulus leads to a different, potentially unexpected, response – this "disintegration and need of reconstitution" is that which causes those potentially different responses. This insight led to his refutation of the stimulus–response theory of behavior well before it would become known and applied widely as behaviorism.

Evolution of the Theory

While Dewey's lab schools would receive great attention, both contemporaneously and contemporarily, it was after his move to Columbia University in 1904 that the majority of his work was published. He spent most of his academic career at Columbia, retiring in 1930 after publishing around 40 books and 700 articles in well over 100 journals. Many of those books are still considered classics in education, including *How We Think* (1910), *Democracy and Education*, (1916), and *Experience in Education* (1938), published eight years after his retirement. In each, he continues to explore the ideas he first considered in 1896, refining and deepening them, clarifying his thoughts, and increasingly incorporating the concept of education being integral to the development and maintenance of a democratic society.

It was previously stated that perhaps the primary difference between cognitivism and constructivism is that the latter recognizes learner reflection as an integral part of the education process. This is supported by Dewey in his 1910 publication: "Learning, in the proper sense, is not learning things, but the *meanings* of things. . ." (Dewey 1910, p. 212, emphasis original). This statement from *How We Think* indicates Dewey's belief in the importance of reflection in education. Although this statement is made within the context of the importance of language and symbols because it was through language that meanings could be learned, it is a clear nod to the difference between cognitivism and constructivism, though it would not be a necessary distinction until half a century after this was penned.

In another prescient nod to what would evolve into constructivism, Dewey concludes *How We Think* by alluding to his discontent with the traditional classroom of his day.

> nor work, drudgery
>
> Exclusive interest in the result alters work to drudgery. For by drudgery is meant those activities in which the interest in the outcome does not suffuse the means of getting the result. Whenever a piece of work becomes drudgery, the process of doing loses all value for the doer; he cares solely for what is to be had at the end of it. The work itself, the putting forth of energy, is hateful; it is just a necessary evil since without it some important end would be missed. Now it is a commonplace that in the work of the world many things have to be done the doing of which is not intrinsically very interesting. However, the argument that children should be kept doing drudgery tasks because thereby they acquire power to be faithful to distasteful duties, is wholly fallacious. Repulsion, shirking, and evasion are the consequences of having the repulsive imposed – not loyal love of duty (Dewey 1910, pp. 263–264).

In his 1916 book, *Democracy and Education*, Dewey would revisit this idea, reinforcing his views that education should not separate learning from real life: "There is the standing danger that the material of formal instruction will be merely the subject matter of the schools, isolated from the subject matter of life-experience," he writes (p. 459). It is obvious that Dewey believes education is what sews humanity and the social conscience together: the education of children to be good citizens is the only way he sees democracy continuing its success.

The integral role education plays in evolving a democratic society was a recurring theme throughout his life, as was his emphatic argument that schooling should be learner-centered, active, and environmentally appropriate. In *Experience in Education* (1938), for example, he states that teaching children "adult standards, subject matter, and methodologies" was unhelpful (Williams 2017, p. 92). Instead, he argued, learning experiences should be socially engaging and developmentally appropriate, a theme seen in even his earliest work, which pointed out Dewey's early thoughts on the value of making learning enjoyable. He writes at length about the importance of not separating work from play, but finding ways to ensure that work and play are incorporated and equally balanced so that children can learn from work while still enjoying it playfully. The seeds of constructivism were sown, though they would not grow in the tall shadow of Thorndike's widely embraced behaviorism; the world was not quite ready for a more abstract, less authoritarian approach to education in the early twentieth century, it would seem.

These themes were the threads tying Dewey's lifetime of work together, though his ideas strongly contradicted the societally accepted approaches to teaching at the time, which believed that children should be treated as little adults, taught by authoritarian teachers charged with filling the empty vessels that children were viewed as. Instead, Dewey argued, teaching children should be approached holistically, taking into consideration student interests, emphasizing project learning to deliver curricular contents, and providing and experience that nurtured the whole child – from intellect to spirit, from physical to emotional, from social to academic (Williams 2017).

But how did Dewey come to these conclusions? He noted – through careful observations – that children seemed to be influenced by other children and the adults with whom they interacted and that the physical environment had some effect on learning as well. As he worked to reconcile his observations of children and their learning with his fervent belief that education was the only way to promote and preserve democracy – defined as a way of life rather than a political ideology – he proposed that schools should be places where children were taught the skills and knowledge to become good, democratic citizens (Williams 2017; Tomlinson 1997; Dewey 1916). "Beings who are born not only unaware of, but quite indifferent to, the aims and habits of the social group have to be rendered cognizant of them and actively interested.

Education, and education alone, spans the gap," he wrote (Dewey 1916, p. 366).

To Dewey, this also meant that teachers should be allowed some freedom in the way they approached their students – no more lockstep delivery of isolated content within a specific curriculum – but rather the flexibility to address the perceived needs and deficiencies of the students as they arose. Curricula, then, needed to be more of an outline of what needed to be covered, with the Roman numerals identified and the capital letters strongly suggested, but the lowercase letters left up to the individual teachers. It would be this radical-for-the-time approach to education that would eventually upend radical behaviorism as the dominant learning theory in the US.

Contemporary Impact

The seeds of constructivism were sown in 1896 with Dewey's ground-breaking publication, which thoughtfully and carefully refuted the idea that learning could be broken into separate entities of stimulus and response. He would continue to evolve the ideas first laid out in 1896 through a career filled with prodigious publications and deep thoughts about psychology, education, and democracy. Although his theory fell on deaf ears for many decades, stunted in their growth and spread as they lay in the shadow of society's ecstatic embrace of Thorndike's behaviorism, they would eventually find their sun, emerge, grow, and be fruitful. Though his ideas are compacted in this very brief summary of his work, the impact his ideas had on education cannot be overstated; not only did he provide a theory consistent with his scientific approach to psychology and education, applied and refined through his lab schools and the opportunities afforded him to conduce educational experiments (Tomlinson 1997), he also provided reasons that theory was important to education some support for the idea that theory is important for both practicing and improving education.

Because Dewey believed that knowledge, no matter its scope or content, was merely an instrument for the control of experience, he also firmly believed that *"theory must be understood as a form of practice"* (Tomlinson 1997, p. 379, emphasis original) and thus, as Tomlinson goes on to point out, "rather than reducing teachers to instruments of theory, Dewey. . . demonstrated that we must learn to see theory as an instrument which teachers can use to improve their understanding of the educational process" (p. 380). Theory, Dewey argued, should be *used*, not just discussed for the sake of discussion. And educational theory should not be created by academics or content matter experts in Dewey's mind; it should be created by teachers because, he argued, teachers should be revered as they are the shoulders upon which rest the very soul of democracy. His consistent and persistent theorizing made a huge impact on educational reform in the US and around the world and continues to influence our educational processes.

For those who follow the waxing and waning of educational theory popularity, you may be aware that Dewey's theory still comes into question (as do all theories, in point of fact). But he has weathered the storms. His ideas have transcended centuries, and will likely continue to do so well into the future.

Maria Montessori [1870–1952]
Early Years and Career Highlights

Maria Montessori was born in Italy in 1870; she would go on to become the first Italian woman to graduate from the University of Rome's medical school and establish an approach to schooling children that is still popular today and carries her name. The Montessori method originated from her interest in children with intellectual disabilities, whom she studied during her volunteer time as assistant physician at her alma mater in the psychiatric clinic; she was not paid as she was not allowed to be paid due to her gender (Thayer-Bacon 2012; Tikkanen 2022a). As part of her duties, she was required to select suitable subjects for the clinic by visiting Rome's asylums for the insane; it was these visits that triggered her interest in the children housed there, who were living with adults in conditions that barely kept them alive (Montessori 1912; Thayer-Bacon 2012). During her ministrations with these "idiot children," based on the interest in children's health she developed during medical school, she began to suspect their perceived mental disabilities might be a problem of teaching rather than one of medicine (Montessori 1912).

From 1897 to 1900, Montessori worked to determine whether other physicians had attempted to educate "feebleminded children," discovering published work by French physician Edouard Seguin, who had written about his and his teacher's, Jean-March-Gaspard Itard, efforts to educate deaf children (Thayer-Bacon 2012). It was through her discovery of Itard's work via Seguin, who were proponents of pedagogy joined with medicine to cure various children's diseases, that she determined "mental deficiency presented chiefly a pedagogical, rather than mainly a medical, problem" (Montessori 1912, p. 31).

During this same time, she was actively studying the children with whom she was working, and while she was a scientist – not an educator and/or philosopher – she felt strongly that "man's cosmic task [was] to continue, collectively, the work of creation on earth, to discover with his intelligence the endless latent possibilities of the world's creations and make them manifest in new forms" (Montessori Jr. 1976, p. 4). This conviction was the basis of her approach to studying children: she felt they were

worthy human beings who deserved to be treated and considered as such. Her training as a physician was science-based, but her beliefs about humanity were based on her strong faith.

Thus, through direct, careful, thorough, and systematic observations, Montessori was able to extract the "basic phenomena relevant to human development" and integrate these phenomena into a vision of humanity that accounted for the complexity of our existence on earth (Montessori Jr. 1976, p. 5). In combination with the techniques published by Seguin, she began formulating her own ideas about how to educate children deemed to have significant intellectual disabilities. By 1900 she was appointed codirector of the State Orthophrenic School of Rome and was allowed to remove the children from the asylum to an empty Roman hospital ward (Thayer-Bacon 2012, Tikkanen 2022a).

In the empty hospital without adult psychiatric patients surrounding them, Montessori was able to teach the children with her unique approach and created educational methods, which consisted of "attractive, self-correcting, and sequential" materials that isolated basic concepts for ease of understanding; she also created multisensory opportunities to learn through materials that incorporated test, touch, sight, and smell (Montessori 1912; Thayer-Bacon 2012, p. 6). Simultaneously, as any good scientist does, she studied her students and continued creating materials based on her findings. Her educational approach worked remarkably well, as several of the children in her program passed state examinations with above-average scores; Montessori's fame was born (Burnett 1962; Thayer-Bacon 2012; Tikkanen 2022a).

With such resounding success in her pocket, Montessori, who felt she had earned her first and "true degree in pedagogy" (1912, p. 33), felt from the beginning that the methods she used to teach her children with disabilities "contained educational principles *more rational* than those in use. . . . . .and. . .I became convinced that similar methods applied to normal children would develop or set free their personality in a marvelous and surprising way" (Montessori 1912, pp. 32–33, emphasis original). This feeling, "so deep as to be in the nature of an intuition" (Montessori 1912, p.32), led her to resign from her directorship with the orthophrenic school and return to school herself, diving deeply into understanding the mind of normal children through the study of philosophy (Montessori 1912; Thayer-Bacon 2012).

Having read Seguin's book in French during her time at the psychiatric clinic, Montessori was unable to find the English book that had been published in New York two decades later (Montessori 1912). Fortunately, she would acquire a copy of his book during her graduate studies in philosophy, and her intuition appeared to have some support: Seguin clearly believed his methods for teaching children with disabilities would also work for normal children (Montessori 1912). It would also be during her tenure as a graduate student that she would study "Pedagogic Anthropology" in elementary schools to better understand the methods used to teach normal children; it was this work that led to her appointment as a teaching professor in Pedagogic Anthropology at the University of Rome (Montessori 1912); she would teach there for about five years.

Her next role, and the one that sealed her educational legacy, would come as a result of an article she had written for a magazine discussing her work with the children she had taken from the asylum (Thayer-Bacon 2012). She was approached by an individual involved with building a housing project for low-income families in one of Rome's slum districts, where children roamed during the day while their parents were at work (Thayer-Bacon 2012). It was determined by the group that the 60 children residing in their new housing project needed someone to supervise them, and Montessori was offered the job; in spite of universal disapproval from her friends and medical colleagues, she accepted the position, which she viewed as the perfect opportunity to test her educational approach on normal children (Thayer-Bacon 2012).

At the *Casa dei Bambini* ("Children's House," so named by her friend Signora Olga Lodi), which catered to children aged three to six years, Montessori set out to determine whether her methods would be effective for normal children who were young enough that most thought they were uneducable. The children spent the entire day in the school, where they were fed lunch and provided a multitude of opportunities to interact with different materials under the supervision of a hired "directress," a woman intentionally selected by Montessori as someone with no educational training, as she wished the person to have no preconceived notions of what a teacher should be doing (Thayer-Bacon 2012). The woman was charged with observing the children, noting their interests, describing their behaviors, and providing feedback about how they functioned within the environment (Thayer-Bacon 2012).

Montessori filled the room with child-sized furniture, provided the materials she had developed for the children who had been placed in the asylums, and placed donated toys into the room, learning quickly that the children gravitated toward her educational materials over the toys, much to the surprise of the adults (Thayer-Bacon 2012). Through it all, Montessori continued designing and testing academic materials, discovering that preschool-aged children desire to and will learn on their own if provided an environment conducive to doing so (Thayer-Bacon 2012).

Educational Theory from a Different Angle

Montessori's approach to educating children was born of a combination of her faith, her commitment to "contribute to a comprehensive science of man," and her medical training (Montessori Jr. 1976, p. 5). She drew upon a variety of disciplines throughout her life as she refined her pedagogy, including medicine, anthropology, psychology, and "pedagogical hygiene" (Montessori 1912, p. 5). She also knew her methods and approach worked; she had tangible evidence in the form of state test scores from children – both mentally challenged and normal – that proved it.

Essentially, Montessori believed – and demonstrated – that children placed in appropriately prepared environments and watched over by an adult who was placed to observe and monitor rather than teach and direct would "discover what they need for their own development at an appropriate time by themselves and absorb it into their mind and body" (Tsubaki and Matsuishi 2008, p. 1; Burnett 1962). The fundamental concept upon which Montessori built her observations of children that grew into a specific educational method was "*the liberty of the pupils in their spontaneous manifestations*" (Montessori 1912, p. 81, emphasis original). Thus, unlike many theorists, who viewed the role of teacher as essential to learning (regardless of their views of teachers as experts or facilitators), Montessori believed that adult interference disrupted learning and child development, thus her emphasis on a patient adult who provided objects for children to focus on, as well as the time, place, and autonomy to do so for themselves (Tsubaki and Matsuishi 2008). This does not mean that adults should not help, it merely means that help should not be provided unless it is requested by the child.

Liberty and spontaneous manifestations did not mean, however, chaos and disorder. On the contrary, Montessori created and maintained in her school system an order that was child-sized, getting rid of desks, designing and having manufactured child-sized furniture, and individual cupboards that contained a variety of teaching materials that students could access at any time for any reason throughout the day (Montessori 1912; Burnett 1962; Tsubaki and Matsuishi 2008). She also hung blackboards at child height and installed carefully selected pictures that represented "simple scenes in which children would naturally be interested" (Montessori 1912, p. 83). This organized, well-stocked, and child-sized environment would become one of the hallmarks of the Montessori method.

In Montessori's mind, the liberty of the child was equivalent to activity (1912). Her views on traditional teaching opposed their view of discipline, stating "We do not consider an individual discipline only when he has been rendered as artificially silent as a mute and as immovable as a paralytic. He is an individual *annihilated*, not *disciplined*" (Montessori 1912, p. 86, emphasis original). Such a prescient observation from a woman over 100 years ago, who clearly believed that corporal punishment or severe consequences intended to curb poor behavior resulted in curbing the student as a learner altogether. Such views, combined with her emphasis on the necessity of activity for children to learn, place her firmly in the constructivist camp and openly opposes behaviorism. For those who might have doubts, you must only open her first book to page 101, where she boldly states that there must be an "ABOLITION OF PRIZES AND EXTERNAL FORMS OF PUNISHMENT" (Montessori 1912, emphasis original). This behaviorist form of discipline contrasted steeply with her definition of discipline, which consisted of the idea that a disciplined child could "master of himself . . . [and] therefore, regulate his own conduct when it shall be necessary to follow some rule of life" (Montessori 1912, p. 87). This concept of self-regulation mirrors that of Piaget, in his discussions of equilibration (covered in an upcoming section).

Montessori's final principle of education was that children must be guided to independence through learning. It was through this last principle that some flashes of her feminism would appear; she spent much of her life working to bring women to the fore, within the confines of her society and times when she was unable to safely stretch them. In the section of her first book discussing the value of teaching independence, however, she pulls no punches.

The grand gentleman who has too many servants not only grows constantly more and more dependent upon them, until he is, finally, actually their slave, but his muscles grow weak through inactivity and finally lose their natural capacity for action. The mind of one who does not work for that which he needs, but commands it from others, grows heavy and sluggish. If such a man should some day awaken to the fact of his inferior position and should wish to regain once more his own independence, he would find that he had no longer the force to do so (p. 99).

She follows this with further explanation of her desire to educate children for independence by stating:

. . . [women] are taught as a part of their education the art of *not moving*. Such an attitude toward woman leads to the fact that man works not only for himself, but for woman. And the woman wastes her natural strength and activity and languishes in slavery. She is not only maintained and served, she is, besides, diminished, belittled, in that individuality which is hers by right of her existence as a human being (Montessori 1912, p. 100).

In concluding her plea to educate for independence, she connects the perils of dependence to helplessness and, ultimately, a degeneration of the normal man, punctuated by her analogy of the dominating man who is, in spirit and behavior, a "task-master toward the slave" and thus, she intones, "We must make of the future generation, *powerful men*, and by that we mean men who are independent and free" (Montessori 1912, p. 101, emphasis original).

These three principles – an orderly and appropriate environment; gently guided activity; and education for independence – form the backbone of Montessori's educational theory, although had you asked her, she would likely have scoffed at the idea that she would be viewed as a theorist. Coming to her views from the trained physician's and anthropologist's views, she was both similar to and different from other theorists discussed in this chapter. It is clear that she was committed to observing, creating, and implementing interventions, assessing those interventions, and determining how to improve them – all hallmarks of a deductively driven scientist and more similar to behaviorists and cognitivists methodologically than to constructivists. But her ultimate goals were different: she wanted to and felt this could not be based on any single discipline; it should be an orderly amalgamation and integration of the findings from scientists in varying disciplines who were studying human beings. And, most importantly, it was centered on the active engagement of a liberated child whose ultimate goal was to gain independence.

Certainly, other educational theorists covered here drew from their understanding of other disciplines, but none of them were so blatant in their willingness to accept the value of interdisciplinary studies of humans to their theories. The vast majority of educational theorists emerged from psychology, a discipline that spent many decades trying to establish itself as a science at all, though it was psychiatry, in an ironic twist, that would ultimately be responsible for the emergence of the Montessori method. And while many of these theorists also grounded their theories in observations, they were focused on elucidating the processes of the mind and its relationship to learning and child development. Montessori wanted action, not musing about processes.

It bears noting that Montessori had a series of unique challenges and opportunities available to her. Being a woman in the late nineteenth and early twentieth centuries, her career choices were limited by society, though she chose to ignore many of them the moment she entered medical school and subsequently earned her medical doctor degree. This did not stop her, however. She took posts that were likely not very palatable to her male counterparts, and from it, she discovered that all children can be taught. In approaching children and their learning the way she approached medicine, Montessori "discovered the world within the child" (Thayer-Bacon 2012, p. 7). Perhaps Montessori's inclusion within a section covering educational theorists is misplaced; rather than being viewed as theorist, it is potentially more accurate to refer to her as a "pedagogical thinker" in terms of her real contributions to education. However, her ideas about teaching, although she never formally referred to them as educational theory, most certainly were.

Contemporary Impact

Potentially one of the most recognizable names in children's education, Montessori is rarely as lauded as her male counterparts of the time. Perhaps this is, as Thayer-Bacon (2012) argues, primarily due to her gender, which prohibited her from achieving the same academic and social roles that men were able to reach. Or, perhaps, it is because "She was not a theoretician. She did not construct a differentiated theoretical framework that paved the way for later applications of her work. On the contrary; in her struggle to give expression to phenomena that did not fit any existing theories, she often borrowed terms from them, dissociating them from their frame of reference and using them in her own context" (Montessori Jr. 1976, p. 4).

Regardless of scholarly labels and opinions, Montessori's impact on education over 100 years later has proven staying power. Within two years of the opening of her first *Case dei Bambino* in1907, several more "Children's Houses" were opened, and in 1909, Italian Switzerland "began to transform its orphan asylums and children's homes. . . into 'Children's Houses,' adopting our methods and materials" (Montessori 1912, p. 44). In 1908, her successes had taken off worldwide, and she resigned from her position at the University to pursue teaching full time (Thayer-Bacon 2012). From there, she cemented her legacy through training teachers, writing (her first book, *The Montessori Method*, extensively quoted and cited in this section, was translated into over 10 languages within three years), and opening low-income children's schools in Italy. Eventually her work would lead to the establishment of over 3000 Montessori schools spanning more than 80 countries, including the US (Thayer-Bacon 2012; Tikkanen 2022a; Montessori Jr. 1976).

Jean Piaget [1896–1980]

Early Years and Career Highlights

Born in Switzerland, in 1896, Jean Piaget was a psychologist who focused on children and was committed to the value of educating them. His father was a professor and his mother, though intelligent, was apparently somewhat neurotic (Boeree 1997). A prolific observer and writer from a young age, he was fascinated by nature and had published numerous papers about mollusks by the time he was 15, garnering much attention from European zoologists (Duignan 2022). At 24, he earned his PhD in biology, but soon after he became interested in psychology, went to Zurich to study under Carl Jung and Eugen Bleuler, then moved on to Paris where he studied and taught at the Sorbonne (Duignan 2022).

While in Paris, Piaget became interested in the types of errors children made on the reading tests he had devised, and this led him to explore their reasoning processes (Duignan 2022). Just two years after he started his work with children, he began publishing his results – that would be the basis of his first five books on child psychology – and simultaneously moved back to Switzerland, where he began his appointment as director of the Jacques Rousseau Institute (Boeree 1997; Duignan 2022).

In 1923, he married Valentine Chatenay, with whom he would have three children and would spend many hours intensely observing them; their research would produce three additional books on the topic of child psychology (Boeree 1997). By 1925, he had begun his academic career as a professor at his alma mater; four years later he joined the University of Geneva as a professor of child psychology and became the director of the International Bureau of Education, a position he held until 1967. During his work with the International Bureau of Education, he conducted large research projects in collaboration with several colleagues, though his primary partner would be Barbel Inhelder, demonstrating his willingness to embrace the work of women in experimental psychology – an anomaly for the times (Boeree 1997).

Piaget's career was marked with achievements and honors, none of which appeared to affect his dedication to his work. By the end of his storied career, he had published over 50 books and contributed to hundreds of articles; given speeches all over the world, and seen his work impact the educational approaches of teachers in numerous countries. His major area of research was always focused on child development, in particular the development of thinking (Boeree 1997). At the time, little had been done in this area (if you recall, behaviorism was the learning theory of the times and it paid no attention to the thinking processes that Piaget was so keen to discover), and thus he labeled his new topic of inquiry *genetic epistemology*, or the study of knowledge development (Boeree 1997; Duignan 2022).

Five years after publishing *Introduction to Genetic Epistemology*, in 1955 Piaget established and became Director of the International Centre of Genetic Epistemology in Geneva (Duignan 2022). It was this work that would resonate most deeply with the world and is, among all his work, the best-known of his theories. This evolution of his work from his early days in Paris would come to full bloom in his theory on the stages of the child's mental development, which he believed started at birth and evolved through a linear set of stages through adulthood.

Observations of Child Development

In 1955, Piaget published a book titled *The Construction of Reality in the Child*, in which he states that children evolve from believing they are the center of a universe they control to understanding that they are simply a piece of a world that does not depend upon them to exist or function. This evolution, he claimed, can only be explained by the development of intelligence (Piaget 1955). Although he contextualizes this evolution only within the confines of sensorimotor intelligence, he would clearly go on to further develop a robust theory of learning based on this work.

Piaget's conclusions about child development were reached through talking with children – his own children and others (Duignan 2022). During these conversations, he asked them "ingenious and revealing questions about simple problems he had devised, and then he formed a picture of their way of viewing the world by analyzing their mistaken responses" (Duignan 2022, n.p.). Through such conversations with and observations of thousands of children, Piaget created a learning theory that provided psychologists and educators alike a more accurate picture of how children developed and learned. In addition to creating an entirely new field of study in the form of genetic epistemology, he also introduced new vocabulary and concepts. It was Piaget who first used the term "schema" in relation to learning, and the evolution of the schema concept being akin to a computer processor was more prescient than even he could have known: current evidence supports the primary principles of the importance of educators organizing and chunking information in this way through neuroscientific studies (Knowland and Thomas 2014; Merriam 2008; Cozolino and Sprokay 2006; Jensen and McConchie 2020).

The basis for all of Piaget's work, however, is rooted firmly in his epistemology. While there is a plethora of information out there outlining the four stages of child development, there is less written about his epistemological stance and how it preceded his ultimate theory of learning. Smith (2001), states this boldly: "Piaget's account of education is dependent on his epistemology. The link between them is knowledge and development as normative facts" (p. 38). What does this mean? It means that because knowledge develops within the context of norms, such knowledge becomes normative facts (Smith 2001) – or facts that establish information upon which further knowledge can be built. Thus, empirical investigations into normative facts can be accomplished through identifying associated *acts of judgment*, with *acts* being due to

psychosocial causes and *judgments* being made due to normative, meaningful implications (Smith 2001).

Additionally, according to Piaget (1964), development and learning were distinct but intimately intertwined issues. Development of knowledge is a spontaneous process tied to the development of the body, nervous system, and mind that ended only in adulthood. Learning, however, was a provoked act – whether by an experiment, a teacher, or some other external situation. It was also a process that was limited, whether to a single problem or a single structure (Piaget 1964). From this separation of development and learning, he concluded that "development explains learning" (p. 176), which went against the behaviorist's view that development was the sum of a series of specific learned items. In other words, Piaget believed that learning was a function of development, not an output that explained it.

> Knowledge is not a copy of reality. To know an object, to know an event, is not simply to look at it and make a mental copy or image of it. To know an object is to act on it. To know is to modify, to transform the object, and to understand the process of this transformation, and as a consequence to understand the way the object is constructed. An operation is thus the essence of knowledge; it is an interiorized action which modifies the object of knowledge (Piaget 1964, p. 171).

To interpret and paraphrase, Piaget is making his case that there is a difference between knowing and learning. To him, the former is to merely register an object (piece of information, element of content), whereas the latter is to register the object and somehow *act* upon it – transform it and use it in a way that both provides insights into how said object (piece of information or thought) was constructed (through the social norming of predecessors) and expands it as an object for others to repeat the process.

The next layer of knowledge (and learning) was the *operation*, which he described as "the essence of knowledge; it is an interiorized action which modifies the object of knowledge" (Piaget 1964, p. 176), or a set of actions that modify and object that allows the learner to "get at the structures of the transformation" (p. 177). Additionally, these operations are always linked together, which means they are each pieces of an overall structure; it is these operational structures, in Piaget's mind, that constitute the basis of knowledge. Thus, the central problem, as he saw it, was to determine how such structures were formed, elaborated upon, organized, and functioned. In attempting to answer these questions, he felt he could empirically identify those *acts of judgment* previously discussed.

It is this idea of the operation, as defined and viewed by him, that undergirded Piaget's theory of the four sequential stages of learning; what he referred to as his stages of the development of the structures that were built from these individual operations. Essentially, Piaget and Inhelder (1969), theorized in *The Psychology of the Child* that "the mental development of a child appears as a succession of three great periods" (location 1286). Each period, they believed, "extends the preceding period, reconstructs it on a new level, and later surpasses it to an even greater degree" (Piaget and Inhelder 1969, location 1286). In other words, there are three distinct periods of mental development in children, each overlapping its predecessor. This overlap provided the genesis for the next level of development, which was then outgrown and moved to the next level. It may be easiest to think of this as three consecutive circles with the edges of the second circle overlapping the edges of both the first and third circles, for those struggling to visualize the concept.

Although Piaget and Inhelder muddied the waters slightly in their 1969 book by referring to only "three great periods" of child development, Piaget's earlier works adhered to a four-stage model of child development (Piaget and Inhelder 1969; Kagan 2000; Piaget 1962; Piaget 1964). In the four-stage model, a stage was added to cover the learning (building of structures) between the toddler and early elementary ages (Piaget 1962, 1964). It is the four-stage model of child development that endures today and is described below, as paraphrased from Piaget's 1964 paper published in the *Journal of Research in Science Teaching*.

Stage 1: the preverbal stage, also referred to as the sensory-motor stage (it would later evolve into the sensorimotor stage), lasted about 18 months. This is when practical knowledge was developed, laying the "substructure of later representational knowledge" (p. 177). Some examples of infants building these substructures include the acquisition of object permanence (knowing something continues to exist even when it cannot be seen); temporal succession (if I cry, then something happens); and elementary sensory-motor causality (when I suck my thumb, I feel better).

Stage 2: the preoperational stage, where language begins to emerge, as well as an understanding of symbolic function, spanned the ages of about two to seven years. In this stage, "there must now be a reconstruction of all that was developed on the sensory-motor level" (p. 177). The child has entered an entirely new phase and must build new operations that incorporate those acquired during the first stage of development. The example provided is that of a child who sees an adult pour liquid from one glass to another that is of a different shape and believes there is now more water in one than was in the other. This lack of understanding of the concept of conservation – or the ability to understand that things can be the same even if they look different – is the hallmark of this stage.

Stage 3: the concrete operations stage is where children are now operating on objects but not yet verbalizing their own ideas about the world. Such operations might include "operations of classification, ordering, the construction of the idea of number, spatial and temporal operations, and all the fundamental operations of elementary logic of classes and relations, of elementary mathematics, and even of elementary physics" (p. 177). In other words, children in this stage can follow preexisting structures, or schemas, but are still unable to create their own. Children in this stage have also acquired the concept of conservation that eluded them in stage 2 and they understand the concept of reversibility or the idea that items can change shapes or states and *be returned* to their original states or shapes.

Stage 4: the hypothetic-deductive operations (later referred to as the formal operational stage) is where the child can "reason on hypotheses, and not only on objects. He constructs new operations, operations of propositional logic, and not simply the operations of classes, relations, and numbers. He attains new structures which are on the one hand combinatorial . . . on the other hand more complicated group structures" (pp. 177–178). Here, children can think abstractly – beyond current time, place, and people. They can create and consider hypothetical situations, generate and test hypotheses, and approach new problems in a logical, systematic way.

Piaget was fond of sequencing and chunking; he uses four factors to explain the progression of children from one stage to the next. Maturation, experience, social transmission, and equilibration – also known as self-regulation – are inherent to the developmental and learning processes. While each is important, he emphasizes equilibration as the most fundamental factor in development:

> Equilibrium, defined by active compensation, leads to reversibility. Operational reversibility is a model of an equilibrated system where a transformation in one direction is compensated by a transformation in the other. Equilibration, as I understand it, is thus an active process. It is the process of self-regulation. I think that this self-regulation is a fundamental factor in development. . . This process of equilibration takes the form of a succession of levels of equilibrium, of levels. . .I call sequential probability, that is, the probabilities are not established *a priori*. There

is a sequence of levels. It is not possible to reach the second level unless equilibrium has been reached at the first level . . . (Piaget 1964, p. 181).

It is here you can see that Piaget firmly believed learning and development were ordered and sequential; this has often been mistaken as him believing that his stages occurred at set ages. It is clear, however, that this is not the case, as he states quite plainly that "although the order of succession is constant, the chronological ages of these stages varies a great deal" (Piaget 1964, p. 178). And it is equilibration, according to Smith (2001), that made its biggest mark on education through two principles: (i) creativity is important because each individual with an active mind has the potential to advance and (ii) teaching can be effective, as long as learning tasks are creatively designed and intended to trigger the transformation required for novel learning (Smith 2001).

Contemporary Impact

Although Piaget started his work in the early twentieth century, it did not take hold in the US until the mid-1960s, when his ideas were "made comprehensible" by John Flavell (Kagan 2000). The esoteric and somewhat wandering nature of his writing is easy to get lost in, and at least for this author, required multiple readings to get at what seemed to be a reasonable understanding of his ideas. Thus, Kagan's (2000) observation feels astute. Those who have studied Piaget extensively, however, have been able to continually clarify his works, a very small portion of which has been presented here.

A contemporary of Vygotsky, the two are closely linked both temporally and intellectually. It would be an interesting exercise in thinking to consider how Vygotsky's views might or might not have evolved in a manner similar to Piaget had he not died so tragically young and made it through the communist Russian revolution in the early twentieth century. Why? Because their ideas were similar enough during their parallel time on earth to wonder if they might have eventually converged. They were different enough, however, that perhaps they would have diverged instead.

That musing aside, it is clear that both Piaget's work – primarily the four stages of learning (which has been criticized by many but still endures) – and Vygotsky's ZPD (discussed later in the chapter) are still quite popular today. It is also clear that much of the work behind Piaget's four stages of learning has been lost in the grand appreciation shown for what has become a staple of US educators. Our K-12 curricula have been created and delivered based on Piaget's stages, and children's books and toys are guided by them as well. He laid the groundwork, along with Vygotsky,

for constructivism as a movement (in spite of his beginning work that seems more aligned with cognitivism).

We see his influence in the work of Bruner, who did ultimately have some divergences of thought from Piaget but certainly saw value in his ideas of schemas and the foundation he laid for the idea of scaffolding (remember Piaget's comments that one could not achieve the next stage of development without first achieving the benchmarks of the stage immediately preceding it?). And if one watches children for any period of time, it is clear that Piaget's work, while startling at the time, is as accurate now as it was then. Perhaps he did not fully explain the process of learning and development, but he certainly injected innovative-at-the-time ideas that continue to impact education as a whole.

In a laudatory article written by John H. Flavell (1996), himself a developmental psychologist (and the one, if you recall, credited with making Piaget's work accessible in the US!), Piaget's many positive impacts are outlined, including changing the questions asked about child development, the idea that children are not empty vessels to be passively filled, and that "children's cognitive behavior is intrinsically rather than extrinsically motivated" (Flavell 1996, p. 200). Additionally, Smith (2001) makes it clear that Piaget impacted classrooms everywhere with his concept of equilibration and its importance in development. To adequately summarize Piaget's impact during his life and beyond is a task not intended to be completed here; there are books upon books and articles upon articles written by and about Jean Piaget that you could peruse to find an array of educational implications for K-12 through undergraduate, graduate, and professional classrooms. The writings are far too numerous to adequately incorporate into a single chapter in a small textbook. For now, let it be sufficient to say that Piaget is generally acknowledged as a significant force within the fields of psychology and education. His legacy endures today and is well ingrained enough into the institution of education that his impacts will continue to influence the practices of educators around the world. In short, though he is not the only titan of educational theory, he is certainly one you cannot ignore if you wish to be considered an informed educator.

Lev Vygotsky [1896–1934]

Katherine Fogelberg and Kimberly S. Cook

Introduction

Lev Vygotsky was a Russian psychologist who is another highly impactful educational theorist, primarily through his sociocultural theory of human learning. His views on human development were that children learn their cultural values, beliefs, and problem-solving strategies through collaborative interactions with those in society who have more knowledge. In contrast to Dewey, who theorized that learning came after development, Vygotsky argued the opposite – that learning was a prerequisite to development. If you have heard of Vygotsky previously, it was likely in reference to his zone of proximal development, or ZPD, which states that there is a zone between the points where students can gain mastery through independent work and where the students need help to gain such mastery – it is this zone that must be recognized and managed for students to reach their learning potential. If left on their own, students will not obtain mastery, but if provided support from a learned other, they can move out of the zone and into a new ZPD that is more advanced than the one they just left. There are echoes of Piaget in this work, and it is with Piaget that Vygotsky is most often paired theoretically when studied.

Vygotsky was a key figure in moving us away from radical behaviorism into cognitivism and constructivism, also paralleling Piaget. However, his ideas still have their roots, at least, in social behaviorism, even if his ultimate teaching approaches were firmly planted in constructivism (DeVries 2000). And, because his work was originally written in Russian, it was not until the early 1960s through an American translation of his *Language and Thought*, prefaced by Jerome Bruner, that his influence truly came into being (Bernicot 1994). Incidentally, Bruner was heavily influenced by Vygotsky, as you may have come to realize in reading about Bruner's SCT earlier in this chapter.

Context and Culture

Lev Vygotsky was born in then Russia, now present-day Belarus, in 1896 to an educated, middle-class, Jewish family who spoke multiple languages (Smidt 2009). Vygotsky's mother was a trained teacher, though her role as a mother kept her from the classroom. She focused on her children's education as the family shared a love of arts and letters fostered by regular family dialogue around things of the mind (Van der Veer 2007). Despite anti-Semitic policies limiting the numbers of matriculating Jewish students, talented Vygotsky pursued higher education in Moscow, considering first medical school, then law school. Ultimately, he settled into a study of arts and letters that kindled his lifelong interest in psychology, majoring in history and philosophy (Ardichvili 2001). He graduated from university as World War I was concluding, and just prior to the Bolshevik Revolution, which completely changed the dynamics of society in Russia and ushered in Marxism and communism – each of which had elements that he had a complicated relationship with, but can be seen in his work (Van der Veer 2007). At a minimum, "Vygotsky at least initially combined an active interest in Marxist theory with a belief in the new Soviet society. Whether and to what extent he

became disillusioned by the events to come remains unknown" (Van der Veer 2007, p. 19).

Vygotsky began his career as a teacher and found connection with like-minded educators to begin researching. He worked with children who were mentally and physically disabled and was invited to Europe to present and study systems of education for students with special needs. In 1924, after delivering a presentation discussing the methodology of psychological studies, he was invited to the Moscow Institute of Psychology to be a research fellow; in 1925, he defended his doctoral thesis, in which he argued that psychology could not limit itself to direct evidence (Ardichvili 2001). One of his most notable developments was including the perspectives of the children with whom he worked in his research (Smidt 2009). In the final decade of his life, he was very active in publishing, teaching, and clinical and governmental work. Unfortunately, also during that final decade, he was gravely ill with tuberculosis, having multiple bouts that constrained his activities, though he remained prolific. He died at age 37 from a fatal bout of tuberculosis.

Vygotsky and the Soviet Union

Being a theorist and a psychologist is sure to be rife with many political considerations. However, being a middle-class, Jewish psychologist in the totalitarian-ruled Soviet Union of the 1920s and 1930s put Vygotsky at odds with Stalin's government in multiple aspects. He had established relationships with a number of individuals that were eventually considered enemies of the state, including Leon Trotsky.

Additionally, as the new lines were being drawn in postrevolution Russia concurrently with the foundations of the field of psychology, the only certainty was that one's work should not run the risk of being labeled anti-Marxist. Those in authority, including university leaders and friendly colleagues active in the governing party, required a Marxist psychology, though what that exactly meant was up for interpretation (Ardichvili 2001). "It took great courage and moral resolve to withstand all this social pressure and to stick to the position that one believed was the scientifically right one and it will come as no surprise that very few people were capable of that" (Van der Veer 2007, p. 23). However, during his career, Vygotsky remained focused on his research, as independent of the political pressures as possible. Though sad, it is highly likely that his early death from tuberculosis prevented later arrest, or even worse, at the hands of the ruling party (Ardichvili 2001).

Sociocultural Theory of Cognitive Development

According to Ardichvili (2001), Vygotsky's appeal in the West is likely due to his encyclopedic knowledge of psychology as a discipline; he had a profound understanding of his immediate research area as well as diverse areas in the field, including the "psychology of art, literary theory, neurology, defectology and psychiatry" (p. 35), which provided him an interdisciplinary slant that appealed to scientists from variety fields. Secondly, and perhaps more pertinent to this text, is his theory that mental functioning in individuals can only be understood by examining the social-cultural processes from which it originates (Ardichvili 2001), which resonates with contemporary social scientists and is the basis of his sociocultural theory of cognitive development.

Vygotsky's sociocultural theory of development, which he originally labeled a cultural-historical theory, viewed the mind, cognition, and memory as functions that could be carried both between others and within an individual (intermental and intramental), and posited that an individual's life activity was determined by the "historical development of culture" (Ardichvili 2001, p. 35). Accordingly, he believed that children learned and developed in large part because of their interactions with others, including adults and other children (Ardichvili 2001; Costley 2012).

Language and Cognitive Development

While studying at the Institute of Psychology from 1926 to 1930, Vygotsky's research looked at the "mechanism of transformation of natural psychological functions into the higher functions of logical memory, selective attention, decision making, learning and comprehension of language" (Ardichvili 2001, p. 34). This demarcation between "lower" and "higher" mental functions was Vygotsky's way of marking the dividing line between humans and other animal species. Lower mental functions included basic responses to the environment and ways of learning, were built-in biological functions, and were exhibited by many species, whereas the higher mental functions, including those listed above, were only exhibited by humans (Costley 2012; Ardichvili 2001). Of the higher mental functions Vygotsky studied, he had a particular interest in the development and progression of language. He felt strongly that language was an important cognitive tool, and that while thought and language were separate until children were about two years old, from there they became increasingly interdependent, with the development of "inner speech" (the silent self-talk we all do when reasoning through a problem or considering new information) being an important cognitive development point in children (Ardichvili 2001; Costley 2012).

While Vygotsky demonstrated some similar thoughts about cognition and learning as behaviorists, the inner speech debate was a definite break from behaviorist views. Whereas behaviorists viewed thought as subvocal speech – mashing together overt speech and thought as a continuum – Vygotsky viewed thought (or "inner speech") and overt speech as two discrete forms of language: overt or spoken language for communicating with others and internal language or inner speech as an internal locus of control for behavior regulation (Ardichvili 2001; Costley 2012; Dastpak et al. 2017).

It may seem odd to be reading about theories of speech development in a section covering theories of learning, but for Vygotsky, it was not possible to separate thought and word, because while inner speech was distinct from overt speech, both were necessary to acquire the social personality required for human development (Dastpak et al. 2017). Additionally, Vygotsky believed that human development is facilitated by social interactions, which require both types of language, and are integral to the development of thought (Dastpak et al. 2017). And finally, it was the aggregation of these theories that produced his most impactful concept, his positing with regard to the ZPD, one of the most influential and well-known learning theories even today.

Zone of Proximal Development

As just stated, one of the most enduring and often applied pieces of Vygotsky's work is his ZPD. This approach to learning is based on the idea that there are two different developmental levels in children, the first being *actual development*, which Vygotsky defines as the "level of development of a child's mental functions that has been established as a result of certain already completed developmental cycles" (Vygotsky 1978, p. 37). This, he further clarifies, is the age often established by using standardized tests, given and taken individually, without the help of others. The second is the *ZPD*, or *"the distance between the actual developmental level as determined by independent problem solving and the level of potential development as determined through problem solving under adult guidance or in collaboration with more capable peers"* (Vygotsky 1978, p. 38; emphasis original). In other words, Vygotsky opined, children might have more or less capability at any given fixed age in years, but this should be determined not by said fixed age and/or based on what learning they demonstrate individually, but by what they are capable of learning with the help of others. It is this zone that determines the true "mental age" of a developing child – this zone that provides the best insight into what they have learned and what they are capable of learning at any given time in their training.

The concept of the ZPD is intimately intertwined with his thoughts on language and speech development. While the concept of the ZPD provides for adult or advanced peer support to help guide learners through acquisition of new knowledge, such support is provided through speech, which plays a critical role in the child's cognitive development (Dastpak et al. 2017). Because Vygotsky viewed thinking as a purposeful activity that is mediated by social interactions (Dastpak et al. 2017; Costley 2012), it is his views on language, social interactions, and the ZPD that combine to fully flesh out what would ultimately be termed his sociocultural theory of cognitive development.

What is truly groundbreaking about this theory – and what may be a primary reason it became so popular – is the prospective nature of the ZPD. In Vygotsky's (1978) own words, "The actual developmental level characterizes mental development retrospectively, while the zone of proximal development characterizes mental development prospectively" (p. 38). Until the point of Vygotsky providing a potential way to imagine – in a scientific manner, of course – what the potential learning capacity of a child was, children were assessed on their learning to the point in time the assessment took place. With the ZPD, Vygotsky provided a new way forward for teaching and considering what children *could* do if provided just the right amount of challenge and the right resources (teachers, advanced peers) to support them as they navigated new waters.

It is this legacy, perhaps more than any other, that defines Vygotsky and enshrined him in educational theory history; we can all remember those times when we felt unable to move forward in learning but, with the help of another, were finally able to push through the frustration and acquire the information or skill we struggled with. This basic premise, which seems so clear to us now, was too long overlooked as theorists strove to answer their questions about mental capacity, learning, and behavior by looking solely at the individual child or learner. With the expansion of the learning universe to expressly acknowledge the important role of the teacher, mentor, or peer, Vygotsky helped educators everywhere realize just how important their roles were. They were no longer fountains of knowledge there to spew forth information for students to absorb; instead, they were now an integral part of the social environment and, therefore, the learning process – a process that could be extended ad infinitum if students, peers, and teachers were willing to continue stretching the learning boundaries of every individual learner.

Contemporary Impact

According to Ardichvili (2001), Vygotsky's influence was far-ranging and too voluminous to adequately summarize; in the course of researching this very small section covering his outsized influence on education, it is easy to see why Ardichvili makes this statement. During Vygotsky's short life, he established himself as a profound and prodigious thinker who provided enormous opportunities for others to take his ideas and stretch them. Through his meticulous work and willingness to put his thoughts on paper for those with interest, Vygotsky encouraged others to break new ground and consider alternatives to the existing thoughts of the day. His influence on psychology, education, linguistics, communication, and others cannot be denied, even almost 100 years after his untimely death.

For educators, in particular, his views on the power and necessity of language combined with the startling idea that learners should be viewed in terms of potential rather than current achievement have become ingrained in school systems worldwide. In taking the perspective of growth and potential for learners, then adding in the concept that teaching could and should promote growth, Vygotsky planted hearty seeds from which many of constructivism's stalks would grow. The prevailing approach to education during his lifetime being rooted in behaviorism, researchers, theorists, and educators viewed children as empty vessels to be filled rather than as inquisitive, capable, motivated learners. This led to those lecture-at approaches that often led to student (and teacher!) frustration when materials were not absorbed and demonstrated later. A simple change of perspective – from student as individual learner who would eventually reach a ceiling, to student as learner with unlimited potential if provided a little help and challenge – was paradigm shifting. He would never have known it then, but his ideas can even be connected to Carol Dweck's work on growth versus fixed mindsets, considered groundbreaking almost a century later!

Section 3: Educational Equity: The Classroom as an Equalizer

Katherine Fogelberg

Part 1: Introduction

"Education, then, beyond all other divides of human origin, is a great equalizer of conditions of men - the balance wheel of the social machinery" (Horace Mann 1848, as cited in Growe and Montgomery 2003).

"To educate as the practice of freedom is a way of teaching that anyone can learn. That learning process comes easiest to those of us who teach who also believe that there is an aspect of our vocation that is sacred; who believe that our work is not merely to share information but to share in the intellectual and spiritual growth of our students. To teach in a manner that respects and cares for the souls of our students is essential if we are to provide the necessary conditions where learning can most deeply and intimately begin" (bell hooks 1994, *Teaching to Transgress*, p. 13).

According to Growe and Montgomery (2003), from its beginnings, public education in the US has put forward the idea that education is the Great Equalizer. From this idealistic perspective, it is surmised that education in the US will provide the opportunities needed to pull oneself out of poverty, overcome the color of our skin, and create spaces where gender is no longer a driving reason behind economic and intellectual success. Unfortunately, it is not a secret that education has been, and continues to be, inequitable in the US and around the world; it has never been equitable and, though we strive toward equity, we have yet to achieve it. As much as we would like to deny it, our gender, our skin color, and our family economics, among other things, have always had – and continue to have – an outsized influence on the opportunities afforded us, starting with our access to education.

Were education truly the path to equity and success, we would not have needed a Brown v. Board of Education. But even with the forced integration of schools that has been in place for almost 75 years, school inequities continue: schools in low-income areas or that serve low-income children have fewer resources in terms of money and people (Growe and Montgomery 2003). And while early childhood education programs focused on low-income children (e.g., Head Start) show significant positive impact on student readiness, such impacts are relatively short-lived and unable to overcome certain parental characteristics, specifically parents who demonstrated depressive symptoms (Puma et al. 2010). Why this is the case is well beyond the scope of this small section, though it would not be far off to hypothesize that poor resourcing once those students transition into school is a likely culprit. When high-quality instruction is consistently demonstrated to be one of the highest impact factors in helping students learn, and knowing that schools serving low-income students have difficulties attracting teachers of any quality, the dots are pretty easy to connect (Puma et al. 2010; Okpala and Ellis 2005). The reality of it all is that while education can certainly support equity, it is in and of itself inequitable and thus, unable to truly bridge the equity gap.

Fortunately, it is not solely education that determines one's financial and/or career success in life, though it certainly contributes to the likelihood that success defined by these parameters will occur; one only has to look at the popular press to periodically find reports that a college degree increases a person's lifetime earnings by X amount over that of someone with "only" a high school diploma, at least in the US. And there are certainly multitudes of studies demonstrating results that support such claims; far too many to include here. But beyond the financial and career success metrics, education contributes to much, much more. It is a door into the world of opportunity and advantage. For those who are illiterate, the door remains tightly closed – not immovable, but certainly opaque and much more challenging to get through than for those who have even a basic level of ability to read and write. For those who cannot perform simple math problems, everyday life can be a minefield, filled with frustrations and opportunities for others to prey upon their lack of skill and knowledge. It is education, then, whether formally or informally gained, that opens those doors wider and lowers the obstacles – the more education achieved, the wider the door opens and the lower the obstacles become. Not always. But it certainly helps. And while it does not, by itself, guarantee "success," it certainly increases access to that heady goal.

However, education is also power, and in this, we see another form of inequity. When authoritarian regimes take over very often the first thing to fall is access to education for girls and women; in the early years of Western societies – including the US – education was only accessible to White males of the upper classes (while Mann may have purported to believe education was the great equalizer, he clearly felt it was only the great equalizer for *men*). And even today, access to education, especially beyond the high school level, is tempered by many things, including finances, experience, geography, and yes, the color of our skin.

For those who obtain access – through high school or beyond – education provides advantages; some are quantifiable, some are not. But all impact one's ability to succeed in the world – whether that means having fewer babies who live longer or earning more money and prestige. It may not be the great equalizer, but it incontrovertibly contributes to decreasing some of the challenges that exist without it.

This section introduces four educational theorists who explicitly take on the issue of educational (in)equity. Perhaps unsurprisingly, none of them are White, in stark contrast to those who have been profiled to this point. Half are female, one openly identified as queer during her lifetime. As with the section just preceding this, these theorists are presented in alphabetical order in a best attempt to not try to prioritize them by importance or impact or any other subjective criterion. Three of the four are more contemporary, also in contrast to the preceding section. While the contemporary educational theorists writ large were not included in the previous section for a variety of reasons, those included here are selected because educational equity theories, with the exception of DuBois, did not gain traction until the latter part of the twentieth century.

Additionally, the idea that educational equity was even needed was somewhat preposterous for many decades – unless you happened to be one of the educated who hailed from a marginalized group, as DuBois did. And even he had a relatively privileged childhood, not experiencing any significant racism until his college years and beyond. While we hail the theorists discussed to this point already, we often gloss over the fact that they were, almost without exception, White males who often had the added privilege of being financially well-to-do. Having already pointed out that Thorndike was a self-proclaimed eugenicist, it is rarely discussed that Dewey, too, had xenophobic beliefs, as his remarks to a Chinese audience in 1919 indicated:

> The simple fact of the case is that at present the world is not sufficiently civilized to permit close contact of peoples of widely different cultures without deplorable consequences. . . [therefore] unrestricted contact through immigration and by similar activities should not take place" (Dewey 1919, as cited in Johnson 2000, p. 74).

Granted, it is difficult to go against the grain in any given time, but this is what makes DuBois so important; his race and experiences, along with his intellect and the good fortune he had to be lifted up by a cadre of well-meaning White men, ensure history would have at least one voice of dissent at the turn of the twentieth century.

One might argue that DuBois cracked the door open for those who followed, whether they were explicitly familiar with his work or not. On the other hand, perhaps it was Maria Montessori who opened the door for female theorists to walk through, as unintentional as her almost theory of education may have been. Tracing the lineage of these theories and theorists is not the purpose of this section, but it is certainly a worthwhile endeavor to consider, given the somewhat rarified company those silhouetted in this chapter inhabit. (One of the books referenced in this chapter, for example, profiles 50 modern thinkers in education, only five of whom are female!)

It is with this background in mind that the educational theorists with their wholly different roots are presented here. Education and understanding learning certainly owes much of its evolution to those paternal, northern European traditions and thinkers, but there is a lot of damage that has also been done, whether intentionally or not. It seems important and appropriate, particularly in a textbook aimed at those in one of the least diverse professions in the US, to give voice to viewpoints that are not the norm. As we strive to increase diversity, equity, and inclusion in higher education and the veterinary profession, perhaps some understanding of the educational theorists who have tackled this issue will help us better understand how to do so in our classrooms, labs, and clinics – the places where every veterinarian begins their journey.

Part 2: Gloria Evangelina Anzaldúa [1942–2004]

Freyca Calderon and Karla O'Donald

Introduction and Overview

Self-described as a "Tejana patlache (queer) nepantlera spiritual activist" (Anzaldúa and Keating 2002, p. 602), Gloria Anzaldúa was born in a small ranchería in the Río Grande Valley in South Texas in September 1942 to a long-standing family of Tejano farm workers. She was the oldest of four children and after graduating from high school in Harlingen, she left the south Texas valley to start university at Texas Women's University. A year later, she returned home with a writing accolade but was unable to pay for tuition. She did not give up on her education and remained near her birth-home, obtaining a Bachelor of Arts in English, Art, and Secondary Education from Texas Pan-American University (now the University of Texas-Rio Grande Valley, or UTRGV). She would move on to graduate school at the University of Texas at Austin, simultaneously starting her teaching career near her family's home with students in every level of schooling.

Upon completing her Master of Arts, Anzaldúa moved to the Midwest to serve as a liaison between migrant families and Indiana's school system. She held this position for a couple of years but decided to move back to Austin to pursue a PhD; it was during this pivotal period that she established relationships with radical Chicanas and LGBTQ activists. After a difficult time in Austin, she moved to California to focus on her writing, where her career as a writer blossomed and produced most of her transcendent work. After many gigs, as Anzaldúa like to call her presentations and talks around the United States, teaching university courses and workshops, and continuous focus on her writing, she passed away from diabetes-related complications in 2004.

Her work is far reaching and in the critical edition of *Borderlands La Frontera: The New Mestiza* (Anzaldúa 2021), an extensive list of fields she influenced is provided; it includes: Feminism, Chicana Feminism; Chicano literature; Poetry, Rhetoric & Writing; Queerness; Disability; and Education & Teaching, among others (p. 515–517). This text also contains a detailed biography that offers a closer understanding of Anzaldúa's life and legacy. *The Gloria Anzaldúa Reader* (Keating 2009), also provides a panoramic timeline of Anzaldúa's work for a quick, but detailed reading. However, Cantú's preface of the critical edition of Borderlands (2021), is the piece that best presents and shares a uniquely personal introduction and understanding of the impact that the life and work of Anzaldúa have had intellectually and on individuals. Reading Cantú's personal and professional relationship with Anzaldúa is a wonderful combination that represents how her work touches those of us that not only have studied her work but have been transformed by it.

> Through its creation of epistemological and ontological frameworks. . . (she) offers a paradigm shift that is sorely needed in this time of political, social, and spiritual transition in our globalized world. From her earlier work to the last piece that was published in her lifetime, Anzaldúa's urgent and visionary goal was "to do work that matters" (Anzaldúa 2021, p. 14)

Answering Anzaldúa's call echoed by Cantú, we embark on this writing endeavor to share Anzaldua's concepts, theories, and methodologies that can help the reader engage the world in a different way, particularly in education. Starting with *Borderlands*, her foundational work, we follow her scholarship through several evolutions. We focus on the work she published and present posthumous pieces that she did not have a chance to see in print, but fortunately were completed by her close friends that worked as her editors. We hope this brief glimpse at her work sparks your interest and energizes you to also engage in "work that matters."

Borderlands La Frontera: The New Mestiza (1987): Culture, Poetry, Language, Identity

Borderlands is Anzaldúa's most renowned work and is where many of her ideas, concepts, and theories are born. *Borderlands La Frontera: The New Mestiza* (Anzaldúa 1987), is divided into two parts. The first includes seven chapters that can be read in any order and can stand alone. They also serve as steps of development culminating in the most important chapter, which alludes to the title, *La conciencia de la mestiza*: Towards a New Consciousness (p. 99). The second part of the book is divided into six sections that offer a collection of poems. The book closes with the transcript of an interview that Anzaldúa had with Karin Ikas, in which she described the connections between her writings and personal life and her development as a critical Chicana scholar. Anzaldúa (2021) describes the book as, "iconic precisely because it voices what has been silenced. . . (it) explores innumerable paths to self-discovery and actualization" (p. 8). Cantú shares with us her personal experience with the book in a way that many of us who have read it have also experienced:

> I recognized it for the life-defining, paradigm-shattering text that it has proven to be. . . it was the first time I found, in an academic setting, a voice that spoke to my own experience and that relied on that experience to theorize about the larger world. . .

a text that opened countless options as it forged a path alongside the familiar academic one giving me permission to speak in my own Spanglish and to reflect on the cultural forces that taught me how to be in the world (2021, p. 7–8).

As border crossers, we can testify to the truth of these words because we have felt the same way. We have studied this foundational text for many years now, have shared it with our students, and theorized with and about it with our colleagues, always seeing new possibilities and messages.

One feature of the book, as Cantú mentions, is Anzaldúa's use of Spanish/Spanglish in her writing. Many times, Anzaldúa writes completely in Spanish, especially her poetry, and leaves the English monolingual speaker to fend for themselves in search of meaning. For us as bilingual speakers, this becomes an extremely personal and familiar moment that is the embodiment of our state as borderlands people. We cross the borders of language constantly, every day. By mixing Spanish and English, we create and dwell in a third space of knowledge and understanding. Is not a secret form of expression. Yet, it is a deeply connective exercise that Anzaldúa, so many years ago, dared to propose, explore, share, and model for us.

By simply reading the book title, Anzaldúa immediately introduces her idea and theory of *Borderlands,* but it is in the chapter's title, *La conciencia de la mestiza*: Towards a New Consciousness (1987, p. 99), where her ideas begin to flourish. Anzaldúa defines **borderlands** as "a vague and undetermined place created by the emotional residual of an unnatural boundary. It is in a constant state of transition" (1987, p. 7). To her, borderlands isf a place where cultures, ideas, nationalities, identities, desires, and many more categories intersect, and even collide. She indicates that "borderlands are physically present wherever two or more cultures edge each other" (1987, p. 19). The intersection(s) in which these categories encounter each other could be smooth, easy to cross, chaotic, difficult, or dangerous to move through; all depending on the structures and dynamics of power between the categories. Anzaldúa's examples for these borderlands include the intersection of race, class, gender, sexual orientation, ethnicity, religion, nationality, language, ability, and any other characteristic or group that does not meet the standards of the dominant culture, namely White, male, Christian, middle/upper class, European-descendent, English language, etc.

Anzaldúa also adds that in the borderlands, "the prohibited and forbidden are its inhabitants" (p. 7). Therefore, she conceives borderlands from the disenfranchised positionality, from a place where individuals feel alienated and divided by socially constructed categories. The dominant culture places minoritized people at the margins when it labels them as "others" and denies them recognition as equals. Then, she explains that *Borderlands* theory aims to recenter the analysis, perception, and acceptance of those borders that are socially constructed and questions its simple view as physical and geographical boundaries.

Borderlands theory is to be understood in a multidimensional way, including ideological and epistemological dimensions of the territorial concept that individuals inhabit. Anzaldúa adds that *Borderlands* theory is a hybrid, nonlinear, and complex construction of an individual's understanding of the world grounded in his/her experiences. This theory begins with an individual's personal experiences and uses counternarratives to express and reflect on the multiple border crossings that occur constantly. To simplify, an individual makes use of his/her stories to recount the trials and tribulations they experience, while traversing the different borderlands they continuously cross. This constant movement in and out of worlds presents both opportunity and loss. We must now discuss the New *Mestiza*; a concept Anzaldúa developed to better understand this complexity.

We start by introducing the concept of *mestizo/a*. The *mestizo/a* is the product of the colonization of the Americas. *Mestizos* are people of mixed race. Anzaldúa classifies herself as a *mestiza* because she is of mixed race; European and Indigenous. She draws upon Vasconcelos' (1958), concept of "*La raza cósmica*" to explain Latin-American peoples' hybrid origin. Vasconcelos' explains that being of mixed blood is positive because it provides the individual with perspective and depth into certain situations and experiences. Still, a close reading of the book shows racist views that Vasconcelos, a Mexican philosopher and educator, had toward people of color, particularly people of African origin. However, Anzaldúa uses this book and Vasconcelos's argument to explain that people of mixed blood have differential perspectives, which gives them the ability to move through borders, and provides them with both the colonizer and the colonized notions of the world.

Next, we explain the use of the feminine and masculine forms of this noun. Spanish is a gendered language; *mestiza* is a female noun, and *mestizo* is the male noun. Anzaldúa uses, exclusively, the female noun of *mestiza*. She does not mean to alienate the masculine, but instead, she aims to integrate particular feminine qualities that any human possesses regardless of their gender. To explain, Anzaldúa values and finds certain pivotal experiences and reactions that are dismissed and disregarded by patriarchal scientific-based narratives. As an example, we can talk about *una corazonada*, which could be translated as a gut feeling. In Spanish, a *corazonada* is an emotion, a sense, or a state, that

people experience when they receive a message. It is like a warning that derives from or is delivered directly to the heart (*corazón*). You can see that this is the same in English, but the body part is different. It is very important to understand that the *mestiza* can be experienced by males and females because any person regardless of the gender can receive these gut feelings. Anzaldúa tells us,

> La *mestiza* constantly has to shift out of habitual formations; from convergent thinking, analytical reasoning that tends to use rationality to move toward a single goal (a Western mode), to divergent thinking, characterized by movement away from set patterns and goals and toward more whole perspective, one that includes rather than excludes. (1987, p. 101)

An individual that is in constant movement between and among borders, and that convenes and utilizes his/her knowledge and experiences to evaluate and reflect on the situation at hand, can develop what she calls "**a new mestiza consciousness**, *una conciencia de mujer*. It is a consciousness of the Borderlands" (1987, p. 99). The *mestiza* consciousness is a kin sense and awareness of complexity. This consciousness is an affinity to view the contradictions and incongruences that reality presents to individuals who do not align with the standards that the dominant culture establishes. The *mestiza* consciousness allows the individual to view multiple and multilevel realities and to uncover the discrepancies of the power structures constructed and sustained by the dominant culture. Consequently, a *mestiza* consciousness produces the courage and agency necessary to confront the hegemonic forces systematically and pervasively embedded in our society that aim to separate and alienate minorities by casting them out to the margins. Also, it symbolizes the ability to identify potential alternatives that bring about solutions to the situation the individual is encountering. Anzaldúa affirms, "The new mestiza copes by developing a tolerance for contradictions, a tolerance for ambiguity. . . She learns to juggle cultures. . . Not only does she sustain contradictions, she turns the ambivalence into something else" (1987, p. 101). The development of *mestiza* consciousness produces inner change, which in turn generates transformations in that person's surroundings because "Awareness of our situation must come from inner changes, which in turn come before changes in society. Nothing happens in the 'real' world unless it first happens in the images in our heads" (1987, p. 109). But borderlands theory and the *mestiza* consciousness are not the only components needed to create change in the world around us.

Another pivotal concept of this book is that of **Nepantla**, which originates from *Náhuatl*, the Aztec language, and describes the experience of living in-between, a liminal or third space. *Nepantla* is the place where the *mestiza* dwells as she encounters and moves in, out, through, and among borders where she can feel "disoriented" (Keating 2009, p. 181). experiencing the turbulence that this fluctuation entails. *Nepantla,* however, is not a place of isolation. Instead, it is a space for growth and personal transformation. *Nepantla* represents and offers a safe space in which a person may reflect, confront, and evaluate possibilities. It is a place to search and find recovery, where a person can find a supportive community that enables both the development of courage and the agency to act. Although many contradictions can be present in this space, *Nepantla* also offers a healing space for reflection which leads to wisdom production and encourages praxis. In *Nepantla*, the individual can reflect on the meaning of the social categories enacted by the dominant culture that hinders personal growth and actualization. *Nepantla* is the space where the individual (re)constructs, (re)considers, and (re)creates possibilities not just for the self but for the world he/she inhabits. Anzaldúa explains that while in *Nepantla*, the *mestiza* consciousness is key since the formation of a new perspective, a new self, allows the individual to make sense of the contradicting messages that the crashing and collapsing borders denote. It is also in this place where a person can become a *Nepantlera*; the concept of becoming a *Nepantlera* is addressed in her later writings. As stated before, it is the feminine form of the noun, but we must remember that this does not signify the gender of the person. The main message is to become this being (male, female, queer, or agender) with a new consciousness. Anzaldúa defines *Nepantleras* as,

> agents of awakening (conocimiento). . .(they) nurture psychological, social, and spiritual metamorphosis. . . Las nepantleras know that each of us is linked with everyone and everything in the universe and fight actively in both the material world and the spiritual realm. . . (Las nepantleras) engaged in the struggle for social, economic, and political justice, while working on spiritual transformation of selfhoods. (2015, p. 83)

Being in *Nepantla* and becoming a *Nepantlera* is a continuous, difficult, and disorienting work, but it is "work that matters" to create change in the world.

Anzaldúa also developed what she calls **La Facultad**, which refers to the ability to tolerate ambiguity and "the capacity to see in surface phenomena the meanings of deeper realities, to see the deep structure below the surface. It is an instant 'sensing' a quick perception arrived at without conscious reasoning" (1987, p. 60). Anzaldúa

identified as a lesbian and she argued that LGBTQ+ people have this *facultad,* since they straddle different worlds and have the advantage of seeing from different positionalities. Anzaldúa explained that *la facultad*, "is an affinity, a kind of sixth sense that makes you have a hyper-awareness for what is not seen in the surface. (Anzaldúa 2000, p. 122). *La facultad* is introduced in the chapter *Entering the Serpent* (1987, p. 60), in *Borderlands*, and explains how this way of knowing that the *facultad* gives us was taken away from individuals by oppressive systems, capitalism, religion, and colonization, but "It is latent in all of us" (p. 61, 1987). *La facultad* works with images and symbols that connect the senses. Therefore, Anzaldúa urges us to focus on (re) acquiring and nurturing *La facultad* by being cognizant of the signs, cues, and clues that our experiences provide.

Anzaldúa's work is taught and studied in diverse fields: Chicano and/or Latino Studies, Rhetoric, Multicultural and Bilingual Education, Women and Gender Studies, and Cultural Studies to name a few. Interweaving poetry and prose, her work is groundbreaking for its denunciation of multilevels of oppression experienced by the marginalized. As a Chicana and postcolonial feminist, Anzaldúa's work portrays the connections between personal, social, and cultural identity, highlighting the inaccuracy of binary thinking, and featuring the importance of making coalitions among marginalized groups. For Anzaldúa, writing was a form of reflecting and making sense of all the experiences, stories, voices, and cultures that intersect within ourselves. Her writings ushered com/passion for others, all of this as she endured physical and emotional pain due to illnesses. She marked a turning point in educational scholarship, particularly for Chicana/Latina feminist scholars in terms of what is considered academic writing. This complex combination of emotions, experiences, and feelings makes her work uniquely inspiring for a wide variety of audiences that have been placed at the margins in one or more social categories. Anzaldúa's work will likely continue to grow since much of her unpublished work will slowly be released, allowing us to explore new ways of studying and expanding knowledge based on her concepts, theories, and methods.

Anzaldúas' Metaphorical Language using Animals

> On our way to a new consciousness, we will have to leave the opposite bank, the split between the two mortal combatants somehow healed so that we are on both shores at once and, at once, see through serpent and eagle eyes (1987, p. 101).

Anzaldúa regularly used metaphors characterized by animals, borrowing this from an indigenist conceptualization of the world. Some of her concepts and theories were heavily influenced by Aztec cosmology, which is filled with deities that have animal characteristics and abilities, as you can read in the quote above. Anzaldúa describes the development of the new mestiza and writes, "She becomes a nahual, able to transform herself into a tree, a coyote, into another person" (1987, p. 105). Zaytoun (2015), offers an extensive study of this term in Anzaldúa's work, explaining that this concept is only introduced in *La conciencia de la mestiza* (1987), but in her later writings it becomes the central piece, surpassing *la mestiza*, *borderlands*, and *Nepantla*, which come together to become the fundamental features of **la naguala**. Again, Anzaldúa used the feminine for this word, but not in reference to gender.

Anzaldúa also takes some liberties and changes the spelling of the word from *nahuala* to *naguala*. *La naguala* is the conduit among worlds, among the various steps needed to travel in the "*Path of Conocimiento*" (Keating 2009, p.181), which is Anzaldúa's most defining theory and method that aims to acquire a higher level of consciousness. Also, Anzaldúa writes a piece titled "*El nagual* in my house" (2015, p. 27), in which she narrates how this ability appears in her. This piece is dreamlike, but that is precisely what the *naguala* is; an in-between-worlds *conocimiento* that allows us to travel, bring, and take from different levels of consciousness. Zaytoun (2015), mentions that Anzaldúa had several stories and writings unpublished that focused on *la naguala*, her abilities, and essence:

> . . . the transformation that la *naguala* invokes extends purpose into the physical world in concrete ways via the imagination, which she viewed as energy-producing and material. *La naguala*, situated both in and beyond the body, shifts the shape and the boundaries of the subject beyond intellectual, humanist frameworks (Zaytoun 2015, p. 70).

For Anzaldúa, *la naguala* is imagination, creativity, and language as concepts that are embodied alive, moving, changing, shifting, and constantly shapeshifting. As Zaytoun (2015), puts it, *la naguala* is "a concept borrowed from indigenous thought, serves as a vehicle that deconstructs and decolonizes embodiment and being" (p. 72). Unfortunately, Anzaldúa did not finish developing this concept in its totality. Still, we can see how her cosmology of the world connects among all forms of life, whether human or nonhuman. Through her use of metaphorical language, she suggests and highlights the importance and the power of animals.

The serpent is an animal of great importance in Aztec cosmology whose most powerful deity was *Quetzalcoatl*, the feathered serpent. For Anzaldúa, the serpent represents the conduit to more than one way of knowing, which transports the individual from one form of consciousness to another. This shift in consciousness she also defined as an awakening, titling it a "serpent movement." In the chapter "Entering the serpent," (Anzaldúa 1987, p. 47), she discusses the trinity of the Mexican/Chicana origin: *la virgen de* Guadalupe (the virgin), *la chingada/Coatlicue* (an Aztec goddess), and *La Llorona* (a legend ghost like female figure). Anzaldúa dives into the role of religion as a tool for the colonization of the Americas and how these three female figures were created to manipulate colonized people's consciousness and push them to assimilate colonial beliefs. Anzaldúa expressed, "We are taught that the body is an ignorant animal; intelligence dwells only in the head" (1987, p. 59). She disputed this belief and encouraged us to pay attention to the body and to the *gut feeling (la corazonada)*. Anzaldúa makes use of the "serpent movement" to explain how it helps to move from place to place, border to border, and into ourselves, to look for the pieces, stories, and memories that were stolen and pushed to be forgotten by colonization. Anzaldúa wrote,

> At some point, on our way to a new consciousness, we will have to leave the opposite bank, the split between the two mortal combatants somehow healed so that we are on both shores at once and, at once, see through serpent and eagle eyes. (1987, p. 78–79)

She incites us to become empowered and shift into the new mestiza, "the serpent, a symbol of absolute alterity, which endlessly deconstruct her self-sovereignty by opening the chasm of her ontological ground" (Yountea and Mena 2014, p. 176). The "serpent movement" leads us to ecdysis and guides us to (re)configure ourselves anew; to be whole again. Anzaldúa used the metaphor of the serpent to invite us to embody an alternative reality when experiencing oppression and marginalization from the dominant culture and move through border crossings that lead us to new "paths of *conocimiento*" (2013).

In her children's book, *Prieta and the Ghost Woman* (1995), she describes the protagonist, *Prieta*, as being a jaguar (p. 283–285). Anzaldúa ties this connection to animals to shamanism, which is prevalent in the creation of other concepts and theories that she was not able to finish developing. The shaman, she explained, shifts and becomes the connection to another world, another consciousness, which guides him/her in finding new ways of seeing and engaging the world. Our spirit animal, whichever that may be, is present in us but colonization forced us to stop listening to him/her. Ultimately, the message Anzaldúa solidifies in her legacy is that those of us who do not fit into the societal normativity of the dominant culture – that is, the colored, the poor, the foreign, the queer, the female, the physically challenged people – we can challenge that ideology and become a new *mestiza*. The power is within us, we just need to listen to those animal insights that guide us to see the world from a different perspective.

We end this section with a list of Anzaldúa's major works.

- This Bridge Called My Back: Writings by Radical Women of Color – 1981
- Borderlands/La Frontera: The New Mestiza – 1987
- Making Face, Making Soul/Haciendo Caras: Creative and Critical Perspectives by Feminists of Color – 1990
- Friends from the other side – 1993 (children's book)
- Prietita and the Ghost Woman – 1995 (children's book)
- Interviews/Entrevistas – 2000
- This Bridge We Call Home: Radical Visions for Transformation – 2002
- The Gloria Anzaldúa Reader – 2009
- Light in the Dark/Luz en lo Oscuro: Rewriting Identity, Spirituality, Reality 2015

Part 3: W.E.B. DuBois [1868–1963]

Katherine Fogelberg

Introduction and Schooling

William Edward Burghardt DuBois (pronounced doo-boys) was born in Massachusetts in 1868. At age 20, he graduated from Fisk University, and seven years later he would become the first Black man to earn a PhD from Harvard, publishing his dissertation titled *The Suppression of the African Slave-Trade to the United States of America, 1638–1870* in 1886 (Rudwick 2023). DuBois, as with several of the theorists discussed in this textbook, did not fancy himself an educational theorist; some might argue that he should not be included in an educational theory section. However, also like others discussed in this text, DuBois was an educator during his career, and saw the value of education – not just for the privileged and "civilized," but also for those whose labor contributed most intimately to the prosperity of the land: the recently freed Black men who "first should be made the intelligent laborer, the trained farmer, the skilled artisan of the South" (DuBois 1932, p. 204).

W.E.B. DuBois, as he would come to be known, grew up in a small town in the US and counted a number of wealthy White children among his friends, with whom he shared a disdain of the immigrant mill workers (Johnston 2000). Somewhat precocious intellectually, DuBois graduated from high school at age 15 with dreams of attending Harvard one day (Johnston 2000).

DuBois's education was rigorous, with his high school courses ranging from Latin to math, English to ancient and US history, and science to music (Broderick 1958). His completion of high school with high honors – along with the financial support and urging from his high school principal – provided him an opportunity to attend Fisk University in Nashville, TN on a scholarship arranged by the local townsmen (Broderick 1958). It was at Fisk that DuBois would first experience overt racial discrimination and would eventually realize his vision of meritocracy was flawed, embittering him as he viewed, for the first time in his life, the very real divisions between Black and White humans (Johnston 2000). He would persevere, however, and complete his Reniassance education at Fisk, where he excelled and would graduate just three years later, having collected a staunch group of supporters – all White men "with a missionary commitment to the uplift of the Negro race" – who would provide the launching pad he needed to enter the hallowed halls of Harvard University (Broderick 1958, p. 11).

He began his studies at Harvard repeating his last two years of undergraduate studies, taking a broad range of courses, including English composition, ethics, economics, and geology (Broderick 1958). Although he performed well, during his second year he turned to philosophy, studying French and German philosophers, as well as logic, psychology, the ethics of social reform, elocution, political economy, a survey or railroads and bimetallism, and US constitutional and political history (Broderick 1958; Johnston 2000). It appears he enjoyed engaging with philosophy more than he did with science, as his musings indicated: "The Infinite – that specious invention foe making something out of nothing" and, "Science is Mathematics. Mathematics is Identity. Science is Identity" (DuBois 1888–1890, as cited in Broderick 1958, p. 13). Ultimately, however, he would wander into political economy and history as his studies continued, cemented by study abroad in Berlin, where a course with Gustav von Schmoller would lead him to research and a mentor who encouraged him to pursue an academic career. In 1895, a year after his return to Harvard from Berlin, DuBois would finally complete his PhD in history while teaching at Wilberforce College (Broderick 1958; Johnson 2000).

In 1897 DuBois earned an academic appointment at Atlanta University, where he began his writings about a heterogeneous cultural system in the US that was not hierarchical (Johnston 2000). In his publications, DuBois put forth the theory that people could be loyal to the US while maintaining their cultural identities, asking, "Am I an American or am I a Negro? Can I be both?" in his article "On the Conservation of Races" and going on to propose the idea of an inclusive Americanism – one where all cultures are embraced and welcomed for their contributions (Johnson 2000, p. 82). This idea of cultural pluralism – a term that would not be coined for almost 20 years after DuBois's initial theory was published – had at its heart the idea that people of cultures other than White America should not be asked to assimilate into the White culture, but appreciated for their uniqueness and viewed as contributors to the American culture; an idea that was in direct contrast to the other well-known and respected Black scholar of his day, Booker T. Washington (Johnson 2000; Rudwick 2023). A seemingly radical idea at the time, it is still resonant with many nonmainstream cultures in the US even today. It also served as the foundation for his educational theories that challenged the eugenic approach to education during his times and refuted the idea that people could not learn to change – whether their skin was Black or White or any shade in between (Johnson 2000).

Educational Theory

As a champion of education, DuBois was committed to a broadly based, general education for all students (Johnston 2000). His focus on the education of Black intellectuals was always at the forefront; however, and he firmly believed in the importance of building a core group of Black intellectuals who could and "would lead the 'Negro' to a state of equality" and, for this reason, felt strongly that the ideal Negro college must be created as much as possible to the meet the same standard as White colleges (Johnson 2000, p. 83).

But though DuBois's acts were at the university level, his educational theory was firmly centered on children. Based on his history training and writings, DuBois was firmly entrenched in the idea that one way to decrease racism in the US was to incorporate social studies into school curricula (Johnson 2000; Graves 1998). It was through social studies, which included the study of all cultures, native and immigrant alike, that DuBois felt that true liberation could be achieved (Graves 1998).

DuBois started his career as an optimist; he strongly believed that people of all colors could be educated to accept equity – that Whites could be taught the value of Black culture and grow to understand the value of a heterogeneous cultural society, while immigrants and freed Black slaves could be educated to understand the predominantly White culture within which they had been embedded with neither having to assimilate themselves to the other (Johnson 2000; Graves 1998). He was adamant that racism was about ignorance more than anything else: "The world was thinking wrong about race, because it did not know. The ultimate evil was stupidity. The cure for it was knowledge based on scientific investigation" (DuBois 1968, as cited in Graves 1998, p. 6).

Unfortunately, as with many idealists, DuBois would learn that racism was not easily educated away. His experiences as a young man in Atlanta reminded him daily that being a Black man in the United States, even a highly intelligent and educated one, did not insulate him from being relegated to "less than" his White counterparts. And while this removal of his rose-colored glasses did awaken him to the size of the challenge he had tackled, he continued to hold out hope that racism could be conquered (Graves 1998). In 1906, DuBois would predate Paulo Freire's concept of critical consciousness in a speech where he described the sudden consciousness of a human being who realized that there are "tremendous powers lying latent within him" causing him to rise "to the powerful assertion of a self, conscious of its might" (DuBois 1906, as cited in Graves 1998, p. 7). But where did this critical consciousness arise from? What prompted it? In DuBois's mind, it was education – a tool that could be used to empower, certainly, but could also be used to stir dissatisfaction and discontent that might then be used to alter the very social fabric of the societies in which one resided (Graves 1998).

It is here that we see the true emergence of DuBois's educational theory focused on educational equity; in his maturity obtained through education and life experience, he determined that education designed for Black people would empower them and enable them to transform American society (Graves 1998). He was fully cognizant of the "Great Fear" that his emancipatory education system would incite in the northern European-centric society that had firmly established itself in the US, but believed the only way to equity was through education. As Graves (1998) eloquently stated: "For DuBois, it was possible for the school to serve as a vehicle for empowerment, but not without struggle" (p. 7).

These ideas well predated the work of Paulo Freire, who is often the first to be brought up in a discussion of critical pedagogy or the concept of critical theory. For those, then, who are willing to go deeper into the historical origins of both these ideas and truly understand what they were intended to do, you must be fully open to the idea that DuBois was likely the true progenitor of critical pedagogy (a teaching approach where educators encourage students to consider, deeply think about, and critique structures of power and oppression), which cannot truly exist without the idea of critical theory, or the importance of using education to help students become aware of and question society's status quo.

Lasting Legacy

Although there are those who argue – and support such arguments – that DuBois's work is firmly situated in the stance that focuses on the work of Black men to the detriment of Black women (Harvey 1998), his legacy should not be denied. Perhaps it is concerning that DuBois chose to eschew the work of Black women during his time, or perhaps it is, in contradiction to his own educational theory, simply a sign of the times in which he was raised. Regardless, Graves (1998), argues convincingly that DuBois and one of his contemporaries, Carter G. Woodson, theorized the concept of critical pedagogy (without calling it such) well before Paulo Freire would do so (and become spectacularly famous and popular as a result). Both had a strong belief that education had the power to transform, with DuBois, as you just read, particularly believing that through education European Americans could be turned away from racist behavior (Graves 1998).

You will see, as you continue to read through the remainder of this section, that Grave's argument certainly rings true, though there are some major differences between DuBois, Freire, and eventually hooks when it comes to the details of critical pedagogy and its sister, critical theory. But all have in common the idea that education should be more than just a deposition of information; it should also be a tool that provides a path to freedom – from racism, sexism, inequitable cultural norms – anything that keeps students locked in a cage of someone else's making. It is this, then, that truly should be part of DuBois's lasting legacy. The color of his skin will always be discussed and viewed as the unique aspect of his educational life, but it is with hope that you go beyond this to see that while his race was important, the ideas he had about education and its purposes are the pieces that should determine his historical stature; his brown skin should only be an aside.

Part 4: Paulo Freire [1921–1997]

Katherine Fogelberg

Introduction, Historical Context, and Influences

Paulo Reglus Neves Freire was born in Brazil in 1921, just a few decades after slavery was officially abolished in 1888 and almost 100 years after Brazil gained its independence from Portugal (Díaz n.d.). The Portuguese colonization was harsh on the country's indigenous people, many of whom died due to forced labor and/or foreign disease, with those who lived being enslaved to work in sugar mills (Díaz n.d.). Sadly, so many of the indigenous people died during colonization that the Portuguese turned to the purchase of African slaves to run their sugar mills, producing Brazil's primary economic export during the 300-plus years of Portugal's control of the country (Díaz n.d.).

Because very few Portuguese moved to Brazil during their centuries of control, the vast majority of the Brazilian population was of Indigenous and African descent, who were kept illiterate for most of that time and viewed merely as cogs in the machine of an economy working to keep pace with some rival European countries (Díaz n.d.). In gaining independence from Portugal in the early nineteenth century, Brazil did finally achieve some significant economic growth, but it would not consistently continue (Díaz n.d.). In fact, during the mid-twentieth century, economic hardships caused many farmers to sell themselves or their family members into slavery to avoid starvation (Díaz n.d.).

It was into this world that Paulo Freire was born, and it was this history, both personal and cultural, which would shape him and his work. He experienced crippling hunger as a child growing up during the economic depression of the 1930s, made worse by the loss of his father during this same time (Díaz n.d.; Freire and Vittoria 2007; Gadotti and Torres 2009). Forced by circumstances to steal food for himself and his family, he ended up leaving elementary school to work so he could help support his family financially (Díaz n.d.). Living this reality provided Freire a connection to the poor that was never broken; one that would shape his desire to improve the conditions of marginalized people throughout his life (Díaz n.d.). Eventually, Freire would manage to finish elementary school and later attend secondary school (Díaz n.d.).

As with so many successful people, Freire had many individuals in his life who significantly influenced him, including his family and several key educators in his early years. Though he lost his father when he was just 13 years old, his mother continued to raise him and his three siblings in a tolerant and loving home (Díaz n.d.). His preschool teacher, Eunice Vasconcelos, instilled in him a love of learning and helped him view school as a place where his curiosity could be explored (Díaz n.d.). And his principal at secondary school, who allowed Freire to study in spite of his inability to pay tuition as long as he committed to being a good student (and who was the father of his future second wife, Ana Maria Araújo Freire), had a significant and lasting impact on Freire the student (Freire and Vittoria 2007; Díaz n.d.). It was at this same secondary school where Freire would begin teaching Portuguese classes in 1942 to repay the kindness, and where he would teach Ana long before she would become his wife (Freire and Vittoria 2007). Ana (called Nita by Paulo) earned her own Doctor of Education degree from the Pontificia Universidade Católica de São Paulo in Brazil; her discussion with Paolo Vittoria, published in 2007, is a peek into his work and mind from someone who knew him very well.

Freire completed his law degree in his hometown law school, graduating in 1947, although he would never practice law, instead choosing to teach; a calling he had started during his studies as a secondary school student (Gadotti and Torres 2009; Díaz n.d.; New World Encyclopedia 2022). He also began working in the Division of Public Relations, Education, and Culture at a government agency known as the Serviço Social da Indústria (SESI), whose goal was to provide health, housing, education, and leisure services to the Brazilian working class (Freire and Vittoria 2007; Gadotti and Torres 2009; Díaz n.d.).

During his 10-year tenure with the SESI, Freire discovered that working-class parents were raising their children in an authoritarian environment replete with harsh physical punishment that appeared to alienate them from each other (Díaz n.d.). He saw this reflected in the teachers' approach to teaching, as well, all of which was in direct contrast to his own upbringing and schooling. Concerned about the disconnect between children, teachers, and parents, Freire engaged in teaching parents and teachers less authoritarian approaches to disciplining children with hopes that student experiences would improve and help increase learning (Díaz n.d.).

Freire's work experiences with the SESI would be the basis for his doctoral studies and dissertation research at the University of Recife and would lay the groundwork for *Pedagogy of the Oppressed*, while simultaneously establishing himself as a progressive educator (Freire and Vittoria 2007; Díaz n.d.). Alongside his first wife, Elza Maia Costa de Oliveira [1924–1986], whom he married in 1944 and had five children with, he initially began working with the Catholic Action Movement, where he developed his methods for addressing illiteracy through applied research (New World Encyclopedia 2022; Gadotti and Torres 2009; Apple et al. 2001; Díaz n.d.). Although they would eventually leave the Catholic organization due to concerns about the contradictions between the lifestyles of its members and the faith they professed to adhere to, Freire and Elza continued to build their own programs and provide services through them, continuing their work aimed at increasing adult literacy in Brazil (New World Encyclopedia 2022; Apple et al. 2001; Díaz n.d.). In 1959, Freire completed and published his doctoral dissertation, titled *Educacão e Actualidade Brazileira* (*Present-day Education in Brazil*).

Commitment to Improving Adult Literacy

Rooted in his own experiences and understandings of the impacts that poverty and hunger had on learning, Freire committed himself early to teaching impoverished adults – mainly peasants in rural northeastern Brazil – how to read (Apple et al. 2001; Díaz n.d.), and it was through this work that he would come to prominence in his own country. As an educator, he also gained rapid notoriety on a global scale through the adult literacy programs he developed, where his core ideas about critical education would emerge (Apple et al. 2001; Freire and Vittorio 2007). These ideas included his belief that learning should be about cooperative decision-making, social participation, and political responsibility; the importance of learners understanding their social problems and discovering themselves as creative agents; and education extending beyond mastering knowledge and skills for professional gain – in other words, education was about more than learning information, it was also about developing as a responsible and informed citizen (Gadotti and Torres 2009; Díaz n.d.). While perhaps not completely new, they certainly were different from the presiding approaches to education in Brazil during the time – of theorists covered in this text, you should see echoes of Dewey in particular, and recognize Freire's ideas and actions as being aligned with the constructivist approach to education in general.

However, there were many intellectuals who influenced Freire's work in and thinking on education, including theorists and philosophers G. W. Hegel, Karl Marx, Anísio Teixeira, John Dewey, Albert Memmi, Erich Fromm, Frantz Fanon, and Antonio Gramsci (Díaz n.d.). Philosophically, existentialism, phenomenology, Christianity, Marxism, and humanism left their marks on him, particularly humanism, according to his second wife, Ana Freire, whom he affectionately called "Nita" (Freire and Vittorio 2007; Díaz n.d.). But he was a true lifelong learner; one who was continually open to intellectual challenges, self-criticism, and a willingness to reconsider his assumptions (Freire and Vittoria 2007; Schugurensky 1998). As such, Freire's early influences remained but would later be added to through postcolonial theory and critical race theory, feminism, and postmodernism (Schugurensky 1998).

In 1961, Freire was asked by the mayor of his home city, Recife, to help develop city programs focused on improving and encouraging literacy of working-class Brazilians, fostering a climate of democracy, and preserving indigenous culture (Gadotti and Torres 2009; Díaz n.d.). Here he was presented with an opportunity to put theories into action, and he did so with resounding success: using what he termed "circles of culture" (to avoid using the term "illiterate, which he felt was pejorative), he taught 300 sugarcane workers to read and write in just 45 days through use of student–coordinator (rather than teacher) conversations, allowing the learners to use their own experiences to help them become literate rather than asking them to learn from traditional reading primers (Gadotti and Torres 2009; Díaz n.d.). It was not just literacy that Freire was aiming for through his educational practice, however; he was also committed to instilling political awareness in his students through both his content and his methods because he ultimately wanted his students to view education as a path to liberation rather than domestication (Díaz n.d.).

In 1961, the populist leader João Goulart was elected president of Brazil and his political stance emboldened a variety of student groups, unions, and peasant leagues, even while an increasing communist presence was emerging (Díaz n.d.). Goulart fully supported Freire after the success of his original literacy experiment, and between June 1963 and March 1964, Freire and his team trained all who were interested in teaching adult literacy in hopes of establishing teaching literacy to five million adults within just two years (Freire and Vittorio 2007; Díaz n.d.). Thousands of his circles of culture were indeed created, and while Freire's goal was not fully reached, he was certainly well on his way before he was interrupted by a coup (Gadotti and Torres 2009).

On 1 April 1964, the Goulart administration was overthrown by the Brazilian military with support from the US (Gadotti and Torres 2009; Díaz n.d.). Subsequently, Recife's mayor was arrested, Freire was removed from his position and his teaching materials were confiscated; Freire himself was interrogated and accused of being a communist (Díaz n.d.; Gadotti and Torres 2009). Subsequently, he would spend about 70 days (the specific number is not clearly reported) in jail, where he would begin writing *Educação como Practica da Liberdade* (Education as the Practice of Freedom), his first book, though it would not be published until 1967, while he was living in Chile (Gadotti and Torres 2009; Díaz n.d.). Ultimately, the new military-controlled government decided that Freire's literacy project was subversive and cut all its funding (Gadotti and Torres 2009; Díaz n.d.). Although Freire was released from jail, he and his family were exiled for the remainder of 1964 through his return to Brazil in 1980; he settled first in Bolivia and then moved to Chile, where he picked up his work of teaching adult literacy to Chilean farmers (Schuguerensky 1998; Gadotti and Torres 2009; Díaz n.d.).

Inspired by his work with both the Brazilian and Chilean peasants, Freire realized that literacy itself was not liberating; many he worked with were landowners, yet even they did not consider themselves "free" (Gadotti and Torres 2009; Díaz n.d.). Armed with this new insight, Freire turned toward helping his students discover themselves as human beings; he wanted his students to have agency as individuals, members of a community, and culture creators (Díaz n.d.).

Conscientização

It is the combination of Freire's childhood experiences, his work with peasant farmers in various South American countries, the influences of his prodigious knowledge of other educational theories and philosophies, and his commitment to improving adult literacy that provided the content and inspiration for his second, and probably most well-known and important book, *Pedagogy of the Oppressed*. First published in 1968 in Portuguese, it became known quickly around the world and is now considered a foundational text in many education studies programs (Schuguerensky 1998; Gadotti and Torres 2009). It has been translated into over 40 languages and recently celebrated its 50th anniversary, with over one million English language copies sold since its translation in 1970 and another 750,000-plus sold worldwide.

It is in *Pedagogy of the Oppressed* that Freire fully forms his experiences and encapsulates his reasons for education in a single term: *conscientização* (pronounced con-scene-che-**zess**-o) or, in loose translation, *critical consciousness*. Conscientização is what happens when a person learns to perceive social, political, and economic contradictions and then, illuminated by this understanding, takes action to overcome their oppressive elements. It is this term that caused this book to be banned by many, himself to be banned from entering several countries in Latin America and Africa, inspired many in education and nongovernmental organizations, resulted in socialist-oriented governments, and incited revolutions (Schuguerensky 1998). It is also this term that has immortalized Freire in the pantheon of highly influential educational theorists.

Freire was not the first to oppose the "banking model" of education – that model was made popular by the positivist movement and behaviorist learning theory in the early 1900s. But he was the first to explicitly connect power and oppression to this banking model in a manner that resonated with the world. In his reflections on his own practices as a teacher who engaged in such an approach, he came to understand that in viewing education and delivering information to students this way, he was unwittingly modeling the behaviors of "an oppressive society in which to be is merely to have" (Schugurensky 1998, p. 19).

In Freire's mind, to counteract this oppression, a new form of teaching needed to occur; one that was emancipatory, based on co-intentionality between teachers and students, critical thinking, and a desire to effect transformative social change (Schugurensky 1998). This shift from a teacher-centered to a learner-centered pedagogy should remind you of constructivism and the basic tenets of its theoretical approach to learning.

Lasting Impact

Overall, Freire's educational theory of *conscientização* continues to hit a chord with educators – and others – globally. While on the surface his central purpose was the literacy education of rural farmers, the more you learn about Paulo Freire the more you understand how much more there was to his educational thoughts and approaches. His theory of critical consciousness was a result of deep thought, life experiences, keen observations, a willingness to continuously self-reflect, and being open to challenge. Freire was, above all, a humanist – a man who believed that, through education, he could teach marginalized adults that not only did they have value, they had power. He was also a man who believed that in that awakening to power through education, those who rose up against the oppressed must not become the oppressors (Freire 1970). More than anything, Freire wanted all people to be humanized, or liberated, and literacy was the first step in this process.

> Because it is a distortion of being more fully human, sooner or later being less human leads the oppressed to struggle against those who made them so. In order for this struggle to have meaning, the oppressed must not, in seeking to regain their humanity (which is a way to create it), become in turn oppressors of the oppressors, but rather restorers of the humanity of both (Freire 1970, p. 26).

Part 5: bell hooks [1952–2021]

Katherine Fogelberg

Introduction and Overview

Born in Kentucky, Gloria Jean Watkins was one of six children; her father was a janitor and her mother was a maid, and segregated schools were the norm during her younger years (Smith 2022). Raised in a rural town culturally closer to the Midwest than the South, Watkins was an avid reader from a young age, and her reading habit would persist throughout her life. Born just two years before the Supreme Court would strike down school segregation via *Brown v. Board of Education*, Watkins experienced school education in segregated elementary schools and lived through the forced desegregation that occurred after the landmark ruling, graduating from a desegregated high school (hooks 1994; Smith 2022). Desegregation would have a lasting impact on hooks's philosophical views of education, likely both because and in spite of her experiences.

Going to an all-Black school was, for young Gloria Jean, a place where she could be and grow into her fullest self; a place to forget the self who existed at home, where conformity and expectations were placed upon her and she struggled daily to meet those expectations (hooks 1994). Unfortunately, the desegregation of schools ended the joy and zeal of her learning experience; integration forced her to worry only about information, disconnected from life and politics; it became more like home – where obedience and measured responses, docility and acceptance were rewarded, except now she was also being forced to learn that she was genetically inferior, less capable than her White peers, and potentially even unable to learn at all (hooks 1994).

Because of the few Black, and even fewer White, teachers who worked against the biased teaching practices that were the norm, Gloria Jean graduated high school still "believing that education was enabling, that it enhanced [their] capacity to be free," a belief that would be tested time and time again as she continued her educational journey (hooks 1994, p. 4). After earning her high school diploma, she moved to California to attend Stanford University on a scholarship, where she discovered that teachers were not excited to teach and that obedience to authority – rather than education as the practice of freedom – was the primary lesson to be learned (hooks 1994). She began to feel as if the classroom were a place of punishment rather than a place of promise, and it was only her writing – she began her first book, *Ain't I a Woman* (finally published 10 years later, in 1981), at age 19 – and her work as a telephone operator alongside a number of other Black women that sustained her (hooks 1994; Smith 2022).

Watkins earned a Bachelor of Arts in English in 1973 and was accepted to graduate school at the University of Wisconsin–Madison, from which she would earn her Master of Arts in English in 1976. She would move back to California shortly thereafter to attend the University of California, Santa Cruz (UCSC) and completed her PhD in English in 1983, where her dissertation work focused on the works of a prominent Black female author, Toni Morrison (Smith 2022). It was in 1978, however, that she published her first book of poetry, *And There We Wept*, under the pseudonym she would become known by and use for the rest of her life: bell hooks (Glikin 1989).

bell hooks borrowed her pseudonym from her grandmother, Bell Blair Hooks, and used the lowercase lettering of her name deliberately. She did this to honor female legacies, to distinguish her name from her grandmother's, and because she wanted to focus attention on her words and the intensity of her message rather than herself (Smith 2022; Tikkanen 2022b). In the end, her lowercase nomenclature did little to decrease focus on her as Black woman intellectual, though it did uniquely distinguish her from her peers and colleagues.

Academic Life

hooks never wanted to become a teacher; from the time she was young she imagined herself as a writer, but in what she termed the "apartheid South," she knew that "black girls from working-class backgrounds had three career choices. We could marry. We could work as maids. We could become schoolteachers. And since, according to the sexist thinking of the time, men did not really desire 'smart' women, it was assumed that signs of intelligence sealed one's fate. From grade school on, I was destined to become a teacher" (hooks 1994, p. 2).

For hooks, teaching was the job; it was how she would earn her living, but writing would be the real work (hooks 1994). From the time she was a child, she envisioned a life of writing and teaching, which was a fundamentally political act because educating was "rooted in antiracist struggle," and it was in her all-black schools that she would come to understand and experience learning as revolution (hooks 1994, p. 2). Such were the echoes of Freire, bouncing through the walls of hooks' childhood school buildings and countless other all-black schools in the US at the time. And it would be Freire whom she would discover later, coming to view him as a guide and mentor from afar, using "his pedagogical paradigms to critique the limitations of feminist classrooms" (hooks 1994, p. 6).

After graduating with her PhD in English, hooks would continue her academic career at UCSC, this time as a member of the faculty, teaching English and Ethnic Studies; she would go on to teach African and Afro-American studies at Yale in the 1980s, move to Oberlin College to teach women's studies in 1988, City College of New York to teach English in 1995, and Berea College in 2004, where she would end her storied career, having been drawn to the school after delivering their convocation in 1999 (Smith 2022; Tikkanen 2022b; Encyclopedia of World Biography n.d.; https://www.berea.edu/bhc/about-bell/ n.d.). It was at Berea, in her home state of Kentucky, that she would establish the bell hooks institute, and where she would donate her letters, manuscripts, and memorabilia in 2015. And it was in the city of Berea, in her home, where bell hooks would pass away of kidney failure in 2021 – a passing that reverberated throughout the academy and was particularly poignant for me, as I was preparing to travel to my alma mater, Texas Christian University, to hear her speak before I heard the news. I will forever be saddened that her life was so short; I will forever regret that I never had the opportunity to learn from the towering intellectual who was bell hooks.

A Pedagogy of Freedom and a Pedagogy of Hope

In her "pedagogy of freedom," addressed explicitly in hooks's text *Teaching to Transgress*, we see the impetus of hooks' work in the classroom. Her lack of joy in learning throughout her university experiences was rooted in her reality as a Black woman among White professors; even those White female professors developing and teaching within Women's Studies programs were more interested in maintaining the status quo than encouraging students to

critically consider and challenge the concepts presented. This was especially true of Black women students – but hooks was unwilling to accept that the classroom should be about assimilation and obedience; she wanted her students to "be better scholars, to live more fully in the world beyond academe" (hooks 1994, p. 6).

Thus, the first time hooks taught at the undergraduate level, she made a commitment to teaching the way she had been taught by her Black teachers in elementary school rather than the White teachers she had suffered through during high school. She based her approaches to teaching on those experiences, "Freire's work, and on feminist thinking about radical pedagogy" (hooks 1994, p. 7). And she incorporated an idea she found in neither of those – that learning should be fun, never boring – a concept explored in elementary schools and occasionally high schools but not yet reaching the university level (hooks 1994). It was in this first undergraduate teaching experience that hooks would cut her teaching teeth, and her book *Teaching to Transgress* would talk in depth about those experiences, presenting a diverse audience with ideas that resonated with many while making others very angry (hooks 2003).

In 2003, hooks published another volume on teaching, this one titled *Teaching Community: A Pedagogy of Hope*. In its preface, she describes the 10 years of her career since the publication of *Teaching to Transgress* as making connections with teachers and students outside her regular classrooms as she "spent more time teaching teachers and students about teaching than [she] spent in the usual English Department, Feminist Studies, or African-American Studies classroom" (hooks 2003, p. x). But she does not write this grudgingly; indeed, she has now expanded her commitment to teaching students as a means to freedom to include the teaching of educators: "I want all passionate teachers to revel in a job well done to inspire students training to be teachers," she writes (hooks 2003, p. x).

It is in *Teaching Community* that we also see hooks' concerns regarding the "academization of feminism" (p. xii). In her eyes, teaching and the art of teaching needed to be accessible to all; the language used needed to speak not only to those creating educational theory in this space but also to those wanting to use such theories in their classrooms, no matter which grade they were teaching. hooks yearned to achieve academic success – alongside her feminist colleagues – through work that connected teachers through inclusive language, rather than divided them through esoteric, academic, and inaccessible verbiage that was often required to climb the tenure and promotion ladder in academe (hooks 2003).

Published 20 years ago, so many of hooks's observations are keenly relevant today; I suspect at her passing she was saddened by the regressive ideas being forwarded and forcibly implemented in both public and private institutions of learning that are growing even as I write this. Her work in the university classroom that was so powerful and progressive almost 20 years ago is seeing pushback and challenges on a daily basis now, but there is still hope. Hope was evident in her pedagogy, in her activism, in her outspoken commitment to education as a means to liberate, and in her writing. It is stated clearly in her title, addressed squarely in her textbooks, and serves as an amplification of her mentor Paulo Freire's educational theory, whom she never knew but always admired and whose ideas she used to forge her own unique path to educational freedom and success.

Lasting Impact

Those of us who have worked both as teachers and students to transform academia so that the classroom is not a site where domination (on the basis of race, class, gender, nationality, sexual preference, religion) is perpetuated have witnessed positive evolutions in thought and actions. We have witnessed widespread interrogation of white supremacy, race-based colonialism, and sexism xenophobia. . .By making the personal political, many individuals have experienced major transformations in thought that have led to changing their lives: the white people who worked to become antiracist, the men who worked to challenge sexism and patriarchy, heterosexists who begin to truly champion sexual freedom. There have been many quiet moments of incredible shifts in thought and action that are radical and revolutionary. To honor and value these moments rightly we must name them even as we continue rigorous critique" (hooks 2003, pp. xiii–xiv).

It is probably fitting that as I write this, the College Board has announced that its advanced placement course for high school students interested in African American studies has been launched, albeit significantly changed from the original curriculum. One individual in one state that is very politically powerful as of this writing has been leading the charge to erase critical theory and accurate African American history from the textbooks and schools in his state, and while the College Board vows they are not bowing to this political pressure, appearances tell us this is not wholly the truth. Several of the changes made to the originally planned curriculum include the editing out of information presenting "a handful of vital Black thinkers and some important subject matter" (Gay 2023) – removing all references to Ta-Nehisi Coates and, importantly for readers of this text – bell hooks. I have spent many words providing you insights into hooks' background and impact on education, especially higher education. It is with a heavy heart that I see attempts at her erasure already beginning, just two short years after her death.

But, as hooks reminds us in all of her work, education is power, and through education, great – even radical – change can be made. She theorized that education can both oppress and empower and that the teacher gets to choose which way that pendulum swings. hooks believed that education should be fun and engaging from kindergarten through the highest levels of the academy and that teaching students to be critical thinkers and questioners was the ultimate goal. She was a Black critical theorist who believed that the classroom could serve political purposes, but her theories transcend her purposes; do we not want our professional students to critically think and question? To use their knowledge and skills to empower others to care for each other, the planet, and its living beings? hooks's theories are suited for far more than anti-racist activism, as the excerpt above makes clear. Yes, she was an Afro-centric educational theorist, but those who view her work as being relevant only in that domain are missing the bigger implications of her work.

It is impossible to fully summarize hooks's work in this small section of a textbook that covers so many topics. But this last quote from her 2003 text comes close; it encapsulates all that she worked for and against in her life while still demonstrating her passion for learning, leading, and teaching. It tells us that she had, above all else, hope that education could continue to help us evolve, grow, and *transgress* boundaries that are placed upon us; a hope that can and should be taught to every student in every classroom. It reminds us that though much work has been done, there is still much to be done. And it reminds us that, above all, education is about more than acquiring pieces of information; it is about learning to think, question, and take action in ways that preserve hope and propel us toward equality while understanding that the hard work is never done.

Summary

From the late 1800s to now, this chapter outlines the ebb and flow of the Big Three educational theories, their little brother (who hangs around and influences them sometimes overtly and other times slyly), as well as the theorists who contributed significantly to each. It provides brief summaries of major educational theorists who were instrumental in supporting and forwarding each theory and gives you a glimpse into, in many cases, the experiences and influences that each theorist came to their understanding with. Additionally, it gives you a strong foundation for exploring more deeply any and all theories and theorists presented here if you so desire, and the language to explore theories and theorists *not* explored here that you might find in your search for additional information.

The chapter ends with a foray into educational theorists of note who are not always acknowledged or explored as deeply as those appearing earlier in the chapter. The idea of education as a political process has always been argued against; schools are ostensibly places of learning, not places of lobbying. However, the four educational theorists highlighted in the last section demonstrate that this is not true; education is, indeed, political, no matter how much we say it is not. When compared and contrasted with behaviorism, cognitivism, and constructivism, theories of educational equity may appear to be more calls to action than learning theories. The former were seeking to determine how individuals learn through observation and hypothesizing about how children absorb information and demonstrate a change as a result; the latter were seeking to determine how that learning effects change at the individual and *societal* levels, flipping the script a bit from the original ideas about learning. These theories are not, as you likely figured out early in your reading of this chapter, mutually exclusive. Nor do they have specific lines of demarcation between them, and this is true of all the theories explored in this chapter, not just the more traditional ones that are leaned upon heavily in the early parts.

There is a lot of material covered in these pages and, combined with the first chapter that introduces you to the philosophy of education, your head may be spinning. This is perfectly reasonable, and you are certainly not alone – much of the information is quite dense and potentially quite new to many of you. It is my hope that it is not so dense that you found yourself having to rest your head on the keyboard and massage your temples as you worked to absorb the information. On the other hand, if you breezed through the information without having to think hard about or look up something here and there, the goal to challenge has not been met, either.

If it helps, you may rest assured that writing this chapter has been a challenge I was not fully prepared to take on when I imagined this textbook; I had high hopes that others with more understanding and insights than I in this area of education would be willing and able to step in and shoulder the burden. It was not to be the case, and while I have struggled to write this chapter, perhaps it is better that it worked out this way; I have learned a ton in my reading (including that I need to do more reading!), and come to realize that I understand educational theories slightly better than I thought but not quite well enough to consider myself fully capable of doing a chapter like this justice. Please know that I have done my very best. I hope that you have found something within it that inspired some thoughtful moments, caused you to do some self-reflection, and/or left you with some answers to questions you may not have realized you had, while moving you to ask some new questions you never thought you would need to ask.

References

Acton, H.B. (1951). Comte's positivism and the science of society. *Philosophy* 26 (99): 291–310. https://www.jstor.org/stable/3747190.

Al-Shammari, A., Faulkner, P.E., and Forlin, C. (2019). Theories-based inclusive education practices. *Education Quarterly Reviews* 2 (2): 408–414.

American Psychological Association (2010). Little Albert experiment. https://www.apa.org/monitor/2010/01/little-albert (accessed 21 September 2022).

Anzaldúa, G. (1987/2007)*Borderlands/La frontera: The New Mestiza*. San Francisco, CA: Aunt Lute Books.

Anzaldúa, G.E. (2000). *Interviews/entrevistas*. New York, NY: Routledge.

Anzaldúa, G. (2021). *Borderlands / la frontera: The new Mestiza* (ed. R.F. Vivancos-Pérez and N.E. Cantú). Aunt Lute Books.

Anzaldúa, G. and Keating, A. (ed.) (2002/2013)*This Bridge We Call Home: Radical Visions for Transformation*. New York, NY: Routledge.

Apple, M., Gandin, L.A., and Hypolito, A.M. (2001). Paulo Freire. In: *Fifty Modern Thinkers on Education: From Piaget to the Present* (ed. J.A. Palmer), 128–132. New York, NY: Routledge.

Ardichvili, A. (2001). Lev Semyonovich Vygotsky. In: *Fifty Modern Thinkers on Education: FromPiaget to the Present* (ed. J.A. Palmer), 33–37. New York, NY: Routledge.

Bandura, A. (1971). *Social Learning Theory*. New York City, NY: General Learning Press.

Beatty, B. (1998). From laws of learning to a science of values: efficiency and morality in Thorndike's educational psychology. *American Psychologist* 53 (10): 1145–1152.

Berea College. (n.d.). Get to know bell hooks: bell and the World. https://www.berea.edu/bhc/about-bell/ (accessed 3 February 2023).

Bernicot, J. (1994). Speech acts in young children: Vygotsky's contribution. *European Journal of Psychology of Education* IX (4): 311–319.

Biesta, G.J.J. (2013). On the idea of educational theory. In: *The Handbook of Educational Theories* (ed. B.J. Irby, G. Brown, R. Lara-Alecio, and S. Jackson), 5–15. Charlotte, NC: Information Age Publishing, Inc.

Boeree, C.G. (1997). Jean Piaget: 1896–1980. http://webspace.ship.edu/cgboer/perscontents.html (accessed 29 December 2022).

Boghossian, P. (2006). Behaviorism, constructivism, and socratic pedagogy. *Educational Philosophy and Theory* 38 (6): 713–722.

Broderick, F.L. (1958). The academic training of W.E.B. DuBois. *The Journal of Negro Education* 27 (1): 10–16.

Bruner, J. (2004). Psychological theories of learning. *Daedalus* 133 (1): 13–20.

Burnett, A. (1962). Montessori education today and yesterday. *The Elementary School Journal* 63 (2): 71–77. https://www.jstor.org/stable/1000044.

Clark, K.R. (2018). Learning theories: cognitivism. *Radiologic Technology* 90 (2): 176–179.

Costley, K.C. (2012). An overview of the life, central concepts, including classroom applications, of Lev Vygotsky. https://files.eric.ed.gov/fulltext/ED529565.pdf (accessed 02 January 2023).

Cozolino, L. and Sprokay, S. (2006). Neuroscience and adult learning. In: *New Directions for Adult and Continuing Education*, no. 110, 11–19. Wiley InterScience.

Dastpak, M., Behjat, F., and Taghinezhad, A. (2017). A comparative study of Vygotsky's perspectives on child language development within nativism and behaviorism. *International Journal of Languages' Education and Teaching* 5 (2): 230–238. https://doi.org/10.18298/ijlet.1748.

DeVries, R. (2000). Vygotsky, Piaget, and education: a reciprocal assimilation of theories and educational practices. *New Ideas in Psychology* 18 (2000): 187–213.

Dewey, J. (1896). The reflex arc concept in psychology. *The Psychological Review* 3 (4): 357–370.

Dewey, J. (1910). *How We Think*. Boston, MA: D.C. Heath & Co.

Dewey, J. (1916). *Democracy and education*. In: *John Dewey: The Collected Works of John Dewey*, 20–461. Pergamonmedia.

Dewey, J. (1938). *Experience and Education*. McMillan: New York, NY.

Díaz, Kim. (n.d.). Paulo Freire. *Internet Encyclopedia of Philosophy*. https://iep.utm.edu/freire/ (accessed 29 January 2023).

DuBois, W.E.B. (1932). Education and work. *The Journal of Negro Education* 87 (3): 202–216.

Duignan, B. (2022). Jean Piaget: Swiss psychologist. *Encyclopedia Britannica online*. https://www.britannica.com/biography/Jean-Piaget (accessed 29 Decmber 2022).

Encyclopedia of World Biography. (n.d.). bell hooks biography. https://www.notablebiographies.com/He-Ho/Hooks-Bell.html (accessed 25 January 2023).

Flavell, J.H. (1996). Piaget's legacy. *Psychological Science* 7 (4): 200–203.

Freire, P. (1970). *Pedagogy of the Oppressed*, translated by Myra Bergman Ramos. London, England: Penguin Books.

Freire, A.M.A. and Vittoria, P. (2007). Dialogue on Paolo Freire. *Interamerican Journal of Education for Democracy* 1 (1): 1–21.

Gadotti, M. and Torres, C.A. (2009). Paulo Freire: education for development. *Development and Change* 40 (6): 1255–1267.

Galef, B.G. (1998). Edward Thorndike: revolutionary psychologist, ambiguous biologist. *American Psychologist* 53 (10): 1128–1134. https://doi.org/10.1037/0003-066X.53.10.1128.

Gardner, H. (2001). Jerome S. Bruner. In: *Fifty Modern Thinkers on Education: From Piaget to the Present* (ed. J.A. Palmer), 90–96. New York, NY: Routledge.

Garnham, A. (2019). *Cognitivism*, 2e. London, England: The Routledge Company.

Gay, M. (2023). Erasing Black history is not the role of the College Board. *New York Times* (4 February).

Glikin, R. (1989). *Black American Women in Literature: A Bibliography, 1976 through 1987*, vol. 10. Jefferson, NC: McFarland & Company.

Gouinlock, J.S. (2022). John Dewey: American philosopher and educator. https://www.britannica.com/biography/John-Dewey (Accessed 2 January 2023).

Graham, G. (2019). Behaviorism. https://plato.stanford.edu/entries/behaviorism/#ThreTypeBeha (accessed 21 December 2022).

Graves, K.L. (1998). Outflanking oppression: African American contributions to critical pedagogy as developed in the scholarship of W.E.B. DuBois and Carter G. Woodson. *Paper presented at the Annual Meeting of the American Educational Research Association*, 13–17 April 1998, San Diego, CA: American Educational Research Association.

Growe, R. and Montgomery, P.S. (2003). Educational equity in America: is education the great equalizer? *The Professional Educator* XXV (2): 23–29.

Hagen, P. (2005). Theory building in academic advising. *NACADA Journal* 25 (2): 3–8.

Harvey, R. (1998). W.E.B. DuBois and the question of Black women intellectuals. *Philosophy of Education* 401–403. https://educationjournal.web.illinois.edu/archive/index.php/pes/article/view/2139.pdf.

Hinchey, P.H. (2010). Chapter three: Rethinking what we know: Positivist and constructivist epistemology. *Counterpoints* 24: 33–55. http://www.jstor.org/stable/42976884.

hooks, b. (1994). *Teaching to Transgress: Education as the Practice of Freedom*. New York, NY: Routledge.

hooks, b. (2003). *Teaching Community: A Pedagogy of Hope*. New York, NY: Routledge.

Jaeger, A.J., Dunstan, S., Thornton, A.B. et al. (2013). Put theory into practice. *About Campus* 12–15. https://doi.org/10.1002/abc.21100.

Jensen, E. and McConchie, L. (2020). *Brain-Based Learning: Teaching the Way Students Really Learn*, 3e. Thousand Oaks, CA: Corwin Press.

Johnson, D. (2000). W.E.B. Dubois, Thomas Jesse Jones and the struggle for social education, 1900-1930. *The Journal of Negro History* 85 (3): 71–95.

Johnston, D. (2000). W.E.B. DuBois, Thomas Jesse Jones and the struggle for social education, 1900–1930. *The Journal of Negro History* 85 (3): 71–95.

Kagan, J. (2000). Foreword. In: *The Psychology of the Child* (ed. J. Piaget and B. Inhelder). Translated from the French by Helen Weaver. The definitive work of the great psychologist's work, ix–viv.

Keating, A. (2009). *The Gloria Anzaldúa Reader*. Durham, NC: Duke UP.

Knowland, V.C.P. and Thomas, M.S.C. (2014). Educating the adult brain: how the neuroscience of learning can inform educational policy. *International Review of Education* 60: 99–122.

Kurbegovic, E. (2022, December 22). Education. https://eugenicsarchive.ca/discover/encyclopedia/54668bd62432860000000001.

Lasley II, T.J. (2022). Bloom's taxonomy. *Encyclopedia Britannica*. https://www.britannica.com/topic/Blooms-taxonomy#ref1200717.

Merriam, S.B. (2008). Adult learning theory for the twenty-first century. In: *New Directions for Adult and Continuing Education*, no. 119, 93–98. Wiley InterScience.

Montessori, M. (1912/2012)*The Montessori Method: Scientific Pedagogy as Applied to Child Education in "The Children's Houses" with Additions and Revisions by the Author*. (A.E. George, Tans.). Frederick A Stokes Company. https://doi.org/10.1037/13054-000.

Montessori, M.M. Jr. (1976). The Contribution of Maria Montessori. In: *Education for Human Development: Understanding Montessori* (ed. P.P. Lillard), 1–16. New York, NY: Schocken Books.

New World Encyclopedia (2022). Paulo Freire. https://www.newworldencyclopedia.org/entry/Paulo_Freire (accessed 16 December 2022).

Okpala, C.O. and Ellis, R. (2005). The perceptions of college students on teacher quality: a focus on teacher qualifications. *Education* 126 (2): 374–383.

Ozdem-Yilmaz, Y. and Bilican, K. (2020). Discovery learning-Jerome Bruner. In: *Science Education in Theory and Practice: An Introductory Guide to Learning Theory* (ed. B. Apkan and T.J. Kennedy), 177–190. Cham, Switzerland: Springer Texts in Education.

Piaget, J. (1955). *The Construction of Reality in the Child: The Elaboration of the Universe (Conclusion)*, M Cook (transl). Routledge and Kegan Paul. https://www.marxists.org/reference/subject/philosophy/works/fr/piaget2.htm.

Piaget, J. (1962). The relation of affectivity to intelligence in the mental development of the child. *Bulletin of the Menninger Clinic* 26 (3): 129–137.

Piaget, J. (1964). Part I: Cognitive development in children: Piaget: development and learning. *Journal of Research in Science Teaching* 2: 176–186.

Piaget, J. and Inhelder, B. (1969/2000)*The Psychology of the Child*. New York, NY: Basic Books, Inc.

Pavlov, I. (1967). *Nobel Lectures, Physiology or Medicine 1901-1921*. Amsterdam: Elsevier Publishing Company. noeblprize.org.

Puma, M., Bell, S., Cook, R., et al. (2010). Head Start Impact Study. Final report. Published by the U.S. Department of Health and Human Services, Administration of Children and Families, 1–35.

Rannikmae, M., Holbrook, J., and Soobard, R. (2020). Social constructivism – Jerome Bruner. In: *Science Education in Theory and Practice: An Introductory Guide to Learning Theory* (ed. B. Apkan and T.J. Kennedy), 259–275. Cham, Switzerland: Springer Texts in Education.

Rudwick, E. (2023). W.E.B. DuBois: American sociologist and social reformer. https://www.britannica.com/biography/W-E-B-Du-Bois (accessed 11 January 2023).

Samelson, F. (1981). Struggle for the scientific authority: the reception of Watson's behaviorism, 1913–1920. *Journal of the History of the Behavioral Sciences* 17: 399–425.

Schneider, S.M. and Morris, E.K. (1987). A history of the term *radical behaviorism*: from Watson to Skinner. *The Behavior Analyst* 10 (1): 27–39.

Schugurensky, D. (1998). The legacy of Paulo Freire: a critical review of his contributions. *Convergence* 31 (1/2): 17–28.

Skinner, B.F. (1959). John Broadus Watson, behaviorist. *Science* 129 (3343): 197–198.

Skinner, B.F. (1963). Behaviorism at fifty. *Science* 140 (3570): 951–958.

Smidt, S. (2009). *Introducing Vygotsky: A Guide for Practitioners and Students in Early Years Education*. London, England: Routledge https://doi.org/10.4324/9781315824185.

Smith, L. (2001). Jean Piaget. In: *Fifty Modern Thinkers on Education: From Piaget to the Present* (ed. J.A. Palmer), 37–44. New York, NY: Routledge.

Smith, C. (2022). bell hooks (1952–2021). *History in the Making* 15 (11): 205–227.

Takaya, K. (2008). Jerome Bruner's theory of education: from early Bruner to late Bruner. *Interchange* 39 (1): 1–19. https://doi.org/10.1007/s10780-008-9039-2.

Thayer-Bacon, B. (2012). Maria Montessori, John Dewey, and William H. Kirkpatrick. *Education and Culture* 28 (1): 3–20. https://doi.org/10.1353/eac.2012.0001.

Thorndike, E.L. (1910). The contribution of psychology to education. *The Journal of Educational Psychology* 1: 5–12.

Tikkanen, A. (2022a). Maria Montessori: Italian educator. *Encyclopedia Brittanica online*. https://www.britannica.com/biography/Maria-Montessori (accessed 31 December 2022).

Tikkanen, A. (2022b). bell hooks: American scholar. *Encyclopedia Brittanica online.* https://www.britannica.com/biography/bell-hooks (accessed 3 February 2023).

Tomlinson, S. (1997). Edward Lee Thorndike and John Dewey on the science of education. *Oxford Review of Education* 23 (3): 365–383.

Tsubaki, M. and Matsuishi, T. (2008). On the pedagogical theory of Maria Montessori. *Journal Of Disability and Medico-Pedagogy* 18: 1–4.

Van der Veer, R. (2007). *Lev Vygotsky.* London, England: Continuum. Bloomsbury.

Vasconcelos, J. (1958). *La raza cósmica: misión de la raza iberoamericana,* 19. Barcelona: Agencia mundial de librería.

Vygotsky, L.S. (1978). Interaction between learning and development. In: *Readings on the Development of Children* (ed. M. Gauvain and M. Cole), 34–40. New York, NY: Scientific American Books.

Watson, J.B. (1925). Behaviorism: A psychology based on reflexes. Presented at the fifty-first annual meeting of the American Neurological Association, Washington, DC: Archives of Neurology & Psychiatry. https://jamanetwork.com.

Watson, J.B. (1994). Psychology as the behaviorist views it. *Psychological Review* 101 (2): 248–253. Originally printed in 1913, 20: 158-177.

Watson, R. and Coulter, J. (2008). The debate over cognitivism. *Theory, Culture & Society* 25 (2): 1–17.

Weegar, M. and Pacis, D. (2012). A comparison of two theories of learning – behaviorism and constructivism as applied to face-to-face and online learning. Open-access online at http://www.g-casa.com/conferences/manila/papers/Weegar.pdf (accessed 03 February 2023).

Williams, M.K. (2017). John Dewey in the 21st century. *Journal of Inquiry & Action in Education* 9 (1): 91–102.

Wortham, S. (2003). Learning in education. In: *Encyclopedia of Cognitive Science Volume 1* (ed. L. Nadel), 1079–1082. New York: Nature Publishing Group.

Yilmaz, K. (2011). The cognitive perspective on learning: its theoretical underpinnings and implications for classroom practices. *The Clearing House* 84 (5): 204–212.

Yountae, A. and Mena, P.A. (2014). Anzaldúa's Animal Abyss: Mestizaje and the Late Ancient Imagination. In: *Divinanimality: Animal Theory, Creaturely Theology* (ed. S.D. Moore), 161–181. Fordham University Press.

Zaytoun, K.D. (2015). "Now Let Us Shift" the subject: tracing the path and posthumanist implications of La Naguala/the shapeshifter in the works of Gloria Anzaldúa. *MELUS: Multi-Ethnic Literature of the United States* 40 (4): 69–88.

3

Cognition and Learning

Peter Doolittle, PhD

Virginia Tech University, School of Education, Blacksburg, VA, USA

Meghan Byrnes, DVM, PhD

Virginia-Maryland College of Veterinary Medicine, Blacksburg, VA, USA

Section 1: Introduction

How do students learn the anatomy and physiology of dogs and cats, cows and horses, and lemurs and dragons? How do students become proficient at typical behavioral procedures such as physical exams, diagnostic testing, and essential surgeries? How do instructors create educational environments that foster long-term, meaningful, and integrated knowledge? These questions are common among veterinary medicine educators and the answer is always the same: **It depends**.

The science of learning and teaching is complicated and has a long history. The modern dawn of the science lies in the late nineteenth and early twentieth centuries, although its historical, educational, ideational, and philosophical roots go back much further. Currently, the science of learning and teaching is often explained through a series of canonical theories of human learning: classical and operant conditioning (behaviorism), social cognitive theory and information processing theory (cognitivism), and the emerging theories associated with cognitive neuroscience. This chapter will focus on cognitivism.

It should be noted, however, that cognitive science is not an "exact" science, as humans tend to be unpredictable and contextually bound, while the brain has yet to give up the wealth of its secrets. As George Ladd, President of the American Psychological Association, stated in the very first issue of *Psychological Review* in 1894, "all human science is but patches of a shallow, superficial stratum, dimly lit through occasional rifts in the clouds, over the fathomless depths of the ocean of reality" (Ladd 1894, p. 8). While Ladd's language is long on metaphor, the intent is clear: there is much yet to learn in human learning science, including cognitive science. Indeed, it is not possible to program a human being the way one might program a computer – the same inputs do not always result in the same outputs. One has only to teach a year or two in the classroom when it becomes apparent that a lesson taught at 10 am may foster significant student learning, while the same lesson taught at 2 pm on the same day, may fall flat. Why? It depends.

While I agree that "it depends" is a wholly unsatisfying refrain, it is accurate. This chapter will address issues of learning, memory, and cognition in general, and how they relate to instruction, in particular. However, it is not possible to state that if an instructor engages veterinary medical students in solving three problems, explaining two concepts, and writing one summary that all students will have learned the relevant content to a deep level – it depends. It will depend on

a) the prior knowledge of the students (i.e., are they novices or experts, is their knowledge well-integrated or fragmented?),
b) the attitudes of the students (i.e., are they fearful or confident in their studies, are they more likely to persistent in the presence of failure or give up?),
c) the engagement of the students (i.e., are they learning rotely or meaningfully, are they thinking and interacting actively or passively and individually or socially?),
d) the nature of the instruction (i.e., is it alienating or engaging, are the students motivated to engage with the learning process?), and,
e) the structure of the content itself (i.e., is the content simple or complex, is the content focused on concepts, procedures, or both?).

Guidelines for learning and teaching always have an "it depends" asterisk because the effectiveness of guidelines always depends on the interactions between the students, the learning environment, and the content.

Finally, and with the greatest emphasis, "it depends" necessitates that instructors maintain an active role in the education of their students. Who knows best the students' backgrounds, prior knowledge, and dispositions; the contents' structure, relationships, and importance; and the instructions' purpose, organization, and delivery? The instructor does. It is the instructors who must make the application of the cognitive theories and findings to their classrooms, labs, and clinics, as well as informal discussions. As the psychologist William James (1899, p. 10), stated regarding the application of psychological theory to educational practice: "An intermediary inventive mind must make the application, by using its originality" – that is you.

Part 1: A Framework

The history of cognitive science is replete with experimental studies demonstrating that there is a relationship between how we think about our experiences (processing) and what we ultimately learn and can do (performance). This processing–performance relationship can be thought of as a framework designed to organize these various experimental findings into a coherent approach to the understanding of learning and the development of instruction. Frameworks are like theories in organization and purpose, but different in that they may be less systematic and less neat and tidy in representing a field. In this chapter, the processing–performance framework will be represented using the following mantra: **What we process we learn.**

Perhaps the best representation of this processing–performance framework is the concept of **depth of processing** proposed by Craik and Lockhart. In their framing paper (Craik and Lockhart 1972; see also Zinchenko 1939), they proposed that the *deeper* we process experiences, the better we remember them. This "depth" is represented by a continuum where processing can be shallower, based on superficial sensory or physical characteristics (attributes), or deeper, based on pattern recognition and meaning making (semantics).

This depth of processing concept was addressed empirically by Craik and Tulving (1975), who asked students to process words based on an *orienting question* designed to foster shallower or deeper processing. Specifically, participants were asked to answer one of three types of questions upon the presentation of a word: *case* questions (Is the word in capital letters?), *rhyme* questions (Does the word rhyme with _____?), or *sentence* questions (Would the word fit in the sentence: He met a _____ in the street.). A different sentence was provided for each word. The

rationale behind the study was that a *case* question focused on a shallow or superficial (attributes) processing of the word, a *rhyme* question focused on an intermediate or phonetic processing of the word, and a *sentence* question focused on a deep or meaning-based (semantic) processing of the word. After answering a series of questions (e.g., case, rhyme, or sentence) in relation to specific words, participants were asked to either recognize or recall the specific words. What Craik and Tulving found (see Experiment 1) was that participants were able to recognize 16% of the case words, 57% of the rhyme words, and 89% of the sentence words. These findings were interpreted as evidence that the case questions fostered shallower processing resulting in less retention, and the sentence questions fostered deeper processing resulting in more retention. That is, how we process an experience influences what we remember from an experience (what we process we learn).

Over the next 50-plus years the concept of depth of processing (or what is sometimes referred to as levels of processing) has been criticized, lauded, expanded, and refined. Almost immediately upon publication, it was realized that there would be a need for an "index of depth" to determine the depth of processing of a particular task with some specificity (Baddeley 1978). For example, to what degree is analyzing a word for appropriateness in a sentence "deeper" than determining if a word rhymes with another? How do we know that problem-based learning is deeper than the use of flash cards? Unfortunately, such an index never materialized and current depth of processing experiments still use shallow and deep as their metric. Another concern regarding the depth of processing approach occurred when it was demonstrated that learning is not solely a function of the initial learning task (encoding), as proposed by Craik and Lockhart (1972), but rather, is also dependent upon the nature of and relationship to the subsequent performance task (retrieval).

This learning–performance (encoding–retrieval) perspective is evident in the research focusing on **transfer appropriate processing** (see Morris et al. 1977), which demonstrated that when the same type of cognitive processing occurs during both initial learning and subsequent performance, performance is enhanced. For example, Agarwal (2018) had students read eight short passages and immediately complete an initial *fact-based* multiple-choice test for four of the readings and an initial *higher-order-based* multiple-choice test for the other four readings. After a two-day delay, half of the students who initially completed a fact-based test completed a delayed fact-based test, while the other half of the students completed a delayed higher-order-based test. In addition, half of the students who initially completed a higher-order-based test after reading the passages completed a delayed higher-order-based test, while the other half of the students completed a delayed fact-based test. Thus, for some students, their immediate test and their two-day delayed test aligned (fact-based/fact-based, higher-order-based/higher-order-based), while for other students their tests misaligned (fact-based/higher-order-based, higher-order-based/fact-based). Students who initially completed a fact-based test after reading a passage did better when completing a delayed fact-based test (78%) than a delayed higher-order test (46%). Similarly, students who initially completed a higher-order-based test after reading a passage did better when completing a delayed higher-order-based test (72%) than a delayed fact-based test (53%). These results indicated that when the type of cognitive processing was the same during learning and performance, performance was enhanced – aligning of the learning and performance processing matters.

Similar to the transfer appropriate processing research, the research focusing on **encoding specificity** (see Tulving and Thomson 1973), demonstrated that when the same context is present at both initial learning and subsequent performance, performance is enhanced. For example, Godden and Baddeley (1975), had individuals learn lists of words either on land (dry) or underwater (wet) with the assistance of scuba gear, and then later recall the learned words either on land (dry) or underwater (wet). This procedure resulted in four conditions, (i) learned on land, recalled on land (dry, dry), (ii) learned on land, recalled underwater (dry, wet), (iii) learned underwater, recalled underwater (wet, wet), and (iv) learned underwater, recalled on land (wet, dry). Godden and Baddeley found that individuals recalled significantly more words when the learning and recall environments aligned (i.e., dry, dry and wet, wet) than when they misaligned (i.e., dry, wet and wet, dry). These results indicated that when the context was the same during learning and performance, performance was enhanced – aligningof the learning and performance context matters.

Taken together, depth of processing, transfer appropriate processing, and encoding specificity research demonstrates that the depth of processing, type of processing, and context of processing at the time of learning and performance matter. However, these concepts of processing depth, type, and context are not exact. There is no formula that mathematically models the effectiveness of their relationship. *What we process we learn* serves as a guide, a framework, to help understand that examining the nature of the learning process and performance matters. Thus, in general, veterinary students will be able to perform well in the clinic (or operating room) to the degree that their learning occurred in a similar situation, involving similar processing, and to a similar degree. As will be seen, learning and performance are impacted by a plethora of mechanisms and conditions. How? Unfortunately, it depends.

Section 2: Social Cognitive Theory

The intimate relationship between learning and performance is clearly evidenced in social cognitive theory. Social *cognitive* theory grew out of social *learning* theory, which had its roots in behaviorism. **Behaviorism** dominated the theoretical landscape of learning in the early twentieth century. Behaviorism focused on the relationship between an individual's environment (stimulus), their behavior (response, and the subsequent outcome of their behavior consequence). Specifically, for a behaviorist, learning occurs when past experiences (stimulus-response-outcome) increase or decrease the frequency of future behaviors, specifically, when positive behavioral outcomes lead to increases in behavioral frequency (e.g., when a veterinary student answers a question in class and is correct or gets praised, the frequency of their question answering behavior is likely to increase), while negative behavioral outcomes lead to decreases in behavioral frequency (e.g., when a veterinary student studies for a quiz in a noisy café instead of at home where it is quiet and performs poorly, the frequency of their café-studying behavior is likely to decrease). This stimulus–response conditioning is seen as deterministic, that is, the environment causes this change in frequency through the consequences of the response, and not that the individual is *choosing* to engage (more or less) in a particular behavior. For more in-depth discussion about behaviorism, revisit Chapter 2.

In the middle of the twentieth century, through the work of Julian Rotter and, later, Albert Bandura, **social learning theory** emerged. Initially, this work was viewed as an extension of behaviorism but later evolved into an alternative to behaviorism. Rotter proposed "social learning," a theory that involved individuals developing subjective interpretations and values of experiences that then led to expectations for future performance. Specifically, according to Rotter (1954, 1966), individuals developed expectancies based on the relationship between their past behaviors and subsequent outcomes. These behavior–outcome expectancies would then result in an increase in the potential of the individual to engage in that specific behavior if the outcome was previously positive, or a decrease in the potential to engage in that specific behavior if the outcome was previously negative. While this relationship may sound behavioristic – positive behavioral outcomes lead to an increase in the frequency of the behavior – the cause of the relationship had shifted from the environment to the person. It is the individual's psychological beliefs (expectancies) that cause the potential increase (or decrease) in the frequency of the behavior, not the existence of factors present in the environment (stimuli).

In addition to these general behavior–outcome expectancies, an individual engaged in a behavior was also influenced by the individual's perceived locus of control (Rotter 1966). That is, whether the individual believed they were in control of their own success or failure due to their own skills and actions (internal control), or if success or failure was out of their control and due to luck, chance, or others' actions (external control). Thus, from Rotter's social learning theory perspective, engaging in specific actions was influenced by perceptions of previous success or failure (expectancies), as well as whether the individual believed that they were able to cause those successes or failures (locus of control).

Part 1: Human Agency

Rotter's social learning theory served as a bridge between the stimulus–response relationships of behaviorism and the learning–performance relationships of cognitivism. Albert Bandura crossed this bridge, expanding and extending social learning theory in the 1970s, and proposing a new, albeit related, **social cognitive theory** (Bandura 1971, 1986, 1997; Bandura and Cervone 2023). Bandura's social cognitive theory of human learning rests on the concept of *emergent interactive agency* (Bandura 2001a). As explained by Bandura, emergent interactive agency means that humans have control or intentionality when it comes to their own actions (agency), these actions exist within and between individual and social systems (interactive), and, over time, the exercise of this control leads to self-development and adaptation (emergent), thus, "agency refers to acts done intentionally" (p. 7).

Agency itself is the ability of an individual to exhibit control over themselves and their environment: "To be an agent is to influence intentionally one's functioning and life circumstances . . . people are self-organizing, proactive, self-regulating, and self-reflecting" (Bandura 2006, p. 164). Bandura's human agency stands in contrast to the determinist behaviorist view where life is a function under environmental control. It is the intentional nature of agency, with its focus on the regulation and control of one's cognition, behavior, and motivation, which leads to humans playing a functional role in the conduct of their lives.

When Bandura refers to agency, he typically is referring to personal agency, although he defines three types of agency (Bandura 2001a, 2006): personal, proxy, and collective. *Personal agency* represents an individual's ability to influence the course of their own action and environment. Through their own cognitive, behavioral, social, and affective choices, individuals are able to exercise control over the quality and direction of their life. That said, there are times when one would like to move their life in a direction over which they have little direct control. In these cases, an individual may engage in *proxy agency*, where one is able to influence others to act on their own behalf. This socially mediated form of agency relies on others who have the power, resources, and means to assist in the achievement of the individual's desired outcomes. Finally, one may be motivated to impact both their own lives and the lives of others through *collective agency*. In collective agency, goals are achieved only through the socially interdependent efforts of multiple people. These are not a group of randomly acting individuals, but rather, the coordinated and conjoint efforts of individuals who share intentions, knowledge, and skills in the pursuit of common goals.

Part 2: Human Agency and Self-Regulation

Bandura (1986), created a contextual model within which emergent interactive agency exists. For Bandura (2001b), human functioning involves the integration of individual, social, and environmental factors, a codetermination of development, adaptation, and change. Thus, individuals are influenced by their own thoughts and the actions of others, as well as contributing to their social sphere that may in-turn impact others as well.

Bandura called his model, at various times, reciprocal determinism, triadic codetermination theory, and reciprocal causation. **Reciprocal causation** emphasizes the interactional nature of personal, environmental, and behavioral factors on learning and behavior (see Figure 3.1). Specifically, *personal factors* include the learner's physical characteristics (e.g., height, weight, eye color), cognitive characteristics (e.g., knowledge, beliefs, self-efficacy), and social/cultural characteristics (e.g., group membership, social reputation, cultural roles), while *environmental factors* include a situation's physical context characteristics (e.g., building attributes, climate), social context characteristics (e.g., group size, others' attitudes), and response characteristics (e.g., positive outcomes, negative outcomes), and *behavioral factors* include an individual's actions (e.g., performance, habits), expressions (e.g., emotions, demeanor), and verbalization (e.g., explanations, exclamations).

Bandura proposed that the relationships between the three factors – personal, environmental, and behavioral – were bidirectional, although personal factors were seen as having primacy, with external influences affecting

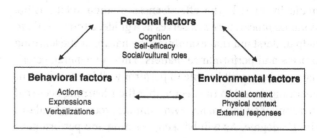

Figure 3.1 Bandura's reciprocal causation and the interaction between personal, environmental, and behavioral factors.

thought and behavior indirectly as the internal factors determine the meaning, importance, and lasting impact of the external influences. Thus, given the interactive nature of reciprocal causation, the proximal causes of one's action depend on the salience and synthesis of the personal, environmental, and behavioral factors: "In human transactions, one cannot speak of 'environment,' 'behavior,' and 'outcomes' as though they were fundamentally different events with distinct features inherent in them" (Bandura 2006, p. 165).

For example, consider Chris, a veterinary student, who volunteers at a small animal veterinary clinic and enjoys interacting with the clients in the clinic. This enjoyment (a personal factor) leads Chris to volunteer in the clinic more often (a behavioral factor), which leads to Chris feeling more confident at the clinic (a personal factor), which leads to Chris being provided additional opportunities within the clinic by the attending veterinarians (an environmental factor) which leads to Chris exhibiting more leadership (a behavioral factor), and so on. Also, consider Dr. Perez, who is discussing risk factors for the progression of renal disease within a class using PowerPoint slides (a behavioral factor) to a group of students (environmental factor). Dr. Perez notices students squinting as they attempt to read the slide's small font and view the slide's small images (an environmental factor), so Dr. Perez makes a mental note (a personal factor) and revises her slides, enlarging the font sizes and images, prior to the next class (a behavioral factor). In both examples, Chris and Dr. Perez are evidencing control (agency) over their lives, choosing to work in the clinic and revising the slides, respectively.

A. Fostering Agency Through Self-Regulation

For Bandura (1986, 2001a, 2018), personal agency is a product of a broad self-regulatory framework. Agency presupposes that individuals have proactive control over their thoughts and actions. This control is governed by the recurring processes of developing expectations, setting challenging goals, and mobilizing one's resources, skills, and knowledge in pursuit of these goals. It is the discrepancy between one's expectations, as expressed in goals, and one's current state, as determined through self-reflection, that motivates one to action. This self-regulatory framework involves four aspects: intentionality, forethought, self-reactiveness, and self-reflectiveness.

1) *Intentionality*. Agency presupposes that humans can self-generate plans to enact future courses of action. Intentionality refers to an individual rationally (as opposed to impulsively) designing and proactively committing oneself to a course of action through *goal setting*. Developing these goals for action involves merging one's desires, values, and strengths with mentally visualizing the possibility of future actions and outcomes. At the planning stage, it is impossible to know the ultimate outcomes of a plan enacted. Individual agency only extends to planning and enacting, as outcomes are beyond one's direct causality. Although, once a plan is enacted, an individual may interpret the outcomes and intentionally reengage with the planning process, a form of self-guidance and self-motivation managed by forethought.

2) *Forethought*. Forethought involves looking ahead in time to consider which courses of action may lead to beneficial outcomes and which to detrimental outcomes. These *outcome expectations* are the amalgam of past experiences resulting in success and failure, current conditions of resources and priorities, and personal efficacy beliefs related to the likelihood of future success or failure (i.e., projected reciprocal causation). This forethought, which may project 10 minutes or 10 years into the future, motivates an individual to move beyond the present, to escape the forces that may be influencing their current behavior, and to intentionally choose and enact a path forward.

3) *Self-Reactiveness*. Although intentionality and forethought may result in a well-defined and highly motivated course of action, influenced by mentally projecting possibilities for success or failure into the future, success is not guaranteed. The benefits of actions are due in part to ongoing self-reactiveness, particularly self-regulation involving consistent and on-going monitoring and evaluation of the current state and progress of one's actions, in relation to one's desired outcomes and personal standards. This self-evaluation provides information upon which to self-regulate one's plans and actions, as well as to sustain internal motivation to act, in continued pursuit of positive outcomes. Thus, agency is a continuous process of self-regulation guided by one's reflective self-consciousness (self-reflectiveness).

4) *Self-Reflectiveness*. While self-reactiveness and self-regulation provide real-time course-of-action correction, self-reflectiveness provides a higher level of self-evaluation focused on long-term, life-scale issues of one's motivations, values, and pursuits. To what degree are one's current life pursuits still valid and aligned with one's values? To what degree is one making progress toward a long-term goal? Overall, are one's collective courses of action being successful in moving one forward? A core aspect of this self-reflective agency is the judgment of one's efficacy in impacting change. This *self-efficacy* belief system, belief in one's ability to successfully engage in specific actions that will yield predictable and positive outcomes, is central to planning, refining, sustaining, and completing a course of action.

Among the mechanisms of personal agency, none is more central or pervasive than people's beliefs in their capability to exercise some measure of control over their own functioning and over environmental events. Efficacy beliefs are the foundation of human agency. Unless people believe they can produce desired results and forestall detrimental ones by their actions, they have little incentive to act or to persevere in the face of difficulties. (Bandura 2001a, p. 1)

Ultimately, self-reflectiveness focuses on an individual's agency in directing the course of one's life.

It should be noted that while listed sequentially, the human agency core features of intentionality, forethought, self-reactiveness, and self-reflectiveness are not linear, but rather integrated in an ongoing lived experience where processing impacts learning. For example, consider a veterinary student with an upcoming equine reproduction test. In demonstrating agency, the student reflects on their past successes and failures related to studying for tests (self-reflectiveness) and develops a plan likely to succeed for their upcoming test studying (intentionality, forethought). The student recognizes that studying in loud, social spaces has been detrimental to their test performance in the past and that studying in a quiet, solitary environment has typically led to success (self-reflectiveness). Therefore, the student elects to study in a small alcove in the library to increase their chances of a successful study session (forethought), as would be evidenced by a successful test performance. In addition, the student recognizes that it would be helpful to bring their course textbook, lecture notes, and computer to support their studying (forethought), as well as water and bananas as they intend to study for several hours, and thirst and hunger have interrupted their study plans previously (forethought, self-reflectiveness). The student gathers their resources, including sustenance, and locates an out-of-the-way alcove in which to study. After a short period of study, the student notices that they are being distracted by a small group of students working on a group project nearby, so they pack up their belongings and find a new quiet, solitary location (self-reactiveness). In addition, as the student continues to study, they recognize that there are concepts and terms in the textbook that are not in their notes and that they do not fully understand (self-reactiveness). To remedy the situation, the student decides to open their computer and search for additional information on the web (intentionality, forethought), a strategy that has been successful in the past so the student believes it will be successful now (self-reflectiveness) to enhance their understanding (self-reactiveness). Over the next several hours, the student monitors their comprehension to identify gaps

in their understanding (self-reactiveness), reflects on strategies that have been helpful for comprehension in the past (self-reflectiveness), devises a new plan to close these comprehension gaps (intentionality, forethought), and enacts that plan. Throughout the study session, the student's self-efficacy for study strategy use will be enhanced when the strategy use facilitates their understanding and diminished when the strategy use does not facilitate their understanding. Ultimately, through this expression of agency, a positive outcome of the study session would be an excellent test performance. Through self-reflectiveness, this positive outcome would likely lead to increased self-efficacy for studying. Thus, intentionality, forethought, self-reactiveness, and self-reflectiveness are intertwined to provide individuals with the agency needed to guide their lives and pursue their interests based, to a large extent, on their efficacy beliefs – their beliefs that they *can* have a positive impact on their own lives.

Part 3: Human Agency and Self-Efficacy

Bandura's concept of agency is intimately related to efficacy beliefs. Personal **self-efficacy** relates to reflections that yield judgments as to one's ability to successfully accomplish a future task. The importance of personal self-efficacy in agency is that self-efficacy provides motivation for an individual to engage in actions they believe will have positive outcomes: "To be an agent is to intentionally produce certain effects by one's actions" (Bandura 2018, p. 130). The belief that one is capable of successfully engaging in actions provides the impetus to regulate one's behavior and persist in the face of challenges, thus representing a core belief of agency.

> Efficacy beliefs influence whether people think self-enhancingly or self-debilitatingly, optimistically or pessimistically; what courses of action they choose to pursue; the goals they set for themselves and their commitment to them; how much effort they put forth in given endeavors; the outcomes they expect their efforts to produce; how long they persevere in the face of obstacles; their resilience to adversity; how much stress and depression they experience in coping with taxing environmental demands; and the accomplishments they realize. (Bandura 2001b, p. 270)

One recurrent question regarding personal self-efficacy is whether self-efficacy is a general trait ("It is easy for me to focus on my goals") or a specific belief ("I can successfully complete a feline ovariohysterectomy"). Bandura (2018) is clear on this point: "Perceived self-efficacy is not a global trait, but a differentiated set of self-beliefs linked to distinct realms of functioning" (p. 133). Indeed, there are robust findings (see Goetze and Driver 2022; Klassen and Tze 2014; Livinți et al. 2021) that higher self-efficacy is related to higher performance in a vast array of specific activities (e.g., exercising, teaching, writing, reading), academic domains (e.g., math, science, medicine, engineering), and academic management (e.g., academic self-regulation, academic motivation, academic self-control, academic judgments), as well as negatively related to specific affect (e.g., mood, depression, anxiety, fear). Therefore, one should think specifically; that is, "self-efficacy for _____." For example, self-efficacy for presenting at conferences, self-efficacy for writing research reports, and self-efficacy for veterinary surgery. The degree to which one specifies depends on the domain, thus self-efficacy for veterinary surgery may better be specified as self-efficacy for orthopedic surgeries and self-efficacy for soft tissue surgeries.

However, there are several general trait self-efficacy measures (i.e., General Self-Efficacy Scale, Self-Efficacy Scale, New General Self-Efficacy Scale; see Scherbaum et al. 2006), and accompanying research examining the relationship between general self-efficacy and a variety of topics, including higher work resilience in veterinarians (McArthur et al. 2021), health care usage in older adults (Whitehall et al. 2021), and life satisfaction (Azizli et al. 2015). Finally, specificity may be functional, that is, while self-efficacy to learn animal anatomy and physiology, and self-efficacy to learn food animal medicine and surgery may be important, it may be equally or more important that one has a high self-efficacy for learning new knowledge. Therefore, is self-efficacy specific or general? It depends.

The last connection is that while personal agency is impacted by perceived personal self-efficacy, the aforementioned collective (group) agency is influenced by perceived collective efficacy. As groups of individuals work together to achieve a collective goal, they develop a shared,

group-level, emergent collective efficacy beyond the sum of the group members' individual self-efficacies: "Members acting on their common beliefs contribute to the transitional dynamics that promote group attainments" (Bandura 2006, p. 166). The collective efficacy represents a shared belief in the group's ability to produce desired change or to achieve group goals. In addition, the quality of the shared collective efficacy positively impacts the quality of the group functioning (Gully et al. 2002; Salanova et al. 2020).

A. Impacts of Self-Efficacy on Action

The relationship between self-efficacy and specific actions has been demonstrated to have interesting impacts on behavior. Self-efficacy impacts not only which tasks are attempted, but also which tasks are completed and how much one learns (see Figure 3.2).

1) *Choices.* Individuals with high self-efficacy for a particular action will tend to choose to engage in that action more often than if they had low self-efficacy. That is, individuals will be more likely to choose activities that they believe will lead to success, rather than failure. In addition, if an individual both believes in the likelihood of their success *and* they value the outcomes of that success, they will be more likely to choose to engage in that action (Wigfield et al. 2016). For example, veterinary students may be more likely to participate in a voluntary rabbit dentistry wet lab if they have high self-efficacy for working with rabbits and/or dentistry and plan to pursue exotic medicine once in practice.

2) *Goals.* Individuals with high self-efficacy for a particular action will tend to set higher goals for the successful completion of that action. In addition, goals that are specific rather than general, short term rather than long term, and challenging rather than easy tend to foster

Figure 3.2 The cyclical nature of the (a) positive effects and (b) negative effects of self-efficacy on task selection, effort and persistence, and achievement.

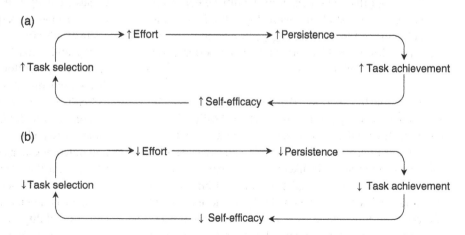

greater motivation and engagement (Locke and Latham 2002, 2015). Further, goal setting and planning (forethought) help to focus an individual's attention and maintain that focus over time (i.e., commitment). This maintenance of attention leads to the self-evaluation of progress (self-reactiveness) which can have a positive impact on motivation from both perceived progress and perceived discrepancies between a goal and one's current outcomes, indicating a greater need for effort and persistence. For example, a veterinary student interested in behavioral medicine may volunteer with the local animal shelter's veterinarian to help with behavioral assessments and modifications. As this takes considerable time and effort, a student with high self-efficacy for the task may set goals to not only help numerous animals but also to design a long-term behavioral modification protocol the shelter can continue to utilize.

3) *Effort and persistence.* Individuals with high self-efficacy for a particular action will tend to put forth greater effort and greater persistence to be successful (Bandura 1997; Komarraju and Nadler 2013). This high self-efficacy includes high outcome expectations, beliefs that they *will be* successful (eventually), which leads to persistence in goals over time (achieving a series of short-term goals leading to the achievement of long-term goals). For example, a veterinary student with high self-efficacy who is interested in pursuing a career in Emergency and Critical Care may put forth effort by working through virtual cases to improve their level of knowledge and preparation regarding critical cases.

4) *Achievement.* Individuals with high self-efficacy for a particular action who set high goals, expend significant effort, and persist in that effort, tend to achieve more often than individuals with lower self-efficacy who expend less effort and are less persistent (Bandura 1977). In addition, the successful achievement of a desired action (goal) strengthens self-efficacy for the action itself, thus increasing the likelihood that the individual will attempt that action again in the future. For example, veterinary students with high levels of self-regulation tend to be more engaged in learning during their clinical clerkships and have higher performance levels (de Jong et al. 2017).

The relationship between these characteristics can be represented cyclically (see Figure 3.2). Specifically, an individual's high self-efficacy may lead an individual to attempt a task more often. In addition, while choosing the task more often, they are also likely to put forth significant effort and persistence to complete the task. Ultimately, this effort and persistence will tend to lead to achievement and an increase in task self-efficacy, which begins the process again (see Figure 3.2a). It should, however, be noted that the cyclical nature of self-efficacy can lead to detrimental effects, where poor self-efficacy leads an individual to select a task less often, put forth minimal effort and persistence, and, predictably, perform poorly (see Figure 3.2b).

B. Fostering Self-Efficacy

Given the cyclical nature of self-efficacy and achievement, and the causal nature of self-efficacy and agency, the development of self-efficacy is essential. Self-efficacy is positively impacted by several different types of experiences, each a different source of information from which an individual may make self-efficacy judgments. That said, it is not the experiences themselves that directly impact one's self-efficacy, rather it is an individual's interpretations of these experiences (Schunk and DiBenedetto 2020).

1) *Performance experiences.* The strongest indicator of future success and failure is past success and failure. These past performance experiences (sometimes referred to as mastery or enactive experiences) serve as the most reliable and authentic source of self-efficacy information – learning through the consequences of one's own actions. Still, judgments of "success" or "failure" may themselves come from several sources based on one's performance, including comparison to peers, progress over time, achievement of established criteria, and completion of tasks. Further, the nature of these judgments is important. For example, if a veterinary student successfully completes a physical examination, the impact that this success has on the student's self-efficacy for conducting physical exams will be influenced by how the student perceives the experience. If the exam is perceived as a routine canine wellness exam, the success may have minimal impact on their self-efficacy, but if the exam is perceived as a challenging diagnostic exam, their self-efficacy may be enhanced.

In addition, as an individual progresses and overcomes challenges, based on effort and persistence, they may develop a **resilient self-efficacy**. Specifically, resilient self-efficacy is the ability, in the presence of difficulty and setback, to (i) maintain an expectation of success, (ii) monitor and reevaluate progress relative to desired outcomes, (iii) modify plans to account for the difficulties and setbacks as new courses of action emerge, (iv) maintain personal standards and criteria for success, and (v) reflect on the challenges, responses, and outcomes to accurately revise one's self-efficacy, as needed. Further, Djourova et al. (2020), indicate that resilient self-efficacy allows for the development of a sense of competence and control during uncertainty, and the ability to reframe challenges as learning experiences. As Bandura (1989) stated, "development of resilient self-efficacy requires some experience in mastering difficulties through perseverant effort" (p. 1179).

2) *Observational experiences.* In addition to experience, self-efficacy can be influenced through the observation of others' actions and their success or failure, sometimes referred to as vicarious experiences. Vicarious experiences include **vicarious reinforcement**, which involves individuals learning to exhibit a known behavior more often after observing another receiving reinforcement (i.e., a positive outcome) for the same behavior, while **vicarious punishment** involves individuals learning to exhibit a known behavior less often after observing another receiving punishment (i.e., a negative outcome) for the same behavior. Bandura (2018) refers to those observed as social models who may be physical, observed through face-to-face encounters, or symbolic, observed through social media or digital technologies, including textbooks. Thus, observing others' behaviors, attitudes, values, and resilience can lead to a change in self-efficacy, based on the positive or negative outcomes associated with the model's performance, without the presence of a direct performance experienced by the observer. This observation of others can serve to change one's motivation to act, standards for action, and self-regulatory capabilities through one's agency. In addition, it has been found that the nature of the modeling matters; individuals are more likely to be influenced by (i) a model who is perceived as similar in abilities, attributes, age, or gender; (ii) a model who is perceived as working hard to be successful, especially models who demonstrate resilience or who are observed when the observer is new to the task; and, (iii) multiple models being observed, rather than just one model (Bandura 1977; Gale et al. 2021; Schunk and Usher 2019). For example, if a veterinary student compares their successful castration of a cat to a (perceived) less skilled peer, the impact of their accomplishment on their self-efficacy for surgery is not likely to be significant; however, if their peer comparison is to a (perceived) highly skilled peer, the impact on their self-efficacy is more likely to be consequential.

Finally, while traditionally an individual tended to interact with a limited number of other people in their day-to-day lives (e.g., family, friends, peers, colleagues), digital technologies have allowed individuals to observe others worldwide engaging in a vast array of behaviors 24 hours a day, including online education and tutorials, thus increasing an individual's potential observational experiences and repertoire of observed actions. Ultimately, while observations of others can influence one's self-efficacy, the impact of observed experiences on self-efficacy tends to be less than with performance experiences, and long-term changes in self-efficacy due to observation generally necessitate some performance experience at some point.

3) *Persuasive experiences.* Usually less impactful and shorter in duration than performance experiences and observational experiences, social persuasive experiences can also affect an individual's self-efficacy. Persuasive experiences include verbal communications (e.g., "excellent effort, try another approach, you'll get this") and behavioral communications (i.e., providing a student with an easier task when they are struggling with a more difficult task potentially communicates that the instructor believes the student is incapable of succeeding at the more challenging task). The impact of persuasive experiences is enhanced when the provider of the persuasion is perceived as credible and when the persuasion is provided frequently (Bandura 1977; Schunk and Usher 2019). Highly credible sources of performance information, such as experts, teachers, and successful peers, typically impact an individual's self-efficacy more than a less credible source and receiving credible messages more often tends to be more effective than less frequent persuasions. For example, a veterinary student may value feedback more from an experienced large animal veterinarian during the examination of a cow than from a veterinary student peer who is also just learning about bovine care.

Also, individuals who are novices and lack a wealth of personal knowledge and experience may heed persuasive messages more than those with significant knowledge and experience. These novices may lack the personal knowledge and experience necessary to make their own judgments regarding their actions, so they may rely more on others' judgments, which may, in turn, impact their self-efficacy. Finally, two unfortunate caveats: negative messages tend to have more of an impact (reducing self-efficacy) than positive messages (increasing self-efficacy) and increases in self-efficacy due to persuasive experiences tend to fade if not verified through performance experiences.

4) *Physiological experiences.* A final source of information regarding one's self-efficacy is their own physiological and emotional reactions, such as excitement, calm, interest, fear, anxiety, and stress. These emotions may be interpreted as indicators of one's beliefs in their likelihood of being successful – "I'm nervous, I'm going to fail this test," or "I'm excited, this lab is going to be fun" – and, thus, increase or decrease one's related self-efficacy. For example, a veterinary student walking to an anatomy lab may feel restless and sweaty and perceive this as "anxiety" and an indication of being ill-prepared, resulting in a lower self-efficacy for completing the lab.

One emerging relationship regarding self-efficacy and physiological experience is the importance of the *interpretation* of one's physiological experience. Reexamining the veterinary student's experience of restlessness and sweating on the way to the anatomy lab, what if the student interpreted their physiological experience not as "anxiety," but rather, as "excitement," or if while they first interpreted the physiological experience as anxiety, they were subsequently able to reappraise the experience as excitement? This reinterpreting of one's physiological response is **cognitive reappraisal**. Cognitive reappraisal of the emotional interpretation of a physiological response or event (sometimes referred to as positive reappraisal) has been demonstrated to have a significant impact on subsequent thought and action (Gross 1998; Neta et al. 2022; Webb et al. 2012). Hanley et al. (2015) found that cognitive reappraisal following perceived academic failure was positively related to academic self-efficacy, in particular, the ability to reinterpret perceived failure as beneficial was associated with higher self-efficacy (i.e., resiliency). Similarly, Riepenhausen et al. (2022) determined that a disposition, or style, toward positive cognitive reappraisal – a tendency or bias toward interpreting or reinterpreting a negative physiological experience in a positive way – was associated with effective resilience. Finally, cognitive reappraisal is subject to its own self-efficacy: cognitive reappraisal self-efficacy is the belief in one's ability to successfully engage in cognitive reappraisal in order to regulate one's emotions (Goldin et al. 2009, 2012). Ultimately, cognitive reappraisal provides an avenue for the development of positive self-efficacy and resilience through the reinterpretation of negative physiological experiences.

C. Self-Efficacy in Academic Settings

Self-efficacy has a powerful impact on functioning within a classroom for both students and teachers. Previous discussions of the sources of self-efficacy (i.e., performance, observation, persuasion, and physiological experiences), impacts on behavior (i.e., choices, goals, effort, persistence, and achievement), as well as the development of agency (i.e., intentionality, forethought, self-reactiveness, and self-reflectiveness) all apply within the classroom.

1) *Student Academic Self-Efficacy*. Overall, high student academic self-efficacy, or the student's belief in their ability to successfully complete academic tasks and achieve academic goals, has a significant impact on the student's overall academic achievement. Academic self-efficacy has been posited as one of the most important factors in students' college success (Robbins et al. 2004). Specifically, higher student academic self-efficacy is associated with:

- increased academic learning, performance, achievement, and transfer;
- increased goal orientation, motivation, and self-regulation;
- increased commitment, effort, and persistence;
- increased problem-solving and self-regulation;
- increased domain-specific achievement (e.g., math, science, writing, and reading);
- increased use of cognitive, metacognitive, and deep processing strategies;
- decreased academic anxiety and stress; and
- decreased academic procrastination.

(Alemany-Arrebola et al. 2020; Bandura 1998; Hayat et al. 2020; Pintrich 2003; Schunk and DiBenedetto 2020; Walker and Greene 2009; Zimmerman and Kitsantas 2005).

2) *Teacher Self-Efficacy*. Similarly, high teaching self-efficacy, a teacher's belief in their ability to positively impact student learning performance, has a significant impact on teacher and student classroom learning performance. Specifically, higher teacher self-efficacy is associated with:

- increased teaching quality, engagement, commitment, and motivation;
- increased teaching enthusiasm, passion, resilience, and retention;
- increased quality of lesson plans, classroom management, assessments, and strategies;
- increased teacher cooperation with students, colleagues, and parents;
- increased student achievement, academic self-efficacy, motivation, and engagement;
- increased teaching satisfaction and well-being; and
- decreased teacher burnout and stress.

(Calkins et al. 2023; Kasalak and Dağyar 2020; Perera et al. 2019; Poulou et al. 2019; Tschannen-Moran et al. 1998; Tschannen-Moran and Woolfolk Hoy 2007; Wang et al. 2015).

The impact of teacher self-efficacy is substantial, resulting in more effective class preparation, teaching practices, student assessment, and, ultimately, student learning. The sources of teaching self-efficacy – performance, observational, persuasive, and physiological experiences – can be seen in the work of Gale et al. (2021), who surveyed and interviewed beginning, novice, and career teachers, with 1-year, 2–3 years, and 4+ years of secondary teaching experience, respectively. Gale et al. found that participants' teaching self-efficacy was most impacted by performance experiences and persuasion experiences, regardless of teaching experience level (beginning, novice, career). Teachers' performance experiences were based primarily on student achievement (e.g., test performance, classroom performance, "light bulb" moments); when students learned, teachers had a higher perception of their own teaching. In addition, teachers identified consistently low student learning and an inability to explain this lower student performance as the main source of information lowering their self-efficacy. Gale et al. also reported that more experienced teachers with high teaching self-efficacy were more likely to reappraise negative teaching experiences as opportunities to learn (resiliency). In relation to social persuasion, the teachers reported the importance of informal comments from administrators and other teachers and the need for persuasive comments to be paired with performance experiences. Finally, while observational experiences were expected to have a greater impact on teachers' self-efficacy, Gale et al. explained that teaching is often a solitary experience. Rarely do classroom teachers observe other teachers and rarely are classroom teachers observed themselves; thus, classroom teachers only infrequently have the opportunity to engage in observational experiences. The impact of affective or physiological experiences on self-efficacy was rarely mentioned by teachers.

3) *Calibration of Self-Efficacy Judgments.* Given the importance of self-efficacy in an individual's task engagement and achievement, it is reasonable to question whether individuals are accurate in estimating their ability to be successful and whether it might matter: Does a high self-efficacy inherently mean high task performance? **Self-efficacy calibration** is the relationship between a student's self-efficacy for a task and their ability to perform that task. For example, imagine a veterinary student learning to complete a canine otoscopic evaluation. If this student has high self-efficacy for performing otoscopy, but their performance is low, they would be overconfident (a self-efficacy that is unwarrantedly high), while if their self-efficacy is low and their performance was high, they would be underconfident (a self-efficacy that is unwarrantedly low), both evidencing a self-efficacy miscalibration.

Does it matter if self-efficacy and task performance are miscalibrated? Given the relationship between self-efficacy and agency, this miscalibration could have significant ramifications. For instance, an overconfident student may choose to engage in procedures for which they lack sufficient skills, neglect to prepare sufficiently for an upcoming procedure, rush or pay inadequate attention during the procedure, fail to seek help when needed, or injure the patient. An underconfident student may spend too much time preparing for the procedure and neglect other important tasks, exude apprehension that is interpreted by the client as a lack of skill, accept inappropriate advice from less-skilled others, or choose not to engage in procedures and thus, diminish their skills (Boekaerts and Rozendaal 2010; Schunk and Pajares 2004; Usher 2009; Zvacek et al. 2015).

Talsma et al. (2019, 2020), examined academic self-efficacy and performance across two studies in which undergraduate psychology students rated their self-efficacy for course-based written assignments and multiple-choice content exams, as well as their self-efficacy for their course performance (i.e., course grade). In addition, Talsma et al. collected students' performance on the written assignments, multiple-choice exams, and course grades. Across both studies, Talsma et al. found that while overall academic self-efficacy was positively related to academic performance, on an individual level, academic self-efficacy and performance were often miscalibrated. Specifically, at the task level, concerning self-efficacy and performance related to written assignments and multiple-choice tests, students tended to be underconfident; that is, their expressed self-efficacy was lower than the assignment/exam performance. However, at the domain level, concerning course grades, students tended to be overconfident; that is, their expressed self-efficacy was higher than their course grades. Finally, across both studies, lower-achieving students tended to be overconfident regarding both written assignments and exams, while high-achieving students tended to be underconfident (Talsma et al. 2019), or appropriately confident (Talsma et al. 2020).

Given these findings, care needs to be taken in interpreting self-efficacy and performance results. Does it matter if self-efficacy and task performance are miscalibrated? It depends. First, the general findings that task self-efficacy and task performance are positively related are based on correlations and should not be interpreted as causal. That is, having a high self-efficacy for a particular task does not directly cause high task performance or indicate definite higher performance. A student can have high self-efficacy and low performance, as well as low self-efficacy and high performance; therefore, general measures of self-efficacy are not enough. It is important to consider the self-efficacy of individual students related to specific tasks. Second, the accuracy of self-efficacy ratings seems to be positively related to experience; therefore, less experienced students should be expected to overrate their performance, while more experienced students should be expected to more appropriately rate their performance.

Part 4: Human Agency and Social Modeling

Social cognitive theory's emphasis on self-regulatory human agency is grounded in the interactions between the individual, the social, and the environment (reciprocal causation), including one's cognition and expectancy beliefs (self-efficacy), and one's interactions with others (social modeling). Social modeling involves learning by observing others and the consequence of their behaviors, where learning can be a new behavior, an increase or decrease in the frequency of a known behavior, or a modification of a known behavior, and where "behavior" may be physical, cognitive, social, or affective. Social modeling provides an avenue of learning that is distinct from the more traditional approach of learning through direct experience (Bandura 2001a, 2006). This observational learning through social models is a source of human agency that simplifies the learning process, allowing for the learning of one's culture – language, behaviors, mores, ideology, and ethics – through social interaction, not formal instruction, and where "culture" may be one's local culture (e.g., family, social club, veterinary clinic) or global culture (e.g., ethnicity, region, country).

Social modeling provides a mechanism for the link between everyday social experiences and cognitive, behavioral, social, and affective functioning. Individuals can learn both formal and informal knowledge, skills, and attitudes through the cognitive processing of social models. For example, a veterinary student can learn informally about animals and veterinary medicine by watching the animals and veterinarians engaging in everyday actions. The student can also learn when engaging in more formal actions, as part of a class or laboratory session. When a veterinarian models procedures as part of a class, they are explicitly articulating what they are doing, why, and the expected outcomes. A benefit of learning through social modeling, rather than direct experience, lies in the access to social models. Where once one needed to be in the presence of a model, one now merely needs to access their smart phone or laptop.

In recent years, the availability of social models has exploded. Traditionally, social models were limited to those present in one's everyday face-to-face experiences, for example, one's parents, siblings, extended family, friends, school peers, work colleagues, and daily acquaintances (e.g., a barista, car mechanic, office assistant, convenience store clerk). Today, however, one has access to models from across the globe, anytime day or night, via the internet. With a few clicks, one can observe the newest social craze being modeled in fashion, reading, pottery, politics, cooking, music, sports, and entertainment, as well as veterinary practice, surgeries, and pharmacology. This global reach of social models can lead to the development of new properties of agency as these models demonstrate emerging, unfamiliar, or infrequently experienced attitudes, values, behaviors, language, and resilience. In addition to socially experiencing these new properties, one is often able to see the outcomes of the knowledge and skills. Observing behaviors and outcomes, and constructing new outcome expectancies, can lead to increases or decreases in one's self-efficacy for the new knowledge and skills. In turn, these new outcome expectancies influence one's motivation, goals, plans, actions, reactions, and reflections – an individual's agency (i.e., intentionality, forethought, self-reactiveness, self-reflectiveness).

A. Characteristics of Effective Social Models

The role of the social model is not always well defined but is often simply an individual doing what they do on a daily basis: parents parenting, teachers teaching, and workers working. That said, there are characteristics that have been identified that make for a more effective model (Bandura 1971, 1986). It is, however, important to understand that these characteristics are perceptions of the observer and not objective attributes of the social model. The effectiveness of a social model depends on perceived:

1) *Competence.* An effective model is perceived by the observer to be competent in the behavior they are modeling. For example, a veterinary student may find a well-published veterinarian conducting antimicrobial resistance research highly competent as a researcher and worth emulating, but a class peer conducting a lab experiment as a less competent researcher and less likely to be emulated.

2) *Prestige and power.* An effective model is perceived by the observer to have power and prestige, in the form of status, respect, influence, reputation, resources, and/or authority. For example, a first-year veterinary student may find a fourth-year veterinary student who has published a paper and received a job offer as reflecting prestige and power and, thus, worthy of emulation.

3) *Socially Acceptable Behavior.* An effective model is perceived by the observe to be engaging in socially or culturally acceptable (often referred to as stereotypical) behaviors. For example, a veterinary student is more likely to mimic veterinary behaviors (e.g., social interactions, dress codes, conflict management) that are deemed more typical of veterinarians.

4) *Relevance.* An effective model is perceived by the observer to be exhibiting behaviors that have some functional value or relevance to the observer or the observer's situation. For example, a veterinary student interested in pursuing a residency in small animal internal medicine is more likely to find a small animal internist worthy of emulation than a public health veterinarian.

B. Observational Learning from Social Models

The process of observational learning through social models involves the interaction between one's social experiences and cognitive functions. Bandura (2001b), identified four cognitive functions, or methods of processing, necessary for effective observational learning: attention, retention, production, and motivation.

1) *Attention.* The first criterion for effective observational learning is that the observer's attention must be focused on the model and the behaviors of importance in which the model is engaging. In addition, this attention needs to be focused on the relevant task features of the performance. The focus of the observer's attention may be influenced by both the actions of the model, such as verbalizations ("See how the dog's leg moves through the full range of motion") and operations (the instructor demonstrates moving the dog's leg through a full range of motion repeatedly), as well as the mindset of the observer, such as prior knowledge and skills (growing up, the student had a pet dog who had hip dysplasia and thus lost much of his range of motion), and value preferences (fostering ethics of care).

2) *Retention.* The observer must encode the model's behaviors, verbally and/or visually, in memory. Memory retention is intricately related to attention in that one's focus of attention influences what and how one learns. In addition, as with attention, retention is influenced by the actions of the model, such as how the model aligns what they are saying with what they are doing, and the processing by the observer, such as how the observer connects new observations to prior knowledge. For example, veterinary students performing their first live animal surgeries might be asked about the methods they used to remember how to perform the procedure once they were standing at the operating table (Langebæk et al. 2015). In this case, the majority of students were able to remember the steps needed by recalling the surgical demonstration videos that were provided by the instructor. Instruction such as assigned reading, lectures, and practicing foundational surgical skills on models or cadavers did not align the instruction to the action as effectively as the demonstration video of a model performing the procedure in its entirety. The students were then able to connect their new observations (their first live animal surgery) to their prior knowledge (the memory of the steps performed in the video). Ultimately, retention is a function of what and how the observer processes the social model – what we process we learn.

3) *Production.* The production of the observed behavior is an essential aspect of observational learning; indeed, it is the reproduction of the observed action that indicates what the observer has learned. However, the observer's first reproductive attempts may be error-prone or simple approximations of the observed behavior; thus, reproducing the observed behavior immediately may help the observer to learn the behavior (the behavioral movement being an additional form of processing) and may allow the model to provide corrective feedback to the observer. For example, Thomson et al. (2019), found that when learning to perform dental extractions, students found the laboratory setting (where they could practice the hands-on skillsets) to be more valuable than lecture time, perceiving that their technical skills development improved most because the instructional setting allowed for immediate feedback and involvement from instructors. However, it may be the case where the observer is simply unable to replicate the observed behavior due to a lack of knowledge or skill. In addition, there are situations where the observer does not attempt to replicate the observed behavior for days, weeks, or years later due to the lack of need to do so.

4) *Motivation.* Finally, while an individual may have attended to, mentally retained, and be capable of exhibiting a new behavior, they may still not engage in the behavior if they are not motivated to act. This is particularly relevant given that veterinary students often struggle to maintain high motivation levels over the course of their studies (Mikkonen and Ruohoniemi 2011). The observer must *want* to perform the modeled behavior. An individual is more likely to be motivated to perform a new action if (i) they have observed others, such as role models or successful classmates, engaging in the action reaping positive consequences; (ii) they see the value of engaging in the new behavior as contributing to or an indication of the achievement of their goals, such as veterinary students maintaining their motivation to study when they deem the course content to be useful in obtaining their future goals (Parkinson et al. 2006); (iii) they view engaging in the new behavior as a challenge that will increase their self-efficacy, specifically, a difficult but attainable challenge, that with effort and persistence will result in success, and (iv) they perceive the new behavior as evidence of or contributing to their membership in a particular group, as indicated by the large number of national and international student clubs and organizations focused on specialties and interests that offer experiential learning opportunities available outside of the veterinary curriculum. Ultimately, Dale et al. (2010) determined that veterinary students with a preference for complexity, or a deep approach to learning, tend to have higher intrinsic, social, and extrinsic motivation.

Part 5: Human Agency and Identity

Human agency, the ability to regulate one's cognitive, behavioral, social, and affective processes in pursuit of individual, social, or environmental change, is built upon intentional self-regulation, efficacy beliefs, and social learning. This human agency also synergistically supports the construction of one's **identity**. Identity, as a self-theory, can be viewed as both a product and process and comprise both individual and social influences (Bandura 2006; Berzonsky 2011; Berzonsky and Kuk 2021; Crocetti et al. 2022). As a *product*, identity is a persistent cognitive structure that provides an *individualized frame of reference* for representing and interpreting past and present experiences, choices, beliefs, and values, as well as projecting these to plan for the future. As a *process*, identity functions to organize and understand one's experiences and identity-relevant information and to motivate and self-regulate one's socio-cognitive strategies to construct, maintain, and revise one's individualized frame of reference. In addition, the experiences, choices, beliefs, and values that give rise to one's identity may have either an individual or social genesis – the interpretation of one's experiences and the influence of one's social groups.

Identity, like agency, is an on-going process of self-regulation through (i) evaluating one's past, present, and future experiences, (ii) consciously and intentionally making life path decisions and commitments, (iii) constructing a sense of control of one's life, and (iv) continuously evaluating one's functioning to strengthen effective actions and beliefs, weaken ineffective actions and beliefs, and initiate change and adaptation as needed. Bandura (2006) explicitly links identity and agency: "As an agent, one creates identity connections over time and construes oneself as a continuing person over different periods of one's life" (p. 170). Similarly, as stated by Berzonsky (2011), from the identity side of the conversation: "Having the cognitive resources to represent the past, and then use transformations of those representations to anticipate the future, enables people to transcend time and maintain a sense of themselves as persistent volitional agents who think, doubt, will, act, desire, and self-regulate" (p. 56). Thus, the development of agency and self-regulation help an individual to construct an identity.

This relationship between identity and agency is embedded in three main identity-processing styles as proffered by Berzonsky: informational identity-processing style, normative identity-processing style, and diffuse-avoidant identity-processing style (Berzonsky 2011; Berzonsky and Luyckx 2008; Berzonsky and Kuk 2021; Crocetti et al. 2022). These identity styles are based on effective (or ineffective) agency and self-regulation, giving rise to effective (or ineffective) identity construction: "Selfhood embodies one's physical and psychosocial makeup, with a personal identity and agentic capabilities operating in concert" (Bandura 2006, p. 170).

1) *Informational identity-processing style*. Individuals with an informational identity-processing style are rational, self-directed, decision focused, and open minded to new ideas and new experiences. They are also flexible in their approach to how they see themselves, as evidenced by well-developed self-reflection and self-awareness, a questioning of their own self-beliefs, and a willingness to entertain values and ideas distinct from their own. The sense of identity of individuals with an informational style tends to represent personal values, beliefs, and goals derived from deliberate self-reflection and self-knowledge (i.e., agency). In general, an informational identity-processing style is associated with a more positive identity construction, including adaptive and problem-focused coping, effective decision-making strategies, and mastery achievement goals.

2) *Normative identity-processing style*. Individuals with a normative identity-processing style are (i) rational, but intuitively so, eschewing the need for engaged cognition; (ii) committed to their ideals, but through premature cognitive closure, unquestioningly adopting the ideals of others; (iii) conscientious and self-disciplined, but unwilling to entertain values and ideas different from their own; and (iv) dedicated to existing structures, but intolerant of ambiguity and changes in the status quo. The sense of identity of individuals with a normative style tends to represent a firm and unquestioning adoption of the collective identities of others, such as a family; a religious, cultural, occupational, or political organization; or specific self-attributes, such as patriotism, inclusivity, or athleticism. In general, a normative identity-processing style is associated with positive and negative identity construction. Specifically, a normative style is positively associated with goal setting, engagement, conscientiousness, and achievement goals, but negatively associated with open-mindedness, tolerance for ambiguity, and need for deliberate cognitive engagement.

3) *Diffuse-avoidant identity-processing style*. Individuals with a diffuse-avoidant identity-processing style attempt to avoid making a conscious and rational choice of identity, seeking instead to procrastinate or vacillate based on the present circumstance or with whomever they are currently associating. When choices are made, they tend to be weak, reactive, hedonistic, and guided by situational demands and the avoidance of stress and conflict. In addition, those with a

diffuse-avoidant style tend to engage in minimal self-discipline and self-awareness and have low self-esteem and academic difficulties. The sense of identity of individuals with a diffuse-avoidant style tends to represent maladaptive coping and dysfunctional decision-making focused on self-satisfying with choices related to furthering one's popularity, reputation, or distinction. In general, a diffuse-avoidant identity-processing style is associated negatively with identity construction, including poor cognition, adaptation, coping, and decision-making.

The overlap between identity and agency is substantial: "As the model of triadic reciprocal causation suggests, a sense of selfhood is the product of a complex interplay of personal construal processes and the social reality in which one lives" (Bandura 2006, p. 170). Berzonsky (2003), Schwartz et al. (2005), and Berzonsky and Kuk (2021) found that agency and self-regulation were positively associated with informational and normative identity-processing styles and negatively associated with a diffuse-avoidant identity-processing style. In addition, Berzonsky and Kuk established that agency and self-regulation mediate the relationship between informational style and depression and loneliness for first-year students, such that information style is positively related to agency and self-regulation, which are negatively related to depression and loneliness. Ultimately, one's identity is at least partially a function of one's agency – poor agency negatively impacts one's identity construction.

A. Personal Identity and Veterinary Medicine

These relationships between identity, agency, and self-regulation are important as one considers the construction of veterinary medical students' professional identities as veterinarians, and also practicing veterinarians' identities as teaching veterinarians. First, it is important to clarify that there is not a single "veterinary identity" or "veterinary educator identity." The identities of a veterinary surgeon and a veterinary epidemiologist and a livestock veterinarian are likely to overlap, yet also differentiate. In addition, each individual has more than a single identity, potentially, including a personal identity, professional identity, cultural identity, and religious identity, to name but a few. Finally, identities are not static, but rather evolve and adapt as one's experiences, values, behaviors, and contexts change, for example, as one's professional life develops from veterinary student to novice veterinarian to experienced veterinarian, or one's job focus changes from clinical practice to academic practice (Armitage-Chan 2020; Armitage-Chan and May 2019; Gardner and Hini 2006).

The construction of a strong and appropriate veterinary identity is essential to the vocational success, career satisfaction, and mental health of the veterinarian. According to Armitage-Chan and May (2019), the development of veterinary identity has three main phases. The initial phase accounts for the development of a naïve self, as one moves from being a college student to a veterinary student. As a college student, the individual will have little or no first-hand experience with veterinary medicine, so their identity is based on conjecture, rather than the exploration of veterinary experiences. As veterinary students engage in their veterinary studies (the second phase), they will experience a multitude of situations and experiences, including exposure to new knowledge and skills, as well as to practicing veterinarians, animals, clients, surgeries, and contexts. Within these situations, the students will experience the integration of self, actions, and environments (Bandura's reciprocal causation) leading to the development of beliefs and values through the necessity of veterinary interpretations and choices. This second phase may extend into a student's early career as they navigate their new professional work environments. While working as a veterinarian (the third phase), individuals become fully responsible for enacting their role as a veterinarian, interpreting their environment, making choices, acting in accordance, and bearing the responsibility for those actions (mental and physical). During this third phase, veterinarians reflect on the development of their identity, determining the alignment between their identity (as represented by their values, choices, and actions) and their environment (the vocational and social pressures inherent in their work). Ultimately, it is the interplay of these individual and social influences, contexts, and processes that lead to professional identity construction, maintenance, and ongoing development.

The result of veterinary identity construction, as depicted by Armitage-Chan and May (2019), may be any of Berzonsky's three identity-processing styles. Although, as mentioned by Armitage-Chan and May, identity construction is "complex and messy" (p. 160), more complex and messier than three phases and three outcomes; however, these phases and outcomes provide a foundation for understanding the challenges that can be faced by new veterinarians and new veterinary educators. A misalignment between one's identity and one's environment, when one's environmentally induced actions do not align with one's values and beliefs (identity dissonance), may lead to poor mental health and job dissatisfaction, increased fatigue and burnout, and decreased resilience (Armitage-Chan 2020; Fawcett and Mullan 2018). This misalignment may be the result of perceived failure in properly supporting an animal's care, differing judgments from colleagues in animal care, lack of instrumentation necessary to complete needed treatments, reduction in animal care due to restricted client finances, and criticisms from clients regarding empathy and care (Armitage-Chan and May 2019; Armitage-Chan 2020; Mossop and Cobb 2013). In the case of misalignment, the solution is frequently an adjustment in one's identity or the pursuit of a new environment.

Fostering a stable identity requires a significant degree of agency, based on an ongoing integration of self-regulation and self-efficacy. Within veterinary education, professional identity construction is recognized essential to the development of fully functioning veterinarians (Armitage-Chan 2020; Mossop and Cobb 2013). The intentional development of a professional identity within veterinary education entails explicit discussions and modeling regarding professionalism, as well as designing opportunities for students to consciously reflect on their experiences, beliefs, choices, and outcomes with the intent of exploring and committing to a sense of identity as a veterinarian. Thus, the combined development of identity and agency involves (i) intentionally planning and committing to goals based on one's values, beliefs, and knowledge, and one's forethought regarding potential outcome expectancies, (ii) deliberately engaging in one's plans, monitoring one's progress in relation to those plans, and making adjustments, as needed, and (iii) reflecting on the overall process (beliefs, goals, actions, outcomes) and creating a deliberate and rational guiding sense of self.

Part 6: Educational Implications of Social Cognitive Theory

Social cognitive theory is a robust and wide-ranging theory addressing learning in an integrated context of the individual and the social. This reciprocal causation is the ether within which the individual processes their experiences and develops their agency and identity. Social cognitive theory is not a narrow, specialized theory with limited application; rather, it is an everyday theory of human functioning, including functioning within the realm of veterinary medical education. The application of social cognitive theory constructs to veterinary medical education are innumerable. What follows are a few implications of social cognitive theory for the classroom, clinic, and lab.

A. Human Agency and Self-Regulation

1) *Students' learning involves the integration of their thoughts and actions, as well as the people and environments around them.* While learning results from processing, that processing may take several forms, including cognitive, behavioral, social, and affective processing. Students may learn cognitively through experiences diagnosing patients, studying class notes and scholarly articles, and making informed decisions; behaviorally through completing procedures, using diagnostic equipment, and emulating veterinary specialists; socially through observing veterinarians, discussing issues with peers, and answering client questions; and, affectively through monitoring and reflecting on their emotional responses, developing and reevaluating their beliefs, and reappraising the cognitive labels they apply to new and prior emotions and experiences. This processing is integrated within a student's individual, social, and environmental experiences (reciprocal causation); thus, a veterinary student's learning environment needs to include deliberately integrated individual, social, and environmental experiences and reflections.

2) *Students' learning is enhanced when they are given opportunities to develop and demonstrate control over their learning and lives.* As students learn through their integrated individual, social, and environmental experiences, they need to develop a sense of agency. This agency is built on the self-regulation of intentionality, forethought, self-reactiveness, and self-reflectiveness. Further, self-regulation is guided by a student's self-efficacy, their belief in their ability to successfully act. Thus, veterinary students need to be given opportunities to self-regulate: to plan, act, succeed, fail, revise, act, succeed, fail, and, ultimately, to self-reflect and self-evaluate, leading to changes in their agency, self-regulation, and self-efficacy, as well as, potentially, their identity.

B. Human Agency and Self-Efficacy

1) *Students' learning is guided and sustained by efficacy beliefs.* Due to the importance of self-efficacy in relation to one's agency, it is important that individuals become aware of its existence and its impacts on their behavior. A greater understanding of self-efficacy beliefs and their influence on one's self-regulation can lead to greater planning, regulating, and performing, and, ultimately, success. Self-efficacy beliefs are the result of a synthesis of informational sources: experience, observation, persuasion, and physiology. Specific information from multiple sources regarding the effectiveness of one's planning, regulating, and performing can lead to more accurate judgments, as well as a better understanding of the need for regulation. Ultimately, healthy self-efficacy beliefs can lead to greater resilience. Thus, veterinary students need to be given authentic and challenging tasks to complete and then receive support in

task completion and accurate feedback on their task performance.

2) *Students' learning is strengthened by focusing on resilience and small successes.* In working on authentic and challenging tasks, some tasks will inevitably lead to unsuccessful task completion. In the face of struggle, two avenues may appear: reduce the difficulty of the situation or raise and maintain one's efforts and expectations for success. Reducing the level of challenge to achieve success is less likely to lead to long-term growth than developing resilience by reevaluating one's expectancies, developing new plans, engaging in greater or redirected effort, and evaluating one's progress continuously. Bandura (1993) emphasized that expectations must remain appropriate and that self-efficacy should be built through intermediate goals. The key to impacting change in self-efficacy, based on the cyclical nature of self-efficacy (see Figure 3.2), is to foster small, but meaningful, achievements. Small achievements may be more attainable than large-scale achievements, nudging one's self-efficacy in a positive direction incrementally. Thus, veterinary students need to be engaged with tasks of varying degrees of difficulty to strengthen known and new knowledge and skills, and to develop the resilience necessary to maintain effort and persistence when challenged, until the task is completed.

3) *Students' learning is aided by the reappraisal of the sources of self-efficacy information.* Engaging in authentic and challenging tasks will tend to lead to various emotional states that are evaluated and labeled – exhilaration, anxiety, joy, stress, triumph, and frustration – which, in turn, may impact one's task performance, and, ultimately, one's self-efficacy. The labels that a student uses to identify an emotion are not automatic and beyond the student's control; thus, veterinary students should be encouraged to reexamine and reevaluate their emotional responses and labels in order to foster greater resilience and self-efficacy.

C. Human Agency and Social Modeling

1) *Students' learning is expanded through the observation of social models.* Learning is not attained simply through first-hand experience, but can also be the result of observational experience. Observing others (models) engaging in actions and the results of those actions (positive or negative) can lead to the development of new actions in the observer. These new actions, however, may not be reproduced immediately, but rather, potentially after a delay from days to months to years, depending on the need or motivation of the observer to engage in those new actions. In addition, these models may be in the observer's immediate environment, or they may be virtual, available online. Thus, veterinary students can be taught not only through direct instruction and problem-solving but through the observation of others engaging in relevant actions.

2) *Students' learning is generated through the cognitive processing of social models.* Observational learning is the result of distinct cognitive processes. Specifically, the observer must focus their attention on an appropriate task and the components of that task, as well as retain the nature, components, and procedures for completing that task. In addition, the observer must be physically able to complete the observed task and be motivated to do so. Thus, veterinary students must not only be provided with appropriate models and the modeling of relevant actions but also be encouraged to cognitively process their observations in the moment to better retain and reproduce them later.

3) *Students' learning is supported by the use of competent, relevant, and resilient social models.* An important component of observational learning is the attributes of those observed. Models are most effective when they are perceived by the observer to be competent in the observed task, socially powerful and prestigious, engaged in socially acceptable behaviors, and relevant to the observer's needs and desires. In addition, in the pursuit of developing resilient students, students can learn resiliency by watching models who struggle, persist, and eventually overcome challenges to be successful. Thus, it is important that veterinary students observe novice, resilient, and expert models whose actions align with their level of knowledge and skill and are relevant to their specific goals and actions.

D. Human Agency and Identity

1) *Students' learning is focused through the development of agency and identity.* Identity provides students with a personal frame of reference for understanding and engaging with themselves and the world around them. Identity is constructed through one's agency – guiding, enacting, interpreting, and reflecting on their own individual and social experiences – leading to the creation and commitment of their own beliefs, values, and actions. A conscious, self-regulated, and flexible identity and agency provide a student with the motivation and vision necessary to guide their own learning path and progress. Thus, veterinary students need to be provided with cognitive, social, behavioral and affective opportunities to develop and execute their agency and self-regulation in order to construct and strengthen their identities.

2) *Students' identity is made conscious through identity-focused curriculum and self-reflection.* The construction of identity is fostered when students consciously align their beliefs and values to the development of their own actions and then reflect on the outcomes and self-satisfaction of those actions. In addition, student identity construction is bolstered from watching others' actions and comparing those actions with their own beliefs and values in order to reflectively examine their relationship. Comparing one's own and others' beliefs and values with actions and outcomes can lead to the development of a conscious, self-regulated, and flexible identity. Thus, veterinary students need a curriculum that provides observational moments where beliefs and values intersect with actions, along with explicit opportunities for students to reflect on their own beliefs, values, and actions.

Social cognitive theory provides a foundation for how people synthesize their individual and social experiences in attempting to construct more adaptive ways of acting and being. Through the self-regulation of one's cognitive, behavioral, social, and affective actions, an individual reflects on who they are, and where they are, in creating a plan for moving forward. As one moves forward, they reflect on their goals and progress in order to have a better understanding of their development. This self-awareness and self-reflection provide information for the review and revision of their goals and actions, as well as a better understanding of their capabilities. Ultimately, how students process their individual and social experiences determines what they learn and who they become, which leads to the importance of processing in learning, memory, and cognition.

Section 3: Learning, Memory, and Cognition

The pursuit of understanding learning, memory, and cognition is a quest to balance the structure and function of the brain with the structure and function of the individual. What is the relation between one's experience, thinking, and action (cognitive, behavioral, social, and affective)?

Mayer (1992) discussed three views of learning and instruction that can help to organize the following discussion: Learning as Response Acquisition, Learning as Knowledge Acquisition, and Learning as Knowledge Construction.

Learning as Response Acquisition focuses on the development of appropriate behaviors as a result of positive consequences for appropriate behaviors (or approximately appropriate behaviors) and negative consequences for inappropriate behaviors – what behaviorism refers to as shaping. In this model, the learner responds, and the teacher provides feedback. Learning as Knowledge Acquisition and Learning as Knowledge Construction are more like Part 1 and Part 2 of the same view, rather than separate views. This knowledge acquisition and construction view emphasizes the roles of memory and cognition in the processing of experience and the development of understanding.

Part 1: A Framework for Memory and Cognition

For decades, discussions of learning, memory, and cognition have been based on a model of **information processing** provided by Atkinson and Shiffrin (1968) that is neat and tidy. The problem, however, is that learning, memory, and cognition are neither inherently neat nor tidy. The Atkinson and Shiffrin *dual-store model* provides a framework, or an organization, for examining learning and performance. What follows is a discussion that uses the dual-store model for organizational purposes but goes beyond the original model with ideas and concepts developed since the model's inception (see Figure 3.3).

Imagine a veterinary student sitting in an animal nutrition lecture. Their lecture experience begins through the **stimulation** of their five senses – seeing (the room, the instructor), hearing (the instructor, other students), touching (their computer, their phone), smelling (the room, the banana in their backpack), and tasting (their gum, the top of the pen they are chewing on) – with these stimulations briefly occupying their **sensory memory** (sometime referred to as sensory store or sensory register). Unfortunately, their senses and brain cannot adequately process all the stimulation they are experiencing, so

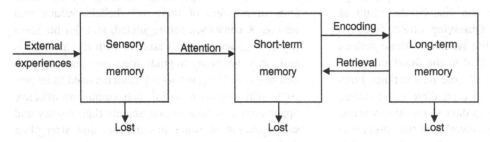

Figure 3.3 A simplified representation of Atkinson and Shiffrin's (1968) dual-store model.

through **attention** the student narrows their field of experience to just a few items, perhaps what the instructor is saying and the computer on which they are typing. The items to which the student is now paying attention enter a form of **short-term memory** – what the instructor has said, the meaning they have constructed from the instructor's words, and what the student is typing – and exist only for a short amount of time. Unfortunately, the student's brain can only maintain the contents of its short-term memory for a very brief period of time. The student must pay attention to what the instructor has said long enough to create meaning and write the ideas down, using their computer. If the student is able to pay enough attention to what the instructor has said, perhaps relating the instructor-expressed concepts to their previous experiences, as well as typing the ideas into their computer, the student may **encode** the ideas discussed by the instructor into **long-term memory**. The student may then **retrieve** these long-term memories, at a later time, to solve a problem, answer a question, or make meaning from new experiences.

As mentioned previously, the Atkinson and Shiffrin model may look neat and tidy, but each aspect of the model is complicated, iterative, cyclical, and integrated. In addition, the processing of information is fragile and subject to interference, leakage, and forgetting. Thus, while the dual-store model appears to have distinct boundaries between sensory memory, short-term memory, and long-term memory the boundaries are overlapping, imprecise and porous. In addition, as will be seen, human information processing is a tale of limited processing resources, where limited processing leads to significant information and knowledge loss and requires distinct strategies to navigate the limits.

There have been several revisions to the Atkinson and Shiffrin model over the intervening years (see Figure 3.4). With regard to sensory memory, originally posited as a very brief retention of sensory information in the form it was first experienced (i.e., visual stimulation retained in a visual format), the concept of sensory memory now includes the influence of existing meanings on how sensations are first perceived, and greater understanding of the relationship between sense receptors and brain function. In addition, one aspect of the model that has undergone significant revision since it was first proposed is the role and nature of short-term memory. Initially, short-term memory was considered an aspect of cognition where a small amount of information or experience was stored or actively maintained for a short period of time (Cowan 2008), and comprised of sensory-specific stores (e.g., visual, auditory, linguistic). That is, short-term memory was considered to have primarily a storage role in cognition, with some limited rehearsal, search, and retrieval processes. Since the model's publication, the role of short-term memory has been subsumed within the larger construct or working memory, which entails a larger role of processing, rather than an emphasis on the storage of a small amount of information or experience. Finally, as proposed by Atkinson and Shiffrin, long-term memory was concerned with the encoding of new information, searching for that information at a later date, and, subsequently, retrieving that information. In this approach, learning was a function of mental rehearsal (more time rehearsing information equals more learning), and forgetting was a function of interference and decay (less interference at learning equals more retention). At present, the methods of encoding have been expanded significantly beyond rehearsal, the organization of knowledge has been recognized as an essential aspect of long-term memory, the relationship between encoding and retrieval has been emphasized, and the role of context in learning and memory has been highlighted. These changes, and others, necessitate an augmented model to facilitate the model's representation of cognition and to provide a better foundation for its use in providing organizational structure to a discussion of learning, memory, and cognition.

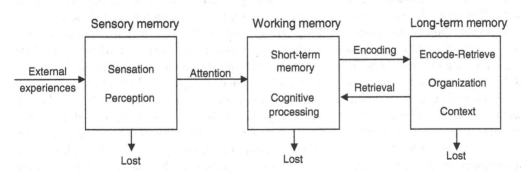

Figure 3.4 A modification of Atkinson and Shiffrin's (1968) dual-store model emphasizing newer theorizing and empirical findings related to learning and memory.

A. Sensory Memory: Sensation and Perception

The first element of the revised learning and memory model is **sensory memory**, comprising sensation and perception (Yorzinski and Whitham 2023). **Sensation** involves the stimulation of any or all of an individual's sense receptors. As a veterinary student examines a cow's eye in a laboratory setting, their visual photoreceptors (rods and cones) will be stimulated by the light reflecting from the cow's eye, their auditory receptors (organ of Corti hair cells) will be stimulated by the sound waves emanating from their lab partner's mouth, their touch receptors (mechanoreceptors) will be stimulated by the cow's eye coming in contact with their fingers, their olfactory receptors (chemoreceptors) will be stimulated by the preservation chemicals wafting in the air and entering their nose, and their taste receptors (taste receptor cells) may be stimulated by the gum they are chewing. These stimulations, from the potentially millions of receptors stimulated, are transduced into neural signals that are then processed by the brain in specialized locations for each sense (e.g., primary visual cortex, primary auditory cortex). This initial sensory processing has a large capacity but a short duration. That is, the veterinary student will experience a multitude of simultaneous and continuous sensations from their environment, but each only briefly, with each sensation typically available for additional processing for less than a second, depending on the sense. This rapid attenuation of sensations is often due to interference where new sensations replace existing sensations, or decay in a simple fading of the original sensation). These sensations will then be further processed by the brain through perception.

This process of **perception** involves recognizing and interpreting raw sensations. For example, in looking at a canine brain metencephalon transection (a raw visual sensation), where does the pyramidal tract end and the trapezoid body begin (i.e., object recognition)? A perception is influenced by both the sensation itself (bottom-up information) and the veterinary student's context, experience, knowledge, and expectations (top-down information). If a student is looking across a field at several horses – four with dark coats and one with a light coat – the light-colored horse is likely to be more noticeable (bottom-up information) as it stands out more (it is distinctive), however, if one of the dark-colored horses is owned and cared for by the student, that horse will be more noticeable (top-down information) as it is more emotionally salient. That said, the degree to which conscious, cognitive processing (e.g., choices, beliefs, motivations) influences perception is uncertain (Cermeño-Aínsa 2020; Stokes et al. 2013). For example, was the student's fondness for their horse a function of the perception itself (i.e., occurring in the primary visual cortex), or was that fondness determined at a higher level of cognition, where the horse perception was mapped to prior knowledge (i.e., prefrontal cortex) and affect (i.e., insular cortex). While the exact nature of how perceptions begin their quest for meaning is unclear, what is clear is that perception requires sensorial interpretations by the brain and that the brain's capacity to sense is far greater than its capacity to perceive and process.

B. Attention: Narrowing of the Field

While sensory memory (sensation and perception) helps to facilitate an individual's interaction with the world around them, the individual is not at the mercy of an autonomously functioning brain, focusing only on shiny objects and meaningful content. Humans have the ability to influence, or self-regulate, what they perceive through attention. **Attention** is a series of processes that allow an individual to select, modify, and sustain a mental focus on various aspects of their external and internal worlds (Narhi-Martinez et al. 2023). The capacity of this focus, however, is limited and leads to two central questions: How many things can we attend to? How long can we attend to them? The exact numbers are not particularly important, although the short answers are (i) beyond a singular point of focus attention becomes less than full on any one of the foci, and (ii) the duration may be a few seconds or much longer during vigilant attention, although the quality of the attention degrades with time. In short, perhaps better answers are "only a few" and "only for a short time." In addition, attention's capacity and duration also depend on the individual, varying from person to person and situation to situation. That said, while the specifics are at least a bit uncertain, the concept that attention has a limited capacity and duration is exceptionally important. Attention represents the first aspect of cognition where limited processing is an issue.

A key function of attention is selection. Relative to selection, *external attention* guides one's focus toward aspects of the world around us, while *internal attention* guides one's focus toward specific cognitive processes and knowledge (van Ede and Nobre, 2023). In addition, *voluntary attention* is under at least partial control of the individual, guided by prior knowledge, values, and emotions, while reflexive or *involuntary attention* is captured as a result of a particularly salient stimulus. These salient stimuli may involve attributes of greater magnitude (e.g., loud noises, noxious odors, fast-moving objects), increased novelty (e.g., unusual smells, unique tastes, odd images), considerable social relevance (e.g., noticing a long line waiting to hear a speaker, people smiling at a newborn animal, reading a book because it is on the best sellers list), or elevated personal meaning (e.g., seeing one's own cat, smelling one's favorite food, hearing one's best friend's voice). A quick note that just as perception may be bottom-up or top-down, so may attention (Leber and Egeth 2006); specifically, a veterinary student may examine an animal's eyes due to their conscious conclusion that the animal's eyes may provide diagnostic information (bottom-up) or due to eye examination being a standard component of a routine physical examination (top-down).

Ultimately, in relation to Atkinson and Shiffrin's model, focusing one's attention on an aspect of the world or the mind makes it more likely that the subject of that attention is moved into working memory and available for further cognitive processing. Of the vast array of stimuli available through sensory memory, most of it is lost as it is never attended to and therefore is either replaced by the next set of sensations, or fades with time.

C. Working Memory: Storage and Processing

As an individual attends to external stimuli and internal processes, these stimuli and processes become resources for **working memory**. For example, if a veterinary student is studying the function of a sheep's heart using a textbook, they are simultaneously engaging several resources: (i) maintaining in memory the purpose of the studying (the form and function of a sheep's heart), (ii) actively examining the material being studied (the text and images in the textbook), (iii) retrieving and maintaining in memory the knowledge already known from previous biology classes (the form and function of a human heart), (iv) processing of the textbook material and prior knowledge to create new knowledge (how the human and sheep hearts are similar and different), and (v) retrieving from and encoding to long-term memory (retrieving prior knowledge of the human heart or sheep's anatomy and physiology, as needed, and encoding new knowledge of the sheep's heart). In addition, and perhaps most importantly, (vi) the student is controlling their attention to manage their resources. Specifically, completing the study effectively involves the ability to actively maintain in memory the textbook information and long-term prior knowledge, while processing the information to construct new understandings and retrieving additional prior knowledge, and storing newly constructed knowledge while suppressing potential distractions (e.g., overheard conversations or the bright sunny day outside the window, internal irrelevant thoughts of lunch or other work to be completed). The engagement of these cognitive resources through *attentional control* occurs in and through working memory, involving significant storing and processing of knowledge. Ultimately, Pavlov and Kotchoubey (2020) have demonstrated that individual differences in working memory capacity (the individual's ability to leverage their working memory resources) are based primarily in differences related to an individual's working memory attentional control and *not* differences in short-term storage capacity.

Miyake and Shah (1999, p. 450), define working memory as "those mechanisms or processes that are involved in the control, regulation, and active maintenance of task-relevant information in the service of complex cognition, including novel as well as familiar, skilled tasks." Thus, working memory involves an integrated effort of various **executive control** *functions* including the focus, control, and maintenance of attention; the maintenance, manipulation, and updating of long-term memory; and the inhibition of attention and long-term memory activation (Miyake and Shah 1999). Neurologically, these functions are distributed broadly across the prefrontal cortex, the anterior cingulate cortex, and the parietal cortex, as well as related perceptual sites (i.e., Broca and Wernicke's areas); thus, working memory is not a specific place or space, but a collection of functions and structures.

Perhaps the most defining feature of working memory, as with attention, is its limited capacity and limited duration. The number of resources that can be consistently brought to bear on a situation is small and the duration short, without continued attention (Cowan 2010; Halford et al. 2007). The estimates of working memory capacity vary from three or four items to eight or nine items, depending on the balance of attention, storage, and processing, as well as new versus prior knowledge, with the duration of items ranging from 10–30 seconds (or more), depending on the maintenance of attention and the presence of distraction (Brady et al. 2016; Broadbent 1975; Cowan 2001; Miller 1956). Specifically, if items in working memory are only attended to briefly, they remain in working memory briefly, but if they are attended to for a longer duration, they will stay in working memory for a longer duration. In addition, distraction, the presence of additional information in working memory from either the mind or the environment, may lead to the shifting of attention and the subsequent loss of working memory resources.

1) *Working Memory Capacity.* Working memory capacity is the ability of an individual to engage efficiently in the attention, storage, and processing functions necessary for working memory to operate effectively (i.e., executive control, attentional control, and memory maintenance). In general, higher working memory capacity is related to higher memory performance – primary memory maintenance, secondary memory search, attentional control, resistance to interference, and long-term memory activation – and higher task performance – reasoning, lecture note-taking, multimedia learning, storytelling, and reading and language comprehension (Conway et al. 2002; Just and Carpenter 1992; Kane et al. 2001; Kiewra and Benton 1988; Lusk et al. 2009; Unsworth and Engle 2007).

Given working memory capacity's role in efficient and effective cognition (bigger is better), can working memory capacity be increased? Yes and no (mostly no).

Working memory training examines the impact of memory training on near and far transfer, where near transfer includes improvement to tasks that are similar to the training task (i.e., Does training on verbal working memory improve verbal short-term memory?) and far transfer is improvement on tasks that are dissimilar to the training task (i.e., Does training on verbal working memory improve reasoning?). Typical results from working memory training studies, across several meta-analyses, include small near-transfer effects and no far-transfer effects (Melby-Lervåg et al. 2016; Sala and Gobet 2017; Soveri et al. 2018; Teixeira-Santos et al. 2019). That is, individuals who engage in working memory training generally get better at the tasks upon which they are trained, but that training does not transfer to a different task. These results indicate that working memory training *does not* improve one's working memory, but rather, reflects a general practice effect where practice leads to specific improvements in the skills practiced.

2) *Cognitive Load Theory.* Cognitive load theory is based on the inherent limitations of working memory capacity and how these capacity limits interact with the instructional process (Sweller 1988; Sweller et al. 2019; Warren and Donnon 2013). Specifically, cognitive load theory posits that each task engaged in by an individual requires a series of cognitive resources in order to complete the task successfully (i.e., attention, storage, long-term memory, and processing requirements). These cognitive resource requirements place a "load" on the memory system and when this load is significantly high, it can negatively impact the learning and performance of the individual. In addition, this cognitive load involves the interaction between the task, the individual, and the environment, and yields two broad categories of load: intrinsic cognitive load and extraneous cognitive load.

Intrinsic cognitive load relates to the essential cognitive resources necessary to complete the task. For example, the task of a veterinary student listening to a cat's heart sounds might generally be interpreted as a lower intrinsic load task (see Figure 3.5a) as it requires minimal cognitive resources: proper placement of the stethoscope, listening to the heart sounds, and interpreting the heart sounds. A higher intrinsic load task may involve a veterinary student interpreting a serum biochemistry panel (see Figure 3.5b) where the student would need to understand the rationale for the panel, the metabolic functions of the liver, the parameters reported, and the parameters' reference values and ranges, as well as how these parameters and animal presentation interrelate. While Figure 3.5a and b indicate that both the heart sound and panel interpretation tasks are within the veterinary student's working memory capacity limits, there may be times when simply completing a task exceeds a student's working memory capacity limits due to the complexity of the task itself (see Figure 3.5c), leading to decreased performance and learning. For example, interpreting a serum biochemistry panel may be a low-load task for an experienced veterinarian, but may induce overload in a novice veterinary student. In this case, the student's performance will be limited, not by a lack of knowledge or external interference, but by an inability to marshal the necessary cognitive resources.

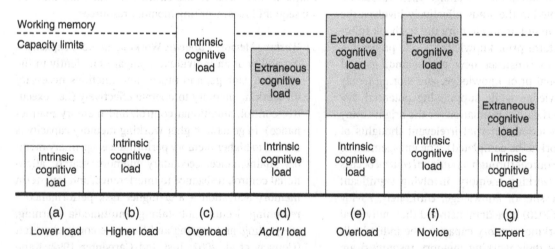

Figure 3.5 Intrinsic and extrinsic cognitive load interact with an individual's working memory capacity, as well as their long-term memory and expertise to influence performance: examples would include (a) a lower intrinsic load task, (b) a higher intrinsic load task, (c) a task where intrinsic load leads to an overload of working memory capacity limits, (d) a task that contains both intrinsic and extrinsic load, (e) a task where the intrinsic and extrinsic loads lead to an overload of working memory capacity limits, (f) a typical intrinsic and extrinsic load of a novice, and (g) a typical intrinsic and extrinsic load of an expert.

Extraneous cognitive load refers to cognitive demands in a situation, presentation, or instruction that negatively impact the individuals' ability to complete the given task. These extraneous cognitive demands are beyond the intrinsic cognitive load required to complete the task itself (see Figure 3.5d), meaning that these extraneous demands are in addition to the intrinsic demands. For example, if the veterinary student's serum biochemistry panel does not include normal or reference ranges for each parameter, the difficulty in interpreting the panel would rise artificially ("artificial" in the sense that a well-articulated panel that includes the normal or reference ranges would not result in extra cognitive load). In addition, if the interpretation was conducted under time duress or if some of the parameter values were unavailable, the difficulty of the task would be unduly increased. Finally, if the combined intrinsic and extraneous cognitive loads approach or exceed an individual's working memory capacity limits (see Figure 3.5e), task performance (learning, performance, and transfer) would likely be impeded.

While intrinsic and extraneous cognitive loads deal primarily with the task and the environment, respectively, cognitive load is also influenced by the individual (Szulewski et al. 2021). Novices, with little knowledge and experience (e.g., new veterinary students), are likely to have higher intrinsic cognitive loads and be more impacted by extraneous cognitive loads than experts with more well-developed and automated knowledge and experience (see Figure 3.5f and g). For example, in considering the serum biochemistry panel, intrinsic cognitive load will be lower for experts as their knowledge of liver function and panel information will be stronger and more easily accessible than a novice's, and the expert's cognitive procedures for interpreting the panel and interrelating the panel information with the animal's presentation will be less demanding (more automated) than a novice's. Finally, the expert is less likely to be distracted or impeded by extraneous cognitive loads (e.g., panel results that are visually hard to read, a hectic clinical environment, unclear animal presentation) than a novice.

3) *Baddeley's Multicomponent Theory of Working Memory*. Theoretically, perhaps the most well-developed model of working memory involves Baddeley's multicomponent model (Baddeley and Hitch 1974; Baddeley et al. 2021). Baddeley's model involves four basic components: the central executive, phonological loop, visuospatial sketchpad, and episodic buffer. The **central executive** controls working memory functions, including executive control, attentional control, and memory maintenance, as well as decision-making and planning.

The central executive provides control over the rest of the working memory system (i.e., the phonological loop, visuospatial sketchpad, and episodic buffer). The **phonological loop** provides a brief (<2 seconds) and capacity limited (≈5 items) memory for verbal information, as well as the ability to extend this memory duration through the *articulatory rehearsal loop* that involves repeating verbal information in subvocalized speech (i.e., nonauditory inner speech). The **visuospatial sketchpad** serves a similar function as the phonological loop (including a limited capacity and duration) except for visual information. This visuospatial sketchpad allows an individual to connect one image to the next, providing a sense of continuity as one changes the focus of their gaze. Finally, the **episodic buffer** provides memory space for the integration of verbal and visual information and the encoding of information into long-term memory. Baddeley's working memory model has been extensively tested both behaviorally and neurologically, providing support for its viability, although gaps in its ability to explain the breadth of human behavior still remain (Baddeley et al. 2019; Logie et al. 2020).

In relation to Atkinson and Shiffrin's model, the theoretical concept of short-term memory has been expanded into working memory to include a far greater role for the control of attention, memory, and behavior (Baddeley et al. 2019). One essential aspect of working memory is the control and maintenance of long-term memory. The interaction between working memory and long-term memory is represented through the concepts of encoding, storage, and retrieval.

D. Long-Term Memory: Encoding, Storage, and Retrieval

The road to remembering is uncertain. As human beings, we sense a great deal in our environment, most of which is lost as we only attend to and perceive a small amount of what we sense. Of the small amount that we attend to and perceive, most of it is lost from our working memory as we use our limited working memory capacity to solve problems, engage with others, and make decisions. For some of our experiences, however, we manage to create memories of knowledge, skills, events, and experiences in long-term memory. When examining the relationship between working memory and long-term memory, we focus on encoding, storage, and retrieval.

1) *Memory Encoding*. Memory **encoding** is the process of transforming sensations into perceptions (sensory memory), perceptions into meaningful representations (working memory), and meaningful representations into stored knowledge, skills, and events (long-term memory).

Encoding is critical to creating useful long-term cognitive resources, including how well memories are stored, how long memories are retained, and how easily memories can be retrieved. Effective encoding can lead to strong and flexible memories, memories that are easily accessible and useful across a multitude of situations. Ineffective encoding can lead to weak and poorly connected memories that may fade quickly or become inaccessible. In addition, encoding may take different forms: semantic encoding (processing the meaning of experiences), visual encoding (processing the visual characteristics of experiences), auditory encoding (processing the auditory characteristics of experiences), and motoric encoding (processing the movement characteristics of experiences). There is also olfactory encoding (smell), tactile encoding (touch), and gustatory encoding (taste), although these have been less well-researched within cognitive science.

Whether one engages in effective or ineffective encoding often depends on the strategy used. Strategies designed to enhance the encoding of long-term memory may involve simple or complex approaches. For example, a simple approach to fostering encoding is the use of **chunking**. Given working memory's storage and processing limitations, it is helpful to have strategies that compact or compress information, making the information more efficient from a processing perspective. Chunking involves organizing smaller elements of information into larger, more meaningful units of information (Miller 1956; Norris and Kalm 2021). For example, "howarewefeelingtoday" comprise 20 elements (letters), where 20 elements fall well outside our working memory capacity and would be difficult to process efficiently. If one has knowledge of the English language, however, "howarewefeelingtoday" can be reorganized into "how are we feeling today." At this point, the 20 letters have been chunked into 5 words, which are easily managed by working memory. In addition, if "how are we feeling today?" is used repeatedly as one's greeting to friends and acquaintances, then it can become a onechunked unit of greeting, "how-are-we-feeling-today?," which would require even fewer cognitive resources to be used. An illustration would include a small animal neurologic examination, entailing the systematic evaluation of the entire central and peripheral nervous system. This can appear to be an overwhelming task for novice veterinary students. By chunking the examination into seven categories (mentation, posture and gait, cranial nerves, postural reactions, spinal reflexes, spinal palpation, and pain perception), experienced veterinarians can efficiently and effectively confirm the existence and localization of neurologic lesions.

It should be noted, however, that chunking is an inside-out process: the benefit of chunking depends on an individual's prior knowledge and not simply what one perceives. For example, while chunking "howarewefeelingtoday" into "how are we feeling today" would seem easy for an English language speaker, chunking "jaksiędzisiajczujemy" into "jak się dzisiaj czujemy" would be impossible unless one already knew Polish ("jak się dzisiaj czujemy" also means "how are we feeling today"). To create the word-based chunks, an individual must already know the words. Thus, when chunking information into meaningful units, the "meaning" aspect comes from within the individual and is not inherent in the experience. This is one of the reasons why more experienced veterinarians will encounter less cognitive load in most veterinary situations than novice veterinary students – more knowledge leads to more efficient chunking, which leads to more efficient processing. For example, an experienced veterinarian can efficiently localize a neurologic lesion during a physical examination appointment, whereas a veterinary student will likely need to consult their notes to recall each of the 12 cranial nerves and how to assess for neurologic deficits.

2) *Memory Storage.* Encoding experiences into long-term memory allows for the accumulation of vast amounts of information that needs to be interpreted, organized, synthesized, and integrated in order to be efficiently accessed and used. The distinction between information, knowledge, and memory is helpful in understanding memory storage and organization. **Information** refers to the fundamental facts and perceptions of experience that may lead to the development of knowledge. **Knowledge** refers to the construction of higher levels of meaning through the connection of new knowledge and experiences with prior knowledge and experiences (or the creation of new connections between existing prior knowledge), resulting in an individual's understanding of information to be developed into concepts and skills. Knowledge may be thought of broadly to include facts, concepts, and events (declarative knowledge); skills, behaviors, and procedures (procedural knowledge); and feelings, beliefs, and values (self-knowledge). In addition, the relationship between information and knowledge is iterative; specifically, new information may be processed into a higher level of meaning and thus become knowledge, yet this new knowledge may be considered information at a newer and more complex level, such that further processing may lead to an even greater understanding and thus a new level of more highly connected knowledge. **Memory** refers to the ability to encode, store, and retrieve information and knowledge, as well as the structures necessary to support these processes.

Thus, the concepts of information, knowledge, and memory are, by definition, interrelated. For example, consider a veterinary student attending an anatomy class where they first experience information, such as the basic facts and imagery of anatomy (e.g., direction terms, names, and forms of bones and muscles). This anatomical information becomes knowledge when it is processed – interpreted, organized, synthesized, and integrated – into a more meaningful form (e.g., skeletal and muscular systems, biomechanics). This new level of meaning can serve as necessary information for the development of more advanced meaning making (e.g., diagnosis, surgery, nutrition). A student's memory then serves to retain their developing information and knowledge for later retrieval and use in thought and action.

Memory itself, however, is not a singular concept, but rather, a collection of different memory systems and types (see Figure 3.6). Long-term memory can be seen as possessing two broad types of memory: explicit memory and implicit memory. **Explicit memory** refers to memory of which an individual is consciously aware and can readily and intentionally retrieve. Knowledge within explicit memory is typically referred to as declarative knowledge, or knowledge that can be declared. To illustrate, if a veterinary student was asked, "What are the four chambers of a dog's heart?," their reply would be declarative knowledge stored in explicit memory. **Implicit memory** refers to memory of which an individual is *not* consciously aware, and retrieval is nonconscious, occurring without the explicit intention of the individual. Since the knowledge, retrieval, and use are not conscious, the presence of implicit memories can be seen only through behaviors, not intentionally recollected. For example, an experienced veterinarian does not think back to their communication skills classes when consoling a grieving pet owner. They simply respond, using appropriate verbal and nonverbal communication techniques to offer an empathetic response. Finally, procedural knowledge may start as an explicit list of steps to be taken in the completion of a task (e.g., a wellness exam), but with practice,

these steps will develop into procedural knowledge where the steps fade as a guide to action and the veterinarian simply moves from action to action without consciously recalling each explicitly.

3) *Explicit Memory.* Explicit memory, involving consciously and intentionally retrieved knowledge, is typically seen as comprising episodic memory and semantic memory. **Episodic memory** involves the remembrance of lived events and experiences (episodes) at specific times and places (Renoult et al. 2019; Rubin 2022). For example, a veterinary student may remember that yesterday they attended epidemiology class and sat in front of the classroom in a seat that made seeing the projection screen difficult. This student is remembering a specific event, not recalling a general conclusion that sitting in the front of the classroom makes seeing the projection screen difficult (i.e., semantic memory, see below). A specific form of episodic memory is *autobiographical memory*, which refers to the memory of lived events that have special meaning for the individual – these are the memories one uses when they describe their lives or their personal history. As such, autobiographical memories typically include high levels of meaning, emotions, and beliefs as part of the event description. Where were you when you found out that you were accepted into veterinary school? Over time, episodic memories tend to fade more quickly than autobiographical memories due to the enhanced meaningfulness of the autobiographical memories (Talarico et al. 2004).

In addition to episodic memory, explicit memory also includes **semantic memory** that involves memory for general knowledge, concepts, and facts that are *not* tied to specific events or experiences. Semantic memory focuses on the meaning of knowledge, concepts, and facts, where the meaning tends to be accumulated over time with repeated experiences. For example, a veterinary student who understands the structures and functions of the circulatory system will have constructed this knowledge through multiple interactions with the circulatory system (via lectures, readings, studying, and conversations), not at a specific time and place (e.g., Tuesday's lecture). In addition, this semantic memory

Figure 3.6 A classification of long-term memory components associated with explicit and implicit memory.

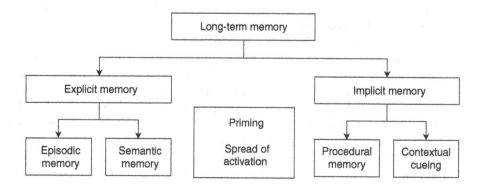

for knowledge, concepts, and facts tends to be organized into various structures or mental frameworks, including categories, networks, schemas, and concepts.

4) *Implicit Memory*. Implicit memory, involving nonconsciously and unintentionally retrieved knowledge, is typically seen as comprising procedural memory and contextual cueing. **Procedural memory**, or procedural learning, involves the learning of skills and habits, typically through extensive practice and experience, resulting in a degree of automaticity. As these skills and habits become more automatic, the individual possessing them begins to lose the ability to articulate what they are doing and why they are doing it. Nevertheless, the development of an automated skill always begins with the conduct of a conscious skill. For example, when a veterinary student first begins to learn how to tie a surgical knot at the beginning or end of a suture line, the experience is highly conscious, challenging, and less than successful; however, watching an experienced surgeon tie a surgical knot can be a bit of a blur. Developing a skill from conscious to automatic requires considerable practice. Early learning is typically slow, error-prone, highly attentional, and thus, more effortful (Anderson 1982; Fitts and Posner 1967). As a result of practice, performance may become more and more automatic such that the performance is faster, increasingly error-free, less attentional, and thus, less effortful. This increase in speed and accuracy is the result of the skill requiring fewer central cognitive resources (i.e., less attentional control, less decision-making), resulting in less cognitive load. While automaticity is generally considered a positive result of practice, developing automaticity can also lead to a lack of awareness and control (Charlton and Starkey 2011; Posner and Snyder 1975).

In addition to procedural learning, learning to use context cues to guide attention can also result in nonconscious and unintentional behavior (Sisk et al. 2019). **Contextual cueing** involves two components: the visual context and the behavioral action. For example, veterinary surgical personnel, after spending considerable time in a surgical suite, will develop a mental map of the visual space so that they nonconsciously know where all of the materials and equipment are located. This mental map will allow the surgical personnel to reach for needed materials or equipment without having to consciously scan or search the room in advance, thus reducing the attentional resources and cognitive load of the procedure itself. In the case of implicit contextual cueing, the awareness of the spatial layout becomes predictive, allowing the individual to unconsciously orient their attention to an appropriate location.

Beyond procedural learning and contextual cueing, priming and spread of activation can connect implicit and explicit memory. Both priming and spread of activation address how the activation of one piece of knowledge can lead unconsciously to the activation of a related piece of knowledge, making that knowledge more accessible and retrievable; thus, the process of activation occurs implicitly, while the knowledge that becomes activated may be explicit. In the case of **priming**, experiencing particular knowledge, such as concepts, thoughts, images, or emotions activates related knowledge, making that related knowledge more available for retrieval (McNamara 2005; Meyer and Schvaneveldt 1971). For example, a veterinary student may overhear a veterinarian talking about the nervous system. In the student's mind, knowledge related to the nervous system may become more active, such as concepts (e.g., neurons, neurotransmitters), images (e.g., an image of a dog's nervous system), or emotions (e.g., fear that they might be asked a question about the nervous system, a system for which their knowledge is uncertain). These concepts, images, or emotions may become more active implicitly, without the student's conscious awareness. Relatedly, **spread of activation** refers to how the activation of one piece of knowledge can unconsciously activate related knowledge, and that the newly activated knowledge can activate additional knowledge related to it (Collins and Loftus 1975; Fazio 2001). In this way, the knowledge activation spreads through a network of related knowledge (the more closely related two pieces of knowledge, the stronger the spread of activation). For example, the student who overhears the veterinarian's discussion of the nervous system may (nonconsciously) activate closely related conceptual knowledge (e.g., neurons, neurotransmitters), and that knowledge may activate further related concepts (e.g., axons, dendrites, synapses, receptors). These activations will make responding to subsequent questions regarding neurotransmitters or synapses easier.

5) *Memory Retrieval*. Memory **retrieval** is the process of accessing, activating, and transferring information stored in long-term memory into working memory for use. Memory retrieval is an uncertain process, as information stored in long-term memory is often partial or interpretive (i.e., not a video of events, or word-for-word transcriptions of discussions) and may involve weak or disorganized storage that results in incomplete or incorrect retrieval. Thus, what is retrieved depends on both the nature of the retrieval and on the strength and accuracy of the encoding. For example, a veterinary student may be examining a lame dog through palpation. The student's prior encoding and storage of the dog's musculoskeletal anatomy and the process for examining a lame dog will influence the quality of the anatomical and procedural information the student retrieves and, ultimately, the quality of their examination and conclusions.

The process of memory retrieval, like memory encoding, often depends on the strategy used. Strategies designed to enhance the retrieval of long-term memory may involve simple or complex approaches. For example, a simple approach to fostering retrieval is the use of **retrieval cues**. Retrieval cues are clues or aspects of the environment that become associated with information when it is learned (or in subsequent learning). These cues can be internal (e.g., emotions, thoughts) or external (e.g., words, images, odors) and influence the ability of an individual to retrieve the encoding information. Cues operate by activating long-term memories that can then be transferred into working memory for use. The smell of an anatomy lab may lead to a flood of memories when lab specimens are placed on display for a final exam, or a funny acronym that an instructor makes up to help students remember the number of taeniae in each section of the equine intestinal tract becomes a mnemonic that stays with the students for years. The more specific and distinctive the cue, the better trigger it may be for activating the encoded memory. This use of retrieval cues is a form of *encoding specificity*, that is, when the context at encoding (learning) is similar to the context at retrieval (performance), retrieval is enhanced (Godden and Baddeley 1975; Tulving and Thomson 1973). Encoding specificity may be broken down into two components: *content-dependent memory* that focuses on the external context present during learning (e.g., location, sounds) and *state-dependent memory* that focuses on the internal context present during learning (e.g., anxiety, mood, fatigue). For example, taking the anatomy exam in the same lab where anatomy class was taught can increase the likelihood of the smells triggering specific details needed for the test.

In relation to Atkinson and Shiffrin's model, memory encoding, storage, and retrieval form a complex inter-relationship of storage and processing that influence an individual's ability to think and act. The interaction between sensory memory, working memory, and long-term memory creates an adaptive system of attentional control, meaning making, and flexible performance. The discussed learning and memory strategies – chunking and retrieval cues – are just the tip of the learning, memory, and cognition iceberg (see the Fostering Deep and Flexible Long-Term Knowledge section below).

Part 2: Conceptual Knowledge

A central aspect of learning, memory, and cognition involves determining patterns in prior knowledge and experience and representing these patterns in a meaningful organization. These organizational representations allow for the integration and synthesis of various aspects of knowledge, including episodic and semantic knowledge, and to a lesser extent procedural knowledge. In addition, these organizational representations – categories, networks, schemas, and concepts – provide benefits beyond simple organization to include: (1) the ability to make inferences and predictions, (ii) the ability to communicate, (iii) the ability to reduce cognitive load, and (iv) the ability to facilitate or inhibit the learning of new knowledge (Carey 2009; Rosch et al. 1976).

1) Conceptual knowledge allows an individual to *infer* from prior knowledge and experience in order to better understand new knowledge and experience. This better understanding may also lead to the ability to *predict* unseen properties of an object or the likelihood of future events.

   For example, a veterinarian who is examining a lame horse may infer from the horse's gait abnormalities that the lameness is associated with the musculoskeletal system or perhaps the nervous system. This inferencing will then guide the veterinarian as they talk to the client, examine and evaluate the horse, and work to narrow the diagnosis. Once the veterinarian determines the cause of the lameness, they can predict the likely needs and courses of action for the client and horse.

2) Conceptual knowledge facilitates *communication* through the use of terms, concepts, and labels that summarize a corpus of knowledge, rather than having to rely on explaining each idea. Domain-based jargon (e.g., ADR means Ain't Doin' Right; HBC means Hit By Car, Fx means Fracture) is often considered in a negative light, but for those that understand the domain knowledge, jargon can lead to significantly easier communication.

   For example, if a veterinarian were to say to a student, "This cat has Grade II periodontal disease and resorptive lesions. Please conduct an oral exam and interpret these dental radiographs," the veterinarian is communicating information about the cat's condition (Grade 2 periodontal disease and resorptive lesions) and the need for assessment (oral exam and interpretation of dental radiographs) without having to explain the knowledge behind the condition and the diagnostics.

3) Conceptual knowledge reduces *cognitive load* by condensing information into packets of knowledge. In addition, since these packets (i.e., schemas and concepts) include regularities of useful knowledge, they help an individual to focus on information that has been demonstrated to be beneficial, rather than a representation of everything one knows or has experienced.

   For example, a veterinary student examining a cat for digestive distress does not need to maintain all of their knowledge regarding the digestive system in working memory all at once; rather, they can begin with relevant questions of the client regarding their cat. These questions may allow the student to narrow the field of interest (e.g., gastroenteritis, colitis, pancreatitis, hair ball) at which point they can focus their knowledge on one or two potential causes in particular, which may represent the symptoms, tests, and treatments for those disorders.

4) Conceptual knowledge can also facilitate or inhibit *learning* and *memory*. To start, conceptual knowledge provides an organized foundation of prior knowledge. However, this foundation of knowledge can both facilitate the learning of new knowledge that can be integrated with the existing conceptual knowledge or inhibit the learning of new knowledge that contradicts existing conceptual knowledge (Alba and Hasher 1983). In both cases, conceptual knowledge influences how an individual interprets and remembers events. This interpretation can negatively influence learning and memory when prior knowledge (for example, in the form of stereotypes toward clients, animals, or approaches) leads to inappropriate and unproductive inferences, predictions, and behaviors, as well as a lack of openness to learning knowledge that is counter to a held stereotype.

Indeed, a veterinary student who has existing knowledge related to normal animal anatomy and physiology is in a better position to learn knowledge regarding general pathology, as they have existing knowledge regarding animal function. They can use this as a foundation upon which to build their new pathology knowledge. Similarly, it would be challenging to learn about neurological diseases if one does not first have knowledge of neurological anatomy and physiology. In addition, while prior knowledge is generally a benefit to learning, it can also impede learning. A veterinary student who has come to believe that animals do not feel pain the way that humans do, or believes that if an animal is not expressing pain auditorily then they are not actually in pain, may be slow to learn new pain management techniques or new knowledge regarding pain management.

The following examples of conceptual knowledge – categorizations, networks, schemas, and concepts – are not discrete or independent of each other. Each type of conceptual knowledge overlaps and may be broadly thought of as hierarchical, and as such, each of these knowledge forms contributes to the four benefits of conceptual knowledge previously mentioned.

A. Categorization

Categorization is the most general term related to the types of conceptual knowledge and can be understood to include networks, schema, and concepts. A categorization provides a grouping of related information (a category, such as cats, dogs, teaching strategies, and learning processes) that also distinguishes this grouping from other groupings. These groupings may involve episodic, semantic, or procedural knowledge. *Concrete categorizations* are well-defined groupings, often defined by observative features, such as birds and squirrels or knowledge of the respiratory or digestive systems. *Abstract categorizations* are less well-defined, often lacking surface feature similarities, such as ethics, happiness, and care. Individuals may begin their conceptual understanding through concrete categorizations and later develop a more abstract understanding (Quinn and Tanaka 2007).

B. Networks

A semantic network of knowledge tends to represent knowledge hierarchically, with superordinate and subordinate categorizations (Collins and Quillian 1969; see Figure 3.7). The most general properties of a category are

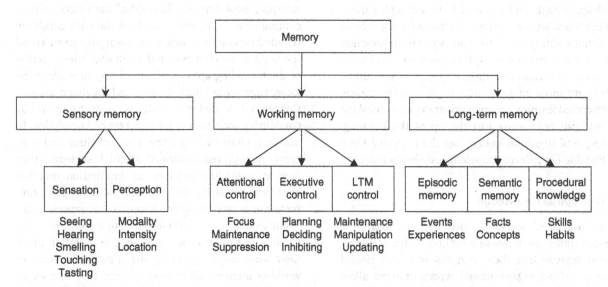

Figure 3.7 An example of a semantic network involving nodes (e.g., sensory memory, sensation, perception) with features (e.g., modality, intensity, location) and organized hierarchically by links (memory " sensory memory " perception).

higher in the structure, while more specific properties are represented lower in the structure. Within the structure exists nodes (attributes), features (elements), and links (relations). Higher nodes generalize to lower nodes such that sensory memory, working memory, and long-term memory are all properties or examples of memory. Nodes closer together tend to be more highly related than nodes farther apart; thus spread of activation will tend to impact nodes that are closer to the originally activated node and dissipate as the spread moves from node to node.

C. Schemas

While a network of categories and their relationships provides organizational information, it does not provide information regarding our general understanding of the categories or specific instances within it. A **schema** is an organizing framework that relies on the abstraction of regularities from a series of specific concept and event experiences (event-based schemas are sometimes referred to as scripts). For example, a veterinary student may be able to read about how to conduct a client consultation, but it is in the repeated experiences of conducting these consultations that the student is able to develop a schema that guides their future consultations. These developed consultation schemas contain the common attributes and behaviors that lead to a successful consultation. Attributes and behaviors that are not common or that do not contribute to a successful outcome do not tend to be included in the schema. Thus, schemas reduce or condense the potentially vast amount of information available in experiences into a more manageable and useful generalization (Bartlett 1932; McVee et al. 2005; Ost et al. 2022).

Once a schema is formed, however, it is not stagnant; instead, it evolves as new relevant experiences are accumulated. New experiences that validate the existing schema will lead to a strengthening of the schema and new experiences that challenge the existing schema or are deemed common and important, but not yet included in the schema, will lead to revisions in the schema. Schemas, developed from prior experience, have a significant impact on current learning, understanding, and experience. Consider a veterinarian entering a new exam room for the first time. They will enter the room with an exam room schema in mind, one that represents a generalization of exam rooms within which they have conducted exams previously. This exam room schema may contain information such as typical room size, lighting options, exam table, small animal scale, seats for clients, sink with running water, artwork, materials cabinets, small equipment, refrigerator, computer, sharps container, and trash can (see Figure 3.8). A veterinarian's schema-based expectations will influence their thoughts and behaviors (e.g., "I don't need to bring exam gloves into the room with me, there will be some in the cabinet"). However, not all elements are equally represented in a schema. Of the elements in the exam room schema, some are more likely to be present (e.g., exam table, seats, materials, and equipment) than others (e.g., lighting options, refrigerator, computer). Finally, schemas may contain other schemas. That is, of the elements listed in a generalized exam room, a veterinarian may have a schema for materials cabinets, a generalized representation of what is likely to be in the materials cabinets, such as gauze, alcohol swabs, scissors, gloves), or the exam room schema may be included itself in a larger schema of a veterinary clinic layout (see Figure 3.8).

An event-based schema, or **script**, condenses the steps typically present in an event or action by focusing on the steps that are typical in the successful completion of the event or action (Bower et al. 1979). These scripts impact an individual's understanding of events or actions, allow for

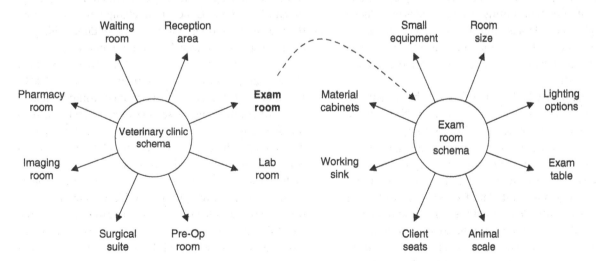

Figure 3.8 Schemas represent a generalization of knowledge and experience, such as typical elements in a veterinary clinic layout. In addition, schemas may contain other schemas, thus the exam room schema is an element of a larger veterinary clinic layout schema.

inference and prediction relative to the events or actions, and influence how they later remember the event or action. A veterinarian, over time, may develop a script for conducting an exam on a cat in respiratory distress that includes several steps: obtain a medical history, perform a physical exam, consider differential diagnoses, develop a diagnostic plan, run and interpret diagnostics, and initiate a treatment plan. It should be noted that not all veterinarians will develop the same script for a respiratory case, although there is likely to be substantial overlap. Finally, while a domain-specific script may be developed and explicitly taught to veterinary students, this official script is likely to be augmented by the individual's personal experiences.

D. Concepts

While categories represent broad labels, networks represent hierarchical organizations, and schemas represent typical elements extracted from experiences, concepts are detailed or concrete representations of objects and events in the world around us that tend to be more defined than schemas (Carey 2009; Nesbit and Adesope 2006). As mentioned previously, categories, networks, schemas, and concepts overlap extensively, so if schemas and concepts seem similar, they are.

Concepts (such as animal, horse, health care, and differential diagnosis) are typically learned through *positive instances* and *negative instances*. A young child with a dog may label a horse and a cow as "dog," since they all have four legs, fur, a face, and a tail. These features are the same as the dog that lives with the child and is perceived as similar, especially from a distance. Ultimately, however, the child will begin to differentiate these animals based on particular defining *features*, such as body size, shape of the face, and movement. This differentiation into separate concepts is facilitated socially when others label a horse a "horse," a cow a "cow," and a dog a "dog." This differentiation is provided by positive and negative examples of each. This differentiation will continue as the child is introduced to sheep, pigs, and llamas, and the veterinary student is introduced to the Clydesdale, the American Quarter Horse, and the Shetland Pony, or the Great Dane, the Golden Retriever, and the Chihuahua.

Beyond features, which can sometimes be difficult to delineate, individuals can represent concepts through the use of exemplars and prototypes. Representing a concept via *exemplars* involves remembering several examples of the concept. For example, remembering "cow" based on remembrances of a Holstein cow, a Hereford cow, and a Black Angus cow at a county fair. Exemplars provide both a sense of the essential features of the concept and the recognition that there is variability in the concept. In addition, there is evidence that we can also represent a concept through a *prototype*, or one typical example of the concept. For example, a veterinary student may have a prototype in

mind for a heart that involves a diagrammatic image of a heart with four neatly drawn chambers, well-labeled valves, and red and blue arteries and veins. Another prototype might be an image of a Rambouillet sheep for "sheep" or a Quarter Horse for "horse."

1) *Developing Concepts.* Individuals can come to develop concepts from the top down, through a teacher-centered process where veterinary students (i) are provided with positive and negative instances of a concept, (ii) extract defining features of the new concept, and (iii) develop a concept definition (concept attainment). Students may also learn concepts from the bottom up, through a student-centered process of (i) generalizing from everyday or known experiences to generate the concept, features, and definition, followed by (ii) using the developed concept to predict, explain, and verify new instances or observations (concept formation). Both concept attainment and concept formation focus on students developing well-defined understandings of concepts, and empirical support exists for both approaches.

Whether using concept attainment or concept formation, concepts are better understood when (i) the defining features are salient and distinct; (ii) the provided definitions are clear and include the defining features, especially when the defining features are subtle or vague; (iii) the concept is explained within the students' prior knowledge of other concepts; (iv) the first examples are simple and clear positive instances, with subsequent instances less clear and more challenging; (v) positive and negative instances are provided simultaneously; and, (vi) both definitions and examples are presented (or developed) during the learning process (Aslin and Newport 2012; Kornell and Bjork 2008).

2) *Conceptual Change.* While developing new concepts can be a challenge, fostering conceptual change is significantly harder. Conceptual change involves more than a slight refinement in one's understanding; it entails a significant transformation in one's representation and application of a concept (Chi and Roscoe 2002; DiSessa and Sherin 1998; Duit and Treagust 2003). Examples of extensive concept change would include a shift from understanding science as a search for facts to the development of an integrative process for expanding understanding of the world around us based on evidence. In veterinary medicine, conceptual change may include a shift from thinking of veterinary medicine as the act of vaccinating puppies and kittens to an understanding of the veterinarian's role in promoting a "One Health" approach, in which veterinarians are integral in ensuring animal health while considering its interdependent relationships with human, public, and environmental health. On a less expansive scale, conceptual

change can also involve the development of knowledge from basic facts and figures to a more sophisticated and nuanced understanding and application.

Fostering conceptual change is a challenge and may vary depending on the concepts to change. The process can be intensive and requires significant engagement on the part of the student and instructor (Dole and Sinatra 1998; Posner et al. 1982; Schnotz and Bannert 2003; Vosniadou 1994; Zuccarini and Malgieri 2022). To engage students in conceptual change, one should attempt to:

- *Foster the identification of preconceptions and engage in the detection of discrepancies.* It is important for students to understand their own knowledge and how they see the world. What do they know, believe, and value? In addition, how do students' understandings, beliefs, and values align with those espoused by the field of veterinary medicine? In general, identifying preconceptions and detecting discrepancies in students' understandings, beliefs, and values are facilitated by (i) student active engagement (e.g., lab and live animal experiences, discussions, problem-solving), (ii) student explicit reflections on new versus prior knowledge (e.g., journaling, discussions, reflection prompts), (iii) student engagement with multiple representations (e.g., data-based graphs and diagram, discussions, readings), (iv) student interactions with peers (e.g., peer feedback, group discussions, group projects), and (v) instructor feedback emphasizing discrepancies (e.g., post-lab notes, discussions, comments based on reflection prompts).
- *Engage students in cognitive conflict supported by explanations and feedback.* One purpose of the identification of preconceptions and the detection of discrepancies is the generation of cognitive conflict, a state of uncertainty and, potentially, discomfort resulting from the realization of discord between one's knowledge, beliefs, and values and those of new information or experiences. This new information needs to be supported by clear explanations of the discrepancies and feedback on the students' understanding of these discrepancies. The rationale for the cognitive conflict is to motivate a student to engage in a reevaluation of their understanding, beliefs, or values in light of the realized discord. Are changes desired and how might these changes be fostered?
- *Foster the accommodation of new knowledge and experiences.* As students become motivated to initiate change, the challenge becomes modifying, or accommodating, one's knowledge representations and personal beliefs and values based on the new knowledge and experiences. Accommodation involves modifying existing or creating new understandings, beliefs, or values that better align with the new experiences. The development of these new representations involves repeated experiences in testing and validating one's understanding through active engagement.
- *Promote active engagement, including practice with feedback and generalization.* In addition to identifying uncertainties and discrepancies, as well as adapting one's knowledge, beliefs, and values based on new information, students should be provided with opportunities to apply and test their new understandings in existing and new contexts or situations through active engagement in problem-solving, peer discussions, client and animal interactions, and lab experiences. It is through these new applications that students can develop new generalized categories, networks, schemas, and concepts.
- *Foster student reflection for the purpose of accommodation and integration.* Conceptual change is an ongoing process of evaluating one's understanding, as well as new information and experiences, in order to identify and address uncertainty and discrepancies. This process, while often initiated by instructors, ultimately should be self-regulated by the student. This self-regulation process can be fostered by encouraging student reflections to identify uncertainty and discrepancies, adjust existing understandings or reframe new knowledge and experience, and integrate or synthesize new and prior knowledge and experiences.

Ultimately, initially expending the effort to learn new concepts accurately, is much easier than trying to change concepts afterward. That said, conceptual change is an important process for students to possess, as a career in veterinary medicine will require continuous adjustments to one's explicit and implicit knowledge.

Part 3: Fostering Deep and Flexible Knowledge

Learning is a function of processing: what we process we learn. This processing, within the idiosyncrasies of human memory, has the potential to result in deep and flexible knowledge, specifically knowledge that is accessible with little or no effort, knowledge that is interconnected with other relevant knowledge, and knowledge that is applicable across a variety of purposes and contexts. Deep and flexible knowledge can be seen when a veterinarian evaluates a horse by asking questions of the client, observing the horse, activating relevant knowledge based on what they have seen and heard, integrating and inferring from what they have seen, heard, and activated, all in order to form a differential diagnosis list. Ultimately, gaining knowledge and experience across a career will lead the veterinarian toward expertise, resulting in faster, more accurate, less effortful, and more applicable knowledge and skills.

As discussed at the beginning of the chapter, learning and performance are intricately linked such that deeper processing during learning generally results in increased levels of performance (depth of processing). Similarly, aligning the type of processing (transfer appropriate processing) or aligning the context of processing (encoding specificity) between the learning and performance situations also generally results in increased levels of performance. This learning–performance relationship can be extended when examining one's intent to learn. Specifically, does it matter if one intends to learn? Yes. No. It depends.

In the 1960s and 1970s, a focus of research evolved to examine whether the **intent to learn** impacted learning (Hyde and Jenkins 1969, 1973; Walsh and Jenkins 1973; see also Craik 2023; Oberauer and Greve 2022). The rationale was based on *depth of processing* (Craik and Tulving 1975), that is, if an individual processed information deeply, they tended to learn more. This led to a related question: Would intent to learn matter if the individual processed information deeply? The short answer is *no*. When individuals process information deeply (meaningfully), it does not matter if the individual intends to learn or not – what we process we learn, whether the processing was intentional or not. Indeed, the intent to learn only matters to the degree that it serves to motivate an individual to engage in deeper processing: "The importance of intentionality lies in its abstract motivational push to perform further processing operations on the event in question" (Craik 2023, p. 302).

This point is significant: Students may learn based on the processing induced through instruction or by the processing initiated by the students themselves. Two revelations: First, *instruction impacts student learning to the degree that the instruction fosters processing*. In the active learning literature (Deslauriers et al. 2019; Freeman et al. 2014; Lombardi et al. 2021), strict lecture instruction (i.e., exposition + note-taking only) is posited as an ineffective method for fostering learning, while student-engaging instruction (e.g., problem-based learning, flipped classroom, small group work) is posited as an effective method. But, why? Why do some instructional strategies foster more learning than others? The answer is processing. The focus on processing helps to address why some strategies, such as flipping the classroom, can be both highly effective and completely ineffective in fostering student learning (see Kapur et al. 2022; Oudbier et al. 2022). Strategies are only effective when their application in the classroom fosters relevant student processing; thus, the effectiveness of instruction has less to do with the strategy itself and more to do with the implementation.

Second, *students' actions impact learning to the degree that these actions foster processing*. For example, students who pay attention during a class and take "good" notes (i.e., making meaning from what the instructor is saying before writing down notes, relating the new notes to prior notes, and highlighting concepts that are still confusing) tend to learn more than students who simply transcribe what the instructor is saying. Students who think about class knowledge outside of class, informally, tend to learn more than students who only think about class prior to an exam. And, students who study across several sessions, talk aloud to themselves during studying, and generate their own summaries will learn more than students who simply reread their notes. Unfortunately, students often engage in learning strategies that have been demonstrated to be ineffective, such as rehearsal or cramming, while eschewing learning strategies that have been demonstrated to be effective, such as summarizing and self-testing (Blasiman et al. 2017; Hartwig and Dunlosky 2012; Morehead et al. 2016).

Thus, while both *intentional* and *incidental processing* may lead to learning, depending on the relevance of the processing to the task to be performed, both are not required. Indeed, previous research has demonstrated that when incidental learning is sufficient for learning a task, additional intentional learning is not beneficial (Evans and Baddeley 2018; Hyde and Jenkins 1969; Oberauer and Greve 2022; Postman and Adams 1956). Just to be clear, the first point here is *not* that intent to learn is unimportant or ineffective, but rather, that **processing is the proximal cause of learning** and that the intent to learn is effective to the degree that it motivates students to engage in effective (meaningful) processing. In addition, the second point is that *teaching matters* and that teaching matters to the degree that it fosters processing that is relevant to the instructor's outcomes for the course.

What follows is a discussion of actions and effects that foster processing and, thus, impact learning. As noted, while these actions and effects foster processing, their effectiveness depends on their implementation. Finally, these actions and effects are not independent and cannot be parsed into individual and discrete boxes – there is significant overlap because learning is neither neat nor tidy. For example, the generation effect, which posits that self-generating meaning leads to greater learning than simply watching a presentation, overlaps with the retrieval practice effect, which posits that retrieving information from long-term memory (which is required to make meaning) also leads to greater learning than simply watching a presentation, which overlaps with the spacing effect, which posits that generating and retrieving information leads to greater learning when they are distributed over time rather than massed in a single session. If you find yourself saying, "This sounds a lot like . . . " or "This seems to be related to . . ., " that is a good thing – you are processing. Finally, everything about to be discussed comes under the depth-of-processing umbrella and the heuristic of, *what we process we learn*.

A. Learning, Forgetting, and Practice

The relationship between learning and performance follows the fairly standard form of a power function (see Figure 3.9a), with more learning early in practice and less learning overtime (Crossman 1959; Snoddy 1926). This ***Power Law of Learning*** relationship is evident across various tasks from language learning (Graves and Garton 2017), to musical instrument proficiency (Lehmann and Ericsson 1997), to memorization (Cepeda et al. 2009). More recently, Heathcote et al. (2000), indicated that while a power function fits the aggregated data across participants, on an individual basis learning follows more of an exponential function. Interestingly, forgetting tends to follow a similarly shaped power function (see Figure 3.9b), decreasing more immediately after the cessation of learning and tapering off less over time forming the ***Power Law of Forgetting***. This relationship is also evident across various functions, such as language learning (Bahrick 1984), skill learning (Walker et al. 2003), and memorization (Wickelgren 1975).

As a general course, when one stops learning, one starts **forgetting**. Unfortunately, the exact details regarding why one forgets are both multifaceted and imprecise (Schacter 2002). In some cases, memories are not forgotten; they were never encoded in the first place. This lack of initial learning may be due to a lack of attention or processing during encoding, or in some cases, due to the presence of memory-impeding pharmaceuticals in the blood, such as alcohol, benzodiazepines, and opioids. If memories are appropriately formed, memory failure may be the result of general decay, poor retrieval, or information interference. First, in the case of ***decay***, the strength of memories may decrease due to a lack of use to the point where the memory become inaccessible (Hardt et al. 2013; Ricker et al. 2016). This does not mean that the memory is completely gone, but only that the memory cannot be activated back to a conscious level. In such cases, relearning the knowledge or skill typically takes less time than the original learning, indicating that the individual was not starting from scratch. Second, forgetting may be due to ***retrieval failure***, where a memory is inaccessible due to the lack of an appropriate cue to activate the memory (Shiffrin 1970). It is common to have a feeling that one knows something (e.g., the name of a piece of equipment or someone's name), but simply cannot seem to retrieve it. In this case, searching for an appropriate cue (e.g., when is the equipment used, or an image of the person's face) may retrieve the memory more effectively than attempting to retrieve the memory directly. Finally, forgetting may be the result of ***interference***, when one memory makes it difficult to retrieve another memory (Barrouillet and Camos 2009; Lewandowsky et al. 2008). For instance, if a person who lived in Louisiana with a 504 area code moves to Virginia with a 540 area code, they may have difficulty upon first moving in retrieving their new area code due to the interference of their old area code. Additionally, veterinary students may struggle to remember the proper way to bandage a catheter in the ICU at the vet school due to interference from the method they were taught at their old clinic, or interference could be caused by a surgical video viewed during vet school which prevents them from learning/recalling new and unfamiliar protocols on a surgical clerkship in their final year.

Beyond initial learning and forgetting, as an individual continues to practice and gain experience, they may develop ***expertise***. Specifically, with practice and experience, they add new knowledge and skills, organize existing knowledge and skills into more effective and integrated formats, generalize knowledge and skills into schemas and concepts, and develop fast and efficient domain-specific skills. The development of expertise is a continuum, with knowledge and skills improving over time. While there have been estimates of how much time it takes to become an expert – 5,000 hours, 10,000 hours, 10 years – there is no magic number and the time it takes will depend on the nature of the practice, the nature of the task, and the nature of the individual. What is known is that expertise takes a lot of practice over a long period of time.

In addition, there are a number of theories associated with the development of expertise, especially skill-based

(a)

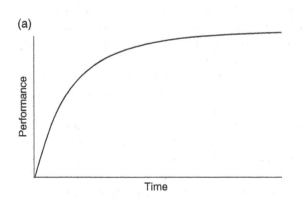

(b)

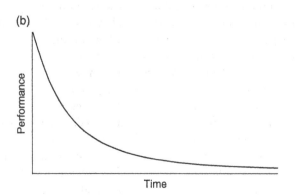

Figure 3.9 A generalized representation of the Power Law of Learning (a) and the Power Law of Forgetting (b).

expertise, and several of them propose three overlapping stages of expertise development (Anderson 1982; Fitts 1964; Kim et al. 2013). The stage names proposed by Anderson (1982) – *declarative, transitional,* and *procedural* – align the development of expertise with the acquisition and refinement of declarative and procedural memory. In this case, the **declarative stage** of expertise involves the acquisition of primarily declarative memory (e.g., facts, concepts, terminology, structures), including processes that are stored in memory as a step-by-step list (this list would be conscious and something the student would write down or talk about). It is common for a novice at the declarative stage to rehearse or talk themselves through the steps of a skill. The declarative stage is typified by slow and error-prone performance that requires high levels of attention and effort. Specifically, for a novice, a new skill generates high cognitive load, as what to focus on is uncertain, decision-making is unreliable, knowledge is poorly organized, and skills are imprecise in execution – all of this effort comes at a high working memory cost that often leads to mistakes.

As an example, a veterinary student learning to spay a cat will need to know the essential reproductive anatomy and physiology of a cat, the basics of instrument and suture handling, soft tissue handling and hemostasis, and the elements involved in preoperative preparation, surgery, and post-op care. A student new to spaying a cat will perform these tasks slowly and intentionally, as they become acquainted with using the instruments and suture on a live animal, learn how much tension they can place on tissue to gain visualization, and work to determine how to properly engage the external rectus fascia and the intradermal layer when closing.

As an individual continues to practice and gain experience, they will enter the **transitional stage,** where they begin to develop more refined declarative memory, in the form of conceptual knowledge (i.e., schemas and concepts) that will entail a better understanding of the context and conditions within which the skill resides. The bulk of the transitional stage, however, will involve *proceduralization*, which involves the refinement of several individual, declaratively driven steps into a single procedural step where the actions become more automated and more accurate. Proceduralization through practice allows the individual to engage in elements of the skill without having to think about them, thus reducing cognitive load.

As the surgical student is given the opportunity to perform multiple cat spays, they gain efficiency and proficiency in this stage, as each individual step in the declarative stage begins to move toward proceduralization. For example, making the initial skin incision, undermining the subcutaneous tissue, identifying the linea alba, making an initial stab incision into the abdomen, and extending the abdominal incision all become "the opening" and are performed more efficiently. However, such skills do not become automated overnight, and skills often become part automated and part conscious.

Finally, the **procedural stage** involves the continued refinement of the skill such that more of the skill becomes proceduralized. As the skill becomes more proceduralized, and with the individual accessing declarative memory less often, the declarative memory upon which the skill was initially built often fades. For example, when one learns to type well, one often forgets where the letters are on the keys. The person can type quickly, but to answer the question, "Where's the W key?," they will need to first type that key in their mind. Ultimately, after practice and proceduralization, the individual will be able to engage in a skill quickly and accurately, and with little cognitive load. For example, the high quality, high volume spay/neuter veterinarian will perform a cat spay in under five minutes and often does not remember the details of the last procedure. Keep in mind, however, that the cost of proceduralization is conscious access to the declarative memory and component skills that led to the expertise. It is this forgetting of the relevant declarative knowledge and component skills that often result in experts becoming poor teachers. Thus, a highly trained veterinarian who begins to teach may need to relearn sets of declarative knowledge or component skills to be better able to explain and model the entire process.

B. Rote, Meaningful, and Elaborative Learning

In the pursuit of learning, meaning is paramount. As previously discussed, engaging new information in a deep and meaningful way (depth of processing) leads to increased retention. This concept that meaningfulness increases learning is present in the concepts of rote, meaningful, and elaborative learning. ***Rote learning*** involves learning through memorization in the absence of significant meaning making or knowledge structure creation such as schemas or concepts (Cho and Powers 2019; Grove and Bretz 2012). This type of learning tends to foster weak memories that are poorly organized and poorly connected to prior knowledge, resulting in more forgetting, less inferencing, and less usefulness in solving new problems (Karpicke and Grimaldi 2012). Consider a veterinary student who is learning anatomy by way of flash cards. On one side of the flash card is a diagram of the canine lymph nodes and vessels, with the nodes and vessels numbered, and on the other side are the names of the nodes and vessels by number. What the student is learning are dissociated facts (which number on the diagram goes with which name) and a simple diagram, not a greater understanding of the function of lymph nodes, how to locate lymph nodes on a live animal, or the diagnosis and treatment of diseases such as lymphoma. Ultimately, if the student is asked a question different from "What are the lymph nodes of the hind limb?," they are likely to be at a loss.

In contrast to rote learning, **meaningful learning** focuses on the generation of understanding through the association of new knowledge and experience with prior knowledge and experience, emphasizing knowledge comprehension, application, and integration (Ausubel 1960; Dochy et al. 2003; Furtak et al. 2012). In creating meaningful associations, the new knowledge is integrated into the existing conceptual knowledge organization, forming relationships that immediately benefit the understanding of the new knowledge. Meaningful learning tends to foster deep and flexible memories that are highly organized and structured, resulting in greater meaning, inferencing, and usefulness. Considering the veterinary student learning the lymphatic system, their understanding would benefit from strategies such as elaborative learning, which emphasizes connections between new and prior knowledge.

Elaborative learning, or sometimes termed *elaboration*, is a generalized approach for developing deep and flexible knowledge that is focused on proactively connecting new and prior knowledge to generate meaningful connections and meaningful learning (Anderson and Biddle 1975; Dunlosky et al. 2013). Specifically, elaborative learning is focused on actively connecting new knowledge with prior knowledge to emphasize the addition of new connections (see Table 3.1). Elaborative learning, however, is not a single strategy, but rather, a generalized approach to fostering meaningful learning that may involve a multitude of strategies, such as summarizing, concept maps, self-explanation, analogical reasoning, and elaborative interrogation (Brod 2021; Chi et al. 1989; Gentner et al. 2003; Pressley et al. 1995).

For example, *elaborative interrogation* involves a student being asked to "interrogate" an idea or concept by providing an explanation or application, often by answering *why* or *how* questions (Froehlich and Rogers 2022), although the nature of the questions may vary. For example, in a presentation addressing kidney function, an instructor may ask, "How does proper kidney function contribute to overall animal health?" In answering this question, the student will need to connect the new knowledge regarding kidney function with their prior knowledge regarding animal health, resulting in meaningful learning (rather than rote learning). In addition, in a unit on feline health, students may be asked, "Why is cat dehydration problematic?" for students to clarify, within themselves, the relationship between hydration, dehydration, and systems functioning. The key in elaborative interrogation is that the questions foster explanation (deeper learning) and connection (flexible learning), not the simple retrieval of answers already provided in class or lab.

Another elaborative learning strategy related to elaborative interrogation is *self-explanation*, where the learner self-generates their own definitions, explanations, inferences, or evaluations. Thus, self-explanations help to connect new

Table 3.1 Definitions and effect sizes for empirically supported learning effects.

Learning effect	Definition	Effect size
Elaboration effect	Learners tend to remember information better when they engage in deeper, more meaningful processing of new information, and actively make connections between new and prior knowledge.	Medium[a] ($g = .55$)
Retrieval effect	Learners tend to remember information better when they actively recall the information from memory, rather than simply rereading or restudying the information.	Medium[b] ($g = .61$)
Generation effect	Learners tend to remember information better when they actively generate it themselves, rather than passively receiving it through reading or a presentation.	Medium[c] ($d = .40$)
Spacing effect	Learners tend to remember information better when they engage in study sessions or practice trials that are spaced out, or distributed, over time, rather than massed into a single session.	Large[d] ($g = .74$)
Interleaving effect	Learners tend to remember closely related information better when they alternate between topics under study, especially when they have similarities that might be confusing, rather than focusing on one topic at a time.	Medium[e] ($g = .42$)
Enactment effect	Learners tend to remember information better when they engage in physical actions related to the information, rather than simply observing or reading about the action.	Large[f] ($g = 1.23$)
Production effect	Learners tend to remember information better when they read words aloud (or type, write, or spell words or phrases), rather than reading words silently.	Medium[g] ($g = .50$)

[a] Citations: Bisra et al. (2018).
[b] Adesope et al. (2017).
[c] Bertsch et al. (2007).
[d] Latimier et al. (2021).
[e] Brunmair and Richter (2019).
[f] Roberts et al. (2022).
[g] Fawcett (2013).

knowledge to prior knowledge, making the knowledge more personally meaningful, and to evaluate the completeness of one's comprehension, monitoring one's understanding, and working to rectify gaps. Self-explanations may include delineating the steps in a procedure, explaining the structure and function of a system, predicting the impact of specific remedies, or clarifying the relationship between observed symptoms and hypothesized causes (Fonseca and Chi 2011). In addition, self-explanation may be individually driven, where a student spontaneously engages in self-questioning or comprehension monitoring or instructor driven, where self-explanations may occur as a result of prompting by the instructor.

Meaningful and elaborative learning both emphasize the importance that meaning and connection make in fostering long-term memories. Specifically, learning is based on meaning, and meaning is created through associating new knowledge and experience with prior knowledge and experience. For example, a veterinary student may take classes on the "normal animal" to begin the process of building knowledge related to the general structure and function of animals, in general, followed by more specific courses designed to integrate a deeper understanding of various animal systems (e.g., circulatory system, musculoskeletal system). However, students need to be encouraged to make connections within and across these courses through the use of elaborative learning strategies, such as elaborative interrogation and self-explanations, so that their knowledge develops into complex conceptual knowledge and well-practiced procedural knowledge.

C. Retrieval Practice Effect and Generation Effect

The ***retrieval practice effect***, sometimes termed (unfortunately) the *testing effect*, indicates that actively retrieving or recalling information from memory, as opposed to simply reexperiencing the information through rereading or a presentation, leads to increased long-term retention, transfer of knowledge, and deeper understanding (Agarwal 2018; Roediger and Karpicke 2006; Zaromb and Roediger 2010). In addition, the retrieval practice effect has been demonstrated to be incredibly robust in its application, resulting in learning increases across subject areas (e.g., STEM, medicine, humanities), student populations (e.g., elementary,

secondary, college students), and simple and complex materials (e.g., facts, concepts, relationships, inferences).

A classic study of the retrieval practice effect was conducted by Roediger and Karpike (2006, Experiment 2), who had students read and learn a passage of approximately 260 words containing 30 idea units. Students were assigned to one of three learning groups, such that one group (SSSS) studied the passage for five minutes ("studying" was defined as rereading the passage and students were able to reread the passage approximately 3.5 times during each five-minute study period), followed by a short two-minute break, four times in a row (i.e., study, break, study, break, study, break, study, break). The second group (SSST) studied the passage three times, followed by taking a recall test where they were given a blank sheet of paper and asked to recall as much information from the passage as possible, in 10 minutes, regardless of wording or order (i.e., study, break, study, break, study, break, test, break). Finally, the third group (STTT) studied the passage once, followed by three testing periods (i.e., study, break, test, break, test, break, test, break). Half of the students from each group completed a final recall test 5 minutes after the completion of their treatment (SSSS, SSST, or STTT), while the other half of the students from each group completed a final recall test one week later.

Roediger and Karpicke found that for the five-minute delayed post-test, the SSSS group recalled more than the SSST group who recalled more than the STTT group (see Figure 3.10). However, for the one-week delayed post-test, the students' performance reversed, such that students in the STTT group recalled more than the SSST group who recalled more than the SSSS group. These findings indicate that while rereading the passage over and over (SSSS) led to significant gains in the short term, retrieving information regarding the passage from memory (STTT) led to longer-term gains. In interpreting these results it is clear in Figure 3.10 that a key finding was that the students who engaged in more information retrieval (STTT) forgot less over time than the students who engaged in more information exposure (SSSS).

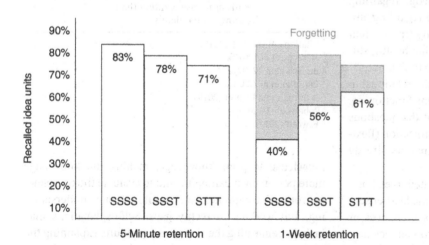

Figure 3.10 Mean recall of idea units on 5-minute delayed and 1-week delayed retention tests for students in each learning condition (SSSS, SSST, STTT). The amount forgotten after one week is represented by the gray bars. *Source:* Original figure, adapted from data reported in Roediger and Karpicke (2006). Copyright 2006 by the Association for Psychological Science.

Considering reviews and meta-analyses of the retrieval practice effect, Adesope et al. (2017; see also Agarwal et al. 2021; Rowland 2014) conducted a meta-analysis of retrieval practice focused on the use of pretesting (i.e., one or more practice tests or quizzes during the learning phase) as a method of retrieving knowledge on students' subsequent test performance. Overall, Adesope et al. found medium to large effect sizes[1] of pretesting during learning on students' subsequent test performance; that is, students who engaged in some form of pretesting retrieval practice outperformed students who did not engage in retrieval practice. Of particular interest, however, are the moderating variables explored by Adesope et al. that help to further explain the robustness of the retrieval practice effect. For example, Adesope et al. found a medium effect when pretesting was compared to rereading or restudying and a large effect when compared to engaging in no activity (no pretesting, no rereading, no restudying). Since rereading is a common study strategy for students (Callender and McDaniel 2009; Karpicke et al. 2009), these findings provide evidence that more active retrieval practice is beneficial to retention and test performance than simply reexperiencing knowledge. Adesope et al. also demonstrated that retrieval practice was robust across instructional settings (classroom and laboratory), educational levels (primary, secondary, and postsecondary), and time interval between the retrieval practice and final test (<1 day delay, 1–6 day delay, >6 days delay) with the effect sizes ranging from medium to large in each case. Finally, Adesope et al. found a transfer-appropriate processing effect; in particular, students' final test performance benefitted most when the pretest and final test were identical in processing (i.e., both addressed the same content in the same format, such as multiple-choice questions or short answer questions).

One challenge in understanding the retrieval practice effect is that the discussion often fixates on "testing." It should be noted that the proximal cause of the retrieval practice effect is the processing involved in retrieving that leads to increases in the strength of the memory, not the "test" itself. As Agarwal et al. (2021) state, "it is the *process* of practicing retrieval (the active attempt) that shapes

learning, not tests" (p. 1412; italics in the original). Within the retrieval practice effect literature, quizzes are often used as they are easy to create, control, and quantify. However, retrieval could be fostered through any number of tasks, such as problem-solving, discussions, concept maps, self-explanations, and writing. The key to the retrieval practice effect is the fostering of the retrieval of knowledge, not the form of the retrieval itself.

The ***generation effect*** indicates that actively creating or generating knowledge, as opposed to passively reading or watching a presentation created by others, leads to increased learning (Jacoby 1978; McCurdy et al. 2020a; Slamecka and Graf 1978). The generation effect has been demonstrated to be robust across various tasks, including problem-solving, study techniques, worked examples, arithmetic, sentence completion, word pairs, and anagrams. Finally, there is evidence that the generation is more effective in fostering learning when fewer constraints are applied to what is generated (e.g., multiple potential solutions or formats), rather than when more constraints are applied (e.g., a single correct answer). Thus, learning is enhanced when the learner is provided with greater latitude in what is produced (Fiedler et al. 1992; McCurdy et al. 2020b).

For example, Foos et al. (1994, Experiment 2) examined the generation effect in relation to student-created study materials. Specifically, students read and studied a 2,300-word text addressing the life and times of bees. The Generate group was asked to generate study questions, of any format (e.g., essay, multiple-choice, fill-in-the-blank), addressing the information in the text and to be used while they studied. The students in the Receive group each received a set of study questions created by a student in the Generate group to be used while they studied. All students were given 30 minutes to read and study (the Generate group also created their questions during this time) for the subsequent 30-item test consisting of 15 multiple-choice items and 15 fill-in-the-blank items, which was administered shortly after the study period. In addition, the ideas from the text that were addressed by both the study materials and the test items were labeled as "target" ideas, while test items that were not also present in the study materials were labeled as "non-target" ideas. Thus, target ideas were "targeted" by the study materials.

The results of Foos et al.'s study (see Figure 3.11) indicate the presence of the generation effect. Specifically, students who generated study materials did better (89%) than students who simply received study materials (72%) when assessed by "target" test items. In cases where the content of test items was not present in the study materials (nontargets), students in both the Generate and Receive groups performed the same, 54%. The results that student learning was better for test items where the content was also present in the study material (targets), as compared to when the

---

1 Meta-analyses synthesize multiple experiments examining specific treatment effects (often a comparison between a control group and a treatment group), using statistical analyses to determine an overall or "absolute" effect, stated in terms of an **effect size**. Meta-analyses typically use the Hedges' g or Cohen's d effect size calculations that express the effect in terms of a standardized mean difference between groups such that a Hedges' $g = 1$ or Cohen's $d = 1$ equates to a group difference of 1 standard deviation. Both Hedges' g and Cohen's d are evaluated as a small effect (0.2), medium effect (0.5), or large effect (0.8). Caution, however, should be taken as the value-laden terms small, medium, and large can be context dependent and vary according to domain.

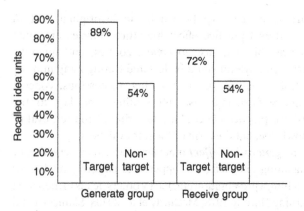

Figure 3.11 Mean test performance for students in both the Generate group and the Receive group for both the targeted ideas (ideas that were present in both the test items and study materials) and the nontargeted ideas (ideas present in the test items that were not present in the study materials). *Source:* Original figure, adapted from data reported in Foos et al. 1994. Copyright 1994 by the American Psychological Association.

test item content was not present in the study material (nontargets), is evidence of transfer-appropriate processing: processing the ideas within the study materials facilitated the processing of the ideas within the test items. Overall, Foos et al. demonstrate that information generated by learners is better remembered than information that is simply read or provided by another.

Considering reviews and meta-analyses of the generation effect, Bertsch et al. (2007; see also MCurdy et al. 2020a) conducted a meta-analysis of the generate effect focused on learning under two broad conditions: read or generate. For example, Peynircioglu and Mungan (1993) used sentence completion, where participants either read the sentence, "Cells of the nervous system are called NEURONS." or generated the end of the sentence, "Cells of the nervous system are called N _ _ _ _ _ _." Pesta et al. (1996) used arithmetic problems, such as "7 x 3 = 21" for the read condition and "7 x 3 = ??" for the generate condition, as well as word pair problems, such as HOT-COLD for the read condition and HOT-C__ for the generate condition. Overall, Bertsch et al. (2007) found a medium effect for the generation effect. Significant moderating variables explored by Bertsch et al. indicated that the generation of responses had a greater effect for meaningful responses (words and numbers) than nonmeaningful responses (nonwords), as well as across all task types (e.g., sentence completion, arithmetic calculations, synonym generation, word completion), except anagrams. Finally, Bertsch et al. found the greatest impact of generation for longer delays in between the generation and the recall test, with immediate and 1-day delays demonstrating a small effect and delays of more than 1-day demonstrating a medium effect.

The retrieval practice effect and the generation effect leverage the fundamental concepts of depth of processing,

transfer-appropriate processing, and encoding specificity. Specifically, they emphasize that accessing long-term memories and using them to create new meanings leads to deep (stronger) and flexible (connected) knowledge, resulting in better overall retention, transfer, and application. For example, veterinary students, as they work their way through a course or over four years of lectures, labs, clinics, and clerkships, need to engage continuously in retrieving prior knowledge and skills in order to create new knowledge and skills and solve new problems and challenges. If students are not learning, they are forgetting.

D. Spacing Effect and Interleaving Effect

The *spacing effect* builds on the concept of retrieval practice. The **spacing effect**, sometimes termed *distributed practice*, indicates that learning is enhanced when retrieval practice is distributed over time, rather than focused on a single session, sometimes termed *massed practice* (Cepeda et al. 2009; Cepeda et al. 2008; Wiseheart et al. 2019). The time span for distributing the retrieval practice can be both shorter (minutes to days) and longer (months to years). In addition, the spacing effect has been demonstrated to have a positive effect on the learning of simple and complex information (Gluckman et al. 2014) for younger children and older adults, including motor and verbal skills, and across various learning tasks, such as science and mathematics concepts, musical performance, and video games (Latimier et al. 2021). Of particular import, relative to the spacing effect, is the time between practice sessions (spacing interval) and the time between the last practice session and the performance session (retention interval). First, it appears that all spacing intervals, from short to long, result in better retention than massed practice. Second, it appears that longer spacing intervals facilitate longer retention intervals. And, third, there is some evidence that massed practice may produce better short-term retention, while distributed practice may produce better long-term retention (Cepeda et al. 2009; Donovan and Radosevich 1999; Greving and Richter 2018; Kapler et al. 2015; Roediger and Karpicke 2011).

Considering reviews and meta-analyses of the spacing effect, Latimier et al. (2021; see also Cepeda et al. 2006; Donovan and Radosevich 1999) conducted a meta-analysis of the memory impacts of the spacing effect – spaced retrieval practice versus massed retrieval practice – focused on semantic and verbal stimuli (i.e., not including perceptual or motor learning). Overall, Latimier et al. (2021) found a large effect for the generation effect.

Intimately related to the spacing effect is the interleaving effect. The **interleaving effect** indicates that learning new information, especially for closely related information, is enhanced when learning different types of information is integrated, rather than focusing on only one type of information at a time. For example, if a veterinary student is learning basic anatomy across several systems – skeletal (S), muscular (M), cardiovascular (C), and neurological (N) – their retention, transfer, and application will benefit from interweaving questions about each system, S-M-C-N-M-C-S-N-S-M-C-N-C-M-S-N, rather than studying each system in isolation, S-S-S-S M-M-M-M C-C-C-C N-N-N-N, a process called blocking. This concept can be counterintuitive for students, and given a choice, students tend to choose blocking over interleaving (Carvalho et al. 2016; Tauber et al. 2013; Yan and Sana 2021), but this interleaving effect has been demonstrated to be effective across a range of tasks, including mathematical procedures, problem-solving, concept identification, and case studies.

The rationale for the interleaving effect, however, is still being debated. One of the two top theoretical contenders is the *discriminative-contrast hypothesis* that posits that students would learn basic anatomy better through interleaving because experiencing different anatomy categories side-by-side (S-M-C-N) would allow the student to better "see" similarities and differences between the categories (Birnbaum et al. 2013; Kang and Pashler 2012). The second theoretical contender is the *distributed-practice hypothesis* that presupposes that students would learn better because interleaving is really spaced practice, such that S-M-C-N-M-C-S-N-S-M-C-N-C-M-S-N (interleaving) is really S-*M*-C-N-*M*-C-S-N-S-*M*-C-N-C-*M*-S-N (spaced practice; Foster et al. 2019). While the rationale for the effectiveness of the interleaving effect is in doubt (Chen et al. 2021; Chen et al. 2022; Sana et al. 2022), the outcome is not.

Considering reviews and meta-analyses of the interleaving effect, Brunmair and Richter (2019) focused on interleaving that involved inductive learning, such as comparing paintings or photographs to determine the names of the painters or the types of birds in the photographs. In addition, their comparisons involved interleaved practice versus massed practice with study materials. Overall, Brunmair and Richter found a medium effect size for interleaving over massed practice. In addition, Brunmair and Richter found a large effect for interleaving involving complex visual materials (e.g., paintings, naturalistic photographs, complex photographs). Finally, Brunmair and Richter found support for the idea that if deductive discrimination between visual materials is the preferred outcome (e.g., learning to interpret blood slides or x-rays), then interleaving works best when materials are presented simultaneously or in close succession, enhancing one's ability to discriminate, rather than spacing the materials out over time.

Rohrer and Taylor (2007) tested both the spacing effect and the interleaving effect. In Experiment 1, addressing the *spacing effect*, students learned how to determine the number of permutations of letter sequences under one of two conditions: massed practice or spaced practice. Students in the *massed practice* group completed four sample problems

(with feedback) and four practice problems (without feedback) during the first week, followed by testing a week later that included completing five novel problems. Students in the *spaced* practice group complete two sample problems and two practice problems their first week, two additional sample and practice problems a week later, followed by testing a week later. Thus, students in both groups completed four sample problems and four practice problems. The massed practice group completed them in one session, while the spaced practice group completed them across two sessions. The results of Rohrer and Taylor's Experiment 1 (see Figure 3.12) indicate the presence of the spacing effect. On the test of permutations, the massed practice group answered 49% of the questions correctly, while the spaced practice group answered 74% of the questions correctly.

In Experiment 2, Rohrer and Taylor (2007) tested the *interleaving effect* by having students learn how to find the volume of four obscure geometric solids (circular wedges, spheroids, spherical cones, and half cones) and then practice under two conditions: massed practice and interleaving practice. Students in the *massed practice* group completed two practice sessions, one week apart. Each session comprised viewing a tutorial on determining the volume of one of the shapes, followed by four practice problems addressing that same shape. This tutorial–practice sequence occurred for each of the four shapes (a tutorial followed by four relevant practice problems). Students in the *interleaving* group also completed two practice sessions, one week apart. Each session comprised viewing a tutorial on determining the volume of each of the shapes, one after the other. After these four tutorials were viewed, all 16 of the practice problems were presented and solved in a random order (interleaved). One week later, the students in both groups complete eight novel problems, two of each shape type in a random order. The results of

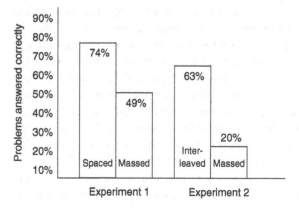

Figure 3.12 Mean correct test performance for students in Experiment 1, spaced versus massed practice of permutation problems, and Experiment 2, interleaved versus massed practice of geometric volume problems. *Source:* Original figure, adapted from data reported in Rohrer and Taylor (2007). Copyright 2007 by Springer Nature.

Rohrer and Taylor's Experiment 2 (see Figure 3.12) indicate the presence of the interleaving effect. On the test of volume computation, the massed practice group answered 20% of the questions correctly, while the interleaved practice group answered 63% of the questions correctly.

The spacing effect and the interleaving effect both provide opportunities for an individual to engage in significant processing as a result of retrieval practice. The spacing effect allows for extended practice over time that leads to greater long-term memory strength, while the interleaving effect allows for comparative practice that leads to greater discrimination in long-term memory. For example, a veterinary student would benefit from distributing their studying across days and weeks, rather than cramming for an exam or surgery. In addition, their knowledge will get stronger as they see more and more clients, necessitating them to naturally activate relevant knowledge over time. Beyond developing strong memories, if they need to learn to differentiate, learning the normal anatomy of multiple species within one semester will allow students to differentiate anatomical features better than if they learn about each individual species in separate courses throughout the curriculum.

E. Enactment Effect and Production Effect

The enactment effect and production effect both involve engagement by the learner that involves some level of physicality. The **enactment effect** indicates that learning is enhanced when an individual physically performs an action associated with information, especially in contrast to only reading the information (Asher 1964; Engelkamp and Krumnacker 1980; Engelkamp 1998). This performative action may be engaging in a whole behavior (e.g., completing a lab experiment, conducting a physical exam, assisting in a surgery), performing the action described by a word (e.g., palpating, otoscopy, intubation), or gesturing (e.g., tapping on the location of a muscle or bone on a live animal while discussing the muscle or bone). The basis of the enactment effect is not entirely certain, although the evidence leans toward multimodal encoding, using multiple sensory and cognitive modalities to engage in information (i.e., visual, auditory, kinesthetic), and embodied cognition, the idea that our cognitive and physical processes are intimately intertwined and mutually contributory (e.g., situated learning, multisensory experiences; Engelkamp 1998; Lakoff and Johnson 1980; Madan and Singhal 2012).

For example, Silva et al. (2015), examined the enactment effect in younger adults and older adults under two conditions, actually engaging in a task (SPT – subject-performed task) or only reading a description of the task (VT – verbal only task). Specifically, 32 action–object sentences were created and written on note cards (e.g., break the toothpick, throw the dice). Participants were shown each sentence card along with the object on the card, one at a time. Participants either performed the action on the card with the object (SPT) or simply read the action–object sentence (VT). Of the 32 action–object sentence cards, each participant enacted 16 (SPT) and read 16 (VT). Following the presentation of all of the action–object sentence cards, participants were asked to recall as many of the action–object sentences as possible. The results of Silva et al.'s experiment (see Figure 3.13) indicate the presence of the enactment effect. For both younger adults and older adults, more of the subject-performed (SPT) action–object sentences were recalled than the verbal only (VT) action–object sentences.

Considering reviews and meta-analyses of the enactment effect, Roberts et al. (2022), focused on how enactment (SPT) compared to watching others perform a task (VT), imagining the completion of a task, and reading or hearing words or descriptions related to tasks. Overall, Roberts et al. found a large effect for the enactment effect. When considering moderating effects, Roberts et al. found that enactment had a large effect on memory and performance when compared to verbal tasks, and a medium effect when compared to watching others engage in the task. So, while reading/hearing about a task or watching others complete a task can improve one's memory and performance related to the task, engaging in the task itself produces significantly greater memory and performance. In addition, enactment has been demonstrated to positively impact memory and performance, whether the recall or performance was immediate or delayed.

While the enactment effect examines the impact of larger-scale physical performances on memory and performance, the production effect examines most smaller physical performances. The **production effect** indicates that information that is read aloud is remembered better than

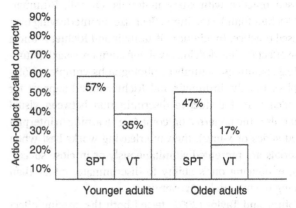

Figure 3.13 Mean correct action–object sentences recalled (e.g., roll the dice) for both younger adults and older adults in both the subject-performed task (SPT) and the verbal only task (VT). *Source*: Original figure, adapted from data reported in Silva et al. (2015). Copyright 2015 CC BY 4.0.

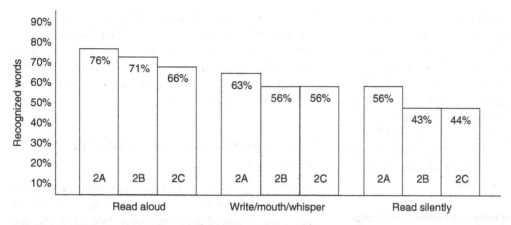

Figure 3.14 Mean correct test performance for students in Experiment 2A (Read Aloud, Write Words, Read Silently), Experiment 2B (Read Aloud, Mouth Silently, Read Silently), and Experiment 2C (Read Aloud, Whisper, Read Silently). *Source:* Original figure, adapted from data reported in Forrin et al. (2012). Copyright 2012 by the Psychonomic Society.

when information is read silently (Fawcett et al. 2022b; Forrin et al. 2012; MacLeod et al. 2010). This reading aloud over reading silently finding has also been extended to studies indicating that writing, typing, drawing, and spelling words or phrases can lead to better learning than simply reading (MacLeod and Bodner 2017). The theoretical foundation for the production effect has been hypothesized as resulting from (i) the read aloud words or phrases becoming "distinctive" against a background of read silently words or phrases or "distinctive" based on the sensorimotor features created during reading aloud (MacLeod et al. 2010), (ii) the read aloud words or phrase becoming more familiar than the read silently words or phrases (Fawcett and Ozubko 2016), or (iii) the read aloud words or phrases becoming more meaningful as they are processed semantically during speech (Fawcett et al. 2022b). It is perhaps most plausible that the production effect is a combination of the three approaches – distinctiveness, familiarity, and semantics – and not dependent on a single process (see Fawcett et al. 2022b).

For example, Forrin et al. (2012, Experiment 2), examined the production effect in relation to reading material aloud, reading material silently, or writing, mouthing (silently), or whispering the material. Specifically, across three experiments (2A, 2B, 2C) students were presented with 90 words, randomly ordered, in one of three colors (blue, white, red) and were told to read aloud the blue words, read silently the white words, and write (Experiment 2A), mouth (Experiment 2B), or whisper (Experiment 2C) the red words. After processing the words, students completed a recognition test where they were presented with 180 words, 30 words they had read aloud, 30 words they had read silently, 30 words they had written, mouthed, or whispered, depending upon the experiment, and 90 new words. The results of Forrin et al.'s Experiment 2 (see

Figure 3.14) indicate the presence of the production effect. Across all three experiments (2A, 2B, 2C), students in the read aloud condition recognized the most words, while students in the read silently condition recognized the least words. Students in the write, mouth, or whisper conditions recognized an intermediate number of words.

Unfortunately, there are currently no meta-analyses examining the impact of production versus only reading (the classic production effect). Fawcett (2013, see also Fawcett et al. 2022a), however, conducted a meta-analysis examining the effect of production between two design approaches: within-subject designs versus between-subject designs. Specifically, the production effect is typically examined using a within-subject design where participants read some words silently and some words aloud, and their remembrance of the silent versus aloud words demonstrates the production effect (aloud words are remembered better than silent words; e.g., Forrin et al. 2012). Early research using a between-subject approach, when one group engages in only reading silently and another group engages in only reading aloud, resulted in no production effect (Dodson and Schacter 2001) and (seemingly) indicating that distinctiveness requires a background (reading silently) against which information becomes noticeable (reading aloud). However, more recent empirical research has demonstrated the presence of between-subject production effects, but at a much lower effect size than within-subject production effect (this finding that between-subject effects are significantly lower than within-subject effects is also evident in the enactment effect literature). Therefore, Fawcett's (2013) meta-analysis' findings of a small-to-medium between-subject production effect are likely indicative of a much larger within-subject production effect, although that analysis had not yet been conducted and published in the literature.

The enactment and production effects involve the fostering of learning through physical engagement, beyond the solely cognitive. These physical approaches can be extremely powerful, especially when combined with more traditional cognitive processing. Being a veterinarian requires a balance of cognitive and physical skills, and encoding specificity and transfer-appropriate processing, along with working memory-based processing, all of which support the use of cognitive + physical enactment and production. Students' learning is enhanced when they "do" and when they talk about the doing.

F. Zooming Out on Fostering Deep and Flexible Knowledge

It is essential to keep in mind our mantra – *what we process we learn*. As indicated previously, processing is neither neat nor tidy. This messiness is evident in the effects just discussed. None of these effects are "process pure," relying on only one or two processes neatly arranged and highly predictive. To be sure, each of these effects involves a diverse set of overlapping and intermixed processes. A veterinary student watching, listening, and assisting a veterinarian in fixing a calf's broken limb will involve retrieval (of prior knowledge regarding bovine anatomy and physiology), elaboration (of the new experiences with the aforementioned prior knowledge), generation (of new calf treatment procedures and behaviors), enactment (of the immobilization and splinting, not simply reading about it), and production (of ongoing comments, questions, and actions). Thus, fostering deep and flexible knowledge involves the making of informed and proactive decisions related to instructional actions and *not* the search for the "best" processing-inducing strategy or activity. For the veterinarian fixing the calf's broken limb, instructionally it would make sense for the veterinarian to (i) verbalize their planning, attention, ongoing actions, and decision-making processes, (ii) ask the student predictive and explanatory questions, and (iii) engage the student in as much of the procedure as possible, without sacrificing the care of the animal. Is this the only way to make this experience educational for the student? Definitely not. The challenge is to make these instructional decisions in an informed and proactive manner for the betterment of the animal, the student, and the profession.

Also, returning to where we started, the idea of "it depends" must be taken seriously. While the previous findings and effects have been discussed with supporting literature and examples, for each of the effects there is literature that finds no effects or even negative effects. These contrary findings do not negate the findings themselves, but rather, they remind us that these effects are not laws that always work for all students, under all conditions. It is common in real-world, real-time educational environments for specific strategies, applied in specific courses, with specific content and students, not to work. Why? It depends. All of the effects mentioned have boundary conditions under which they no longer seem to apply. Making informed and proactive instructional decisions is more like dealing with an elusive internal medicine case than vaccinating a happy, healthy puppy.

Part 4: Implications of Memory and Cognition for Learning

This chapter provides the foundation for understanding the concept of active learning. **Active learning**, while having no formal or agreed-upon definition, focuses on the students' processing of their knowledge and experiences for the purpose of meaningful learning. While Freeman et al. (2014), and Theobald et al. (2020), both provide evidence that engaging students in active learning leads to increased learning, Bernstein (2018) laments that not enough specific guidance is provided to instructors. Hopefully, this chapter and the implications below provide some of that guidance.

A. Students' Learning Is a Function of Meaning Making

To do, to think, to understand, to solve, to evaluate, to interpret, to reason, to apply . . . all require that one first makes meaning. The making of meaning necessitates connecting new knowledge to prior knowledge (meaningful learning) and wrapping prior knowledge around the new knowledge (elaborative learning). In addition, to increase the level of meaning making, new knowledge should be integrated into existing knowledge structures (i.e., schemas, scripts, concepts, procedures) through the application of knowledge and experience to problems.

Learning without meaning (rote learning) results in weak, disconnected, and poorly applicable knowledge, which can lead to inert knowledge. *Inert knowledge*, knowledge that one possesses but cannot use, can result from a lack of context (learning without an understanding of its relevance), rote learning (learning through meaningless repetition), fragmented knowledge (learning without connections to existing knowledge), lack of practice (learning without opportunities to apply knowledge in various context and for various purposes), and a lack of awareness and control of knowledge (learning without an understanding of how and when to apply the knowledge). Rote learning tends to result in more forgetting, less inferencing, and less usefulness in applying the knowledge to new situations.

To encourage meaningful learning, veterinary students' education should include:

1) Providing meaningful contexts and real-world applications of the knowledge and experiences students develop during their education.

2) Encouraging the development of deep learning, critical thinking, and integrated understandings of the underlying concepts that make the knowledge meaningful and useful.

3) Helping students make connections between conceptual and procedural knowledge, promoting the simultaneous organization and usefulness of their knowledge and skills.

4) Engaging students in multiple opportunities to practice and explain their knowledge and skills under varying conditions.

5) Fostering an understanding of what they know, including when, why, and how to leverage their knowledge and skills for the attainment of goals through reflection, self-assessment, and self-regulation.

B. Students' Learning Is Fostered by Their Active Processing of Knowledge and Experience

Learning, the making of meaning, and the application of knowledge entail that students engage in the active processing of their knowledge and skills. Processing covers a wide spectrum of engagement, including perceiving one's environment; attending to relevant aspects of the environment (including one's internal environment); connecting and integrating the objects of one's attention with one's prior knowledge; organizing, integrating, and synthesizing this experience and meaningful knowledge; and applying this knowledge and understanding to current situations, problems, or goals.

Processing is the proximal cause of learning: no processing, no learning. Processing may take many forms, including the conscious and proactive focusing of attention, the deliberate connecting of new and prior knowledge, and the intentional engagement of specific cognitive and behavioral strategies. While processing is not directly observable, its effects are – learning and performance. When a veterinary student engages in self-questioning, creates their own summaries of lectures, explains their understandings of physiological functions to peers, or thinks through the symptoms of diseases while driving to campus, their learning improves. When a veterinary student practices otoscopy on a model or live animal, engages in a client consultation in a clinic setting, or performs a spay under the direction of a veterinarian, their performance improves.

To motivate effective processing, veterinary students should be encouraged to:

1) Engage in deeper, more meaningful processing of new information, and actively make connections between new and prior knowledge (elaboration effect).

2) Recall knowledge and skills from memory, rather than simply rereading or restudying the information (retrieval effect).

3) Generate knowledge and skills themselves, rather than passively memorizing the knowledge and skills from readings or presentations (generation effect).

4) Engage in formal and informal study and practice sessions that are distributed over time, rather than crammed into a single session just prior to an assessment or activity (spacing effect).

5) Alternate between topics under study, especially when the topics have similarities that might be confusing, rather than focusing on just one topic at a time (interleaving effect).

6) Perform physical actions related to new knowledge and skills, rather than simply observing the actions of others or reading about them (enactment effect).

C. Students' Learning Is Constrained by Their Processing Limitations

The human memory system is replete with "bottlenecks" that constrain processing. First, while the human body may sense many sounds, sights, smells, tastes, and touches, it may only perceive, or attend to, a few. Second, the human memory system can only maintain simultaneous activation of a few short-term memories and process a limited amount of information in working memory. Unfortunately, split-attention (a form of multitasking) and high cognitive load have been associated with decreased performance, decreased comprehension, slower task completion, and higher error rates.

With extensive practice and the cunning use of strategies, individuals can mitigate some of the negative impacts of human information processing limitations. Some of these include:

1) *Chunking.* Grouping information into smaller meaningful clusters allows one's memory to operate on the whole chunk or cluster, rather than the smaller individual components, decreasing cognitive load and increasing working memory functioning.

2) *Practice.* Practicing leads to increased efficiency and accuracy in activating knowledge (declarative knowledge) or performing skills (procedural knowledge), as well as the conversion of step-by-step actions into automated skills.

3) *Organization.* Increasing levels of knowledge organization, such as schemas, scripts, and concepts, as well as proceduralized actions, leads to increased efficiency in knowledge access and decreased cognitive load in knowledge processing.

4) *Prioritization.* Focusing on the most critical knowledge and skills, consciously and proactively, will reduce the likelihood of becoming distracted or engaging in multitasking.

5) *Simplification*. Breaking complex knowledge and skills into component parts, especially when one is a novice, will lead to increased organization and decreased cognitive load.

6) *Offloading*. Using external resources to "store" needed knowledge – checklists, Post-It notes, visual aids (charts, diagrams), and voice memos – leads to increased decision-making and decreased cognitive load.

7) *Breaks*. Taking short breaks that include light exercise or routine mental distractions that require a low, but not zero, level of attention (e.g., driving, walking, crossword puzzles, reading news) can help to prevent mental fatigue, improve cognitive function, improve attentional focus, and improve creative thought.

D. Students' Learning Is Facilitated by Instructional Strategies that Encourage Processing

In pursuit of cognitive processing focused on meaning making, instructional strategies provide an effective mechanism for motivating student engagement. That said, understanding the relationship between strategies, processing, and learning is essential. Specifically, the goal of strategy use is to motivate students to engage in cognitive processing that is focused on learning: strategy → processing → learning. These instructional strategies may be formal or informal (cooperative learning versus casual pre-class conversation), large or small (problem-based learning versus think-pair-share), or resource-intensive or resource-efficient (design-based problem-solving versus small-group discussion). The focus on processing is key as instructional strategies are often undertaken with the assumption that the strategies themselves will lead directly to learning, they do not. In using an instructional strategy, instructors must be mindful of how the strategy is employed so that the strategy leads to processing.

For example, the *think–pair–share* strategy involves (i) instructors asking a question or providing a problem, (ii) students thinking about a response or solution to the question or problem, and (iii) students discussing their responses or solutions with other students. The strategy itself is fairly straightforward, but how the strategy is implemented determines its usefulness in fostering learning. If the instructor asks a yes/no question, then the students will have little to think about or discuss. If the instructor asks a question that is too easy or too hard, students will be unwilling or unable to respond adequately. If the instructor asks a question that is deemed irrelevant or trivial by the students, they will be unmotivated to give it much thought. A good think–pair–share question is (i) open-ended, encouraging multiple perspectives or solutions, (ii) higher-order, involving the application of knowledge or the consideration of multiple knowledge sources, (iii) relevant, connecting to the current discussion, class, or course, and (iv) appropriate,

challenging for the students but attainable. After a suitable think–pair–share question is asked, there needs to be a sufficient "wait time" for students to process the question, consider various answers, make decisions, and formulate a response. Finally, students must be provided the time and impetus to share their own thoughts and conclusions, as well as listen to and respond to their partner's thoughts and conclusions. Processing, or the reason for the strategy and the cause of the learning, takes time. Two or three minutes of silence will seem like a long time in the middle of class, but this time is necessary for students to process and signals to the student that their responses should be well thought out and not off-the-cuff. To further foster processing, instructors should provide directions as to how students should "share." For example, "Explain your diagnosis and treatment to your partner, and if you're the partner, provide some feedback on the appropriateness of their response. Then, switch roles." Again, it is important that the students are provided with sufficient time to discuss.

E. Students' Learning Is Subject to Individual Differences in Knowledge, Experience, and Processing

Students are not widgets and do not all respond similarly to the same instruction or instructional materials. Students with little veterinary knowledge and experience will need more time, examples, and explanations to begin the process of building conceptual knowledge and engaging in procedural knowledge. In addition, they will tend to respond slowly, with poorly integrated knowledge and error-prone procedures. Everyone begins their veterinary careers as novices, constructing meaning and understanding over time with experience and feedback. With continued class, project, lab, and clinical experiences fostering real-world, complex processing, students will develop integrated knowledge structures and automated skills. Novices become experts as they process their knowledge and experience across a multitude of classes, discussions, readings, clients, and animal interactions, procedures, and surgeries, including successes and failures. **There is no shortcut to expertise**.

Summary

It seems appropriate to end where we started, searching for meaning through processing that depends on the individual, the experience, and the goals for learning. Applying the principles of learning and integrating the elaboration, retrieval, generation, spacing, interleaving, enactment, and production effects into instruction can result in deep and flexible knowledge and performance. Ultimately, the concepts addressed in this chapter provide a rationale for how and why learning occurs, as well as guidance for effective teaching.

References

Adesope, O., Trevisan, D., and Sundararajan, N. (2017). Rethinking the use of tests: a meta-analysis of practice testing. *Review of Educational Research* 87 (3): 659–701. https://doi.org/10.3102/0034654316689306.

Agarwal, P. (2018). Retrieval practice & Bloom's taxonomy: do students need fact knowledge before higher order learning? *Journal of Educational Psychology* 111 (2): 189–209. https://doi.org/10.1037/edu0000282.

Agarwal, P., Nunes, L., and Blunt, J. (2021). Retrieval practice consistently benefits student learning: a systematic review of applied research in schools and classrooms. *Educational Psychology Review* 33: 1409–1453. http://doi.org/10.1007/s10648-021-09595-9.

Alba, J.W. and Hasher, L. (1983). Is memory schematic? *Psychological Bulletin 93* (2): 203–231. http://doi.org/10.1037/0033-2909.93.2.203.

Alemany-Arrebola, I., Rojas-Ruiz, G., Granda-Vera, J., and Mingorance-Estrada, Á. (2020). Influence of COVID-19 on the perception of academic self-efficacy, state anxiety, and trait anxiety in college students. *Frontiers in Psychology* 11: 570017. https://doi.org/10.3389/fpsyg.2020.570017.

Anderson, J.R. (1982). Acquisition of cognitive skill. *Psychological Review* 89 (4): 369–406. https://doi.org/10.1037/0033-295X.89.4.369.

Anderson, J. and Biddle, W. (1975). On asking people questions about what they are reading. *Psychology of Learning and Motivation* 9: 89–132. https://doi.org/10.1016/S0079-7421(08)60269-8.

Armitage-Chan, E. (2020). Best practice in supporting professional identity formation: use of a professional reasoning framework. *Journal of Veterinary Education* 47 (2): 125–135. https://doi.org/10.3138/jvme.0218-019r.

Armitage-Chan, E. and May, S. (2019). The veterinary identity: a time and context model. *Journal of Veterinary Education* 46 (2): 153–162. https://doi.org/10.3138/jvme.0517-067r1.

Asher, J.J. (1964). Toward a neo-field theory of behavior. *Journal of Humanistic Psychology* 4 (2): 85–94. https://doi.org/10.1177/002216786400400202.

Aslin, R.N. and Newport, E.L. (2012). Statistical learning: from acquiring specific items to forming general rules. *Current Directions in Psychological Science* 21 (3): 170–176. https://doi.org/10.1177/0963721412436806.

Atkinson, R.C. and Shiffrin, R.M. (1968). Human memory: a proposed system and its control processes. In: *Psychology of Learning and Motivation*, vol. 2 (ed. K.W. Spence and J.T. Spence), 89–195. Academic press https://doi.org/10.1016/S0079-7421(08)60422-3.

Ausubel, D.P. (1960). The use of advance organizers in the learning and retention of meaningful verbal material. *Journal of Educational Psychology* 51 (5): 267–272. https://doi.org/10.1037/h0046669.

Azizli, N., Atkinson, B., Baughman, H., and Giammarco, G. (2015). Relationships between general self-efficacy, planning for the future, and life satisfaction. *Personality and Individual Differences* 82: 58–60. https://doi.org/10.1016/j.paid.2015.03.006.

Baddeley, A. (1978). The trouble with levels: a reexamination of Craik and Lockhart's framework for memory research. *Psychological Review* 85: 139–152. https://doi.org/10.1037/0033-295X.85.3.139.

Baddeley, A.D. and Hitch, G. (1974). Working memory. In: *Psychology of Learning and Motivation*, vol. 8 (ed. G. Bower), 47–89. Academic press https://doi.org/10.1016/S0079-7421(08)60452-1.

Baddeley, A.D., Hitch, G.J., and Allen, R.J. (2019). From short-term store to multicomponent working memory: the role of the modal model. *Memory & Cognition* 47: 575–588. https://doi.org/10.3758/s13421-018-0878-5.

Baddeley, A., Hitch, G., and Allen, R. (2021). A multicomponent model of working memory. In: *Working Memory: State of the Science* (ed. R.H. Logie, V. Camos, and N. Cowan), 10–43. Oxford University Press https://doi.org/10.1093/oso/9780198842286.003.0002.

Bahrick, H.P. (1984). Semantic memory content in permastore: fifty years of memory for Spanish learned in school. *Journal of Experimental Psychology: General* 113 (1): 1. https://doi.org/10.1037/0096-3445.113.1.1.

Bandura, A. (1971). *Social Learning Theory*. Morristown: General Learning Press.

Bandura, A. (1977). Self-efficacy: toward a unifying theory of behavioral change. *Psychological Review* 84 (2): 191–215. https://doi.org/10.1037/0033-295X.84.2.191.

Bandura, A. (1986). *Social Foundations of Thought and Action: A Social Cognitive Theory*. Prentice Hall.

Bandura, A. (1989). Human agency in social cognitive theory. *American Psychologist* 44 (9): 1175–1184. https://doi.org/10.1037/0003-066X.44.9.1175.

Bandura, A. (1993). Perceived self-efficacy in cognitive development and functioning. *Educational Psychologist 28* (2): 117–148. https://doi.org/10.1207/s15326985ep2802_3.

Bandura, A. (1997). *Self-Efficacy: The Exercise of Control*. Freeman.

Bandura, A. (1998). Personal and collective efficacy in human adaptation and change. In: *Advances in Psychological Science, Vol. 1. Social, Personal, and Cultural Aspects* (ed. J.G. Adair, D. Bélanger, and K.L. Dion), 51–71. Taylor & Francis.

Bandura, A. (2001a). Social cognitive theory: an agentic perspective. *Annual Review of Psychology* 52: 1–26. https://doi.org/10.1146/annurev.psych.52.1.1.

Bandura, A. (2001b). Social cognitive theory of mass communication. *Media Psychology* 3: 2655–2299. https://doi-org.ezproxy.lib.vt.edu/10.1207/S1532785XMEP0303_03.

Bandura, A. (2006). Toward a psychology of human agency. *Perspectives on Psychological Science* 1 (2): 164–180. https://doi.org/10.1111/j.1745-6916.2006.00011.x.

Bandura, A. (2018). Toward a psychology of human agency: pathways and reflections. *Perspectives on Psychological Science* 13 (2): 130–136. https://doi.org/10.1177/1745691617699280.

Bandura, A. and Cervone, D. (2023). *Social Cognitive Theory: An Agentic Perspective on Human Nature*. Wiley.

Barrouillet, P.N. and Camos, V. (2009). Interference: unique source of forgetting in working memory? *Trends in Cognitive Sciences* 13 (4): 145–146. http://doi.org/10.1016/j.tics.2009.01.002.

Bartlett, F. (1932). *Remembers: A Study in Experimental and Social Psychology*. Cambridge.

Bernstein, D.A. (2018). Does active learning work? A good question, but not the right one. *Scholarship of Teaching and Learning in Psychology* 4 (4): 290–307. https://doi.org/10.1037/stl0000124.

Bertsch, S., Pesta, B., Wiscott, R., and McDaniel, M. (2007). The generation effect: a meta-analytic review. *Memory & Cognition* 35 (2): 201–210. https://doi.org/10.3758/BF03193441.

Berzonsky, M.D. (2003). Identity style and well-being: does commitment matter? *Identity* 3 (2): 131–142. https://doi.org/10.1207/S1532706XID030203.

Berzonsky, M.D. (2011). A social-cognitive perspective on identity construction. In: *Handbook of Identity Theory and Research*, vol. 1 (ed. S.J. Schwartz, K. Luyckx, and V. Vignoles), 55–76. Springer https://doi.org/10.1007/978-1-4419-7988-9_3.

Berzonsky, M.D. and Kuk, L. (2021). Identity styles and college adaptation: the mediational roles of commitment, self-agency and self-regulation. *Identity* 4: 310–325. https://doi.org/10.1080/15283488.2021.1979552.

Berzonsky, M.D. and Luyckx, K. (2008). Identity styles, self-reflective cognition, and identity processes: a study of adaptive and maladaptive dimensions of self-analysis. *Identity* 8: 205–219. https://doi.org/10.1080/15283480802181818.

Birnbaum, M.S., Kornell, N., Bjork, E.L., and Bjork, R.A. (2013). Why interleaving enhances inductive learning: the roles of discrimination and retrieval. *Memory & Cognition* 41: 392–402. https://doi.org/10.3758/s13421-012-0272-7.

Bisra, K., Liu, Q., Nesbit, J.C. et al. (2018). Inducing self-explanation: a meta-analysis. *Educational Psychology Review* 30: 703–725. https://doi.org/10.1007/s10648-018-9434-x.

Blasiman, R.N., Dunlosky, J., and Rawson, K.A. (2017). The what, how much, and when of study strategies: comparing intended versus actual study behaviour. *Memory* 25 (6): 784–792. https://doi.org/10.1080/09658211.2016.1221974.

Boekaerts, M. and Rozendaal, J. (2010). Using multiple calibration indices in order to capture the complex picture of what affects students' accuracy of feeling of confidence. *Learning and Instruction* 20 (5): 372–382. https://doi.org/10.1016/j.learninstruc.2009.03.002.

Bower, G.H., Black, J.B., and Turner, T.J. (1979). Scripts in memory for text. *Cognitive Psychology* 11 (2): 177–220. https://doi.org/10.1016/0010-0285(79)90009-4.

Brady, T.F., Störmer, V.S., and Alvarez, G.A. (2016). Working memory is not fixed-capacity: more active storage capacity for real-world objects than for simple stimuli. *Proceedings of the National Academy of Sciences of the United States of America* 113 (27): 7459–7464. https://doi.org/10.1073/pnas.1520027113.

Broadbent, D.E. (1975). Cognitive psychology and education. *British Journal of Educational Psychology* 45 (2): 162–176. https://doi.org/10.1111/j.2044-8279.1975.tb03241.x.

Brod, G. (2021). Predicting as a learning strategy. *Psychonomic Bulletin & Review* 28 (6): 1839–1847. https://doi.org/10.3758/s13423-021-01904-1.

Brunmair, M. and Richter, T. (2019). Similarity matters: a meta-analysis of interleaved learning and its moderators. *Psychological Bulletin* 145 (11): 1029–1052. https://doi.org/10.1037/bul0000209.

Calkins, L., Wiens, P., Parker, J., and Tschinkel, R. (2023). Teacher motivation and self-efficacy: how do specific motivations for entering teaching relate to teacher self-efficacy? *Journal of Education* https://doi.org/10.1177/00220574221142300.

Callender, A.A. and McDaniel, M.A. (2009). The limited benefits of rereading educational texts. *Contemporary Educational Psychology* 34 (1): 30–41. https://doi.org/10.1016/j.cedpsych.2008.07.001.

Carey, S. (2009). *The Origin of Concepts*. Oxford.

Carvalho, P.F., Braithwaite, D.W., de Leeuw, J.R. et al. (2016). An in vivo study of self-regulated study sequencing in introductory psychology courses. *PloS one* 11 (3): e0152115. https://doi.org/10.1371/journal.pone.0152115.

Cepeda, N., Pashler, H., Vul, E., and Wixted, J. (2006). Distributed practice in verbal recall tasks: a review and quantitative synthesis. *Psychological Bulletin* 132 (3): 354–380. https://doi.org/10.1037/0033-2909.132.3.354.

Cepeda, N., Vul, E., Rohrer, D. et al. (2008). Spacing effects in learning: a temporal ridgeline of optimal retention. *Psychological Science* 19 (11): 1095–1102. https://doi.org/10.1111/j.1467-9280.2008.02209.x.

Cepeda, N., Coburn, N., Rohrer, D. et al. (2009). Optimizing distributed practice: theoretical analysis and practice implications. *Experimental Psychology* 56 (4): 2236–2246. https://doi.org/10.1027/1618-3169.56.4.236.

Cermeño-Aínsa, S. (2020). The cognitive penetrability of perception: a blocked debate and a tentative solution. *Consciousness and Cognition* 77: 102838. https://doi.org/10.1016/j.concog.2019.102838.

Charlton, S.G. and Starkey, N.J. (2011). Driving without awareness: the effects of practice and automaticity on attention and driving. *Transportation Research Part F: Traffic Psychology and Behaviour* 14 (6): 456–471. https://doi.org/10.1016/j.trf.2011.04.010.

Chen, O., Paas, F., and Sweller, J. (2021). Spacing and interleaving effects require distinct theoretical bases: a systematic review testing the cognitive load and discriminative-contrast hypotheses. *Educational Psychology Review* 33: 1499–1522. https://doi.org/10.1007/s10648-021-09613-w.

Chen, Y., Zhang, M., Xin, C. et al. (2022). Effect of encoding of prospective memory. *Frontiers in Psychology* 12: 1–10. https://doi.org/10.3389/fpsyg.2021.701281.

Chi, M.T. and Roscoe, R.D. (2002). The processes and challenges of conceptual change. In: *Reconsidering Conceptual Change: Issues in Theory and Practice* (ed. M. Limón and L. Mason), 3–27. Kluwer https://doi.org/10.1007/0-306-47637-1_1.

Chi, M.T., Bassok, M., Lewis, M.W. et al. (1989). Self-explanations: how students study and use examples in learning to solve problems. *Cognitive Science* 13 (2): 145–182. https://doi.org/10.1016/0364-0213(89)90002-5.

Cho, K.W. and Powers, A. (2019). Testing enhances both memorization and conceptual learning of categorical materials. *Journal of Applied Research in Memory and Cognition* 8 (2): 166–177. https://doi.org/10.1016/j.jarmac.2019.01.003.

Collins, A.M. and Loftus, E.F. (1975). A spreading-activation theory of semantic processing. *Psychological Review* 82 (6): 407–428. https://doi.org/10.1037/0033-295X.82.6.407.

Collins, A.M. and Quillian, M.R. (1969). Retrieval time from semantic memory. *Journal of Verbal Learning and Verbal Behavior* 8 (2): 240–247. https://doi.org/10.1016/S0022-5371(69)80069-1.

Conway, A.R., Cowan, N., Bunting, M.F. et al. (2002). A latent variable analysis of working memory capacity, short-term memory capacity, processing speed, and general fluid intelligence. *Intelligence* 30 (2): 163–183. https://doi.org/10.1016/S0160-2896(01)00096-4.

Cowan, N. (2001). The magical number 4 in short-term memory: a reconsideration of mental storage capacity. *Behavioral and Brain Sciences* 24 (1): 87–114. https://doi.org/10.1017/S0140525X01003922.

Cowan, N. (2008). What are the differences between long-term, short-term, and working memory? *Progress in Brain Research* 169: 323–338. https://doi.org/10.1016/S0079-6123(07)00020-9.

Cowan, N. (2010). The magical mystery four: how is working memory capacity limited, and why? *Current Directions in Psychological Science* 19 (1): 51–57. https://doi.org/10.1177/0963721409359277.

Craik, F. (2023). The role of intentionality in memory and learning: comments on Popov and dames (2022). *Journal of Experimental Psychology: General* 152 (1): 301–307. https://doi.org/10.1037/xge0001329.

Craik, F. and Lockhart, R. (1972). Levels of processing: a framework for memory research. *Journal of Verbal learning and Verbal Behavior* 11: 671–684. https://doi.org/10.1016/S0022-5371(72)80001-X.

Craik, F. and Tulving, E. (1975). Depth of processing and the retention of words in episodic memory. *Journal of Experimental Psychology: General* 104 (3): 268–294. https://doi.org/10.1037/0096-3445.104.3.268.

Crocetti, E., Albarello, F., Meeus, W., and Rubini, M. (2022). Identities: a developmental social-psychological perspective. *European Review of Social Psychology* https://doi.org/10.1080/10463283.2022.2104987.

Crossman, E.R. (1959). A theory of the acquisition of speed-skill. *Ergonomics* 2 (2): 153–166. https://doi.org/10.1080/00140135908930419.

Dale, V.H., Pierce, S.E., and May, S.A. (2010). The role of undergraduate research experiences in producing veterinary scientists. *Journal of Veterinary Medical Education* 37 (2): 198–206. https://doi.org/10.3138/jvme.37.2.198.

Deslauriers, L., McCarty, L.S., Miller, K. et al. (2019). Measuring actual learning versus feeling of learning in response to being actively engaged in the classroom. *Proceedings of the National Academy of Sciences of the United States of America* 116 (39): 19251–19257. https://doi.org/10.1073/pnas.1821936116.

DiSessa, A.A. and Sherin, B.L. (1998). What changes in conceptual change? *International Journal of Science Education* 20 (10): 1155–1191. https://doi.org/10.1080/0950069980201002.

Djourova, N.P., Rodríguez Molina, I., Tordera Santamatilde, N., and Abate, G. (2020). Self-efficacy and resilience: mediating mechanisms in the relationship between the transformational leadership dimensions and well-being. *Journal of Leadership & Organizational Studies* 27 (3): 256–270. https://doi.org/10.1177/1548051819849002.

Dochy, F., Segers, M., Van den Bossche, P., and Gijbels, D. (2003). Effects of problem-based learning: a meta-analysis. *Learning and Instruction* 13 (5): 533–568. https://doi.org/10.1016/S0959-4752(02)00025-7.

Dodson, C.S. and Schacter, D.L. (2001). If I had said it I would have remembered it: reducing false memories with a distinctiveness heuristic. *Psychonomic Bulletin & Review* 8 (1): 155–161. https://doi.org/10.3758/BF03196152.

Dole, J.A. and Sinatra, G.M. (1998). Reconceptalizing change in the cognitive construction of knowledge. *Educational Psychologist* 33 (2–3): 109–128. https://doi.org/10.1080/00461520.1998.9653294.

Donovan, J.J. and Radosevich, D.J. (1999). A meta-analytic review of the distribution of practice effect: now you see it, now you don't. *Journal of Applied Psychology* 84 (5): 795. https://doi.org/10.1037/0021-9010.84.5.795.

Duit, R. and Treagust, D.F. (2003). Conceptual change: a powerful framework for improving science teaching and learning. *International Journal of Science Education* 25 (6): 671–688. https://doi.org/10.1080/09500690305016.

Dunlosky, J., Rawson, K.A., Marsh, E.J. et al. (2013). Improving students' learning with effective learning techniques: promising directions from cognitive and educational psychology: promising directions from cognitive and educational psychology. *Psychological Science in the Public Interest: A Journal of the American Psychological Society* 14 (1): 4–58. https://doi.org/10.1177/1529100612453266.

van Ede, F. and Nobre, A.C. (2023). Turning attention inside out: how working memory serves behavior. *Annual Review of Psychology* 74 (1): 137–165. https://doi.org/10.1146/annurev-psych-021422-041757.

Engelkamp, J. (1998). *Memory for Actions*. Taylor & Francis (UK).

Engelkamp, J. and Krumnacker, H. (1980). Image- and motor-processes in the retention of verbal materials. *Zeitschrift für Experimentelle und Angewandte Psychologie* 27 (4): 511–533.

Evans, K.K. and Baddeley, A. (2018). Intention, attention and long-term memory for visual scenes: it all depends on the scenes. *Cognition* 180: 24–37. https://doi.org/10.1016/j.cognition.2018.06.022.

Fawcett, J. (2013). The production effect benefits performance in between-subject design: a meta-analysis. *Acta Psychologica* 142: 1–5. https://doi.org/10.1016/j.actpsy.2012.10.001.

Fawcett, A. and Mullan, S. (2018). Managing moral distress in practice. *In Practice* 40 (1): 34–36. https://doi.org/10.1136/inp.j5124.

Fawcett, J.M. and Ozubko, J.D. (2016). Familiarity, but not recollection, supports the between-subject production effect in recognition memory. *Revue Canadienne de Psychologie Experimentale [Canadian Journal of Experimental Psychology]* 70 (2): 99–115. https://doi.org/10.1037/cep0000089.

Fawcett, J., Baldwin, M., Whitridge, J. et al. (2022a). Production improves recognition and reduces intrusions in between-subject design: an update meta-analysis. *Canadian Journal of Experimental Psychology* 77 (1): 35–44. https://doi.org/10.1037/cep0000302.

Fawcett, J., Bodner, G., Paulewicz, B. et al. (2022b). Production can enhance semantic encoding: evidence from force-choice recognition with homophone versus synonym lures. *Psychonomic Bulletin & Review* 29: 2256–2263. https://doi.org/10.3758/s13423-022-02140-x.

Fazio, R.H. (2001). On the automatic activation of associated evaluations: an overview. *Cognition & Emotion* 15 (2): 115–141. https://doi.org/10.1080/0269993004200024.

Fiedler, K., Lachnit, H., Fay, D., and Krug, C. (1992). Mobilization of cognitive resources and the generation effect. *The Quarterly Journal of Experimental Psychology A, Human Experimental Psychology* 45 (1): 149–171. https://doi.org/10.1080/14640749208401320.

Fitts, P.M. (1964). Perceptual-motor skill learning. In: *Categories of Human Learning* (ed. A.W. Melton), 243–285. Academic Press.

Fitts, P. and Posner, M. (1967). *Human Performance*. Brooks/Cole https://doi.org/10.1016/B978-1-4832-3145-7.50016-9.

Fonseca, B. and Chi, M.T.H. (2011). Instruction based on self-explanation. In: *Educational Psychology Handbook: Handbook of Research on Learning and Instruction* (ed. R.E. Mayer and P.A. Alexander), 296–321. Routledge.

Foos, P.W., Mora, J.J., and Tkacz, S. (1994). Student study techniques and the generation effect. *Journal of Educational Psychology* 86 (4): 567–576. https://doi.org/10.1037/0022-0663.86.4.567.

Forrin, N.D., Macleod, C.M., and Ozubko, J.D. (2012). Widening the boundaries of the production effect. *Memory & Cognition* 40 (7): 1046–1055. https://doi.org/10.3758/s13421-012-0210-8.

Foster, N., Mueller, M., Was, C. et al. (2019). Why does interleaving improve math learning? The contributions of discriminative contract and distributed practice. *Memory & Cognition* 47: 1088–1101. https://doi.org/10.3758/s13421-019-00918-4.

Freeman, S., Eddy, S.L., McDonough, M. et al. (2014). Active learning increases student performance in science, engineering, and mathematics. *Proceedings of the National Academy of Sciences of the United States of America* 111 (23): 8410–8415. https://doi.org/10.1073/pnas.1319030111.

Froehlich, A. and Rogers, E.B. (2022). Four keys to unlocking equitable learning: retrieval, spacing, interleaving, and elaborative encoding. In: *Teaching and Learning for Social Justice and Equity in Higher Education* (ed. L. Parson and C. Ozaki), 142–163. Palgrave https://doi.org/10.1007/978-3-030-88608-0_10.

Furtak, E.M., Seidel, T., Iverson, H., and Briggs, D.C. (2012). Experimental and quasi-experimental studies of inquiry-based science teaching: a meta-analysis. *Review of Educational Research* 82 (3): 300–329. https://doi.org/10.3102/0034654312457206.

Gale, J., Alemdar, M., Cappelli, C., and Morris, D. (2021). A mixed methods study of self-efficacy, the sources of self-efficacy, and teaching experience. *Frontiers in Education* 6: 1–16. https://doi.org/10.3389/feduc. 2021.750599.

Gardner, D. and Hini, D. (2006). Work-related stress in the veterinary profession in New Zealand. *New Zealand Veterinary Journal* 54 (3): 119–124. https://doi.org/10.1080/00480169.2006.36623.

Gentner, D., Loewenstein, J., and Thompson, L. (2003). Learning and transfer: a general role for analogical encoding. *Journal of Educational Psychology* 95 (2): 393–408. https://doi.org/10.1037/0022-0663.95.2.393.

Gluckman, M., Vlach, H.A., and Sandhofer, C.M. (2014). Spacing simultaneously promotes multiple forms of learning in children's science curriculum: spacing, memory, and generalization. *Applied Cognitive Psychology* 28 (2): 266–273. https://doi.org/10.1002/acp.2997.

Godden, D.R. and Baddeley, A.D. (1975). Context-dependent memory in two natural environments: on land and underwater. *British Journal of Psychology (London, England: 1953)* 66 (3): 325–331. https://doi.org/10.1111/j.2044-8295.1975.tb01468.x.

Goetze, J. and Driver, M. (2022). Is learning really just believing? A meta-analysis of self-efficacy and achievement in SLA. *Studies in Second Language Learning and Teaching* 12 (2): 233–259. http://doi.org/10.14746/ssllt.2022.12.2.4.

Goldin, P.R., Manber-Ball, T., Werner, K. et al. (2009). Neural mechanisms of cognitive reappraisal of negative self-beliefs in social anxiety disorder. *Biological Psychiatry* 66 (12): 1091–1099. https://doi.org/10.1016/j.biopsych.2009.07.014.

Goldin, P.R., Ziv, M., Jazaieri, H. et al. (2012). Cognitive reappraisal self-efficacy mediates the effects of individual cognitive-behavioral therapy for social anxiety disorder. *Journal of Consulting and Clinical Psychology* 80 (6): 1034–1040. https://doi.org/10.1037/a0028555.

Graves, K. and Garton, S. (2017). An analysis of three curriculum approaches to teaching English in public-sector schools. *Language Teaching* 50 (4): 441–482. https://doi.org/10.1017/s0261444817000155.

Greving, S. and Richter, T. (2018). Examining the testing effect in university teaching: retrievability and question format matter. *Frontiers in Psychology* 9: 2412. https://doi.org/10.3389/fpsyg.2018.02412.

Gross, J.J. (1998). The emerging field of emotion regulation: an integrative review. *Review of General Psychology* 2 (3): 271–299. https://doi.org/10.1037/1089-2680.2.3.271.

Grove, N.P. and Lowery Bretz, S. (2012). A continuum of learning: from rote memorization to meaningful learning in organic chemistry. *Chemistry Education Research and Practice* 13 (3): 201–208. https://doi.org/10.1039/c1rp90069b.

Gully, S.M., Incalcaterra, K.A., Joshi, A., and Beaubien, J.M. (2002). A meta-analysis of group efficacy, potency, and performance: interdependence and level of analysis as moderators of observed relationships. *Journal of Applied Psychology* 87 (5): 819–832. https://doi.org/10.1037//0021-9010.87.5.819.

Halford, G.S., Cowan, N., and Andrews, G. (2007). Separating cognitive capacity from knowledge: a new hypothesis. *Trends in Cognitive Sciences* 11 (6): 236–242. https://doi.org/10.1016/j.tics.2007.04.001.

Hanley, A., Palejwala, M., Hanley, R. et al. (2015). A failure in mind: dispositional mindfulness and positive reappraisal as predictors of academic self-efficacy following failure. *Personality and Individual Differences* 86: 332–337. https://doi.org/10.1016/j.paid.2015.06.033.

Hardt, O., Nader, K., and Nadel, L. (2013). Decay happens: the role of active forgetting in memory. *Trends in Cognitive Sciences* 17 (3): 111–120. https://doi.org/10.1016/j.tics.2013.01.001.

Hartwig, M.K. and Dunlosky, J. (2012). Study strategies of college students: are self-testing and scheduling related to achievement? *Psychonomic Bulletin & Review* 19 (1): 126–134. https://doi.org/10.3758/s13423-011-0181-y.

Hayat, A., Shateri, K., Amini, M., and Shokrpour, N. (2020). Relationships between academic self-efficacy, learning-related emotions, and metacognitive learning strategies with academic performance in medical students: a structural equation model. *BMC Medical Education* 20: 76. https://doi.org/10.1186/s12909-020-01995-9.

Heathcote, A., Brown, S., and Mewhort, D.J. (2000). The power law repealed: the case for an exponential law of practice. *Psychonomic Bulletin & Review* 7 (2): 185–207. https://doi.org/10.3758/bf03212979.

Hyde, T.S. and Jenkins, J.J. (1969). Differential effects of incidental tasks on the organization of recall of a list of highly associated words. *Journal of Experimental Psychology* 82 (3): 472–481. https://doi.org/10.1037/h0028372.

Hyde, T.S. and Jenkins, J.J. (1973). Recall for words as a function of semantic, graphic, and syntactic orienting tasks. *Journal of Verbal Learning and Verbal Behavior* 12 (5): 471–480. https://doi.org/10.1016/s0022-5371(73)80027-1.

Jacoby, L.L. (1978). On interpreting the effects of repetition: solving a problem versus remembering a solution. *Journal of Verbal Learning and Verbal Behavior* 17 (6): 649–667. https://doi.org/10.1016/s0022-5371(78)90393-6.

James, W. (1899). *Talks to Teachers on Psychology: And to the Students on Some of Life's Ideals.* Holt.

de Jong, L.H., Favier, R.P., Van der Vleuten, C.P., and Bok, H.G. (2017). Students' motivation toward feedback-seeking in the clinical workplace. *Medical Teacher* 39 (9): 954–958. https://doi.org/10.1080/0142159X.2017.1324948.

Just, M.A. and Carpenter, P.A. (1992). A capacity theory of comprehension: individual differences in working memory. *Psychological Review* 99 (1): 122–139. https://doi.org/10.1037/0033-295X.99.1.122.

Kane, M.J., Bleckley, M.K., Conway, A.R., and Engle, R.W. (2001). A controlled-attention view of working-memory capacity. *Journal of Experimental Psychology. General* 130 (2): 169–183. https://doi.org/10.1037/0096-3445.130.2.169.

Kang, S.H. and Pashler, H. (2012). Learning painting styles: spacing is advantageous when it promotes discriminative contrast. *Applied Cognitive Psychology* 26 (1): 97–103. https://doi.org/10.1002/acp.1801.

Kapler, I.V., Weston, T., and Wiseheart, M. (2015). Spacing in a simulated undergraduate classroom: long-term benefits for factual and higher-level learning. *Learning and Instruction* 36: 38–45. https://doi.org/10.1016/j.learninstruc.2014.11.001.

Kapur, M., Hattie, J., Grossman, I., and Sinha, T. (2022). Corrigendum: fail, flip, fix, and feed-rethinking flipped learning: a review of meta-analyses and a subsequent meta-analysis (front). *Frontiers in Education* 7: https://doi.org/10.3389/feduc.2022.956416.

Karpicke, J.D. and Grimaldi, P.J. (2012). Retrieval-based learning: a perspective for enhancing meaningful learning. *Educational Psychology Review* 24 (3): 401–418. https://doi.org/10.1007/s10648-012-9202-2.

Karpicke, J.D., Butler, A.C., and Roediger, I. (2009). Metacognitive strategies in student learning: do students practice retrieval when they study on their own? *Memory* 17 (4): 471–479. https://doi.org/10.1080/09658210802647009.

Kasalak, G. and Dağyar, M. (2020). The relationship between teacher self-efficacy and teacher job satisfaction: a meta- analysis of the Teaching and Learning International Survey (TALIS). *Educational Sciences: Theory and Practice* 20 (3): 16–33. http://doi.org/10.12738/jestp.2020.3.002.

Kiewra, K.A. and Benton, S.L. (1988). The relationship between information-processing ability and notetaking. *Contemporary Educational Psychology* 13 (1): 33–44. https://doi.org/10.1016/0361-476x(88)90004-5.

Kim, J.W., Ritter, F.E., and Koubek, R.J. (2013). An integrated theory for improved skill acquisition and retention in the three stages of learning. *Theoretical Issues in Ergonomics* 14 (1): 22–37. https://doi.org/10.1080/1464536x.2011.573008.

Klassen, R. and Tze, V. (2014). Teachers' self-efficacy, personality, and teaching effectiveness: a meta-analysis. *Educational Research Review* 12: 59–76. https://doi.org/10.1016/j.edurev.2014.06.001.

Komarraju, M. and Nadler, D. (2013). Self-efficacy and academic achievement: why do implicit beliefs, goals, and effort regulation matter? *Learning and Individual Differences* 25: 67–72. https://doi.org/10.1016/j.lindif.2013.01.005.

Kornell, N. and Bjork, R.A. (2008). Learning concepts and categories: is spacing the "enemy of induction"?: is spacing the "enemy of induction"? *Psychological Science* 19 (6): 585–592. https://doi.org/10.1111/j.1467-9280.2008.02127.x.

Ladd, G.T. (1894). President's address before the New York meeting of the American Psychological Association. *Psychological Review* 1 (1): 1–21. https://doi.org/10.1037/h0064711.

Lakoff, G. and Johnson, M. (1980). Conceptual metaphor in everyday language. *The Journal of Philosophy* 77 (8): 453. https://doi.org/10.2307/2025464.

Langebæk, R., Toft, N., and Eriksen, T. (2015). The SimSpay—student perceptions of a low-cost build-it-yourself model for novice training of surgical skills in canine ovariohysterectomy. *Journal of Veterinary Medical Education* 42 (2): 166–171. https://doi.org/10.3138/jvme.1014-105.

Latimier, A., Peyre, H., and Ramus, F. (2021). A meta-analytic review of the benefit of spacing out retrieval practice episodes on retention. *Educational Psychology Review* 33 (3): 959–987. https://doi.org/10.1007/s10648-020-09572-8.

Leber, A.B. and Egeth, H.E. (2006). It's under control: top-down search strategies can override attentional capture. *Psychonomic Bulletin & Review* 13 (1): 132–138. https://doi.org/10.3758/bf03193824.

Lehmann, A.C. and Ericsson, K.A. (1997). Research on expert performance and deliberate practice: implications for the education of amateur musicians and music students. *Psychomusicology* 16 (1–2): 40–58. https://doi.org/10.1037/h0094068.

Lewandowsky, S., Geiger, S.M., and Oberauer, K. (2008). Interference-based forgetting in verbal short-term memory. *Journal of Memory and Language* 59 (2): 200–222. https://doi.org/10.1016/j.jml.2008.04.004.

Livinți, R., Gunnesch-Luca, G., and Iliescu, G. (2021). Research self-efficacy: a meta-analysis. *Educational Psychologist* 56 (3): 215–242. https://doi.org/10.1080/00461520.2021.1886103.

Locke, E.A. and Latham, G.P. (2002). Building a practically useful theory of goal setting and task motivation: a 35-year odyssey. *The American Psychologist* 57 (9): 705–717. https://doi.org/10.1037/0003-066x.57.9.705.

Locke, E.A. and Latham, G.P. (2015). Breaking the rules: a historical overview of goal setting theory. In: *Advances in Motivation Science*, vol. 2 (ed. A.J. Elliot), 99–126. Elsevier https://doi.org/10.1016/bs.adms.2015.05.001.

Logie, R.H., Camos, V., and Cowan, N. (2020). *Working Memory: The State of the Science*. Oxford: Oxford University Press.

Lombardi, D., Shipley, T.F., and Astronomy Team, Biology Team, Chemistry Team, Engineering Team, Geography Team, Geoscience Team, and Physics Team (2021).

Thecurious construct of active learning. *Psychological Science in the Public Interest* 22 (1): 8–43. https://doi.org/10.1177/1529100620973974.

Lusk, D.L., Evans, A.D., Jeffrey, T.R. et al. (2009). Multimedia learning and individual differences: mediating the effects of working memory capacity with segmentation. *British Journal of Educational Technology* 40 (4): 636–651. https://doi.org/10.1111/j.1467-8535.2008.00848.x.

MacLeod, C. and Bodner, G. (2017). The production effect in memory. *Current Directions in Psychological Science* 26 (4): 390–395. https://doi.org/10.1177/0963721417691356.

MacLeod, C.M., Gopie, N., Hourihan, K.L. et al. (2010). The production effect: delineation of a phenomenon. *Journal of Experimental Psychology. Learning, Memory, and Cognition* 36 (3): 671–685. https://doi.org/10.1037/a0018785.

Madan, C.R. and Singhal, A. (2012). Using actions to enhance memory: effects of enactment, gestures, and exercise on human memory. *Frontiers in Psychology* 3: 507. https://doi.org/10.3389/fpsyg.2012.00507.

Mayer, R.E. (1992). *Thinking, Problem Solving, Cognition*. Freeman.

McArthur, M.L., Learey, T.J., Jarden, A. et al. (2021). Resilience of veterinarians at different career stages: the role of self-efficacy, coping strategies and personal resources for resilience in veterinary practice. *Veterinary Record* 189 (12): e771. https://doi.org/10.1002/vetr.771.

McCurdy, M.P., Viechtbauer, W., Sklenar, A.M. et al. (2020a). Theories of the generation effect and the impact of generation constraint: a meta-analytic review. *Psychonomic Bulletin & Review* 27 (6): 1139–1165. https://doi.org/10.3758/s13423-020-01762-3.

McCurdy, M., Sklenar, A., Frankenstein, A., and Leshikar, E. (2020b). Fewer generation constraints increase the generation effect for item and source memory through enhanced relational processing. *Memory* 28 (5): 598–616. https://doi.org/10.1080/09658211.2020.1749283.

McNamara, T.P. (2005). *Semantic Priming: Perspectives from Memory and Word Recognition*. Psychology Press.

McVee, M.B., Dunsmore, K., and Gavelek, J.R. (2005). Schema theory revisited. *Review of Educational Research* 75 (4): 531–566. https://doi.org/10.3102/00346543075004531.

Melby-Lervåg, M., Redick, T.S., and Hulme, C. (2016). Working memory training does not improve performance on measures of intelligence or other measures of "far transfer": evidence from a meta-analytic review: evidence from a meta-analytic review. *Perspectives on Psychological Science: A Journal of the Association for Psychological Science* 11 (4): 512–534. https://doi.org/10.1177/1745691616635612.

Meyer, D.E. and Schvaneveldt, R.W. (1971). Facilitation in recognizing pairs of words: evidence of a dependence between retrieval operations. *Journal of Experimental Psychology* 90 (2): 227–234. https://doi.org/10.1037/h003156.

Mikkonen, J. and Ruohoniemi, M. (2011). How do veterinary students' motivation and study practices relate to academic success? *Journal of Veterinary Medical Education* 38 (3): 298–304. https://doi.org/10.3138/jvme.38.3.298.

Miller, G.A. (1956). The magical number seven, plus or minus two: some limits on our capacity for processing information. *Psychological Review* 63 (2): 81. https://doi.org/10.1037/h0043158.

Miyake, A. and Shah, P. (1999). *Models of Working Memory*. Cambridge: Cambridge University Press.

Morehead, K., Rhodes, M.G., and DeLozier, S. (2016). Instructor and student knowledge of study strategies. *Memory* 24 (2): 257–271. https://doi.org/10.1080/09658211.2014.1001992.

Morris, C., Bransford, J., and Franks, J. (1977). Levels of processing versus transfer appropriate processing. *Journal of Verbal Learning and Verbal Behavior* 16: 519–533. https://doi.org/10.1016/S0022-5371(77)80016-9.

Mossop, L. and Cobb, K. (2013). Teaching and assessing veterinary professionalism. *Journal of Veterinary Medical Education* 40 (3): 223–232. https://doi.org/10.3138/jvme.0113-016R.

Narhi-Martinez, W., Dube, B., and Golomb, J.D. (2023). Attention as a multi-level system of weights and balances. *Wiley Interdisciplinary Reviews. Cognitive Science* 14 (1): e1633. https://doi.org/10.1002/wcs.1633.

Nesbit, J.C. and Adesope, O.O. (2006). Learning with concept and knowledge maps: a meta-analysis. *Review of Educational Research* 76 (3): 413–448. https://doi.org/10.3102/00346543076003413.

Neta, M., Harp, N., Tong, T. et al. (2022). Think again: the role of reappraisal in reducing negative valence bias. *Cognition and Emotion*. https://doi.org/10.1080/02699931.2022.2160698.

Norris, D. and Kalm, K. (2021). Chunking and data compression in verbal short-term memory. *Cognition* 208: 104534. https://doi.org/10.1016/j.cognition.2020.104534.

Oberauer, K. and Greve, W. (2022). Intentional remembering and intentional forgetting in working and long-term memory. *Journal of Experimental Psychology. General* 151 (3): 513–541. https://doi.org/10.1037/xge0001106.

Ost, J., Udell, J., Dear, S. et al. (2022). The serial reproduction of an urban myth: revisiting Bartlett's schema theory. *Memory* 30 (6): 775–783. https://doi.org/10.1080/09658211.2022.2059514.

Oudbier, J., Spaai, G., Timmermans, K., and Boerboom, T. (2022). Enhancing the effectiveness of flipped classroom in health science education: a state-of-the-art review. *BMC Medical Education* 22 (1): 34. https://doi.org/10.1186/s12909-021-03052-5.

Parkinson, T.J., Gilling, M., and Suddaby, G.T. (2006). Workload, study methods, and motivation of students within a BVSc program. *Journal of Veterinary Medical Education* 33 (2): 253–265. https://doi.org/10.3138/jvme.33.2.253.

Pavlov, Y.G. and Kotchoubey, B. (2020). The electrophysiological underpinnings of variation in verbal working memory capacity. *Scientific Reports* 10 (1): 16090. https://doi.org/10.1038/s41598-020-72940-5.

Perera, H., Calkins, C., and Part, R. (2019). Teacher self-efficacy profiles: determinants, outcomes, and generalizability across teaching level. *Contemporary Educational Psychology* 58: 186–203. https://doi.org/10.1016/j.cedpsych.2019.02.006.

Pesta, B.J., Sanders, R.E., and Nemec, R.J. (1996). Older adults' strategic superiority with mental multiplication: a generation effect assessment. *Experimental Aging Research* 22 (2): 155–169. https://doi.org/10.1080/03610739608254004.

Peynircioglu, Z. and Mungan, E. (1993). Familiarity, relative distinctiveness, and the generation effect. *Memory & Cognition* 21 (3): 367–374. https://doi.org/10.3758/BF03208269.

Pintrich, P.R. (2003). A motivational science perspective on the role of student motivation in learning and teaching contexts. *Journal of Educational Psychology* 95 (4): 667–686. https://doi.org/10.1037/0022-0663.95.4.667.

Posner, M. and Snyder, C. (1975). Facilitation and inhibition in the processing of signals. In: *Attention and Performance* (ed. P. Rabbitt and S. Dornic), 231–249. Academic.

Posner, G.J., Strike, K.A., Hewson, P.W., and Gertzog, W.A. (1982). Accommodation of a scientific conception: toward a theory of conceptual change. *Science Education* 66 (2): 211–227. https://doi.org/10.1002/sce.3730660207.

Postman, L. and Adams, P.A. (1956). Studies in incidental learning: IV. The interaction of orienting tasks and stimulus materials. *Journal of Experimental Psychology* 51 (5): 329–341. https://doi.org/10.1037/h0043781.

Poulou, M.S., Reddy, L.A., and Dudek, C.M. (2019). Relation of teacher self-efficacy and classroom practices: a preliminary investigation. *School Psychology International* 40 (1): 25–48. https://doi.org/10.1177/0143034318798045.

Pressley, M., Brown, R., El-Dinary, P.B., and Allferbach, P. (1995). The comprehension instruction that students need: instruction fostering constructively responsive reading. *Learning Disabilities Research & Practice* 10 (4): 215–224.

Quinn, P.C. and Tanaka, J.W. (2007). Early development of perceptual expertise: within-basic-level categorization experience facilitates the formation of subordinate-level category representations in 6-to 7-month-old infants. *Memory & Cognition* 35 (6): 1422–1431. https://doi.org/10.3758/BF03193612.

Renoult, L., Irish, M., Moscovitch, M., and Rugg, M.D. (2019). From knowing to remembering: the semantic-episodic distinction. *Trends in Cognitive Sciences* 23 (12): 1041–1057. https://doi.org/10.1016/j.tics.2019.09.008.

Ricker, T.J., Vergauwe, E., and Cowan, N. (2016, 2014). Decay theory of immediate memory: from Brown (1958) to today. *Quarterly Journal of Experimental Psychology (2006)* 69 (10): 1969–1995. https://doi.org/10.1080/17470218.2014.914546.

Riepenhausen, A., Wackerhagen, C., Reppmann, Z.C. et al. (2022). Positive cognitive reappraisal in stress resilience, mental health, and well-being: a comprehensive systematic review. *Emotion Review* 14 (4): 310–331. https://doi.org/10.1177/17540739221114642.

Robbins, S.B., Lauver, K., Le, H. et al. (2004). Do psychosocial and study skill factors predict college outcomes? A meta-analysis. *Psychological Bulletin* 130: 261–288. https://doi.org/10.1037/0033-2909.130.2.261.

Roberts, B.R.T., MacLeod, C.M., and Fernandes, M. (2022). The enactment effect: a systematic review and meta-analysis of behavioral, neuroimaging, and patient studies. *PsyArXiv* http://doi.org/10.31234/osf.io/b8qps.

Roediger, H.L. III and Karpicke, J.D. (2011). Intricacies of spaced retrieval: a resolution. In: *Successful Remembering and Successful Forgetting* (ed. A.S. Benjamin), 41–66. Psychology.

Roediger, H.L. and Karpicke, J.D. (2006). Test-enhanced learning: taking memory tests improves long-term retention: taking memory tests improves long-term retention. *Psychological Science* 17 (3): 249–255. https://doi.org/10.1111/j.1467-9280.2006.01693.x.

Rohrer, D. and Taylor, K. (2007). The shuffling of mathematics problems improves learning. *Instructional Science* 35 (6): 481–498. https://doi.org/10.1007/s11251-007-9015-8.

Rosch, E., Mervis, C.B., Gray, W.D. et al. (1976). Basic objects in natural categories. *Cognitive Psychology* 8 (3): 382–439. https://doi.org/10.1016/0010-0285(76)90013-x.

Rotter, J. (1954). *Social Learning and Clinical Psychology*. Prentice Hall.

Rotter, J. (1966). Generalized expectancies for internal versus external control of reinforcement. *Psychological Monographs: General and Applied* 80 (1): 1–28. https://doi.org/10.1037/h0092976.

Rowland, C.A. (2014). The effect of testing versus re-study on retention: a meta-analytic review of the testing effect. *Psychological Bulletin* 140 (6): 1432–1441. https://doi.org/10.1037/a0037559.

Rubin, D.C. (2022). A conceptual space for episodic and semantic memory. *Memory & Cognition* 50 (3): 464–477. https://doi.org/10.3758/s13421-021-01148-3.

Sala, G. and Gobet, F. (2017). Does far transfer exist? Negative evidence from chess, music, and working memory training. *Current Directions in Psychological Science* 26 (6): 515–520. https://doi.org/10.1177/0963721417712760.

Salanova, M., Rodriguez-Sanchez, A., and Nielsen, K. (2020). The impact of group efficacy beliefs and transformational leadership on followers' self-efficacy: a multilevel-longitudinal study. *Current Psychology* 41: 2024–2033. https://doi.org/10.1007/s12144-020-00722-3.

Sana, F., Yan, V.X., and Carvalho, P.F. (2022). On rest-from-deliberate-learning as a mechanism for the spacing effect: commentary on Chen et al. (2021). *Educational Psychology Review* 34 (3): 1843–1850. https://doi.org/10.1007/s10648-022-09663-8.

Schacter, D.L. (2002). *The Seven Sins of Memory: How the Mind Forgets and Remembers*. HMH.

Scherbaum, C., Cohen-Charash, Y., and Kern, M. (2006). Measuring general self-efficacy: a comparison of three measures using item response theory. *Educational and Psychological Measurement* 66: 1047–1063. https://doi.org/10.1177/0013164406288171.

Schnotz, W. and Bannert, M. (2003). Construction and interference in learning from multiple representation. *Learning and Instruction* 13 (2): 141–156. https://doi.org/10.1016/s0959-4752(02)00017-8.

Schunk, D. and DiBenedetto, M. (2020). Self-efficacy and human motivation. *Advances in Motivation Science* 8: 1–27. https://doi.org/10.1016/bs.adms.2020.10.001.

Schunk, D.H. and Pajares, F. (2004). Self-efficacy in education revisited: empirical and applied evidence. In: *Big Theories Revisited* (ed. D.M. McInerney and S.V. Etten), 115–138. Information Age.

Schunk, D. and Usher, E. (2019). Social cognitive theory and motivation. In: *The Oxford Handbook of Human Motivation*, 2e (ed. R. Ryan), 11–26. Oxford: Oxford University Press https://doi.org/10.1093/oxfordhb/9780190666453.013.2.

Schwartz, S.J., Côté, J.E., and Arnett, J.J. (2005). Identity and agency in emerging adulthood: two developmental routes in the individualization process. *Youth & Society* 37 (2): 201–229. http://doi.org/10.1177/0044118X05275965.

Shiffrin, R.M. (1970). Forgetting: trace erosion or retrieval failure? *Science* 168 (3939): 1601–1603. https://doi.org/10.1126/science.168.3939.1601.

Silva, A., Pinho, M., Souchay, C., and Moulin, C. (2015). Evaluation the subject-performed task effect in healthy older adults: relation with neuropsychological tests. *Socioaffective Neuroscience & Psychology* 5: 1–12. https://doi.org/10.3402/snp.v5.24068.

Sisk, C.A., Remington, R.W., and Jiang, Y.V. (2019). Mechanisms of contextual cueing: a tutorial review. *Attention, Perception, & Psychophysics* 81: 2571–2589. https://doi.org/10.3758/s13414-019-01832-2.

Slamecka, N.J. and Graf, P. (1978). The generation effect: delineation of a phenomenon. *Journal of Experimental Psychology. Human Learning and Memory* 4 (6): 592–604. https://doi.org/10.1037/0278-7393.4.6.592.

Snoddy, G.S. (1926). Learning and stability: a psychophysiological analysis of a case of motor learning

with clinical applications. *The Journal of Applied Psychology* 10 (1): 1–36. https://doi.org/10.1037/h0075814.

Soveri, A., Antfolk, J., Karlsson, L.C. et al. (2018). Working memory training revisited: a multi-level meta-analysis of N-back training studies. *PsyArXiv* https://doi.org/10.31234/osf.io/fvyra.

Stokes, M.G., Kusunoki, M., Sigala, N. et al. (2013). Dynamic coding for cognitive control in prefrontal cortex. *Neuron* 78 (2): 364–375. https://doi.org/10.1016/j.neuron.2013.01.039.

Sweller, J. (1988). Cognitive load during problem solving: effects on learning. *Cognitive Science* 12 (2): 257–285. https://doi.org/10.1016/0364-0213(88)90023-7.

Sweller, J., van Merriënboer, J.J.G., and Paas, F. (2019). Cognitive architecture and instructional design: 20 years later. *Educational Psychology Review* 31 (2): 261–292. https://doi.org/10.1007/s10648-019-09465-5.

Szulewski, A., Howes, D., van Merriënboer, J.J.G., and Sweller, J. (2021). From theory to practice: the application of cognitive load theory to the practice of medicine: the application of cognitive load theory to the practice of medicine. *Academic Medicine: Journal of the Association of American Medical Colleges* 96 (1): 24–30. https://doi.org/10.1097/acm.0000000000003524.

Talarico, J.M., LaBar, K.S., and Rubin, D.C. (2004). Emotional intensity predicts autobiographical memory experience. *Memory & Cognition* 32 (7): 1118–1132. https://doi.org/10.3758/bf03196886.

Talsma, K., Schuz, B., and Norris, K. (2019). Miscalibration of self-efficacy and academic performance: self-efficacy ≠ self-fulfilling prophecy. *Learning and Individual Differences* 69: 182–195. https://doi.org/101016/j.lindif.2018.11.002.

Talsma, K., Norris, K., and Schuz, B. (2020). First-year students' academic self-efficacy calibration: differences by task type, domain specificity, student achievement level, and over time. *Student Success Journal* 11 (2): 109–120. https://doi.org/10.5204/ssj.1677.

Tauber, S.K., Dunlosky, J., Rawson, K.A. et al. (2013). Self-regulated learning of a natural category: do people interleave or block exemplars during study? *Psychonomic Bulletin & Review* 20 (2): 356–363. https://doi.org/10.3758/s13423-012-0319-6.

Teixeira-Santos, A.C., Moreira, C.S., Magalhães, R. et al. (2019). Reviewing working memory training gains in healthy older adults: a meta-analytic review of transfer for cognitive outcomes. *Neuroscience and Biobehavioral Reviews* 103: 163–177. https://doi.org/10.1016/j.neubiorev.2019.05.009.

Theobald, E.J., Hill, M.J., Tran, E. et al. (2020). Active learning narrows achievement gaps for underrepresented students in undergraduate science, technology, engineering, and math. *Proceedings of the National Academy of Sciences of the United States of America*

117 (12): 6476–6483. https://doi.org/10.1073/pnas.1916903117.

Thomson, A., Young, K.M., Lygo-Baker, S. et al. (2019). Evaluation of perceived technical skill development by students during instruction in dental extractions in different laboratory settings—A pilot study. *Journal of Veterinary Medical Education* 46 (3): 399–407. https://doi.org/10.3138/jvme.0717-096r1.

Tschannen-Moran, M. and Woolfolk Hoy, A. (2007). The differential antecedents of self-efficacy beliefs of novice and experienced teachers. *Teaching and Teacher Education* 23 (6): 944–956. https://doi.org/10.1016/j.tate.2006.05.003.

Tschannen-Moran, M., Hoy, A.W., and Hoy, W.K. (1998). Teacher efficacy: its meaning and measure. *Review of Educational Research* 68 (2): 202–248. https://doi.org/10.3102/00346543068002202.

Tulving, E. and Thomson, D. (1973). Encoding specificity and retrieval processes in episodic memory. *Psychological Review* 80 (5): 352–373. https://doi.org/10.1037/h0020071.

Unsworth, N. and Engle, R.W. (2007). The nature of individual differences in working memory capacity: active maintenance in primary memory and controlled search from secondary memory. *Psychological Review* 114 (1): 104–132. https://doi.org/10.1037/0033-295X.114.1.104.

Usher, E.L. (2009). Sources of middle school students' self-efficacy in mathematics: a qualitative investigation. *American Educational Research Journal* 46 (1): 275–314. https://doi.org/10.3102/0002831208324517.

Vosniadou, S. (1994). Capturing and modeling the process of conceptual change. *Learning and Instruction* 4 (1): 45–69. https://doi.org/10.1016/0959-4752(94)90018-3.

Walker, C. and Greene, B. (2009). The relations between student motivational beliefs and cognitive engagement in high school. *Journal of Educational Research* 102 (6): 463–472. https://doi.org/10.3200/JOER.102.6.463-472.

Walker, M.P., Brakefield, T., Seidman, J. et al. (2003). Sleep and the time course of motor skill learning. *Learning & Memory (Cold Spring Harbor, N.Y.)* 10 (4): 275–284. https://doi.org/10.1101/lm.58503.

Walsh, D.A. and Jenkins, J.J. (1973). Effects of orienting tasks on free recall in incidental learning: "difficulty," "effort," and "process" explanations. *Journal of Verbal Learning and Verbal Behavior* 12 (5): 481–488. https://doi.org/10.1016/s0022-5371(73)80028-3.

Wang, H., Hall, N., and Rahimi, S. (2015). Self-efficacy and causal attributions in teachers: effects on burnout, job satisfaction, illness, and quitting intentions. *Teaching and Teacher Education* 47: 120–130. https://doi.org/10.1016/j.tate.2014.12.005.

Warren, A.L. and Donnon, T. (2013). Optimizing biomedical science learning in a veterinary curriculum: a review. *Journal of Veterinary Medical Education* 40 (3): 210–222. https://doi.org/10.3138/jvme.0812-070R.

Webb, T., Miles, E., and Sheeran, P. (2012). Dealing with feeling: a meta-analysis of the effectiveness of strategies derived from the process model of emotion regulation. *Psychological Bulletin* 138 (4): 775–808. https://doi.org/10.1037/a0027600.

Whitehall, L., Rush, R., Gorska, S., and Forsyth, K. (2021). General self-efficacy of older adults receiving care: a systematic review and meta-analysis. *Gerontologist* 61 (6): e302–e317. https://doi.org/10.1093/geront/gnaa036.

Wickelgren, W.A. (1975). Age and storage dynamics in continuous recognition memory. *Developmental Psychology* 11 (2): 165–169. https://doi.org/10.1037/h0076457.

Wigfield, A., Tonks, S.M., and Klauda, S.L. (2016). Expectancy-value theory. In: *Handbook of Motivation at School*, 2e (ed. K.R. Wentzel and D.B. Miele), 55–74. Routledge.

Wiseheart, M., Küpper-Tetzel, C.E., Weston, T. et al. (2019). Enhancing the quality of student learning using distributed practice. In: *The Cambridge Handbook of Cognition and Education* (ed. J. Dunlosky and K.A. Rawson), 550–583. Cambridge.

Yan, V.X. and Sana, F. (2021). The robustness of the interleaving benefit. *Journal of Applied Research in Memory and Cognition* 10 (4): 589–602. https://doi.org/10.1016/j.jarmac.2021.05.002.

Yorzinski, J.L. and Whitham, W. (2023). Sensation, perception, and attention. In: *The Routledge International Handbook of Comparative Psychology* (ed. J.L. Yorzinski and W. Whitham), 61–70. Routledge.

Zaromb, F.M. and Roediger, H.L. 3rd. (2010). The testing effect in free recall is associated with enhanced organizational processes. *Memory & Cognition* 38 (8): 995–1008. https://doi.org/10.3758/MC.38.8.995.

Zimmerman, B.J. and Kitsantas, A. (2005). The hidden dimension of personal competence: self-regulated learning and practice. In: *Handbook of Competence and Motivation* (ed. A.J. Elliot and C.S. Dweck), 509–526. Guilford.

Zinchenko, P. (1939). Problema neproizvol'nogo zapominaniia. *Nauchnye zapiski Khar'kovskogo pedagogicheskogo instituta inostrannykh iazykov* 1: 145–187.

Zuccarini, G. and Malgieri, M. (2022). Modeling and representing conceptual change in the learning of successive theories: the case of the classical-quantum transition. *Science & Education* 1–45. http://arxiv.org/abs/2108.06919.

Zvacek, S.M., de Fátima Chouzal, M., and Restivo, M.T. (2015). Accuracy of self-assessment among graduate students in mechanical engineering. *Proceedings of the International Conference on Interactive Collaborative Learning (ICL)* 1130–1133. https://doi.org/10.1109/ICL.2015.7318192.

4

Andragogy

Katherine Fogelberg, DVM, PhD (Science Education), MA (Educational Leadership)
Virginia-Maryland College of Veterinary Medicine, Blacksburg, VA, USA

Section 1: Introduction

Andragogy as a formally recognized term has not been around that long in education, but in the latter half of the twentieth century, it really began to take hold and is now a permanent fixture in the education lexicon – love it or hate it. In fact, there are advanced degree programs based on the principles of andragogy, or adult learning, as it has come to be known, and while there is still some negotiation in the discipline, the term appears to be here to stay.

This chapter will cover a brief history of pedagogy, a more detailed history of andragogy, describe andragogy's features and foundations, discuss the challenges to and promises of this educational theory, look briefly at the literature supporting it, and end with some thoughts on its applications to veterinary – or indeed, any professional – education program.

Section 2: A Very Brief History of Pedagogy

There can be no discussion of andragogy without first talking about pedagogy, because it was pedagogical assumptions that gave birth to theories of learning, upon which education is built. These assumptions, however, were based on observations by monks in teaching simple skills to children (Holmes and Abington-Cooper 2000), with no initial thought given to how, and indeed even whether, adults learned. Thus, we will begin with a brief history of pedagogy and complete this section with andragogy's emergence.

According to Holmes and Abington-Cooper (2000), pedagogy evolved in European monastic schools from the seventh to the twelfth centuries. Etymologically, the term is derived from the Greek *paidagōgia*, "education, attendance on boys," from *paidagōgos*, "teacher" (Etymology n.d.,

accessed 13 September 2022). Today, pedagogy is generally – and somewhat literally – defined as "the art and science of teaching children." The assumptions made by the monks about how children learned were further adopted and reinforced with the spread of elementary schools in Europe and North America in the eighteenth and nineteenth centuries, and endured until educational psychologists started studying learning around the turn of the twentieth century (Knowles 1988).

Educational psychology limited its research mostly to children's and animal's reactions to systematic instruction, which reinforced the pedagogical model (Holmes and Abington-Cooper 2000; Knowles 1988). It was these observations made by the monks teaching children that formed the basis of education, shaped the scientific studies of learning, and formed the foundations of the educational theories upon which much our education system was built for centuries.

Unfortunately, pedagogy as a field did not address potential differences in learning by children and adults (Knowles 1988). It has also recently become generally perceived as being *teacher-centered*, or more concerned with the transmission of information and skills from a "sage on the stage" to students who are forced to "sit and get." This positivist approach has fallen out of favor in both K-12 and higher education classrooms as new research supports a more student-centered, active learning approach.

The evolution of pedagogy is a beautiful illustration of how science works: observation leads to theories and research that inform practice, all the while constructing a discipline through evolution and refinement of that research and those theories. This is clearly evident in the emergence, and evolution, of the three Big Theories of education: behaviorism, cognitivism, and constructivism. These three theories were introduced in Chapter 2 of this text, along with a variety of theorists who created and/or were influential in forwarding these theories. As a quick review, they have been summarized here to provide context and to help make the connections between pedagogy and andragogy more explicit.

Behaviorism is rooted in the work of Pavlov and reached its height through BF Skinner, who did much of his work on lab animals and which eventually evolved into what you may know today as operant conditioning, a behavioral approach used more explicitly in animals than humans, though one could argue that humans still experience this without intention in school systems. Grades, for example, are a reward for good behavior – studying hard, answering enough questions correctly, performing a task well, etc. At its very basest conceptually, behaviorism is the theory that punishment and reward shape the learning of students.

Cognitivism emerged as a reaction to behaviorism and rejected the idea that learning is simply a stimulus-response process. Instead, it focuses on how information is received, organized, stored, and retrieved. A good analogy for cognitivism is to view the mind as a computer processor, which means that learning is a series of internal mental processes, so learners are actively involved in the way information is processed. Just like behaviorism, behavior changes are observed but, unlike behaviorism, such changes are viewed as indicators of what is going on in the learner's mind rather than reactions to rewards or punishments. In short, cognitivists are concerned with what learners know and how they come to acquire it.

Constructivism theorizes that learning is an active process; it occurs through the learner creating meaning and connecting this learning with previous experiences, which leads to internal representations of knowledge that are constantly open to change as the experience of the learner changes. Constructivists believe that during the learning process, learners' personal interpretations of the world are based on their experiences and personal interactions in various contexts according to what they consider relevant and meaningful. Thus, social interactions and cultural context play an important role in the construction of knowledge. Think about children playing – or, if you prefer to stay academic – consider the Montessori method, a pedagogical approach that predated the formalizing of constructivism as a learning theory.

As you read through each of these summaries of the Big Three learning theories, you should also recall how each had identified shortcomings that gave rise to a different view of learning, resulting in a new theory. It is this evolution that likely influenced the emergence of andragogy as a concept; a concept that would eventually evolve into a theory; a theory that would be influential enough to warrant an entire chapter being dedicated to it in this textbook.

Section 3: History and Emergence of Andragogy

Draper (1998) informs us that adult education and andragogy were not always one and the same; this is borne out by the others as well, including the arguably most well-known and influential andragogue, Malcolm Knowles. Draper (1998), however, makes the case explicitly, noting that many informal efforts to educate children, *and adults*, were evident in the 1700s and 1800s as a response to a number of societal changes. Such changes included "the industrial revolution and the mobility of people from rural to urban areas. . .the increasing technological sophistication of navigation, war, and commerce; the number of private societies that were established to educate the masses of society, many of whom were illiterate" (p. 5).

Specifically, opportunities to increase literacy among adults – at least to the extent that they were able to read scripture – caused a rapid increase in adult education programs (Draper 1998). Such programs provided many opportunities to observe how adults learned, though the vast majority still used pedagogical approaches in the most teacher-centered sense. Draper (1998) completes his history lesson by discussing Thomas Pole's 1814 lament that many had worked hard to educate children, but few had done so in the service of adults. It was not until 1833 that the term andragogy would be coined by Alexander Kapp; a term that would eventually come to be synonymous with the phrase "adult education" (Henschke 2009; Loeng 2017).

Draper's (1998) assertions somewhat support Henschke's (2011) view that andragogy was a concept long before Kapp's presentation of it. Henschke (2011) posits that the idea originated in the times before Jesus Christ with the Hebrew prophets, arguing that various Hebrew words and their Greek counterparts provided the first foundations of adult education as a scientific discipline of study. Whether this is accurate or not, the first documented use of andragogy as a term is by Kapp, a German educator who studied at Pestalozzi's institute and subsequently published a book on education, in which he dedicated an entire section to adult education, calling it andragogy (Henschke 2011; Loeng 2017). As was the norm during his time, Kapp excluded women from this idea, as "only through a man can a woman be part of the state" (Kapp 1833, p. 6, as reported in Loeng 2017). As annoying as this is today, it was not a lie at the time – and his ideas of andragogy, which emphasized reason and classical Greek philosophy, justified the necessity of education for adult men, describing the qualities he felt were important to develop in adult male learners and laying the foundations for modern-day theorists in this area. While not a theory in itself, nor a guide for how such learning should occur, andragogy at the time at least provided an outline for why attention to the education of man was important.

As with pedagogy, andragogy etymologically derives from Greek. It is a term that takes the stem of *andr-*, a Greek noun meaning man, and combines it with *-gogy*, or guide, resulting in a word that literally translates to "education of man" (Knowles 1988). Fortunately, this term has evolved in its meaning as it has gained traction and been massaged throughout the decades; this will be covered throughout this chapter.

A cursory glance into the literature via a Google Scholar search for "andragogy" is likely to turn up far more hits referring to Malcolm Knowles than Alexander Kapp. But Kapp is the original andragogue, while Knowles is the celebrity (albeit also an expert) andragogue. Let's start with Kapp, then, and work our way up to Knowles.

Kapp's advocacy of self-education and lifelong learning, in particular, is something we see in our modern-era education approaches. As veterinary professionals, this concept is part of our core professional values. In the veterinarian's oath, we see the line: *I accept as a lifelong obligation the continual improvement of my professional knowledge and competence* (AVMA, accessed online 13 September 2022). And in the veterinary technician's oath, we see this included: *I accept my obligations to practice my profession conscientiously and with sensitivity, adhering to the profession's Code of Ethics, and furthering my knowledge and competence through a commitment to lifelong learning* (NAVTA, accessed 13 September 2022).

It is hard to imagine that the social happenings of the 1800s did not heavily influence Kapp's thinking. Humanism, or the idea that humans had dignity and autonomy (discussed more in detail in an earlier chapter of this text) and thus should be less managed and more encouraged, was sweeping through the Western world in rebellion against the strict authoritarian regimes in place (Draper 1998). The Enlightenment was also in full swing, and these forces moved education from an authoritarian, teacher-centered practice to a more holistic, student-centered one (Draper 1998). We see echoes of this movement in Kapp's firm belief that understanding one's character was central to learning – "know yourself" might have been his motto, were he alive today (Loeng 2017). By knowing oneself, he stated, you could better figure out where you fit in the world and that helped you work toward the greater social good – you knew what you should and should not spend your time learning (Loeng 2017). And working toward the greater social good also meant you needed to learn the importance of outer, objective competencies – not just learning for learning's sake, per se, but also for figuring out how your learning would help you reach specific, socially oriented goals (Loeng 2017).

As for how learning happened, Kapp felt that for adults it was a combination of being taught, reflecting on the self, and through lived experiences, though the latter was less emphasized than the first two (Loeng 2017). He also strongly believed that education occurred through conversation and talking; delivering information via text was not the best way to teach adults, according to Kapp (Loeng 2017).

In spite of the work done in this area by Kapp in the late 1800s, andragogy did not quite take off during his time. There was actually quite a long break between Kapp's use of andragogy and its subsequent recognition – in Europe, that is, and specifically in Germany – by Eugen Rosenstock-Huessy (pronounced *hew-sy*) in 1925 (Henschke 2009).

Rosenstock-Huessy was opposed to rationalism, dualism, and idealism, and felt that those who would not or could not let their knowledge be changed by events should not be part of andragogy. In his view, those who are mere men of "book knowledge, the dogmatist, the professional man, the philosopher and the rationalist" (Loeng 2017, p. 638) fell into this category. He additionally believed that learning history was imperative to avoid past mistakes, and that past and present work together to move us to the future. Lastly, he argued that the process of creating theory was cyclical – theory becomes practical deed, becomes the stuff for theory, and that andragogy was a necessity for this process (Loeng 2017).

It seemed as if andragogy was finally having its day, as in 1926, Eduard Lindeman, inspired by Rosenstock-Huessy, furthered the idea of andragogy by putting experiences in the center, saying that discovering the meaning of our experiences is what learning is about (Loeng 2017; Henschke 2011). Lindeman was the first to bring the idea of andragogy to the US, and following in Kapp's footsteps, asserted that discussion was the best method for teaching adults. In spite of its introduction in the US early in the twentieth century, however, we would not see it gain a true foothold here until past the mid-century mark (Henschke 2011; Loeng 2017; Zmeyov 1998).

Andragogy reemerged in Great Britain in the early 1960s with the idea that andragogy was a title that could be used by those attempting to "identify a body of knowledge relevant to the training of those concerned with Adult Education" (Simpson 1964, as cited in Henschke 2011, p. 6). A few years later, in 1968, it was Malcolm Knowles who would reintroduce andragogy in the US. He would be responsible for it becoming a mainstay in the discipline of education and was its fiercest proponent. Even in the face of significant criticism, Knowles persevered in working toward having andragogy viewed as a unifying theory of adult learning.

Section 4: Features and Foundations of Knowles's Andragogy

Knowles was introduced to the term andragogy by Dusan Savicevic, a Yugoslavian adult educator who, along with several other Europeans, was instrumental in pushing andragogy as an autonomous field of study beginning in the 1950s (Henschke 2011; Knowles 1988). It should be noted that, according to Zmeyov (1998), the origins of this field were influenced by Maslow's hierarchy of individual needs and Rogers' idea that the individual had the leading role in the process of his or her learning and convalescence (Rogers was a physician).

After learning about it from Savicevic, Knowles developed his own philosophy and meaning of andragogy, basing it on research that emerged in the 1960s that "focused on the internal processes of adult learning" (Knowles 1988, p. 42). Interestingly, Knowles (1988) attributes the term andragogy to European adult educators whom he states "felt the need for a label for this new theoretical model that would enable them to talk about it in parallel with pedagogy" (p. 42). Regardless of this error, Knowles's at-the-time emergent theory posited that adults accumulate experiences that become increasingly rich sources for their learning as they mature (Henschke 2011; Loeng 2017).

The idea of experiences being important to learning was not necessarily a new concept – remember that Kapp included this in his original concept as well. In his earliest work on the theory, however, Knowles believed andragogy was different than pedagogy in four crucial ways: adults are independent, rather than dependent, learners; adults have personal experiences that contribute to their learning; their readiness to learn is increasingly oriented to the developmental tasks of their social roles; and they need an immediate application of their learning for it to be worthwhile (Henschke 2011). Knowles, along with others, would later provide additional differences and ideas about what andragogy was and why it was important, but these original tenets were the origins of the separation between teaching children and teaching adults. Knowles was the first to explicitly separate pedagogy from andragogy, and it was this separation that apparently led to the popularization of the American version after 1970 (Henschke 2011).

Interestingly, while andragogy as we know it has been most widely associated with higher education, Knowles created his definition of andragogy and first applied it in leadership training with the Girl Scouts. It would not be until a little later that he would also employ its principles in his undergraduate courses at Boston University, where he held a faculty position. His approach was group and self-directed learning (SDL), in keeping with his ideas that

experiences and exploring these experiences were important for adult learning (Henschke 2011).

Knowles continued to refine and evolve his theory throughout his career, as he worked hard to create his ultimate goal of putting forth a viable unifying theory of adult education. One of his first steps in this process was to change from the literal definition of andragogy to one that was more palatable and descriptive, thus he ultimately defined andragogy as "the art and science of helping adults learn" (Knowles 1988, p. 43). Whether intentionally or not, this is certainly a much more inclusive definition, and it provides a far more education-focused slant than the original, literal definition.

Andragogy and the man himself quickly became the study of graduate students and other education scholars – just a few years after his original premise was published, he became the subject of research himself and was referred to as a "field builder" by Henschke in 1973, the first known dissertation on the topic (Henschke 2011). Though Knowles was faculty through the late 1970s, he cast a wide net for applying his adult education theory. By 1973, he had pivoted to applying his theory to human resources development (HRD), signaling his recognition that adult learning took place in a variety of industries outside of education (Henschke 2011). It was in HRD that he would do much of his work and later action research.

In 1975, just a few years before he retired from academia, Knowles published his first guide on SDL, a hallmark of andragogy. This is the first instance where he refers to pedagogical as teacher-directed and andragogical as self-directed, a differentiation that is often lost in modern applications of andragogy. It was here that he also presented andragogy as more than a theory; he refers to it also as a philosophy – another step on his way to creating a unifying theory of adult education. In this guide, he argues that SDL is *how* the philosophy is implemented, while andragogy itself remains the overarching theory of learning. Because SDL was the action portion, he initially proposed nine competencies of SDL in his text, *Self-Directed Learning*, originally published in 1975 (paraphrased):

1) An understanding of the differences in assumptions about learners and the skills required for learning under teacher- and self-directed learning, and being able to explain these differences to others.
2) A concept of self as a nondependent and self-directing person.
3) Being able to relate to peers collaboratively and to view them as resources for diagnosing needs, planning learning, and learning; and both giving help to and receiving help from them.

4) Realistically diagnosing individual learning needs with help from teachers and peers.

5) Being able to translate learning needs into learning objectives in a manner that makes accomplishments assessable.

6) Being able to relate to teachers as facilitators and taking the initiative to make use of their resources.

7) Being able to identify human and material resources needed to achieve different types of learning objectives.

8) Being able to select effective strategies for using learning resources, taking the initiative to do so, and using such strategies skillfully.

9) Being able to collect and validate evidence demonstrating achievement of various types of learning objectives.

You can see here that Knowles did not include the idea that adults needed a reason to learn something – a reason that makes sense to them – in this original outline of SDL; this was not incorporated until 15 years or so after he first began the US's andragogy movement. However, with current knowledge of the neuroscience of learning's contributions to learning theory, this appears to be one of his most important – and potentially overlooked – additions to the theory.

It is highly likely that all adult – and probably even young and teenaged – students have experienced those moments in the classroom where the question of "how is this information relevant to me?" has popped up (perhaps more than once). Lack of understanding the "why" often leads to frustration and lack of motivation to learn the material, which then leads to a lot of wasted effort on the instructor's part when delivering information that students question the applicability of. These instances are also lost opportunities to engage students with content that *is* truly relevant, because students are busy worrying about other information they know is applicable. As a result, this sixth assumption, added by Knowles in 1995 during his later career (Henschke 2011), seems to be an imperative for adult educators – children will often accept that what you tell them is important because you are viewed as an authority figure. Adults, on the other hand, have learned to question your authority to varying extents – which means there must be a reason other than "because I'm your teacher" to encourage and motivate them to learn.

We see a softening of Knowles's stance on the rigid separation between pedagogy and andragogy in later versions of his text, *The Modern Practice of Adult Education: From Pedagogy to Andragogy, Revised and Updated* (1988). In Chapter 4 we see this clearly when he states:

> Originally I defined andragogy as the art and science of helping adults learn, in contrast to pedagogy as the art and science of teaching children. Then an increasing number of teachers in elementary and secondary schools (and a few in colleges) began reporting to me that they were experimenting with applying the concepts of andragogy to the education of youth and finding that in certain situations they were producing superior learning. So I am at the point now of seeing that andragogy is simply another model of assumptions about learners to be used alongside the pedagogical model of assumptions, thereby providing two alternative models for testing out the assumptions as to their "fit" with particular situations. *Furthermore, the models are probably most useful when seen not as dichotomous but rather as two ends of a spectrum, with a realistic assumption in a given situation falling in between the two ends* (p. 43; emphasis this author's).

He also stated, however, that diehard pedagogues are committed to keeping their students dependent upon them because this is where they feel most rewarded in their efforts – meaning, those who teach with pedagogical techniques get a teaching "buzz" from knowing their students are dependent upon them for learning (Knowles 1988). This is a whole other topic of discussion, but hopefully it does lead you to reflect on why *you* like to teach; understanding your motivations will contribute significantly to your understanding of the types of approaches you choose to deliver your content, the teaching and learning theories that personally resonate with you, and the underlying philosophy(ies) of education that define your overall educational approaches.

If you recall, Knowles published his original guide to SDL in 1975; in 1991 he published a document outlining updates he made to the skills of the self-directed learner and shared his vision of the competencies needed to perform life roles; all within the context of his goal of facilitating lifelong learning. Although the original writing is no longer accessible online, Henschke (2011) reports that Knowles identified life roles for adults, including "learner, being a unique person, friend, citizen, family member, worker, and leisure-time user" (n.p.) and eight skills of the self-directed learner (paraphrased below) for adults to be lifelong learners. The ability to:

1) Think divergently.

2) Objectively reflect on oneself and take feedback positively.

3) Understand one's learning needs within the context of the competencies required to perform life roles.

4) Create learning objectives that describe performance outcomes.

5) Identify appropriate resources needed to accomplish various types of learning objectives.

6) Design and use a plan of strategies that appropriately and effectively uses learning resources.
7) Successfully carry out a learning plan, which is indicative of being able to think convergently.
8) Document evidence that learning objectives have been met and validate evidence through performance.

In this same document, Knowles also presented his views of how SDL might operate in the twenty-first century – certainly a prescient discussion given the huge boom in virtual learning that occurred not long after his death; a boom that enabled millions more adults to access formal and informal education. It is in the same year that Peters and Jarvis – Jarvis being one of the vocal earlier detractors, as you will see later in the chapter – pay homage to Knowles's work by calling him "one of the best-known and most respected adult educators of all time" (Henschke 2011, n.p.) Malcolm S. Knowles died in 1997, before he was able to see how his almost 30 years of work would play out in the twenty-first century. An idea that started as a theory that spawned an entire discipline, andragogy appears to be here to stay. And no matter who else comes along, Knowles will likely continue to be viewed as the single biggest influence in the creation, evolution, and sustainment of this discipline – at least in the United States.

Andragogy, as with any theory – especially one that looks to be a unifying theory – continued to evolve through the early aughts and is still evolving today, even though its tour de force is no longer with us. We see Knowles' profound and continuing influence in direct and indirect ways. Take, for example, a concept such as contract learning, where students and instructors create a contract outlining the goals and benchmarks for learning that arise from an agreement between the teacher and the students. Student participation in the process is imperative in this alternative approach to learning because it provides students an opportunity to have a say in both what is learned and how their learning will ultimately be assessed, providing buy-in from the student and, theoretically, contributing to motivation. This is clearly an offshoot of the andragogy movement, stemming from the idea that adult learners are self-directed and, as such, their outcomes should be measured differently. Other versions of contract learning have since been developed, so if and when you come across them, know that they, too, have roots in Knowles' theory.

Section 5: Challenges to Andragogy

Knowles' contemporaries lost no time in jumping on the andragogy bandwagon in the early 1970s, with Furter proposing that universities formally recognize the field of andragogy in 1971, the first guide to using andragogy by Ingalls coming out in the same year after it was developed and tested by the US government, and Knowles recognizing the growing interest in andragogy by industry in 1972, when he also first suggested that it applied to any form of adult learning (Henschke 2011). Andragogy and its supporters continued to grow and expand through the mid-1980s before receiving any real pushback, but inevitably, the pushback did come. The following sections are based on Henschke's (2011) comprehensive review of Knowles's work unless noted otherwise.

Among the many detractors, some more strongly dissented than others, with some criticisms aimed at Knowles's lofty ambition of providing a unified adult learning theory and others working to erase the term – and thus the theory – altogether. On the more moderate side, for example, Allman (1983) proposed that a more comprehensive theory of andragogy could be created if the concept of neuroplasticity and her ideas of group learning were combined with both Knowles's current theory of andragogy and Mezirow's (1981) reframing of Habermas's critical theory as an adult learning theory comprised of three generic domains: work, practical, and emancipatory.

On the more extreme dissenting side, Hartree and Jarvis would come forward as the two biggest detractors, using arguments that were viewed as legitimate within the academy. In light of Knowles's desire to make andragogy a viable comprehensive learning theory for adult education, Hartree argued that he had failed to establish andragogy as a true learning theory because it lacked a coherent discussion of the different dimensions of learning. It also fell short philosophically, she said, because it failed to incorporate an epistemology, demonstrating a lack of insight into how Knowles viewed learning about learning.

Jarvis added to Hartree's concerns in the 1980s with one less convincing reason and one very convincing reason. Arguing that andragogy was explicitly tied to romanticism and this movement was fading, Jarvis posited that the theory was losing its appeal. However, he also pointed out that there was little to no empirical support for the theory, which was a much stronger criticism and one that should generally be well-heeded.

Although retired from academia by the time these criticisms were levied, Knowles responded by publishing the third edition of his original book, *The Adult Learner*, focused on HRD. He additionally published a book of case examples of andragogy in action, discussing what worked and what did not. The cases covered a large group of settings where adult learners existed, although none were specified as research studies, nor were any peer-reviewed, leaving only anecdotal evidence from the originator of the US version of andragogy to rely on.

Others in the US were also beginning to question the theoretical soundness of Knowles's ideas. Brookfield cautioned that the theory was unproven so one should avoid believing that it accurately represented the unique characteristics of adult education practice. Davenport jumped into the fray by stating that rather than clarity, the term andragogy was increasing confusion due to assumptions that lacked clarity and solid empirical support; he went so far as to say that many adult educators of the time felt it would be better to drop the term altogether. And Pratt, an early supporter of andragogy, grew less so over time. On a philosophical level, it appeared to Pratt that there was tension between freedom and authority, human agency, and social structures presented in the theory – creating a roadblock to Knowles' original conception of andragogy. He asked, if teaching learner independence leads to freedom, how does authority come into play? If one is learning independence to perform social tasks, then how do those social structures affect the agency of the learner? These tensions are interesting and are certainly worth reflecting upon and exploring.

Through it all, Knowles continued to fight for and refine his theory, and we see that his efforts have not gone unrewarded. Even today, his name continues to be almost synonymous with the term he co-opted and spent most of his career committed to refining and working to disseminate. While those in academia may have been split about the theoretical and philosophical aspects of andragogy, those in the business sector more willingly supported it, especially those in the HR fields. This is evidenced by Nadler's 1989 comment that "every HRD practitioner should have an understanding of the theories of Adult Learning" (Henschke 2011, n.p.).

Given the lack of empirical evidence and the enduring criticisms regarding a lack of epistemological stance and inclusion of other potential pieces of the theory, why has andragogy as an approach, or theory, or philosophy (depending on your own views) persisted in the US? Long (1991, as cited in Henschke 2011) suspected there were five reasons for its survival:

1) The appeal of its underlying humanistic ideals to adult educators in general.
2) The research refuting andragogy is weak in its evidence.
3) Knowles's flexibility in reacting to his critics, allowing him to incorporate criticisms levied at him into his revised versions of the theory.
4) A high level of respect and renown within the field for other contributions.
5) The inclusion of Knowles's andragogy into the adult education knowledge base provided a framework for integrating several potentially useful ideas, one of which is the concept of SDL.

Other benefits of this poorly supported learning theory, from this author's perspective, include its recognition and inquiry into some potential differences between teaching adults and teaching children, which had not explicitly been previously addressed. With such recognition and the opening of inquiry into this possibility, educators were provided a guide for engaging adult learners that, at the time of the theory's publication, was very different in its approach from how children were taught.

Another benefit was, and still is, its wide applicability. Knowles believed it would work as well in industry and business as it did in the more formal classroom, and he went to great lengths to demonstrate this. Lastly, it gave those focused on adult education a new field of inquiry and scholarship, as well as gave rise to degree-granting adult education programs, which have expanded greatly over the last few decades. While there is nothing to empirically support the next statement, it seems like a logical conclusion: the creation of a new field of inquiry and new degree-granting programs in the area were likely to have not happened unless someone had proposed this theory. And there does appear to be need for specializing in teaching adults that just was not recognized prior to Knowles's untiring efforts to work toward his unifying theory of adult education.

As with any new idea, discovery, or wide-ranging thought, andragogy had many supporters and detractors. As with any negative reaction, some is smoke and some is legitimate. The primary concern swirled – and to some extent continues to swirl – around the lack of empirical evidence supporting the theory. As we gain a small understanding of the neuroscience of learning, this concern carries a little less weight, but at least in the empirical education literature, there still is not a whole lot of evidence supporting it – and there is still a whole lot of controversy.

Section 6: Support of Andragogy

Although Knowles was inspired to build his theory of andragogy because of advances being made in the study of adult learning specifically, scientific support of his initial core assumptions about adult learners (recall that these included SDL, prior experience, learning readiness, and need for immediate application) has come from an area less traditionally connected to education: neuroscience. Recent advances in neuroimaging and other modalities have helped illuminate what happens during learning itself, and studies using such technology are beginning to shed light (both literally and figuratively!) on the science of learning through watching the brain in action.

As a result of such research, we have found that, contrary to a long-held belief, brains are constantly changing in response to stimuli. Some brain changes are temporary, and some are permanent – but these changes are occurring *throughout life*. This means that our brain plasticity, aka neuroplasticity, is not, as was once thought, limited to the childhood years. Rather, we are capable of continuous learning and in doing so, we change the neural landscapes of our brains (Cozolino and Sprokay 2006; Jensen and McConchie 2020).

While this seems somewhat intuitive now – we all clearly continue to learn throughout life, although mostly outside of formal learning institutions – it should be easy to see why this was such a breakthrough at the time. We often fail to think about learning outside the formal institution, in spite of the fact that well over 90% of our learning during life actually occurs outside the walls of a schoolhouse or university.

With the awareness that neuroplasticity continues throughout life, you may be wondering how you can prime and/or enhance it in your students (and maybe even yourself) – no matter their (or your) age. A three-step process has been suggested that has the potential to help improve neuroplasticity in students – aka, growing new neural networks and increasing the capacity for such growth, which generally results in deeper, more meaningful learning. These steps, taken from Jensen's and McConchie's 2020 *Brain-Based Learning: Teaching The Way Students Really Learn, Third Edition,* are outlined and summarized below, with additional references incorporated as appropriate.

Readiness is the structural framework for enhancing students' neuroplasticity. It involves ensuring students are emotionally and psychologically ready to learn new information through adding, modifying, or priming the brain to create new neural networks. To do this, you must first understand how much students already know about the content to be delivered. Clearly, the more students already know, the faster they can learn more about the topic. However, it is important to determine what they know correctly versus what they think they know, which means finding out what their misconceptions are is an important part of building this structural framework.

Some ways to figure out what students already know or have misconceptions about include using ungraded pre-tests, engaging in a classroom discussion, and/or having students work in small groups to list or write out what they have learned. This serves a couple of purposes: first, it provides pre-exposure to the information to come and primes the students for learning the material. Second, it provides a foundation for the material to be delivered and projects for the students the content for the day. Finally, it provides the instructor an opportunity to connect the information to be delivered with real-world problems, situations, cases, and the like. In other words, it provides behavioral relevance for the students.

It should be jumping off the page at you that this stage of brain-based learning (often used interchangeably with neuroscience of learning) is fully consistent with at least two of the four basic premises Knowles put forth in andragogy: prior experience and learning readiness. One could argue that it might also incorporate a third premise of his, which is the need for immediate application. You might also be investigating the book being referenced here and realize that it was written primarily for K-12 educators; yet another example of Knowles's prescience when he brought up the continuum of learning theory from pedagogy to andragogy (1980), something he appeared somewhat reluctant to admit but did fully embrace once it was apparent.

The next step in teaching students to enhance their neuroplasticity is to provide **coherent construction**. It is here that you must organize the learning into appropriately sized pieces, or "chunks," of information so students can absorb it. Based on your understanding of their prior learning and current misconceptions, such chunks should be modified to fit the depth of their prior knowledge. Bigger chunks of information (and bigger can mean more detailed or more) can be delivered when students know more, and smaller chunks when there is less. During this stage, it is important to address biases – both your students' and your own. Important note: biases are not necessarily just those we consider within the context of diversity, equity, and inclusion as we know it today, but also those we often completely forget about, such as being a large animal practitioner and not remembering that some students have never seen – much less touched – a pig, cow, chicken, or other production or farm animal. And vice versa, of course – small animal folks might forget that some students have never handled a cat or are afraid of dogs.

Returning to the purposes of this step, however, this is the place where *content delivery* is the focus. Not only the act of content delivery, but the physical aspects of it. Through using multimodal and multisensory instruction, students are provided more opportunities to learn in a way that supports neuroplasticity and increases their ability to recognize and retain the "important stuff." Research tells us that about 80% of sensory inputs are visual, so use of videos, photos, illustrations, and the like increases the likelihood that students will not only pay attention, but also learn better (Jensen and McConchie 2020). Sound is also an important instructional tool – it has been found that the effect size of classroom discussion is 0.82, for example, and that the sense of touch can be impactful when it comes to the temperature of the learning environment, which should ideally be between 68 and 73 °F (Jensen and McConchie 2020).

The physicality of learning and the learning process also aligns with the impact that being physically active outside the classroom has. Most of us are probably keenly aware that being physically fit can improve cognition, but just being physically active alters brain chemistry and the adult brain's responsiveness to learning (Ratey and Loehr 2011). And research clearly demonstrates that physical exercise is associated with better performance on IQ tests in young adults; better task performance, planning, scheduling, inhibition, and working memory; improved information processing and decision-making; better processing speeds and mental flexibility; and increased hippocampal volume in the elderly (Ratey and Loehr 2011).

What might be novel, and potentially surprising, is that neuroscience supports that in-person and active learning may be more important for adults than for children. Why? Well, according to Merriam (2008), physical responses to sensory data are recorded by the brain as experience, and therefore, able to be accessed and reconstructed as memory. In other words, without experience, our brains have no basis for constructing meaning (Merriam 2008). Additionally, neuroscience supports that learning is strengthened through the use of multimodal teaching approaches incorporating experiences that appeal to emotions, the senses, and provide kinesthetic engagement (Merriam 2008).

It is important in this step to remember that optimal learning is achieved during a moderate state of arousal, what some might call a state of "safe emergency" – in other words, a state of high attention without an accompanying, debilitating anxiety. Students pushed into a learning environment they perceive to be unsafe or too stressful can shut down. Fear and anxiety can literally physically inhibit a student's ability to talk, something we may have seen first-hand and not fully appreciated or realized when it was occurring. Upon reflection, however, it makes sense, and it aligns with how we are neurally wired. It is obvious to us, for example, that our brains are wired to respond to urgent needs first – hence the reason someone who is hungry, tired, or *feeling unsafe* generally performs less well than those without those immediate concerns.

For students who are well-fed and well-rested (among other things) in a classroom that is designed to challenge and stretch them without pushing them outside their state of safe emergency, the brain is going to similarly prioritize. Thus, those concepts or ideas that appear to be most urgent or important are going to be dealt with first; the rest will be stored, fairly imperfectly as it so happens, to be revisited when the opportunity arises.

When this revisitation of content occurs, the brain sifts through information to determine what needs to be retained with the intent to protect itself from information overload. Those items that are deemed high enough priority to be retained will be shifted to long-term memory while the rest will drift away over varying degrees of time. How the brain determines the information to be transferred to that long-term memory is generally related to how well the information ties to their experience and allows them to expand on their existing knowledge (well aligned with the concept of *scaffolding*, which you read about in an earlier chapter).

This step in supporting and nurturing neuroplasticity can best be summed up by the observation that learning is currently viewed as involving the body, emotions, spirit, and mind (Jensen and McConchie 2020) – which certainly harkens back to Kapp's first use of the term andragogy and supports the original four premises of Knowles. Keeping in mind, of course, that these findings are not exclusive to adults alone.

Consolidation is the accuracy and transferability of learning. This is where the student is creating the pathways for moving information from short- to long-term memory. It involves three principles: *correct conclusions, spaced learning,* and *relevant transfer.* Each is discussed in more depth below.

Correct conclusions mean that students receive immediate, formative feedback during the learning process. However, they are also strongly encouraged to practice *retrieving* the information *without the use of aids* intermittently outside of the classroom. In other words, old-fashioned flashcards (which can now be created in the electronic ether), oral questioning in peer groups, and fill-in-the-blank (FITB) type questions are most useful for consolidating of learning.

Another aspect of helping students come to correct conclusions is that they should be *unexpectedly challenged* with the new information. While the student may leave the classroom and be willing/able to work on their learning through retrieval practice, educators have a responsibility to provide opportunities in the classroom to aid in that retrieval practice. Pop quizzes – which can be either very low or no stakes – along with "clicker" questions or some other form of in-class, anonymous questioning system that requires retrieval rather than recognition (i.e., FITB or flashcard questions rather than multiple choice questions) is incredibly helpful in this stage – to both consolidate learning and enhance neuroplasticity.

One last note on the correct conclusions part of consolidation: likely unsurprisingly, this aspect of consolidation is especially impacted by poor sleep. Students who are tired (and stressed or hungry or. . .) are going to struggle more than those who are well-rested, less stressed, and satiated. While this is not surprising to anyone reading this text, and is not likely to be surprising to students, either, it is still important to note. Sometimes seeing such common-sense things in black and white can really help drive home its meaning. It also clearly ties back to the earlier parts of this chapter that highlight the idea that learning is a physical, mental, and emotional process.

Spaced learning helps with consolidation of learning through *chunking and revisiting*. While this may seem the same as the correct conclusions piece covered just previously, it is slightly different in that this refers to creating "chunks" of information that the student can then revisit as larger pieces. For example, in the correct conclusions part of learning, students might be focused on new vocabulary (caudal, cranial, proximal, distal, origin, and insertion), specific details (tendons connect muscles to bones, ligaments connect bones to bones, superficial digital flexor muscle, and common calcanean tendon), and/or individual concepts (flexion means to contract and extension means to relax).

In the spaced learning part of learning, students should be focused on connecting the individual pieces of knowledge into bigger, conceptual *chunks*. Here, for example, the learning should be evolving into something similar to: *the common calcanean tendon, which is made up of tendons from several muscles, extends distally from the gastrocnemius to where it inserts on the calcaneus. This is an anatomical feature of the hindlimb of the dog.* You can see here that such a student has moved from knowledge and recall of bits and pieces to connecting those bits and pieces into relevant and larger chunks; this allows the brain to process the information contextually and in a way that no longer requires recall of many pieces, but rather a single piece that can then be identified more quickly and easily. This is not only a step in the process of consolidating learning, but is also a recognized evolution in the movement from novice to expert.

The final step in consolidation is the *relevant transfer* of the acquired information. This step also overlaps a bit with the step before it – this time as it demonstrates the student connecting the dots (viewed as chunking in the previous step) – but expanding beyond the boundaries of the specific content area. Here is where students are connecting hindlimb anatomy to radiographic images, normal and abnormal neural processes, and the like. It is also where students should be trying different bias filters and finding new areas that tie into the new learning. A good example for this might be a student who has seen hindlimb lameness primarily in horses, so how is that affecting their understanding of hindlimb lameness in other species, such as cats, dogs, or cows? It is here that students can truly solidify their learning through demonstration of how well they are able to transfer learning from a familiar setting to an unfamiliar setting. In the previous example, this would be a student successfully using what they know about horse lameness (familiar) to apply appropriate diagnostics to a lame cat (unfamiliar).

The connections between training for neuroplasticity and Knowles's original four premises of andragogy are pretty clear: true learning is not just a passive transfer of information from one human to another. Rather, it is an entire experience; one that encompasses all aspects of the student – mental, emotional, and physical. This experiential aspect of learning is imperative for adult learners because it gives them context and something to build upon; it also recognizes that they have something to bring to the table – sometimes accurate and sometimes inaccurate. Regardless, however, there is legitimization of the experience when it is related to the learning that is being nurtured in the classroom or laboratory.

Section 7: Applications to the Veterinary Classroom

Knowles was perhaps the most outspoken about andragogy and the differences between children and adult learners, but others have supported several of his original premises over the decades as well, including the idea that adults generally do better when concepts and principles tie to their experience and allow them to expand existing knowledge (Cozolino and Sprokay 2006; Taylor 2006; Jensen and McConchie 2020). Additionally, some of the neuroscience of learning findings go back to Kapp's ideas that talking with adults is preferable to them receiving information via text. As Cozolino and Sprokay (2006) point out, "brains grow best in [the] context of interactive discovery and through cocreation [sic] of stories that shape and support memories of what is being learned" (p. 11). They go on to point out that in light of these findings, classroom discourse is important to learning because narratives constructed in dialogue support memory function. Such discourse also provides guidance to students for future behavior through introduction to context and the provision of relevance of the information being delivered, both of which support and enhance learning (Cozolino and Sprokay 2006).

With this in mind, it is likely good to be reminded that setting high expectations and encouraging help-seeking behaviors is excellent teaching practice regardless of the age of the learner – but especially so in professional program classrooms. Many students attending veterinary school, as with other professional programs, are extremely high-achieving and goal-oriented. They have spent their entire young lives earning high grades and doing the activities that are important to gain admittance to the school of their choice, often from undergraduate, or even high school, on. It is inevitable, then, that many students who get into professional programs find themselves in very unfamiliar territory – earning Bs, Cs, and even, occasionally, Ds and Fs. For those who have never experienced a B, let alone being below the average or failing, the impact can be devastating.

One way to help counteract this is to nurture neuroplasticity, as just discussed. Another extremely important one is to set high – but achievable – expectations. There is a large body of work supporting that teacher expectations can impact student learning either positively or negatively, which started in the late 1960s with Rosenthal and Jacob's article titled "Pygmalion in the classroom" (1968). Rosenthal partnered with Rubin (1971) a few years later in reaffirming his original findings (in a firm rebuttal to criticism levied at his original study) that teachers who expressed high or low student expectations were generally rewarded with student successes or failures aligned with such expectations, and a number of subsequent studies supported these findings (Feldman and Prohaska 1979). Rosenthal's (1968, 1971) research went beyond achievement, demonstrating empirical support for his premise that teacher expectations could potentially alter student achievement and actual measurable intellectual ability (i.e., IQ score).

Although there is now research calling the true and lasting effects of teacher expectations on student IQ, (Jussim and Harber 2005), there is little evidence to support that the Rosenthal (aka Pygmalion) effect does not impact student achievement, particularly in the short term. It is probably important to point out here that there is also a robust body of research supporting that high-quality and effective teaching has one of the biggest effect sizes when evaluating learner achievement (Wright et al. 1997). Within the context of supporting neuroplasticity, it is important to also remember that not only is this good, evidence-based teaching practice, it is also contributing to you being as effective and high quality in your teaching as possible, which is another intentional way that you can support student learning!

It is also important – especially for our veterinary/professional program students – to both model and encourage help-seeking behaviors. This includes admitting you when you don't have the answer to a question, asking questions regularly, and telling stories of times when you had to seek help to answer questions or solve a problem. Modeling this behavior undermines the often-held belief that asking questions makes one appear stupid and demonstrates to students that even the most expert among us cannot possibly know the answer to every question. Especially for those students who are experiencing academic challenges for the first time, it is imperative to encourage help-seeking behaviors. Research has shown that adaptive help-seeking behavior (i.e., realization by the student of the need for help and finding resources that provide such support) is positively correlated with higher achievement (Fong et al. 2023), which is likely not surprising. What is also likely not surprising is that lower-performing students are often the least likely to seek help; thus the importance of modeling such behaviors and creating a culture that normalizes adaptive help-seeking so that lower-achieving students view this as valuable rather than shaming.

Summary

Pedagogy and andragogy are a continuum that informs teaching practices. Widely viewed as highly teacher-centered, "sage on the stage," pedagogy has been challenged by andragogy, which has leaned more toward learner-centered, "guide on the side" approaches. Pedagogy and its attendant theories were rooted in somewhat crude observational studies, but such studies and the learning theories they spurred have helped evolve teaching practices for children over the years.

Andragogy got its start in either the ancient times of Jesus Christ or a bit more recently in the 1700–1800s, depending on who you choose to believe. What is agreed upon, however, is that Alexander Kapp was the first to coin the term andragogy in the early 1800s and, from there, it would flourish and languish until Malcolm Knowles resurrected it for good in the United States in the latter half of the twentieth century. As the first to declare andragogy separate from pedagogy, Knowles stirred much debate for decades, with prominent scholars on both sides. Ultimately, this has been generally resolved as Knowles acknowledged in 1980 that perhaps the demarcation was not necessary, noting that many teachers were discovering his premises of learning for adults were finding success when applied to children, as well.

Ultimately, emerging neuroscience of learning studies do support several of Knowles's assertions, including that learning is a multifocal process that relies on the physical, social, experiential, and applicability of information being learned. As such, a multimodal, active approach to teaching is desirable, especially given that neuroscience also seems to indicate that adults require as much or more social interaction for learning than do children.

The idea that neuroplasticity is not limited to children and can be nurtured and supported throughout the lifespan means that it can and should be supported in the classroom – starting with young children and continuing through the entire educational experience. Such insights into the brain and the way it learns might lead us to view both Kapp and Knowles as prescient educators who were way ahead of their times, and while this is certainly partially true, it is also important to remember that Knowles specifically backtracked in his firm demarcation between pedagogy and andragogy. His evolution in thought did not negate the idea that we need to pay attention to differences in how children and adults learn, but rather added in the previously lacking acceptance that what is good for adults is often also good for children and vice versa.

Finally, it is important to understand that Knowles's impact is not any less now that he has formally recognized that teaching children and adults is more of a continuum than it is a hard break. His insistence on the value of incorporating the learner's experiences and emphasis on SDL

has been well-supported by recent research in the neuroscience of learning, and there continues to be support for his idea that adults need social interaction to most effectively learn as well. While it is true that younger learners also benefit from some of these teaching practices, one has to wonder if this would have come to light as quickly if Knowles had not made the bold statement he did. Regardless, the implications for the professional school classroom remain the same: incorporating multimodal teaching approaches, setting and maintaining high expectations, making learning relevant, and bringing in students' prior experiences remain high-quality teaching practices that result in high-quality learning.

References

Allman, P. (1983). The nature and process of adult development. In: *Education for Adults: Adult Learning and Education*, vol. 1, chapter 2.5 (ed. M. Tight), 107–123. London: Croom Helm & the Open University.

Cozolino, L. and Sprokay, S. (2006). Neuroscience and adult learning. In: *New Directions for Adult and Continuing Education, no. 110*, 11–19. Wiley InterScience.

Draper, J.A. (1998). The metamorphoses of *andragogy. Cjsac/RCEEA* 12 (1): 3–26.

Etymology (n.d.). Online etymology dictionary. https://www.etymonline.com/search?q=pedagogy&utm_campaign=sd&utm_medium=serp&utm_source=ds_search (accessed September 2022).

Feldman, R.S. and Prohaska, T. (1979). The student as Pygmalion: effect of student expectation on the teacher. *Journal of Educational Psychology* 71 (4): 485–493.

Fong, C.J., Gonzales, C., Hill-Troglin Cox, C., and Shinn, H.B. (2023). Academic help-seeking and achievement of postsecondary students: a meta-analytic investigation. *Journal of Educational Psychology* 115 (1): 1–21. https://doi.org/10.1037/edu0000725.

Henschke, J.A. (2009). *Beginnings of the History and Philosophy of Andragogy 1833–2000. IACE Hall of Fame Repository.*

Henschke, J.A. (2011). Considerations regarding the future of andragogy. *Adult Learning,* 22(1): 34-37. https://doi.org/10.1177/104515951102200109

Holmes, G. and Abington-Cooper, M. (2000). Pedagogy vs. andragogy: a false dichotomy? *The Journal of Technology Studies* 26 (2): 50–55.

Jensen, E. and McConchie, L. (2020). *Brain-Based Learning: Teaching the Way Students Really Learn*, 3e. Thousand Oaks, CA: Corwin Press.

Jussim, L. and Harber, K.D. (2005). Teacher expectations and self-fulfilling prophecies: knowns and unknowns, resolved and unresolved controversies. *Personality and Social Psychology Review* 9 (2): 131–155.

Knowles, M.S. (1975). *Self-Directed Learning*. Chicago, IL: Associated Press.

Knowles, M.S. (1988). The modern practice of adult education: from pedagogy to andragogy. Revised and updated. *Cambridge Adult Education* 40–59. https://pdfs.semanticscholar.org/8948/296248bbf58415cbd21b36a3e4b37b9c08b1.pdf.

Loeng, S. (2017). Alexander Kapp – the first known user of the andragogy concept. *International Journal of Lifelong Education* 36 (6): 629–643. https://doi.org/10.1080/02601370.2017.1363826.

Merriam, S.B. (2008). Adult learning theory for the twenty-first century. In: *New Directions for Adult and Continuing Education no. 119*, 93–98. Wiley InterScience.

Mezirow, J. (1981). A critical theory of adult learning and education. *Adult Education* 32 (1): 3–24.

Ratey, J.J. and Loehr, J.E. (2011). The positive impact of physical activity on cognition during adulthood: a review of underlying mechanisms, evidence, and recommendations. *Reviews in the Neurosciences* 22 (2): 171–185.

Rosenthal, R. and Jacobson, L. (1968). Pygmalion in the classroom. *The Urban Review* 3 (1): 16–20.

Rosenthal, R. and Rubin, D.B. (1971). Pygmalion reaffirmed. In: *Pygmalion Reconsidered* (ed. J.D. Elashoff and R.E. Snow), 16–20. Worthington, OH: Jones.

Taylor, K. (2006). Brain function and adult learning: implications for practice. In: *New Directions for Adult and Continuing Education no. 110*, 71–85. Wiley InterScience https://doi.org/10.1002/ace.221.

Wright, S.P., Horn, S.P., and Sanders, W.L. (1997). Teacher and classroom context effects on student achievement: implications for teacher evaluation. *Journal of Personnel Evaluation in Education* 11: 57–67.

Zmeyov, S.I. (1998). Andragogy: origins, developments, and trends. *International Review of Education* 44 (1): 103–108.

5

Understanding the Professional Program Student

Bobbi J. Conner, DVM, DACVECC
Virginia-Maryland College of Veterinary Medicine, Blacksburg, VA, USA

Lawrence Garcia, MS, DVM
University of Florida College of Veterinary Medicine, Gainesville, FL, USA

Matthew Schexnayder, DVM, MS, DACVP
IDEXX Laboratories, Inc., Baton Rouge, LA, USA

Section 1: Introduction and Overview

Bobbi J. Conner

In this chapter, we aim to provide information that will help the reader better understand students in a veterinary professional program. We do this with the knowledge that a book chapter cannot fully capture the essence of an individual, let alone the many thousands of students enrolled in various veterinary schools and colleges throughout the world. We recognize that, as authors, we introduce our own perspectives and biases: we each are veterinary educators working in the United States. As a consequence, this chapter was written through that lens; our colleagues throughout the world may identify significant gaps and divergent perceptions. We encourage veterinary educators to keep in mind the distinct perspectives of each student and to remember that the forthcoming chapter is meant to provide some context and, we hope, a useful starting point for educators to better understand their students with the aim of continually improving veterinary education. We will highlight some specific themes that have been identified, emphasize commonalities that arise, and shed light on areas that have not received much attention. We lament that not all will be represented fully in the coming pages and, as such, strongly encourage educators to do the additional work necessary to gain deeper insight and understanding of their students.

Section 2: Who Are Our Students?

Lawrence Garcia

Part 1: Introduction

Veterinary medical colleges and the graduates they produce are a unique resource as healthcare professionals trained in multispecies comparative medicine (Hoblet et al. 2003). In total, there are currently 30 accredited veterinary medical colleges in the United States, five in Canada, and 14 others around the world that are American Association of Veterinary Medical Colleges (AAVMC) members.

As students apply for admission to these various veterinary medical programs, demographic data is collected by each of the 30 veterinary medical colleges in the United States. The AAVMC then captures this data by way of an annual survey completed by each college, which they then pool, analyze, and publish in an annual report. This data has been collected since 1980, with the demographics captured expanding over the years, and has served as a valuable tool highlighting both successes and areas of opportunity in the veterinary admissions processes, as well as helping to inform veterinary curricula. For example, the data highlights a lack of racial and ethnic diversity in the application pool and the profession as a whole, resulting in efforts focused on how best to recruit underrepresented minorities (URM). The likelihood is that URM applicants may have different resources and support to be successful in pursuit of a career in the field. Furthermore, this information may be used as a stimulus to evaluate and update veterinary curricula in ways that best serve a racially and ethnically diverse pool of applicants.

Overall, veterinary medical applicants bring class cohort and college identity through educational, socioeconomic, experiential, and cultural backgrounds. Veterinary colleges must work to be more inclusive to diversify the field.

Part 2: Motivation and Experience

When considering applicant pool background, it is also important to understand what life and veterinary experiences motivate individuals to pursue a career in the field. In a survey of veterinary students and veterinarians, Ilgen and associates (2003) found that having a pet, other animal experiences, and working with a veterinarian were the three strongest influences on pursuit of Veterinary Medicine as a career. In addition, Ilgen and associates (2003) found that in-depth interpersonal experiences with a veterinarian, living on a farm, interacting with a friend or family member who was a veterinarian, or even a teacher in a course, had a greater influence on selection of Veterinary Medicine than any other form of exposure to the field. This is important, as some individuals may never have exposure to these influences and, therefore, might not even consider the field as an option; although, there are those who do pursue the field without these experiences.

Exposure to and experience in this field can be very helpful in preparing potential applicants for the joys and rigors of the work. This is important when considering the difficulty associated with gaining acceptance into an accredited program, as well as the potential accumulation of significant debt. Furthermore, Ilgen and associates (2003) found that those who identify as female report being attracted to the field through pet ownership, while those who identify as male report being attracted by the status of the field or the rigors of the educational environment. Understanding this information may explain to some degree the gender identity disparities noted in applicant demographic data. We will continue the deep dive into this demographic data to gain a better understanding of the applicant pool.

As previously mentioned, prior animal experiences can be very influential in applicant awareness of, interest in, and pursuit of the profession. Historically there has been variation in the recommendations/requirements for veterinary, animal, and research-related experience for acceptance to veterinary colleges. This variation is likely the result of no available evidence to suggest that a certain amount and kind of previous experience guarantees

successful matriculation through the curriculum and effectiveness as a veterinarian.

The AAVMC data for the class of 2026 revealed that the overall mean and median experiential hours for veterinary, other animal exposure, and research background of applicants to be greater than 3000 hours, greater than 2500 hours, and less than 700 hours respectively (Figure 5.1). Since 2020, the number of experiential hours has significantly decreased as a result of the COVID-19 global pandemic.

The Impacts of the COVID-19 Pandemic

In December of 2019, the first case of COVID-19 (SARS-CoV-2) was identified in Wuhan, China. The virus was highly contagious and characterized by severe acute respiratory symptoms (Saniasiaya et al. 2021). Symptoms tended to be variable but included fever, cough, headache, fatigue, breathing difficulties, and loss of taste and smell (Saniasiaya et al. 2021; Saniasiaya and Kulasegarah 2021; Agyeman et al. 2020). The World Health Organization (WHO) declared a Public Health Emergency of International Concern on 30 January 2020 and a pandemic on 11 March 2020. As of 18 January 2022, there were over 300 million cases and over 5.5 million deaths worldwide, making it one of the deadliest pandemics in history. The pandemic triggered severe social and economic disruptions globally, with widespread supply and food shortages, as well as ongoing supply chain disruptions. The resultant near-global lockdowns caused educational institutions and public areas to be partially or fully closed with many major events canceled. The impacts of COVID-19 caused variability in applicant experience portfolios as well as classroom-based and clinical veterinary students having to convert to majority or completely online instructional delivery. Admissions committees have had to take these circumstances into consideration while evaluating applicant portfolios.

Part 3: Financial Considerations

Individuals applying to veterinary colleges are competing for a limited number of seats and can incur high educational debt loads without proper financial planning prior to and during veterinary school. Starting veterinary college with minimal debt can be very helpful in eliminating debt as a stressor in veterinary candidates upon graduation. Ilgen and associates (2003) hypothesized that the cost of veterinary education would deter applicants, but noted that it did not seem to have an impact. This is fairly striking when studying the high debt-to-income ratios for recent graduates.

There can be various reasons for high debt loads, especially for those attending private and offshore veterinary colleges, which tend to have higher tuition costs when

Figure 5.1 Mean and median experiential hours. *Source:* Reproduced with permission of American Association of Veterinary Medical Colleges (2022).

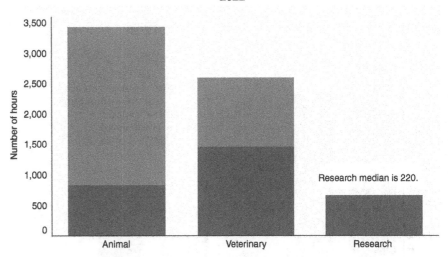

The mean experiential hours shown here should **not** be interpreted as recommendations by prospective applicants. Application requirements regarding experiential hours vary widely across the colleges of veterinary medicine, and applicants may be successful in earning admission with a portfolio of experiences that differ greatly than what is shown here.

This data simply represents the mean number by experience type reported by applicants to the class of 2026.

The total number of applicants to the Class of 2026 was 10,834.

compared to U.S. colleges. Additionally, offshore veterinary students must relocate for their clinical year and pay international tuition. Students are given the opportunity to list their top desired colleges to fill their clinical requirements but often do not get their first choice. In addition, some private and other veterinary colleges in the United States do not have a teaching hospital. In these cases, students generally must relocate frequently to fulfill their clinical requirements. Thus, collecting previous educational debt data on applicants can be helpful in creating resources, pathways, and support for those interested in pursuing the profession.

When surveyed about how they would fund their professional curriculum, approximately 60% of the class of 2024 reported having no prior educational debt, while 40% reported some level of prior debt according to the American Association of Veterinary Medical Colleges 2019–2020 annual data report (retrieved 30 November 2021). The mean level of debt for candidates entering the professional curriculum was approximately US$ 24,000. Figure 5.2 illustrates the sources of professional curriculum funding reported by the class of 2026 with low or no undergraduate debt. This is valuable information and may reveal areas where financial support and resource pathways could be created prior to and during the professional curriculum to support greater diversity and inclusion. According to

Chisolm and associates, educational debt has been known to contribute to significant stress and hardships in the profession (2019); finding ways to provide financial guidance, resources, and support will help to eliminate barriers and minimize the hardships.

Part 4: Applicant Community of Origin

Community of origin (CO) can have a strong impact on candidate development, experience, and interests, and is one of the many factors and influences that contribute to a candidate's decision to pursue veterinary medicine. AAVMC's data divides community types into rural, urban, and suburban (Figure 5.3). CO influences exposure, experiences, and perceptions of the field. In addition, CO likely influences the candidate's inclination toward a practice type and location. It is possible that candidates will return to their home community or desire one similar to that from which they originated, simply based on familiarity; others may prefer a community intentionally different from their home community, as a means of exploring alternate or unfamiliar places. In fact, many factors may influence this choice and it would be interesting to identify such specific influences and how they are prioritized by applicants.

The AAVMC survey of the class of 2026 found that approximately 10–20% of the applicants came from rural

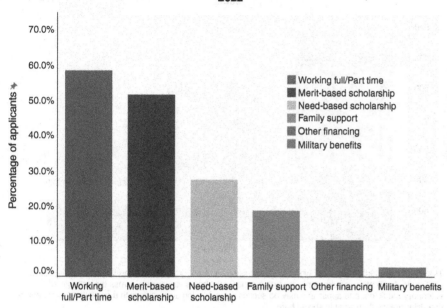

Figure 5.2   Sources of aid. *Source:* Reproduced with permission of American Association of Veterinary Medical Colleges (2022).

Applicants were allowed to select multiple sources of anticipated aid.

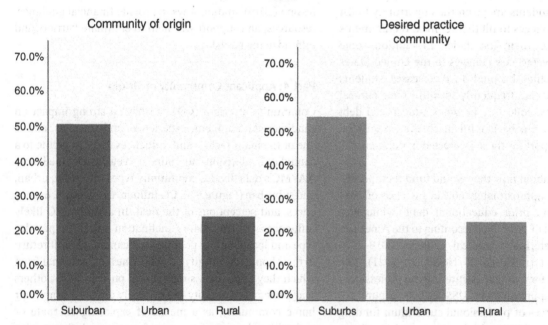

The total number of applicants to the Class of 2026 was 10,834.

Figure 5.3   Community of origin. *Source:* Reproduced with permission of American Association of Veterinary Medical Colleges (2022).

areas, 20–30% from urban areas, and 50% from suburban areas. It is not surprising that suburban and urban are the higher percentages, having higher population densities, when compared to rural areas. Additionally, animal experience opportunities can vary significantly from one community to another, with large animal exposure being available in all three types. In general, large animal opportunities tend to be more common in rural areas, while small animal opportunities can be more common in urban and suburban areas, although large and small animals can be found in all areas. For example, horses used by police, as well as horse and buggy rides, are common in urban areas; likewise, cats, dogs, and other small pets can be found in rural areas. CO is clearly important as it represents influences that may have encouraged this career path, but more research needs to be done here to gain a better understanding of its influence.

During the application process as part of the query about CO, applicants are also asked where they would like to practice. This same group of applicants identified the following as their preferred areas for practice: 20% rural, 10–20% urban, and greater than 60% suburban. In general, urban and suburban areas tend to provide higher salaries and more predictable hours, therefore it is not surprising to note the greater desire to practice in these areas when compared to rural locations. Based on the data, approximately 20% of applicants originate from rural areas and about 20% of applicants desire to practice in a rural area. The data does not differentiate whether those who originated from rural areas are the same as those who desire to return there, although there tends to be anecdotal evidence that with individual variability, there would be some crossover between groups. In the author's experience, many students prefer communities that are familiar, while a smaller cohort seeks an entirely different community experience from their CO. However, most veterinary candidates change their desired career path at least once as they matriculate through the curriculum. More work is needed in this area to determine if this information might provide valuable insights into strategies to better serve areas of need and create awareness and interest in URM communities.

Part 5: Preprofessional Education

Based on unpublished data collected by the University of Florida College of Veterinary Medicine (UFCVM) Office of Admissions, veterinary applicants often have multiple preprofessional degrees. In some cases, it appears to be the result of a career path change during undergraduate studies and the need to meet veterinary prerequisite requirements. For others, demonstrating abilities with a more

difficult course load similar to that of the veterinary curriculum can be quite helpful. Furthermore, additional coursework can be valuable in improving overall grade point average. Unfortunately, the reasoning behind the multiple degrees is not currently captured; it would be interesting to see if having multiple degrees positively influences acceptance and if so, if it also positively influences matriculation and effectiveness in the field. Examples of preprofessional degrees acquired by applicants to the University of Florida College of Veterinary Medicine include Associate of Arts, Associate of Arts and Sciences, Associate of liberal Arts, Associate of Science, Bachelor of Applied Science, Bachelor of Arts, Bachelor of Arts and Science, Bachelor of Engineering, Bachelor of Liberal Arts, Bachelor of Music, Bachelor of Science, Other Bachelor's, Master of Science, Doctor of Science, Master of Arts, Master of Medical Science, Master of Business Administration, and Master of Public Health. This list clearly illustrates a wide variety of preprofessional degrees seen as valuable by those seeking admission and highlights diversity in educational background of the applicant pool. It is also important to note that an Associate's degree alone will not qualify a candidate for acceptance to veterinary school, and therefore is often accompanied by a Bachelor's degree. There is little to no research demonstrating whether educational background diversity contributes significantly to class character and career pathway choice; it would be an interesting topic to study.

Based on unpublished UFCVM demographic data (obtained from and with the permission of the UFCVM Office of Admissions), there is significant variability in percentage of first-generation college applicants, ranging from 10% to 30% in a given year. According to Carr and Greenhill (2015), a first-generation applicant is defined as someone whose parents did not attend or complete a four-year college or university program. It would be interesting to study the cause of this variability, but this too may illustrate some of the diversity in socioeconomic or other background of applicants. The diversity of educational background, regardless of reason, does appear to create a more balanced class dynamic.

Part 6: Application Process

The process of applying to veterinary college has been somewhat streamlined over the years through the Veterinary Medical College Application Service (VMCAS). Through this process applicants submit all personal, academic, and other pertinent information via a single electronic portal. The applicant can then request to distribute their application to multiple veterinary colleges for a fee, some of whom request more specific supplemental information. It is important to note that while the majority of veterinary programs in the United States participate in this VMCAS, there are still a small number who do not, so students wishing to apply to those programs must apply directly to the school or go through a different system.

Although the process can be quite expensive and tedious, it is the standard process for most U.S. veterinary colleges. Due to the limited number of available seats annually, and the highly competitive nature of the field, veterinary applicants may not gain admission on the first attempt. Figure 5.4 illustrates that nearly 80% of the class of 2026 were first time applicants, less than 20% were second time applicants, less than 5% were third time applicants, and less than 2% were fourth or more time applicants. With a majority being first time applicants, it would be interesting to see what percentage of the first-time applicants gain acceptance. This is another area that could benefit from further study, to elaborate on which applicants are likely to reapply until they get in, what steps applicants take if they are not admitted the first time, and common reasons for not being accepted the first time.

Part 7: Class Size Demographic

Increasing class size plays an integral role in producing more veterinarians and provides for growth and development of the programs in veterinary colleges. According to AAVMC data, U.S. veterinary class cohorts have increased at a steady rate of approximately 2% annually over the last 42 years (Figure 5.5). This speaks to the strengths of veterinary programs and their ability to grow. It is not fully clear whether the increasing class size is the result of an increasing number of applicants, a deficiency of veterinarians in the field, or veterinary school funding models. Work in this area has been plagued by inconsistent response rates or tracking of this type of information. Additionally, the factors driving the increase in class size are not well known at this time. From an educational perspective, increased class size means increasing the size of educational spaces and the need for additional faculty and staff to meet student needs. However, it is not certain that the increase in tuition dollars associated with class size increases has matched the increased need for resources. Although the increase in class size could contribute to program growth and advancement, this information is not necessarily captured or studied at a global level.

Increasing veterinary class size has contributed to a substantial increase in the overall number of students enrolled in veterinary programs and increased graduate numbers. Based on data from the AAVMC 2020–2021 academic year, there were approximately 13,000 students enrolled in veterinary medical colleges throughout the United States, a number that is more than double compared to reports from 1980. Factors that might affect enrollment status throughout the curriculum include students leaving voluntarily or involuntarily prior to program completion, the need for a student to be held back and delay graduation, and cases where students might complete graduate work within the rigorous veterinary curriculum. To gain perspective, enrollment data were evaluated and revealed a lack of direct

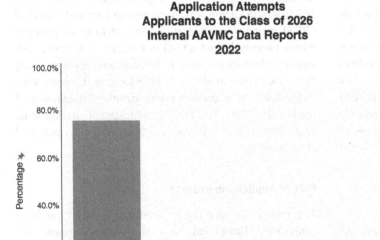

**Application Attempts
Applicants to the Class of 2026
Internal AAVMC Data Reports
2022**

The total number of applicants to the Class of 2026 was 10,834.

Figure 5.4 Application attempts.
Source: Reproduced with permission of American Association of Veterinary Medical Colleges (2022).

Figure 5.5 Total enrollment. *Source:* Reproduced with permission of American Association of Veterinary Medical Colleges (2022).

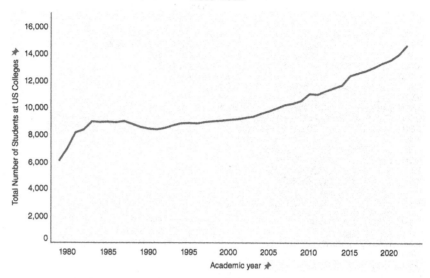

Total Enrollment at U.S. Colleges of Veterinary Medicine
Internal AAVMC Data Reports
1980–2022

On average, seats have increased 2.0% per year since 1980. During the last decade (2011–2022), the number of first year seats at US colleges of veterinary medicine have increased an average of 2.6% per year

Figure 5.6 Matriculation to graduation correlation. *Source:* Reproduced with permission of American Association of Veterinary Medical Colleges (2022).

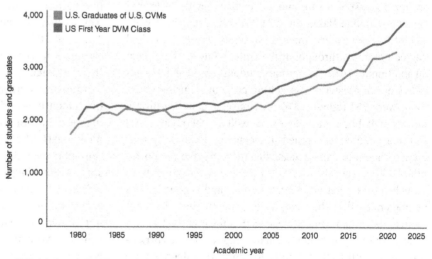

First Year and Graduation Classes
at U.S. Colleges of Veterinary Medicine
Internal AAVMC Data Reports
1980–2022

Although the relationship between first year seats and graduation is expected to be a direct one, there are numerous reasons that explain perceived lags in graduation of DVM students. Numerous dual-degree options allow DVM students to step in and out of the professional curriculum.

correlation between first-year and graduation class sizes (Figure 5.6). Overall, this data demonstrated a perceived lag in graduation times for a proportion of veterinary students, which is one strong reason that there are more students in the curriculum overall and fewer losses due to departure from the program.

Part 8: Professional Dual Degree Programs

Dual degree programs within the veterinary curricula have become increasingly popular, as they help prepare students for additional career pathways. In some cases, students can complete these programs without additional cost (Figure 5.7).

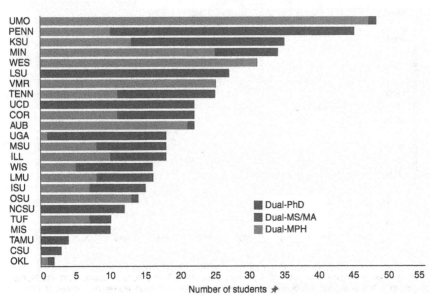

DVM Student Enrolled in Dual Degree Programs by U.S. College of Veterinary Medicine Internal AAVMC Data Reports 2022

Figure 5.7 Dual degree enrollment. *Source:* Reproduced with permission of American Association of Veterinary Medical Colleges (2022).

There are currently 492 DVM students enrolled in dual degree programs in the United States. There are 79 veterinary students also enrolled in MS/MA programs; while there are 254 students who are also earning an MPH program. Finally, 159 veterinary students are also enrolled in PhD programs across the U.S.

These opportunities may help candidates with interests particular to the college, and gain additional training in preparation for, exposure to, and more focus on their desired career discipline. Based on 2022 AAVMC data, there were 492 (4.5%) veterinary medical students enrolled in dual degree programs throughout the United States. There were an additional 79 (0.7%) veterinary students enrolled in Master of Science or Master of Agriculture programs. Furthermore, there were 254 (about 2.3%) veterinary students earning a Master of Public Health degree, as well as 159 (about 1.5%) veterinary students enrolled in Doctor of Philosophy programs. These numbers indicate that there are many opportunities within veterinary medical programs for students to branch out and get additional training and education and demonstrates that the delay in graduation time does not seem to deter applicants. It appears that the many veterinary colleges offering such additional training within the curriculum (e.g., professional certificates and MPH degrees) are valued by veterinary students, even with many programs requiring an early commitment and some also requiring research and course work during lighter course loads or summers so that students can remain on track for graduation.

Part 9: Class Cohort Population Demographic

Multiple studies have illustrated that most veterinary applicants are white (Cannedy 2004; Chubin and Mohamed 2009; Elmore 2003; Lowrie 2009). This highlights the need

to recruit more URM to the field. More research is needed in this area to establish how and when to expose URM populations to and begin recruiting these individuals, as well as helping them create their path to the profession. There should also be pathways to provide support and resources to URM within the curriculum and as they join the workforce.

Admissions processes can and should be more inclusive of all identities and URM. AAVMC aggregate data regarding racial and/or ethnic under representation in veterinary medicine (URVM) does reveal a gradual increase in representation over the years, from approximately 2% to 22% since 1980 (Figure 5.8). While this is good news, it highlights the need to seek out and address the causes of underrepresentation. Examples of URVM groups include, but are not limited to Latinx/Hispanic, Asian, Multi-Racial/Multi-Ethnic, African American/Black, Unknown, Foreign National, American Indian/Native Alaskan, Native Hawaiian/Pacific Islander, or other race.

Admissions data from the University of Florida College of Veterinary Medicine (UFCVM) reveal that anywhere from 11% to 26% of applicants identify as Latin-X/Hispanic, 0.8% to 2% American Indian, 4% to 7% Asian, 2% to 5% Black, 0% to 0.8% Pacific Islander, and 84% to 90% Caucasian, which is consistent with national data showing that overall URVM groups generally represent less than 10% of the veterinary medical student population in the United States. This is an area of ongoing opportunity and

Figure 5.8 Underrepresented minority representation. *Source:* Reproduced with permission of American Association of Veterinary Medical Colleges (2022).

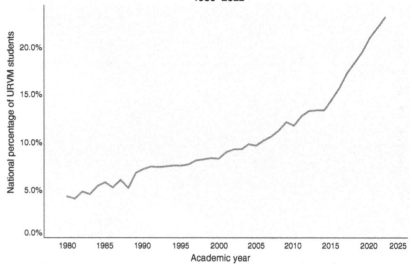

Aggregate Racial/Ethnic URVM Representation at U.S. Colleges of Veterinary Medicine Internal AAVMC Data Reports 1980–2022

URVM: *Underrepresented in Veterinary Medicine.*
In this visualization, URVM is specific to race and ethnicity.

Total DVM student enrollment at the U.S. Colleges of Veterinary Medicine is 14,503.

one of the primary focuses of the Diversity, Equity, and Inclusion (DEI) movement.

When considering disparities in the applicant pool, it is also important to consider gender. The AAVMC gender representation data from 1980 through 2022 illustrated that those individuals identifying as nonbinary represented only 0.1% of the overall veterinary medical student population, although this information has only been collected since 2017. In 1980, demographic data from U.S. veterinary medical colleges revealed that those identifying as female represented approximately 35% of the veterinary medical student population, while currently, those identifying as female represent approximately 85% nationwide (Figure 5.9). While there are certainly many factors that have led to this shift, it would be interesting to study the contributing factors.

Unpublished admissions data (obtained from and with the permission of the UFCVM Office of Admissions) for the UFCVM classes of 2021–2025 revealed the proportion of the female student population to be 73–89%, with an average of 11–25% males. The class of 2022 had the largest proportion of females at 89% and the class of 2023 had the largest proportion of males at 25%. According to Watson (2011), some reasons for this disparity include the result of elimination of discrimination based on gender, improvements in large animal chemical restraint, increased numbers of female role models in the profession, the reluctance of men to enter professions with low or stagnant incomes, loss of autonomy in the profession as corporate practice

predominates, and a trend effect in which the fact that because males no longer predominate, the profession holds less prestige for them.

Inclusivity is very important in our society; self-identified orientation is apparently equally important, as AAVMC found that the in the class of 2024, greater than 80% of applicants identified as female while fewer than 20% identified as male, and fewer than 10% identified as transgender spectrum, gay or lesbian, prefer not to answer, or orientation not listed (Figure 5.10). All veterinary schools should be inclusive of all gender identities. To ensure inclusivity within the application process, it might be helpful to provide the opportunity for applicants to self-identify if they wish to and feel comfortable doing so. This first step is a major one that could help some of the underrepresented groups feel more welcome and likely to apply. Additionally, it would be helpful to determine the ideal time frame in which to expose underrepresented groups to the field to encourage, empower, and create pathways for them to consider pursuit of the profession.

Section 3: Neurodivergence

Matthew Schexnayder

As we continue our discussion of class cohort demographic, we would be remiss if we did not consider neurodivergence. The discussion centered around neurodevelopmental disorders

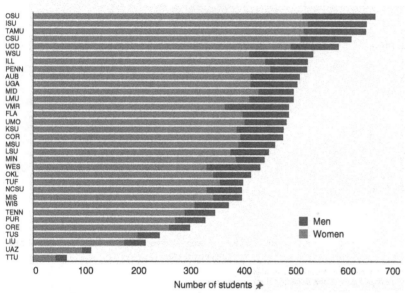

Figure 5.9 Enrollment by gender.
Source: Reproduced with permission of American Association of Veterinary Medical Colleges (2022).

Total DVM student enrollment at the U.S. Colleges of Veterinary Medicine is 14,503.

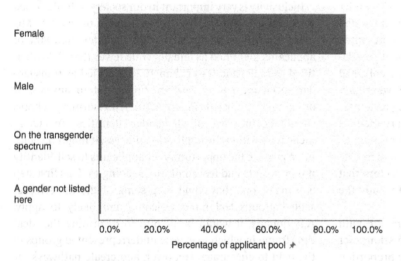

Figure 5.10 Gender identity of applicants.
Source: Reproduced with permission of American Association of Veterinary Medical Colleges (2022).

The total number of applicants to the Class of 2026 was 10,834.

identified by the American Psychiatric Association has witnessed a grassroots humanitarian vernacular shift in recent decades that has grown alongside incidence. The use of "neurodivergent" as an inclusive term generally encompassing Attention-Deficit/Hyperactivity Disorder (ADHD), Autism Spectrum Disorder (ASD), and Specific Learning Disorder (SLD), the latter of which includes dyslexia and

dyscalculia, challenges the traditional paradigm that "different" equates "disorder." Proponents for neurodiversity argue that society can adapt to include individuals with different brain function and behavioral traits, rather than limit their potential by forcing them to fit the neurotypical mold. In concert with primary and secondary schools, institutions of higher education, including veterinary and human medical schools, have begun to recognize their role in meeting the unique needs of neurodivergent students.

The number of students in higher education self-disclosing neurodivergent conditions has increased and overall perceptions have improved (White et al. 2019). While no data has been published regarding American veterinary medical students, survey data collected from participating Association of American Medical Colleges accredited medical schools between the years 2014 and 2016 revealed the two largest categories of self-disclosed disabilities among medical students to be ADHD (33.7%) and "learning disability" (21.5%), the latter of which was not further specified (Meeks and Herzer 2016). A follow-up survey of the same reporting institutions revealed an overall increase in students self-disclosing disabilities, from 2.7% in 2016 to 4.6% in 2019, with absolute increases in each of the previously mentioned categories (Meeks et al. 2019).

The reason for increasing numbers of neurodivergent students is likely multifactorial. For instance, there has been an expansion of diagnostic criteria and increasing awareness of ASD, contributing to a reported 30 to 40-fold increase in incidence over the past two decades (Graf et al. 2017). Moreover, the likelihood of self-reporting increases when students feel secure in doing so. Increasing disclosure may partly serve as an indicator of improving perceptions of neurodivergence; however, recognizing the historical stigma of these conditions will help educators facilitate a safe and inclusive educational environment.

Foremost, it should be noted that neurodivergent students matriculating into veterinary medical programs, by default, have achieved a degree of academic adaptation and success. Throughout primary, secondary, and undergraduate educational programs, these students will have – consciously or subconsciously – taken extra efforts to meet the standard goalposts that neurotypical students routinely achieve. As it is currently believed neurodivergent conditions penetrate along a spectrum of severity, it follows that the compensatory mechanisms students employ will reach their limits at varying stages of academic stress. For some students, compensation is so thorough they might not identify a neurodivergent condition until facing the extreme pressures of the veterinary curriculum. As educators, we should embrace such students with heightened appreciation for what they have been able to achieve and support their decision should they elect to receive academic accommodation.

By the combined effects of the Rehabilitation Act of 1973 and the Americans with Disabilities Act (ADA) of 1990, educators must broadly ensure their content is equally accessible to all learners and neurodivergent students may seek reasonable accommodation aimed at mitigating the challenges of neurotypical educational norms. Institutional accommodations for neurodivergent students range based on the academic program, though they generally include extended examination time, access to a testing area that is either private or less stimulating compared with standard testing facilities, and designated note takers. Board examinations such as the North American Veterinary Licensing Examination (NAVLE) and specialty veterinary boards also comply with ADA standards. However, some neurodivergent medical students elect to abstain from extra examination time, as they feel it would serve as an eventual crux (Miller et al. 2009). Perhaps the most universally helpful accommodation that educators can provide is earlier access to course materials such as lectures or reading assignments, given that the most common adaptive tactic neurodivergent students develop is increased study time. Not only does early access to course materials benefit both neurodivergent and neurotypical learners, but such universal strategies also accommodate neurodivergent students that choose to forgo formal accommodation, which would otherwise require self-identification.

Unfortunately, not all neurodivergent students disclosing their status are met with understanding, and competitive educational environments, such as veterinary and human medical schools, can prove particularly hostile. A study by Bottema-Beutel and Miele (2019) found that neurotypical undergraduate students were prone to justifying exclusion of neurodivergent students in the educational setting when a grade was at stake, especially when the neurodivergent student had ASD. Some neurodivergent medical students elect not to receive accommodations to avoid detection by and resentment from their neurotypical classmates (Pirttimaa et al. 2015). Beyond peer discrimination, a study published in 2020 reported that 11.9% of adolescent students with ASD experienced harassment from their teachers, further identifying that these students were at an increased risk for low self-esteem, drug or alcohol abuse, and suicidal tendencies (Lin et al. 2021). In the medical educational setting specifically, such authority figures extend to medical staff and preceptors, whose biases can negatively impact neurodivergent medical students, interns, and residents. Despite having resoundingly successful examples of neurodivergent practitioners in both veterinary and human medicine, there are those that believe neurodivergence prevents the successful study of medicine. Miller et al. (2009) found that 12% of medical students with disabilities reported discrimination that discouraged them from asking for help, including derogatory comments from medical staff regarding disabilities.

It is critical to understand that neurodivergent conditions are not necessarily associated with intellectual deficits, though they may occur concurrently. In general, affected students can be expected to reach the same intellectual heights as their neurotypical peers, albeit often with more time and effort. To better inform veterinary educators, preceptors, and residency coordinators in positions of authority over veterinary students and trainees, a brief discussion of neurodivergent conditions is provided below.

Part 1: Attention-Deficit/Hyperactivity Disorder

ADHD is defined by the "Diagnostic & Statistical Manual of Mental Disorders, 5th Edition" (DSM-V; American Psychiatric Association 2013) as "impairing levels of inattention, disorganization, and/or hyperactivity-impulsivity" and is often noted to persist into adulthood. While the signs of ADHD are frequently appreciated in childhood, it is not uncommon for students to receive an initial diagnosis in college, when their compensatory mechanisms for keeping up with their coursework are exceeded (Vekaria and Peverly 2018). Postsecondary students with ADHD are more likely than their neurotypical peers to withdraw from courses, struggle with working memory, underachieve academically, and report lower levels of life satisfaction (Nugent and Smart 2014). Students with ADHD commonly struggle to maintain focus throughout long lectures or consecutive lecture periods and may require more frequent breaks or increased levels of engagement. This lack of focus can bleed into their study habits as well, leading to difficulty keeping up when large amounts of material must be learned in short periods of time.

Students with ADHD may be on medications to aid their focus, but specific learning strategies may help them as well. Foremost, ADHD students must strive to always remain fully aware of their pending tasks. A tendency toward inattention can lend itself to missed assignments and falling behind on studying; therefore, staying organized is paramount. Utilizing checklists and introducing routine study habits is recommended. Modern smartphone applications can help ADHD students manage their workloads in a dynamic way that they are more likely to adhere to. Furthermore, scheduling shorter, more frequent study sessions can help ADHD students preempt distractions. As with neurotypical students, group study sessions may help or hurt academic progress and should be considered on a case-by-case basis, keeping in mind that the student should not hesitate to study alone if groups prove too distracting. On the other hand, a study of postsecondary students with ADHD revealed lower levels of resilience toward meeting academic goals, which implies peer and educator encouragement may help ADHD students visualize their own success (Gray et al. 2016).

Part 2: Autism Spectrum Disorder

ASD has undergone changes in diagnosis and naming convention over recent years. Asperger's Syndrome, previously recognized as a form of high-functioning autism, is now included within the general term of ASD. Current characterization based on DSM-V favors the use of specifiers to relay information between healthcare professionals regarding details such as severity, age of onset, and additional deficit areas. The baseline diagnostic criteria for ASD consist of persistent deficits in social communication and interaction, as well as restricted and/or repetitive patterns of behavior that are present during early development. It is important for educators to realize that language and intellectual deficits are not ubiquitous to individuals with ASD, but rather may be tacked on as modifiers under the current diagnostic guidelines. To the contrary, students with ASD may display intense interest in and unusual aptitude for specific subjects. Studies have found ASD individuals develop alternative cortical networks for auditory processing and multisensory integration (Brandwein et al. 2015), resulting in benefits as well as drawbacks. For instance, ASD students may exhibit enhanced visual perception and pattern recognition as compared to neurotypical students (Plaisted et al. 1998; Caron et al. 2004; Shah and Frith 1983), though they might find separating speech from background noise more difficult (Foxe et al. 2015). ASD students may be more easily overstimulated than their neurotypical peers, as multisensory integration is reduced (Zhang et al. 2019).

Relative to ADHD and SLD, the social differences generally observed with ASD are more prone to making affected individuals stand-out among neurotypical groups. Students with ASD are less likely to maintain eye contact or uphold the social norms of body language. They may fail to perceive and adapt to social contexts that neurotypical individuals integrate subconsciously, often coming off as rigid and disconnected. Literal interpretation of language and a failure to appreciate sarcasm are common, along with difficulty initiating and maintaining casual "small talk" conversations. The tendency of ASD individuals to have restrictive and intense interests can periodically lead to decreased social engagement, which, in a training scenario, might be perceived as active disinterest by neurotypical clinicians or preceptors. Furthermore, those with ASD frequently adhere to rigid routines and may become overwhelmed or react negatively to sudden or drastic changes to their schedules, especially if the changes are spontaneous or disciplinary in nature. For veterinary students, interns, and residents with ASD, experiencing unplanned shifts in roles and responsibilities may be particularly challenging. Despite these inclinations, high functioning individuals with ASD often respond to societal feedback over time, with the effect of reducing social deficits to a degree, occasionally to the point of blending in with neurotypical societies.

Strategies that facilitate the success of ASD students may mitigate their social deficits or degree of sensory overload, while leaning into their natural inclination toward rigid routines. Veterinary students may consciously or subconsciously ostracize their ASD peers based on perceptions of social inadequacy or misconceptions of intellectual deficits. Therefore, graded group activities may prove particularly traumatic for ASD students, proportional to their inability to pass as neurotypical. Ideally such assignments would be avoided, however, early intervention in the form of non-graded collaborative group work may alleviate negative implicit bias and potentially pave the way to atraumatic group experiences for ASD students. This use of low-stakes group contact time to improve peer acceptance of ASD students is an application of intergroup contact theory and is further supported by White et al. (2019), who demonstrated knowledge of ASD alone did not predict positive attitudes of postsecondary students toward ASD peers.

Minimizing sensory overload can be particularly challenging for ASD students and trainees in a clinical setting, as veterinary clinical environments are intrinsically stimulatory. An ASD student may need additional time to adjust to the bright lighting, beeping fluid pumps, and barking dogs of a busy intensive care unit prior to being questioned by a preceptor. Reserving clinical case discussions for a quieter environment may make the difference between a successful interaction with an ASD student and an ineffectual one. While ASD students may struggle adjusting to the clinical environment, they will typically excel in maintaining a methodical routine; i.e., meeting their routine daily responsibilities. In both the clinical and didactic phases, ASD students may be among the most organized. Their tendency toward developing intense areas of interest may even correlate with uncommon aptitude in a specific veterinary niche with potential for specialization.

Part 3: Specific Learning Disorder

SLD includes any component or combination of difficulty reading, difficulty spelling, deficient reading comprehension, reduced number sense, and poor mathematical reasoning. Per DSM-V, the deficit should be substantial in comparison to the individual's peer group and should persist for greater than six months despite corrective interventions. Currently, SLD is diagnosed and further specified with which deficit components it is associated with. Alternatively, the terms dyslexia or dyscalculia may be used when the deficits relate specifically to accurate or fluent word recognition or to processing numerical information, respectively. Additionally, the severity of SLD varies and is graded as mild, moderate, or severe. As with ADHD, affected individuals may not receive a diagnosis until academic expectations and stressors exceed their capacity to keep pace with their neurotypical peers, which may occur in childhood or as an adult learner. It should be reiterated that students with SLD, as those with other neurodivergent conditions, can be expected to exhibit the same eventual content mastery as their neurotypical peers.

Given that the content of the veterinary curriculum is largely filtered through reading rather than numerical analysis, students with dyslexia are more prone to struggle with maintaining their progress as compared to those with dyscalculia. Slower reading speeds and the need to potentially read content many fold more times than their neurotypical peers correlate with longer time to concept mastery for dyslexic students. Some students with dyslexia report persistent feelings of underachievement and may even alter their intended career paths if they perceive the required reading assignments as insurmountable (Pirttimaa et al. 2015). Like other neurodivergent students, dyslexic students commonly compensate with increased study time expenditure, however, specific strategies such as the use of text-to-audio software applications and visually mapping course material may reduce the strain of large reading assignments. Educators can aid SLD students by incorporating visual learning elements such as concept maps into their course material, providing students with content outlines that reduce the burden of unnecessary verbiage, and offering lasting access to lecture recordings.

Section 4: Personality Types

Bobbi J. Conner

Despite what one may assume, there is no evidence to support the idea that certain personality types or characteristics predominate amongst veterinary professionals in general, nor amongst veterinary students in particular (Doherty and Nugent 2011; Haight et al. 2012; Mohammadreza et al. 2013). Because the student body of any given veterinary class will be made up of individuals from various backgrounds, experiences, and dominant personality traits, no single teaching style or technique will be ideal for all students or situations. Understanding that each student comes with their own perspectives, needs, and ideas, educators must be prepared with a diverse arsenal of teaching strategies and approaches.

Although veterinary medical students will all have their own unique challenges and perspectives, there have been some commonalities and peculiarities identified in some of these cohorts. For example, Killinger et al. (2017) reported rates of stress and depression amongst over 1200 North American veterinary medical students that were higher than is reported for the general population. Higher than average suicide rates have also been reported for veterinary professionals (Reisbig et al. 2012). While the reasons for these issues are not yet well established, it is reasonable to assume there are many contributing factors. Veterinary educators are encouraged to consider the external and programmatic factors that may impact students' well-being and efforts to ameliorate contributing factors wherever possible is of paramount importance.

Part 1: Misunderstandings About Learning Styles

It can be tempting when trying to understand the veterinary medical student to consider learning styles. The term "learning styles" has become commonplace in educational settings and there are thousands of publications (both scholarly works and lay publications) dedicated to the discussion, and often promotion, of learning styles, including veterinary-specific works (Neel and Grindem 2010) and other healthcare-specific publications (Mohanna et al. 2007). The concept suggests that individuals intrinsically have certain methods of learning that work best for them. As a result, the recommendation is often made that teachers (and administrators) should first identify the learning styles of their students and then adjust the delivery of content to match their students' style. On its face, this seems quite reasonable. The problem lies in the fact that there is little to no evidence that teaching to a student's learning style leads to improved outcomes; that is to say, teaching to specific learning styles does not yield improved understanding or long-term retention (Cuevas 2015; Nancekivell et al. 2020), nor is it associated with academic success (Kamal et al. 2021). Additionally, assessing students using methods that match their style are not supported by the available literature (Pashler et al. 2009).

Learning styles might be better understood as learning preferences. That is to say, when asked, individuals will report preferences for learning under certain conditions. And there is likely a benefit to all students if teachers can vary the methods with which they provide instruction, however, the instructional method should match the content being taught, not the preferences of the learners.

Part 2: Stressors Impacting Veterinary Students

While it can be challenging, if not impossible, to parse out which stressors are impacting our students' well-being,

Table 5.1 Academic and external stressors affecting veterinary medical students.

Academic stressors	Nonacademic stressors
• Academic performance/ grades • Workload • Time spent studying • Unclear expectations • Difficulty understanding material	• Homesickness • Financial concerns • Family illness/death • Personal illness • Personal/relationship conflicts • Transportation challenges • New environment/moving • Perceived difficulty fitting in

it can also be helpful to consider specific factors and how educators can be helpful in mitigating their impact (Kogan et al. 2005; Hafen et al. 2008). For the purposes of this chapter, we will divide the various stressors into two categories: academic stressors and nonacademic stressors (Table 5.1).

Educators can have a direct impact on some of the academic stressors faced by students. Ensuring expectations for students are clearly communicated, repeated and reinforced, consistent, and readily available via multiple means is a relatively simple way to reduce some sources of stress for students. Ensuring students are aware of academic resources (tutors, study guides, faculty office hours, etc.) can lessen the workload for students in other cases. Because the volume of content for veterinary medical students is often significantly larger and more complex than they had experienced during their undergraduate education, specific training or courses on effective study practices may be a worthwhile addition to veterinary curricula. Some researchers have proposed that pass/fail or satisfactory/unsatisfactory grading schemes may reduce the academic performance stress many students experience in a traditional A–F or numerical grading scale (Nahar et al. 2019).

While it may not be possible or appropriate for educators to have an impact on many of the external stressors students often face, a general awareness that students' lives outside of the academic setting can be a source of additional and significant stress, such as in the case of a death in the family. Empathy and understanding of these external factors might be incredibly helpful for some students. Ensuring easy, ideally on-site, access to counseling and other mental health support structures should be of paramount importance for administrators, and educators should become very familiar with the resources available to their students and encourage their use.

Section 5: How Our Students Fit into Our Structures

Lawrence Garcia

Although we have discussed data regarding student identities, backgrounds, experiences, perspectives, challenges, and gifts, we still have an incomplete picture. Recognizing that the context in which our students are learning strongly influences their educational experience/success, underscores the aims of the next part of our chapter. Below we will discuss curricular and para-curricular factors that impact our students.

Part 1: Veterinary Curricula

Veterinary curricula are divided into preclinical and clinical concentrations, with the preclinical portion being more information uptake while the clinical portion is more application focused. The preclinical and clinical segments embedded in each college's curriculum may vary. For some colleges, the preclinical segment completely precedes the clinical portion, while for others, the preclinical and clinical segments may occur in various mixes where students will alternate between the two as they matriculate through the curriculum. An example of this would be where students spend the first two of four years focused on lecture and lab-based preclinical concentration, then transition directly to six months of clinical concentration, return to preclinical concentration for a year to complete upper-level medicine and surgery courses, then return to the clinic for the final six months prior to graduation. For this particular format, students anecdotally report that entering the clinical concentration after two years of foundational preclinical curriculum helps them to assimilate and apply the knowledge they have acquired to that point more effectively in the clinical setting. Students also report that having the clinical segment earlier in their curriculum helps them to focus their study in the upper-level preclinical concentration in specialty-based medicine and surgery courses.

Another benefit of the described split curriculum is that it allows students to prepare for and take the NAVLE while they are off clinics. In formats where the preclinical segment is completed prior to starting the clinical segment, students take the NAVLE during their clinical rotations. Students on rotations, especially those with overnight duties leading up to the examination, might be at a disadvantage with this format, although being in the midst of the clinical segment could be considered an advantage as well. In colleges where students are in clinics for the examination, accommodations are made to give students limited time leading up to their examination date for preparation.

Although curricular formats may differ, research is needed to determine if or how each format impacts pass rates and if there are any notable trends in either area. In general, the preclinical environment tends to be more structured and predictable, while the clinical environment can be more dynamic, requiring significant adaptability on the part of both the instructors and students. During the COVID pandemic most, if not all, institutions went to completely or largely virtual platforms for instructional delivery for both aspects of the curriculum. Although not ideal, especially for clinical application, this provided continuity of curricular delivery so that students could fulfill their requirements for graduation, especially those graduating in 2020. In this author's experience, some students did find significant difficulty with the lack of in-person instruction. Many students returned to their home during this time, where there were family distractions, competition for internet bandwidth, and a total change in study habits and environment.

Many in the class of 2020 missed out on the last eight to ten weeks of clinical experiences altogether. For the classes of 2021, 2022, and 2023, their schedules had to be modified and rearranged to make up missed labs, especially surgery labs. For some clinical clerkships, prerequisite requirements had to be waived to help students to continue matriculating through the curriculum without issue. More research is necessary to evaluate the impacts of these instructional changes due to COVID-19 to help address and anticipate concerns that may occur in future similar disasters. For the purposes of this chapter, we will discuss the preclinical and clinical portions separately, with the recognition that there is often significant overlap between the two.

Part 2: The Preclinical Curriculum

The preclinical segment of the curriculum may be delivered via lecture- or activity-based methods. This portion of the veterinary medical program is generally delivered in a group setting, such as a classroom, auditorium, or laboratory environment with a relatively large student-to-instructor ratio. Additionally, interactions between instructors and students often range in duration and frequency. For example, a course might meet once daily or several times each week.

Lecture-based delivery is still quite common in the classroom and can be extremely effective depending on the instructor's skill and the content being covered. However, active learning techniques are increasingly becoming incorporated into veterinary curricula in preclinical courses, including problem-based learning, case-based learning, the flipped classroom model, interactive polling and quizzes, and others. Although the instructor to student ratio is the same, it often requires students to engage in some learning prior to the class session so that during class time they are applying their knowledge and asking questions of the instructor and each other to solidify their learning. The flipped classroom model is a good example of active learning; it posts materials to study which students are expected to learn prior to the class meeting. During class, rather than engaging in an instructor-led lecture or review of the materials, students are asked to share information they've learned with one another in a small group, followed by a large group discussion guided by the instructor. Such interactions can be recorded and made available for students who could not attend, as well as for use as an additional study tool.

Additionally, although the COVID-19 pandemic caused many disruptions socially and within the academy, the forced use of virtual teaching platforms led to more (forced) instructor flexibility in terms of content delivery. This resulted in many moving to a hybrid lecture format that involved some students attending virtually while others were in-person. Another very common adaptation was to have students alternate in-person with virtual attendance, thus allowing all to have equal opportunity for in-person instruction. Those who attended in-person interacted in the typical ways, while those who attended virtually interacted via chat within the platform utilized.

The recordings included both in-person and chat interactions, which was very helpful for those watching the recording as it helped them to have a more complete experience. The chat feature worked best if there was someone monitoring it while the instructor monitored the in-person audience; this also allowed all students to have equal opportunity to ask questions. This hybrid format has proven to be somewhat successful and will likely continue as class sizes expand. Importantly, for some portions of the preclinical segment, such as laboratory work, because of larger class sizes (100–150 students), it can be helpful to break the class into smaller groups. Although beneficial for students, such smaller groups do require more instructors and support staff to deliver information and assessment of student mastery and retention of information. Regardless of the format and modality used to deliver the curriculum, it is important to evaluate and update it regularly for relevance and effectiveness.

To gain a better understanding of the preclinical segment, Magnier and associates, as reported in Schoenfeld-Tacher et al. (2015), surveyed students' perceptions of the preclinical curriculum. They found that students perceived the preclinical concentration to be both academically and personally challenging. The preclinical concentration requires students to assimilate large volumes of foundational

information in a relatively short period of time, which can be a great challenge for some students. Some courses are delivered in their entirety over a period of two weeks, with multiple daily meetings during that period. This can be a great deal of information to process, retain, and master for most students, although, for testing purposes, the information may be fresher when compared to testing over the entire semester. In addition, most veterinary curricula involve in excess of 20 credit hours per semester. Within the large course loads, there will be varying credit values, requiring the students in some cases to strategize and focus their efforts on the courses worth the most to maintain their grade point average. In the author's experience, students tend to find this to be almost an ethical dilemma, as in some cases, this approach may go against previous study habits. Many students report anecdotally that the greatest adjustment they had to make when entering the veterinary curriculum was related to previous study habits. This is not surprising as the veterinary curriculum is extremely rigorous and time-intense, usually requiring course work, lab work, and/or class attendance Monday through Friday from 8 a.m. to 5 p.m., which is quite different from a typical undergraduate semester. The overarching goal for the preclinical curriculum is to establish the knowledge foundation for success in the clinical curriculum.

Part 3: The Clinical Curriculum

The clinical part of the curriculum requires students to have a solid foundational knowledge base from their preclinical phase. During clinical rotations, in a traditional veterinary teaching hospital (VTH) model, students function in a much smaller student-to-instructor ratio and have frequent opportunities for one-on-one interaction in an apprenticeship-style format (Magnier et al. 2011). Students are generally assigned to specific cases scheduled for the next receiving day and are expected to study and gain a working knowledge of common differentials for the presenting concerns and history. Often the clinician will round with students about the incoming cases in the morning on the day of the appointment to evaluate the student's level of preparedness for the case; this also provides the student an opportunity to demonstrate their knowledge and ask questions they may not have been able to answer through their own precase studies.

At the appointment time, the student is expected to collect a comprehensive history and perform a thorough physical examination (PE). Upon completion of these tasks, the student normally meets with the supervising clinician(s) and house officers to discuss the history and exam findings, as well as provide differentials and propose diagnostic and treatment plans. The clinician(s) and house officers provide feedback and coaching; the team then meets with the owner(s) to discuss a diagnostic plan. Through this process, the clinicians and students work as a team to diagnose and create a treatment plan for the case. Through these steps, clinicians also illustrate to the student the key steps for evaluating and critically thinking through a case, as they would in practice on their own.

These opportunities are both experiential and practice-based. Magnier and associates (2011) also reported that students find this environment to be more authentic for teaching and learning. This is likely because they are given the opportunity to work through a case as they would in practice, but with the safety net of faculty oversight. The overarching goal of the clinical rotations is to develop the student's ability to think critically in a systematic and logical manner, make sound, safe clinical judgments, and develop clinical reasoning and diagnostic skills (Magnier et al. 2011). This may seem daunting but is very achievable with proper planning and preparation on the part of both the clinician and the student, despite the ever-changing dynamics of the clinical environment.

It is important to remember that within the clinical rotations, caseload variability can significantly impact learning, both in terms of case volume and types of cases. For example, students might experience multiple similar cases or have a very light caseload as a result of holidays (or other reasons). The clinical curriculum at a traditional, VTH-model program occurs in a tertiary referral facility where the caseload may include a large proportion of complex, specialty-level cases that students would not normally see and/or treat in general clinical practice. As a result, students often experience a predominance of tertiary referral level cases in contrast to common presentations in a general practice. Although some of these cases may require more advanced skills than those needed for day-one practice readiness, they do provide an opportunity for students to learn how to provide superior care. In addition, students gain understanding of how general practitioners identify cases that require specialty care and should be referred to a referral hospital.

It is important to point out that newer veterinary programs within the United States are increasingly relying on private and corporate general practices, as well as private and corporate specialty hospitals for clinical year rotations. These are referred to as either distributive or hybrid distributive models, and they do not have an associated VTH. But regardless of caseload or teaching environment, every case exposure is an opportunity for students to gain critical thinking skills and reinforce foundational knowledge. Additionally, regardless of clinical rotation location, the experience of each student will be unique and help to form their overall clinical proficiency. Therefore, it is imperative that faculty and practicing clinicians functioning as faculty help students recognize that they likely will not see every possible case to prepare them for practice, but that each case they do see serves as an opportunity to further develop their problem-solving abilities and clinical proficiency. The clinical curriculum is vital in preparing students for the profession by providing them with hands-on experiences with high-quality coaching in a safe environment. Day one clinical proficiency is the overarching goal of all aspects of veterinary curricula.

Section 6: Expectations

Lawrence Garcia

Setting expectations is extremely important in all aspects of the curriculum, as it brings a common level of understanding and security among students, faculty, and staff. However, setting expectations can be difficult, especially when working as part of a team, due to differences in personalities, ideas, approaches, perspectives, and the like. Thus, when setting expectations there must be clear and consistent communication to ensure that all involved agree upon and understand the stated goals, all of which should mirror those for daily practice from the first day or orientation to the day or graduation.

Part 1: Professional Behavior

All pieces of the curriculum should include the setting of expectations for professionalism, accountability, and duties. This can be done in various ways, including requiring professional dress throughout the curriculum, setting specific behavioral expectations, and having a committee of peers help with mutual accountability. The expectation for appropriate interpersonal interactions, accomplishing learning objectives, assignment submissions, and meeting deadlines should be embedded throughout. This can be addressed and reinforced through team exercises, encouraging collegiality, professional dress, and setting expectations for assignments exacting consequences when standards are not met. This can be done by including professionalism and teamwork as part of a grading rubric, especially during the clinical portion of the curriculum.

Modeling of professionalism also helps encourage appropriate behavior and builds mutual respect, two essential elements for a successful professional career after graduation. Anecdotally, this is an area of opportunity, as faculty, staff, and house officers may not be very good about demonstrating the expectations and standards we talk to our students about. For example, the movement toward well-being is currently quite strong, but although those in mentoring and teaching roles may verbally emphasize its importance, our actions often do not support our words. Another example centers on collegiality or lack thereof. If we speak poorly of colleagues in front of students, we can certainly expect students to do the same, so this type of behavior must be avoided and pointed out to colleagues (in private). By demonstrating that we are living these values, we not only model these behaviors for the students, but we also provide valuable insights into how they can overcome barriers to self-care and quality of life-based on our individual experiences. One way we can accomplish these goals is to remember that we were all in the student role at some point; this will help us be more understanding and willing to coach them based on our journeys within the profession.

Part 2: Client and Patient Care

Providing excellent care to patients and clients is another crucial expectation. Based on experience, defining what excellent patient care means and describing what it looks like on the first day of a rotation is key. It is also imperative to provide regular feedback and guidance to students as they collect histories, perform PE, and communicate with clients throughout the rotation. Feedback can come in a variety of ways including verbal, written, and through repetition of a skill. For example, sometimes it is more helpful to ask a student to repeat a PE than to tell them what they missed during their initial PE. This allows the student to find what they missed and provides the clinician the opportunity to encourage the student to reflect on why the issue was missed the first time, which should help the student better understand how to avoid missing the same or similar findings in the future. However, it is also important to help students understand that they will miss more by not looking or by not being thorough than not knowing.

Evaluating students with regard to both their client interactions and communications are key to providing excellent care. As such, modeling again comes into play. Faculty, staff, and house officers should speak respectfully with and about clients and set the example for students while holding themselves and their students accountable in this area. Setting the expectation for excellent client and patient care is key to the success of a practicing veterinarian. Those who master this skill are set up for longer success in the field.

The Importance of Lifelong Learning

Lifelong learning and ongoing curiosity are essential to success in this ever-growing and changing field. The expectation should be set that intellectual curiosity is vital to success in the field and supports growth and development of ourselves and our profession. With the current ease of access to technology and diagnostics, it is easy to become too dependent on outside resources. This could be a significant problem in the event of a natural or man-made disaster where such infrastructure is lost. Students should be able to navigate such technology and ensure they are relying on credible sources, but also need to be encouraged to question, challenge, and always be looking for the answer in a way that emphasizes the process rather than the outcome. Intellectual curiosity is also key to professional fulfillment and should be encouraged by our up-and-coming veterinarians. In the end, lifelong learning is key to the growth and sustainability of our profession (Table 5.2).

Section 7: Student Factors

Bobbi J. Conner

Part 1: Fixed Versus Growth Mindset

Students' mindset, that is, their beliefs about themselves and their qualities, can have a profound impact on their educational outcomes. In her book on mindset, Carol Dweck (2006) describes two mindsets: fixed and growth. Briefly, people with a fixed mindset believe their underlying traits and abilities (e.g., personality and intelligence) are inherent and cannot really be changed. Those with a growth mindset believe these traits are malleable and can be changed throughout life. There is evidence that the mindset of a veterinary student correlates with their self-reported anxiety (Whittington et al. 2017; Bostock et al. 2018), which is supported by evidence from other fields (He and Hegarty 2020; Cribbs et al. 2021; Schroder 2021). The reported proportion of students with a growth versus fixed mindset varies (Whittington et al. 2017; Armitage-Chan and Maddison 2019; Royal 2020) and may be at least partly attributed to students' cultural backgrounds. As educators, there is much that we can do to change our students' mindsets (Dweck 2006; Guttin et al. 2021).

The way we provide feedback to our students can have an important impact on how they view their own ability to learn and grow: comforting students when they fail and reducing their workload may seem like a kindness when it may, in fact, demotivate students (Rattan et al. 2011). Educators should provide assistance and help students strategize methods to improve and overcome failure – many of them will be experiencing failure in ways they had not experienced prior to veterinary school and may be ill-prepared for. Developing students' mindsets to be more growth-oriented may better prepare them for the ubiquitous uncertainties associated with the healthcare professions (Moffett et al. 2021).

Table 5.2 Example of some of the expectations made of students throughout veterinary curricula.

Expectations of the veterinary profession		
Professionalism	Expected and emphasized in verbal and nonverbal communication, includes attire, attitude, and respect	Throughout the curriculum
Self-care and balance	Dividing weekend duties and case responsibilities, expectation of life outside the profession, and professional obligations can be met through a collegial team approach, organizational strategies, family activities, community service, hobbies, and physical recreation	Throughout the curriculum
Treating colleagues with respect	As colleagues we should learn about each other's backgrounds, goals, and styles in order to understand our differences and treat each other with respect, through this we develop trust and cohesiveness	Throughout the curriculum
Patient care	Pets should be treated as if they are our own, multitasking, interpersonal and relationship-building skills, self-management skills, leadership, knowledge of practice and business management, innovative thinking with sound judgment	Clinical concentration
Client care	The responsibility for final decisions about therapy is shared between the veterinarian, who has medical and scientific expertise, and the client, who has expertise with a specific animal and knowledge of his or her own lifestyle that will affect his or her ability to care for the pet. This type of relationship is desired by many pet owners and, in many cases, results in greater client and veterinarian satisfaction	Clinical concentration
Intellectual curiosity	Knowing the correct answer is important, but understanding the process of getting to said answer is more important as is ongoing curiosity throughout their professional life	Throughout the curriculum

Source: Adapted from Howell et al. (2002).

Part 2: Learning to Fail

Failure is a tricky concept. We do not like making mistakes and failure is often considered something that should be avoided at all costs. However, despite our deep dislike of failure, there is a large body of evidence supporting the idea that circumstances that promote challenges, difficulties, and errors will lead to better long-term retention and ability to transfer knowledge to new situations (Bjork 1994; Eva 2009). Importantly, one must know that they have made a mistake for the error to be beneficial to learning – without coaching and feedback, lack of proficiency can be perpetuated (Jowett et al. 2007; Kornell and Metcalfe 2006). However, too much feedback can, perhaps paradoxically, hinder long-term retention if the feedback is too immediate and too constant. That is, learners must be challenged – perhaps even induced to make errors – and given feedback after a delay to improve. Unfortunately, the ideal amount and timing of feedback remain elusive. The main point is for educators to recognize that mistakes can be powerful tools in the learning process and the avoidance

of all mistakes is not something that should be encouraged or, perhaps, even rewarded. Failure's beneficial role in the learning process may not be fully realized unless students believe that they can master new skills and information with practice.

Section 8: Practical Tips for Safely Incorporating Failure into Veterinary Education

Bobbi J. Conner

To balance the power of mistake-making for the learning process with the negative impact too much failure can have on students' well-being, educators should be thoughtful about how to incorporate challenges into their instruction. Creating challenging but low-stakes assignments, where the instructions are explicit that mistakes are likely to occur, might be one option for striking such a balance. Creating opportunities for retrieval (not just review) of material can increase the likelihood that learners' recall will be erroneous, but – with appropriate feedback – can significantly improve long-term retention. Therefore, quizzes and exams are particularly important to the learning process. Being explicit about the importance of exams for learning, not just for evaluation, might also help. Assignments or exams where students must *generate* the required information rather than recognize it (i.e., short answer questions versus multiple choice) will also likely lead to greater learning. These need not all be high stakes, however. Creating conditions that will enhance learning will, necessarily, be challenging for students; instructors must be aware of the mental and cognitive load being placed on their students. One option to help is to provide some flexibility and autonomy into the students' workloads. The timing of assignments or assessments could conceivably be flexible to account for students' varied stressors outside of the learning environment; offering multiple opportunities for various assignments; or plenty of chances to revise and resubmit coursework can help.

Any practicing veterinarian also knows that mistakes are inevitable; sometimes those mistakes can be devastating. Medical errors in the clinical setting are a leading cause of morbidity and mortality in human medicine (Anderson and Abrahamson 2017). Although such numbers are not known in veterinary medicine, it is reasonable to suspect they might be similar. We want our students to make errors under the right conditions (e.g., during a communication simulation, while practicing surgical knot-tying, when making a diagnosis in a supervised clinical scenario, etc.) to enhance their learning. However, for the safety of our patients, we want to reduce the chances that practicing veterinarians will make errors. How we train veterinarians to think about errors can have far-reaching impacts on their abilities to become life-long learners as well as their abilities to become resilient, successful veterinarians.

Summary

Veterinary educators can be more effective instructors by understanding their students and the systems in which they teach. The previous sections have outlined some of the demographics of veterinary students, some of the themes that are unique to the profession, and some of the common systems that are utilized in education. But what should an educator *do* with this information? While some tips have been discussed throughout this chapter, more specific discussions of veterinary educators' responsibilities are discussed in other chapters within this text.

References

Agyeman, A.A., Chin, K.L., Landersdorfer, C.B. et al. (2020). Smell and taste dysfunction in patients with COVID-19: a systematic review and meta-analysis. *Mayo Clinic Proceedings* 95 (8): 1621–1631. https://doi.org/10.1016/j.mayocp.2020.05.030. Epub 2020 Jun 6. PMID: 32753137; PMCID: PMC7275152.

American Association of Veterinary Medical Colleges (2022, May). AAVMC 2021–2022 annual data report. https://www.aavmc.org/about-aavmc/public-data/ (accessed 12 August 2022).

American Psychiatric Association, DSM-5 Task Force (2013). *Diagnostic and Statistical Manual of Mental Disorders: DSM-5™*, 5e. American Psychiatric Publishing, Inc. https://doi.org/10.1176/appi.books.9780890425596.

Anderson, J.G. and Abrahamson, K. (2017). Your health care may kill you: medical errors. *Student Health and Technology Information* 234: 13–17.

Armitage-Chan, E. and Maddison, J. (2019). The influences of curriculum area and student background on mindset to learning in the veterinary curriculum: a pilot study. *Veterinary Medicine and Science* 5: 470–482.

Association of American Veterinary Medical Colleges (2020, January). AAVMC 2019–2020 annual data report. http://www.aavmc.org/about-aavmc/public-data/ (accessed 30 November 2021).

Bjork, R.A. (1994). Memory and metamemory considerations in the training of human beings. In: *Metacognition: Knowing about knowing* (ed. J. Metcalfe and A. Shimamura), 185–205. Cambridge, MA: MIT Press.

Bostock, R., Kinnison, T., and May, S.A. (2018). Mindset and its relationship to anxiety in clinical veterinary students. *Veterinary Record* 183: 623.

Bottema-Beutel, K. and Miele, D.B. (2019). College students' evaluations and reasoning about exclusion of students with autism and learning disability: context and goals may matter more than contact. *Journal of Autism and Developmental Disorders* 49 (1): 307–323.

Brandwein, A.B., Foxe, J.J., Butler, J.S. et al. (2015). Neurophysiological indices of atypical auditory processing and multisensory integration are associated with symptom severity in autism. *Journal of Autism and Developmental Disorders* 45 (1): 230–244.

Cannedy, A.L. (2004). Veterinary Medical Colleges' diversity awareness. *Journal of Veterinary Medical Education* 31 (4): 417–420. https://doi.org/10.3138/jvme.31.4.417.

Caron, M.-J., Mottron, L., Rainville, C., and Chouinard, S. (2004). Do high functioning persons with autism present superior spatial abilities? *Neuropsychologia* 42 (4): 467–481.

Carr, M.M. and Greenhill, L.M. (2015). Veterinary school applicants: financial literacy and behaviors. *Journal of Veterinary Medical Education* 42 (2): 89–96. https://doi.org/10.3138/jvme.1114-113r.

Chisholm-Burns, M.A., Spivey, C.A., Stallworth, S., and Zivin, J.G. (2019). Analysis of educational debt and income among pharmacists and other health professionals. *American Journal of Pharmaceutical Education* 83 (9): 7460. https://doi.org/10.5688/ajpe7460.

Chubin, D.E. and Mohamed, S. (2009). increasing minorities in veterinary medicine: national trends in science degrees, local programs, and strategies. *Journal of Veterinary Medical Education* 36 (4): 363–369. https://doi.org/10.3138/jvme.36.4.363.

Cribbs, J., Huang, X., and Piatek-Jimenez, K. (2021). Relations of mathematics mindset, mathematics anxiety, mathematics identity, and mathematics self-efficacy to STEM career choice: a structural equation modeling approach. *Math Education* 121: 275–287.

Cuevas, J. (2015). Is learning styles-based instruction effective? A comprehensive analysis of recent research onlearning styles. *Theory and Research in Education* 13: 308–333.

Doherty, E.M. and Nugent, E. (2011). Personality factors and medical training: a review of literature. *Medical Education* 45: 132–140.

Dweck, C.S. (2006). *Mindset: The New Psychology of Success*. New York: Random House.

Elmore, R.G. (2003). The lack of racial diversity in veterinary medicine. *Journal of the American Veterinary Medical Association* 222 (1): 24–26. https://doi.org/10.2460/javma.2003.222.24.

Eva, K.W. (2009). Diagnostic error in medical education: where wrongs can make rights. *Advances in Health Sciences Education* 14: 71–81.

Foxe, J.J., Molholm, S., Del Bene, V.A. et al. (2015). Severe multisensory speech integration deficits in high-functioning school-aged children with Autism Spectrum Disorder (ASD) and their resolution during early adolescence. *Cerebral Cortex (New York, N.Y.: 1991)* 25 (2): 298–312.

Graf, W.D., Miller, G., Epstein, L.G., and Rapin, I. (2017). The autism "epidemic". *Neurology* 88 (14): 1371–1380.

Gray, S.A., Fettes, P., Woltering, S. et al. (2016). Symptom manifestation and impairments in college students with ADHD. *Journal of Learning Disabilities* 49 (6): 616–630.

Guttin, T., Light, T.P., and Baillie, S. (2021). Exploring the mindset of veterinary educators for intelligence, clinical reasoning, compassion, and morality. *Journal of Veterinary Medical Education* https://doi.org/10.3138/jvme-2021-0057.

Hafen, M., Reisbug, A.M.J., White, M.B., and Rush, B.R. (2008). The first-year veterinary student and mental health: the role of common stressors. *Journal of Veterinary Medical Education* 35: 102–109.

Haight, S.J., Chibnall, J.T., Schindler, D.L., and Slavin, S.J. (2012). Associations of medical student personality and health/wellness characteristics with their medical school performance across the curriculum. *Academic Medicine* 87: 476–485.

He, C. and Hegarty, M. (2020). How anxiety and growth mindset are linked to navigation ability: impacts of exploration and GPS use. *Journal of Environmental Psychology* 71: 1–12.

Hoblet, K.H., Maccabe, A.T., and Heider, L.E. (2003). Veterinarians in population health and public practice: meeting critical national needs. *Journal of Veterinary Medical Education* 30 (3): 287–294. https://doi.org/10.3138/jvme.30.3.287.

Howell, N.E., Lane, I.F., Brace, J.J., and Shull, R.M. (2002). Integration of problem-based learning in a veterinary medical curriculum: first-year experiences with application-based learning exercises at the University of Tennessee College of Veterinary Medicine. *Journal of Veterinary Medical Education* 29 (3): 169–175. https://doi.org/10.3138/jvme.29.3.169.

Ilgen, D.R., Lloyd, J.W., Morgeson, F.P. et al. (2003). Personal characteristics, knowledge of the veterinary profession, and influences on career choice among students in the veterinary school applicant pool. *Journal of the American Veterinary Medical Association* 223 (11): 1587–1594. https://doi.org/10.2460/javma.2003.223.1587.

Jowett, N., LeBlanc, V., Xeroulis, G. et al. (2007). Surgical skill acquisition with self-directed practice using computer-based video training. *American Journal of Surgery* 193: 237–242.

Kamal, I., Karim, M.K.A., Awang Kechik, M.M. et al. (2021). Evaluation of healthcare science student learning styles based VARK analysis technique. *International Journal of Evaluation and Research in Education* 10: 255–261.

Killinger, S.L., Flanagan, S., Castine, E., and Howard, K.A.S. (2017). Stress and depression among veterinary medical students. *Journal of Veterinary Medical Education* 44: 3–8.

Kogan, L.R., McConnell, S.L., and Schoenfeld-Tacher. (2005). Veterinary students and non-academic stressors. *Journal of Veterinary Medical Education* 32: 193–200.

Kornell, N. and Metcalfe, J. (2006). Study efficacy and the region of proximal learning framework. *Journal of Experimental Psychology* 32: 609–622.

Lin, J.E., Asfour, A., Sewell, T.B. et al. (2021). Neurological issues in children with COVID-19. *Neuroscience Letters* 743: 135567. https://doi.org/10.1016/j.neulet.2020.135567. Epub 2020 Dec 19. PMID: 33352286; PMCID: PMC7831718.

Lowrie, P.M. (2009). Tying art and science to reality for recruiting minorities to veterinary medicine. *Journal of Veterinary Medical Education* 36 (4): 382–387. https://doi.org/10.3138/jvme.36.4.382.

Magnier, K., Wang, R., Dale, V.H.M. et al. (2011). Enhancing clinical learning in the workplace: a qualitative study. *Veterinary Record* 169 (26): 682. https://doi.org/10.1136/vr.100297.

Meeks, L.M. and Herzer, K.R. (2016). Prevalence of self-disclosed disability among medical students in us allopathic medical schools. *Journal of the American Medical Association* 316 (21): 2271–2272.

Meeks, L.M., Case, B., Herzer, K. et al. (2019). Change in prevalence of disabilities and accommodation practices among us medical schools, 2016 vs 2019. *Journal of the American Medical Association* 322 (20): 2022–2022.

Miller, S., Ross, S., and Cleland, J. (2009). Medical students' attitudes toward disability and support for disability in medicine. *Medical Teacher* 31 (6): 272–277.

Moffett, J., Hammond, J., Murphy, P., and Pawlikowska, T. (2021). The ubiquity of uncertainty: a scoping review on how undergraduate health professions' students engage with uncertainty. *Advances in Health Sciences Education* 26: 913–958.

Mohammadreza, H., Erdmann, J.B., and Gonnella, J.S. (2013). Personality assessments and outcomes in medical education and the practice of medicine: AMEE Guide No. 79. *Medical Teacher* 35: e1267–e1301.

Mohanna, K., Chambers, R., and Wall, D. (2007). Developing your teaching style: increasing effectiveness in healthcare teaching. *Postgraduate Medical Journal* 83: 145–147.

Nahar, V.K., Davis, R.E., Dunn, C. et al. (2019). The prevalence and demographic correlates of stress, anxiety, and depression among veterinary students in the Southeastern United States. *Research in Veterinary Science* 125: 370–373.

Nancekivell, S.E., Shah, P., and Gelman, S.A. (2020). Maybe they're born with it, or maybe it's experience: toward a deeper understanding of the learning style myth. *Journal of Education Psychology* 112: 221–235.

Neel, J.A. and Grindem, C.B. (2010). Learning-style profiles of 150 veterinary medical students. *Journal of Veterinary Medical Education* 37: 347–352.

Nugent, K. and Smart, W. (2014). Attention-deficit/hyperactivity disorder in postsecondary students. *Neuropsychiatric Disease and Treatment* 10: 1781–1791.

Pashler, H., McDaniel, M., and Rohrer, D. (2009). Learning styles: concepts and evidence. *Psychological Science in the Public Interest* 9: 105–119.

Pirttimaa, R., Takala, M., and Ladonlahti, T. (2015). Students in higher education with reading and writing difficulties. *Education Inquiry* 6 (1).

Plaisted, K., O'Riordan, M., and Baron-Cohen, S. (1998). Enhanced visual search for a conjunctive target in autism: a research note. *Journal of Child Psychology and Psychiatry, and Allied Disciplines* 39 (5): 777–783.

Rattan, A., Good, C., and Dweck, C.S. (2011). "It's ok — Not everyone can be good at math": Instructors with an entity theory comfort (and demotivate) students. *Journal of Experimental Social Psychology* 48: 731–737.

Reisbig, A.M.J., Danielson, J.A., Wu, T.F. et al. (2012). A study of depression and anxiety, general health, and academic performance in three cohorts of veterinary medical students across the first three semesters of veterinary school. *Journal of Veterinary Medical Education* 39: 34–358.

Royal, K. (2020). Exploring veterinary medical students' mindset about intelligence, personality, attitude, and skills and abilities. *Education in the Health Professions* 3: 33–35.

Saniasiaya, J. and Kulasegarah, J. (2021). Dizziness and COVID-19. *Ear, Nose & Throat Journal* 100 (1): 29–30. https://doi.org/10.1177/0145561320959573. Epub 2020 Sep 15. PMID: 32931322; PMCID: PMC7492824.

Saniasiaya, J., Islam, M.A., and Abdullah, B. (2021). Prevalence and characteristics of taste disorders in cases of COVID-19: a meta-analysis of 29,349 patients. *Otolaryngol Head Neck Surgery* 165 (1): 33–42. https://doi.org/10.1177/0194599820981018. Epub 2020 Dec 15. PMID: 33320033.

Schoenfeld-Tacher, R.M., Kogan, L.R., Meyer-Parsons, B. et al. (2015). Educational research report: changes in students' levels of empathy during the didactic portion of a veterinary program. *Journal of Veterinary Medical Education* 42 (3): 194–205. https://doi.org/10.3138/jvme.0115-007r.

Schroder, H.S. (2021). Mindsets in the clinic: applying mindset theory to clinical psychology. *Clinical Psychology Review* 83: 1–16.

Shah, A. and Frith, U. (1983). An islet of ability in autistic children: a research note. *Journal of Child Psychology and Psychiatry, and Allied Disciplines* 24 (4): 613–620.

Vekaria, P.C. and Peverly, S.T. (2018). Lecture note-taking in postsecondary students with attention-deficit/hyperactivity disorder. *Reading and Writing* 31 (7): 1551–1573.

Watson, P. (2011). Gender and veterinary medicine. *Canadian Veterinary Journal* 168 (24): 649. https://doi.org/10.1136/vr.d3733.

White, D., Hillier, A., Frye, A., and Makrez, E. (2019). College students' knowledge and attitudes towards students on the autism spectrum. *Journal of Autism and Developmental Disorders* 49 (7): 2699–2705.

Whittington, R.E., Rhind, S., Loads, D., and Handel, I. (2017). Exploring the link between mindset and psychological well-being among veterinary students. *Journal of Veterinary Medical Education* 44: 134–140.

Zhang, J., Meng, Y., He, J. et al. (2019). McGurk effect by individuals with autism spectrum disorder and typically developing controls: a systematic review and meta-analysis. *Journal of Autism and Developmental Disorders* 49 (1): 34–43.

6

Roles of the Professional Program Instructor

Philippa Gibbons, BVetMed(Hons), MS, DACVIM (LA), MRCVSm PGDipVetED
Texas Tech School of Veterinary Medicine, Amarillo, TX, USA

Dawn M. Spangler, DVM, MS, DACVPM
Richard A. Gillespie College of Veterinary Medicine, Lincoln Memorial University, Harrogate, TN, USA

Lynda M.J. Miller, DVM, PhD, DACT
Richard A. Gillespie College of Veterinary Medicine, Lincoln Memorial University, Harrogate, TN, USA

Erik H. Hofmeister, DVM, DACVAA, DECVAA, MA, MS
College of Veterinary Medicine, Auburn University, Auburn, AL, USA

Lisa M. Greenhill, MPA, PhD
American Association of Veterinary Medical Colleges, Washington, DC, USA

Sraavya M. Polisetti, BS
American Association of Veterinary Medical Colleges, Washington, DC, USA

Kendall P. Young, MPA
American Association of Veterinary Medical Colleges, Washington, DC, USA

Shelly Wu, PhD (Science Education)
Peter O'Donnell Jr. School of Public Health, University of Texas Southwestern Medical Center, TX, USA

Gabriel Huddleston, PhD
Texas Christian University, Fort Worth, TX, USA

Ryane E. Englar, DVM, DABVP (Canine and Feline Practice)
University of Arizona College of Veterinary Medicine, Oro Valley, AZ, USA

Micha C. Simons, VMD, MVEd
Virginia-Maryland College of Veterinary Medicine, Blacksburg, VA, USA

Stephanie Thomovsky, DVM, DACVIM (Neurology), MS (Health Professions Education)
Purdue College of Veterinary Medicine, West Lafayette, IN, USA

Section 1: Classroom Learning

Philippa Gibbons

Part 1: Introduction

Veterinary education has traditionally been delivered largely by large group classroom learning, i.e., "the lecture." But over the past few decades, veterinary education has evolved significantly, with two key changes being the promotion of a competency-based curriculum and the ever-expanding volume of information in veterinary medicine. The development of competency-based veterinary education (CBVE) and formulation of entrustable professional activities (EPAs) have emphasized the need for new graduates to have clinical reasoning ability, alongside clinical and professional skills.

Clinical reasoning requires students to have basic science and clinical medicine knowledge, and the ability to apply that knowledge to deductively solve a clinical problem. In the traditional lecture, where the teacher/lecturer imparts expert knowledge (Parmelee et al. 2020), there is often minimal student engagement; it also commonly results in students developing recall level knowledge, or learning at the lower tier of Bloom's Taxonomy. Such learning has been defined as "fragile knowledge," where the information is only reproducible in the short term for examinations (May and Silva-Fletcher 2015).

As educators, we desire students to develop the ability to become self-regulated learners and wish to stimulate deep learning that will sustain them out into their chosen career tracks, while also encouraging them to be life-long learners. Deep learning has been associated with instructors who encourage students to be critical thinkers, integration of course material in other disciplines, courses that encourage thinking and reading about the learning material, and books and articles that challenge students while providing explanations beyond the lecture material (Chigerwe et al. 2011). Parmelee et al. (2020), identified six principles to develop these skills based on cognitive neuroscience. These include: retrieval learning that is meaningful, thereby developing long term learning; spaced repetition where deliberate retrieval of knowledge is required after a gap; interleaving, by incorporation of multiple concepts at the same time; increasing testing – both high and low stakes with feedback; elaborative interrogation and self-exploration by the instructor by asking students to justify their answer; and metacognition, thereby enabling life-long learners by using inquiry based and collaborative learning. Introduction of active learning in the classroom has been promoted to achieve these needs and can be described as all formats that promote student engagement (May and Silva-Fletcher 2015).

Active learning, contrary to the beliefs of many, is achievable in both large group teaching and small group learning activities. It often requires collaborative learning, group work, and public speaking. These are skills that veterinary students often lack; therefore, students should be prepared for, and trained to receive, these types of sessions for effective learning to occur (Thurman et al. 2009).

Challenges presented to active learning include the delivery of large volumes of information that are required for students to pass licensing examinations; the need to integrate clinical medicine into basic science courses, which can be challenging for non-veterinarians and vice versa; and the physical structure of the classroom (Parmelee et al. 2020). However, veterinary educators should not become overwhelmed at the need to substantially change their courses: active learning goals simply include analysis, reflection, and problem-solving. These interventions can be varied, from introduction of peer instruction within a traditional lecture, such as think–pair–share activities and audience response systems

(ARS), to changing one or multiple lecture-based courses to team or problem-based learning (PBL), to development of clinical reasoning active learning sessions alongside traditional lectures. The other unique aspect of active learning is that multimodal integration can be developed in a course (Berrian et al. 2021).

Harden and Cosby (2000), described the 12 roles of the teacher in higher education in 2001. The roles that specifically correspond to classroom learning include those of information provider, role model in teaching, learning facilitator, examiner, and resource developer. In an active learning classroom, more emphasis can be placed on the learning facilitator and resource provider roles.

However, even with encouragement to develop more active learning activities, traditional lectures are still often maintained as the principal method of content delivery. It is inevitable that much of the veterinary curriculum is still likely to be delivered by the traditional large group (>25 students) due to restraints on faculty time, faculty and other facilitator numbers, class size, and practical building restrictions. Therefore, there are some recommendations for making lectures more engaging for students (Brown and Manogue 2001). In particular, there are two aspects that enable effective lecturing. One is introducing an aspect of active learning, and the second is effectively delivering the lecture material. Brown and Manogue (2001), described the different styles of lecturers and what students feel occurs in a weak lecturer's classroom. Box 6.1 describes the qualities to consider for a good lecture, keeping in mind that students learn from lectures by listening, observing, summarizing, and note-taking (Brown and Manogue 2001). This chapter will introduce active learning interventions that can be used in veterinary education and the evidence supporting their use in the veterinary classroom.

Part 2: Lecture Capture

One relatively recent introduction in the classroom, which has been controversial, is the implementation of recorded

---

Box 6.1   Qualities to consider for a good lecture.

- Audibility
- Coherence
- Speed
- Audiovisual aids
- Balance volume of material
- Use of summaries
- Assumption of prior knowledge level and preparation
- Timing
- Summarizing.

Source: Adapted from Brown and Manogue (2001).

lectures. Faculty report concerns about lecture recording reducing student attendance, but this has actually not been supported in the literature. Other concerns include not being conducive to interactive styles of lecturing, intellectual property rights, poor recording quality, and lack of IT support or technological ability of the faculty (Kwiatkowski and Demirbilek 2016). However, advantages of lecture recording include allowing students to watch lectures they would otherwise have missed due to excused absences, the ability to rewatch lectures for exam preparation, assistance for students who are not being taught in their native language, and for students with disabilities (Nkomo and Daniel 2021). Future changes coming to the veterinary classroom, fueled by the issues of decreasing faculty numbers along with increasing student numbers, are opportunities for online courses delivered across institutions that can be used as part of a blended classroom or as a primary method of course delivery (Dooley et al. 2018).

Part 3: Active Learning

Many courses in the veterinary curriculum are team-taught and, as a result, changing course design requires buy-in from multiple faculty and administration. The active learning interventions listed in Box 6.2 can be implemented by individual faculty at the lecture level, giving flexibility to each instructor rather than requiring a full curricular overhaul.

Many active learning strategies have been employed in the veterinary classroom; Box 6.2 lists some that have been reported in the literature (Bucklin et al. 2021), and best lend themselves to integration into a traditional lecture learning

---

Box 6.2   List of examples of active learning.

- Case-based discussion
- Panel discussion
- Simulation exercises
- Audience response polling
- Large group discussion
- Small group discussion
- Self-reflection exercises
- Think–pair–share
- Flipped classroom
- Peer observation and feedback
- Turn and talk
- Pause procedures during lecture
- One minute paper
- Bulleted breaks during lecture
- Gaming
- Group reflection
- Role-playing.

---

environment. The list does not include PBL, team-based learning (TBL), and integrated case-based approaches, which, to be done well, typically require course or curriculum redesign. Such teaching approaches *can* be implemented in individual lectures within a course, but this is often challenging and some, in particular team- and PBL, require students to understand the pedagogical principles behind them to be truly effective. The list also does not include mood induction procedures (e.g., short breaks integrated into the lecture showing funny images or videos). While not defined as active learning per se, these approaches were utilized in a pharmacology course and reported to positively affect students' mood, interest in material, and self-reported understanding of material (Kogan et al. 2018).

Part 4: Classroom Discussion

High-quality classroom discussion is needed to achieve the goals of deep learning and the development of critical thinking skills in students, and many examples of active learning involve classroom discussion. Hines et al. (2005), defined some features of high-quality discussion, including participation of students, students asking insightful questions, accepting criticism and other points of view by creating a safe environment, and ability to adapt to new information.

The instructor's role for such discussions is that of facilitator, which may be unfamiliar, and therefore one key to introduction of group discussion and success is instructor training. Becker et al. (2020), describe an effective faculty training session on delivery of a self-directed, inquiry-based course in human medical education in which the goals for the facilitators were to: provide constructive feedback to enhance the learning environment and improve group process; assist students in developing areas for self-improvement; improve peer to peer teaching; integrate foundational knowledge; create a safe learning environment; and identify learning objective and resources to address knowledge gaps. Facilitator training was enabled by the faculty participating in an example course, using a veterinary topic (neurological horse case). Use of a veterinary example ensured participants were unfamiliar with the content, thus placing them in the position of their students. Feedback from the training session indicated that it was well received by faculty. Students were taught in courses by facilitators trained using this case, and students thought their facilitators were well prepared.

Part 5: Flipped Classroom

The flipped classroom approach is a method where the students complete preparatory material in their own time, while the in-class, face-to-face (F2F) session is dedicated to active learning, typically small or large group discussion. In a flipped classroom, the students are presented with the required course material prior to the F2F session. This may be in the form of narrated Powerpoints™, videos, podcasts, provided reading materials, etc. (Matthew et al. 2019). The in-class session may be small group activities, case-based, labs or practical's, or class discussion (Matthew et al. 2019).

This approach allows for flexible and learner-centered teaching. However, for a flipped classroom to be successful, it requires students to be self-directed learners. As with many classroom interventions that are unfamiliar to the student, effective course delivery will be enabled by giving students clear expectations, consistent feedback, and explaining the rationale of the course (Dooley et al. 2018). This approach can be integrated into one or more sessions within a traditional lecture-based course, which means that not every session need be designed this way.

One concern with implementing the flipped classroom is that preparatory work for a session is overly onerous to the student, therefore care must be taken to balance the course content of both preparatory material and in-class time relative to the credit/course hours. Timing of release of preparatory material is also important, as adequate time must be given for the students to prepare. However, if the goal for the F2F classroom time is group discussion, not releasing case information until the session begins prevents students from working individually ahead of time. For the instructor to evaluate whether students have adequately prepared for the in-class session, a quiz may be delivered before the session begins. Using ARS in this manner allows for either formative or summative assessment and real-time evaluation of students' understanding if the anonymized responses are displayed on the screen for all to see. This may be followed by a period built into the session where the instructor can review areas that the questions and responses have identified the students are struggling in.

In a study comparing a traditional lecture course with small group sessions compared to a flipped classroom in a large preclinical curriculum course titled "Foundations of Animal Health" for undergraduate veterinary students, flipped classroom students had improved grades for a written exam, but not a multiple-choice exam, and student satisfaction was higher with the flipped classroom (Dooley et al. 2018). In this example, preclasswork material for the flipped model included multiple videos and short formative questions with feedback. The in-class session consisted of small group case-based learning (CBL) activities. Challenges reported by the students were that they felt less engaged with the lecturer and lacked the ability to ask questions in real time as their only interaction was via video. Students did appreciate the resources for repeat learning and the ability to rewind and rewatch for parts they needed to digest slower and for exam study. They also appreciated the feedback provided by online learning activities and the interactive nature of the videos (Dooley et al. 2018).

Part 6: Case-Based Learning

CBL can be considered a model of course instruction in its own right, but often it is blended with other forms of active learning or within a traditional lecture-based course (Crowther and Baillie 2016). CBL typically involves the students working through a (preferably real) clinical case with emphasis on developing their clinical reasoning skills.

The process of developing clinical reasoning skills is usually emphasized as the hypothetico-deductive reasoning method. Translated practically for clinicians this involves the following process: problem identification; problem analysis; development of a differential diagnosis list; justification of the list based on lesion, pathophysiology, signalment, and history; diagnostic plan; interpretation of diagnostic tests; refinement of differential list; and treatment plan (Hines et al. 2005). Integration of case-based material into a course also highlights the concept that there is not just one correct answer (Berrian et al. 2021), allows for demonstration of evidence-based veterinary medicine, and gives insight into the teacher's own critical thinking thought processes (Harden and Cosby 2000).

Case-based instruction can be utilized in the classroom in a multitude of ways, with large groups using think–pair–share and ARS (Berrian et al. 2021), small group learning activities (Dooley et al. 2018), group work out of class time followed by in-class discussion delivered either as a computer-based program or on paper (Hines et al. 2005; Krockenberger et al. 2007; Alvarez and Reinhart 2020), or individual work out of class time and turned in for a homework grade.

CBL can also be delivered by low-stakes methods (few or no points assigned), such as audience polling during a traditional lecture (Berrian et al. 2021), or high-stakes methods as part of course assessment (Dooley et al. 2018). One study, for example, used an online case-based module to provide case material for students to write a SOAP (subjective-objective-assessment-plan medical note) that was then assessed (Alvarez and Reinhart 2020). Veterinary students in China preferred integration of case material into a traditional lecture course of histology and had improved exam scores (Li and Chen 2011). And an online case-based program was used in a cardiology elective, where students moved through a case at a pace guided by an instructor, followed by time for small group discussion to answer questions posed (Tayce et al. 2021).

CBL can also be incorporated into clinical years, and involve professional and clinical skills (Malher et al. 2009). Examples of CBL across the veterinary curricula span courses as diverse as pathology (Hines et al. 2005; Krockenberger et al. 2007; Patterson et al. 2007), small animal urinary tract disease (Grauer et al. 2008), one health (Franco-Martínez et al. 2020), and dairy herd consultancy (Malher et al. 2009).

Studies describing CBL in the literature have found that students liked a computer-based program (Hines et al. 2005), although many felt the time invested was high relative to their learning. Additionally, faculty felt that the discussion was not of the quality they anticipated or expected, which indicates that discussion is a skill students need to develop throughout the entire curriculum. Another challenge of CBL for faculty is the time needed to develop cases of the appropriate level that are realistic, although this can be mitigated somewhat by drawing from real-life cases the instructor or colleagues have previously seen.

CBL can be incorporated across all years of the curriculum, with the understanding that clinical reasoning, evidence-based veterinary medicine, and critical thinking skills are key competencies for new graduates and that it takes time to develop them. While clinical students can typically take a case from history to treatment plan and prognosis, a first-year student does not have the skills or knowledge to do so. And regardless of year, complicated referral cases may not be effective as students may get too bogged down in minor problems or bloodwork abnormalities outside of normal ranges.

Where in the curriculum institutions introduce certain courses, e.g., diagnostic imaging and clinical pathology, may influence where diagnostic testing interpretation should be introduced in a CBL session. Current thinking is the "ideal" case is likely one that effectively reinforces previous and current course knowledge and is common enough that students will see it in general practice (Crowther and Baillie 2016). Cases may also be selected to emphasize particular clinical or professional skills; for example, a welfare case or ethical conundrum. Both clinicians and basic science instructors should be involved in developing the case, as well as involved in session facilitation. This ensures that material is reinforced as it is first taught.

Finally, CBL sessions or courses allow for effective horizontal and vertical integration of material. Teaching case-based or other clinical reasoning courses alongside preclinical and clinical courses allows students to understand the relevance of the material they are learning. In addition, it can improve students' professional skills in the areas of communication, teamwork, and leadership (Gordon et al. 2022).

Part 7: Problem-Based Learning

PBL was developed at McMaster University, Canada in their medical school. PBL in its purest form has been described as "student-centered, problem-based, inquiry-based, integrated, collaborative, reiterative, learning" (Newman 2019).

Practically, it is a small group learning technique with a facilitator who uses a clinical case as a starting point to integrate preclinical and clinical knowledge. The exact formation of the student groups is also key to effective PBL development, with the intent to create a diverse mix of genders, cultures, and personalities (Lane 2008). The development of group dynamics and stages (forming, storming, norming, performing, and adjourning) is key to a successful PBL course. The emphasis is on student-led inquiry starting with the development of their own learning objectives.

The process for performing PBL can vary, with some courses utilizing Maastricht's seven-step model and others the eight tasks of PBL (Newman 2019); the eight tasks are shown in Box 6.3. There are several examples of entire veterinary curricula that are PBL, including, for example, Western University of Health Sciences. Other institutions may deliver individual courses via the PBL method, with still others continuing to be delivered in the more traditional lecture format, for example, Cornell University College of Veterinary Medicine.

Training both students and faculty to learn and teach within a PBL course is essential (Lane 2008; Davis 1999). The evidence to support PBL in improving student outcomes, rather than student opinions, is variable, largely due to the varied nature of study outcomes and intervention quality (Newman 2019; Lane 2008).

Part 8: Team-Based Learning

TBL draws on the flipped classroom method for student preparation and delivery of materials; it is a system that allows for small-group active learning with larger numbers of students. The teams (groups) are structured by the instructor to allow for different levels of students in each

---

Box 6.3   8 steps of PBL.

1) Explore the problem: clarify terms and concepts that are not understandable, create hypotheses, identify issues
2) Identify what you know already that is pertinent
3) Identify what you do not know
4) As a group, prioritize learning needs, set learning goals and objectives, allocate resources, members identify which task they will do
5) Engage in a self-directed search for knowledge
6) Return to the group and share your new knowledge effectively so all members learn the information
7) Apply the knowledge; try to integrate the knowledge acquired into a comprehensive explanation
8) Reflect on what has been learned and the process of learning.

group, and the teams remain the same throughout the course. Teamwork is only during class time, and peer evaluation is part of the course. TBL is arranged into preclass preparation, readiness assurance (in-class individual assessment followed by group assessment using the same questions based on the preparatory material), and then group work to solve a problem and whole class discussion (Michaelsen et al. 2004).

The students are provided with learning objectives to guide their preparatory material. The individual readiness assessment test (IRAT) provides an opportunity for each student to demonstrate their level of preparation in a low-stakes situation. This is followed by a team readiness assessment test (TRAT), which allows students to discuss the answers as a group before submitting their final answers. This can be done in hard copy but is primarily being delivered electronically, as the IF-AT cards have been out of print for some time now. Another key aspect is that each group works on the same problem at the same time and reports their findings. There are veterinary institutions where TBL is the primary method of content delivery, such as the University of Arizona, and others where it is utilized exclusively in one course or as part of a course, for example, Texas Tech School of Veterinary Medicine. See Parmelee et al. (2012), for more details on effective delivery of TBL courses in medical education.

In a study investigating TBL use for teaching anatomy, students participating in a focus group reported that TBL allowed for increased feedback, reinforced concepts, and promoted life-long learning. The negative feedback included students' challenges and dislikes about group work (Diamond et al. 2020). Another study reported that peer learning was a positive aspect in a course that included TBL, traditional lectures, and laboratories in a behavior, welfare, and ethics course (Hazel et al. 2013). From the instructor's perspective, TBL classes that include the in-class readiness test also appeared to ensure that class attendance was high and increased faculty enthusiasm for teaching (Hazel et al. 2013). However, there is limited evidence that TBL delivered material results in equivalent or improved outcomes in medical education (Parmelee et al. 2012).

Part 9: Audience Response Systems

ARS have been shown to enhance student engagement, observation, motivation, and reflection (Doucet et al. 2009; Rush et al. 2013). Inserting ARS questions into a lecture around the 15-to-20-minute mark can maintain interest, as students are typically unable to focus well for more than 20 minutes (Gibbs et al. 1987). ARS can be used for formative feedback in real time, or linked to a learning platform for summative assessments. However, the evidence supporting the positive effects of using ARS on short- and long-term retention has been variable (Plant 2007; Doucet et al. 2009; Rush et al. 2013).

ARS technology is widely used in veterinary education. In the literature, the implementation of ARS in veterinary education has been reported for a third-year radiology course (Hecht et al. 2013), small animal medicine, small animal surgery, and food animal courses (Rush et al. 2013), a dermatology course (Plant 2007), a medicine and surgery course (Mariani and Roe 2021), a pharmacology course (Doucet et al. 2009), and an anesthesia course (Duret and Senior 2015).

There are many software companies that provide this service, some of which are cloud-based, both for a fee and free when using a basic model. The variability of systems available ensures that institutions, and even individual faculty, have choices depending on which system works best in their scenario. For all ARS, students use handheld "clickers," their smartphones, tablets, or computers to respond.

ARS have replaced the classic "show of hands" scenario in a large group lecture, and encourages a safe space for students to respond, as responses are typically anonymous and do not require them to speak in public, which can be daunting (Moffett et al. 2014). Faculty most commonly employ ARS to ask multiple choice or short answer/one-word answers to build a word cloud. Questions can be asked at the start of class to assess recall or understanding from previous lectures or may be used to deliver a summative quiz.

For formative assessments, faculty can assess student understanding in real time. Additional time can be built into the lecture plan to allow for review of any material that may be needed based on student responses. ARS can also be used for students to pose anonymous questions to the teacher, again providing a safe space to ask questions. It can also be paired or grouped with other active learning interventions, including think–pair–share, CBL, and small group discussions.

ARS may also benefit faculty, as real-time session evaluations can be delivered; this allows faculty to adapt future sessions without having to wait for whole course evaluations that may be time delayed. Concerns with using technology in the classroom are that students may become distracted as they have their devices out to use as part of the class and the time required for faculty to learn the system, which varies between products (Duret and Senior 2015; Doucet et al. 2009).

Part 10: Gaming and Other Active Learning Strategies

Games can be incorporated into the classroom to emphasize the experiencing and doing parts of Kolb's learning cycle (Buur et al. 2013). Games can be custom-designed card or board games where students play the game in small groups (Buur et al. 2013), or computer-based games (Mauldin Pereira et al. 2018). Examples in veterinary education include card games for learning antimicrobial drugs and hypersensitivity reactions, and a board game for one health disease outbreaks (Buur et al. 2013). Computer (CD rom)-based interactive activities for animal health outbreaks have also been described (Conrad et al. 2007). Second Life gaming is where students take on an avatar and interact with other students in their group in an "island." Second life has been used to develop clinical reasoning skills in a clinical environment (Mauldin Pereira et al. 2018), and in disaster management (Bissett et al. 2013).

Geocaching apps have also been used to teach clinical reasoning skills using neurology cases (Nessler et al. 2021). Virtual reality has been used in clinical rotations and small group sessions, but could also be used in larger, classroom-based educational settings (McCaw et al. 2021). One example of virtual reality is a virtual web-based dairy herd (based on a real herd) where veterinary students interact with a program to "run" their own dairy herd to learn dairy management (Calsamiglia et al. 2020). Other methods of active learning interventions reported in the veterinary literature include seminar learning (Spruijt et al. 2013), and project-based learning for a veterinary anatomy course (Borroni et al. 2021).

Part 11: Summary

In summary, classroom learning is evolving toward incorporation of active learning. However, this does not mean that the lecture model of knowledge delivery in the veterinary curriculum is gone. Active learning spans from parts of individual lectures, individual teaching session activities, to whole course or curriculum design. Active learning can be high or low-tech, making it easy to implement for a variety of courses. The goal of classroom learning in whichever method of delivery is to ensure that students are interactive, engaging, and employing higher-order learning skills.

Section 2: Laboratory and Clinical Skills Instruction

Dawn M. Spangler and Lynda MJ. Miller

Part 1: Overview

The course director for a clinical skills program plays an integral role in the progression of a veterinary learner to a day-one competent veterinarian upon graduation. While mentoring is still important and necessary for the newly graduated veterinarian in clinical practice, they should have the knowledge and skills to think and act independently to provide basic medical care to their patients. To achieve this outcome, the role of course director encompasses a wide range of tasks to implement and maintain a successful program year after year. Aside from the obvious focus on the delivery of approved curriculum, the role is broad and involves duties such as determination of model and live animal needs for laboratories, oversight and development of assessments, oversight of lab leaders, training of instructors, and supervision of students.

Part 2: Delivery of Curriculum

First and foremost, the course director's role in the delivery of curriculum involves working with the faculty and curriculum designers to ensure that the content of material delivered in the laboratories aligns with the didactic curriculum and core educational competencies of the institution. Horizontal and vertical alignment of the curriculum are necessary to enable the students to better assimilate coursework rather than the random delivery of concepts throughout the curriculum. D'Souza et al. (2018), saw added student acceptability and satisfaction with an integrated curriculum.

Modeled after competency-based human medical education, veterinary medical education competencies were constructed by the American Association of Veterinary Medical Colleges Competency-Based Veterinary Education (AAVMC CBVE) working group which was assembled in 2015. These competencies were designed to "prepare graduates for professional careers by confirming their ability to meet the needs of animals and the expectations of society" (Molgaard et al. 2018, n.p.). The AAVMC CBVE framework design includes nine domains of competence with 32 sub competencies. In addition to the domains and competencies, the group developed EPAs, defined as "an essential task of a discipline that a learner can be trusted to perform with limited supervision in a given context and regulatory requirements, once sufficient competence has been demonstrated" (Molgaard et al. 2018, n.p.). The competencies developed encompass all facets of veterinary medicine with clinical skills and EPAs woven throughout. Sub competencies utilized by an institution can be tailored to meet specific program goals. Skill-based competencies and EPAs can and should be taught during the preclinical curriculum to enable the learner to further practice and refine these skills while completing their training in the clinical year versus postgraduation.

To further support the need for teaching these skills in the curriculum, the American Veterinary Medical

Association Council on Education (AVMA COE) policy requires institutions to meet certain educational standards of performance to maintain accreditation. Accreditation standard 11 (AVMA COE 2021) requires veterinary programs to assess students both formatively and summatively, and collect and analyze the data based on nine competencies, which are notably similar to the AAVMC CBVE domains. This data is then to be used to improve the program which will keep the institution's curriculum current and relevant to new practices and research in the veterinary field. This standard also ensures that the students are held accountable for their learning and performance during their tenure in the program. The standard states that a remediation program must be in place for those students who are found to lack competence which may include repetition of a course(s) or additional training and assessment in a specific skill area. The course director takes the responsibility to see that the curriculum stays current with the core competencies and that data collected is used to continually improve the program.

Part 3: Animal Use in Laboratories

While it is important to utilize models for teaching and consider the 3Rs – replacement, reduction, and refinement – to minimize animal use (Hubrecht and Carter 2019; Nagy et al. 2016), there are certain skills that are more meaningful and better learned when incorporating a live animal into a laboratory session. Laboratories that teach skills such as physical exam, phlebotomy, the neurologic exam, and the orthopedic exam are best taught using live animals. Students practice these skills with instructor oversight, which affords them the opportunity to ask questions and receive constructive feedback on their technique to help them achieve proficiency. This also gives students more occasions to practice and hone their handling and restraint skills.

Because use of live animals is critical to a veterinary student's learning, the course director must ensure that the live animal requirements can be met for the labs. Live animals that may be used include university-owned animals, privately-owned animals, and shelter-owned animals. Privately-owned animals should be reserved for labs that are noninvasive, such as a physical exam lab, rather than an invasive one, such as a phlebotomy lab. When using privately-owned animals, to protect the institution and ensure the owner understands how the animal will be used, it is important to have the owner sign a waiver and verify their behavior and vaccine status.

It is important to note that the use of animals in educational programs requires oversight by the Institutional Animal Care and Use Committee (IACUC) as directed by The Animal Welfare Act and Regulations (AWA;

USDA-APHIS n.d.). The AWA is a law regulated by the United States Department of Agriculture Animal and Plant Inspection Services (USDA APHIS). The regulations are found in the "Blue Book," which outlines these regulations as they pertain to animal use in "research, teaching, testing, exhibition, transport" (USDA-APHIS n.d., n.p.). Any tasks that are not medically necessary require an approved animal use protocol from the IACUC.

All laboratories utilizing animals must have a written protocol that includes information such as a literature review for alternatives, animal housing, training of staff involved, and the step-by-step procedure(s) that will be performed including the frequency of occurrence. For example, a laboratory using dogs for an anesthesia induction would need to have every step from physical exam to recovery and any drugs being used in the animal use protocol for the IACUC to review and approve. With multiple laboratories using live animals, it is ideal to write an IACUC protocol specific to the species being used. For example, laboratories involving dogs or cats would be included within the same protocol, but horses and cattle would be on different protocols. While the AWA does not cover all species (e.g., rodents) or owned animals, most institutions still require protocols to be approved for their use to ensure the humane use and general welfare of all animals used for teaching are maintained. The course director is generally in the best position to write and submit the protocols yearly due to their intricate involvement in the maintenance of the laboratory's objectives; they are also most knowledgeable about the need for live animals used in laboratories for the upcoming academic year. An important responsibility for the course director is to continue to review the literature for alternatives to living animal use and be actively involved in the development of new models and educational research to support the 3Rs (Picture 6.1).

Part 4: Models

Without models, teaching clinical skills would be a very challenging task. Psychomotor skills are learned very differently than facts and require "deliberate practice, which is defined as repetitive performance of psychomotor skills with rigorous assessment, specific feedback, and progressive increase in level of difficulty" (Hunt et al. 2022, p. 53). Models in the laboratory give the veterinary learner the ability to practice the psychomotor skills necessary for them to be competent upon graduation. Models also help simulate real-life situations that students may encounter as practitioners, such as a patient who has coded and requires CPR. A canine mannikin is commercially available that enables students to do chest compressions, intubate, give respirations, and place an IV catheter. This is an excellent model to use in a clinical skills lab; one that gives students the opportunity to practice the

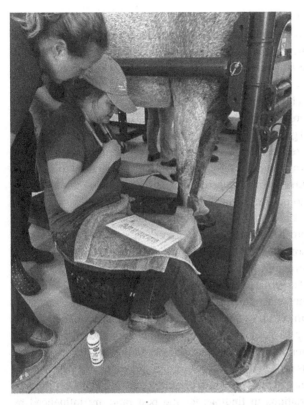

Picture 6.1 Student learning to use the ultrasound to image tendons in live horse.

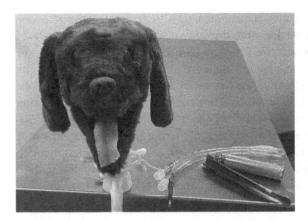

Picture 6.2 K9 Intubation Trainer from RescueCritters! ® Brand.

necessary clinical skills, as well as those related to communication and working as a team member. CPR is high stress because it is a life-or-death situation, so using this model to practice a code can help students be more confident and prepared when faced with the situation in real life.

Models can be bought from vendors who specialize in medical models, or they can be created within your own laboratory. Purchasing models from vendors can be quite costly and could have a significant impact on the budget. For this reason, institutions often develop and build many of their own models, which can significantly reduce the cost of the program, while producing an acceptable model to accomplish the teaching task. Both low-fidelity and high-fidelity models can be incorporated into the curriculum, although Massoth et al. (2019), state that high-fidelity models are not superior to low-fidelity models and can lead to student overconfidence. The course director should work with lab leaders to identify or create models that can be successfully used as part of the course (Picture 6.2).

Part 5: Assessments

As directed by the AVMA COE, assessment of veterinary students is required for institutions to maintain their accreditation. Assessments enable instructors to gauge the progress and learning of their students. They help course

directors identify students who may be struggling to master a skill or practicing a skill incorrectly. Identification of such students allows for provision of additional resources and/or instruction to the learner to help improve their skills. Assessments enhance student motivation and achievement (Woytek 2005), in the classroom and they are more engaged in their learning (Näsström et al. 2021).

Assessments in clinical skills courses can be both formative and summative, with formative generally focusing on the individual tasks and summative being more cumulative. An example of a formative assessment in a skills-based laboratory is a student performing a two-handed surgical hand tie or safely picking up a horse foot to use hoof testers for no grade. Feedback should be provided immediately after the skill has been completed, and viewed as an opportunity for the instructor to provide both positive feedback and corrective feedback that the student can use to improve their skill moving forward.

Providing high-quality feedback is critical to the student's learning. Cantillon and Sargeant (2008), indicated that students receiving high-quality feedback can cause students to over self-evaluate while students receiving high-quality negative feedback were related to a more accurate self-evaluation of their performance. They additionally note that positive remarks give the student the opportunity to reflect on their performance and improve their skill (Cantillon and Sargeant 2008). Therefore, it is important to help instructors understand the need to provide high-quality negative feedback, as this can help prevent students from being overconfident in their skills.

Other formative assessments that can be used in clinical skills laboratories are quizzes, case-based assignments, and group projects. Each can be employed as active learning exercise where students engage more deeply with the material, which can contribute significantly to a student's ability to retain information (Wolff et al. 2015). Summative laboratory assessments may be written (exams, quizzes, identification of items, etc.) or active, as with an objective structured clinical exam (OSCE). Both categories of assessments are more explicitly discussed in other chapters of this text (see Chapters 10–12).

While clinical skills are not specifically assessed on the North American Veterinary Licensing Exam (NAVLE), labs and content should be designed to develop critical thinking skills and reinforce concepts and facts learned in the classroom during the lecture-based coursework. Repetition of facts and skills will help the student retain information, which will help them when taking the exam during their final year of veterinary school (Augustin 2014).

Part 6: The Role of the Lab Leader

The course director's role is not to teach every lab and skill in the curriculum, rather, it is to identify subject matter experts within the institution and coordinate these individuals to lead laboratories in the skills curriculum. Lab leaders are pivotal in developing and delivering the content of the laboratory(s) and formative assessments of the skills the students learn. The lab leader(s) should work closely with the course director to determine the appropriate learning objectives for the laboratory and to ensure content is aligned with the curriculum. To maintain consistency from year to year, it is advised to have the lab leader develop a written plan that includes presentation materials, supply lists, and assessment strategies. Putting a written lab plan in place protects the course in the event there is faculty turnover or another instructor is needed to lead due to an emergency or other acute situation. It is helpful to have a dedicated support staff to maintain models, order supplies, and set up/break down laboratories.

Part 7: Student Preparation

Limiting the amount of pre-lab preparation materials students are expected to review is advised. As with all professional students, veterinary students carry heavy course loads and a large amount of prework may result in students not completing it prior to the session, which leaves them unprepared and facilitates poor learning. Alternatively, because many students enjoy being in a laboratory more than sitting in a classroom, they may choose to concentrate their efforts on preparing for laboratories, to the detriment of their lecture-based courses. Thus, consistency among lab leaders should be maintained; with the guidance of a course director who sets a prep:lab time ratio, lab leaders will be better able to manage the amount of material they present.

As students are learning new skills, it is important to present skills in the most consistent manner possible. While there is an accepted way to do most skills, seasoned veterinarians often develop preferential methods for performing some tasks, especially surgical tasks. When students hear these different methods during a laboratory, it creates frustration and often negatively affects their attitude toward learning the skill. Therefore, the lab leader should have a pre-lab meeting with all instructors teaching in the laboratory to review the skill and ensure that all instructors are teaching the skills using consistent techniques. Although there may be more than one way to complete a skill, the initial goal should be for students to achieve competency in one correct method to avoid confusion and frustration.

To provide an effective and efficient laboratory session, the course director must be cognizant of the instructor-to-student ratio needed during scheduling. This ratio will vary depending on the difficulty of the task being taught and whether there is use of live animals versus models in the session. Dubrowski and MacRae (2006), determined the optimal instructor-to-student ratio at 1 : 4 when teaching suturing skills. While this might be the ideal number, it can be difficult to obtain a ratio that is low due to faculty and staff limitations. Hunt et al. (2021), found that "good educational outcomes may be reached with a 1 : 10 instructor-to-student ratio or, potentially, fewer instructors, depending on the educational aids present in the laboratory and students' prior level of experience" (p. 556), when teaching suturing skills on models. Variations in findings for the best ratio are influenced by many factors, including experience level of the student and resources required and available to teach the skills.

Part 8: Rater/Grader Training

The course director also plays a key role in training that focuses on delivery of feedback and rater training for the OSCE. The in-lab feedback should include defining a "hawk" (harsh) versus a "dove" (soft) rater and ensure that the instructors are providing detailed high-quality positive and negative feedback that is fair across students. It is common for instructors to neglect giving positive feedback and this can negatively impact a student's learning and motivation. DePasque and Tricomi (2015) research "suggests that motivation modulates neural responses to performance-related feedback and that changes in motivation facilitate processes in areas that support learning and memory" (p. 175). High-quality feedback is important for students to assess their progress as they proceed with self-directed learning, as Marteau et al. (1990), discovered in their study, which demonstrated that repeating skills unsupervised and without feedback increases confidence but does not improve competence. For these reasons, rater training should be completed yearly for all instructors participating in assessments, particularly for those who support OSCEs. Such training should emphasize the fair grading of students, adherence to the rubrics, and assessing down the middle rather than being a "hawk" or a "dove." It is critical to reinforce consistency between raters and provide guidance to those who have not previously functioned as raters. The course director can also ensure that the raters understand expectations with regard to prompting and feedback during an exam.

Part 9: Student Supervision

The clinical skills course director plays a vital role in the development of the veterinary learner into a well-rounded professional. In addition to learning hands-on skills, both with models and live animals in the laboratories, students should also be addressing deficiencies in their professionalism throughout their courses. Expectations should be set at the onset of their schooling regarding attendance, tardiness, dress, and communication; these expectations should be demonstrated and assessed during their laboratory sessions as well. Students generally take these expectations seriously when there are consequences for their actions, such as an impact on their grades. Therefore, it is up to the course director to establish what those consequences entail to help shape the veterinary learner for their professional career.

To ensure optimal learning opportunities, it is highly recommended that all laboratory sessions are mandatory. Repeated absences by a student will prevent the progression of their skills because so many clinical skills build upon one another. Thus, if early labs are missed, students may struggle to obtain the skill level of their peers. In a busy program, it can be difficult to schedule makeup labs for students who have legitimate excused absences, but in these cases, the course director should work with administration to determine an acceptable period a student can be absent without limiting their ability to pass the course.

The course director must address academic deficiencies in a timely manner to provide resources, such as counselors or tutors, to help the student progress and achieve success. There is often a wide range of skill sets between students, whether due to differences in experiences, psychomotor, fine, and gross motor skills, or other reasons. Regardless, it is necessary for the course director to have an open line of communication with the lab leaders and instructors, as they spend many hours working with the students and may be better able to identify deficiencies early on. This gives the course director an opportunity to address the concerns with the student and refer them for additional help if necessary.

Section 3: Teaching Personal Finances

Erik H. Hofmeister

Personal finances are those aspects of finances that are directly affected by an individual (or family), as opposed to business finances, which affect a company. Since money is the mechanism society uses to exchange goods and services, it is an essential aspect of everyone's life. Finances have significant psychological impact, as financial stress can lead to psychological distress (Hafen et al. 2022). Veterinary students continue to accrue greater degrees of debt than other health professions students, with recent graduates having an approximate 2 : 1 debt-to-income ratio (Bain et al. 2020).

Depending on the institution, median student debt ranges from US\$ 80,000 to US\$ 240,000, and pre-veterinary students may decide to attend veterinary school even in the face of a massive tuition and debt burden (Britt-Lutter and Heckman 2020). Twenty-eight percent of veterinary students with a credit card carry a credit card balance (Carr and Greenhill 2015). Although veterinary students report having a high degree of confidence in their personal finance knowledge, their actual knowledge is quite poor (Jones et al. 2019).

Given these deficiencies, veterinary education programs have identified the importance of teaching personal finances in the curriculum (Lane and Strand 2008). There is a significant relationship between financial literacy and debt levels and retirement planning (Lusardi and Tufano 2009). Unfortunately, simply providing general personal finance education may not lead to behavior change (Fernandes et al. 2014). In one study, there was no difference in financial knowledge between medical students who had and had not received counseling or information (Jayakumar et al. 2017). And in general, education does not seem to affect short-term financial behaviors, such as budgeting and timely debt payments (Wagner and Walstad 2019). In contrast, there is evidence that long-term behaviors, such as retirement planning, can be influenced by education (Wagner and Walstad 2019; Poon et al. 2022; Bar-Or et al. 2018).

An effective educational intervention for personal finance needs to be timely, repetitive, accessible, engaging, and use technology effectively (President's Advisory Council on Financial Capability 2013). Timing education with the students' needs is also important and helps connect the information with action (Jones et al. 2019). Elective and required core courses, individual lectures within existing courses, weekend programs, and a series of weekly workshops have all been used to provide personal finance education (Grewal and Sweeney 2021; Poon et al. 2022; Bar-Or et al. 2018; Jones et al. 2019; Sewell and Rogers 2022). There is some evidence that even providing personalized, "just-in-time" education achieved behavior change in 59% of veterinary students (Jones et al. 2019).

There is no consensus regarding the curriculum for personal finances that should be taught to veterinary students. However, some suggested topics are listed in Table 6.1, keeping in mind that suitable topics likely depend upon where a student is in their training. For example, veterinary school

Table 6.1 Proposed curricular topics for personal finance education to veterinary students and house officers.

General topic	Specific topics	General topic	Specific topics
Basics	Emergency Fund	Retirement planning	Expense Tracking
	Choosing a Financial Advisor		Safe Withdrawal Rates
	Time Value of Money		Tax-Deferred Accounts
	Credit Rating		Tax-Free Accounts
Taxes	Progressive Tax System		Social Security
	State Taxes		Pensions
	FICA and Medicare Taxes		Taxable Account
	Capital Gain Taxes	Managing debt	Reducing Debt
Budgeting	Expenses (housing, food, transportation, pets, etc.)		Refinancing Debt
			Repayment Strategies
	Creating a Budget	Student loans	Repayment Options
	Applying a Budget		Federal versus Private
Interest	Simple Interest		Debt : Income Ratio
	Compound Interest		Estimated Repayment Time
	Amortization		Tax on Forgiveness Plans
Credit cards	Costs	Capital purchases	Planning/Saving
	Interest Expenses		House
	Penalties		Business
	Cash Advances		Auto
	Fringe Benefits (miles, points, etc.)		Loans/Mortgages
Insurance	Disability	Scholarships	Application
	Life		Availability
	Malpractice		Taxes
	Health	Family contributions	Spouse IRA
	Auto		Spouse Insurance Coverage
	Home		Education Payment Planning
	Umbrella		529 Plans
	Avoiding Whole Life	Employment	Enrolling in Retirement Accounts
Savings	Bucket Strategy		Noncompete Clauses
	Bank Accounts (checking, saving, CDs)	Negotiation	Contracts
	Banks versus Money Market Accounts versus Credit Unions	Employment benefits	Insurance (health, malpractice, disability)
	Cash Flow Management		Retirement Plans
	Writing Checks		Vacation
	Debit Cards		Sick Leave
Investing	Risk Return	Psychology	Bias
	Investing versus Speculation		Barriers to Decision-Making
	Stocks		Evidence versus Emotion
	Index Investing		Market Timing
	Investment Fees		Pay Off Debt versus Invest
	Bonds		Delayed Gratification
	Real Estate		Life Values
			Simple Living
			Lifestyle Creep

applicants would benefit most from psychology, budgeting, student loans, scholarships, and simple living. Veterinary students would additionally benefit from learning about interest and managing debt. And as students approach graduation, taxes, insurance, savings, investing, retirement planning, capital purchases, employment benefits, contract negotiation, and employment topics become important. Interns and residents need specialized advice for managing student loans, particularly if they are pursuing Public Service Loan Forgiveness.

Educational activities around personal finance should be as individualized and engaging as possible. Helping students address their specific personal challenges regarding finances should be a hallmark of teaching activities. Having students participate, when their knowledge may be quite low and given the challenge of talking about money in the culture of the United States, may be difficult. This can often be mitigated by being transparent about one's own finances, encouraging an open environment, and ensuring a nonjudgmental attitude.

Small class sizes may also facilitate interaction and openness. Some suggested assignments and activities are in Table 6.2. These assignments can be completed by students

Table 6.2 Assignments related to personal finance.

Budget	Students create a budget for their household and practice applying it for at least one month
Net worth	Students calculate their net worth
Repayment plan	Students create a loan repayment plan
Reflection	Students reflect on what they have learned and how it will impact them moving forward
Online discussion	Students participate in online discussion forums with questions posed by the instructor
Quiz	Instructor-made or external (e.g., FINRA Financial Literacy Quiz)
Expense tracking	Track all expenses for three months
Financial goals	Develop and reflect on personal goals
Investor policy statement	Create an IPS
Credit card comparison	Evaluate the average percentage rate, how interest is calculated based on average daily balance, fees, punitive interest rate, rebates or frequent miles available, and versatility
Debt reduction	Summarize all debts and practice applying debt snowball techniques to the balances
Tax return	Complete a tax return as if a newly graduated doctor or a doctor who had been in practice for some time

individually or in a group and can be graded, done for a completion grade, or be ungraded, minimizing the burden on faculty instructors to grade them. Students may also select assignments that are most relevant to them, allowing their content to be personalized to their individual financial circumstances. For example, some students without student loan debt may not see the point in completing a student loan repayment plan but may be interested in comparing renting versus buying a house.

An ideal outcome goal for teaching students personal finance is that they will take control of their money and make decisions that enhance their financial stability and health. Given the breadth of topics available, education efforts need to be focused on problems that are most pertinent to students at the time. Changing behaviors is challenging, but education is an essential foundation and is associated with financial literacy (Lusardi and Tufano 2009). A wide variety of educational interventions are available, and any effort is better than no effort to improve students' financial knowledge.

Section 4: Including Cultural Humility, Cultural Competency, and Cultural Fluency in the Veterinary Medical Curriculum

Lisa M. Greenhill, Sraavya M. Polisetti, and Kendall P. Young

Part 1: Changing Demographics

There has always been a significant need for diversity, equity, and inclusion (DEI) content within the veterinary curriculum. content should be seen as fundamental to professional and skill development, but also a notable contributor to an inclusive institutional climate, work environment, positive health outcomes, and community engagement. Continued demographic shifts in the US and abroad also demonstrate a need for greater attention and commitment to preparing new veterinarians for work in far more diverse spaces than ever before.

For example, although the most recent United States Census marked a slowdown in total population growth, the data revealed much greater racial and ethnic diversity than in previous census data. The country's primary growth remains in communities of color with individuals identifying as multiracial growing by 276%, while the American White population declined by nearly 9% between 2010 and 2020 (US Census Bureau 2023).

These changes are reflected in an increasingly diverse complement of DVM professional students. In 2000, the cumulative representation of students who identified as non-White sat at only 8.4%; today, the percentage is 23.2% (AAVMC 2022). Similarly, the percentage of underrepresented faculty has doubled during the same period. While there is still much work to be done with respect to the relative lack of diversity writ large (the profession is estimated to be only 10–15% non-White), colleges of veterinary medicine are increasingly committed to recruiting, admitting, and educating increasing numbers of Black, Indigenous, and other People of Color (BIPOC) and creating pathways to similar growth among their faculty ranks.

Part 2: Changing Relationships with the Owners/Pet Parents/Caregivers

BIPOC individuals and families continue to own pets at a lower rate than their White counterparts (AVMA n.d.); however, there is evidence that racialized minorities own a wide variety of animals as do individuals from lower-income brackets. Pet ownership in these communities has long been assumed to be very different, suggesting that BIPOC owners are less likely to seek out veterinary services for their animals and fundamentally have a different kind of human–animal bond than their White counterparts.

The reality is that seeking veterinary medical services is often hindered by "structural barriers embedded with racial inequalities" (Decker et al. 2018, p. 1). Such barriers include but are not limited to housing discrimination, sexual orientation identity-based discrimination, racism, and economic inequality (Applebaum et al. 2021). These barriers often result in members of marginalized communities making difficult decisions about food, housing, and other necessities so that they can maintain ownership of their animals in the face of persistent marginalization. There is no difference in racial/ethnic demographics in willingness to seek out care for animals (Park et al. 2021), and when structural barriers are removed, there is no racial or ethnic difference in veterinary service-seeking behaviors.

What does this mean for the teaching of veterinary medicine? It means that even with the growth in racial and ethnic diversity among students and professionals, there is a need to ensure that new veterinary graduates are culturally competent and aware of the myriad of barriers that historically marginalized populations experience in seeking out care for their animals. Newly minted veterinarians (and seasoned professionals for that matter) should be competent at working in increasingly diverse practice settings and some of the cultural and interpersonal challenges that naturally arise in these settings.

Continued reliance on increasing various kinds of diversity in order to overcome the barriers to veterinary care is shortsighted in terms of cultural competence; this solution assumes that veterinarians with marginalized identities are inherently culturally competent. Increased diversity simply increases the likelihood of more culturally relevant care for communities that are represented in that diversity, but increased diversity cannot ensure that *all* new veterinarians are equipped to meet the needs of a changing society. Further expecting professionals from historically underrepresented and marginalized backgrounds to exclusively shoulder the burden of meeting those population needs absolves a large part of the profession from collectively working to reduce barriers to veterinary medical care. In short, everyone must learn how to work interculturally.

The profession has a greater responsibility to the animal-owning public to deliver culturally competent care that is also underpinned by a constant quest for cultural humility at the individual level.

Part 3: What Should New Graduates Know?

To meet current and future client expectations, new veterinary graduates should have a range of measurable skills related to DEI. From a practical perspective, new graduates should have a basic understanding of the ways in which the lived experiences of clients shape their relationship with and decision-making regarding their animals. There should be a sociological understanding of the ways in which policies and procedures may limit physical access to veterinary medical services, present barriers to affording such care, or even how such things shape the ability of individuals to own an animal.

Often, curriculum efforts related to DEI have centered on good communication strategies and the driver of being good professionals. This is and should remain an important part of the curriculum; however, it is also important that future veterinary professionals understand why such strategies are necessary. There is a greater likelihood of adherence to positive communication strategies if individuals understand how sociocultural and demographic characteristics shape approaches to medical care decision-making. These understandings reposition communication strategies as an output of understanding rather than simply good talk. Examples of such understandings might include the willingness to bridge communication gaps caused by language dialects and idioms, the use of digital language tools, de-escalation techniques, and knowing when to refer cases to another veterinarian when the relationship is unsalvageable.

At the center of so much of veterinary education is problem-solving and new graduates should be able to apply those skills beyond clinical problems presented in clinical settings. Veterinary professionals must show an ability and willingness to meet clients where they are. Referrals to supportive services, and the ability to consider clinical climate – how do clients feel in this space? How do employees truly feel here? Do compensation packages reflect a practice that believes in diversity and inclusion? How do you know?

From a much broader perspective, the inclusion of DEI content in the veterinary medicine curriculum relies on the development of three interconnected competencies: cultural humility, cultural competence, and cultural fluency. Cultural humility is often described as an ongoing process that emphasizes openness, self-awareness, and reciprocity of knowledge in differing communities with sensitivity to that community's cultural context (Campinha-Bacote 2019). Although some may consider it as somewhat of an intrinsic mindset, cultural humility can be developed through the teaching of certain key "building blocks" (Habashy and Cruz 2021), which are discussed in more detail below. Cultural competence is commonly defined as "a set of consistent behaviors, attitudes, and policies that enable a system, agency or individual to work within a cross-cultural context or situation effectively" (Cross 1989; Watt et al. 2016).

While cultural humility is more process-focused, cultural competence is outcomes-focused and institutionally supported. Cultural competence requires education from cultural mentors, training to identify unconscious biases, and anti-racism training, without perpetuating stereotypes. Developing cultural fluency helps a student adapt to new cultural situations. While a student may be an expert in one cultural context, it is likely that they will be a novice in another. Cultural fluency utilizes guidance from mentors and prior expertise to easily transition into new cultural contexts (Peisachovich 2015). Cultural humility, cultural competence, and cultural fluency describe the "who, what, and how" necessary for a student to be able to engage with their community in a way that includes DEI principles.

Part 4: Cultural Humility

A crucial aspect of cultural humility is maintaining an attitude of openness and non-judgment toward becoming familiar with new cultural environments. Cultural humility is often observed as a life-long commitment to learning and reciprocal partnership with members of the new cultural community (Campinha-Bacote 2019). There are several frameworks through which students can develop cultural humility, but there are a few key points that overlap. Self-evaluation and identification of personal biases are widely considered integral to developing the open, empathic attitude needed to practice cultural humility (Masters et al. 2019). Students must be willing to cultivate multiple perspectives within themselves. They should also be able to identify which personally held "truths" are the result of a cultural influence and *unconscious* bias and

are not necessarily true among other cultures (Habashy and Cruz 2021). Recognition of areas of ignorance as well as inviting collaboration from members of the cultural community is equally important. In fact, it is likely that an individual client is more likely to be an expert in their specific cultural context than the practitioner (Habashy and Cruz 2021).

It is just as important for a veterinarian to consider the experiences, boundaries, and cultural knowledge of their client when developing treatment plans as it is for a client to follow the agreed-upon plan. Additionally, service providers should make themselves aware of a client's personal preferences and choices and develop plans that respect them (Masters et al. 2019). The final key element in developing cultural humility is resilience and adaptability (Masters et al. 2019), especially when faced with ambiguity or personal ignorance (Habashy and Cruz 2021). During the process of self-evaluation, a student will likely identify many areas of cultural ignorance, or instances where the current method of education will not be sufficient to fully understand the cultural context. Students should be able to recognize when a topic is outside their level of expertise or beyond the limitations of their institution. The ability to practice self-empathy and openness in these situations will help foster resiliency and allow students and practitioners to better adapt to new cultural contexts.

Part 5: Cultural Competence

Cultural competence can be best developed through the institutional implementation of policies, guidance, and education to help individuals practice the necessary skills for competence in real-world settings. A culturally competent student can help to remove health inequities between groups, while a lack of competence among practitioners during their client interactions results in a lower quality of care and worse health outcomes (Watt et al. 2016). Important aspects to consider while educating for cultural competency include the recognition of potential internal and external barriers to cross-cultural communication and care. Often veterinarians claim to be knowledgeable about culturally competent practices but express difficulty engaging with clients from different cultures (Shepherd et al. 2019). New graduates should understand the need to utilize resources, such as interpreters or cultural mentors from the community to enhance their own competency levels, as opposed to shifting the work to avoid personal discomfort.

It is also important to be aware of different cultural practices and acknowledge that alternative cultural approaches to healthcare can and should be considered and incorporated into existing Western methods of care (Shepherd et al. 2019). Additionally, institutions should support the importance of cultural competence by incorporating competency frameworks and utilizing the expertise of cultural mentors because individuals are often unable to recognize personal biases in professional settings. Training can be helpful to help a practitioner apply intersectional frameworks to a clinical situation; however, care must be taken to avoid perpetuating myths or stereotypes about other communities. Educators, students, and practitioners should refer to the expertise of cultural mentors and allow their guidance to develop relationships with the communities in consideration (Watt et al. 2016).

Part 6: Cultural Fluency

While cultural humility and cultural competence represent one's awareness of and ability to incorporate and respect the practices of different cultures, cultural fluency is the ability to adapt to and gain expertise in new cultural contexts. The main methods of developing cultural fluency are familiarity with the levels of proficiency, awareness of the continuum of regression and progression through those levels, and the importance of instructor guidance and experiential learning to effectively transition through the levels of proficiency (Peisachovich 2015). Proficiency in cultural fluency exists on a continuum from novice to expert. Progression along the continuum is "multidirectional and dependent on the social, cultural, or sociocultural context of a situation" (Peisachovich 2015, p. 53). The novice end of the spectrum is only able to follow predetermined rules and guidelines. They utilize a step-by-step method of problem-solving and have limited ability to conceptualize unfamiliar outcomes. Experts are defined as practitioners who can intuitively and automatically respond to a situation (Peisachovich 2015).

When developing cultural fluency, it is important to understand that not everyone will regress to a novice level in new cultural contexts. Over time, it is likely that gaining expertise will allow a student to adapt more easily. Even if one is considered an expert, there will likely still be a regression in new situations, but building the skill of cultural fluency will reduce the time it takes to transition through proficiency levels in new cultural contexts. This increased proficiency will help to promote a shared understanding with the members of the new culture (Broughten et al. 2021). Ultimately, for a student to effectively develop expertise and adaptability, they need instructors to provide guidance to smoothly transition through the levels of proficiency. Learning environments should generate situations where students need to utilize their knowledge with discretion and develop a way to see "the bigger picture" in a situation. Strengthening this judgment through experiential learning will help a student adapt to new cultural contexts,

instead of just memorizing predetermined cultural norms (Peisachovich 2015).

The development of these competencies relies on the creation of an educational environment that supports personal exploration, learning, and growth about oneself in society. Much of this work is about personal development – identifying and understanding conscious and unconscious biases, personal values, empathy, and compassion for both the animal and the client. This personal development leads to a cultivated thirst for specific areas of knowledge that create scaffolding for cultural humility, competence, and fluency. It is understandably a challenge to consider how and where to fit such personal work in such a demanding curriculum.

Much like their human medical counterparts, new veterinary graduates should be on the path to developing an adequate level of cultural fluency or an understanding of the sociocultural and demographic characteristics of marginalized and/or minority populations. Such development can be demonstrated by asking clients, for example, whether spiritual faith has an impact on veterinary care decisions. Other examples might include whether a family is unwilling to euthanize because of cultural beliefs or cultural norms around how to care for the elderly, humans, and animals alike. New graduates should also be well on their way to successfully navigating potentially conflictual conversations about the importance of meat protein in animal nutrition to vegan pet owners.

This may sound like more than the veterinary curricula are traditionally designed to handle; there also is the reality that many veterinary faculty may not be equipped to deliver this content within the curriculum. Both positions may be true, and Colleges of Veterinary Medicine may elect to modify admissions requirements to require prerequisite coursework that creates a baseline from which the professional program can continue competency development. What is increasingly clear, however, is that it is critical that new graduates achieve an entry-level of cultural competence, fluency, and humility prior to entering the workforce.

Part 7: Methodologies for Inclusion

Lecture

At most institutions, lecture remains a significant instructional approach in the early years of the professional veterinary curriculum. It certainly can be used for teaching cultural fluency and humility with positive effects. Over the last two decades, veterinary faculty have leaned into lectures, usually offered by guests with personal experiences or expertise on DEI content, in practice management, and professional overview courses. Some schools have created curriculum requirements that students engage in certain activities on or around campus related to DEI and submit short reflection papers. Additionally, institutions have developed parallel certificate programs on DEI to supplement traditional curriculum content. Each of these approaches has had a positive impact on the development of personal awareness for new veterinarians. However, there must be numerous opportunities for different approaches to the inclusion of this content because didactic cultural learning is not sufficient to truly improve competence to the point of changing behavior (Choi and Kim 2018).

Increased diversity within DVM classes provides an opportunity for students to learn and practice working in more culturally diverse environments. Colleges should facilitate intercultural learning and competence development throughout the curriculum (Markey et al. 2020), during which time DVM students can learn more about other populations and themselves. These efforts should not burden underrepresented or otherwise marginalized students to "teach" about their larger cultures but should nurture curiosity and commitment to mutual respect across the cohorts of students.

Teaching approaches that include opportunities for experiential learning, either through case studies, role-play, or service learning, are seen as more effective strategies for improving cultural competence among students (Newman et al. 2019; Forsyth et al. 2017). There is a need to improve student knowledge about sociocultural differences as well as, to explicitly bolster "confidence and commitment" to the delivery of culturally competent care (O' Brien et al. 2021). This typically cannot be achieved through more passive learning approaches, such as unidirectional lectures. Additional opportunities for experiential learning are essential for optimal learning.

Role-Play

Role-play is recognized as a useful teaching strategy for these purposes. Like the ways in which colleges simulate veterinarians' interactions with client actors for communication skill development, role-play can be a useful exercise for veterinary students to practice engaging clients in culturally appropriate ways or experiences when culturally relevant care is or is not provided. Role-play learning should be highly structured with specific learning objectives and assessment criteria. Strong classroom management skills are needed for this instructional approach as participants may demonstrate a wide range of responses. This approach, like others, also requires a time for group debriefing and a period for reflection for students to consider what was gleaned from the exercise as it relates to the delivery of intercultural care (Shearer and Davidhizar 2003).

Service-Learning

Service-learning provides meaningful learning opportunities for veterinary students to learn humility and cultural competence and to immediately operationalize those lessons. Service-learning provides students the opportunity to experience delivering care in broader environments and in places where they may have previously had minimal exposure. Research exploring student perspectives on diversity pre and post learning experiences show they have a positive impact on a student's ability to notice institutional discrimination, feel more comfortable working with diverse populations (Melchor 2015), to increase cultural awareness and skill related to cultural competence (Kohlbry 2016), and to appropriately self-evaluate their own levels of cultural competence (Short et al. 2020). Some benefits of service-learning approaches do decay over time. It is important to ensure students have a basis of understanding of cultural humility and competency and methods to adequately debrief and process the experience are provided (Short et al. 2020). Faculty should also strongly encourage regular continuing education and/or dedicated opportunities for future community-based experiences to guard against loss of knowledge and sensitivity.

It is critical that these experiences be highly supervised with faculty giving guidance in real time. Students should understand that service-learning is an engaging learning experience in which they are delivering care in marginalized and/or underserved communities and should be briefed on the ethics involved. Additionally, it is important for faculty to understand their specific role in educating students pre, peri, and post-experience. Service-learning experiences play an important role in professional identity development. Faculty supervisors should be modeling appropriate behavior, ensuring that the client recipients are receiving the best possible care and that there is a high level of engagement and dialogue among students and with those supervising them (Wiese and Bennett 2018).

Asynchronous Learning Modules

Online learning modules are increasingly popular in providing educational content on DEI in veterinary medicine. For nearly a decade, Purdue University College of Veterinary Medicine has offered an online certificate program in DEI in veterinary medicine; several other colleges in the United States and abroad have also developed similar offerings. The benefits are numerous in that these offerings allow students and professionals to engage in the content at their own pace, they can vary in length and cover a wide range of topics related to cultural humility and competency. Unfortunately, the programs do not provide real-time feedback or student/colleague engagement with one another to discuss the content, both of which can assist learning and retention greatly.

Despite this limitation, asynchronous learning modules provide good opportunities for basic knowledge about diverse concepts in general and specific applications in veterinary medicine. This approach may make it easier for faculty facilitators to identify knowledge gaps as students move through the content and supplement with other teaching modalities when appropriate. Ultimately online learning modules can convey important information, again, increasing student knowledge about culture, cultural humility, and cultural competence, but because it is a passive learning approach, it is unlikely to improve skill development (Trinh et al. 2021). This approach is best used when introducing content and should be supplemented with approaches such as role-play and/or service learning to have a more positive effect on the delivery of care.

Part 8: Assessment

Assessment must be a part of the learning exercises associated with the development of cultural competence, cultural humility, and cultural fluency. Three kinds of assessment are recommended for consideration.

Reflective Writing

Reflective writing is a frequent tool used during the assessment of cultural competencies and cultural humility. This approach supports the development of reflective capacity in students, which is key to eventually demonstrating competency related to cultural content. It is useful in considering how feedback is received, determining what content students may struggle to grasp fully, how they see themselves as veterinarians in relation to the content, and how they can emotionally self-manage medicine's complexity, especially when considering issues like DEI (Schei et al. 2018).

Using reflective writing specifically for grading purposes poses a few challenges. There is a need for a clear working definition of reflection that is clearly communicated by faculty to students (Wald and Reis 2010). Reflective writing can pose difficulties in achieving quantitatively valid and reliable data on student development, meaning one essay may not predict performance in a future essay (Moniz et al. 2015). However, it is important to note that a new scale, the GRE-9, has shown positive inter-rater reliability in objectively grading reflective essays (Makarem et al. 2020). Finally, with the average veterinary school class being approximately 100 students, grading reflective writings can be very labor-intensive.

Despite the challenges, there is value in reflective writing that is ungraded, yet still requires submission. The assignment creates designated time and guidance for reflective practice, which is critical to professional identity development. Time is needed for students to explore new knowledge and ponder its relevance to practice more deeply than a classroom setting allows. The lack of a specific grade reduces the likelihood of students parroting what may be perceived as the *right* answer but also creates an opportunity for students to self-evaluate their understanding of the material. Essays need not be lengthy, and they should be framed with a prompt from the instructor. Essays may be used to frame future classroom discussions about how students are experiencing the process of developing cultural humility, competency, and fluency.

Pre/Post Testing

Pre and posttesting approaches to assessing cultural humility and competency are used across health professions education as a means of determining the efficacy of diversity content in the curriculum. The Intercultural Development Inventory (IDI; Hammer et al. 2003), is a frequently used tool due to the strength of its construct validation (Jankowski 2019), although there are limitations to the use of this tool. Critiques of the IDI include an absence of content related to structural inequality in multicultural environments and questionable assessment validity when measuring the competence of black, indigenous, and other people of color (Punti and Dingle 2021). Using the IDI or other similar tools pre–post curriculum content coverage can show the impact on veterinary students' movement toward becoming culturally competent. As colleges of veterinary medicine continue to become more racially and ethnically diverse, there may be a need to supplement the use of tools like the IDI with other assessment tools discussed in this chapter.

Client Interaction Assessment

Assessment of interactions with clients during the clinical component of professional education provides a meaningful opportunity for students to be assessed on cultural humility and cultural competence. As many institutions situate clinical rotations near the end of the curriculum, these opportunities may be viewed through a capstone lens. Students will have exposure to relevant content during the didactic portion of the curriculum; clinical faculty should include a brief refresher of this content as students move into the clinical phase of programming. Students who have been exposed to DEI content and a refresher ahead of clinical rotations are more likely to demonstrate behaviors associated with cultural humility and cultural competence; additionally, there is evidence that students with this exposure and refresher intervention demonstrate greater clinical competency (Khoury et al. 2022). Faculty doing the evaluations should also demonstrate appropriate behaviors in the clinical setting and have sufficient training in cultural humility and competence to be best prepared for evaluating students within the clinical environment.

Part 9: Conclusion

The development of cultural humility, competence, and fluency is crucial to inclusion of DEI content in the DVM curriculum. These skills not only create opportunities for increased professional growth for students, but they are essential to providing relevant and holistic care to the increasingly diverse population being served by the veterinary community. While it may be challenging to incorporate these teachings into the already rigorous curriculum, utilizing multiple strategies and resources can reduce the burden on both instructors and students. Lecture, role-play, service-learning, and asynchronous learning modules can be used in conjunction to create an atmosphere of learning for the veterinary student that promotes the practice of cultural competency skills.

It is also important to use adequate assessment models for these strategies to ensure that coursework is suitable, and to adjust methodologies when needed. Graded and ungraded methods of assessment that can be useful are reflective writing, pre/post testing such as the IDI, and client interaction assessments are useful tools for evaluating the effectiveness of a DEI-inclusive curriculum. The skills of cultural humility, competency, and fluency rely heavily on self-reflection and self-assessment to develop an attitude of openness and awareness. Assessment materials must also be able to assess and promote growth in those areas, in addition to assessing an understanding of policies and practices related to DEI content and cultural competency.

Section 5: Teaching Empathy and Ethics

Shelly Wu and Gabriel Huddleston

Ethics aims to understand morality, which includes "how we should conduct our lives and, especially, how we should interact with others" (Noddings 2016, p. 145). With this in mind, and as educators are expected to uphold ethical obligations at various scales, an understanding of morality is essential in various pedagogical settings. For example, on the broader scale of the teaching profession, the National Education Association (NEA) has established codes of ethics with statements regarding how educators should demonstrate their commitment to the profession (National Education Association 2020). In the field of veterinary education, educators teach professional values, such as principles of veterinary medical ethics and applicable regulations for animal care (Kipperman et al. 2021). On a smaller scale, with daily encounters in the classroom, educators also have moral responsibilities toward their interactions with students. For example, educators decide how to enact the curriculum to reconcile ethical dilemmas that occur between and with their students (Blackley et al. 2021; Brophy 2010; Bullough 2011).

In addition to professional codes of ethics, educators draw upon different ethical frameworks to guide their decisions. For example, consequentialist ethics bases a decision on the consequences to maximize the benefit for the greatest number of individuals. Another common framework is non-consequentialist ethics, which focuses on respect for persons as moral agents (Strike and Soltis 2009). While these ethical frameworks may provide some guidance for an educator's decision-making, it is sometimes difficult to apply generalized principles when the decision-making process does not account for specific, ethical contexts (Cahn 2009). The goal of this section is to promote an awareness of an educator's ethics in teaching and to consider implementing care ethics in education. The rationale for advocating for care ethics as a framework is that it does not rely on abstraction, but rather takes a relational approach to ethics to consider the specific context to best enhance caring for students. As such, we believe that veterinary educators can benefit from an understanding of care ethics and apply it to their own teaching.

A key responsibility of educators is to make decisions regarding curriculum, such as deciding what knowledge is taught and the learning methods that will be used. The nature of knowledge and instructional methods used are value-laden with underlying beliefs that have implications for an educator's teaching practices (Nouri and McComas 2021). Ethical values are embedded in a paradigm, which are the assumptions that an individual holds about the world, including what constitutes knowledge and how that knowledge is generated; these, in turn, inform our actions (Lincoln and Guba 2003). In the teaching profession, the paradigm to which an educator ascribes impacts their decision-making, including their learning goals, how they teach, and the nature of their relationship with students (McManus 2001). For example, a dominant paradigm in science is positivism, which assumes that knowledge can be obtained in an objective manner to generalize a singular truth about reality (Park et al. 2020). Previous research has suggested that a positivist epistemology influences the way students might learn objective, positivist knowledge, such as "whole class lectures, textbook readings, related assignments, and application problems that require mathematical manipulation to describe an event. Common to each of these pedagogical choices is the transmittance of some privileged, objective knowledge about the world" (Yerrick et al. 1998, p. 621). For example, preservice teachers with positivist beliefs perceived their role as communicating authoritative knowledge for students to acquire factual information (Bryan 2012).

The lack of student agency in the knowledge-building process may reinforce the idea that students only need to learn the canonical knowledge reinforced by the teacher (Miller et al. 2018). A teacher-centered approach might result in a more impersonal teacher–student relationship if students are only responsible for recalling knowledge (McManus 2001). It has also been acknowledged that large lecture-based courses in veterinary education may not meet the learning needs of every student (Fletcher et al. 2015). The positivist way of teaching is problematic because it occurs primarily through teacher-directed communication. Education philosopher Paulo Freire (2000), criticized what he termed the "banking model of education," which occurs when teachers presume to have the authority of knowledge that they deposit in each student's mind. The banking model of education reflects an oppressive education system where students are expected to comply. If communication is mostly teacher-directed and aims to reaffirm positivist knowledge, students lack participation in the learning process. The premise of a caring relationship is that it "requires a contribution from both parties," such as educators allowing students to contribute to their own learning in the curriculum (Noddings 2005, 2017, p. 317). Therefore, an ethical stance of teaching absolute knowledge only through transmissive methods could exclude students from equitable participation in their learning and, furthermore, prevent students and their teachers from building a caring relationship.

Alternative paradigms to positivism acknowledge that truth claims to the world are not free of bias and knowledge is constructed in sociocultural contexts (Lemke 2001; McComas 1996). The sociocultural perspectives that students bring to the class should be considered in the curriculum, as previous research has suggested that veterinary students' and professional's viewpoints toward animals will vary by factors, such as their societal upbringing, gender, or work experiences (Menor-Campos et al. 2019; Tzioumis et al. 2018). Leveraging the learner's lived experiences and perspectives might enrich student learning.

Education philosopher John Dewey recognized learning as a social process and criticized learning through passive methods of absorbing knowledge. He believed learning should occur through experience, which can help learners make meaning of the world. Dewey also viewed educational institutions as places for preparing students for democratic life, affording students opportunities to communicate shared interests and values through joint participation

(Dewey 2007). Simpson (2017), further describes Dewey's view of community "as part of engaged living, school involves thinking with and learning with and from others and expanding each person's life through interactions that include both inquiry and creative problem solving" (p. 242).

Deweyan approaches to student-centered learning can vary greatly, from students having agency in developing learning objectives to an educator building a community of learners, to facilitation of student-led conversations in the classroom on topics relevant to society (Noddings 2016; Williams 2017). A teaching stance that includes diverse student perspectives could contribute to more equitable participation in student learning. To foster democratic participation in schools, Dewey (2007), envisioned that "All education which develops power to share effectively in social life is moral. . .Interest in learning from all the contacts of life is the essential moral interest" (p. 259). This view suggests that developing relationships with others is important for moral growth and may enhance an ethic of caring.

In reflection thus far, an educator makes a combination of pedagogical and ethical choices, including the use of specific learning conditions to reflect their end goals. As discussed earlier, if an educator takes a pedagogical stance of positivist teaching, the learning environment would be set up such that students are ". . .passively listening to the teacher at the front, and writing down what is heard for the purpose of memorization and recitation" (English 2017, p. 121). Teaching in this manner is also an ethical choice to prioritize achieving academic objectives over creating the conditions for caring in the classroom (Noddings 2005). In contrast, creating a learning environment that aims for moral development empowers students to learn collaboratively and contribute to the curriculum. Taking a student-centered approach to teaching also reflects an educator's intentional, ethical stance to create opportunities for caring relations to develop (Noddings 2005, 2016).

Education philosopher Nel Noddings (2013), describes care ethics as a relationship between the "one-caring" and the "cared-for" (p. 4). For example, the "one-caring" in the context of education can be an educator, and the "cared-for" can be students. An important distinction from patriarchal ethical frameworks is that an ethic of care moves beyond abstraction of ethical principles toward a concrete, caring relationship that focuses on a relational and contextual approach to ethics. The "one-caring" moves beyond natural caring to an ethic of care to consider the perspectives of the cared-for(s) and that the relationship is reciprocal, such as an educator accounting for the expressed and inferred learning needs of their students (Noddings 2013, 2016). An educator that takes an ethical stance of caring ethics would be attentive to each student's individual talents, capabilities, and interests to promote their moral development (Noddings 2005). Noddings (2013), contends that "as we build an ethic of caring and examine education under its guidance, we shall see that the greatest obligation of educators, inside and outside formal schooling, is to nurture the ethical ideals with whom they come in contact" (p. 49). In other words, a moral education shifts beyond merely teaching toward genuinely caring for each student's personal growth to become the best version of themselves (Noddings 2005, 2013). Helping students achieve their ethical ideals might begin with Noddings' four components for a moral education.

The first component of Noddings' moral education is the use of dialogue to understand each other's views. Dialogue is important to shift the teacher–student model from a top-down authoritarian approach to a more balanced relationship in the learning process. In alignment with her ideas, Paulo Freire advocated for an education system that respects students as individuals by using transformative pedagogies that value their perspectives, such as critical inquiry and dialogue. Dialogue can foster open-ended discussion in which both educators and students co-participate in the process of problem-solving (Freire 2000). The second component of a moral education is modeling to demonstrate caring for cared-for(s). In the context of education, modeling care has also been described as "exemplifying a caring disposition to students" (Velasquez et al. 2013, p. 165). The third component of a moral education is practicing care ethics, such as students implementing caring actions toward their relationships with animals and the environment. Lastly, the confirmation of care in education is when an educator takes an intentional stance to confirm the best in their students, such as helping students achieve their goals (Noddings 2013, 2016; Velasquez et al. 2013).

Although there are various ways an educator can implement components of a moral education, an educator may consider fostering students' epistemic agency as one way to facilitate care ethics. Epistemic agency is the idea of facilitating student autonomy in the learning process, such as "...identifying problems to work on, deciding how to pursue these investigations, and partnering with teachers to reach consensus about what has been figured out" (Zivic et al. 2018, p. 25). Instead of teachers dictating the knowledge, students are positioned as an epistemic agent, taking ownership in making decisions individually and collectively with peers during the learning process that contribute to their understanding of the knowledge being investigated (Kawasaki and Sandoval 2020). For example, if students are engaged in scientific inquiry, students with epistemic agency might decide how they will approach an investigation that might include posing research questions, the methodology of the study, and interpretation of results to develop student-led explanations (Ko and Krist 2018).

One valuable aspect of providing students with epistemic agency is that they can understand how knowledge is created and communicated, which reflects how scientists operate in reality. This contrasts traditional learning methods that do not reflect how scientific knowledge is generated if the educator only deposits knowledge (Stroupe 2014). More importantly, the process of engaging in epistemic agency may contribute to caring ethics, such as students feeling valued and being engaged in critical-thinking skills that will prepare them for their future profession.

In summary, an educator's underlying ethics can shape their methods of teaching, their disposition toward students, and ultimately, student learning outcomes. In veterinary ethics, educators identified several important reasons for teaching ethics, including the development of students' ethical awareness of issues in veterinary practice, ethical knowledge, ethical reasoning skills, and lastly, students' ethical viewpoints and identity, which has implications for their veterinary practice (Magalhães-Sant'Ana et al. 2014). It is important to recognize that teacher-centered approaches might limit students' abilities to engage in moral reasoning and identify their own ethical perspectives. However, embedding an ethic of caring in teaching with student-centered approaches might offer opportunities for students to be epistemic agents in the construction of their own moral development.

Section 6: Teaching and Practicing Foundational Communication Skills

Ryane E. Englar

Prior to the 1990s, healthcare education largely excluded clinical communication from curricular design, and exploring the interpersonal aspects of the consultation was seen as a "soft skill" that could be acquired through on-the-job training (Englar 2017). However, when researchers Byrne, Long, Maguire, Fairbairn, and Fletcher assessed postgraduate success in human healthcare settings, they identified deficiencies in provider–patient communication (Byrne 1976; Maguire et al. 1986a,b). Maguire et al concluded that:

> Some young doctors do discover for themselves how best to give patients information and advice, but most remain extremely incompetent. This is presumably because they get no training as students in this important aspect of clinical practice. This deficiency should be corrected, and competence tested before qualification to practise *[sic]*. (Maguire et al. 1986b, p. 1576)

This recognition of the need to train proficiency in communication gave rise to curricular reform to develop guidelines for teaching professional skills in human healthcare training programs (Batalden et al. 2002; Duffy et al. 2004; Englar et al. 2016; Rider et al. 2006). In 1999, Brown and Silverman identified similar needs within veterinary medical education (Brown and Silverman 1999). Perceived deficits in nontechnical skills, knowledge, and abilities were identified and addressed based upon recommendations put forth by the executive summary of the Brakke study (Cron et al. 2000), the National Commission on Veterinary Economic Issues (Cron et al. 2000; Lewis and Klausner 2003; Lloyd and King 2004; Volk et al. 2005), and a 2002 proposal by Lloyd and Walsh for curricular revision (Lloyd and Walsh 2002). By 2004, 23 of the (then) 27 veterinary colleges within the United States self-reported that coursework had been remodeled to include team building and interpersonal skills (Lloyd and King 2004).

Veterinary stakeholders, including employers and paraveterinary staff, agree that communication competence is key to employability (Bell et al. 2019, 2021; Haldane et al. 2017; Kurtz 2006; McDermott et al. 2015; Meehan and Menniti 2014; Reinhard et al. 2021; Rhind et al. 2011; Show and Englar 2018). Because of the growing evidence that communication drives patient outcomes and provider–consumer satisfaction with healthcare services, the AVMA Council on Education (COE) now requires that communication be taught and assessed by all accredited colleges of veterinary medicine (COE Accreditation Policies and Procedures: Requirements 2021; Show and Englar 2018).

Part 1: Communication Models and the Calgary–Cambridge Guide

To facilitate communication training, healthcare educators have designed a variety of models that incorporate communication skills into the structure of the consultation. These include the Three-Function Model (Cohen-Cole 1991), the E4 model for physician–patient communication (Keller and Carroll 1994), the SEGUE framework (Makoul 2001), the Patient-Centered Care Model (Levenstein et al. 1986), the Model of the Macy Initiative in Health Communication (Kalet et al. 2004), and the Calgary–Cambridge Guide [CCG] (Kurtz et al. 2003; Kurtz and Adams 2009). The CCG is the primary model in North and South America as well as the United Kingdom (Burt et al. 2014; Dohms et al. 2021; Gillard et al. 2009). It has been translated into Spanish, Portuguese, Japanese, Nepali, and Indonesian (Dohms et al. 2021; Ishikawa et al. 2014; Kurtz 2006; Moore 2007) and has been modified as needed to reflect global cultural differences (Pun 2021).

The CCG is a systematic approach to healthcare consultations that emphasizes procedural tasks (Denness 2013; Englar 2020e; Kurtz 2006; Kurtz et al. 1998, 2003; Kurtz and Silverman 1996; McDermott et al. 2015; Riccardi and Kurtz 1983; Silverman et al. 2008, 2013):

- initiating the session
- gathering information
- explaining and planning
- closing the session.

Physical examination of the patient takes place between *gathering information* through history-taking and the *explaining and planning* stage of the consultation (Denness 2013; Englar 2020e; Kurtz 2006; Silverman et al. 2008). Two additional tasks, *building the relationship* and *providing structure*, span the entire consultation (Denness 2013; Englar 2020e; Kurtz 2006; Silverman et al. 2008). *Building the relationship* emphasizes the need for veterinarians to partner with clients because patient advocacy roles overlap and both parties contribute to decision-making (Englar 2020e). *Providing structure* reminds veterinarians to clarify the flow of the consultation so that clients know how each visit will progress (Englar 2020e).

In addition to these sequential tasks, the CCG builds over 70 communication process steps into its framework ((Englar 2020e; Kurtz 2006; Kurtz et al. 1998, 2003; McDermott et al. 2015; Silverman et al. 2013). These steps include inviting the client to speak, listening attentively, gathering essential data, confirming the sequence of events in the patient history, and checking for understanding. Such steps, in concert with sequential tasks, establish and maintain relationship-centered care (Englar 2020e; Kurtz et al. 2004).

Radford et al. adapted the CCG to veterinary practice in 2002 (Adams and Ladner 2004; Englar et al. 2016; Radford et al. 2006). This adaptation has been successfully incorporated into some veterinary medical curricula in the United States, Canada, and the United Kingdom (Englar et al. 2016; Radford et al. 2003; Silverman et al. 2013). The author (Englar) and colleague Teresa Graham Brett have expanded upon the original visual representation of the CCG by Kurtz, Silverman, and Draper in a novel diagrammatic representation of the feline skeleton, where correlated tasks are depicted from left to right, as seen in the Figure 6.1 below.

Unfortunately, curricular time constraints often limit the breadth and depth of communication training, including which skills can be taught (Englar et al. 2016). It is impossible to insert the 70-plus CCG process steps into any curriculum. Rather than teach it all, educators can concentrate on foundational skills, which are fundamental and transferrable, meaning that they are carried with learners throughout their careers and can be applied to any position

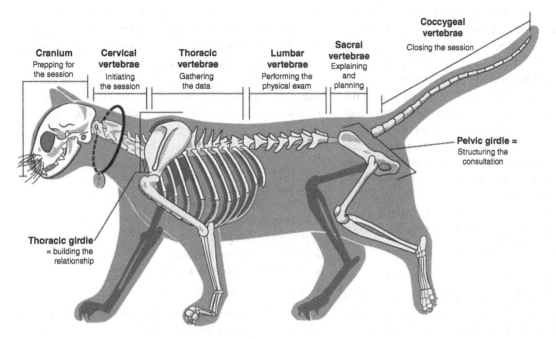

Figure 6.1 Anatomical Representation of the CCG, in which spinal segments correspond to key sequential tasks. *Source:* Courtesy of Dr. Ryane E. Englar and Teresa Graham Brett, with support from Multimedia Specialist Eric Beasley.

held. Foundational skills also serve as scaffolding upon which complimentary and/or advanced communication skills can be developed.

The following sections will look more in-depth at a process to incorporate and teach communication skills in veterinary programs. It relies on the CCG, which has been studied primarily within the context of canine and feline practice. It is important to note, however, that additional client communication strategies specific to equine and production animal medicine are actively being researched (Blach 2009; Kleen et al. 2011; MacDonald-Phillips et al. 2022; Ritter et al. 2018, 2019; Svensson et al. 2019).

Part 2: The TONERR Model for Teaching Communication Skills

Research consistently demonstrates that open-ended questions, nonverbal cues, empathy, and reflective listening enhance the client experience (Hafen et al. 2013; Latham and Morris 2007; Stevens and Kedrowicz 2018). In addition, companion animal owners seek transparency and unconditional positive regard in the consultation room (Englar et al. 2016). Collectively, these six communication skills are foundational.

To facilitate student learning, the author has incorporated foundational communication skills into the acronym, TONERR:

- T = transparency
- O = open-ended questions
- N = nonverbal cues
- E = empathy
- R = reflective listening
- R = regard

Part 3: Transparency

Conversations about transparency in healthcare intensified nearly two decades ago when the Institute of Medicine (IOM) released a controversial report in 1999 about human deaths due to preventable medical errors (Kohn et al. 2000). This publication was among the first of its kind to publicly acknowledge that medicine is imperfect, and that risk can be mitigated by sharing medical mistakes openly (Englar 2020d). In 2021, IOM published a follow-up report, *Crossing the Quality Chasm: A New Health System for the 21st Century*, in which transparency was said to drive accountability (Englar 2020d).

When errors are addressed, standard operating procedures (SOPs) can be developed or refined to improve safety (Wachter et al. 2015). Disclosure of medical errors also allows the entire healthcare team to pivot when unexpected challenges arise. Allowing human patients and veterinary clients to weigh in on decision-making builds trust and reinforces partnership (Wachter et al. 2015).

Medical mistakes are just one aspect of healthcare transparency. Companion animal owners have expressed the need for veterinarians to be transparent about patient diagnosis, prognosis, and quality of life (Englar 2020d; Englar et al. 2016).

Dog owners do not want information withheld, even if the news is grim, as demonstrated by one participant in a focus group study, who emphasized the importance of veterinarians being direct: "Get right to it. Don't soften things up. I want to know exactly what's happening with the dog and what the worst outcome could be" (Englar et al. 2016). Failure on the veterinarian's part to disclose a poor prognosis offended dog-owning focus group participants, who assumed the veterinary team felt they could not handle bad news. Dog owners also felt that they were denied the opportunity to make informed decisions about patient care because they were not privy to all the facts (Englar et al. 2016).

Cat owners also prefer a direct approach, particularly with respect to uncertainty during the diagnostic process. One focus group participant shared that:

> I want [veterinarians] to say, "no, I really don't know." The test for [diagnosing this condition] is US$ 300, the medicine is US$ 100, let's just give the medicine and see what happens. And if it doesn't work, we'll move on to something else. Be open to saying, "I don't know, but this is the best course to try." (Englar et al. 2016)

There is comfort in receiving honest answers about the unknown. Focus group participants shared that it is okay if the veterinary team is uncertain about the patient's health if the team shares their plan for finding a solution. Similarly, when clients ask veterinarians, "What would you do if my pet were yours?," they want honest answers (Englar et al. 2016). Clients value the veterinary perspective even if it is not what they want to hear.

Transparency is not always easy to demonstrate, particularly in cases involving bad news delivery. In these instances, clients may benefit from a preparatory statement or "warning shot" (Ptacek et al. 2004), which helps set the tone. The author prefers to refer to this statement in class as a "heads up." It is a verbal cue to the client that the team has serious news to share. Examples of effective "preparatory statements" include:

- "I need to talk to you about something serious."
- "I have some difficult news to share with you about. . ." (Garrett 2013)
- "I know that what I'm about to share with you will be very hard to hear."
- "What I'm about to say may come as a shock. . ."

Part 4: Open-Ended Questions

The successful practice of veterinary medicine begins with gathering information, through history-taking and eliciting the client's perspective. In practices that model relationship-centered care, the client is invited to share their story (Englar 2019d, 2020f). Knowing how to prompt the client for pertinent details requires a mix of closed and open-ended questions or statements.

Closed-ended questions minimize storytelling because the client's answers are typically limited to a "yes" or "no" (Shaw 2006). Consider, for example, the following question set:

- Is Foxy sneezing?
- Is Foxy coughing?
- Is Foxy vomiting?
- Is Foxy having diarrhea?
- Is Foxy eating?
- Is Foxy limping?
- Is Foxy using the litterbox?
- Is there blood in Foxy's stool?
- Is Foxy acting painful?

Closed-ended questions may also ask the client to provide a numerical answer. For example:

- How many meals has Vulpes skipped in the last 24 hours?
- How many times has Vulpes vomited?
- How often is Vulpes having diarrhea?

Closed-ended questions are essential when a definitive answer is needed. However, closed-ended questions are restrictive for those clients who may wish to share additional details. In these cases, clients benefit from being asked open-ended questions or statements that begin with (Adams and Kurtz 2017; Kurtz et al. 2004; Shaw 2006; Silverman et al. 2008):

- Tell me
- Help me
- Show me
- Share with me
- Describe

For example:

- Tell me more about Lowell's litterbox habits.
- Help me to picture how Lowell's litterboxes are set up in your home.
- Show me how Lowell's litterboxes are arranged in your household.
- Share with me what concerns you most about Lowell's litterbox habits.
- Describe what you are noticing about Lowell's litterbox habits.

Open-ended questions can also begin with "what?" or "how?". For example:

- "What do you think is causing Cheeto to gain weight?"
- "How do you feel about getting Cheeto spayed?"

Although "why?" is also a lead-in for an open-ended question, the author tends to steer clear of it only because "why?" is often associated with judgment. For example, the following questions may stir up defensiveness even if the clinician is asking to ask, rather than judge:

● "Why didn't you bring Brie in sooner?"
● "Why are you declining to vaccinate Brie?"

These questions could be reworded in a way that achieves the same purpose:

● "What prompted you to bring Brie in today?"
● "What makes you reluctant to vaccinate Brie?"

This shift in phraseology may be subtle; however, the client may be more willing to express themselves openly if they feel that the clinician is receptive to their perspective.

Part 5: Nonverbal Cues

Not all communication requires words and, in fact, nonverbal communication is the primary way by which we express emotion (Carson 2007). How we feel is often displayed on our faces and is reinforced by how we carry ourselves (Roter et al. 2005).

There are four categories of nonverbal cues (Carson 2007; Englar 2020b):

● Kinesics
● Proxemics
● Paralanguage
● Autonomic shifts

Kinesics is the study of how we gesture and move our body to communicate safety, fight, or flight (Carson 2007; Englar 2020b). Clients communicate important messaging through body language (Carson 2007), which includes (Caris-Verhallen et al. 1999; Carson 2007; Duggan and Parrott 2001; Endres and Laidlaw 2009; Englar 2020b; Gabbott and Hogg 2001; Marcinowicz et al. 2010; Myers 2009; Roter et al. 2005; Shaw 2006; Verderber and Verderber 1980):

● Body movement
  – Whole body
  – Body part isolations
● Body position and posture
  – Open versus closed body posture
  – Forward versus backward lean
● Body tension
● Eye contact
● Facial expressions
● Gestures
● Touch (Caris-Verhallen et al. 1999; Cocksedge et al. 2013; Connor and Howett 2009; Edwards 1998; Estabrooks and Morse 1992; Peloquin 1989)

Open body postures, such as uncrossed arms and legs, in concert with relaxed facial expressions, communicate safety and security (Carson 2007). As challenging conversations arise, clients may reflect their discomfort through one or more of the following cues:(Carson 2007; Englar 2020b):

● Taut mouth
● Tight jaw
● Clenched fists
● Lowered brow
● Reluctance to sit down or to remain seated
● Narrowed palpebral fissures
● Whole body leans away
● Crossed arms or legs
● Increasing personal space
● Breaking eye contact.

As clinicians, it is our responsibility to pick up on these nonverbal cues and respond in a way that promotes psychological safety (Englar 2020b). Only clients who feel safe and secure in the consultation room are able to partner with us so that we can effectively deliver high-quality healthcare (Englar 2020b).

Proxemics is how we make use of space to meet our needs (Carson 2007; Englar 2020b). This requires us to consider physical distance and barriers between clients and veterinary team members, including but not limited to, the exam room table (Argyle 1988; Carson 2007; Hall 1973; Shaw 2006). In clinical practice, "one wall" rooms are becoming increasingly popular, meaning that the veterinarian's workspace, the exam table, and client seating are all along one wall (Chapel 2017). This visually enhances partnership because the veterinarian is no longer hidden behind the exam room table. Veterinarians who practice in consultation rooms with more traditional designs can achieve the same effect by coming around the table to talk to clients.

Paralanguage is how we speak rather than the words we use. Paralanguage emphasizes the volume and pacing of speech, pitch, tone, and the strategic use of pauses (Carson 2007).

Autonomic shifts are those aspects of nonverbal communication that are largely outside of our control. They arise in response to our perception that we are under attack (Carson 2007; Englar 2020b):

● facial flushing or blanching
● sweaty palms
● shallow or rapid breathing
● holding one's breath.

Although these are internally triggered changes, we are responsible for tuning into ourselves and reflecting upon what initiated the reaction so we can transition from reaction to response.

Part 6: Empathy

There is no universal definition of empathy (Halpern 2003; Hojat 2007; McMurray and Boysen 2017; Pedersen 2009; Preusche and Lamm 2016; Shaw 2006; Shea 1998; Singer and Lamm 2009). For some, empathy is a demonstration of perspective-taking, the ability to identify with and develop a conscious awareness of how someone else experiences the world (McMurray and Boysen 2017), a skill that has been coined *cognitive* empathy (Adams and Kurtz 2017). Cognitive empathy allows us to tune into another person's situation (Englar 2020a), allowing us to recognize that someone feels a certain way and make an effort to understand why (Adams and Kurtz 2017). We may not agree with their perspective (Silverman et al. 2008), but we can accept and acknowledge the real impact of their perceptions (Adams and Kurtz 2017). This form of empathy is purely cerebral and can be used by veterinarians to understand their client's point of view (McMurray and Boysen 2017).

Emotional empathy is the capacity to feel as others, instead of feeling for them (Adams and Kurtz 2017; Preusche and Lamm 2016). This figure of speech implies that, through empathy, we can feel what another being feels (Englar 2020a). Emotional empathy is raw (Englar 2020a); it connects us to our clients as we ourselves take on their emotional state to better appreciate what they are going through (Kurtz et al. 2004; McMurray and Boysen 2017; Shaw 2006; Shea 1998; Silverman et al. 2008).

Emotional empathy humanizes medicine and strengthens the veterinarian-client-patient relationship (VCPR) by communicating that "I get you," "I feel you," and "We are one" (Englar 2020a). In human healthcare, this connectivity is associated with the following positive outcomes (Bertakis et al. 1991; Decety and Fotopoulou 2014; Goodchild et al. 2005; Graugaard et al. 2004; Halpern 2012; Maguire et al. 1996; McMurray and Boysen 2017; Norfolk et al. 2007; Ong et al. 2000; Riess et al. 2012; Schoenfeld-Tacher et al. 2015, 2017; Shaw et al. 2004a; Shaw et al. 2012; Stewart 1995):

- Improved rapport between healthcare provider and patient
- Increased physician and patient satisfaction with healthcare delivery
- Greater accuracy of history-taking and diagnosis
  - Patients are more likely to share fuller histories
  - Patients are likely to disclose pertinent details
- Increased patient compliance and adherence to healthcare recommendations
- Reduced risk of board complaints and lawsuits alleging malpractice.

The veterinary profession experiences similar benefits when empathy is applied to the VCPR (Kanji et al. 2012; McArthur and Fitzgerald 2013; Schoenfeld-Tacher et al. 2017; Shaw et al. 2012).

Part 7: Reflective Listening

It has been estimated that each clinician conducts over 100,000 consultations during the course of their career (Keifenheim et al. 2015; Morrisey and Voiland 2007; Nichols and Mirvis 1998) and that 60–80% percent of diagnoses in human healthcare can be made from data obtained through history-taking (Hampton et al. 1975; Kassirer 1983; Lichstein 1990; Peterson et al. 1992; Sandler 1980; Takemura et al. 2007). Accuracy of diagnosis stems from attentive listening by healthcare professionals to their patients' verbal and nonverbal cues. Attentive listening is an active, reflective process in which the clinician checks their understanding of what the client shared to clarify the message (Devito 2007; Levitt 2001; Simon 2018; Trenholm and Jensen 2004; van Dulmen 2017; Weger et al. 2010). For this reason, attentive listening is often called reflective or active listening.

Active listening requires the speaker to have undivided attention. As the speaker shares their thoughts, concerns, experiences, and perspectives with the listener, the listener may convey attentiveness through minimal verbal feedback, such as "hmm," "uh-huh," "yeah," "ok," and "right," or nonverbal feedback, as through a head-nod. When the speaker has concluded, they and the listener trade roles, and the new speaker paraphrases, restates or otherwise reflects what they heard. This process invites the client to clarify any gaps in understanding and to share additional details as needed.

Reflective listening implies that the listener is fully engaged, which requires mental preparation in advance of entering the consultation room (Englar 2020c). It may be helpful for clinicians who are wrapping up a case to take a deep breath before beginning another. They may also close their eyes to shut out distractions, literally and figuratively, and picture themselves setting other tasks to the side so that they can start over with the next case.

Reflective listening is particularly essential in veterinary practice because providers oversee the care of nonhuman patients who cannot speak for themselves as to their needs, wants, and expectations. Veterinarians must therefore rely heavily upon the client's perspective to gain insight into the patient's presenting complaint(s).

Part 8: Regard

Regard – short for unconditional positive regard – is a mental health construct (Amadi 2013). The concept suggests that each patient is an individual who should be accepted for who they are (Englar 2020d; Englar et al. 2016). Rather than label human patients or veterinary clients as "difficult," healthcare team members should remind themselves that life circumstances, *not people*, challenge team dynamics (Englar 2020d). Instead of focusing on good versus bad traits, healthcare teams must find common ground by asking what both patient and provider wish to achieve and how to achieve those goals together (Gibson 2005).

It can be challenging for healthcare providers to set aside judgment because judging others' beliefs, perceptions, and misperceptions is inherently human (Englar 2020d). However, regard is worth the investment. When human patients and veterinary clients fear being judged, they limit information-sharing as a self-protective mechanism, and the resulting limited exchange of data may challenge providers to make diagnostic and/or therapeutic recommendations (Englar 2020d).

Being respected rather than judged is critical to the maintenance and growth of the VCPR. In a 2015 focus group study, cat-owners shared the importance of being understood. They do not always do what is right, but they want to be recognized as having good intentions even if their actions were unintentionally wrong (Englar et al. 2016). In the words of one participant, "[When] the cat [eats] a cardboard box and [swallows] it, [vets] don't say, 'why on earth did you let him eat the cardboard box?'" (Englar et al. 2016).

Being accepted by the veterinary team strengthens the bond between healthcare providers and clients and paves the way for respect (Patterson and Joseph 2006). Respect is a two-way street. If clients feel respected, they are more likely to respect the veterinary team. For respect to blossom, demonstrations of regard must come across as being sincere.

Part 9: Teaching and Practicing Communication Skills

How to embed and scaffold communication skills within curricula varies tremendously between healthcare programs, as is evidenced by the list of commonly employed techniques and practices below (Baile and Blatner 2014; Barrows 1993; Bucklin et al. 2021; Chun et al. 2009; Egnew et al. 2004; Englar 2017; Englar 2019b; Hafen et al. 2013; Hafen et al. 2009; Kurtz et al. 2004; Radford et al. 2003; Rickles et al. 2009; Root Kustritz et al. 2017; Shaw et al. 2004a; Tan et al. 2021; Veterinary Communication 2019):

- Didactic methods
  - Readings
  - Narrated or Recorded Lectures
  - Seminars
  - Presentations
  - Podcasts
  - Demonstrations
- Interactive methods
  - Flipped classroom
  - Think–pair–share
  - Turn and talk
  - Gallery walks
  - Facilitated workshops
  - Group discussions
  - Case studies
  - Simulation
    o In-person Role-Play
    o Telephone Role-Play (Hamilton et al. 2014)
    o Virtual Role-Play (Hamilton et al. 2014)
    o Action Methods Role-Play (Baile and Blatner 2014)
      ▪ Warm-up exercises to prepare students to engage in role-play
      ▪ Role-creation
        □ Learners take on the role of characters that they create
      ▪ Doubling
        □ Learners engage in perspective-taking to consider and share aloud what each character might be thinking or feeling, but not saying. One of the characters may be the learner's "inner self"
      ▪ Role-Reversal
        □ Learners take on the opposite role (e.g., the patient, instead of the doctor) to experience what it is like to be on the other side of the consultation table
      ▪ Group-processing
        □ Learners debrief about their experiences taking on another's role to reflect upon lessons learned
  - Direct observations of student doctor interactions with human patients and/or veterinary clients in the form of clinical evaluation exercises (CEXs)
  - Reviews of video-recorded interactions with real human patients and/or veterinary clients
  - Objective Structured Clinical Examinations (OSCEs)

Lecture-based practices have been the traditional vehicle by which content is delivered to learners because they allow for a high volume of foundational knowledge to be delivered efficiently (Bucklin et al. 2021). Lessons are largely teacher-centered and structured around how much content can be covered in one sitting. The educator takes on an authoritative figure, meaning that the expert drives the content, which the learner passively receives. The delivery of factual content lends itself well to this approach; however, opponents of this method of instruction have criticized it for promoting passive students who are surface learners. Learners expect to be given what they need to know rather than deepening their approach to content by building skills for independent problem-solving.

When learners are instead tasked to actively engage with content through interactive teaching methods, they are provided with the context by which they can attach relevance to learning (Bucklin et al. 2021). Students who see value in what they are learning are more likely to retain knowledge and apply it to real-life clinical situations (Bucklin et al. 2021; McMahon 2016; Prober and Heath 2012; Prober and Khan 2013). In other words, their knowledge is transferable. The role of the educator in active learning environments, therefore, transitions from the proverbial "sage on the stage" to "guide on the side" (Englar 2020c). Teaching becomes less about imparting knowledge and more about training students how to engage in critical thinking (Bucklin et al. 2021).

Active learning is related to, but not synonymous with, experiential learning, which has been defined as the "common pathway that converts understanding, knowledge, and attitude into behavior and action" (Miller 2005). Students learn by doing, then apply lessons learned to future experiences (Kolb 1984). Reflective observation plays a critical role in self-discovery as learners consider both content (what) and process (how) to increase awareness of internal thoughts, feelings, values, beliefs, and biases that influence their behavior (Adams et al. 2006).

Because experiential learning concentrates on the learning process, students have opportunities to move beyond hearing and/or reading about others' experiences and instead create their own. Learners are encouraged to make discoveries through first-hand observations and interactions with others as well as their surroundings. Not all outcomes are predictable when learning is approached in this manner, and students can potentially develop misconceptions about content. However, the ability to test the waters and reflect upon past experiences to shape future interactions lends itself well to communication training.

Simulation has increasingly played a role in developing communication skills among human medical and veterinary students (Adams and Ladner 2004; Bagnasco et al. 2014; Englar 2017, 2018, 2019a,c; Grevemeyer et al. 2016; McCool and Kedrowicz 2021; Rauch et al. 2022). Simulated client (SC) encounters, in which actors engage with student doctor-in-training to practice consultations, offer the opportunity to practice dialogic communication in safe, supportive environments. Cases are scripted, and SCs are trained to deliver their lines as they would in clinical practice (Englar 2018, 2019c). Although the authenticity of simulations has been criticized by some, students who have interacted with SCs have self-reported a range of emotions, including anxiety, fear, and grief as they experiment with word choice and the impact that phraseology has on others (Englar 2019c). Many students have expressed that cases feel real, as demonstrated by a comment that was made (Englar 2018, 2019c) in a debriefing from a simulation on death notification:

> . . .he really "just wanted to take the client's pain away." He realized after the fact that his words

"implied that [the patient] had no intrinsic value or was replaceable." This was not his intent. He had simply wanted to "apply a Band-Aid to an open wound". (Englar 2019c)

SC encounters can cover any aspect of any consultation but typically focus on history-taking, explaining, and planning. As students develop proficiency in foundational communication skills, simulations advance in difficulty to include such topics as cost of care and economic euthanasia, anticipatory grief, team conflict, and animal cruelty reporting (Englar 2017, 2018; R. E. Englar 2019c). The University of Arizona College of Veterinary Medicine currently has the most extensive simulation program for SCs among North American veterinary colleges, requiring students to individually complete 30 SC encounters over six consecutive preclinical semesters (Table 6.3).

Student access to clinical cases in preclinical curricula increases transference of conceptual knowledge and shifts learners toward deep learning (Kurtz et al. 2005; Washburn et al. 2016). Additionally, interactions with SCs prompt students to develop the skills and processes to explore the lens through which they see the world; develop an understanding of their own assumptions, beliefs, values, and experiences; stretch beyond their own sense of self to recognize and suspend judgments; critically examine where biases come from; and address power imbalances inherent in the VCPR to develop and sustain mutual, equitable partnerships with clients (Tsimaras et al. 2022). Such training fosters personal and professional growth because it is learner-centered (Makoul et al. 1998; Makoul and Schofield 1999; Novack et al. 1997).

Students can be tasked to set their own communication-based objectives for each SC encounter. After each event, they are required to reflect on both their strengths – referred to as "what worked well" (WWW) at the University of Arizona College of Veterinary Medicine – and their "opportunity areas for growth" (OAG). Learning is grounded in prior experiences and how the learner interprets experiences from the past to guide future actions (Taylor 2008).

Teaching communication in healthcare curricula is the first step toward integrating medical knowledge with appreciation for the patient's experience in a way that translates to enhanced healthcare delivery (Makoul and Schofield 1999). However, teaching communication is not enough. As outlined in Standard 11 of the AVMA COE Accreditation Policies and Procedures, all accredited colleges of veterinary medicine must develop and deliver formal processes by which students are assessed in nine competencies. The eighth competency combines clinical communication and perspective seeking to solicit and understand individual narratives across a diverse

Table 6.3 Outline of Simulated Client (SC) encounters at the University of Arizona College of Veterinary Medicine.

Year	Semester	Event #	Name of Patient	Species	Name of Client	Stage(s) of Consultation
Year 1	FALL	1	Tango	Feline	Bailey Wright	Greeting the Client & History-Taking
						New Patient/New Client/ Wellness Visit/Preventative Medicine
Year 1	FALL	2	Equine Trio - Mambo, Salsa, and Samba	Equine	Peyton Ford	Greeting the Client & History-Taking
						New Client/Multiple Patients - "Herd Health"
Year 1	FALL	3	Tango Returns	Feline	Bailey Wright	Greeting the Client & History-Taking
						Returning Client/Patient has Presenting Complaint/Taking a Dermatological History
Year 1	FALL	4	Jive	Canine	Quinn Caldwell	Explaining and Planning Good Prognosis, but condition is zoonotic
Year 1	SPRING	5	Quickstep	Equine	Alex Martinez	Explaining and Planning Poor Prognosis. Patient will not return to function
Year 1	SPRING	6	Paso Doble	Canine	Jaylen Brunt	Explaining and Planning Discussing Abnormal Physical Exam Finding
Year 1	SPRING	7	Lindy Hop	Canine	Shiloh Parker	Explaining and Planning Relaying Results of a Diagnostic Test and Recommendations for Preventative Care
Year 1	SPRING	8	Peabody	Canine	Jamie Billough	Explaining and Planning Relaying Results of a Diagnostic Test and Recommendations for Referral
Year 1	SUMMER	9	Zouk	Canine	Chris Wheaton	History-Taking
Year 1	SUMMER	10	Charlie	Canine	Devin Amari	Explaining and Planning
Year 1	SUMMER	11	Foxy	Feline	Phoenix Garcia	Explaining and Planning
Year 1	SUMMER	12	Milonga	Canine	Aspen Frankel	Explaining and Planning
Year 1	SUMMER	13	Cumbia	Feline	Ash Cheung	Explaining and Planning
Year 2	FALL	14	PS (Short for Promenade Swivel)	Feline	Blake Ng	Explaining and Planning
Year 2	FALL	15	Do-Si-Do	Canine	Zain Ito	Greeting the Client & History-Taking
Year 2	FALL	16	Do-Si-Do	Canine	Zain Ito	Explaining and Planning
Year 2	FALL	17	AC (Short for Abrazo Cerrado)	Equine	Amit Patterson	Greeting the Client & History-Taking

(Continued)

Table 6.3 (Continued)

Year	Semester	Event #	Name of Patient	Species	Name of Client	Stage(s) of Consultation
Year 2	FALL	18	AC (Short for Abrazo Cerrado)	Equine	Amit Patterson	Explaining and Planning
Year 2	FALL	19	Gancho	Reptile - Iguana	Ren Rodriguez	Greeting the Client & History-Taking
Year 2	FALL	20	Gancho	Reptile - Iguana	Ren Rodriguez	Explaining and Planning
Year 2	SPRING	21	Raas	Avian - Budgerigar ("Budgie")	Arbor Donovan	Explaining and Planning
Year 2	SPRING	22	Kabuki	Small Mammal - Guinea Pig	Grey Vasquez	Explaining and Planning
Year 2	SPRING	23	Shishimai	Feline	Natori Coleman	Explaining and Planning
Year 2	SPRING	24	Pizzica	Feline	Kai Alvarez	Explaining and Planning
Year 2	SPRING	25	Two-Step	Caprine	Dakari Abrams	Greeting the Client & History-Taking
Year 2	SUMMER	26A	Wes	Canine	Emi Turla	Explaining and Planning
Year 2	SUMMER	26B	Cossack (kaa-suhk)	Canine	Devin Moretti	Explaining and Planning
Year 2	SUMMER	27	Alemana	Feline	Jovi Arceo	Explaining and Planning
Year 2	SUMMER	28	Gurrunga	Canine	Kyan Svendsen	Explaining and Planning
Year 2	SUMMER	29	Chaal (ch-all)	Canine	Darcy San Juan	Explaining and Planning
Year 2	SUMMER	30	Tango	Feline	Bailey Wright	Greeting the Client & History-Taking

Courtesy of Dr. Ryane E. Englar and Teresa Graham Brett.

clientele (COE Accreditation Policies and Procedures: Requirements 2021). Assessments are imperative for students to receive constructive feedback, as well as critical interventions when they require additional support (Makoul and Schofield 1999).

A variety of communication assessment instruments have been developed for use in healthcare education and to assess postgraduate performance, including the CCG, which has been validated (Burt et al. 2014; Englar 2020e; Englar et al. 2016; Scheffer et al. 2008). Other assessment pathways for communication include:

- Self-assessment
- Real-time assessment by an observer
  - Peer
  - Instructor
- Standardized Patient (SP) or SC-assessment
- Audio transcript analysis
- Video transcript analysis
- Human patient/veterinary client post-visit evaluation questionnaire.

Self-assessments are vital to the learning process. Becoming self-aware is essential if the learner is to step outside of their own thoughts and feelings and relate to another person through perspective-taking (Batson et al. 1997; Gerace et al. 2017). Taking on another's perspective is a critical element of relationship-centered care as student doctors-in-training learn how to acknowledge and be responsive to the needs of patients (Makoul et al. 1998; Makoul and Schofield 1999; Novack et al. 1997).

The reliability and validity of SPs in human healthcare education have both been called into question by some studies; however, others have cited the benefits of being coached by actors who can provide immediate feedback. A 2015 cross-sectional study by Gude et al. compared SP assessment scores to outside observers' scores and found that the SP scores had strong predictive power. Because of this, the National Board of Medical Examiners (NBME) continues to make use of SPs to lead OSCEs that students must pass to be eligible to practice medicine.

SCs are not required elements of most veterinary medical education programs. However, the first-ever outcomes assessment study that tracked student growth between the first and last SC encounter at Midwestern University CVM demonstrated that communication exercises with SCs increased student confidence and student use of CCG communication skills. Additionally, in one study SC evaluations of student performance confirmed that in the final simulation as compared to the first, students were more likely to take a comprehensive patient history and build rapport with their client (Englar 2019a).

How best to assess communication training in veterinary medical education remain to be determined. At the University of Arizona CVM (UA CVM), SCs provide both oral and written feedback. Oral feedback is delivered by the SC to the student learner immediately following the event after asking for permission to share. Written feedback is provided to the student learner in the form of a completed rubric that summarizes which skills met expectations, which represented OAG, and which were not observed and/or not applicable (Table 6.4).

Within the UA CVM program, SC feedback does not equate to a letter grade or pass/fail. The instructional team has elected to grade students based on their post-encounter self-reflection assignments rather than their performance. This allows students to approach each simulation as a learning laboratory in which they can actively try out new skills, test hypotheses, and refine techniques.

This is not the only approach to communication assessment. Colleges of veterinary medicine are encouraged to explore pedagogical strategies that complement the design of their program and teach goal-focused communication. Students benefit from learning how to prioritize their own goals, determine which steps they need to take to achieve their goals and provide feedback to themselves

Table 6.4 Example of Rubric for Simulated Client (SC) Encounter #4: Jive, the Dog.

Explaining the diagnosis	Meets expectations	Opportunity area for growth (OAG)	Did Not Observe or Not Applicable
Student clinician shared the diagnosis with the client			
Student clinician elicited the client's perspective, i.e., "are you familiar with mange?" to establish client's baseline of knowledge			
Student clinician explained the diagnosis in an easy-to-understand fashion, limiting use of medical jargon. The student clinician tailored their explanation to the client's level of baseline knowledge.			
Student clinician explained the zoonotic potential of this type of mange.			
Student clinician advised client to seek advice from a human healthcare provider if the client acknowledged having any sort of skin lesions, including rash.			
Student clinician did not provide medical advice even if the client asked for it.			
Student clinician asked if the client had any questions and/or gave the client the opportunity to ask questions about the diagnosis.			
Forward-Planning			
Student clinician outlined their proposed treatment plan for Jive.			
Student clinician asked if the treatment plan is feasible/possible for the client? i.e., can the client medicate Jive?			
Student clinician asked if there are other pets in the household or if Jive has been around other dogs/cats			
Student clinician explained that Jive's condition is contagious to other pets in the household and other dogs/cats elsewhere			
Student clinician explained that other pets in the household will need to be examined.			
Student clinician explained that they are not legally allowed to treat the other pets in the household without a veterinarian-client-patient relationship (VCPR)			
Student clinician asked if the client had any questions and/or gave the client the opportunity to ask questions about treatment recommendations			

(Continued)

Table 6.4 (Continued)

Explaining the diagnosis	Meets expectations	Opportunity area for growth (OAG)	Did Not Observe or Not Applicable
Gathering information through history-taking (as needed) to establish treatment recommendations			
Student clinician delivered an open-ended question to clarify the patient's history, i.e., "Tell me what you've been noticing at home."			
Student clinician asked appropriate clarifying questions to follow-up (as needed) on the client's concern(s) about Jive's itch, i.e., what is the perceived severity of the itch? Where is he itchy (localized itch vs whole body itch)? Is the itch spreading? Is the itch getting worse? Is the itch associated with any other skin lesions on the dog?			
Student clinician asked the client if they are noticing any skin lesions on their own body.			
Student clinician asked if Jive is on any medications to manage the itch (prescription, over the counter, supplements) and whether it appeared to be helping			
Student clinician asked if Jive is on any additional medications – i.e., flea/tick and/or heartworm preventative			
Communication skills for history-taking			
The student clinician used nonverbal cues appropriately			
The student clinician used easy-to-understand language			
The student clinician used an appropriate tone throughout the encounter			
The student clinician used an appropriate volume throughout the encounter			
The student clinician spoke at an appropriate pace throughout the encounter			
Overall assessment			
What worked well (WWW)	[Free text response]		
Opportunity Areas for Growth (OAG)	[Free text response]		

as they reflect upon the progress that they are making toward meeting these goals (Denness 2013; Englar 2020e). Such learning fosters self-awareness, which is essential, because before learners can provide relationship-centered care to others, they must first care for and understand themselves.

Section 7: Teaching on the Clinical Floor – Veterinary Students and House Officers

Micha C. Simons and Stephanie Thomovsky

Part 1: Introduction

Teaching in a clinical setting has been previously defined by Spencer (2003), as teaching and learning focused on, and usually directly involving, patients and their problems. Clinical settings can be complex environments to navigate. Delivery of clinical care provides educational opportunities while at the same time that care can eclipse the learner's needs (Harden and Cosby 2000). Teaching in the clinical setting often takes place during the specific time frame of a clinical rotation, and the teaching is focused on specific patient cases and rationale for clinical decision-making. Students are able to focus on skills essential to their careers including, but not limited to: history-taking, physical examination, patient communication, professionalism, and the appropriate application of medical knowledge to a patient.

Effective clinical teaching is multidimensional. Clinical teachers must possess a wide range of knowledge, skills, and personal attributes and know when and how to apply them. Irby et al. have outlined numerous skills necessary for a clinical educator, listed in Figure 6.2. Historically, it has been assumed that professionals who have graduated from health professional programs are qualified to teach

Skill necessary for excellent clinical teaching:

- a passion and enthusiasm for teaching
- organization and clarity of content presented
- knowledge and clinical reasoning ability
- professionalism
- group interaction skills
- clinical supervision skills

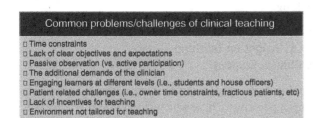

Figure 6.2 Essential skills for clinical teaching. *Source:* Adapted from Irby and Rakestraw (1981) and Irby and Papadakis 2001).

others upon graduation. However, veterinary education has recently experienced some paradigm shifts that are moving toward competency-based education and the modernization of veterinary education through a more student-centered approach. Concurrent with this movement, it is becoming a more common expectation that veterinary educators possess both clinical and educational expertise. The profession is also starting to see the formation of formalized organizations supporting the discipline of veterinary education (e.g., various regional academic educational consortia and the Academy of Veterinary Educators, formed in 2022).

Supporting the learning paths of students, house officers, and potential veterinary assistants and/or technicians requires veterinary educators to capitalize on a combination of planned, opportunistic, formal, and informal teaching (and learning) while balancing the needs of patients, learners, and available resources. Spencer (2003), identified several unique challenges specific to the clinical teaching in medical environments (Figure 6.3).

Despite these challenges, clinical teaching remains quite rewarding as it allows educators to witness the transformation of learners into colleagues.

Part 2: Applicable Educational Theories

The theories discussed in Chapter 2 provide the necessary foundation when preparing for teaching, in general,

Common problems/challenges of clinical teaching

- Time constraints
- Lack of clear objectives and expectations
- Passive observation (vs. active participation)
- The additional demands of the clinician
- Engaging learners at different levels (i.e., students and house officers)
- Patient related challenges (i.e., owner time constraints, fractious patients, etc)
- Lack of incentives for teaching
- Environment not tailored for teaching

Figure 6.3 Common problems and/or challenges of clinical teaching. *Source:* Adapted from Spencer 2003.

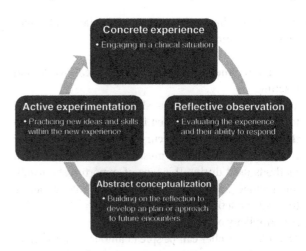

Figure 6.4 Kolb's Cycle of Experiential Learning.

with some of this foundational material more applicable to clinical teaching. Here we will discuss several theories specific to teaching-learning methods, strategies, and assessments appropriate for clinical environments.

Experiential learning describes the idea of a student learning by the act of doing. Kolb's Cycle of Experiential Learning (1984), further outlines this process (Figure 6.4).

To be considered experiential learning the encounter should provide the following:

1) Opportunities for reflection, critical analysis, and synthesis of knowledge.
2) Opportunities for students to demonstrate their knowledge, show initiative, and take responsibility.
3) Opportunities assessment and feedback; space to learn from their mistakes and successes.

A subset of this experiential learning is termed *work-based learning*. Work-based learning can be defined as opportunities provided within a learning program to link classroom learning to authentic workplace experiences. The clinical time of veterinary students and house officer (i.e., interns and residents) training are great examples of this form of learning.

In these workplace settings, the educator must (i) ensure they are providing experiences at a learner-appropriate level, (ii) help facilitate learner recognition of problems and subsequent application of knowledge, (iii) create opportunities for spontaneous learning that do not compromise the appropriate delivery of medical care, and (iv) provide space for reflection along with timely and specific feedback.

Steinert et al. (2017), proposed that the unique intersection between clinical care and teaching is an example of work-based learning and thus introduced the concept of work-based teaching. These authors identified the following three themes intrinsic to physician-lead teaching while on clinical rotations:

1) The interconnectedness between clinical work and teaching

   Teaching in the clinical year should be inextricably tied to the clinical care provided in a teaching hospital. In these settings, teaching occurs constantly; the needs of the patient and learners must be balanced. Common methods used during this type of opportunistic teaching include spontaneous questioning, role-modeling thoughts or activities, and rounding.

2) A multiplicity of teachers

   The role of teacher can be spread among various members of the team. This concept of scaffolding occurs when more senior members of the team are asked to assess their junior colleagues (i.e., a resident assessing the knowledge of an intern or student).

3) Influence of space and artifacts

   It is well known that environment can dramatically affect learning. Clinical educators also need to be cognizant of the environments created in teaching hospitals and work to identify and minimize potential barriers to learning within those spaces.

Part 3: The Environment

A supportive and organized learning environment with sufficient space, appropriate numbers of students, house officers, and faculty necessary to deliver care, should be considered and arranged, to capitalize on all learning opportunities (Kilminster et al. 2007). Clinical year students benefit from active participation in patient management and exposure to a high volume of relevant and diverse clinical cases (Löfmark and Wikblad 2001). Active involvement and, the space to perform under supervised independence, increase student motivation and improve professional and clinical skills (Kilminster et al. 2007). These experiences, coupled with specific, timely, and constructive feedback, have been shown to have a positive effect on performance and clinical year examinations (Châtenay et al. 1996).

Part 4: Outcomes and Assessment

At its core, clinical teaching is an important, and final, piece of veterinary education where the knowledge gained in the classroom setting can be applied to real-life situations. Students are expected to demonstrate, not only their cognitive abilities, but also their skills pertaining to problem-solving, critical thinking, clinical reasoning, clinical judgment and decision-making.

Similar to any other form of teaching, clinical instructors need to assess the impact of their teaching. Historically, we have relied heavily on student evaluations as the primary measure of teaching effectiveness. While informative, the student perspective is incomplete and often lacking in objective measurements. Information gathered from learners and clinical teachers should be used to improve teaching and learning quality and clinical teaching roles (Snell et al. 2000).

The authors propose 15 potential sources of evidence to document effective teaching. These include: (i) student ratings; (ii) peer observations; (iii) peer review of course materials; (iv) external expert ratings; (v) self-ratings; (vi) videos; (vii) student interviews; (viii) exit/alumni ratings; (ix) employer ratings; (x) mentor guidance; (xi) administrator ratings; (xii) teaching scholarship; (xiii) teaching awards; (xiv) learning outcome measures; and (xv) teaching portfolio. Additionally, self-reflection on teaching encounters is an essential part of professional development. Considering questions like: what went well? what did not go well? could anything have been improved? what would have to be done to make learning better? – can help educators improve their effectiveness.

Some medical educators are investigating standardized questionnaires and rubrics to better streamline the documentation of clinical teaching effectiveness (Copeland and Hewson 2000). Such tools may be a useful additions to existing evaluation methods (Parsell and Bligh 2001; Copeland and Hewson 2000). To the authors' knowledge, no such tools have been described or evaluated in veterinary clinical education. It is imperative to acknowledge that the learning process is a complex one and that the clinical environment introduces many unique factors. It is important to consider multiple sources and evaluations for assessing effectiveness of both the educator and the environment (Berk 2013).

It has been suggested that using multiple sources of evidence can help decrease bias and create a more complete picture of an educator's effectiveness (Berk 2013). Additional research is needed to determine which combinations and/or weighing of evidence is the most accurate representation of truly successful and high-quality teaching.

Part 5: Insight on Teaching the Clinical Student

Teaching in the academic veterinary setting is a very interesting opportunity. Those who instruct veterinary students, in their clinical clerkships, generally have little formal training in instruction or teaching (Carr et al. 2021). However, they are typically individuals who work in an academic setting because they enjoy teaching and want to inspire future generations of veterinarians. Those who teach in the clinical year are faculty clinicians, residents, interns, staff, and nurses. It does truly take a village of individuals to foster growth and encourage learning in veterinary clinical practice. Making clinical teaching exciting and also challenging is that teaching moments are peppered throughout every aspect of the veterinary student's clinical day (Smith and Lane 2015).

The Block Begins...

The clinical year begins with day 1 of a block. That block may be neurology, clinical pathology, shelter medicine or equine community practice, but whatever the block, there is always a "day 1"! It is on *day 1* that the mood for the clinical block is set. It is good to start the block with an organized, clear, and concise outline of block expectations. A block can be very difficult, exhausting, and carry a heavy time burden, but if expectations are set ahead of time, students will be more apt to engage and participate.

One way to set expectations is to give orientation materials or an orientation packet to students ahead of day 1. The packet should lay out the student's responsibilities for the block. Be clear and concise, but do not overload the students. If orientation is too verbose, the students will tune out and not remembering the most important points. Guidelines are key and expectations need to be clear. A brief overview of the orientation package is a recommended way of beginning block 1. The first meeting with the group is crucial – you want to make sure students feel comfortable and ready to learn.

Begin the meeting with an icebreaker. As the instructor, you want to make yourself human to the students, while also maintaining the authority of head instructor. It is good to ask the students about themselves and their experience with veterinary medicine to date, and even within the hospital itself. Ask them what rotations they were on prior to your block. This gives you two pieces of information – (i) it gives you critical information on whether they had blocks with or without patient care and (ii) it makes the student understand that you care about them as an individual and about their journey through the clinical year. Once the ice is broken it is good to discuss a brief overview of block expectations – hit the high points of the orientation packet. Discuss patient care, the student's role in appointments, how to divide up appointments between students. It is good to try to analyze the dynamic of your group – paying attention to the quieter students, as they may need

encouragement to speak up and participate as the block moves forward.

Around and Around We Go

Following introductions, day 1 typically continues with rounds. There are two varieties of rounds commonly practiced on the clinic floor: case rounds and topic rounds. It is best to perform case rounds twice a day, in the morning and the evening, so the team is unified with respect to hospitalized case decision and management. The students, house officers, and staff all need to know what needs to be accomplished with a patient. These rounds foster teamwork and further solidify the critical roles each member of the team plays. In addition to learning the how and why of a disease process and learning how to recognize and treat disease, students also need to learn the role of a veterinary nurse versus veterinarian, and these roles can be solidified in case rounds.

Often the day does not allow for thorough morning and evening case rounds, so a quicker more concise round is done once a day and the more thorough, extensive rounds are done at the opposite time of day. After a long, arduous day, attention spans can lapse as fatigue mounts, so the lead clinician may need to adapt rounds to accommodate. While it is a good idea to encourage students to teach their fellow block mates what they have learned through admitting and caring for a particular case, during rounds, if one student is nodding off in the corner and the other speaking gibberish out of fatigue, it may be best to assign a learning objective about a particular topic for discussion at tomorrow's session. Students should always be encouraged to shared information learned with their classmates, however if your students are not alert or focused enough to absorb information, then it is always best for discussion to take place the following day when the team is fresh.

The second type of rounds performed on the clinic floor is topic rounds. These rounds, during a busy rotation, are typically the first to be skipped. Nevertheless, these rounds are critical to learning, especially in the age of preprocessed, PowerPoint. There remains a place for in person, live, and "off-the-cuff" teaching. If nothing else, these rounds allow for an ease that encourages live, and in the moment, student questions. As a clinician, you will likely never forget the first time a student says something similar to, ".....wait so you mean central vestibular literally means disease of the medulla...?!" These moments of true understanding cannot be replicated in the classroom.

Topic rounds participation is best when students have been given a chance to prepare. Students who prepare for expected rounds topics will excel during these sessions. For example, when entering dermatology it is understood that you will probably round about the causes of pruritus, or on critical care, you will discuss fluid therapy. Therefore, it should be expected that a student comes prepared for basic topics on day one. Nevertheless, it is good practice to give them an outline of topics to be discussed throughout the block as it progresses and, at the day's end, to remind the students what the following day's topic of choice will be.

A *round-robin* technique can also be quite effective in rounds; using this technique you alternate between students calling on each student during rounds. This helps students keep and maintain attention; it also encourages them to appropriately prepare for rounds and learn the material. This technique also serves to make sure each student is treated equally, forces the quieter, shy students to participate, and ensures that the louder, more confident students still share their thoughts but at the appropriate time. If all parties are struggling, you can make a question multiple choice – this technique engages students and is fun! Not to mention that by the fourth year of veterinary school, all students are familiar with multiple choice testing and have a certain comfort level with this type of quizzing.

It is also always a good idea to diversify student's learning – have each doctor (including house officers on the block) lead topic rounds. This gives the residents on the block investment in learning and teaches them what teaching is like. If you have a visiting resident on the block, encourage them to lead a round topic of their choice. This can help push him or her out of his or her comfort zone and learn a topic in greater depth.

The same can be said for a visiting intern – as the clinician, you can assign the intern a topic they are responsible for teaching during the block. The clinician should use this opportunity to meet with the intern, guiding them on proper lecture creation and ensuring the intern understands what information is most crucial for a student to learn. When it comes to their day to lead topic rounds, the intern can also learn from the experience as the clinician can critique their presentation and teaching style.

Appointments

New appointments are often a great place for the fourth-year veterinary students to sink their teeth into a case and, it is often during these appointments, that they become most invested. Students are often able to follow the case from entrance to exit, along the way becoming bonded to both the client and the patient. But for this to occur, the student should be allowed to go into the exam room and obtain the history from their client, when a student is able

to meet an owner, take a history, perform a physical exam, and develop a problem list, their investment in the case, patient, owner, and ultimately their learning, exponentially improves (Lane 2008).

The physical examination can be done in front of the client in the exam room, or the patient can be removed from the room and the exam done in the back, away from the client. The former is best for emulating "real practice," as many veterinarians do not have time, during short appointments, to remove the patient from the client to perform the exam. It also builds trust with the client, as they are able to see what they are paying for, in a way. The downside to students doing patient exams in the room with the clients is that it can be intimidating to this young, learning doctor. It also prevents classmates from engaging in and learning from each other's examinations and patients. Removal of the patient from the exam room allows multiple students to learn from the examination process. It also allows for a real-time case discussion without pressure from the client's presence, allows for proper gait analysis, and can make it easier for nursing staff to help assist the students with their examination. Removal of the patient does, however, create separation from the client and their pet which can be off-putting to clients.

During the initial case discussion and exam, you should be able to determine the student's overall foundational knowledge, their observational skills, and their approach to diagnostic interpretation and diagnosis (Lane 2008). To help support student learning and clinical growth, make sure to allow the clinical student to be present and to listen when you talk with owners and present your diagnostic and treatment plan. Demonstrating active listening can be a wonderful source of learning and growth, as the communication techniques a seasoned veterinarian uses when talking to clients and explaining disease processes can be invaluable.

As previously mentioned, another of the student's learning is understanding how their staff can help facilitate their efficiency with appointments. It is good to encourage the nurses to oversee a particular case to make sure that samples and other diagnostics, such as radiographs, are obtained in an efficient manner leaving the student to think about the case and his or her examination findings and diagnostic results. New appointments are fresh/untainted ground for the student. They should be encouraged to interpret diagnostics and determine a treatment plan for their cases. Having their voice heard facilitates the ownership the student has for the case, patient, and client. It also helps foster an environment where the student feels like they are part of the team and part of the decision-making.

Recheck appointments are a different learning process. Here there is often already a diagnosis; a treatment plan has usually already been instituted, but there is still much that can be learned. For example, students can learn a targeted way to obtain information from the client in an efficient and effective manner. The focus of these appointments is typically response to treatment and taking note of any salient changes to patient exam or condition since the previous examination. Recheck appointments also teach students tools that the vast majority of them will require when they go out into veterinary practice – sharing cases with a colleague and co-managing cases. The majority of veterinarians will work in a multi-doctor practice and need to learn how to share case management with a colleague.

Recheck appointments also allow clinicians to observe how successful a student is at discerning what is important from an often extensive medical record, and assess clinical student case preparation. Has the student read the record? Is he or she aware of the chronology of the case? Has he or she taken the time to work on the case the night before its arrival? Has he or she looked to the literature for clarification of a topic or examination finding? How effective the student is at organizing his or her thoughts during a case presentation. Is he or she able to prioritize different aspects of a case?

It is best to discuss previous salient imaging and bloodwork results with the student prior to the patient's arrival. This in addition to giving the student a short case synopsis prior to the recheck's arrival – encourages student case involvement. It is also important in helping students view you as being invested in the case, because the more invested you are in a particular case, the more involved the student will feel and the more invested they will be in learning. Even if an exam finding or diagnosis seem mundane, to the clinical student, it will be the very opposite. Though it may be your one hundredth heat stroke, it will be the student's first or second. These "typical" or "bread and butter" cases are vital to building a student's foundational knowledge, solidifying, and teaching basic pathophysiology.

Transfer cases can be the most difficult cases to use for teaching. A case that is transfered on an already busy morning often is least prioritized by the student. As mentioned earlier, the student is able to meet clients and patients for new appointments. Transfers, meanwhile, are partially completed cases. There is a faceless client behind a phone; the student often does not meet the client until a patient visitation, or perhaps not even until discharge. When the case is transferred, the exam, diagnostics, and sometimes even treatments have already been initiated.

As a result, true case ownership is less natural and less easy. To increase investment in such cases, one approach is to make sure to give the student time to ascertain information from the record or client. Take time to examine the patient together. Do not just tell the student you heard a grade IV systolic heart murmur, find the murmur and allow the student to hear it, as well. If your investment in the case and in the student is tangible, learning will be facilitated.

Carr et al.'s (2021), Five Microskills Model of teaching, also known as the one-minute preceptor model of clinical teaching, states that the instructor should start by getting a commitment from the student. Make them commit to what they found on the history, what they think is abnormal on physical exam, and ultimately, what they want to do with the case. Probe the student for evidence to support said commitment. Use the opportunity to then teach general rules pertaining to a case, diagnosis, or physical exam finding, then reinforce what the student did well with a case, and what part of the clinical thinking process was to be commended. Lastly, take the opportunity to correct any mistakes that were observed or any places the student became off track or erred in his or her thought process (Carr et al. 2021).

Evaluations and Grading

Perhaps the ultimate opportunity to correct mistakes takes place during the evaluation and grading phase of the clinical rotation. The rotation grade is the last teaching moment that a clinician has with his or her student, so it is important for this moment to be productive. Grading should be consistent, fair, and based on a rubric to decrease bias as much as possible, and students should be provided both positive and constructive feedback; they should not be coddled. You are working to produce veterinarians who are competent, which includes being aware of their shortcomings. Remember that these are professional graduate students who are about to become doctors. They are about to counsel owners, treat patients, and make life-and-death decisions on a weekly, if not daily, basis. Evaluations should be different at the start of the clinical year as compared to the last few months of final year to compensate for the growth that is expected during a year of clinical training. All students have areas at which they can improve and areas at which they excel, and ensuring that students have a realistic understanding of their skills and knowledge at all times is imperative to the learning process.

Keys that Make for a Good Instructor

There are four main keys that, when adopted, make for an effective instructor.

Provide Structure

Providing structure, delegating to your team, being involved, and leading by example are important. It is imperative to provide structure and clear standards for the student. As previously presented, from the onset of day one, lay out block expectations. Much like composing visit instructions for a client, you must provide the students with an outline for the block. When expectations are clear and there is structure, it is much easier for a student to adapt to his or her role and flourish. Similarly, even in the midst of a very busy block, it is imperative that structured topic rounds are not left by the wayside. Structured teaching gives the team time to loosen up, relax, and just learn. The team that is allowed allotted time to relax, recharge, and learn together will work more effectively and cohesively. Think of this as similar to the busy family who makes sure to sit down and share a meal at the end of a busy day; this act is critical to fostering the family bond.

Delegate

It is critical to remember that your support staff is also part of the team. Part of the last year of veterinary school is meant to instruct students on their roles versus the roles of their support staff. Many students have not worked with skilled nurses, so take this time to delegate and lead by example, showing students how to effectively use their support staff. As the leader, the students will need to know how to perform certain "technical tasks," such as urinary catheterization, jugular blood draw, or nasogastric tube placement. Licensed or credentialed veterinary technicians can teach many of these technical aspects of veterinary medicine (refer to your individual state's scope of practice guidelines to ensure you are not over or underutilizing your credentialed technicians). This garners respect for the technical staff while simultaneously teaching the student what they can expect their trained staff to be able to accomplish while out in practice.

Similarly, teach students to delegate among themselves. If you have taught a student how to express a urinary bladder, encourage them to delegate – there is no reason the learned student cannot teach their student colleague the same task. This "teach others" mentality allows for peer feedback, and is part of a TBL approach that has been shown to be an effective tool aimed at skills acquisition and knowledge retention between cases (Carr et al. 2022). Encouraging students to teach each other also allows both the student teacher and the student learner to build on foundational knowledge (Carr et al. 2022). And overall, maximizing the skills of your team allows for improved student teaching and learning (Lane 2008).

Lead by Example

At the end of the day, you are the teacher, the authority figure, and the lead clinician. Like it or not, you are setting an example with each of your actions. Stay positive, remain upbeat, and create an environment others want to share. Role modeling is an important teaching tool for the clinical veterinary teacher (Smith and Lane 2015).

Some ways to intentionally model good clinical practice include such practices as "thinking aloud" during a case discussion. This technique can be used to provide the student with the literal framework the instructor uses in his or her mind to organize thoughts or ideas about a case (Smith and Lane 2015). Both of these techniques can teach students how to use evidence, experience, and foundational knowledge to work through a clinical situation or discern the meaning of abnormal physical exam findings (Smith and Lane 2015). Other techniques include using referral cases, diagnostic tests, or treatments performed pre-referral as teaching moments – this provides an opportunity for you to both command respect and shows respect to students, clients, pets, and other veterinarians. Make sure to point out things that were done well while also providing open discussion about other, more appropriate ways to have diagnosed or treated a certain patient or disease process. It is okay and appropriate to use the consultation case as a time to teach and instruct. Students should understand that even when they leave the four walls of your teaching hospital the learning does not cease. You can also use yourself as an example; students should not be afraid or nervous about referring cases to you, but you also want to use real-world examples to do real-time teaching. Never forget that when you are around students, they are learning from you – both from your actions and your behaviors. Therefore, it is important to teach them in a positive manner. If you are on the phone with a referring veterinarian or consulting on a case within the hospital from a different department – be respectful.

Get Your Hands Dirty

Team is vital. Every student will work to his or her full capacity if he or she is invested and part of the team. The leader of the team, the captain of the army who commands respect, is the person who is in the trenches with his or her soldiers. Similarly, when the block leader works shoulder to shoulder with his or her students, the students will work harder and learn more. Patient care is key – students need to learn that it is critical for a veterinarian to take care of his or her patient. This may mean wiping dried food off the e-collar of an anemic puppy, or giving a paralyzed dog a rear-end bath, or cleaning the medial canthus of a kitten's eyes with *Herpes* virus. If the students realize teamwork is important, that patient care is key, and that you respect not only them, but also the patients, clients, and staff, the students will respect you. With that respect, comes effort, time, learning, and success.

Part 6: Considerations for House Officers

While postgraduate studies may not be the primary focus of this text, we would be remiss to not consider house officers and their impact on clinical teaching, especially in academic settings. In keeping with the American Veterinary Medical Association's (AVMA) American Board of Veterinary Specialties (ABVS), the following terms have been defined (AVMA n.d.) below.

An *internship* is a one-year clinical training program that emphasizes mentorship, direct supervision, and learning experiences including rounds, seminars, and formal presentations. It provides practical experience in applying knowledge gained during the professional curriculum and an opportunity to obtain additional training in the clinical sciences. The primary goal of an internship is the education and preparation of a veterinarian for high-quality service in general practice or for advanced specialty training.

A *specialty internship* provides experiences and education related to an AVMA-recognized veterinary specialty organization or AVMA-recognized veterinary specialty.

A *residency* is advanced training in an AVMA-recognized veterinary specialty conducted under the supervision of a board-certified specialist. Such programs are intended to lead to board certification in an AVMA-recognized veterinary specialty organization.

Being able to balance the teaching needs of the clinical year student and those of the house officer is a constant struggle for faculty clinicians. Rather than completely separating the two tasks, it is not uncommon that house officers are expected to share in the teaching experience. While there appears to be some overlap in the skills needed to produce good clinicians and effective teachers, there is a large body of literature in medical education examining this relationship. More recently Smith et al. (2018), identified four skills domains of proficient resident teachers that appear to also enhance their development as clinicians: development of interpersonal skills, improving communication skills, self-awareness, and commanding a deeper understanding of the knowledge. Additionally, some studies have suggested a positive association between teaching and postgraduate training examinations (Seely et al. 1999). While we could assume similar relationships exist, information relating directly to veterinary education and specialty training programs is lacking.

Despite these proposed benefits, the question remains: What is the best way to teach a house officer? While many of the same theories and clinical educator attributes can be brought to house officer training, here the experiential and workplace-based learning is even more important. Considerations for deliberate practice and learning curves may also be helpful when discussing resident training. Are we allowing sufficient opportunities for our learners to practice a skill and/or its components safely (i.e., deliberate practice)? And what do we know about the number of repetitions of a given skill necessary to expect proficiency (i.e., learning curve)? There have been very few studies in the veterinary literature exploring these ideas (Fink et al. 2017; Freeman et al. 2017). Like most areas in veterinary education, additional research is warranted on this topic to determine the best pedagogical approach to training our postgraduate veterinarians.

Part 7: Summary

This chapter has covered a broad range of topics, beginning with classroom instruction, moving through laboratory and skills instruction, touching on personal finance and how to embed DEI into the curriculum, discussing the how and why of teaching empathy, ethics, and morality, delivering information about the current good practices in teaching communication skills, and leaving you with a brief discussion of clinical teaching – both for veterinary students and house officer. If this feels like a huge spectrum of skills and information, it should – because it is. We touched upon some of the biggest and most obvious responsibilities of the professional (veterinary) program instructor, but to truly cover all of these topics in great depth would be a separate text of its own. Thus, the hope is that this chapter provides you some level of insight and guidance for the challenges and joys of delivering content within a professional program, while also pushing you to consider how much or little you truly know about the complexities of teaching in higher education broadly and within a professional program specifically.

References

AAVMC (2022). *Annual Data Report 2021–2022* [Internet], 1–67. Washington, DC: American Association of Veterinary Medical Colleges https://www.aavmc.org/wp-content/uploads/2022/08/2022-AAVMC-Annual-Data-Report-8.8Update.pdf.

Adams, C.L. and Kurtz, S.M. (2017). *Skills for Communicating in Veterinary Medicine*. Otmoor Publishing and Dewpoint Publishing.

Adams, C.L. and Ladner, L.D. (2004). Implementing a simulated client program: bridging the gap between theory and practice. *Journal of Veterinary Medical Education* 31 (2): 138–145. https://doi.org/10.3138/jvme.31.2.138.

Adams, C.L., Nestel, D., and Wolf, P. (2006). Reflection: a critical proficiency essential to the effective development of a high competence in communication. *Journal of Veterinary Medical Education* 33 (1): 58–64. https://doi.org/10.3138/jvme.33.1.58.

Alvarez, E.E. and Reinhart, J.M. (2020). Use of an interactive online teaching module improved students' ability to write a clinically appropriate SOAP Note. *Journal of Veterinary Medical Education* 47 (6): 700–708. https://doi.org/10.3138/jvme.0918-107r.

Amadi, C. (2013). Clinician, society and suicide mountain: reading Rogerian doctrine of unconditional positive regard (UPR). *Psychological Thought* 6 (1): 75–89.

Applebaum, J.W., MacLean, E.L., and McDonald, S.E. (2021). Love, fear, and the human-animal bond: on adversity and multispecies relationships. *Comprehensive Psychoneuroendocrinology* 7: 100071. https://doi.org/10.1016/j.cpnec.2021.100071.

Argyle, M. (1988). Spatial behavior. In: *Bodily Communication*, 2e, 168–187. International Universities Press.

Augustin, M. (2014). How to learn effectively in medical school: test yourself, learn actively, and repeat in intervals. *The Yale Journal of Biology and Medicine* 87 (2): 207–212. PMID: 24910566; PMCID: PMC4031794.

AVMA (n.d.). *American Board of Veterinary Specialties.* Definitions: Policy and Procedures Appendix https://www.avma.org/sites/default/files/2021-04/ABVS-PP-Appendix-6.pdf.

AVMA COE Accreditation Policies and Procedures: Requirements. (2021) https://www.avma.org/education/accreditation-policies-and-procedures-avma-council-education-coe/coe-accreditation-policies-and-procedures-requirements

Bagnasco, A., Pagnucci, N., Tolotti, A. et al. (2014). The role of simulation in developing communication and gestural skills in medical students. *BMC Medical Education* 14: 106. https://doi.org/10.1186/1472-6920-14-106.

Baile, W.F. and Blatner, A. (2014). Teaching communication skills: using action methods to enhance role-play in problem-based learning. *Simulation in Healthcare* 9 (4): 220–227. https://doi.org/10.1097/SIH.0000000000000019.

Bain, B., Hansen, C., Ouoedraogo, F., Radich, R., and Salois, M. (2020). 2020 AVMA report on economic state of the veterinary profession.

Bar-Or, Y.D., Fessler, H.E., Desai, D.A., and Zakaria, S. (2018). Implementation of a comprehensive curriculum in personal finance for medical mellows. *Cureus* 10 (1): e2013. https://doi.org/10.7759/cureus.2013.

Barrows, H.S. (1993). An overview of the uses of standardized patients for teaching and evaluating clinical skills.

AAMC. *Academic Medicine* 68 (6): 443-451; discussion 451-443. https://www.ncbi.nlm.nih.gov/pubmed/8507309.

Batalden, P., Leach, D., Swing, S. et al. (2002). General competencies and accreditation in graduate medical education. *Health Affairs (Millwood)* 21 (5): 103–111. https://www.ncbi.nlm.nih.gov/pubmed/12224871.

Batson, C.D., Early, S., and Salvarani, G. (1997). Perspective taking: imagining how another feels versus imagining how you would feel. *Personality and Social Psychology Bulletin* 23 (7): 751–758.

Becker, A.S., Friedrichs, K., Stiles, M. et al. (2020). The clumsy horse: a professional development tool for facilitators of self-directed, case-based learning. *MedEdPORTAL* 16: 10901. https://doi.org/10.15766/mep_2374-8265.10901.

Bell, M., Cake, M., and Mansfield, C. (2019). Success in career transitions in veterinary practice: perspectives of employers and their employees. *Veterinary Record* 185 (8): 232. https://doi.org/10.1136/vr.105133.

Bell, M.A., Cake, M., and Mansfield, C.F. (2021). International multi-stakeholder consensus for the capabilities most important to employability in the veterinary profession. *Veterinary Record* 188 (5): e20. https://doi.org/10.1002/vetr.20.

Berk, R.A. (2013). Top five flashpoints in the assessment of teaching effectiveness. *Medical Teacher* 35 (1): 15–26.

Berrian, A.M., Feyes, E., Hsiao, C.J., and Wittum, T.E. (2021). Multimodal integration of active learning in the veterinary classroom. *Journal of Veterinary Medical Education* 48 (5): 533–537. https://doi.org/10.3138/jvme.2019-0127.

Bertakis, K.D., Roter, D., and Putnam, S.M. (1991). The relationship of physician medical interview style to patient satisfaction. *Journal of Family Practice* 32 (2): 175–181. https://www.ncbi.nlm.nih.gov/pubmed/1990046.

Bissett, W.T., Zoran, D.L., Clendenin, A. et al. (2013). How a disaster preparedness rotation helps teach the seven NAVMEC professional competencies: the Texas A&M University Experience. *Journal of Veterinary Medical Education* 40 (4): 378–388. https://doi.org/10.3138/jvme.1212-114R1.

Blach, E.L. (2009). Customer service in equine veterinary medicine. *The Veterinary Clinics of North America. Equine Practice* 25 (3): 421–432. https://doi.org/10.1016/j.cveq.2009.07.001.

Blackley, C., Redmond, P., and Peel, K. (2021). Teacher decision-making in the classroom: the influence of cognitive load and teacher affect. *Journal of Education for Teaching* 47 (4): 548–561. https://doi.org/10.1080/02607476.2021.1902748.

Borroni, C., Pimentel-Ávila, A., Stoore, C. et al. (2021). A unique approach to project-based learning (PjBL) in a

Veterinary Anatomy Course. *Medical Science Educator* 31 (2): 511–517. https://doi.org/10.1007/s40670-021-01205-1.

Britt-Lutter, S. and Heckman, S.J. (2020). The financial life of aspiring veterinarians. *Journal of Veterinary Medical Education* 47 (1): 117–124. https://doi.org/10.3138/jvme.0218-017r1. Epub 2019 Apr 22. PMID: 31009300.

Brophy, J. (2010). Classroom management as socializing students into clearly articulated roles. *The Journal of Classroom Interaction* 45 (1): 41–45.

Broughten, R., Hearst, O., M., and Dutton, L. (2021). Developing a framework for interprofessional collaborative practice, cultural fluency, and ecological approaches to health. *Journal of Interprofessional Care* 35 (sup1): 3–8. https://doi.org/10.1080/13561820.2021.1981837.

Brown, G. and Manogue, M. (2001). AMEE Medical Education Guide No. 22: Refreshing lecturing: a guide for lecturers. *Medical Teacher* 23 (3): 231–244. https://doi.org/10.1080/01421590120043000.

Brown, J.P. and Silverman, J.D. (1999). The current and future market for veterinarians and veterinary medical services in the United States. *Journal of the American Veterinary Medical Association* 215 (2): 161–183. https://www.ncbi.nlm.nih.gov/pubmed/10416465.

Bryan, L.A. (2012). Research on science teacher beliefs. In: *Second international handbook of science education*, 2e (ed. B.J. Fraser, K. Tobin, and C.J. McRobbie), 477–495. Dordrecht: Springer.

Bucklin, B.A., Asdigian, N.L., Hawkins, J.L., and Klein, U. (2021). Making it stick: use of active learning strategies in continuing medical education. *BMC Medical Education* 21 (1): 44. https://doi.org/10.1186/s12909-020-02447-0.

Bullough, R.V. Jr. (2011). Ethical and moral matters in teaching and teacher education. *Teaching and Teacher Education* 27 (1): 21–28. https://doi.org/10.1016/j.tate.2010.09.007.

Burt, J., Abel, G., Elmore, N. et al. (2014). Assessing communication quality of consultations in primary care: initial reliability of the Global Consultation Rating Scale, based on the Calgary-Cambridge Guide to the Medical Interview. *BMJ Open* 4 (3): e004339. https://doi.org/10.1136/bmjopen-2013-004339.

Buur, J.L., Schmidt, P.L., and Barr, M.C. (2013). Using educational games to engage students in veterinary basic sciences. *Journal of Veterinary Medical Education* 40 (3): 278–281. https://doi.org/10.3138/jvme.0113-014R.

Byrne, P.S. (1976). *Doctors Talking to Patients: A Study of the Verbal Behaviour of General Practitioners Consulting in their Surgeries*. London: H. M. Stationery Off.

Cahn, S.M. (2009). *Exploring Philosophy: An Introductory Anthology*, 4e. Oxford University Press.

Calsamiglia, S., Espinosa, G., Vera, G. et al. (2020). A virtual dairy herd as a tool to teach dairy production and management. *Journal of Dairy Science* 103 (3): 2896–2905. https://doi.org/10.3168/jds.2019-16714.

Campinha-Bacote, J. (2019). Cultural competemility: a paradigm shift in the cultural competence versus cultural humility debate – Part I. *Online Journal of Issues in Nursing* 24 (1): https://doi.org/10.3912/OJIN.Vol24No01PPT20.

Cantillon, P. and Sargeant, J. (2008). Giving feedback in clinical settings. *BMJ* 337 (7681): 1292–1294. https://doi.org/10.1136/bmj.a1961.

Caris-Verhallen, W.M., Kerkstra, A., and Bensing, J.M. (1999). Non-verbal behaviour in nurse-elderly patient communication. *Journal of Advanced Nursing* 29 (4): 808–818. https://www.ncbi.nlm.nih.gov/pubmed/10215971.

Carr, M.M. and Greenhill, L.M. (2015). Veterinary school applicants: financial literacy and behaviors. *Journal of Veterinary Medical Education* 42 (2): 89–96. https://doi.org/10.3138/jvme.1114-113R. Epub 2015 May 7. PMID: 25872561.

Carr, A.N.M., Kirkwood, R.N., and Petrovski, K.R. (2021). Using the five-microskills method in veterinary medicine clinical teaching. *Veterinary sciences* 8 (6): 89.

Carr, A.N.M., Kirkwood, R.N., and Petrovski, K.R. (2022). Effective veterinary clinical teaching in a variety of teaching settings. *Veterinary sciences* 9 (1): 17.

Carson, C.A. (2007). Nonverbal communication in veterinary practice. *Veterinary Clinics of North America: Small Animal Practice* 37 (1): 49–63. abstract viii. https://doi.org/10.1016/j.cvsm.2006.10.001.

Chapel, D. (2017). Exam rooms that shine. DVM360. Retrieved August 14, 2022, from https://www.dvm360.com/view/exam-rooms-shine (accessed 14 August 2022).

Châtenay, M., Maguire, T., Skakun, E. et al. (1996). Does volume of clinical experience affect performance of clinical clerks on surgery exit examinations? *American Journal of Surgery* 172 (4): 366–372.

Chigerwe, M., Ilkiw, J.E., and Boudreaux, K.A. (2011). Influence of a veterinary curriculum on the approaches and study skills of veterinary medical students. *Journal of Veterinary Medical Education* 38 (4): 384–394. https://doi.org/10.3138/jvme.38.4.384.

Choi, J.S. and Kim, J.S. (2018). Effects of cultural education and cultural experiences on the cultural competence among undergraduate nursing students. *Nurse Education in Practice* 29: 159–162.

Chun, R., Schaefer, S., Lotta, C.C. et al. (2009). Didactic and experiential training to teach communication skills: the University of Wisconsin-Madison School of Veterinary Medicine collaborative experience. *Journal of Veterinary*

Medical Education 36 (2): 196–201. https://doi.org/10.3138/jvme.36.2.196.

Cocksedge, S., George, B., Renwick, S., and Chew-Graham, C.A. (2013). Touch in primary care consultations: qualitative investigation of doctors' and patients' perceptions. *British Journal of General Practice* 63 (609): e283–e290. https://doi.org/10.3399/bjgp13X665251.

COE Accreditation Policies *and Procedures: Requirements.* (2021). COE Accreditation Policies and Procedures: Requirements. https://www.avma.org/education/accreditation-policies-and-procedures-avma-council-education-coe/coe-accreditation-policies-and-procedures-requirements (accessed 14 March 2022).

Cohen-Cole, S.A. (1991). *The Medical Interview: A Three-Function Approach.* Mosby-Year Book.

Connor, A. and Howett, M. (2009). A conceptual model of intentional comfort touch. *Journal of Holistic Nursing* 27 (2): 127–135. https://doi.org/10.1177/0898010109333337.

Conrad, P.A., Hird, D., Arzt, J. et al. (2007). Interactive computerized learning program exposes veterinary students to challenging international animal-health problems. *Journal of Veterinary Medical Education* 34 (4): 497–501. https://doi.org/10.3138/jvme.34.4.497.

Copeland, H.L. and Hewson, M.G. (2000). Developing and testing an instrument to measure the effectiveness of clinical teaching in an academic medical center. *Academic Medicine : Journal of the Association of American Medical Colleges* 75 (2): 161–166.

Cron, W.L., Slocum, J.V. Jr., Goodnight, D.B., and Volk, J.O. (2000). Executive summary of the Brakke management and behavior study. *Journal of the American Veterinary Medical Association* 217 (3): 332–338. https://doi.org/10.2460/javma.2000.217.332.

Cross, T.L. (1989). Towards a culturally competent system of care: a monograph on effective services for minority children who are severely emotionally disturbed.

Crowther, E. and Baillie, S. (2016). A method of developing and introducing case-based learning to a preclinical veterinary curriculum. *Anatomical Sciences Education* 9 (1): 80–89. https://doi.org/10.1002/ase.1530.

D, Souza, R.F., Mathew, M., D, Souza, D.S.J., and Palatty, P. (2018). Novel horizontal and vertical integrated bioethics curriculum for medical courses. *Medical Teacher* 40 (6): 573–577. https://doi.org/10.1080/0142159X.2018.1442921.

Davis, M.H. (1999). AMEE Medical Education Guide No. 15: Problem-based learning: a practical guide. *Medical Teacher* 21 (2): 130–140. https://doi.org/10.1080/01421599979743.

Decety, J. and Fotopoulou, A. (2014). Why empathy has a beneficial impact on others in medicine: unifying theories. *Frontiers in Behavioral Neuroscience* 8: 457. https://doi.org/10.3389/fnbeh.2014.00457.

Decker, J.L., Sparks, B.C., Tedeschi, P., and Morris, K.N. (2018). Race and ethnicity are not primary determinants in utilizing veterinary services in underserved communities in the United States. *Journal of Applied Animal Welfare Science* 21 (2): 120–129. https://doi.org/10.1080/10888705.2017.1378578.

Denness, C. (2013). What are consultation models for? *InnovAiT* 6 (9): 592–599.

DePasque, S. and Tricomi, E. (2015). Effects of intrinsic motivation on feedback processing during learning. *NeuroImage* 1 (119): 175–186. https://doi.org/10.1016/j.neuroimage.2015.06.046.

Devito, J.A. (2007). *The Interpersonal Communication Book.* Pearson.

Dewey, J. (2007). *Democracy and Education.* Echo Library.

Diamond, K.K., Vasquez, C., Borroni, C., and Paredes, R. (2020). Exploring veterinary medicine students' experiences with team-based learning at the Universidad Andrés Bello. *Journal of Veterinary Medical Education* 47 (4): 421–429. https://doi.org/10.3138/jvme.0518-062r.

Dohms, M.C., Collares, C.F., and Tiberio, I.C. (2021). Brazilian version of Calgary-Cambridge Observation Guide 28-item version: cross-cultural adaptation and psychometric properties. *Clinics (São Paulo, Brazil)* 76: e1706. https://doi.org/10.6061/clinics/2021/e1706.

Dooley, L.M., Frankland, S., Boller, E., and Tudor, E. (2018). Implementing the flipped classroom in a veterinary pre-clinical science course: student engagement, performance, and satisfaction. *Journal of Veterinary Medical Education* 45 (2): 195–203. https://doi.org/10.3138/jvme.1116-173r.

Doucet, M., Vrins, A., and Harvey, D. (2009). Effect of using an audience response system on learning environment, motivation and long-term retention, during case-discussions in a large group of undergraduate veterinary clinical pharmacology students. *Medical Teacher* 31 (12): e570–e579. https://doi.org/10.3109/01421590903193539.

Dubrowski, A. and MacRae, H. (2006). Randomised, controlled study investigating the optimal instructor: student ratios for teaching suturing skills. *Medical Education* 40 (1): 59–63. https://doi.org/10.1111/j.1365-2929.2005.02347.x. PMID: 16441324.

Duffy, F.D., Gordon, G.H., Whelan, G. et al. (2004). Assessing competence in communication and interpersonal skills: the Kalamazoo II report. *Academic Medicine* 79 (6): 495–507. https://www.ncbi.nlm.nih.gov/pubmed/15165967.

Duggan, A.P. and Parrott, R.L. (2001). Physicians' nonverbal Rapport building and patients' talk about the subjective component of illness. *Human Communication Research* 27 (2): 299–311.

van Dulmen, S. (2017). Listen: When words don't come easy. *Patient Education and Counseling* 100 (11): 1975–1978. https://doi.org/10.1016/j.pec.2017.06.021.

Duret, D. and Senior, A. (2015). Comparative study of three different personal response systems with fourth-year undergraduate veterinary students. *Journal of Veterinary Medical Education* 42 (2): 120–126. https://doi.org/10.3138/jvme.0814-079R2.

Edwards, S.C. (1998). An anthropological interpretation of nurses' and patients' perceptions of the use of space and touch. *Journal of Advanced Nursing* 28 (4): 809–817.

Egnew, T.R., Mauksch, L.B., Greer, T., and Farber, S.J. (2004). Integrating communication training into a required family medicine clerkship. *Academic Medicine* 79 (8): 737–743. https://www.ncbi.nlm.nih.gov/pubmed/15277128.

Endres, J. and Laidlaw, A. (2009). Micro-expression recognition training in medical students: a pilot study. *BMC Medical Education* 9: 47. https://doi.org/10.1186/1472-6920-9-47.

Englar, R.E. (2017). A novel approach to simulation-based education for veterinary medical communication training over eight consecutive pre-clinical quarters. *Journal of Veterinary Medical Education* 44 (3): 502–522. https://doi.org/10.3138/jvme.0716-118R1.

Englar, R.E. (2018). Using a standardized client encounter in the veterinary curriculum to practice veterinarian-employer discussions about animal cruelty reporting. *Journal of Veterinary Medical Education* 45 (4): 464–479. https://doi.org/10.3138/jvme.0117-001r1.

Englar, R.E. (2019a). Tracking veterinary students' acquisition of communication skills and clinical communication confidence by comparing student performance in the first and twenty-seventh standardized client encounters. *Journal of Veterinary Medical Education* 46 (2): 235–257. https://doi.org/10.3138/jvme.0917-117r1.

Englar, R.E. (2019b). Using a standardized client encounter to practice death notification after the unexpected death of a feline patient following routine ovariohysterectomy. *Journal of Veterinary Medical Education* 46 (4): https://doi.org/10.3138/jvme.0817-111r1.

Englar, R.E. (2019c). Using a standardized client encounter to practice death notification after the unexpected death of a feline patient following routine ovariohysterectomy. *Journal of Veterinary Medical Education* 46 (4): 489–505. https://doi.org/10.3138/jvme.0817-111r1.

Englar, R. (2019d). The role of the comprehensive patient history in the problem-oriented approach. In: *Common Clinical Presentations in Dogs and Cats*, 11–18. Wiley.

Englar, R.E. (2020a). Defining entry-level communication skills: empathy. In: *A Guide to Oral Communication in Veterinary Medicine* (ed. R.E. Englar), 98–120. 5m Publishing.

Englar, R.E. (2020b). Defining entry-level communication skills: non-verbal cues. In: *A Guide to Oral Communication in Veterinary Medicine* (ed. R.E. Englar), 121–148. 5m Publishing.

Englar, R.E. (2020c). Defining entry-level communication skills: reflective listening. In: *A Guide to Oral Communication in Veterinary Medicine* (ed. R.E. Englar), 85–97. 5m Publishing.

Englar, R.E. (2020d). Defining two new skills that companion-animal clients value: compassionate transparency and unconditional positive regard. In: *A Guide to Oral Communication in Veterinary Medicine* (ed. R.E. Englar), 282–296. 5m Publishing.

Englar, R.E. (2020e). How can we structure the consultation from the vantage point of clinical communication? The Calgary-Cambridge Guide as a blueprint for a collaborative consultation. In: *A Guide to Oral Communication in Veterinary Medicine* (ed. R.E. Englar), 49–64. 5m Publishing.

Englar, R. (2020f). Defining entry-level communication skills: open-ended questions and statements. In: *A Guide to Oral Communication in Veterinary Medicine*, 149–162. 5m Publishing.

Englar, R.E., Williams, M., and Weingand, K. (2016). Applicability of the Calgary-Cambridge guide to dog and cat owners for teaching veterinary clinical communications. *Journal of Veterinary Medical Education* 43 (2): 143–169. https://doi.org/10.3138/jvme.0715-117R1.

English, E.R. (2017). Experience and thinking: transforming out perspective on learning. In: *John Dewey's Democracy and Education: A Centennial Handbook* (ed. L.J. Waks and A.R. English), 99–107. Cambridge University Press.

Estabrooks, C.A. and Morse, J.M. (1992). Toward a theory of touch – the touching process and acquiring a touching style. *Journal of Advanced Nursing* 17 (4): 448–456. https://doi.org/10.1111/j.1365-2648.1992.tb01929.x.

Fernandes, D., Lynch, J.G., and Netemeyer, R.G. (2014). Financial literacy, financial education, and downstream financial behaviors. *Management Science* 60 (8): 1861–1883. https://doi.org/10.1287/mnsc.2013.1849.

Fink, O.T., Boston, R.C., Wu, T. et al. (2017). The learning curve for veterinary surgery residents performing hemilaminectomy surgeries in dogs. *Journal of the American Veterinary Medical Association* 250 (2): 215–221.

Fletcher, O.J., Hooper, B.E., and Schoenfeld-Tacher, R. (2015). Instruction and curriculum in veterinary medical education: a 50-year perspective. *Journal of Veterinary Medical Education* 42 (5): 489–500.

Forsyth, C.J., Irving, M.J., Tennant, M. et al. (2017). Teaching cultural competence in dental education: a systematic review and exploration of implications for indigenous populations in Australia. *Journal of Dental Education* 81 (8): 956–968.

Franco-Martínez, L., Martínez-Subiela, S., Cerón, J.J. et al. (2020). Teaching the basics of the One Health concept to undergraduate veterinary students. *Research in Veterinary Science* 133: 219–225. https://doi.org/10.1016/j.rvsc.2020.09.022.

Freeman, L.J., Ferguson, N., Fellenstein, C. et al. (2017). Evaluation of learning curves for ovariohysterectomy of dogs and cats and castration of dogs. *Journal of the American Veterinary Medical Association* 251 (3): 322–332.

Freire, P. (2000). *Pedagogy of the Oppressed*, 30th anniversarye. Continuum.

Gabbott, M. and Hogg, G. (2001). The role of non-verbal communication in service encounters: a conceptual framework. *Journal of Marketing Management* 17: 5–26.

Garrett, L.D. (2013). CVC Highlight: How to break bad news to veterinary clients. *DVM 360*: http://veterinarymedicine.dvm360.com/cvc-highlight-how-break-bad-news-veterinary-clients?id=&sk=&date=&pageID=2.

Gerace, A., Day, A., Casey, S., and Mohr, P. (2017). I think, you think': understanding the importance of self-reflection to the taking of another person's perspective. *Journal of Relationships Research* 8: 1–19.

Gibbs, G., Habeshaw, S., and Habeshaw, T. (1987). Improving student learning during lectures. *Medical Teacher* 9 (1): 11–20. https://doi.org/10.3109/01421598709028976.

Gibson, S. (2005). On judgment and judgmentalism: how counselling can make people better. *Journal of Medical Ethics* 31 (10): 575–577. https://doi.org/10.1136/jme.2004.011387.

Gillard, S., Benson, J., and Silverman, J. (2009). Teaching and assessment of explanation and planning in medical schools in the United Kingdom: cross sectional questionnaire survey. *Medical Teacher* 31 (4): 328–331. https://doi.org/10.1080/01421590801953018.

Goodchild, C.E., Skinner, T.C., and Parkin, T. (2005). The value of empathy in dietetic consultations. A pilot study to investigate its effect on satisfaction, autonomy and agreement. *Journal of Human Nutrition and Dietetics* 18 (3): 181–185. https://doi.org/10.1111/j.1365-277X.2005.00606.x.

Gordon, S.J.G., Bolwell, C.F., Raney, J.L., and Zepke, N. (2022). Transforming a didactive lecture into a student-centered active learning exercise – teaching equine diarrhea to fourth year veterinary students. *Education in Science* 12 (68): 1–14.

Grauer, G.F., Forrester, S.D., Shuman, C., and Sanderson, M.W. (2008). Comparison of student performance after lecture-based and case-based/problem-based teaching in a large group. *Journal of Veterinary Medical Education* 35 (2): 310–317. https://doi.org/10.3138/jvme.35.2.310.

Graugaard, P.K., Holgersen, K., and Finset, A. (2004). Communicating with alexithymic and non-alexithymic patients: an experimental study of the effect of psychosocial communication and empathy on patient satisfaction. *Psychotherapy and Psychosomatics* 73 (2): 92–100. https://doi.org/10.1159/000075540.

Grevemeyer, B., Betance, L., and Artemiou, E. (2016). A telephone communication skills exercise for veterinary students: experiences, challenges, and opportunities. *Journal of Veterinary Medical Education* 43 (2): 126–134. https://doi.org/10.3138/jvme.0315-049R1.

Grewal, K. and Sweeney, M.J. (2021). An innovative approach to educating medical students about personal finance. *Cureus* 13 (6): e15579. https://doi.org/10.7759/cureus.15579.

Habashy, N. and Cruz, L. (2021). Bowing down and standing up: Towards a pedagogy of cultural humility. *International Journal of Development Education and Global Learning* 13 (1): 16–31. https://doi.org/10.14324/IJDEGL.13.1.02.

Hafen, M. Jr., Rush, B.R., and Nelson, S.C. (2009). Utilizing filmed authentic student-client interactions as a communication teaching tool. *Journal of Veterinary Medical Education* 36 (4): 429–435. https://doi.org/10.3138/jvme.36.4.429.

Hafen, M., Drake, A.A., Rush, B.R., and Nelson, S.C. (2013). Using authentic client interactions in communication skills training: predictors of proficiency. *Journal of Veterinary Medical Education* 40 (4): 318–326. https://doi.org/10.3138/jvme.0113-019R.

Hafen, M., Drake, A.S., and Elmore, R.G. (2022). Predictors of psychological well-being among veterinary medical students. *Journal of Veterinary Medical Education* 19: e20210133. https://doi.org/10.3138/jvme-2021-0133. Epub ahead of print. PMID: 35587522.

Haldane, S., Hinchcliff, K., Mansell, P., and Baik, C. (2017). Expectations of graduate communication skills in professional veterinary practice. *Journal of Veterinary Medical Education* 44 (2): 268–279. https://doi.org/10.3138/jvme.1215-193R.

Hall, E. (1973). Space speaks. In: *The Silent Language*, 162–185. Anchor Press.

Halpern, J. (2003). What is clinical empathy? *Journal of General Internal Medicine* 18 (8): 670–674. https://doi.org/10.1046/j.1525-1497.2003.21017.x.

Halpern, J. (2012). Clinical empathy in medical care. In: *Empathy: From bench to bedside* (ed. J. Decety), 229–244. The MIT Press.

Hamilton, G., Ortega, R., Hochstetler, V. et al. (2014). Teaching communication skills to hospice teams: comparing the effectiveness of a communication skills laboratory with in-person, second life, and phone role-playing. *The American Journal of Hospice & Palliative Care* 31 (6): 611–618. https://doi.org/10.1177/1049909113504481.

Hammer, M.R., Bennett, M.J., and Wiseman, R. (2003). Measuring intercultural sensitivity: The intercultural development inventory. *International Journal of Intercultural Relations* 27 (4): 421–443. https://doi.org/10.1016/S0147-1767(03)00032-4.

Hampton, J.R., Harrison, M.J., Mitchell, J.R. et al. (1975). Relative contributions of history-taking, physical examination, and laboratory investigation to diagnosis and management of medical outpatients. *British Medical Journal* 2 (5969): 486–489. https://doi.org/10.1136/bmj.2.5969.486.

Harden, R.M. and Cosby, J. (2000). AMEE Guide No 20: The good teacher is more than a lecturer - the twelve roles of the teacher. *Medical Teacher* 22 (4): 334–347.

Hazel, S.J., Heberle, N., McEwen, M.M., and Adams, K. (2013). Team-based learning increases active engagement and enhances development of teamwork and communication skills in a first-year course for veterinary and animal science undergraduates. *Journal of Veterinary Medical Education* 40 (4): 333–341. https://doi.org/10.3138/jvme.0213-034R1.

Hecht, S., Adams, W.H., Cunningham, M.A. et al. (2013). Student performance and course evaluations before and after use of the Classroom Performance System ™ in a third-year veterinary radiology course. *Veterinary Radiology & Ultrasound* 54 (2): 114–121. https://doi.org/10.1111/vru.12001.

Hines, S.A., Collins, P.L., Quitadamo, I.J. et al. (2005). ATLes: the strategic application of Web-based technology to address learning objectives and enhance classroom discussion in a veterinary pathology course. *Journal of Veterinary Medical Education* 32 (1): 103–112. https://doi.org/10.3138/jvme.32.1.103.

Hojat, M. (2007). *Empathy in Patient Care: Antecedents, Development, Measurement, and Outcomes.* Springer.

Hubrecht, R. and Carter, E. (2019). The 3Rs and humane experimental technique: Implementing change. *Animals* 9 (10): 754. https://doi.org/10.3390/ani9100754.

Hunt, J.A., Anderson, S.L., Spangler, D., and Gilley, R. (2021). Influence of instructor-to-student ratio for teaching suturing skills with models. *Veterinary Surgery* 50: 556–563. https://doi.org/10.1111/vsu.13585.

Hunt, J.A., Simons, M.C., and Anderson, S.L. (2022). If you build it, they will learn: A review of models in veterinary surgical education. *Veterinary Surgery* 51 (1): 52–61. https://doi.org/10.1111/vsu.13683.

Irby, D.M. and Papadakis, M. (2001). Does good clinical teaching really make a difference? *The American Journal of Medicine* 110 (3): 231–232.

Irby, D. and Rakestraw, P. (1981). Evaluating clinical teaching in medicine. *Journal of Medical Education* 56 (3): 181–186.

Ishikawa, H., Eto, M., Kitamura, K., and Kiuchi, T. (2014). Resident physicians' attitudes and confidence in communicating with patients: a pilot study at a Japanese university hospital. *Patient Education and Counseling* 96 (3): 361–366. https://doi.org/10.1016/j.pec.2014.05.012.

Jankowski, P.J. (2019). A construct validation argument for the intercultural development inventory. *Measurement and Evaluation in Counseling and Development* 52 (2): 75–89. https://doi.org/10.1080/07481756.2018.1497428.

Jayakumar, K.L., Larkin, D.J., Ginzberg, S., and Patel, M. (2017). Personal financial literacy among U.S. medical students [version 1]. *MedEdPublish* 6 (35): doi: 10.15694/mep.2017.000035.

Jones, C., Fouty, J.R., Lucas, R.B., and Frye, M.A. (2019). Integrating individual student advising into financial education to optimize financial literacy in veterinary students. *Journal of Veterinary Medical Education* 46 (4): 562–572. https://doi.org/10.3138/jvme.1117-156r1. Epub 2019 Jun 13. PMID: 31194629.

Kalet, A., Pugnaire, M.P., Cole-Kelly, K. et al. (2004). Teaching communication in clinical clerkships: models from the macy initiative in health communications. *Academic Medicine* 79 (6): 511–520. https://doi.org/10.1097/00001888-200406000-00005.

Kanji, N., Coe, J.B., Adams, C.L., and Shaw, J.R. (2012). Effect of veterinarian-client-patient interactions on client adherence to dentistry and surgery recommendations in companion-animal practice. *Journal of the American Veterinary Medical Association* 240 (4): 427–436. https://doi.org/10.2460/javma.240.4.427.

Kassirer, J.P. (1983). Teaching clinical medicine by iterative hypothesis testing. Let's preach what we practice. *New England Journal of Medicine* 309 (15): 921–923. https://doi.org/10.1056/NEJM198310133091511.

Kawasaki, J. and Sandoval, W.A. (2020). Examining teachers' classroom strategies to understand their goals for student learning around the science practices in the Next Generation Science Standards. *Journal of Science Teacher Education* 31 (4): 384–400. https://doi.org/10.1080/1046560X.2019.1709726.

Keifenheim, K.E., Teufel, M., Ip, J. et al. (2015). Teaching history taking to medical students: a systematic review. *BMC Medical Education* 15: 159. https://doi.org/10.1186/s12909-015-0443-x.

Keller, V.F. and Carroll, J.G. (1994). A new model for physician-patient communication. *Patient Education and Counseling* 23 (2): 131–140. https://doi.org/10.1016/0738-3991(94)90051-5.

Khoury, N.M., Suser, J.L., Germain, L.J. et al. (2022). A study of a cultural competence and humility intervention for third-year medical students. *Academic Psychiatry* 46 (4): 451–454. https://doi.org/10.1007/s40596-021-01518-8.

Kilminster, S., Cottrell, D., Grant, J., and Jolly, B. (2007). AMEE Guide No. 27: Effective educational and clinical supervision. *Medical Teacher* 29 (1): 2–19.

Kipperman, B., Rollin, B., and Martin, J. (2021). Veterinary student opinions regarding ethical dilemmas encountered by veterinarians and the benefits of ethics Instruction. *Journal of Veterinary Medical Education* 48 (3): 330–342. https://doi.org/10.3138/jvme.2019-0059.

Kleen, J.L., Atkinson, O., and Noordhuizen, J.P. (2011). Communication in production animal medicine: modelling a complex interaction with the example of dairy herd health medicine. *Irish Veterinary Journal* 64 (1): 8. https://doi.org/10.1186/2046-0481-64-8.

Ko, M. and Krist, C. (2018). Redistributing epistemic agency: How teachers open up space for meaningful participation in science. In: *Rethinking learning in the digital age: Making the learning sciences count, 13th International Conference of the Learning Sciences*, vol. 1 (ed. J. Kay and R. Luckin), 232–239. International Society of the Learning Sciences.

Kogan, L.R., Hellyer, P.W., Clapp, T.R. et al. (2018). Use of Short Animal-Themed Videos to Enhance Veterinary Students' Mood, Attention, and Understanding of Pharmacology Lectures. *Journal of Veterinary Medical Education* 45 (2): 188–194. https://doi.org/10.3138/jvme.1016-162r.

Kohlbry, P.W. (2016). The impact of international service-learning on nursing students' cultural competency. *Journal of Nursing Scholarship* 48 (3): 303–311.

Kolb, D.A. (1984). *Experiential Learning: Experience as the Source of Learning and Development*. Englewood Cliffs, NJ: Prentice-Hall.

Krockenberger, M.B., Bosward, K.L., and Canfield, P.J. (2007). Integrated Case-Based Applied Pathology (ICAP): a diagnostic-approach model for the learning and teaching of veterinary pathology. *Journal of Veterinary Medical Education* 34 (4): 396–408. https://doi.org/10.3138/jvme.34.4.396.

Kurtz, S. (2006). Teaching and learning communication in veterinary medicine. *Journal of Veterinary Medical Education* 33 (1): 11–19. https://doi.org/10.3138/jvme.33.1.11.

Kurtz, S.M. and Adams, C.L. (2009). Essential education in communication skills and cultural sensitivities for global public health in an evolving veterinary world. *Revue Scientifique et Techique* 28 (2): 635–647. https://doi.org/10.20506/rst.28.2.1911.

Kurtz, S.M. and Silverman, J.D. (1996). The Calgary-Cambridge Referenced Observation Guides: an aid to defining the curriculum and organizing the teaching in communication training programmes. *Medical Education* 30 (2): 83–89. https://www.ncbi.nlm.nih.gov/pubmed/8736242.

Kurtz, S.M., Silverman, J., Draper, J., and Silverman, J. (1998). *Teaching and Learning Communication Skills in Medicine*. Radcliffe Medical Press.

Kurtz, S., Silverman, J., Benson, J., and Draper, J. (2003). Marrying content and process in clinical method teaching: enhancing the Calgary-Cambridge guides. *Academic Medicine* 78 (8): 802–809. https://doi.org/10.1097/00001888-200308000-00011.

Kurtz, S.M., Silverman, J.D., and Draper, J. (2004). *Teaching and Learning Communication Skills in medicine*. Radcliffe.

Kurtz, S., Silverman, J., and Draper, J. (2005). The "why": A rationale for communication skills teaching and learning. In: *Teaching and Learning Communication Skills in Medicine* (ed. S. Kurtz, J. Silverman, and J. Draper), 13–27. Radcliffe Publishing.

Kwiatkowski, A.C. and Demirbilek, M. (2016). Investigating veterinary medicine faculty perceptions of lecture capture: issues, concerns, and promises. *Journal of Veterinary Medical Education* 43 (3): 302–309. https://doi.org/10.3138/jvme.0615-090R1.

Lane, E.A. (2008). Problem-based learning in veterinary education. *Journal of Veterinary Medical Education* 35 (4): 631–636. https://doi.org/10.3138/jvme.35.4.631.

Lane, I.F. and Strand, E. (2008). Clinical veterinary education: insights from faculty and strategies for professional development in clinical teaching. *Journal of Veterinary Medical Education* 35 (3): 397–406.

Latham, C.E. and Morris, A. (2007). Effects of formal training in communication skills on the ability of veterinary students to communicate with clients. *Veterinary Record* 160 (6): 181–186. https://doi.org/10.1136/vr.160.6.181.

Lemke, J.L. (2001). Articulating communities: Sociocultural perspectives on science education. *Journal of Research in Science Teaching* 38 (3): 296–316.

Levenstein, J.H., McCracken, E.C., McWhinney, I.R. et al. (1986). The patient-centred clinical method. 1. A model for the doctor-patient interaction in family medicine. *Family Practice* 3 (1): 24–30. https://doi.org/10.1093/fampra/3.1.24.

Levitt, D.H. (2001). Active listening and counselor self-efficacy: Emphasis on one micro-skill in beginning counselor training. *The Clinical Supervisor* 20: 101–115.

Lewis, R.E. and Klausner, J.S. (2003). Nontechnical competencies underlying career success as a veterinarian. *Journal of the American Veterinary Medical Association* 222 (12): 1690–1696. https://doi.org/10.2460/javma.2003.222.1690.

Li, E. and Chen, Y. (2011). An experimental teaching-learning program in histology. *Journal of Veterinary Medical Education* 38 (4): 414–416. https://doi.org/10.3138/jvme.38.4.414.

Lichstein, P.R. (1990). The Medical Interview. In: *Clinical Methods: The History, Physical, and Laboratory Examinations* (ed. H.K. Walker, W.D. Hall, and J.W. Hurst), 29–36. Butterworths.

Lincoln, Y.S. and Guba, E.G. (2003). Paradigmatic controversies, contradictions, and emerging confluences, revisited. In: *The SAGE Handbook of Qualitative Research*, 2e (ed. N.K. Denzin and Y.S. Lincoln), 253–291. Sage Publications, Inc.

Lloyd, J.W. and King, L.J. (2004). What are the veterinary schools and colleges doing to improve the nontechnical skills, knowledge, aptitudes, and attitudes of veterinary students? *Journal of the American Veterinary Medical Association* 224 (12): 1923–1924. https://doi.org/10.2460/javma.2004.224.1923.

Lloyd, J.W. and Walsh, D.A. (2002). Template for a recommended curriculum in "Veterinary Professional Development and Career Success". *Journal of Veterinary Medical Education* 29 (2): 84–93. https://doi.org/10.3138/jvme.29.2.84.

Löfmark, A. and Wikblad, K. (2001). Facilitating and obstructing factors for development of learning in clinical practice: a student perspective. *Journal of Advanced Nursing* 34 (1): 43–50.

Lusardi, A. and Tufano, P. (2009). *Debt Literacy, Financial Experiences, and Over-Indebtedness*. Working paper,. Cambridge, MA: National Bureau of Economic Research.

MacDonald-Phillips, K.A., McKenna, S.L.B., Shaw, D.H. et al. (2022). Communication skills training and assessment of food animal production medicine veterinarians: A component of a voluntary Johne's disease control program. *Journal of Dairy Science* 105 (3): 2487–2498. https://doi.org/10.3168/jds.2021-20677.

Magalhães-Sant, Ana, M., Lassen, J., Millar, K.M. et al. (2014). Examining why ethics is taught to veterinary students: A qualitative study of veterinary educators' perspectives. *Journal of Veterinary Medical Education* 41 (4): 350–357. https://doi.org/10.3138/jvme.1113-149R.

Maguire, P., Fairbairn, S., and Fletcher, C. (1986a). Consultation skills of young doctors: I--Benefits of feedback training in interviewing as students persist. *British Medical Journal (Clinical Research Ed.)* 292 (6535): 1573–1576. https://doi.org/10.1136/bmj.292.6535.1573.

Maguire, P., Fairbairn, S., and Fletcher, C. (1986b). Consultation skills of young doctors: II--Most young doctors are bad at giving information. *British Medical Journal (Clinical Research Ed.)* 292 (6535): 1576–1578. https://doi.org/10.1136/bmj.292.6535.1576.

Maguire, P., Faulkner, A., Booth, K. et al. (1996). Helping cancer patients disclose their concerns. *European Journal of Cancer* 32A (1): 78–81. https://www.ncbi.nlm.nih.gov/pubmed/8695247.

Makarem, N.N., Saab, B.R., Maalouf, G. et al. (2020). Grading reflective essays: The reliability of a newly developed tool- GRE-9. *BMC Medical Education* 20 (1): 331–331. https://doi.org/10.1186/s12909-020-02213-2.

Makoul, G. (2001). The SEGUE Framework for teaching and assessing communication skills. *Patient Education and Counseling* 45 (1): 23–34. https://doi.org/10.1016/s0738-3991(01)00136-7.

Makoul, G. and Schofield, T. (1999). Communication teaching and assessment in medical education: an international consensus statement. Netherlands Institute of Primary Health Care. *Patient Education and Counseling* 37 (2): 191–195. https://doi.org/10.1016/s0738-3991(99)00023-3.

Makoul, G., Curry, R.H., and Novack, D.H. (1998). The future of medical school courses in professional skills and perspectives. *Academic Medicine* 73 (1): 48–51. https://doi.org/10.1097/00001888-199801000-00011.

Malher, X., Bareille, N., Noordhuizen, J.P., and Seegers, H. (2009). A case-based learning approach for teaching undergraduate veterinary students about dairy herd health consultancy issues. *Journal of Veterinary Medical Education* 36 (1): 22–29. https://doi.org/10.3138/jvme.36.1.22.

Marcinowicz, L., Konstantynowicz, J., and Godlewski, C. (2010). Patients' perceptions of GP non-verbal communication: a qualitative study. *British Journal of General Practice* 60 (571): 83–87. https://doi.org/10.3399/bjgp10X483111.

Mariani, C.L. and Roe, S.C. (2021). Use of top hat audience response software in a third-year veterinary medicine and surgery course. *Journal of Veterinary Medical Education* 48 (1): 27–32. https://doi.org/10.3138/jvme.1117-171r.

Markey, K., Sackey, M.E., and Oppong-Gyan, R. (2020). Maximising intercultural learning opportunities: Learning with, from and about students from different cultures. *British Journal of Nursing* 29 (18): 1074–1077. https://doi.org/10.12968/bjon.2020.29.18.1074. PMID: 33035086.

Marteau, T.M., Wynne, G., Kaye, W., and Evans, T.R. (1990). Resuscitation: experience without feedback increases confidence but not skill. *BMJ* 300 (6728): 849–850: https://doi.org/10.1136/bmj.300.6728.849.

Massoth, C., Röder, H., Ohlenburg, H. et al. (2019). High-fidelity is not superior to low-fidelity simulation but leads to overconfidence in medical students. *BMC Medical Education* 19 (1): 29. https://doi.org/10.1186/s12909-019-1464-7.

Masters, C., Robinson, D., Faulkner, S. et al. (2019). Addressing biases in patient care with the 5Rs of cultural humility, a clinician coaching tool. *Journal of General Internal Medicine* 34: 627–630 (2019). https://doi.org/10.1007/s11606-018-4814-y.

Matthew, S.M., Schoenfeld-Tacher, R.M., Danielson, J.A., and Warman, S.M. (2019). Flipped classroom use in veterinary education: a multinational survey of faculty experiences. *Journal of Veterinary Medical Education* 46 (1): 97–107. https://doi.org/10.3138/jvme.0517-058r1.

Mauldin Pereira, M., Artemiou, E., McGonigle, D. et al. (2018). Using the virtual world of second life in veterinary medicine: student and faculty perceptions. *Journal of Veterinary Medical Education* 45 (2): 148–155. https://doi.org/10.3138/jvme.1115-184r4.

May, S.A. and Silva-Fletcher, A. (2015). Scaffolded active learning: nine pedagogical principles for building a modern veterinary curriculum. *Journal of Veterinary Medical Education* 42 (4): 332–339. https://doi.org/10.3138/jvme.0415-063R.

McArthur, M.L. and Fitzgerald, J.R. (2013). Companion animal veterinarians' use of clinical communication skills. *Australian Veterinary Journal* 91 (9): 374–380. https://doi.org/10.1111/avj.12083.

McCaw, K., West, A., Duncan, C. et al. (2021). Exploration of immersive virtual reality in teaching veterinary orthopedics. *Journal of Veterinary Medical Education* e20210009: https://doi.org/10.3138/jvme-2021-0009.

McComas, W.F. (1996). Ten myths of science: Reexamining what we think we know about the nature of science. *School Science and Mathematics* 96 (1): 10–16. https://doi.org/10.1111/j.1949-8594.1996.tb10205.x.

McCool, K.E. and Kedrowicz, A.A. (2021). Evaluation of veterinary students' communication skills with a service dog handler in a simulated client scenario. *Journal of Veterinary Medical Education* 48 (5): 538–548. https://doi.org/10.3138/jvme.2019-0140.

McDermott, M.P., Tischler, V.A., Cobb, M.A. et al. (2015). Veterinarian-client communication skills: current state, relevance, and opportunities for improvement. *Journal of Veterinary Medical Education* 42 (4): 305–314. https://doi.org/10.3138/jvme.0115-006R.

McMahon, G.T. (2016). What do i need to learn today?--The evolution of CME. *New England Journal of Medicine* 374 (15): 1403–1406. https://doi.org/10.1056/NEJMp1515202.

McManus, D.A. (2001). The two paradigms of education and the peer review of teaching. *Journal of Geoscience Education* 49 (5): 423–434. https://doi.org/10.5408/1089-9995-49.5.423.

McMurray, J. and Boysen, S. (2017). Communicating empathy in veterinary practice. *Veterinary Ireland Journal* 7 (4): 199–205.

Meehan, M.P. and Menniti, M.F. (2014). Final-year veterinary students' perceptions of their communication competencies and a communication skills training program delivered in a primary care setting and based on

Kolb's Experiential Learning Theory. *Journal of Veterinary Medical Education* 41 (4): 371–383. https://doi.org/10.3138/jvme.1213-162R1.

Melchor, M. (2015). Perceptions of senior dental students regarding cultural diversity before and after community service-learning rotations (Doctoral dissertation). http://hdl.handle.net/10657/2176.

Menor-Campos, D.J., Knight, S., Sánchez-Muñoz, C., and López-Rodríguez, R. (2019). Human-directed empathy and attitudes toward animal use: A survey of Spanish veterinary students. *Anthrozoös* 32 (4): 471–487. doi: 10.1080/08927936.2019.1621518.

Michaelsen, L.K., Knight, A.B., and Fink, D.L. (2004). *Team-Based Learning*, 1e. Stylus Publishing.

Miller, D. (2005). Teaching and Learning Communication Skills in Medicine Kurtz Suzanne, Silverman Jonathan and Draper Juliet Teaching and learning communication skills in medicine Publisher Radcliffe No. of pages: 392 Price£35.0018577565841857756584. *Primary health care* 15 (10): 10–10. https://doi.org/10.7748/phc.15.10.10.s13.

Miller, E., Manz, E., Russ, R. et al. (2018). Addressing the epistemic elephant in the room: Epistemic agency and the next generation science standards. *Journal of Research in Science Teaching* 55 (7): 1053–1075. https://doi.org/10.1002/tea.21459.

Moffett, J., Berezowski, J., Spencer, D., and Lanning, S. (2014). An investigation into the factors that encourage learner participation in a large group medical classroom. *Advances in Medical Education and Practice* 5: 65–71. https://doi.org/10.2147/amep.S55323.

Molgaard, L.K., Hodgson, J.L., Bok, H.G.J. et al. (2018). *Competency-Based Veterinary Education: Part 1 - CBVE Framework. AAVMC Working Group on Competency-Based Veterinary Education*. Washington, DC: Association of American Veterinary Medical Colleges.

Moniz, T., Arntfield, S., Miller, K. et al. (2015). Considerations in the use of reflective writing for student assessment: Issues of reliability and validity. *Medical Education* 49 (9): 901–908. https://doi.org/10.1111/medu.12771.

Moore, M. (2007). What does patient-centred communication mean in Nepal? *Medical Education* 42: 18–26.

Morrisey, J.K. and Voiland, B. (2007). Difficult interactions with veterinary clients: working in the challenge zone. *Veterinary Clinics of North America: Small Animal Practice* 37 (1): 65–77. abstract viii. https://doi.org/10.1016/j.cvsm.2006.09.009.

Myers, W.S. (2009). *Nonverbal Communication Speaks Volumes: Building Better Client Relationships*, 3–5. *Exceptional Veterinary Team*.

Nagy, A.L., Oros, N.A., Farcal, L. et al. (2016). 3Rs in Education. *Alternatives to Animal Experimentation* 33 (2): 85–86: https://doi.org/10.14573/altex.1602011.

Nässtrom, G., Andersson, C., Granberg, C. et al. (2021). Changes in student motivation and teacher decision making when implementing a formative assessment practice. *Frontiers in Education* 6 (616216): 1–17. https://doi.org/10.3389/feduc.2021.616216.

National Education Association (2020). *Code of Ethics for Educators*. https://www.nea.org/resource-library/code-ethics-educators (accessed 12 October 2022).

Nessler, J., Schaper, E., and Tipold, A. (2021). Proof of concept: game-based mobile learning-the first experience with the app action bound as case-based geocaching in education of veterinary neurology. *Front Vet Sci* 8: 753903. https://doi.org/10.3389/fvets.2021.753903.

Newman, I. (2019). When saying 'go read it again' won't work: multisensory ideas for more inclusive teaching and learning. *Nurse Education in Practice* 34: 12–16. https://doi.org/10.1016/j.nepr.2018.10.007.

Newman, T., Trimmer, K., and Padró, F.F. (2019). The need for case studies to illustrate quality practice: Teaching in higher education to ensure quality of entry level professionals. In: *Ensuring Quality in Professional Education*, vol. *I*, 1–17. Cham: Palgrave Macmillan.

Nichols, L.O. and Mirvis, D.M. (1998). Physician-patient communication: does it matter? *Tennessee Medicine* 91 (3): 94–96. https://www.ncbi.nlm.nih.gov/pubmed/9523501.

Nkomo, L.M. and Daniel, B.K. (2021). Sentiment analysis of student engagement with lecture recording. *TechTrends* 65 (2): 213–224. https://doi.org/10.1007/s11528-020-00563-8. Epub 2021 Jan 6.

Noddings, N. (2005). *The Challenge to Care in Schools: An Alternative Approach to Education*, 2e. Teachers College Press.

Noddings, N. (2013). *Caring: A Relational Approach to Ethics and Moral Education*, 2e. University of California Press.

Noddings, N. (2016). *Philosophy of Education*, 4e. Westview Press.

Noddings, N. (2017). Dewey, care ethics, and education. In: *John Dewey's Democracy and Education: A Centennial Handbook* (ed. L.J. Waks and A.R. English), 314–324. Cambridge University Press.

Norfolk, T., Birdi, K., and Walsh, D. (2007). The role of empathy in establishing rapport in the consultation: a new model. *Medical Education* 41 (7): 690–697. https://doi.org/10.1111/j.1365-2923.2007.02789.x.

Nouri, N. and McComas, W.F. (2021). History of science (HOS) as a vehicle to communicate aspects of nature of science (NOS): Multiple cases of HOS instructors' perspectives regarding NOS. *Research in Science Education* 51 (1): 289–305.

Novack, D.H., Suchman, A.L., Clark, W. et al. (1997). Calibrating the physician. Personal awareness and effective patient care. Working Group on Promoting Physician Personal Awareness, American Academy on Physician and Patient. *Journal of the American Medical Association* 278 (6): 502–509. https://doi.org/10.1001/jama.278.6.502.

O' Brien, E.M., O, Donnell, C., Murphy, J. et al. (2021). Intercultural readiness of nursing students: An integrative review of evidence examining cultural competence educational interventions. *Nurse Education in Practice* 50: 102966. https://doi.org/10.1016/j.nepr.2021.102966.

Ong, L.M., Visser, M.R., Lammes, F.B., and de Haes, J.C. (2000). Doctor-patient communication and cancer patients' quality of life and satisfaction. *Patient Education and Counseling* 41 (2): 145–156. https://www.ncbi.nlm.nih.gov/pubmed/12024540.

Park, Y.S., Konge, L., and Artino, A.R. (2020). The positivism paradigm of research. *Academic Medicine* 95 (5): 690–694. doi: 10.1097/ACM.0000000000003093.

Park, R.M., Gruen, M.E., and Royal, K. (2021). Association between dog owner demographics and decision to seek veterinary care. *Veterinary Sciences* 8 (1): 7.

Parmelee, D., Michaelsen, L.K., Cook, S., and Hudes, P.D. (2012). Team-based learning: a practical guide: AMEE guide no. 65. *Medical Teacher* 34 (5): e275–e287. https://doi.org/10.3109/0142159x.2012.651179.

Parmelee, D., Roman, B., Overman, I., and Alizadeh, M. (2020). The lecture-free curriculum: Setting the stage for life-long learning: AMEE Guide No. 135. *Medical Teacher* 42 (9): 962–969. https://doi.org/10.1080/0142159x.2020.1789083.

Parsell, G. and Bligh, J. (2001). Recent perspectives on clinical teaching. *Medical Education* 35 (4): 409–414.

Patterson, T.G. and Joseph, S. (2006). Development of a self-report measure of unconditional positive self-regard. *Psychology and Psychotherapy* 79 (Pt 4): 557–570. https://www.ncbi.nlm.nih.gov/pubmed/17312871.

Patterson, J.S., Stickle, J.E., Thomas, J.S., and Scott, M.A. (2007). An integrative and case-based approach to the teaching of general and systemic pathology. *Journal of Veterinary Medical Education* 34 (4): 409–415. https://doi.org/10.3138/jvme.34.4.409.

Pedersen, R. (2009). Empirical research on empathy in medicine-A critical review. *Patient Education and Counseling* 76 (3): 307–322. https://doi.org/10.1016/j.pec.2009.06.012.

Peisachovich, E. (2015). The importance of intercultural fluency in developing clinical judgment. *GSTF Journal of Nursing Health Care* 2 (20): https://doi.org/10.7603/s40743-015-0020-8.

Peloquin, S.M. (1989). Helping through touch: The embodiment of caring. *Journal of Religion and Health* 28 (4): 299–322. https://doi.org/10.1007/BF00986067.

Peterson, M.C., Holbrook, J.H., Von Hales, D. et al. (1992). Contributions of the history, physical examination, and laboratory investigation in making medical diagnoses. *Western Journal of Medicine* 156 (2): 163–165. https://www.ncbi.nlm.nih.gov/pubmed/1536065.

Plant, J.D. (2007). Incorporating an audience response system into veterinary dermatology lectures: effect on student knowledge retention and satisfaction. *Journal of Veterinary Medical Education* 34 (5): 674–677. https://doi.org/10.3138/jvme.34.5.674.

Poon, E., Bissonnette, P., Sedighi, S. et al. (2022). Improving financial literacy using the medical mini-MBA at a Canadian medical school. *Cureus* 14 (6): e25595. https://doi.org/10.7759/cureus.25595.

President's Advisory Council on Financial Capability (2013). *Final report President's Advisory Council on Financial Capability [Internet]*. Washington, DC: US Department of the Treasury https://www.nefe.org/_images/partnerships/PACFC%20final%20report%20Feb%2019%202013.pdf (accessed 7 October 2022).

Preusche, I. and Lamm, C. (2016). Reflections on empathy in medical education: What can we learn from social neurosciences? *Advances in Health Sciences Education: Theory and Practice* 21 (1): 235–249. https://doi.org/10.1007/s10459-015-9581-5.

Prober, C.G. and Heath, C. (2012). Lecture halls without lectures--a proposal for medical education. *New England Journal of Medicine* 366 (18): 1657–1659. https://doi.org/10.1056/NEJMp1202451.

Prober, C.G. and Khan, S. (2013). Medical education reimagined: a call to action. *Academic Medicine* 88 (10): 1407–1410. https://doi.org/10.1097/ACM.0b013e3182a368bd.

Ptacek, J.T., Leonard, K., and McKee, T.L. (2004). "I've got some bad news . . .": Veterinarians' recollections of communicating bad news to clients. *Journal of Applied Social Psychology* 34 (2): 366–390. https://doi.org/10.1111/j.1559-1816.2004.tb02552.x.

Pun, J. (2021). A study of Chinese medical students' communication pattern in delivering bad news: an ethnographic discourse analysis approach. *BMC Medical Education* 21 (1): 286. https://doi.org/10.1186/s12909-021-02724-6.

Punti, G. and Dingel, M. (2021). Rethinking race, ethnicity, and the assessment of intercultural competence in higher education. *Education Sciences* 11 (3): 110.

Radford, A.D., Stockley, P., Taylor, I.R. et al. (2003). Use of simulated clients in training veterinary undergraduates in communication skills. *Veterinary Record* 152 (14): 422–427. https://doi.org/10.1136/vr.152.14.422.

Radford, A., Stockley, P., Silverman, J. et al. (2006). Development, teaching, and evaluation of a consultation structure model for use in veterinary education. *Journal of Veterinary Medical Education* 33 (1): 38–44. https://doi.org/10.3138/jvme.33.1.38.

Rauch, M., Bettermann, V., Tipold, A. et al. (2022). Use of actors or peers as simulated clients in veterinary communication training. *Journal of Veterinary Medical Education* e20210055: https://doi.org/10.3138/jvme-2021-0055.

Reinhard, A.R., Hains, K.D., Hains, B.J., and Strand, E.B. (2021). Are they ready? Trials, tribulations, and professional skills vital for new veterinary graduate success. *Frontiers in Veterinary Science* 8: 785844. https://doi.org/10.3389/fvets.2021.785844.

Rhind, S.M., Baillie, S., Kinnison, T. et al. (2011). The transition into veterinary practice: opinions of recent graduates and final year students. *BMC Medical Education* 11: 64. https://doi.org/10.1186/1472-6920-11-64.

Riccardi, V.M. and Kurtz, S.M. (1983). *Communication and Counselling in Health Care*. Charles C. Thomas.

Rickles, N.M., Tieu, P., Myers, L. et al. (2009). The impact of a standardized patient program on student learning of communication skills. *American Journal of Pharmaceutical Education* 73 (1): 4. https://www.ncbi.nlm.nih.gov/pubmed/19513141.

Rider, E.A., Hinrichs, M.M., and Lown, B.A. (2006). A model for communication skills assessment across the undergraduate curriculum. *Medical Teacher* 28 (5): e127–e134. https://doi.org/10.1080/01421590600726540.

Riess, H., Kelley, J.M., Bailey, R.W. et al. (2012). Empathy training for resident physicians: a randomized controlled trial of a neuroscience-informed curriculum. *Journal of General Internal Medicine* 27 (10): 1280–1286. https://doi.org/10.1007/s11606-012-2063-z.

Ritter, C., Adams, C.L., Kelton, D.F., and Barkema, H.W. (2018). Clinical communication patterns of veterinary practitioners during dairy herd health and production management farm visits. *Journal of Dairy Science* 101 (11): 10337–10350. https://doi.org/10.3168/jds.2018-14741.

Ritter, C., Adams, C.L., Kelton, D.F., and Barkema, H.W. (2019). Factors associated with dairy farmers' satisfaction and preparedness to adopt recommendations after veterinary herd health visits. *Journal of Dairy Science* 102 (5): 4280–4293. https://doi.org/10.3168/jds.2018-15825.

Root Kustritz, M.V., Lowum, S., Flynn, K. et al. (2017). Assessing Communications Competencies through Reviews of Client Interactions and Comprehensive Rotation Assessment: A Comparison of Methods. *Journal of Veterinary Medical Education* 44 (2): 290–301. https://doi.org/10.3138/jvme.1116-184R.

Roter, D.L., Frankel, R.M., Hall, J.A., and Sluyter, D. (2005). The expression of emotion through nonverbal behavior in medical visits: mechanisms and outcomes. *Journal of General Internal Medicine* 21 (Suppl 1): S28–S34.

Rush, B.R., White, B.J., Allbaugh, R.A. et al. (2013). Investigation into the impact of audience response devices on short- and long-term content retention. *Journal of Veterinary Medical Education* 40 (2): 171–176. https://doi.org/10.3138/jvme.1012-091R.

Sandler, G. (1980). The importance of the history in the medical clinic and the cost of unnecessary tests. *American Heart Journal* 100 (6 Pt 1): 928–931. https://www.ncbi.nlm.nih.gov/pubmed/7446394.

Scheffer, S., Muehlinghaus, I., Froehmel, A., and Ortwein, H. (2008). Assessing students' communication skills: validation of a global rating. *Advances in Health Sciences Education: Theory and Practice* 13 (5): 583–592. https://doi.org/10.1007/s10459-007-9074-2.

Schei, E., Fuks, A., and Boudreau, J.D. (2018). Reflection in medical education: Intellectual humility, discovery, and know-how. *Medicine, Health Care, and Philosophy* 22 (2): 167–178. https://doi.org/10.1007/s11019-018-9878-2.

Schoenfeld-Tacher, R.M., Kogan, L.R., Meyer-Parsons, B. et al. (2015). Educational research report: changes in students' levels of empathy during the didactic portion of a veterinary program. *Journal of Veterinary Medical Education* 42 (3): 194–205. https://doi.org/10.3138/jvme.0115-007R.

Schoenfeld-Tacher, R.M., Shaw, J.R., Meyer-Parsons, B., and Kogan, L.R. (2017). Changes in affective and cognitive empathy among veterinary practitioners. *Journal of Veterinary Medical Education* 44 (1): 63–71. https://doi.org/10.3138/jvme.0116-009R2.

Seely, A.J., Pelletier, M.P., Snell, L.S., and Trudel, J.L. (1999). Do surgical residents rated as better teachers perform better on in-training examinations? *The American Journal of Surgery* 177 (1): 33–37.

Sewell, J. and Rogers, S. (2022). Assessing the impact of a personal finance elective course on student attitudes and intentions. *American Journal of Pharmacy Education* 27: 8942. https://doi.org/10.5688/ajpe8942. Epub ahead of print. PMID: 35477516.

Shaw, J.R. (2006). Four core communication skills of highly effective practitioners. *The Veterinary Clinics of North America. Small Animal Practice* 36 (2): 385–396. vii. https://doi.org/10.1016/j.cvsm.2005.10.009.

Shaw, J.R., Adams, C.L., and Bonnett, B.N. (2004a). What can veterinarians learn from studies of physician-patient communication about veterinarian-client-patient communication? *Journal of the American Veterinary Medical Association* 224 (5): 676–684. https://www.ncbi.nlm.nih.gov/pubmed/15002804.

Shaw, J.R., Adams, C.L., Bonnett, B.N. et al. (2004b). Use of the roter interaction analysis system to analyze veterinarian-client-patient communication in companion animal practice. *Journal of the American Veterinary Medical Association* 225 (2): 222–229. https://www.ncbi.nlm.nih.gov/pubmed/15323378.

Shaw, J.R., Adams, C.L., Bonnett, B.N. et al. (2012). Veterinarian satisfaction with companion animal visits. *Journal of the American Veterinary Medical Association* 240 (7): 832–841. https://doi.org/10.2460/javma.240.7.832.

Shea, S.C. (1998). *Psychiatric Interviewing: The Art of Understanding*, 2e. WB Saunders Company.

Shearer, R. and Davidhizar, R. (2003). Using role play to develop cultural competence. *Journal of Nursing Education* 42 (6): 273–276.

Shepherd, S.M., Willis-Esqueda, C., Newton, D. et al. (2019). The challenge of cultural competence in the workplace: Perspectives of healthcare providers. *BMC Health Services Research* 19 (1): 1–11.

Short, N., St Peters, H., Almonroeder, T. et al. (2020). Long-term impact of international service learning: Cultural competence revisited. *Journal of Occupational Therapy Education* 4 (1): 1–14.

Show, A. and Englar, R.E. (2018). Evaluating dog- and cat-owner preferences for calgary-cambridge communication skills: results of a questionnaire. *Journal of Veterinary Medical Education* 45 (4): 534–543. https://doi.org/10.3138/jvme.0117-002r1.

Silverman, J., Kurtz, S., and Draper, J. (2008). *Skills for Communicating with Patients*. Radcliffe Medical Press.

Silverman, J., Kurtz, S.M., and Draper, J. (2013). *Skills for Communicating with Patients*, 3e. Radcliffe Publishing.

Simon, C. (2018). The functions of active listening responses. *Behavioural Processes* 157: 47–53. https://doi.org/10.1016/j.beproc.2018.08.013.

Simpson, D.J. (2017). The consciously growing and refreshing life. In: *John Dewey's Democracy and Education: A centennial Handbook* (ed. L.J. Waks and A.R. English), 237–244. Cambridge University Press.

Singer, T. and Lamm, C. (2009). The social neuroscience of empathy. *Annals of the New York Academy of Sciences* 1156: 81–96. https://doi.org/10.1111/j.1749-6632.2009.04418.x.

Smith, J.R. and Lane, I.F. (2015). Making the most of five minutes: the clinical teaching moment. *Journal of Veterinary Medical Education* 42 (3): 271–280.

Smith, C.C., Newman, L.R., and Huang, G.C. (2018). Those who teach, can do: characterizing the relationship between teaching and clinical skills in a residency program. *Journal of Graduate Medical Education* 10 (4): 459–463.

Snell, L., Tallett, S., Haist, S. et al. (2000). A review of the evaluation of clinical teaching: new perspectives and challenges. *Medical Education* 34 (10): 862–870.

Spencer, J. (2003). Learning and teaching in the clinical environment. *BMJ* 326 (7389): 591–594.

Spruijt, A., Wolfhagen, I., Bok, H. et al. (2013). Teachers' perceptions of aspects affecting seminar learning: a qualitative study. *BMC Medical Education* 13: 22. https://doi.org/10.1186/1472-6920-13-22.

Steinert, Y., Basi, M., and Nugus, P. (2017). How physicians teach in the clinical setting: The embedded roles of teaching and clinical care. *Medical Teacher* 39 (12): 1238–1244.

Stevens, B.J. and Kedrowicz, A.A. (2018). Evaluation of fourth-year veterinary students' client communication skills: recommendations for scaffolded instruction and practice. *Journal of Veterinary Medical Education* 45 (1): 85–90. https://doi.org/10.3138/jvme.0816-129R1.

Stewart, M.A. (1995). Effective physician-patient communication and health outcomes: a review. *Canadian Medical Association Journal* 152 (9): 1423–1433. https://www.ncbi.nlm.nih.gov/pubmed/7728691.

Strike, K. and Soltis, J.F. (2009). *The Ethics of Teaching*. Teachers College Press.

Stroupe, D. (2014). Examining classroom science practice communities: How teachers and students negotiate epistemic agency and learn science-as-practice. *Science Education* 98 (3): 487–516. https://doi.org/10.1002/sce.21112.

Svensson, C., Emanuelson, U., Bard, A.M. et al. (2019). Communication styles of Swedish veterinarians involved in dairy herd health management: A motivational interviewing perspective. *Journal of Dairy Science* 102 (11): 10173–10185. https://doi.org/10.3168/jds.2018-15731.

Takemura, Y., Atsumi, R., and Tsuda, T. (2007). Identifying medical interview behaviors that best elicit information from patients in clinical practice. *Tohoku Journal of Experimental Medicine* 213 (2): 121–127. https://doi.org/10.1620/tjem.213.121.

Tan, X.H., Foo, M.A., Lim, S.L.H. et al. (2021). Teaching and assessing communication skills in the postgraduate medical setting: a systematic scoping review. *BMC Medical Education* 21 (1): 483. https://doi.org/10.1186/s12909-021-02892-5.

Tayce, J.D., Saunders, A.B., Keefe, L., and Korich, J. (2021). The creation of a collaborative, case-based learning experience in a large-enrollment classroom. *Journal of Veterinary Medical Education* 48 (1): 14–20. https://doi.org/10.3138/jvme.2019-0001.

Taylor, E.W. (2008). Transformative learning theory. *New Directions for Adult and Continuing Education* 119: 5–15.

Thurman, J., Volet, S.E., and Bolton, J.R. (2009). Collaborative, case-based learning: how do students actually learn from each other? *Journal of Veterinary Medical Education* 36 (3): 297–304. https://doi.org/10.3138/jvme.36.3.297.

L.T. Kohn, J.M. Corrigan, M.S. Donaldson (Eds.) (2000). To Err is Human: Building a Safer Human System. http://www.nationalacademies.org/hmd/~/media/Files/Report%20Files/1999/To-Err-is-Human/To%20Err%20is%20Human%201999%20%20report%20brief.pdf

Trenholm, S. and Jensen, A. (2004). *Interpersonal Communication*. Oxford University Press.

Trinh, N., O, Hair, C., Agrawal, S. et al. (2021). Lessons learned: Developing an online training program for cultural sensitivity in an academic psychiatry department. *Psychiatric Services (Washington, D.C.)* 72 (10): 1233–1236. https://doi.org/10.1176/appi.ps.202000015.

Tsimaras, T., Wallace, J.E., Adams, C. et al. (2022). Actualizing cultural humility: an exploratory study of veterinary students' participation in a northern community health rotation. *Journal of Veterinary Medical Education* e2021013: https://doi.org/10.3138/jvme-2021-0130.

Tzioumis, V., Freire, R., Hood, J. et al. (2018). Educators' perspectives on animal welfare and ethics in the Australian and New Zealand veterinary curricula. *Journal of Veterinary Medical Education* 45 (4): 448–463. https://doi.org/10.3138/jvme.0117-017r.

US Census Bureau (2023). National population by characteristics: 2020–2022. Census.gov. https://www.census.gov/data/datasets/time-series/demo/popest/2020s-national-detail.html.

Velasquez, A., West, R., Graham, C., and Osguthorpe, R. (2013). Developing caring relationships in schools: A review of the research on caring and nurturing pedagogies. *Review of Education* 1 (2): 162–190. doi: 10.1002/rev3.3014.

Verderber, R.F. and Verderber, K.S. (1980). *Inter-Act: Using Interpersonal Communication Skills*. Wadsworth.

Veterinary Communication. (2019). Institute for Healthcare Communication (IHC). https://healthcarecomm.org/veterinary-communication/ (accessed 23 June 2022).

Volk, J.O., Felsted, K.E., Cummings, R.F. et al. (2005). Executive summary of the AVMA-Pfizer business practices study. *Journal of the American Veterinary Medical Association* 226 (2): 212–218. https://doi.org/10.2460/javma.2005.226.212.

Wachter, R., Kaplan, G.S., Gandhi, T., and Leape, L. (2015). You can't understand something you hide: Transparency as a path to improve patient safety. *Health Affairs Blog* http://healthaffairs.org/blog/2015/06/22/you-cant-understand-something-you-hide-transparency-as-a-path-to-improve-patient-safety/.

Wagner, J. and Walstad, W.B. (2019). The effects of financial education on short-term and long-term financial behaviors. *Journal of Consumer Affairs* 53: 234–259. https://doi.org/10.1111/joca.12210.

Wald, H.S. and Reis, S.P. (2010). Beyond the margins: Reflective writing and development of reflective capacity in medical education. *Journal of General Internal Medicine* 25 (7): 746–749. https://doi.org/10.1007/s11606-010-1347-4.

Washburn, S.E., Posey, D., Stewart, R.H., and Rogers, K.S. (2016). Merging clinical cases, client communication, and physiology to enhance student engagement, learning, and skills. *Journal of Veterinary Medical Education* 43 (2): 170–175. https://doi.org/10.3138/jvme.1015-177R.

Watt, K., Abbott, P., and Reath, J. (2016). Developing cultural competence in general practitioners: An integrative review of the literature. *BMC Family Practice* 17 (1): 158. https://doi.org/10.1186/s12875-016-0560-6.

Weger, H., Castle, G.R., and Emmett, M.C. (2010). Active listening in peer interviews: the influence of message paraphrasing on perceptions of listening skill. *The International Journal of Listening* 24: 34–49.

Wiese, K.C. and Bennett, D. (2018). Supervised workplace learning in postgraduate training: A realist synthesis. *Medical Education* 52 (9): 951–969. https://doi.org/10.1111/medu.13655.

Williams, M.K. (2017). John Dewey in the 21st century. *Journal of Inquiry and Action in Education* 9 (1): 91–102.

Wolff, M., Wagner, M.J., Poznanski, S. et al. (2015). Not another boring lecture: Engaging learners with active learning techniques. *Journal of Emergency Medicine* 48 (1): 85–93. https://doi.org/10.1016/j.jemermed.2014.09.010. Epub 2014 Oct 13. PMID: 25440868.

Woytek, A. (2005). Utilizing Assessment to Improve Student Motivation and Success. *Essays in Education*, 14(1):1–6. https://openriver.winona.edu/eie/vol14/iss1/22, https://www.aphis.usda.gov/aphis/ourfocus/animalwelfare/sa_awa, https://www.aphis.usda.gov/aphis/ourfocus/animalwelfare/sa_publications/ct_publications_and_guidance_documents, https://www.nal.usda.gov/legacy/aglaw/what-are-regulations-using-animals-educational-programs.

Yerrick, R.K., Pedersen, J.E., and Arnason, J. (1998). "We're just spectators": A case study of science teaching, epistemology, and classroom management. *Science Education* 82 (6): 619–648. https://doi.org/10.1002/(SICI)1098-237X(199811)82:6<619::AID-SCE1>3.0.CO;2-K.

Zivic, A., Smith, J.F., Reiser, B.J. et al. (2018). Negotiating epistemic agency and target learning goals: Supporting coherence from the students' perspective. In: *Rethinking learning in the digital age: Making the learning sciences count, 13th International Conference of the Learning Sciences (ICLS)*, vol. 1 (ed. J. Kay and R. Lukin), 25–32. International Society of the Learning Sciences.

7

Technology in the Classroom

Shane M. Ryan, BS, M.Ed., PhD Candidate
Medical University of South Carolina College of Pharmacy, Charleston, SC, USA

Sarah A. Bell, MEd, EdD
University of Florida College of Veterinary Medicine, Gainesville, FL, USA

Micha C. Simons, VMD, MVEd
Virginia-Maryland College of Veterinary Medicine, Blacksburg, VA, USA

Sarah Baillie, PhD, Principal Fellow of the Higher Education Academy (PFHEA); Member of the Royal College of Veterinary Surgeons (MRCVS)
Bristol Veterinary School, Bristol, UK

Section 1: Introduction

Shane M. Ryan and Sarah A. Bell

As technology evolves, so too does our excitement for what the college classroom of the future is going to look like. Our visions of its possibilities will be realized in the actions we take today to become skilled digital educators who embrace the changing environments we teach in and understand the needs and preferences of our students. Many of the students entering our classrooms today live as much in the digital world as they do in the physical one. Education technologies offer a bridge for instructors to connect the student's physical and digital realities and reach students where they prefer to be.

Students have expectations for how they should receive all their services and content, such as financial and entertainment. Their expectation is clearly digital or technology-enhanced in a meaningful way, and the expectations for their educational services and content are no different. They do not go into a bank to deposit their checks; they snap an image of it on their phone and deposit it digitally. They have that same expectation when it comes to submitting an assignment for a college course.

However, with each advancement comes more challenges and the need for systematic processes for integrating technology into our teaching and designing learning experiences that harness the benefits of the technology or digital modality, seek to avoid negative side effects, and continually guarantee equitable experiences for all students. Toward that end, veterinary educators need to gain a deep understanding of the trends, models, strategies, and systems necessary to support learners and assist in overcoming barriers to student success in the digital age.

Part 1: Learning Management Systems

The transaction of information has a great impact on the learning that occurs in any environment, and the act of such is composed of many different tasks. Learning management systems (LMS) provide a platform for educational functions such as administrative duties, the delivery of content, the monitoring of learning, communication, and student assessment (Cavus 2014). These web-based solutions provide the capabilities and services necessary to complete the transaction, thus enhancing the likelihood for learning to occur.

Most LMS come equipped with a variety of features that can be used to support our educational functions. Administrative tasks, such as record and attendance keeping, are compiled digitally for ease of access. LMS can aid in the delivery of content by providing organizational structures, such as containers or folders for corresponding content that can be grouped into modules or units of study. Programmatic reporting, individual student performance monitoring, and outcomes achievement tracking can be gathered and accessed through the system's gradebook and related toolsets, and communications can be facilitated through virtual inboxes and online discussion boards (Cavus 2014). Differences between LMS and their functions exist, but most offer similar features.

As these LMS are deployed, data is collected to help provide feedback to their creators to help offer a smoother and more efficient product. Similarly, as LMS features are accessed by users, they can provide informative feedback to administrators, instructors, and students through learning analytics.

Part 2: Learning Analytics

Learning analytics is the term used to describe the wealth of data that is collected regarding student learning and engagement with course content and assignments. Learning analytics is a representation of data related to student activity in a digital environment. Educators can use this data to improve content organization, features of instruction, and student learning (Viberg et al. 2018).

Most LMS offer basic resources and features for learning analytics. Often, educators can view the last time a student accessed their course and/or see how active they are in the course over time. They can also use gradebook features to determine how often students are completing assignments and whether the completions are timely. Other features common to learning analytics include opportunities for educators to review how often pages of content are viewed and the number of times documents or files are downloaded. Videoconferencing and recording software often allow educators or administrators access to see who has been viewing videos, how many times an individual viewed a particular recording, and the amount of time spent viewing the recording.

Such information can be used to improve the student learning experience. Files or documents that are downloaded more often than others can be highlighted or moved to more prominent locations for ease of use. Videos that are viewed repeatedly by students may need an accompanying document explaining complex concepts, a diagram representing a system or structure, or other accompaniments to help students better understand the material. Files that are never downloaded or viewed may need to be reorganized, highlighted to demonstrate their importance, or removed entirely if they are not relevant to the learning objectives that support student outcomes.

Student-friendly learning analytics dashboards have also become popular. Like those analytics available to faculty, students can view which resources are accessed by their peers most often, track their progress toward course completion, and monitor the distribution of grades within the course. These features are made available for students to support and promote self-regulated learning (Viberg et al. 2020). Students can see that their classmates are downloading a particular file, which may indicate the file's importance for the class. Students can observe their progress toward completing course assignments to gauge their pace, and they can compare their scores with the whole class grade distribution on a particular exam to monitor their own standing and make necessary adjustments to how they study or approach the course.

Part 3: Learning Tools

Learning tools act as aids in the acquisition and application of knowledge and skills. As such, they can serve a variety of needs in both the classroom and digital learning environment. Most commonly, learning tools are selected to improve the educational experience for both educators and student learners. Learning tools can be used to present information and facilitate interactions with content, connect individuals and teams, and provide opportunities for collaboration, practice, and assessment.

Section 2: Presenting Information and Interactions with Content

Shane M. Ryan and Sarah A. Bell

The expression of knowledge and distribution of content can be facilitated in several ways. Educators can deliver information to and distribute content via video capture software. Video capture software is typically purchased and maintained by governing institutions, each with tutorials for live and prerecorded lecture styles tailored specifically to that software and its corresponding features.

Part 1: Considerations for Cognitive Learning Theories

Mayer and Moreno (2003) define *meaningful learning* as "the deep understanding of material, which includes attending to important aspects of the presented material, mentally organizing it into a coherent cognitive structure, and integrating it with relevant existing knowledge" (p. 43). For students to fully understand a concept, or develop meaningful learning, they must utilize their cognitive capacity – their ability to transfer information from what is gathered through their auditory and visual processing channels, through working memory, and into long-term memory for the purpose of later recall. All human cognitive capacity is limited as to how much information can be processed by the brain at the same time. Instructional designers refer to stress on cognitive capacity as the cognitive load.

When the learner's cognitive processing limits have been reached, this is considered the point of cognitive overload.

Mayer and Moreno (2003) suggest several ways educators can reduce cognitive load and avoid cognitive overload. When presenting material on screen, it is important to consider the amount of visual and auditory processing necessary to understand the material. For example, an instructor using slides that are heavily laden with text might reduce paragraphs of text on screen and into summarized bullet points that are immediately read off by the instructor, eliminating the cognitive load of extensive on-screen text being read by the student while simultaneously trying to listen to the instructor lecture on the topic.

In instances where large amounts of information are presented in both visual and auditory channels, such as during prerecorded lectures, a useful strategy would be pretraining, or introducing difficult terms or concepts before the start of the lesson, to help students make smoother connections with the information as it is presented. Weeding out or eliminating material that is not essential to the learning objectives of the lesson also creates a more coherent presentation for students and reduces cognitive load. Adding cues or signals, such as arrows pointing to important concepts or adding a star beside essential information, additionally can support student visual processing.

Part 2: Considerations for Constructivist Learning Theory

Constructivists view learning as the point at which a student has constructed or built their own knowledge for themselves (see Chapter 2 for a more in-depth explanation of this learning theory). They learn by creating meaning from information they are given. "Constructivism argues that interactive activities in which learners play active roles can engage and motivate learning more effectively than activities where learners are passive" (Zhang et al. 2005, p. 16). It is important to remember that for students to construct their own knowledge, they will need opportunities to engage with you and your course content.

Educators can encourage learner interactions and engagement with content using learning tools. Virtual meeting spaces and video capture and conferencing software can facilitate these exchanges via embedded self-assessments, participant polling, and on-screen coded action triggers such as prompts to click a button to learn more. Other applications promote collaborative interactions through various forms of media, including documents, images, and presentations.

Creating meaningful student interactions with course content is a useful strategy to help students achieve learning outcomes. In instances where educators are using prerecorded content, such as videos or voice-over presentations, signposts, or stopping points for interactions can be built directly into the videos themselves. Most of the popular video recording software typically comes equipped with features that allow for embedded interactions and other options for student engagement activities. Educators can record their content and segment it with stopping points, intentional breaks, or interactive activities at specific points in time within their recorded video, such as at the end of a specific section of the lecture or after introducing a complex concept. Signposts may be the inclusion of a slide that prompts students to stop and summarize the section in their notes, a question aimed at reflection and prior knowledge recall, or a bulleted list referencing important information from the segment.

Educators can also encourage student engagement during live presentations of content. The incorporation of audience polling or audience response systems can facilitate student interactions and increase student satisfaction and attention in sessions (Plant 2007; Rush et al. 2010). Videoconferencing software is often already equipped or easily integrated into polling features, and polls can be used very much like signposts and stopping points in prerecorded material. For example, after the introduction of complex terms or concepts, educators can add a quick poll to gauge student understanding, identify misconceptions, and facilitate discussions surrounding the information presented.

It is common for educators to use non-video materials to introduce content to their students, including images, animations, diagrams, documents, and research articles. Various applications now also allow students to collaboratively engage with these materials, as they allow students to communicate and interact with peers and instructors asynchronously by inserting reactions, comments, or questions at specific time stamps on media recordings, on a specific section of static document, or even a spatial location on a static image or diagram. In turn, instructors can use learning tools that incorporate student reactions and comments to engage students and support their meaningful and collaborative learning goals.

Part 3: Connect and Collaborate

Learning tools that connect learners with their peers and instructors can help foster collaboration and group learning. Davidson and Major (2014) attempted to discriminate between collaborative, cooperative, and problem-based group learning styles within existing literature. While collaborative and cooperative learning had been used synonymously in some instances, the two approaches demonstrated the differences in the amount of guidance and structure provided by the instructor. Educators employing a cooperative learning strategy were more active in their facilitative roles and structured groups more strictly by assigning each group member specific duties. Educators using a collaborative model were still facilitating group tasks but provided more flexibility in group arrangements and structure. In problem-based group learning, depending on the needs of their students, instructors still serve as a facilitator of the task as they would in collaborative and cooperative learning groups. However, in problem-based learning, students are typically intentionally divided into heterogenous groups with differing levels of experience. Additionally, the task itself must be a problem for the group to solve together (Davidson and Major 2014). Group learning, as described by Pickrell et al. (2002), provides students the opportunity to share resources and experiences. These collaborative environments promote the development of knowledge and skills and enhance meaningful learning by refining currently understood constructs or correcting misconceptions with content. Today's LMS and virtual meeting spaces are often equipped with collaborative features that can be used synchronously or asynchronously.

Virtual meeting software and videoconferencing software typically include features for whole group and small group learning. Breakout rooms, for example, divide whole group sessions in virtual meetings into smaller, more intimate sub-sessions. These can be used to foster the collaborative connection between students, and instructors can provide problem-based or case-based activities with questions or prompts for groups to work through in their small group space.

LMS also frequently offer discussion boards for both large and small groups to collaborate asynchronously. Discussion boards are comparable to mini social networks focused on specific topics or questions. Instructors can post educational materials, problems, or example cases to the board and ask students to share their reactions, questions, comments, or arguments. Students can summarize sections of a research article, document the steps in a procedure, and share experiences related to the content. By requiring students to respond to one or more of their group mates, faculty can facilitate connections between peers.

Additionally, dynamic online bulletin boards can be used to facilitate group learning. Online bulletin boards allow students to work together, both synchronously and asynchronously, on a blank canvas. Educators can provide students with a topic, question, or case to guide their learning. Students then scour electronic resources to find images, diagrams, research articles, videos, and other media to pin on the board. The board itself could serve as their final product for this activity, or students can use their bulletin board to summarize information learned, structure a short answer essay, or inform the work of a larger product, such as a poster to share in a poster session or gallery walk.

Some popular examples of online bulletin boards or related products that can accomplish collaborative learning include Google Docs™ and Microsoft's suite of tools that allow students to collaborate in drafting PowerPoint™ slides and Excel™ documents. Dropbox Paper™ is another popular cloud-based collaboration tool that allows multiple users to work on the same document and view changes dynamically. These tools provide students with the ability to work on projects in real time, regardless of their physical location. They allow for easy collaboration, version control, and provide a centralized platform for student teams to communicate and share information.

Part 4: Practice and Self-Assessment

Learning tools can be used to foster opportunities for practice, student self-assessment, and evaluative assessment of student learning. Merrill (2002) lists five principles that are common in most instructional theories: real-world problem-solving, the activation of existing knowledge, modeling or demonstrations of new knowledge or skills, the application of knowledge, and the integration of knowledge into practice. Students require real-world problems to solve and opportunities to practice what they are learning for meaningful learning to occur.

Assignment and quiz features embedded in an LMS can be used to provide opportunities for students to apply and practice what they are learning. Self-assessment activities can also help facilitate the application of knowledge. Learning tools, such as built-in quiz features or polling applications, can help students gauge their own learning in a low-stakes activity. The tools can be used to promote self-reflection and help guide student learning and study time. Instructors often use self-assessment to determine which students may require additional instruction to make them successful (Tobias and Bailey 2020). Self-assessment quizzes can consist of a variety of question types, including multiple choice or select multiple answer options. Case-based questions can be provided, and self-assessments could be created to mimic other real-world problems or issues that students may encounter in practice.

A wide variety of learning tools and analytics are available through an LMS for use by administrators, instructors, and students. LMS can host content and engagement activities, as well as serve as a vehicle for communication, collaboration, and assessment. These robust platforms can be utilized for face-to-face (F2F), blended, and fully online courses to support both faculty and students in the processes of teaching and learning.

Section 3: Online and Blended Learning

Shane M. Ryan and Sarah A. Bell

Stakeholder needs and priorities, in addition to global trends and events, are leading veterinary medical education to begin exploring online and blended learning models as possible permanent features to their professional degree programs. As more of these programs integrate partial or fully online components to their preclinical and clinical curriculums, educators must be equipped to teach across a continuum of modalities – specifically, technology-enhanced F2F, blended, and fully online. This begins with an adequate understanding of the affordances and challenges that each modality presents.

This section of the chapter will start with a review of the stakeholder needs and priorities that will likely inform changes to our teaching and learning environments over the coming years. Next, we will introduce you to the online and blended delivery modes, including two blended learning models: hybrid and HyFlex. For each modality, we will provide a cursory review of the terminology, theories, design choices, and quality standards that define it. We will also mention some practical good teaching practices that you can use to get started in your own online and blended teaching.

Part 1: Instructional Delivery Modes

There are three widely accepted instructional delivery modes in higher education: F2F, online learning, and blended learning (Blau and Drennan 2017). These three modes exist on a continuum, as shown in Figure 7.1, with "F2F" on one side, and "fully online" on the other end. Blended learning is everything between the two that is not 100% traditional, F2F teaching, nor 100% fully online teaching. Blended learning systems at the furthest end of the continuum achieve some degree of technology-enhanced learning (Bonk and Graham 2012), while blended learning systems at the opposite end of the continuum use hybrid or other similar models that shift some amount of structured student contact time to online, internet-based delivery. Within each modality, there are

commonly accepted and adapted models of instruction, such as the hybrid and HyFlex models of blended learning that we will discuss in this section. An instructional model consists of a common pairing of a modality with other specific design choices that when applied and modeled in an appropriate context should produce predicted and desired results.

Part 2: Stakeholder Needs and Priorities

Stakeholder needs and priorities determine to what degree these three modes are used in the delivery of veterinary medical education. Administrators and college leaders are seeking to make students more competitive in the veterinary workforce while also keeping tuition costs from swelling. They are also looking to diversify the profession, which starts with attracting and retaining new types of students (Bonnaud and Fortané 2021). Expanding access and reducing the cost of veterinary programs means that our leaders are exploring innovative models for training students. Models that remove some of the burdens of space and time and provide cost savings through efficiencies and economic-minded methods, such as resource sharing, are increasingly being explored. While remote teaching served as a quick fix to an emergency situation during the COVID-19 pandemic, many leaders now recognize opportunities to capitalize on the work done to enhance infrastructure and train faculty in teaching remotely. For many leaders, it seems like a good time to make some meaningful shifts in how our educational programs are delivered and structured (Sutton and Jorge 2020).

The other important stakeholder group whose needs and priorities cannot be ignored are our students. Any of these three modalities may provide authentic benefits and value to some students, while at the same time presenting major challenges and barriers for others. Hybrid and online learning are often cited by students as being flexible and providing them with control and choices that empower them to be self-directed learners (Mamattah 2016). However, if there is one thing the COVID-19 pandemic made clear, it is that there is a subset of students who do not want remote instruction, and, perhaps counterintuitively, these are not always the poorer performing students; they simply prefer F2F contact with instructors and any alternative is not acceptable to them (Abbasi et al. 2020). These students rightly feel that they "signed up" for a F2F program, and what they received during the pandemic was not always that. If a program were intentionally designed to be online or hybrid and marketed itself as such, then it should attract and admit students that better align with that instructional model, and so this may not be much of a problem beyond the unique situation presented during the

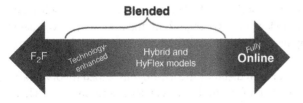

Figure 7.1 Continuum of instructional delivery modes.

COVID-19 pandemic, but student preferences and needs can change unexpectedly, and expectations do not always match reality.

Other learners who often do fall on the weaker end of the performance spectrum can also experience negative outcomes of certain design decisions in online and hybrid learning, such as heavily asynchronous instruction, which is often associated with procrastination and further agitation of poor time management and study habits (Berge and Huang 2004). In the design of online and hybrid instruction, a student-centered, personalized support approach should be taken to provide each student with the individualized care they will need to be successful (Tyler-Smith 2006).

The last but equally important stakeholder group whose needs and priorities will not only shape decision-making but also heavily determine success of any modality choices is that of the educators and educational support specialists. Educators are the boots on the ground and the engine of the curriculum. Other educational specialists may include Licenced Veterinary Technicians (LVTs) with teaching responsibilities, instructional designers, nonfaculty trainers and academic/educational coordinators, assessment specialists, and so forth. Educators, like students, often cite flexibility, choice, and control as reasons for wanting to develop an online or hybrid course (Hubbard 1998).

Preplanning and preproducing some or all of a course prior to implementing it provides many benefits to instructors in allowing them to manage the many other professional and personal responsibilities in their lives during a semester while they may be delivering two to three courses at once. Allocating six months to a year prior to the first day of classes to develop strategy, design the course, and record some or all the content gives an educator much more freedom and less time pressure to create a quality course that better reflects their unique style and teaching philosophy. Front-loading much of the work of teaching a course and spreading it over a longer period not only provides richer opportunities for collaboration and quality control, but it also provides more time during the delivery of the course for the educator to meaningfully engage with students and provide individualized care and support to students who need it.

In reviewing the needs and priorities of various stakeholder groups, it is likely pretty clear that the relationships between these groups can be complex and context-specific, and priorities can often be competing. For these reasons, decisions related to instructional modality should always be considered in the context of the larger system. Later in this chapter, we will explore instructional systems design (ISD) for digital learning and the importance of thinking about teaching in the context of the larger educational systems within which they exist.

Part 3: Online Learning

Online learning as a delivery mode is often referred to as fully online to distinguish it from blended or hybrid learning, although a definition for what technically qualifies a fully online course may vary from one university to another. One often defining characteristic of a fully online course is that there is usually zero required F2F, in-person contact between the students and instructors or students and peers.

There are several design options for fully online courses that can make one online course very different from another. One of the most well-known design decisions to make in the development of a fully online course is communication synchrony: should it be asynchronous, synchronous, or somewhere in between? Asynchronous communication allows the student to interact with instructors and peers outside of a specific and required timeframe. Examples of asynchronous activities include discussion boards or email, which allow students to communicate with each other on their own time, while using videoconferencing tools like Zoom™ or Skype™ during a set time are examples of a synchronous communication tools.

Another well-known design decision is pacing. Determining if the instruction will be self-paced, class-paced, or some mixture of both is important. Self-paced offers several benefits for certain situations; for example, if you are designing an online course for residents to freshen up on basic science or procedural knowledge and want something they can easily fit into their busy schedules, you might choose to make it a fully asynchronous, self-paced online course. If you are designing a fully online course for first-year Doctor of Veterinary Medicine (DVM) students to take at home over the summer prior to the start of the program as a form of orientation to the program, you may choose to make it class-paced to hold them accountable for making progress and introduce them to working at pace with a cohort, and you may decide to build in some synchronous activities to give them a chance to start building relationships with each other.

Part 4: Research and Theory

Researchers have been studying distance and online learning for decades and therefore we have quite a bit of knowledge in the form of theories, principles, and guidelines for designing online and blended instruction. We will focus our review on two important theories that have major implications for student success: cognitive load theory, which we have already touched on a bit in this chapter, and transactional distance theory. Cognitive load theory, again, cautions us of the limitations of short-term memory. There are several well-validated guidelines that use cognitive science principles to help design quality online instruction that seeks to avoid cognitive overload.

One principle says that students learn and recall better when information is provided to them in "chunks" that help to condense separate bits of information into categories or meaningful groups (Morena and Mayer 1999). In the design of an online course, we support student learning by chunking our courses into meaningful units or modules. This allows students to learn a concept within an expertly formed category that groups similar concepts and knowledge, thereby making learning more efficient and connected.

This principle also states that students can more easily process and remember information when it is broken into smaller chunks or segments, rather than presented as a long and continuous stream of information (Morena and Mayer 1999). This is because the human brain has limitations in its ability to process and store large amounts of information at once, and therefore benefits from having the information divided into smaller, more manageable pieces. We accomplish this by creating asynchronous, self-paced content for online courses that are between 3 and 10 minutes long and have a meaningful start and end point. Simply splicing a long lecture does not necessarily accomplish this principle, as you would want to divide the lecture into several mini lectures, each of which should stand on its own as an instructional resource.

Other cognitive learning principles say that students learn and recall better when instructional materials feature an on-screen presenter who is using a conversational speaking style (Moreno and Mayer 1999). When developing fully online courses, it is very important to humanize the instruction and materials as much as possible, which segues us to the second theory that we will cover, transactional distance theory. This theory cautions us of the impact of isolation on motivation in online learning. According to this theory, transactional distance is the psychological or communicative space between student and instructor (Moore 2005). The key construct of transactional distance is dialogue. As the amount of dialogue increases, transactional distance decreases, and as transactional distance decreases, a student's sense of isolation decreases.

How do we increase dialogue in our online courses? Firstly, we can host live events. If live lectures or active learning events are not required, then hosting virtual office hours can provide opportunities for online students to ask questions and voice opinions. Secondly, we can foster a communicative learning culture in the course. Building opportunities and requirements into the course that actively seek to create and sustain a community of support and learning is hard work but vitally important for avoiding student feelings of isolation in an online course. One tip would be to use a discussion board and put in the time

to make it successful. This means the instructors of the course need to be active in facilitating peer-to-peer discussion, and written prompts should be attention-grabbing, interesting, and relevant.

A third way to increase dialogue in an online course is to build opportunities for frequent and personalized feedback. Some LMS offer features that make it easy for instructors to provide personalized feedback or utilize toolsets that mimic personalized contact. One example is formative quizzes that allow instructors to preprogram encouraging feedback (or notes that are released upon submission) to motivate continued practice. Instructors can also share feedback in the form of the learning analytics that we discussed earlier, such as activity hours logged into the LMS or time on task in watching videos or taking practice assessments. Connecting with students and informing them that you are not only paying attention to their individual contributions but are sincerely concerned with their success and progress is an excellent use of dialogue.

Quality Standards for Online Learning

As mentioned above, we know quite a bit about what makes for quality online learning. This abundance of information means that there are several solidly agreed-upon standards for developing a fully online course. While many organizations and universities use and share their own internally developed frameworks and rubrics for evaluating the quality of online courses, if you take some time to review the dozens of commonly referenced sources in the literature, you will quickly notice a few common themes that exist across most of them. Firstly, a quality online course will make sure that students are clear on how to engage with, navigate, and use the course. Most quality standards state specifically how you should accomplish this, such as through an introduction video that covers a detailed overview and demonstrated walkthrough of the course. When new technology tools are introduced to the course, students must be thoroughly trained on how to use them, provided with opportunities for practice, and supported in a timely manner. The learning objectives and a topic map of the course should be presented and explained, providing details of required deadlines, meeting dates, and other structured components of the course's organization. A student should get a sense from day-1 that this is a very organized and well-planned course, know how and where to get started, know what it takes to be successful, and know what to do when they do not feel that they are meeting the outcomes or getting the support they would like.

Other common quality standards involve the development of instructional strategies and materials. Among other best practices in education, these standards seek to keep you compliant with ADA and copyright laws and apply several guidelines for avoiding cognitive overload in students. Quality Matters™ is an organization that provides professional development, rubrics, and a peer review process for quality assurance in online learning. Their most current higher education rubric can be found on their website (Quality Matters 2022) and would be a good example of what basic standards to use for developing your online course or reviewing an existing online course. If your college or university has adopted their own standards for what they have determined their online courses should strive to become, then that would be your best tool to use.

Part 5: Blended Learning

As a veterinarian who works on a clinic floor, working an alternative career in government, or as a corporate executive, the day-to-day activities of most veterinary graduates exist in a blended environment, which integrates the digital world with the physical one. A veterinarian often jumps from an operating room to a Zoom™ room in a matter of minutes. Smartphones are permanent fixtures to our bodies which serve to keep us connected to the internet indefinitely. We might be conversing with a client while simultaneously browsing treatment options on our phones or laptops, chatting with a product specialist through instant messaging in the sidebar. This hybrid work environment was a reality even before the COVID-19 pandemic and has only accelerated since.

Some academics consider technology-enhanced F2F teaching as being on the spectrum of blended learning, and if you accept that definition then that would provide a strong argument for the case that the F2F instructional modality is all but dead, and all that remains is blended and fully online modes of teaching and learning. For the purpose of this chapter, we will not debate where F2F instruction ends and blended learning begins, and instead, we will focus on a couple of prescriptive models of blended learning that are easier to define and conceptualize.

Part 6: Hybrid Learning

The first is the hybrid model. Hybrid courses reduce the amount of F2F in-person time and replace that time with online learning activities (Bonk and Graham 2012). This can look like a course where all lectures are shifted to synchronous or asynchronous online delivery and F2F in-person time is used for small group active learning, or it can look like a course where all class time except for hands-on labs are eliminated and replaced with online course work. There are many ways you can make the hybrid model work as an individual course instructor, but arguably its biggest potential lies in programmatic strategies, which

may be used to tackle some of the major administrative and system problems we are facing in veterinary medical education. Using a hybrid model for an entire curriculum can result in systems and processes that are powerful, reliable, and flexible enough to support all stakeholders, providing benefits across the college.

Hybrid Model Case Example

The fictitious College of Veterinary Medicine at Hogwarts™ University decided to fully redesign their veterinary medical curriculum from the ground up. They decided on a new block-based curriculum that uses integrated and spiraling organization and team-taught courses. Their curriculum design presented challenges and considerations, some of which they determined could be solved through program-wide adoption of hybrid learning. One challenge is that their program and each cohort of students are split across three residential campuses. While most of their primary faculty members are located at their flagship campus, constant travel between campuses is not feasibly an option, and the college is committed to providing an equal quality experience for students housed at all three campuses. Another challenging consideration is the integrated nature of their large team-taught courses. Courses that are taught by 20–30 faculty members require a great deal of communication and collaboration to develop and deliver in a way that fully accomplishes the intended outcomes of an integrated and spiral curriculum.

The college decided to adopt a hybrid model for all courses in the preclinical curriculum that shifts much of the core content delivery to asynchronous online modules and uses in-person contact time with students for small group active learning that occurs regularly at strategically set intervals throughout the curriculum. Active learning strategies are used that help students apply and build upon the knowledge received in the online modules. The hybrid model requires faculty members to prepare all their lecture-based instruction well in advance of the course being delivered, in a format that can be shared with other faculty members that allows for the collaboration, communication, and planning that is crucial for the success of their new curriculum. Interactive videoconferencing technology is used to connect campuses in active learning and ensure equal experiences for all students regardless of campus. Success for this college was dependent on the college's ability to gain faculty buy-in to fully implement this hybrid model for all courses and provide institutional-level support in the form of technology infrastructure, staff support, and faculty training, but in the end, it proved to be a successful model that met their needs and aligned with their college's unique goals and priorities.

Part 7: HyFlex Learning

The term HyFlex has been used inconsistently in the literature. It has been used to describe working and learning spaces, a strategy, and a blended learning model (Eyal and Gil 2022; Naffi 2020; Abdelmalak and Parra 2016). The term as a blended learning model refers to courses and programs that allow students to attend learning events F2F (in-person) or online (synchronously or asynchronously). The idea is that in a HyFlex course a student will have a choice at any given point in time to engage with the course as a F2F student or as an online student. Perhaps attending a live, in-person lecture on Monday; watching the Wednesday lecture live, but remotely from home; then on Friday, if they miss the lecture all together, having the ability to watch a recording of it (or a prerecorded/asynchronous equivalent to the lecture) sometime over the weekend. While HyFlex might seem fairly straightforward in concept, it can be extremely challenging to successfully implement. The biggest and most important challenge lies in guaranteeing whichever choice a student makes (synchronous F2F, synchronous remote, or asynchronous online) is of equal quality. None of the alternative experiences a student may select should be of lesser educational value or perceived to be so by the student. Obviously quantifying this and ensuring exact quality is impossible, but the idea is to strive for equal experiences in the strategy and design of the course and in the technical infrastructure to support it.

What many universities see as a need to correct course and realign with their missions as residential institutions, obligates them to mandate F2F teaching to resume to pre-pandemic standards in all but the most strategically and intentionally planned online and blended programs. Therefore, residential veterinary programs that wish to provide the flexibility and benefits of online or blended learning may need to accomplish this through the HyFlex model.

To accomplish this, a program must invest in technical infrastructure, such as classroom-based interactive video-conferencing systems and the underlying network infrastructure to support it. They must also invest in training instructors to teach in the HyFlex environment. Facilitating discussions F2F and virtually at the same time without leaving either group feeling neglected is just one of the skills instructors will need training in.

Lastly, the biggest investment a DVM program must make for the HyFlex model to be successful is that of teams of people to support this model of teaching. Teams of learning design specialists who can partner with instructors to design the learning experiences and overcome the challenges of developing instructional strategies that bridge multiple delivery modes, and A/V and educational technologies professionals to maintain the technical infrastructure and operate the complex connections. The job of this team of professionals is akin to that of a wedding planner. Taking care of the logistical and operational tasks behind the scenes, attending to urgent troubleshooting needs, and managing the smooth delivery of a HyFlex course so that instructors and students can engage with each other, focusing on the learning objectives of the activity, all but forgetting that digital technology is facilitating the encounter.

When using the HyFlex model the goals of good teaching still remain, most notably promoting individual involvement and active participation in the learning events. HyFlex teaching presents new challenges to this endeavor, but also new opportunities. To best harness the opportunities and overcome the challenges, active learning strategies should be used. Following are some common strategies you may want to explore while using your HyFlex teaching.

Firstly, simply pausing during lectures to gain feedback and allow students to ask questions is a simple form of active learning. You may want to use an audience polling system to optimize this technique, but this is an easy one that works well during synchronous activities and can accommodate students that attend F2F or are synchronously online. For students who elect to watch the lecture asynchronously, many of the content creation tools you may have available will allow you to embed pausing points within the video to quiz the student on a particularly complex section or prompt the student to reflect and review/post questions to a discussion board to mimic the encounter you provide in the synchronous delivery.

Many other active learning strategies often require small group work during class time or for students to collaborate on their own time toward some final project or product. Out-of-class group work is not unique problem for the HyFlex model, but for small group activities that need to be facilitated by an instructor (in-class setting), technical infrastructure will need to be set up to allow the instructor to form students into groups digitally and physically and to jump from the digital classroom to the physical classroom to guide and support the various groups. Groups that are preformed and consist of a mix of online and F2F will prove especially challenging for bringing together for in-class collaboration in active learning, but with practice and the expert support we discussed already, it can be accomplished with minimal technical headaches.

As we move deeper into the "new normal" of postpandemic veterinary education, it is important that we continue to explore different blended learning models and their application at the program, course, or instructional activity levels. The hybrid or HyFlex models discussed or some modification of them may work in the context of your course or program, or you may need to look at other models that have proven to be successful elsewhere. This chapter should provide you with a foundational understanding of the options available in online or blended learning environments and empower you to further evaluate models and design decisions that accomplish your unique pedagogical needs in addition to the needs and priorities of the other stakeholders involved.

Section 4: Instructional Systems Design for Digital Learning

Shane M. Ryan and Sarah A. Bell

Instructional systems design (ISD) is also frequently called instructional design or educational technology as a field of study. The premier professional organization in the field is the Association for Educational Communications and Technology (AECT). Their formal definition is "the study and ethical application of theory, research, and best practices to advance knowledge as well as mediate and improve learning and performance through strategic design, management and implementation of learning and instructional processes and resources" (Association for Educational Communications and Technology 2022).

Instructional design as a profession and practice takes a systematic approach to curriculum development. It involves systems thinking or solving problems in complex systems, such as educational systems in veterinary medical education. When we are dealing with curriculum development in professional degree programs, the instruction we create for a course, no matter how isolated from the rest of the curriculum we would like to believe it is, is a part of the veterinary student experience; a part of their complete and complex environment of learning in the veterinary medical program. Therefore, if we try to create instruction that ignores the systems around it, we increase the chances of negative outcomes for our students.

Using a systematic approach to creating instruction ensures that we account for the impact our instruction has on the larger system and the impact the larger system has on our own instruction. There are five commonly accepted phases of ISD, represented using an acronym called ADDIE: Analysis, Design, Development, Implementation, and Evaluation. ADDIE is often considered a basic instructional design model and therefore it is an example of one of the simplest forms of taking a systematic approach to creating instruction. Depending on your situation and circumstances, there exist a plethora of more prescriptive models for instructional design, most of which incorporate the five ADDIE phases in

some form or another. For the purposes of this chapter, we will not explore any of the more elaborate instructional design models; however, we will focus broadly on the five phases of the ADDIE model.

While ISD is an important approach to creating any type of instruction, it becomes especially important in the creation of digital learning. Unlike traditional F2F learning, fully online or blended learning requires a great deal of logistical coordination, presetting, and planning of the digital environment (Lockee 2020). When instructors attempt to create instructional materials and activities for digital learning without using some form of structured and systematic process, it often culminates in stress, confusion, and an unsatisfactory experience for instructors and students alike (Puzziferro and Shelton 2008).

When you hear reports from instructors and students who absolutely detest digital learning, have had horrible experiences with it, and believe it simply cannot work, it is often the case that the curriculum developer did not know how to, or chose not to, use an ISD approach to the process. I tried to bake a cake once, without using a recipe. It went horribly. I did not swear off baking, however. I recognized that if I want a decent cake, then I need to devote the time to learning the appropriate process for how to do it correctly. Even though I made amazing soups my entire life without using recipes, making a cake is not the same as making soup, and teaching digitally is not the same as teaching F2F.

Part 1: Analysis

ADDIE begins with an analysis of the problem to be solved. It is especially the case in veterinary medical education that we are not teaching for the sake of teaching. We are preparing students for a professional practice. There are specific skills and core competencies that our students need to gain and foundational knowledge that will get them to where they need to be.

The analysis phase of the ADDIE model involves gaining a deep understanding of what exactly we need to accomplish in the instruction we are creating. If we are developing a new lecture for an existing course, why is the new lecture being added? Simply because we had some extra time that needed to be used up? Did we recognize a gap in student knowledge that needed to be addressed? At this phase of the ADDIE model, instructional designers sometimes conclude that instruction is not necessary. However, if there is a determined need, the analysis phase also involves gaining a deep understanding of your learners and the context in which the instruction will be delivered. By the end of the analysis phase, you should be able to answer the following questions before you begin designing your instructional intervention:

1) What are the learning objectives for the students?
2) What prior knowledge and experiences do your students have related to the learning objectives?
3) What are the structural characteristics of the larger system this instruction is nested in?
4) What are the physical and organizational constraints that you will need to operate within?
5) What are the technical requirements necessary to address the context and constraints?

Part 2: Design

Following the analysis phase is the design of the instruction. This is where we work out all details of what the instruction will look like. A final product of the design phase could be as simple as a lesson plan document or, depending on the scope of the project, a detailed blueprint that outlines a plan for development complete with storyboards for interactive content to be developed.

After the analysis phase, you should have a clear understanding of where you need to go, and the design phase will determine how you get there. How will you know when students have achieved your learning objectives? What strategies will you use to engage students? How and when will you provide them with practice opportunities and formative assessment? What are your methods of delivering content? How will you chunk, structure, and sequence your content?

If digital learning is determined to be necessary and appropriate, you will need to make design decisions that we discussed in the earlier sections related to online and blended learning. The design phase could also be called the planning phase because that is a key word here. You should have a plan for all aspects of the instruction, and a detailed action plan for how to get students from point A to point B, for each learning objective.

In earlier sections of the chapter, we discussed the importance of using quality standards for online and blended learning. This is the phase in which you will begin to employ those standards. If the instruction is going to be fully online for example, you need to identify a reliable set of quality standards for fully online instruction and use that to guide your design.

Most lists of quality standards are in the form of rubrics and are designed to be used in the design of an entire course, but you can focus on a subsection of the rubric if you are only designing a single lecture or learning activity as a part of a larger course. The important takeaway here is to use some form of guiding criteria for what you seek to accomplish.

Here are three examples of criteria related to course design similar to what you may find on a quality standards rubric, along with comments for how you may want to address each in the design of your own online instruction (Table 7.1).

Again, these are only three examples of how quality standards could be used to guide you through this phase of the ADDIE model, but the takeaway here is that you should be using some quality framework you can trust and defend in the design and development of your instruction.

Table 7.1 Example quality standards for online learning.

Example quality standard	Consideration for design
Students engage with course content in a variety of ways (UF Standards and Markers of Excellence 2022)	The design phase is when you will determine how you will achieve this quality standard. Providing readings, prerecorded lecture videos, and discussion sessions? Your strategy for how students will receive and engage with your course content needs to be fully outlined. This outline becomes an action plan that you will use in the development phase to prepare the instruction for delivery
Instructional materials and learning activities encourage critical thinking skills when appropriate (UF Standards and Markers of Excellence 2022)	This standard would require you to audit your learning objectives to determine which, if any, requires students to use critical thinking skills to achieve. Next, you would determine which strategies you will use to encourage critical thinking and achieve deeper learning. The planning for how the instructional strategies are integrated into the course are fleshed out in the design phase. Using the Team-Based Learning (TBL) strategy, for example, would require further design and additional planning to pull off successfully, especially if it is being used in the context of an online or blended course
The instructor uses formal and informal student feedback in an ongoing basis to help plan instruction and assessment of student learning throughout the semester (UF Standards and Markers of Excellence 2022)	Preplanning when student feedback is to be collected and how it will be used should be a part of the course design. Have a plan for how you intend to collect feedback, motivate participation, incorporate the feedback, and communicate changes: all within a timeframe that allows any changes to be meaningful

Part 3: Development

The analysis phase determined and framed your need, the design phase put it all in perspective and determined your approach and strategy, and now it is time to bring it all to life. The development phase is where ISD for digital learning really begins to function quite differently from ISD for traditional F2F instruction. In F2F instruction, it is common for the development phase and the implementation phase to be somewhat blurred, as various components of development of the instruction occur as the instruction is being administered to students, especially the bulk of the traditional lecture content. However, when developing online and blended courses, it is extremely important for the instructional materials to be fully created and play-tested prior to administering it to students. This is necessary since we are dealing with technical systems that require preprogramming and careful setup.

Recording quality video content (at home or in a studio), developing a course website, integrating third-party tools such as peer collaboration software for a group project, writing assessment items, and creating the assessment forms within an electronic testing platform are just a few of the development activities you may need to work on during this phase of the ADDIE model. If you try to develop these materials and set up these tools while you are simultaneously administering the course, it is akin to building a plane while flying it, and not surprisingly it will not go well. Fully developing the course and having it 95–100% built and ready before the first day of the course will provide you the ability to deliver a quality designed and developed digital learning experience. When dealing with digital technology, inevitably there will be surprises; you want to discover those surprises well in advance of students being exposed to technology-based instruction.

Project management is an important part of the development phase. Depending on the scope of the project, there may be hundreds of contact hours of content that need to be created. If your design phase produced some form of design document, you will want to elaborate on that document and begin to transition it into a work breakdown structure (WBS). A WBS would provide a granular itemized list of what needs to be physically created and setup for students to access. The WBS document lists all that needs to be accomplished and the timeframe within which it needs to be done. If this is a project in which multiple instructors or a production team is collaborating, then this document becomes even more important in holding each member of the team accountable for their pieces of the puzzle. The WBS documentation details who is responsible for what and when they should be expected to complete their responsibilities.

Part 4: Implementation

Managing the delivery of the instruction needs to be well-planned and scheduled. You should have a plan for when and how you intend to communicate and interact with students. Courses and other instructional activities delivered through LMS allow for a great deal of the implementation tasks to be preprogrammed, which can and should be set up during the development phase. However, there is much that still needs to be coordinated daily by the course coordinators. There should be a prepopulated daily calendar or schedule to remind you of not only each event or activity that needs to be administered, such as a live videoconference Q&A or a proctored exam, but should also outline each communication and asynchronous interaction you will have with your students. It is helpful to schedule reminders for yourself to send emails to the class before an upcoming quiz that includes a few words of encouragement. Similarly, you may want to schedule a reminder to check the discussion board, respond to questions or comments, and to stir discussion; another to grade assignments and provide timely formative feedback. Again, this should all be preplanned and scheduled so that it does not become something you are reactively responding to as students pressure you for it during the delivery of the course. If your students are contacting you en masse a day or two before a quiz, worried because they saw on the syllabus that there was an assessment quickly approaching but they have not received any additional details, then you have room for improvement in how you are administering your course.

Communication and feedback should be a core focus during the implementation phase. If the prior three phases were conducted appropriately, then much of the course should be well planned, and depending on the modality, it may be somewhat automated. This should free up time for frequent outreach to students. It is your responsibility to be regularly active and present during the offering of the course using email, chat, video posts, discussion boards, or any other communication channels you have available in the course. It is also your responsibility to proactively address and be responsive to student concerns as they arise. Feedback should be provided to students in sufficient time for students to progress. Lastly, it is your responsibility to demonstrate ongoing changes and improvements based on the feedback you receive from students. Here are some examples of reflective questions to ask yourself during the implementation phase:

1) Do my students know when they can expect assignments to be graded?
2) If the timeline for grading or other schedule changes occur, can my students trust that I will inform them immediately?

3) Are my students getting the online technical support they need in my course?

4) Are students posing questions on the discussion board or sending emails that are not getting answered in a timely manner?

5) Do my students know that I am actively monitoring my online course? If not, how can I convince them that I am?

Part 5: Evaluation

The ADDIE model, as with many other instructional design models, should be considered an iterative process. While evaluation may be the last letter of the acronym, it is not necessarily the last phase of the process. Evaluation should continually inform just-in-time revisions to your course and instruction in progress. Based on the evaluation and assessment you conduct you may need to revisit any one of the first three phases. The phase that may be most informed by evaluation is the implementation phase, however. Implementation of the instruction will never be perfect, especially the first time, and there will always be room for improvement. Additionally, as your instruction evolves over several years, your design decisions will change, development tools will change, your goals and objectives may change, and as you make changes, your results will vary. Evaluation will always be necessary to continually maintain and improve your instruction.

It is important to be purposeful and targeted with your evaluation. Evaluation should not be ignored until after implementation of your instructional activity or course is complete. It should be premeditated, fully planned, and executed with the same importance as the instruction itself.

Formative evaluation of the instruction should begin no later than the development phase of the ADDIE model. Ideally, the designed course will be reviewed by some form of convened experts or by a group of prospective students to gain insight and gather feedback prior to entering the development phase. You may believe you have a content delivery strategy that students will be pleased with, but before you invest hundreds of hours in creating content and spend an entire semester delivering a course, you may want to get some feedback from students to confirm that your strategy will be well received. For example, if you are considering the use of a new lecture capture tool, you may want to solicit a handful of students to review a sample lecture that you record as a demo, then ask them to attend a 30-minute focus group meeting to share their experience with the tool. They may provide information that would lead you to ditch the tool altogether, although the more likely case is that they

will share information informing how you use the tool, through tips, tricks, and best practices, which may have otherwise taken you an entire semester of delivering a course to gather.

Evaluating consequential decisions prior to the development phase is important, and another important time to conduct major formative evaluation is at the end of the development phase, just prior to implementation. The entirety of the instruction that has been created, whether an entire course or a single learning event, such as a two-hour workshop, should be reviewed in its final state prior to being administered to students. This should be done with enough time to make necessary changes and corrections before the formal delivery begins. Since you will have conducted formative evaluation throughout the design and development of the course, however, this final review prior to launch is less likely to result in any core deficiencies and instead will shed light on last-minute tweaks or settings, which slipped your mind and need to be completed.

When preparing to launch an online or blended course, even if it is the third or fourth year you have done so, there tend to be so many last-minute details to remember, that if you do not have some form of final evaluation rubric, or prelaunch checklist, you are bound to forget something. Having a fresh set of eyes, such as a faculty colleague, review the course in its entirety prior to launching can serve as a fail-safe in addition to your own final reviews.

Part 6: Essential Elements

The ADDIE model and many other instructional design models present distinct stages for analysis, design, development, implementation, and evaluation. However, in practice, and especially in the case of professional degree program curriculum development, our curriculum development projects do not always unfold in a nice and tidy linear fashion. In other words, it is often impractical to methodically follow an instructional design model one phase at a time.

Instead, we often simply reference the model and roughly use it as a guiding framework, while our actual process becomes more-or-less a continuous refinement of our understanding of five essential elements of instructional design: our learners, the outcomes, our assessments, the instructional activities, and the evaluation of our instruction. Having a deep understanding of an instructional design model, however, is important for understanding what ultimately needs to be accomplished in the development and delivery of digital learning.

Section 5: Veterinary Student Success in Technology-Enhanced Learning

Shane M. Ryan and Sarah A. Bell

The use of technology in education can be both encouraging and frustrating. As different populations face different barriers, different circumstances prompt different responses. It is important to consider all students; their learning, well-being, and safety; as well as the security of your content when developing and implementing technology-enhanced content.

Part 1: Equity and Accessibility Considerations

The development of online education has previously been theorized to be the solution to some forms of educational inequity because the use of online learning theoretically provides access to education for students who would not typically have physical access to the same opportunities afforded brick-and-mortar schooling (Meier 2015). However, it is imperative to understand that accessible solutions are not always equitable for the diverse student populations we now serve (Lee 2017).

What Is Accessibility?

According to Merriam-Webster's Dictionary, the term *accessible* refers to something "capable of being reached, capable of being used or seen, capable of being understood or appreciated, and capable of being influenced." To make education accessible is to put what needs to be learned (e.g., the content) and the acts of teaching and learning (i.e., the transaction of knowledge) within reach for *all* students. Accessibility is unique for each individual, based on their personal situations, abilities, conditions, and environments.

Disability and Accessibility

The Americans with Disabilities Act of 1990 (ADA) provided a national mandate to eliminate discrimination and provide enforceable standards for individuals with disabilities (Americans with Disabilities Act 1990). While initially created to address physical barriers in the world, such as curbs and sets of stairs that disadvantage individuals with limited mobility, it quickly became obvious that other barriers existed, including those of a cognitive and social nature. Barriers that relate to information technology and information sharing profoundly affect students with disabilities in today's digital age of education.

According to the Center for Disease Control and Prevention (CDC), more than one-fourth of the US adult population lives with a disability (Center for Disease Control and Prevention 2022). The degree of inaccessibility depends on the disability. Students with visual impairments may struggle with font size or contrasting colors on images. Students who are color-blind may have difficulty discerning between colors or shades of certain colors. Blind students may use screen readers, a technology specifically designed to address visual impairments by reading text on the screen to the student aloud. Students with auditory disabilities may not be able to hear spoken words or audible sounds on recordings. Typing or using touch-screen devices may present challenges for students with physical impairments. Cognitive disabilities can limit a student's ability to attend to specific items on crowded visual sources or focus on small details within large documents (WebAIM 2020). Addressing such barriers benefits all students, not just those with identified disabilities.

Physical and Financial Accessibility

COVID brought to light further inequality when it comes to accessible internet connections for students from rural areas. While internet connectivity may be a requirement to enter professional- and graduate-level programs, the inequity between broadband speed and connection became even more apparent when the option to use physical, on-campus university resources was revoked. Rural areas are more likely to have weaker infrastructures than urban centers and suburban communities (Lai and Widmar 2021). When universities transitioned to remote-only instruction, students living in rural areas during the COVID shutdown struggled to attend videoconference sessions or live-stream events due to inadequate internet speeds.

Access to necessary devices and software is also a barrier for some students. Although students are typically required to acquire an electronic device upon admission to a professional- or graduate-level program, some students may not be able to afford or have the previous experience to know how to maintain or effectively use such devices. Hardware requirements, software licenses, and anti-malware programs require fundamental skills for effective use and maintenance.

Part 2: Creating Accessible Online Environments

Assisting students with overcoming potential barriers is a core responsibility of educators. With the help of assistive technology, instructors and course designers can help support learning for all students. Web Accessibility in Mind (WebAIM 2022) is a great resource for learning and assisting with breaking down barriers associated with online environments.

Accessible Visual Components

There are several layers to visual impairment. Students with visual impairments may require corrective lenses.

Others may be completely or legally blind with limited vision if any at all. Individuals with visual disabilities use assistive technologies to help navigate daily tasks, including educational activities.

Consider a blind student who wants to review online lecture materials. While being legally blind impedes their ability to use a computer mouse to navigate a web page on their school's LMS, keyboard commands assist this student in navigating the page, as long as appropriate web design rules are followed that allow assistive technologies such as screen readers to recognize and parse through the content on the page. Screen reader software can help the student identify links on the screen, and alternative text (or ALT text) can substitute images and diagrams that are non-text features within the page. Logically organized web pages and online documents are essential for screen reader technologies. Such software typically moves by command or keystroke down the page – top to bottom, left to right. Screen readers also use coded headings and subheadings to navigate through dense content. Items such as animations or widgets that require a touchpad or mouse navigation should be avoided for compatibility reasons unless the products you are considering offer ADA-accessible alternatives or assistive features to guarantee an equal experience for all students.

A student with visual impairment may present with a low vision condition. These students may struggle with font size or color contrast in images and texts. Screen magnifiers and zoom features could help students with low vision conditions to see content more clearly. However, it is important to test these enlargement features for functionality. Certain images can become pixelated when zoomed in, and certain text or fonts can become too distorted to read when expanded to larger sizes. Students with low vision often struggle with low-contrast content (i.e., content with text or images that compete with background colors). Red text on a black background might be lost on a student with visual impairment. It is important to confirm any text or images used in educational materials have high contrast. Educators and designers can use free online *contrast checkers* to ensure their content is ready for all learners. Some good examples include WebAIM Color Contrast Checker, Adobe Color Contrast Analyzer, and a color contrast analyzer that is shared free by Deque University.

Other students may have color blindness, a visual condition that inhibits their ability to discern between different shades of color. Depending on a person's type of color blindness, various colors can affect afflicted populations differently. While most individuals have a misconception of color blindness as seeing with a total lack of color or seeing only in gray tones, most individuals with color blindness can still see some form of color and only struggle with specific colors such as red or green. Keeping this in mind, educators need not remove color entirely from their course content but should instead avoid relying on color to communicate essential information. Requiring students to differentiate between the red arrow and the green arrow on a diagram, for example, should be avoided. Instead, accompanying text should be associated with each arrow to ensure full disclosure of the information provided and provide discernment between the two important points.

Accessible Auditory Components

Students with auditory impairments have difficulty hearing spoken words and sounds. While some students may not be able to hear at all, others may retain some level of hearing. Some individuals with hearing impairments use sign language to communicate and receive information. Others might rely on reading lips while they are speaking to people. Depending on the severity of hearing loss, individuals may struggle to hear speakers over background noise. Learners with auditory impairments or those who are deaf benefit from written transcripts and captions on recorded videos and media. Care should be taken when creating video content as well to ensure that irrelevant background noise is eliminated.

It is important to note, students who are deaf or hard of hearing typically do not label the inability to hear as a disability. Where much of the world considers deafness a deficit condition or lack of a particular trait, individuals who are deaf consider deafness a proud attribute that conveys strength and perseverance and consider themselves part of a community or culture that chooses to communicate with their own visual language – sign language (Hladek 2014).

Accessible Manipulative Components

Students with motor disabilities may not have the fine or gross motor control needed to access certain materials. Navigation of online environments can prove to be difficult for students who are unable to move a mouse fluidly or type on a keyboard with accuracy.

Keyboard controls are often used by students who are unable to use a mouse, but for students who are unable to use keyboards, assistive devices, such as voice-activated software, may be used to ease navigation. It is important to note that students with motor impairments can become fatigued by the amount of energy it takes to navigate digital resources. It is important to ensure a logically organized structure is used to relieve some of the burden of fatigue.

Accessible Cognitive Components

Cognitive disabilities include trouble with memory, problem-solving, comprehension, and attention. Issues with memory might include issues with either working memory, short-term memory, or long-term memory and retrieval of information. Difficulties with problem-solving, comprehension, and attention can exacerbate strains on cognitive load. Poorly organized online content can frustrate students who struggle with cognitive issues. By providing an online environment that is simplified and easy to navigate, instructors can support these students and their learning.

Attention disorders make it difficult for some individuals to complete tasks. This is not usually because of inability to learn or process information. Instead, the most common cause is distraction. Students with Attention Deficit Hyperactivity Disorder (ADHD), for example, are often distracted by cluttered and disorganized content. When students are required to search for items deep in their online environment that are meaninglessly scattered across separate locations, frustration can quickly exhaust their efforts. While ADHD manifests differently for every individual, researchers who have studied students with ADHD have found that issues with executive functioning (i.e., brain functions that help an individual with motivation, prioritization, etc.) can and often do affect progress in digital learning environments. These students can struggle with meeting deadlines and completing long-term projects. Instructors can help to support students by providing a clear schedule of deadlines, sending weekly reminders of coursework and assignments, and scaffolding long-term projects, or requiring students to complete a large project in segments. The segments can be mini-assignments that are later compiled into the final product at the end of the term (Friel 2018).

Part 3: Universal Design for Learning

The diversity of learners can be difficult to address in education. Edyburn and Edyburn (2021) use the story of *Goldilocks and the Three Bears* as a catchy metaphor for the diverse needs of learners. The Three Bears in the story have specific needs. When it comes to nourishment, papa likes porridge that is piping hot, Mama likes cold porridge, and Baby Bear enjoys the in-between. Our students are similar, they are all seeking to acquire the same knowledge, but what it will take for them to get there with best results will look different for each student.

Universal Design for Learning (UDL) is a framework that supports a proactive approach to meeting the needs of all students. Developed by CAST, this framework is focused on instruction and is founded on three principles that enhance learning through recognition, strategic, and affective networks of the brain. Recognition learning focuses on the specific content or *what* students are learning, strategic learning focuses on the act of learning or *how* students are learning, and affective learning or "learning motivation"

focuses on *why* students are learning. The UDL Framework uses these three networks as the foundation for its three principles. Just as the Three Bears' meals were tailored to the family's needs, so can we design our courses to support student needs using UDL principles (Boothe et al. 2018; CAST 2018; Edyburn and Edyburn 2021).

The first UDL principle supports recognition learning through multiple means of representation. This principle focuses on *what* students are learning and removes barriers between students and content. Instructors who provide multiple means of representation of their content are providing students with flexible ways to access the information. Instructors can support learning by providing the same content through different modes and media. For example, instructors can include audio recordings, animations, and physical models depicting abstract concepts to support learning through visual, auditory, and tactile channels. Using methods of delivery that are flexible is also a way to strengthen representation of material. Instructors can provide electronic versions of slide presentations and documents that can be digitally enlarged or provide recordings of sounds that can be digitally amplified or slowed to meet this principle. Another way to provide multiple means of representation may include the use of recording transcripts or close captions. Close captions benefit more than just those students with auditory impairments. Captioning can help language learners connect spoken speech to written words and clarify statements made orally for other students. Illustrations, tables, or graphs that demonstrate spoken or written concepts can also help learners comprehend abstract concepts.

The second UDL principle supports the strategic learning network by providing multiple means of expression. This principle focuses on *how* students learn and how they demonstrate that their learning has occurred. All students are different in the ways that they learn, and similarly, all students express what they know in different ways. By providing multiple ways for students to respond to and interact with content, instructors can support connections with the content and with their classmates. Students may face many barriers in their ability to navigate the physical or digital environment. Instructors can help students overcome these barriers by proactively providing tools or technologies to all students, regardless of receiving documented requests for special accommodations. We have all heard the saying: *there is more than one way to solve a problem*. In this principle of UDL, students can demonstrate their learning in a variety of ways if those paths are open for them. Unless the learning objective explicitly requires the student to perform a task a certain way (i.e., use the Pythagorean theorem to solve this problem), it would be helpful, especially for those with specific needs or disabilities, for instructors to offer flexibility in student submissions in response to assignments or questions. Web-based options for course assignments could include a blog post, web design, video presentation, or discussion boards for online chats. This principle of UDL can also be used to support students who struggle with executive functioning. Many students struggle with self-governance, but instructors can help support students by providing opportunities for practice goal setting. They may also support these learners by developing scaffolded assignments and by providing authentic feedback to help guide students toward the learning goals.

The final UDL principle is that of engagement – the *why* behind student learning. The reasons for "motivation to learn" or "engagement" in learning are different for every student and likely linked to physiological, cultural, environmental, and/or personal factors. With this knowledge, it becomes necessary to offer multiple means of engagement to help all students succeed. Student interest, sustained effort, and self-regulation are some areas of focus for the engagement principle. Where possible, it is important to offer choices to help recruit student interest. While we may not be able to change learning objectives based on student interests, it is possible to provide opportunities for creative control. For instance, if students are expected to create a presentation in your course, try providing them with flexibility in choosing the topic or presentation method. By allowing students the opportunity to research and present on a topic of their choosing, they are more likely to remain engaged with the content. Another way to motivate student engagement is by creating relevance. Students are more likely to attend to information and content when they can relate to what is being presented. Provide a variety of activities or sources of information to cover all of your bases and increase the odds that what you are providing is culturally or socially relevant to most (hopefully all) students. In terms of sustaining effort and supporting self-regulation: goal setting, explaining explicit expectations, and providing opportunities for collaboration can help to increase student persistence, promote efforts for task sustainability, and support self-regulation.

Section 6: Safety and Security Considerations

Shane M. Ryan and Sarah A. Bell

Much of our lives now exist in the digital realm. In just a few clicks of a computer mouse, or the tap of a phone screen, we can go from lounging on the couch to socializing with friends or participating in an online class. A few moments later, we can be shopping for shoes, reviewing our financial and health records, or googling images of cats in hats. That which provides us this ease of quick movement through the digital world, however, also puts us at increased risks from many different dangers, both accidental and of malice. It is important to *lock the digital door* to protect ourselves and our property, and as educators using the digital environment to teach in, we must become experts in the threats that exist for our students so that we can prepare our students for navigating those threats and so that we can design our instruction to actively avoid putting our students anywhere near harm's way.

Part 1: Cyber Threats

While students today have access to a wider range of electronic and web-based technology, they are also more vulnerable to cyber threats than those in previous generations. With today's technology, individuals can access anything with the swipe of a finger. Online banking and bill-pay is the new standard. In the education realm, students can access their registration, grades, transcripts, and financial aid statements with ease. Keeping up with the latest trends is even more accessible with social media, online shopping, and digitized entertainment. While these online features make daily life more convenient, they also make our lives more susceptible to threats.

There are several ways that individuals can become victims of cyber threats. Phishing is one of the most common forms of cyberattack. Hackers use phishing scams to collect personal or financial information from their victims to steal their identity or use malicious software (malware) to collect important information from their devices. Phishing scams typically begin with a fake email or text message that asks the receiver to provide specific information or prompts the target to click on a hyperlink. Even just accidentally clicking a link in a phishing email can activate malware installation, which can block the user's access to business networks, copy information from the user's hard drive, or even disable the user's device making their operating systems and programs inaccessible (Commonwealth of Massachusetts 2022; National Cyber Security Alliance 2022; United States Government 2022). Often, identity theft goes unnoticed for some time. The US government recognizes several forms of identity theft, including tax identity theft, medical identity theft, and unemployment identity theft. An identity thief may use your information to file taxes, apply for credit or loans, obtain medical services, or make purchases using your personal information. Understanding how these threats occur can help instructors and students position themselves in a more secure stance against cyberattacks. The National Cyber Security Alliance (2022) offers tips to stay safe online:

1) *Maintain your device.* Keep all your devices up to date with software updates. Many of these can be set to automatically update to help expedite this process. As you consider adopting new technology tools for your teaching, a core consideration in evaluating the various product options on the market should be their level of security and how their security applications will configure with the various devices our students may be using. Educational technology vendors may communicate software updates to you as a vendor client, and it will be your responsibility to quickly pass that along to your students if it requires action on their parts to update software or you may need to help them navigate device incompatibility.

2) *Use unique passwords every time.* It can be difficult to remember dozens of passwords, but this action also is the best prevention against those who would use your passwords against you. The burden of managing passwords can be helped through password manager software, which collects and manages your login and password information digitally on your mobile device. Most browsers and device operating systems offer password manager software as well, so you need not remember all those unique passwords. As an instructor who may be serving as an administrator for a technology tool that you are using in your course, you may be responsible for helping students troubleshoot forgotten passwords. Encouraging them to use unique passwords, use a password manager, and of course not share their passwords with others is something you should repeat over and over to them.

3) *Use multifactor authentication.* Multifactor authentication, or 2-factor authentication, adds additional and robust security to your accounts. Many financial and educational institutions already require this level of security when attempting to access your information; other services may provide it optionally. The most common form of multifactor authentication is via passcode sent to your email or phone number associated with your account. If it is an option for any products that you intend to use in your teaching, go with it. Students may consider it an extra headache, but it does add an important layer of security.

4) *Slow down and think about it.* If you get a request for information, why are they asking? When it comes to emails or unfamiliar websites, it is important to think before clicking any links or attachments. Consider the source; would this sender have requested this information through an email? What are they asking for? Big institutions are aware of phishing scams and therefore they will not ask you for sensitive, personal information such as account information or passwords via email.

Always err on the side of caution, and get a second opinion from an IT expert, or contact the sender by searching for their contact information yourself (not using what was provided in the email or text message). The importance of critically thinking through the risks and approaching all aspects of the digital world with caution is a skill we should impress upon our students over and over again. Most of our current students have been raised from childhood on the internet and most have no expectations of privacy. This can have the negative effect of causing them to be lax when it comes to cyber risks. We should not confuse the younger generations' life-long experiences with the internet with being meaningful experts in navigating cyber threats.

5) *Report phishing scams.* At work or school? Report suspicious emails and communications to the IT department. At home? Most email providers have a way to report emails as spam. Be sure to delete the email after reporting it. Remind your students of this and inform your students of how you will communicate with them. Convey to them what you may and what you will not be asking for via email or other forms of communication you may be using in your course.

6) *Use secure Wi-Fi connections.* Unsecured hotspots and wi-fi connections, such as those at your local coffee shop, can leave you and your device susceptible to cyberattack. Be sure to use your institution's secure wi-fi connection when on campus and a VPN (virtual private network) when off campus. Most institutions provide free VPN services that can be downloaded to your personal device for extra security.

7) *Back up your device.* Malware can affect your device's applications and files. Be sure to retain copies of your files, especially important data. The 3-2-1 rule could help save later heartache: keep at least 3 copies, on at least 2 different forms of storage, with at least 1 of them in a different location than your primary device. The most common forms of data storage are cloud-based, USB, or external hard drives.

8) *Use and update privacy settings.* Anytime you open a new account or download a new software or application, check the privacy settings to ensure they are set to a level you are comfortable with. Regularly check these, as companies often push out new features on privacy settings with their updates. When considering the degree of privacy settings you are comfortable with, and before you provide or post (via social media or other platforms) any personal information about yourself, consider who will see it and what they could do with the information. If you are asking your students to post information about themselves on a public-facing platform, you must be careful to never force students to

share information that makes them feel uncomfortable. In most cases, the use of social media in courses should be avoided since it can require students to share content publicly they may not have otherwise put out there.

Part 2: Reporting Incidents

Since 2005, there have been more than 1,800 data breaches in US schools, including K-12 and colleges/universities. Of these, 87% were breached at institutions of higher education. The largest breach on record is that for the Maricopa County Community College District in 2013 where more than 2.49 million records were affected. In this case, several school databases were breached with alumni, student, and staff information published publicly to the internet. 2020 saw the most cyber security breaches in the last 15 years during the height of the pandemic (Cook 2021).

According to the National Cyber Security Alliance (2022), it can be difficult to investigate individual cyberattacks. However, it is important to report situations to your institution's IT department to help prevent actions against others. If you have received a phishing email and believe your device or information has been compromised, notify your supervisor and the institution's IT department immediately. On a personal device, you should check to see that your device is up to date, and then you can use antivirus software to scan your device for malware. If you believe someone has hacked into your accounts, you should change your passwords, and follow up with the institution to report the breach. In cases of identity theft, your local law enforcement agency can help you file a formal report and provide contact information for other agencies that can assist you.

Part 3: Intellectual Property Integrity

Safeguarding intellectual property can be a difficult task. Intellectual property is any product of the mind. Schools and colleges of veterinary medicine engage in education and research and therefore are major producers and consumers of intellectual property (Warenzak 2018). As content is created and distributed, the transfer of such property is often difficult to police. Ownership of such property can vary as most institutions have their own policies and procedures for maintaining the integrity of intellectual property. Policies for items with patents, copyrights, or trademarks are often very specific. However, a gray area exists pertaining to course materials, videos, manuals, and other property developed for educational purposes by faculty. In some cases, university faculty can claim ownership of their content, but in other instances, the university may retain ownership of all materials developed for the education of university students. In the online learning environment, students can access, download, reproduce, or distribute content rather easily. While students have the right to retain content for personal use, distributing content to other students typically falls under an institution's academic integrity policies and the monetization of another's intellectual property is considered unlawful due to copyright laws. Institutions can develop and implement ethical behavior codes that hinder such behavior and enforceable policies with consequences for offenders.

Part 4: Academic Integrity and Security of Assessments

As instructors and institutions attempt to safeguard course content in online environments, there is a substantial buzz around online assessment. As online assessment gained popularity with the widespread use of online learning, the steep growth in academic integrity violations is discouraging, and the security of student assessments and test items has become hot topic as of late.

Violations of academic integrity are widespread and not limited to any one subject of study. Violations include individual academic dishonesty and the lack of reporting of the dishonest behaviors of others. Students often justify dishonest behavior for high-stakes activities (Hamlin et al. 2013). Students who demonstrate dishonest behavior may plagiarize assignments by copying source material, knowingly omit proper references, copy some or all of another student's work, submit the work of other students to pass it off as their own or provide invalid excuses for missed assignments. With regard to assessment, students who engage in academic dishonesty may access exam materials before the exam is administered, or study from stolen copies of the exam in question. During an exam, students may communicate answers to other test takers, copy test items to pass on to others or locate answers to questions in online material or through internet searches when such use is prohibited.

Universities can combat academic dishonesty by developing honor codes and specific policies regarding academic integrity violations. Furthermore, by applying communication strategies to support policy implementation, and forming committees that focus on the enforcement of those policies. Academic integrity committees can take the pressure and ambiguity of policy enforcement off the instructor (Hamlin et al. 2013).

In online environments, applications can be enabled in your LMS to search documents for plagiarism. A product called Turnitin™, for example, uses artificial intelligence technology that scans student assignment submissions and compares sentences and phrases to existing articles, reference materials, and even other student documents that have been submitted to Turnitin™ partnered systems.

Online proctoring of exams can help deter academic dishonesty. Web-based proctoring is universally available at a cost. Instructors can often determine the level of security with these programs. Most products provide an identity verification step, a browser lock that limits the student's access to only the exam file, and a recording of the student's screen, keystrokes, and camera. While these programs may go as far as to offer a full student room scan to ensure test-takers do not have access to notes or other study materials, this feature has come under recent scrutiny. In August 2022, an Ohio judge ruled in favor of a student who filed a complaint against Cleveland State University's use of the room scan for a chemistry exam. The student claimed that the scan of the room violated his right to privacy and the judge concurred, stating that the student's right to privacy trumps an institution's interest in academic integrity (Holpuch and Rubin 2022). Regardless of outcomes of recent legal challenges to remote proctoring, it will likely remain an option for testing to combat the demands of proctoring, even if the practice of students taking exams from their own homes is no longer permitted.

Part 5: Reputable Sources

The COVID-19 pandemic brought new attention to the rapid spread of misinformation. At the start of the pandemic, individuals in the public and private sectors were hungry for more information about the virus, and the call was answered. A vast number of publications were submitted and published regarding the virus, its clinical presentation, case management strategies, and treatments, many of which were non-peer-reviewed and some shared as preprint resources. A study published in the *Journal of the American Medical Association* reviewed preprint articles published before the pandemic and found the number of preprint articles was increasing, and papers that were published first as preprint papers were more likely to have higher Altmetric scores (i.e., a measure of the amount of attention or mentions of the article) and more likely to have a greater number of citations than papers that were not run first as preprints (Serghiou and Ioannidis 2018).

However, it is important to note, preprint resources have often not gone through peer-review processes and remain unverified until the processes are complete. Peer-review processes work to ensure high-quality and high-validity research. COVID-19 and the flood of preprint research that surrounded it is a prime example of how dangerous preprint work can be without the checks involved in the peer-review process. Specific examples of problematic preprint works were two highly publicized articles on hydroxychloroquine as a treatment for COVID-19 and cardiovascular disease and COVID-19 mortality. These articles were preprint published and then later retracted after it was discovered that the researchers had used fabricated data to complete their reports (Kaul et al. 2020; Mehra et al. 2020a,b).

Reliable sources are those that "provide a thorough, well-reasoned theory, argument, discussion, etc. based on strong evidence" (University of Georgia 2022, n.p.). Most often, reliability is established through the peer-review process when articles are submitted for scholarly books or journals. Articles are chosen based on topic, quality, and urgency and then distributed to subject matter experts for an evaluation of thoroughness and validity. While subject matter experts are those who determine whether a source is credible, editorial reviews often occur in instances where articles are submitted to magazines geared toward the general public, practitioner or trade-based magazines, or professional newspapers (University of Georgia 2022).

Journal articles and other online readings are a tempting addition to online courses. It is easy to find current and targeted content related to topics when we conduct a Google Scholar search, but we need to remain vigilant about the quality and authority of the resources we identify and pass along to our students. We also must pass along to them the skills to critically assess the reputability and rigor of research and other topic material that they find online. As programs engage in more problem-based and self-guided learning strategies, the concerns of access to and ability to assess reputable sources are more important than ever.

Part 6: Conclusion

Veterinary educators who are just entering the teaching profession or those with years of experience who would like to make a transition into online and blended learning should now have a fundamental understanding of the key considerations involved. Becoming an expert digital educator, like teaching in general, requires years of practice and development. Getting active in education-focused groups at your college or university, or taking courses or full degree programs that prepare you for or expose you to digital learning is important to gain the skills necessary to be successful. College administrators seeking to transform educational systems through technology should now have a clear understanding of the many layers of stakeholder considerations and challenges that must be navigated and fully appreciated, but also the possibilities for realizing the visions for a better future for veterinary medical education that will keep us modern and relevant for decades to come.

Section 7: Present and Future Technologies to Enhance Learning

Micha C. Simons and Sarah Baillie

Part 1: Introduction

Veterinary education is constantly evolving in an effort to incorporate the growing body of medical knowledge and to utilize new educational methodologies as they arise. With the ever-changing backdrop of the digital age, many new educational initiatives rely on technology. Various technological applications have been presented in response to some of the common challenges arising in veterinary education, such as increased class sizes, limited resources, variable caseloads, and limited opportunities for practice and/or repetition.

The educational goals of using technology in veterinary education include facilitating basic knowledge acquisition, improving clinical reasoning and professional skills, practicing key psychomotor skills, and training for rare or critical events (Guze 2015). A new charge of veterinary educators is to select and use the best technologies to encourage a more collaborative, yet personalized learning experience for all learners.

Educational technologies have the potential to offer a safe, appropriate, and in some cases, cost-effective training setting in which realistic training tasks can be practiced. In such controlled environments, learners can make errors without adverse consequences, and educators can focus on learners rather than patients.

This section explores some of the common terminology used when discussing educational technologies and presents some examples of these technologies in veterinary education.

Part 2: Relevant Terms and Definitions

As previously defined, *constructivism* is a learning theory that asserts that individuals best learn by adding new ideas and experiences to an existing framework of knowledge and experiences to form new or enhanced understanding. Various models have been proposed over time, with some of the most common theories proposed by Dewey, Piaget, Vygotsky, Gagne, and Bruner (see Chapter 2). Therefore, any educational technology that promotes active learning is supported by this epistemology.

E-learning is the delivery of learning, training, or education programs by electronic means. Common applications in medical and surgical education include online learning portals, social media forums, various games, and simulators. *E-learning theory* (David 2015) uses principles from cognitive science to demonstrate how the use and design of educational technology can enhance effective learning.

Within the development of many of these educational technologies is the consideration for learners to practice a given skill or task. *Deliberate practice* is a form of training directed at improvement of a skill using highly structured, repetitive activity (Ericsson et al. 1993). Specific tasks are used to overcome weaknesses in performance, and the activities are carefully monitored to provide feedback on ways to achieve further improvement before progressing to the next task. The end goal of this deliberate practice is attaining competency and eventually expertise.

Section 8: Common Forms of Educational Technologies

Micha C. Simons and Sarah Baillie

Part 1: Adaptive Learning

Closely related to e-learning theory, *adaptive learning* is a process or processes that facilitate an individualized learning experience with technologies designed to identify a learner's strengths and weaknesses (Sharma et al. 2017). Once recognized, these technologies can modify the content to direct time and focus to improve those weaknesses. Adaptation strategies can also account for learner preferences, aid in navigation through course content, and combine multiple learning resources to create a more efficient learning experience (Paramythis et al. 2004; Sharma et al. 2017).

Part 2: Game-Based Learning Versus Gamification Versus Serious Gaming

The use of games in the classroom is by no means a new concept, but with the rapidly occurring technological advances, the use of games as educational tools has increased.

Game-based learning describes some form of gameplay with defined learning outcomes (Shaffer 2006). These games can be in any format, although in the current landscape, this often refers to digital games. More specifically, *gamification* refers to the use of game-based rules, mechanics, and thinking in various educational contexts to motivate learners to apply or acquire knowledge and problem-solve (Kapp 2012). It is the integration of game elements and thinking into activities that are not actually games. Examples include leaderboards, progress bars, and the use of badges.

Although the term gamification is used often, there are several other terms that may be more appropriate substitutes. *Serious games* are games designed specifically for the purpose of learning and/or training. *Simulators* fall under the category of serious games, and their setting allows the learner to experience realistic training environments.

The use of games and game mechanics in education has been reported to improve some skills by as much as 40% (Giang 2013). Additional reports have shown games to lead to increased engagement and motivation in activities and processes in which they are involved (Kiryakova et al. 2014). Few studies looking at the use of games in veterinary medicine have been conducted to date (de Bie and Lipman 2012), but it can be assumed that the role of such games will increase with the continued technological advances occurring peripherally.

Part 3: Immersive Technology (The Realities)

Several immersive technologies are discussed when considering simulation-based learning. The two most common are virtual and augmented reality (AR). These realities are often customizable, objective and standardized, and repeatable (Pottle 2019). However, the cost tends to be a barrier to their use in veterinary education.

Virtual reality (VR) is the use of digital programs to create a completely simulated and immersive environment (Pottle 2019). Users wear a head-mounted display which facilitates the experience and allows users to engage with the environment and any virtual characters.

Augmented reality (AR), a type of mixed reality, is a real-world-based experience that is enhanced by digital objects or information. Barsom et al. (2016) describe AR as " . . . an interactive virtual layer on top of reality" (p. 4174). The setting is typically augmented using a headset, smartphone, or tablet device to add features to the existing surroundings. In addition to visual digital stimuli, the reality can also be enhanced by introducing auditory, haptic (touch), and even olfactory information or feedback (Eckert et al. 2019).

Section 9: Review of Examples of Technologies Used in Veterinary Education

Sarah Baillie and Micha C. Simons

There are benefits of using innovative technologies to support learning and complement traditional F2F teaching activities, and there is extensive literature to support this in medical education. While still emerging in veterinary medicine, there are some veterinary-specific examples

exploring potential uses. The contexts are quite broad and range from anatomy to clinical skills with the common goal of preparing students for career competency.

Numerous factors have driven the increased adoption of advanced technologies in veterinary education, including the need to complement, or even replace, animal use in education and, most recently, the COVID-19 pandemic. Accreditation standards have also provided impetus for continued innovation as veterinary students are required to gain increasing experiences relevant to their future roles and responsibilities spanning the promotion of public health, limiting the spread of disease, and protecting animal welfare and the environment as outlined by the various governing bodies (e.g., OIE, AVMA, RCVS, EAEVE).

Part 1: Applications in Anatomy

Advances in technology have presented new options for teaching and learning anatomy, with the potential to address some of the challenges encountered with traditional approaches and enhance student learning. A systematic review in medicine comparing virtual and AR with traditional teaching for basic science subjects, including physiology and anatomy, found the different approaches resulted in equivalent test performance (Moro et al. 2021). There is potential for veterinary education to capitalize on the innovation and learn from the evidence generated in medicine. A variety of veterinary examples are described below.

A long-term project has led to the development of the virtual canine anatomy program (Linton et al. 2005, 2022). The program combines photos, diagrams, videos, and 3D models to complement traditional anatomy teaching and has been shown to have beneficial effects on student learning when used as preparation for dissection classes. Another example, driven by challenges during the pandemic, is an AR simulation of the anatomy of the canine head specifically designed for use on mobile devices, and the impact on student learning is being investigated (Xu et al. 2021).

A virtual anatomy dissection table with interactive features to explore anatomical specimens has been created using photographs, CT, and MRI images (Anatomage Inc., San Jose, CA). A veterinary version is now available, and a student can visualize structures from the skin inwards, or by a system with specific labeled structures, and perform a virtual dissection. There is ongoing work in medical education to evaluate the potential contributions of such innovations to learning (Bork et al. 2019).

There is increasing interest in the use of 3D AR in this setting. Some early examples of 3D animations include

The Glass Horse (Moore 2001) to visualize normal gastro-intestinal anatomy and movement of structures in colic scenarios, which has been followed by additional equine and canine examples, and a bovine simulation of normal abdominal anatomy and abomasal displacement (Desrochers et al. 2002). More recently, another anatomy 3D AR has been developed. For example, an AR heart program (IVALA®) was used to guide students through a dissection of this complex 3D organ (Little et al. 2021). When compared to traditional guidance using a textbook, the resulting knowledge improvement was similar, although students had a clear preference for learning using AR. Similar results were found with 3D equine sinuses resources when compared to 2D lecture-based learning, with greater student satisfaction and confidence after using the 3D model; MCQ scores were similar for both groups (Canright et al. 2022).

In medical education, evidence syntheses have identified benefits of the higher fidelity offered by 3D visualization technology compared to 2D on anatomical and spatial knowledge acquisition (Yammine and Violato 2015) and further benefits occur when 3D models are presented stereoscopically (Bogomolova et al. 2021). Whatever the approach to anatomy teaching (innovative, technological, or traditional), it is important that the content focuses only on clinically relevant information as this will foster long-term retention of anatomical knowledge by students (Baker 2022).

Part 2: Clinical Experiences

Technology can also help provide environments for students to develop and practice key clinical skills. Such programs can complement and integrate with the traditional clinical experiences to increase student exposure to given scenarios.

Second Life is a program that has been used to create a virtual veterinary clinic. This innovation replicates a waiting room, reception area, and a consulting room and uses avatars to represent clients, staff, a dog, and the veterinarian (Pereira et al. 2018). The virtual clinic allows students to experience a clinical setting and develop clinical reasoning skills while working in small groups. Student and faculty feedback has indicated that the environment was novel yet authentic and had potential as an effective learning experience (Pereira et al. 2018). When compared to a traditional classroom-based equivalent teaching, students in Second Life demonstrated enhanced skills in history taking, physical examination, and prioritization of a problem list (Pereira et al. 2019).

Another approach is to create a 360° experience by combining still images that are "stitched" together, resulting in a simulation that can include interactive features and hotspots. The user can look around the environment scrolling from side to side and up and down. For veterinary students, it has been used for familiarization with a new location, such as a clinical skills laboratory, a consulting room, anesthetic equipment, a tour of a veterinary medical teaching hospital, or a surgical theater.

Lastly, there are a few examples of VR and AR being used to teach specific clinical skills to students. These include 3D touch technology (haptics) for palpation of a virtual bovine reproductive tract (Baillie et al. 2005) and a virtual abdominal cavity of a horse with colic (Baillie and Rendle 2008), mixed reality where palpable 3D virtual objects are superimposed on a physical model (Parkes et al. 2009), and AR where virtual graphical simulation was superimposed on a physical model to create an intravenous injection simulator (Lee et al. 2013).

Part 3: Challenging Environments

There are some veterinary working environments that are inherently challenging to access, particularly some farming enterprises and abattoirs. This has led to the development of VR and advanced video techniques to reinforce the student experience in these areas.

An example is the Virtual Slaughterhouse Simulation (Seguino et al. 2014). The simulation is based on software normally used in building design and provides students with a 3D, real-time, dynamic "walk through" of an abattoir from the lairage through to postmortem inspection and all stages in between. There are interactive features that integrate aspects of an Official Veterinarian's role, such as legal requirements and auditing, as well as case scenarios that allow students to develop problem-solving skills related to specific veterinary public health learning outcomes, including animal welfare, food hygiene, biosecurity, and one health. The first simulation was developed for a red meat abattoir (Seguino et al. 2014) and new versions are being developed for white meat plants (pigs and poultry; Seguino et al. 2022).

A collaboration of French veterinary schools developed a solution to the lack of access to farms during the pandemic (Delsart et al. 2021). A virtual visit to a pig farm was designed to allow students to experience the farm visit remotely. It was created using 360° video and students can experience arriving on the farm, the biosecurity system to enter the facility, and then explore various areas including where the sows farrow. Students can wear a VR headset or use a laptop and the virtual visit is typically followed by a debriefing session in small groups. Although designed for a specific need associated with the pandemic, as there are challenges accessing some facilities due to biosecurity and large cohorts, the virtual pig farm provides a useful long-term resource to complement real visits. With better preparation through a virtual visit and awareness of what to expect, students can optimize the on-farm learning opportunities. Another option being explored is for students on the farm to wear special glasses and transmit the live feed to students in the classroom with both groups interacting.

There are other examples where 360° videos have been used in farming and could be applicable to veterinary students. A virtual tour of a pig fattening unit has been created for members of the public using a tablet or VR glasses (Schütz et al. 2022). User feedback has indicated that there is potential to use the simulation for the public to gain better insight into farming processes and therefore the industry could use such technology for knowledge transfer and improved transparency around production systems. At an agricultural college a student-led project used 360° videos to allow other students to prepare for a visit to a dairy farm with a virtual walk among the cows in the cubicles and collecting area as well as being in the milking parlor (JISC 2019).

The benefits of virtual visits to farms and other challenging environments include enabling students to experience these environments in a safe and structured way, while having a reasonably realistic and immersive experience, and preparing for visits and work placements. However, if exploring the virtual environment involves wearing 3D headsets, there are a few well-recognized issues with motion sickness that affect some users, and solutions are still being explored to remove this as a barrier to use (Nie et al. 2020).

Part 4: Other, Non-simulation Technologies

As well as the more sophisticated technologies and simulations, it is useful to remember the many open-access educational resources available to veterinary students (Gledhill et al. 2017). There are popular, long-established, and high-quality examples. WikiVet (n.d.) is an international collaboration that utilizes the open-source software platform MediaWiki (as does WikiPedia). Over the years contributors have created a repository of peer-reviewed content that represents the breadth of the veterinary curriculum, searchable by discipline, system, or species. Other examples of open-access resources are those designed specifically for clinical skills and include videos hosted on a YouTube channel (Schaper et al. 2014) and an online repository of instruction booklets (Bristol Veterinary School n.d.); such resources can be used by students in class, for revision, and when learning in the workplace to support skill development (Baillie et al. 2020; Müller et al. 2019).

Social media platforms have also been harnessed and applied to veterinary education. Examples include a project using Twitter to provide an annual event to assist students in studying for final exams (Whiting et al. 2016). Students join a Twitter forum using a hashtag and interact online to discuss a case with a faculty member, with questions, answers, and feedback provided. The sessions are archived to create an online repository to further support student revision. Another example has capitalized on the popularity of Instagram among students and utilizes the information available on veterinary practitioner accounts (with permission) from first opinion and referral settings to enhance the curriculum (Sherwin et al. 2022). It allows students to connect theory to practice and incorporates quizzes, interactive features, and decision-making.

Part 5: Summary and Future Direction

The COVID-19 pandemic created a necessity to quickly adopt alternatives to F2F teaching. The widespread development of more online resources both drove innovation in blended learning and increased the associated skill level of faculty and students. This presented a unique opportunity and provided the catalyst to conversations and advancements in veterinary education technologically while reflecting on how to best integrate such learning into veterinary curricula. A careful balance is required between the cost of such innovations and their overall contribution to learning. Informed decisions will need to be made and it has been noted that enhanced digital literacy among senior decision-makers (i.e., senior faculty and administrators) is needed to ensure that the most cost-effective and educationally valuable technologies are adopted (Watermeyera et al. 2021).

Overall, there are only a handful of examples of advanced technologies being used in veterinary education, and most have not yet been widely adopted or validated. Although there is great potential to harness VR and there are applications where its advantages and ability to complement teaching have been documented in other educational disciplines, there are still significant challenges and barriers relating to cost of development and implementation. Additionally, the veterinary education community and developers have a responsibility to place a greater emphasis on generating more robust research to confirm the benefits of learning as reported in other health professions education. This will make strides in justifying the financial investment and subsequent integration within the veterinary curriculum. Progress in generating evidence has been achieved in other veterinary fields such as using simulation and models to complement clinical skills training and has resulted in recent systematic reviews to illustrate the growing body of evidence (Hunt et al. 2022; Noyes et al. 2022; Valliyate et al. 2012).

References

Abbasi, S., Ayoob, T., Malik, A., and Memon, S.I. (2020). Perceptions of students regarding E-learning during Covid-19 at a private medical college. *Pakistan Journal of Medical Sciences* 36 (COVID19-S4): S57.

Abdelmalak, M.M.M. and Parra, J.L. (2016). Expanding learning opportunities for graduate students with HyFlex course design. *International Journal of Online Pedagogy and Course Design* 6 (4): 19–37.

Americans With Disabilities Act of 1990, Pub. L. No. 101-336, 104 Stat. 328.

Association for Educational Communications and Technology (2022). *The Definition and Terminology Committee*, (3 August). https://aect.org/news_manager.php?page=17578 (3 August 2022).

Baillie, S. and Rendle, D. (2008). A virtual reality simulator for training veterinary students to perform rectal palpation of equine colic cases. *Simulation in Healthcare* 2 (4): 248–283. https://doi.org/10.1097/SIH.0b013e31815e698c.

Baillie, S., Mellor, D.J., Brewster, S.A., and Reid, S.W. (2005). Integrating a bovine rectal palpation simulator into an undergraduate veterinary curriculum. *Journal of Veterinary Medical Education* 32 (1): 79–85. https://doi.org/10.3138/jvme.32.1.79.

Baillie, S., Christopher, R., Catterall, A. et al. (2020). Comparison of a silicon skin pad and a tea towel for learning a simple interrupted suture. *Journal of Veterinary Medical Education* 47 (4): 516–522. https://doi.org/10.3138/jvme.2018-0001.

Baker, K.G. (2022). Twelve tips for optimising medical student retention of anatomy. *Medical Teacher* 44 (2): 138–143. https://doi.org/10.1080/0142159X.2021.1896690.

Barsom, E.Z., Graafland, M., and Schijven, M.P. (2016). Systematic review on the effectiveness of augmented reality applications in medical training. *Surgical Endoscopy* 30 (10): 4174–4183.

Berge, Z.L. and Huang, Y.P.J.L. (2004). Model for sustainable student retention: a holistic perspective on the student dropout problem with special attention to e. *Learning* 13 (5): 97–108.

Blau, G. and Drennan, R. (2017). Exploring differences in business undergraduate perceptions by preferred classroom delivery mode. *Online Learning* 21 (3): 222–234.

Bogomolova, K., Hierck, B.P., Looijen, A.E.M. et al. (2021). Stereoscopic three-dimensional visualisation technology in anatomy learning: a meta-analysis. *Medical Education* 55 (3): 317–327. https://doi.org/10.1111/medu.14352.

Bonk, C.J. and Graham, C.R. (2012). *The Handbook of Blended Learning: Global Perspectives, Local Designs*. Wiley.

Bonnaud, L. and Fortané, N. (2021). Being a vet: the veterinary profession in social science research. *Review of Agricultural, Food and Environmental Studies* 102 (2): 125–149.

Boothe, K.A., Lohmann, M.J., Donnell, K.A., and Hall, D. (2018). Applying the principles of Universal Design for Learning (UDL) in the college classroom. *The Journal of Special Education Apprenticeship* 7 (3): 1–13.

Bork, F., Stratmann, L., Enssle, S. et al. (2019). The benefits of an augmented reality magic mirror system for integrated radiology teaching in gross anatomy. *Anatomical Sciences Education* 12 (6): 585–598. https://doi.org/10.1002/ase.1864.

Bristol Veterinary School (n.d.). Clinical Skills Instruction Booklets. http://www.bristol.ac.uk/vetscience/research/comparative-clinical/veterinary-education/clinical-skills-booklets/ (accessed 26 July 2022).

Canright, A., Bescoby, S., and Dickson, J. (2022). Evaluation of a 3D computer model of the equine paranasal sinuses as a tool for veterinary anatomy education. *Journal of Veterinary Medical Education* 24: e20210134. https://doi.org/10.3138/jvme-2021-0134.

CAST (2018). *Universal Design for Learning Guidelines version 2.2*. Retrieved from http://udlguidelines.cast.org (accessed 18 September 2022).

Cavus, N. (2014). Distance learning and learning management systems. *Procedia-Social and Behavioral Sciences* 191: 872–877.

Center for Disease Control and Prevention (2022). *Disability impacts all of us*. https://www.cdc.gov/ncbddd/disabilityandhealth/infographic-disability-impacts-all.html (accessed 18 September 2022).

Commonwealth of Massachusetts (2022). *Know the types of cyber threats*. https://www.mass.gov/service-details/know-the-types-of-cyber-threats (accessed 18 September 2022).

Cook, S. (2021). US schools leaked 28.6 million records in 1,851 data breaches since 2005. https://www.comparitech.com/blog/vpn-privacy/us-schools-data-breaches/ (accessed 18 September 2022).

David, L. (2015). E-learning Theory (Mayer, Sweller, Moreno). Learning Theories, (December). https://www.learning-theories.com/e-learning-theory-mayer-sweller-moreno.html (accessed 14 October 2022).

Davidson, N. and Major, C.H. (2014). Boundary crossings: Cooperative learning, collaborative learning, and problem-based learning. *Journal on Excellence in College Teaching* 25 (3&4): 7–55.

De Bie, M.H. and Lipman, L.J. (2012). The use of digital games and simulators in veterinary education: an overview with examples. *Journal of Veterinary Medical Education* 39 (1): 13–20.

Delsart, M., Chateau, H., Belloc, C. et al. (2021) Virtual visits of pig farms in times of COVID. *34th EAEVE General Assembly*, Torino, Italy (1 October 2021).

Desrochers, A., Harvey, D., Roy, F. et al. (2002). Surgeries of the abomasum in cattle. Laboratory for the Integration of Computer Technologies in Medical Sciences, Faculty of Veterinary Medicine, Université de Montréal.

Eckert, M., Volmerg, J.S., and Friedrich, C.M. (2019). Augmented reality in medicine: systematic and bibliographic review. *JMIR mHealth and uHealth* 7 (4): e10967.

Edyburn, K. and Edyburn, D.L. (2021). Classroom menus for supporting the academic success of diverse learners. *Intervention in School and Clinic* 56 (4): 243–249.

Ericsson, K.A., Krampe, R.T., and Tesch Römer, C. (1993). The role of deliberate practice in the acquisition of expert performance. *Psychological Review* 100: 363–406.

Eyal, L. and Gil, E. (2022). Hybrid learning spaces – a three-fold evolving perspective. In: *Hybrid Learning Spaces*, Understanding Teaching-Learning Practice (ed. E. Gil, Y. Mor, Y. Dimitriadis, and C. Köppe), 11–23. Cham: Springer https://doi.org/10.1007/978-3-030-88520-5_2.

Friel, C.L. (2018). Experiences of students with attention deficit/hyperactivity disorder (ADHD) in online learning environments: a multi-case study. Doctoral dissertation. University of Missouri-Columbia.

Gledhill, L., Dale, V.H.M., Powney, S. et al. (2017). An international survey of veterinary students to assess their use of online learning resources. *Journal of Veterinary Medical Education* 44 (4): 692–703. https://doi.org/10.3138/jvme.0416-085R.

Guze, P.A. (2015). Using technology to meet the challenges of medical education. *Transactions of the American Clinical and Climatological Association* 126: 260–270.

Hamlin, A., Barczyk, C., Powell, G., and Frost, J. (2013). A comparison of university efforts to contain academic dishonesty. *Journal of Legal, Ethical, and Regulatory Issues* 16 (1): 35–46.

Hladek, G.A. (2014). Cochlear implants, the deaf culture, and ethics. *Monash Bioethics Review* 21: 29–44. https://doi.org/10.1007/BF03351265.

Holpuch, A. and Rubin, A. (2022). Remote scan of student's room before test violated his privacy, Judge rules. *The New York Times*. (Published August 25, 2022).

Hubbard, A. (1998). What it means to teach online. *Computers & Geosciences* 24 (7): 713–717.

Hunt, J.A., Simons, M.C., and Anderson, S.L. (2022). If you build it, they will learn: a review of models in veterinary surgical education. *Veterinary Surgery* 51 (1): 52–61.

Joint Information Systems Committee (JISC) (2019). Getting students ready for the changing world. https://www.jisc.ac.uk/membership/stories/getting-students-ready-for-the-changing-workplace-18-nov-2019 (accessed 21 July 2022).

Kapp, K.M. (2012). *The Gamification of Learning and Instruction: Game-Based Methods and Strategies for Training and Education*. Wiley.

Kaul, V., Gallo de Moraes, A., Khateeb, D. et al. (2020). Medical education during the COVID-19 pandemic. *Education and Clinical Practice: Chest Reviews* 159 (5): 1949–1960. https://doi.org/10.1016/j.chest.2020.12.026.

Kiryakova, G., Angelova, N., and Yordanova, L. (2014). Gamification in education. *Proceedings of 9th International Balkan Education and Science Conference*. https://www.researchgate.net/profile/Gabriela-Kiryakova/publication/320234774_GAMIFICATION_IN_EDUCATION/links/59d6514eaca27213df9e77e4/GAMIFICATION-IN-EDUCATION.pdf (accessed 14 October 2022).

Lee, K. (2017). Rethinking the accessibility of online higher education: a historical review. *The Internet and Higher Education* 33: 15–23. https://doi.org/10.1016/j.iheduc.2017.01.001.

Lee, S., Lee, J., Lee, A. et al. (2013). Augmented reality intravenous injection simulator based 3D medical imaging for veterinary medicine. *The Veterinary Journal* 196 (2): 197–202. https://doi.org/10.1016/j.tvjl.2012.09.015.

Linton, A., Schoenfeld-Tacher, R., and Whalen, L.R. (2005). Developing and implementing an assessment method to evaluate a virtual canine anatomy program. *Journal of Veterinary Medical Education* 32: 249–254.

Linton, A., Garrett, A.C., Ivie, K.R. Jr. et al. (2022). Enhancing anatomical instruction: impact of a virtual canine anatomy program on student outcomes. *Anatomical Sciences Education* 15 (2): 330–340. https://doi.org/10.1002/ase.2087.

Little, W.B., Dezdrobitu, C., Conan, A., and Artemiou, E. (2021). Is augmented reality the new way for teaching and learning veterinary cardiac anatomy? *Medical Science Educator* 31 (2): 723–732. https://doi.org/10.1007/s40670-021-01260-8.

Lockee, B.B. (2020). Designing forward: Instructional design considerations for online learning in the COVID-19 context. *The Journal of Applied Instructional Design* 9 (3): https://doi.org/10.51869/93bl.

Mamattah, R.S. (2016). Students' perceptions of e-learning. [Unpublished Master's thesis]. Linköping University.

Mayer, R.E. and Moreno, R. (2003). Nine ways to reduce cognitive load in multimedia learning. *Educational Psychologist* 38 (1): 43–52.

Mehra, M.R., Desai, S.S., Kuy, S. et al. (2020a). Retraction: Cardiovascular disease, drug therapy, and mortality in Covid-19. *The New England Journal of Medicine* 382 (26): 2582.

Mehra, M.R., Desai, S.S., Ruschitzka, F., and Patel, A.N. (2020b). Retracted: Hydroxychloroquine or chloroquine with or without a macrolide for treatment of COVID-19: a multinational registry analysis [published online ahead of print May 22, 2020]. *The Lancet* https://doi.org/10.1016/S0140-6736(20)31180-6.

Merrill, D.A. (2002). First principles of instruction. *Educational Technology Research and Development* 50 (3): 43–59.

Moore, J.N. (2001). The glass horse. http://www.sciencein3d.com/products.html (accessed 22 July 2022).

Moreno, R. and Mayer, R.E. (1999). Cognitive principles of multimedia learning: the role of modality and contiguity. *Journal of Educational Psychology* 91 (2): 358.

Moro, C., Birt, J., Stromberga, Z. et al. (2021). Virtual and augmented reality enhancements to medical and science student physiology and anatomy test performance: a systematic review and meta-analysis. *Anatomical Sciences Education* 14 (3): 368–376. https://doi.org/10.1002/ase.2049.

Müller, L.R., Tipold, A., Ehlers, J.P., and Schaper, E. (2019). TiHoVideos: veterinary students' utilization of instructional videos on clinical skills. *BMC Veterinary Research* 15: 326. https://doi.org/10.1186/s12917-019-2079-2.

Naffi, N. (2020). The Hyber-Flexible Course Design Model (HyFlex): a pedagogical strategy for uncertain times. *Revue Internationale des Technologies en Pédagogie Universitaire* 17 (2): 136–143.

National Cyber Security Alliance (2022). *Online safety + privacy basics.* (Published May 26, 2022). https://staysafeonline.org/resources/online-safety-privacy-basics/ (accessed 18 September 2022).

Nie, G.-Y., Duh, H.B.-L., Liu, Y., and Wang, Y. (2020). Analysis on mitigation of visually induced motion sickness by applying dynamical blurring on a user's retina. *IEEE Transactions on Visualization and Computer Graphics* 26 (8): 2535–2545. https://doi.org/10.1109/TVCG.2019.2893668.

Noyes, J.A., Carbonneau, K.J., and Matthew, S.M. (2022). Comparative effectiveness of training with simulators versus traditional instruction in veterinary education: Meta-analysis and systematic review. *Journal of Veterinary Medical Education* 45 (1): 25–38.

Paramythis, A., Loidl-Reisinger, S., and Kepler, J. (2004). Adaptive learning environments and e-Learning standards. *Electronic Journal of eLearning* 1: 369–379.

Parkes, R., Forrest, N., and Baillie, S. (2009). A mixed reality simulator for feline abdominal palpation training in veterinary medicine. *Studies in Health Technology and Informatics* 142: 244–246.

Pereira, M.M., Artemiou, E., McGonigle, D. et al. (2018). Using the virtual world of Second Life in veterinary medicine: student and faculty perceptions. *Journal of Veterinary Medical Education* 45 (2): 148–155. https://doi.org/10.3138/jvme.1115-184r4.

Pereira, M.M., Artemiou, E., McGonigle, D. et al. (2019). Second Life and classroom environments: comparing small group teaching and learning in developing clinical reasoning process skills. *Medical Science Educator* 29 (2): 431–437. https://doi.org/10.1007/s40670-019-00706-4.

Pickrell, J.A., Boyer, J., Oehme, F.W. et al. (2002). Group learning improves case analysis in veterinary medicine. *Journal of Veterinary Medical Education* 29 (1): 43–49.

Plant, J.D. (2007). Incorporating an audience response system into veterinary dermatology lectures: effect on student knowledge retention and satisfaction. *Journal of Veterinary Medical Education* 34 (5): 674–677.

Pottle, J. (2019). Virtual reality and the transformation of medical education. *Future Healthcare Journal* 6 (3): 181–185. https://doi.org/10.7861/fhj.2019-0036.

Puzziferro, M. and Shelton, K. (2008). A model for developing high-quality online courses: integrating a systems approach with learning theory. *Journal of Asynchronous Learning Networks* 12: 119–136.

Quality Matters (2022). *QM Rubrics & Standards.* https://www.qualitymatters.org/qa-resources/rubric-standards (accessed 4 August 2022)

Rush, B.R., Hafen, M. Jr., Biller, D.S. et al. (2010). The effect of differing audience response system question types on student attention in the veterinary medical classroom. *Journal of Veterinary Medical Education* 37 (2): 145–153.

Schaper, E., Ehlers, J.P., Dilly, M., and Crowther, E. (2014). Using YouTube to share teaching resources. *Journal of the American Veterinary Medical Association* 245 (4): 372–373. https://doi.org/10.2460/javma.245.4.372.

Schütz, A., Kurz, K., and Busch, G. (2022). Virtual farm tours – virtual reality glasses and tablets are suitable tools to provide insights into pig husbandry. *PLoS One* 17 (1): e0261248. https://doi.org/10.1371/journal.pone.0261248.

Seguino, A., Seguino, F., Eleuteri, A., and Rhind, S.M. (2014). Development and evaluation of a virtual slaughterhouse simulator for training and educating veterinary students. *Journal of Veterinary Medical Education* 41 (3): 233–242. https://doi.org/10.3138/jvme.1113-150R.

Seguino, A., Bettini, G., and De Cesare, A. (2022). UNA Europa project "The Virtual Slaughterhouse Simulator": demo and student feedback. In: *25th Graz European Conference on Veterinary and Medical Education*, 29. University of Budapest, Hungary https://graco2022.univet.hu/ (accessed 21–23 April 2022.

Serghiou, S. and Ioannidis, J.P.A. (2018). Altmetric scores, citations, and publication of studies posted as preprints. *Journal of the American Medical Association* 319 (4): 402–404. https://doi.org/10.1001/jama.2017.21168.

Shaffer, D.W. (2006). Epistemic frames for epistemic games. *Computers & Education* 46: 223–234. http://doi.org/10.1016/j.compedu.2005.11.003.

Sharma, N., Doherty, I., and Dong, C. (2017). Adaptive learning in medical education: the final piece of technology enhanced learning? *The Ulster Medical Journal* 86 (3): 198–200.

Sherwin, G., Payne, E., and Cobb, K. (2022). Can Instagram be used as an educational tool in veterinary medicine? *12th VetEd Conference*, School of Veterinary Medicine and Science, University of Nottingham, UK (6th–8th July 2022).

Sutton, M.J. and Jorge, C.F.B. (2020). Potential for radical change in Higher Education learning spaces after the pandemic. *Journal of Applied Learning and Teaching* 3 (1): 124–128.

Tobias, K.M. and Bailey, M.R. (2020). Veterinary student self-assessment of basic surgical skills as an experiential learning tool. *Journal of Veterinary Medical Education* 47 (6): 661–667.

Tyler-Smith, K. (2006). Early attrition among first time eLearners: a review of factors that contribute to drop-out, withdrawal and non-completion rates of adult learners undertaking eLearning programmes. *Journal of Online Learning and Teaching* 2 (2): 73–85.

University of Florida (2022). UF Standards and Markers of Excellence. https://cals.ufl.edu/content/pdf/faculty_staff/UF_Standards_Markers_Of_Excellence.pdf (accessed 20 September 2022).

United States Government (2022). Identity theft. https://www.usa.gov/identity-theft (accessed 18 September 18 2022).

University of Georgia, University Libraries (2022). Finding reliable resources. https://guides.libs.uga.edu/reliability (accessed 18 September 2022).

Valliyate, M., Robinson, N.G., and Goodman, J.R. (2012). Current concepts in simulation and other alternatives for veterinary education: a review. *Veterinární Medicína* 57 (7): 325.

Viberg, O., Hatakka, M., Balter, O., and Mavroudi, A. (2018). The current landstape of learning analytics in higher education. *Computers in Human Behavior* 89: 98–110.

Viberg, O., Khalil, M., and Baars, M. (2020). Self-regulated learning and learning analytics in online learning environments: a review of empirical research. In: *Tenth International Conference on Learning Analytics & Knowledge (LAK '20)*, 524–533. New York, NY, USA: Association for Computing Machinery https://doi.org/10.1145/3375462.3375483.

Warenzak, M. (2018). Universities and intellectual property law. https://www.sgrlaw.com/wp-content/uploads/2018/09/24-25_Summer2018_TTL_Intellectual-Property_Web_Spreads.pdf (accessed 18 September 2022).

Watermeyera, R., Crick, T., and Knight, C. (2021). Digital disruption in the time of COVID-19: learning technologists' accounts of institutional barriers to online learning,

teaching and assessment in UK universities. *International Journal for Academic Development*, Ahead-of-print, 1–15. https://doi.org/10.1080/1360144X.2021.1990064.

WebAIM (2020). *Introduction to accessibility*, (18 September). https://webaim.org/intro/.

Whiting, M., Kinnison, T., and Mossop, L. (2016). Developing an intercollegiate Twitter forum to improve student exam study and digital professionalism. *Journal of Veterinary Medical Education* 43 (3): 282–286. https://doi.org/10.3138/jvme.0715-114R.

WikiVet (n.d.). Veterinary Education Online. https://en.wikivet.net/Veterinary_Education_Online (accessed 25 July 2022).

Xu, X., Pan, X., Kilroy, D. et al. (2021). Augmented Reality for Veterinary self-learning during the pandemic: a holistic study protocol for a remote, randomised, cross-over study. *34th British HCI Workshop and Doctoral Consortium* (HCI2021-WDC) (20, 21 July 2021). Burlington: USAScienceOpen.

Yammine, K. and Violato, C.A. (2015). A meta-analysis of the educational effectiveness of three-dimensional visualization technologies in teaching anatomy. *Anatomical Sciences Education* 8 (6): 525–538. https://doi.org/10.1002/ase.1510.

Zhang, D., Zhou, L., Briggs, R.O., and Nunamaker, J.F. Jr. (2005). Instructional video in e-learning: assessing the impact of interactive video on learning effectiveness. *Information & Management* 43: 15–27.

Moore, M. (2005). Theory of transactional distance. In: *Theoretical Principles of Distance Education* (ed. D. Keegan), 22–38. Routledge.

Meier, E. (2015). Beyond a digital status quo: re-conceptualizing online learning opportunities. *Occasional Paper Series*, 34. https://doi.org/10.58295/2375-3668.1000

Lai, J. and Widmar, N.O. (2021). Revisiting the digital divide in the COVID-19 era. *Applied Economic Perspectives Policy* 43 (1): 458–464. https://doi.org/10.1002/aepp.13104. Epub 2020 Oct 12. PMID: 33230409; PMCID: PMC7675734.

WebAIM (2022). WebAIM (accessed 18 September 2022). https://webaim.org/

Giang, V. (2013). "Gamification" techniques increase your employees' ability to learn by 40%. Retrieved from Business Insider. https://www.businessinsider.com/gamification-techniques-increase-your-employees-ability-to-learn-by-40-2013-9.

Additional Resources

Deque Color Contrast Analyzer: https://dequeuniversity.com/color-contrast

Adobe: https://color.adobe.com/create/color-contrast-analyzer
WebAIM: https://webaim.org/resources/contrastchecker/

8

The Syllabus

Katherine Fogelberg, DVM, PhD (Science Education), MA (Educational Leadership)

Virginia-Maryland College of Veterinary Medicine, Blacksburg, VA, USA

Section 1: Introduction

What is a syllabus? Why do we have to wrestle, wrangle with, and write them? How do we use them appropriately – and why are they, at times, used inappropriately? Why do students not read them? Where did they come from and are they really that important?

We have all – at some point or another – in our careers as university students and, for some of us, as university professors, come in contact with a syllabus. We are all indoctrinated into the apparent value of the syllabus and are told that syllabi are important, but from personal experience as a student, I was never taught why syllabi are important; I had to figure it out on my own.

Similarly, those who go into academia and teach are either handed a syllabus or told to put one together. Much like instruction on how to teach, which is pretty nonexistent at the postsecondary level, instruction on how to put a syllabus together, what its purpose is, and why it is important is rarely – if ever – provided.

This chapter will first define what a syllabus is, then discuss the purposes of a syllabus, suggest approaches to creating effective syllabi, and offer some ideas for how to create and use syllabi in ways that increase student engagement, support student learning and faculty development, and invite students of all backgrounds, abilities, and the like into the learning process. Links to syllabus templates are provided throughout.

Part 1: Defining the Syllabus

Oxford Languages (used by Google for its English dictionary) presents the etymology of the word syllabus as originating in Greek from the word *sittuba*, meaning title slip, label. In modern Latin, it was a misreading of the Latin term *sittybas*, which was the accusative plural of *sittyba*;

sometime during the mid-seventeenth century, it evolved into the term *syllabus*, meaning a concise table or heading of a discourse. Today, however, the term is defined as "a summary outline of a discourse, treatise, or course of study or of examination requirements" according to the Merriam-Webster online dictionary.

Where, when, and by whom the syllabus as we know it in our classrooms today was first used is still a bit of a mystery – even after an extensive search of the literature and through general searches on Google. There is some indication that Cicero used it in his writings to Atticus in 58 BCE, shortly after he returned from his exile and as a request for aid in arranging his library, although how the term syllabus itself was derived from *sittybas* is somewhat obfuscated; it could have been a scribe error or Cicero's direct error, according to the only online source found that discusses a history other than the known etymology of the word (http://www.inrebus.com/blog/syllabusetymology).

Regardless of where it started or how the word evolved, syllabi or syllabuses, are currently ubiquitous in higher education; they have spawned a decent body of literature and, of course, lots of opinions about their uses, usefulness, and necessity. The next section will cover the purposes of a syllabus, some of which may surprise you and some of which you are likely already aware.

Section 2: Syllabus Purposes

"At the very least, the syllabus sends a symbolic message to the student regarding your personality as a teacher and the amount of investment you have made in the course. First impressions are so important that it would be foolhardy to ignore the opportunity to make the impression favorable…the syllabus is…a manageable, profound first impression" (Matejka and Kurke 1994, p. 115).

According to Parkes and Harris (2002), the history of the syllabus is somewhat ambiguous in both its origins and its meanings over time, which is not surprising given the brief section that precedes this one. What might surprise you, however, is that the purposes of a syllabus and its uses continue to be somewhat unclear. Additionally, as you may have gleaned from your own experiences as a student and/or a faculty member, there is no universally accepted template or guide for creating syllabi, although there are elements in common to most, if not all, of them.

In an attempt to better define the purposes of a syllabus, Parkes and Harris (2002), reviewed over 200 syllabi from 11 colleges and schools at a single university, from which they concluded that syllabi varied in two fundamental areas: (i) the reasons for writing the syllabus and (ii) the syllabus content. This study led the authors to posit three purposes of a syllabus: (i) it serves as a contract; (ii) it serves as a permanent record; and (iii) it aids student learning. These three purposes are proposed in support of their position that while syllabus content is important, it is the syllabus's purpose that should drive that content.

While there has been some additional research into syllabi and their purposes recently, there was little to no research on this topic previous to the turn of the twenty-first century, although there are several others who had reported that the syllabus serves as a contract, of sorts, between the instructor and the student (Cooper and Cuseo 1989; Lowther et al. 1989; Matejka and Kurke 1994). However, the majority of studies regarding syllabi have looked more at how to create and what makes a good syllabus; recent research seems to be continuing in this vein rather than looking specifically at the syllabus's purpose. For example, Habanek (2005), stated that the syllabus functions as a "major communication device" (p. 62), Bowers-Campbell (2015), published a study "Investigating the Syllabus as a Defining Document," and Thompson (2007), provided advice on using the syllabus as a communication document by outlining how to construct and present a syllabus. Additional work has been done on how to use the syllabus to document the scholarship of teaching and learning (Albers 2003), and its usefulness in promoting diversity, equity, and inclusion (DEI; Fuentes et al. 2020). It is interesting that of all the peer-reviewed documents reviewed and/or used for this chapter, over half cited Parkes's and Harris's "The Purposes of a Syllabus" as the guide used to justify their recommendations for creating a good syllabus; it would appear, then, that their stated purposes are generally accepted, making their three seemingly simple suggestions a great place to begin.

Part 1: Serves as a Contract

"That atmosphere of litigation and accountability that increasingly constrains the educational process has placed a new emphasis on the syllabus as an agreement between students and the instructor" (Albers 2003, p. 61). Although this was written early in the century, it still holds today and is one of the many reasons a syllabus is such a useful tool. Unfortunately, due to this rather cynical view of the syllabus, the document itself has also emerged as an authoritarian, often harsh outline of requirements, consequences, and demands (sometimes masked as expectations). The syllabi of today are often one-way communications – a telling of students what the instructor will do and how the students will (attempt to) achieve their grades in the course.

It is easy to understand why this approach has come about, as increasingly students and parents want to know what their tuition dollars are "purchasing" in higher education, and a syllabus is one way to indicate what they are, ostensibly, receiving in exchange for their dollars. And while we still view the syllabus as a contract, keep in mind that it is not actually a legal contract; rather, it is an agreement that may be referred to should some sort of dispute arise.

At its most basic, the syllabus should provide some information that lays out the plan for a course and helps hold both the instructor and the students accountable for various activities. Matejka and Kurke (1994), recommend that you provide, at minimum, the following elements:

instructor's name
course [title]
location
time
office hours
phone number/contact information
required and recommended textbooks
required and recommend other readings
instructional methods
course objective(s)
assessments
grading
attendance and participation policies
schedule of the class activities.

Das, in a 2012 manuscript, recommends 13 elements be included in the syllabus:

Introductory information
Complete course title
Course description
Course overview and prerequisites
Course competencies and/or objectives
Required and optional texts and supplies

Class delivery methods/attendance/class behavior
Withdrawal policy/reinstatement policy
Student responsibilities
Evaluation/examination
Final grade options
Other information
Syllabus acknowledgment.

Parkes and Harris (2002), summarize the elements of a syllabus they feel should be included this way:

Clear and accurate course calendar
Grading policies, including components and weights
Attendance policy
Late assignment policy
Makeup exam policy
Policies on incompletes and revisions
Academic dishonesty policy
Academic freedom policy
Accommodation of disabilities policy.

Note that there are some big differences between the recommendations on the first two lists and this last list; this is an excellent demonstration of the wide variety of interpretations and thus, approaches, to writing a syllabus. The first two lists are much more focused on specific information – course title and instructor, date, time, location of the course, etc. Whereas the last list is viewing the syllabus more as a contract, recommending mostly policy and procedural content. As someone who has worked extensively with individual faculty on all aspects of teaching, including syllabus preparation, this author finds the Parkes and Harris list to be the most helpful guide. It is, in this author's experience, common for students to quibble about grades, late assignments, and the need for makeup exams far more often if those are not explicitly addressed in the syllabus. In a decade plus of higher education instruction, this author has never had a formal grade complaint filed because of the clarity of these policies in the syllabi.

However, the contents of a syllabus may be left up to the individual instructor and sometimes the institution, individual program, or school has a template that must be followed. For those with a template, while this can get frustrating at times, it is nice to know there is consistency from course to course for both students and faculty. It is also important to remember that templates are still only guides; yes, you must include everything the template asks for, but it does not prohibit you from adding on. There is always some leeway to add in such things as your teaching approach or philosophy, any policies you feel are omitted (e.g., your makeup exam/assignment policies), or other information you feel is important to include.

For those without a template, it can be overwhelming to consider what should be included. Keeping in mind the general recommendations provided above, remembering that the syllabus is an agreement between the students and the instructor, as well as a record of what was taught and how it was assessed, creating a basic syllabus, should be slightly less intimidating.

Creating a syllabus that does more than tell students what to do and when to do it can become a bit more complicated. This will be explored a bit further in another section of this chapter, but suffice it to say that there are numerous approaches to creating high-quality syllabi; it is up to the individual instructor to determine their goals for the syllabus, how much they wish to communicate to the student up front, and how the syllabus may be used to support the students and the instructor throughout the course.

For some examples of different types of syllabi covering a variety of topics and some general syllabi templates, see the additional resources at the end of the reference section in this chapter. There you will find a couple of links to sites that provide strong samples of both.

Part 2: Becomes a Permanent Record

If you have spent any time in academia as a faculty member at any level, you have likely had a student or two request a syllabus from you so they can decide whether or not to sign up for a class, to see if they might be able to transfer credit from one school to another, or to determine if they are eligible to take your course. This is more an undergraduate and graduate than professional program phenomena, although with increasing numbers of students transferring from one professional program to another, it is becoming more common than it once was.

Likewise, faculty often ask others for their syllabi for a variety of reasons. Perhaps you have found yourself in one of these situations:

1) You are teaching a course for the first time that someone else used to teach and you are curious to see how the other faculty member constructed and delivered the course.
2) You are a new professor – either in your first faculty position or at a new institution – and you would like to see how syllabi are constructed at your university.
3) You are thinking about creating a new course and would like to see examples of other new courses that have been created, perhaps that are related to yours but not the same.

There are certainly other reasons that faculty – you – might ask to see a syllabus, but these are the most common ones that come to mind. Regardless of the reason, however, you can see that whether it is for student or faculty purposes, syllabi become permanent records of the information delivered and the assessments made of student learning during your course at that institution and in that period of time. Thus, a syllabus maintains importance during the delivery of your course and, in many cases, for years after the course has concluded, even if you have moved on or no longer teach the course.

To this end, it is imperative that you create a syllabus that accurately documents your expectations for student learning, how you achieve that learning, and how you assess that learning. You must provide enough information to the reader that they can determine at what level the content is being delivered, how many student contact hours were achieved, and the specific topics covered during the course, among the many other items that a syllabus contains. If you have never thought about the importance and impact of a syllabus, you should do so from here on out. Parkes and Harris see the permanent record as the place where many of the recommended elements in the previous section should be considered. In their 2002 manuscript, they see the following as essential elements of a syllabus to ensure the permanent record is complete:

Title of date(s) of the course
Department offering the course
Credit hours earned
Title and rank of the instructor(s)
Pre or corequisites
Required texts and other materials
(Recommended texts and other materials)[1]
Course objectives, linked to professional standards
Description of course content
Description of assessment procedures.

In short, the syllabus is a document for the past, the present, and the future. Once it is prepared, it relays a variety of important information to your present students, including who you are, when you will be accessible, where and when your course will meet, what your expectations are of them for success in the course, and how they will be assessed, among other things. Once you have delivered the course, the syllabus stands as a past reminder of what you did or did not do and provides a glimpse into your course that help others determine whether the information is transferable to other institutions or fulfills the prerequisites for other courses. It also serves as documentation to support accrediting bodies and may, at other times, support you in your quest to be promoted, tenured, or hired at

another institution. As a document of the future, your syllabus helps guide you in future course preparations. If your courses are similar, you can use it as a template and make changes as appropriate; if they are completely different, they can serve as a template as you create a new syllabus. But each iteration of an existing syllabus is an important document to help you understand where you started, where you have been, and where you are going.

Part 3: Is a Learning Tool

In creating syllabi it is highly uncommon for instructors – and administrators – to address the syllabus as anything other than a contract or guide for the students. It is emphasized as an important document but mostly as a document to help with possible student issues during the semester. However, Parkes and Harris make it clear – as do a spate of other studies – that syllabi should also be viewed as a *learning tool* – for the students, certainly, but also potentially for the instructor. As such, we are seeing a movement toward a more inviting syllabus; one that encourages students, provides guidance with a defter hand, establishes the teacher–student dyad as collaborators rather than superior–subordinate, and enhances the learning experience. The contract aspect referred to in the previous section still remains, but more and more we are seeing it evolve as a contract into which both parties enter having participated in its creation, earning buy-in from students and instructors alike.

Parkes and Harris (2002), state that the syllabus as a learning tool should direct students in the following ways:

Helping them to plan and improve self-management skills
Suggesting how much time they will need to spend on the course outside of class
Providing tips for success on assessments
Presenting common misconceptions or mistakes
Specifying study strategies for success
Informing them of instructor(s) and assistant(s) availability
Providing campus resources
Specifying contacts or offices that support students with disabilities
Supplying the relevance and importance of the course
Providing a model of high-quality work.

Other researchers and instructors have discussed using the syllabus as a learning tool as well, and not always solely for the student. In approaching the syllabus as a learning tool, it is important to have the foundations of the syllabus as a contract and the syllabus as a permanent record solidly intact (Eberly et al. 2001). From those foundations – as previously stated – you can add to the syllabus in ways that can enhance its usefulness beyond these purposes.

---

1 This is not included on the original list by Parkes and Harris but was added by this author as a reminder that many courses are increasingly recommending resources and that these should also be recorded.

It is also important to understand your personal teaching philosophy and approach to content delivery. Think about the syllabus of an instructor who is more lecture-based versus one who is more activity based; what might those look like? What similarities and differences might you see if you were to put those syllabi side by side? Now consider which type of instruction you most closely align with; this will help you as you construct your own syllabi.

If you are a more lecture-based instructor, your syllabus is likely to focus more on the document as a contract and as a permanent record. There are still opportunities to use it as a tool for learning, as those are somewhat embedded in the expectations set forth by these two purposes, but explicitly using it as a learning tool is less likely. The language of purely lecture-based syllabi tends to be more authoritarian, telling rather than conversing with or inviting students into the course. This is not an indictment of these types of syllabi; they can be effective and functional and may even be needed in some courses.

For those who lean more toward constructivism and/or active learning in their teaching approach, however, there are many opportunities to use the syllabus as a contract and permanent record while also being intentional about its use as a learning tool. Having students cocreate the syllabus with you is one way to do this (Hudd 2003; McDevitt 2004; Parkes and Harris 2002); other methods include incorporating your educational or teaching philosophy (Das 2013; Parkes and Harris 2002), and using inviting and inclusive language (Fuentes et al. 2020; Helmer 2018; Harnish and Bridges 2011; Ludy et al. 2016).

Syllabus cocreation can be accomplished in a number of ways. McDevitt (2004), for example, discussed her approach to cocreation of a syllabus as a way to span the cultural differences in her constructivist teaching philosophy with those of her Omani students, who were raised in a strictly positivist environment. Her coconstruction consisted of beginning the course with a series of tasks well within the capabilities of her students to help them gain confidence and to establish rapport. From there, class discussions were used to create the remaining expectation – student and instructor – for the course, from assignments to grading. Thus, in this process, McDevitt was able to help her adult English Language Learners (ELL) learn English more effectively and efficiently while simultaneously exposing them to an entirely new paradigm of teaching and learning, e.g., constructivism.

In her paper, McDevitt (2004), writes that her students had been raised in a purely positivist system, where instructors were viewed as superior in knowledge and that they, as students, could only learn by listening and memorizing the wisdom provided by their teachers. Through the process of coconstructing the syllabus, McDevitt was able

to demonstrate that teachers can be experts and not be authoritarian; and that teachers can value and adjust to the needs of their students and still be effective in their delivery. Admittedly, the syllabus negotiations were "not a complete success. I suspect that from the group of 18 students, three or four of them never really saw the point of the whole exercise" (McDevitt 2004, p. 8). However, for about 50% of her students, their English language gains "were considerable. These students presented written and oral projects of a very high standard, and their sense of achievement was very gratifying" (McDevitt 2004, p. 8). Thus, cocreation of a syllabus, even in a classroom filled with students from a significantly different cultural background, can be a successful tool in helping both the learner and the instructor gain benefits.

As with all educational approaches, this is not a one-size-fits-all method. Syllabus cocreation is generally best used for more advanced students, students in smaller classes (less than 30), and/or in courses aimed at middle to higher-level thinking skills, as classified by Bloom's taxonomy. That is not to say that, for instance, a cocreated syllabus would be inappropriate for a first-year undergraduate course, it just may be much more difficult to achieve due to potentially large class sizes and/or a lack of understanding on the part of the less seasoned students about what syllabi are supposed to do. Thus, should you choose to work with your students to create a syllabus, you should carefully consider your students and the content you are delivering.

Cocreation of syllabi does not need to be a true 50/50 split, either. Perhaps you are working with a large group of students or a group of younger and/or less knowledgeable students but would still like them to have some input into the syllabus. In these cases, you may consider having students select the types of assessments they would prefer, help determine how many and when summative assessments should be scheduled, or even develop one or more of the assignments they would need to complete to be successful in the course. In other words, syllabus cocreation is not an all-or-nothing approach. Do not be afraid to dabble in it a little bit to see what does and does not work for you and your particular teaching style.

Incorporating your educational or teaching philosophy first requires that you *have* such a philosophy. While it was rare to be asked about such a thing even a few decades ago, there are a few academics who are asking faculty candidates about their teaching experiences and, perhaps more importantly, their views on education (Vaidya and Urias 2008). Thus, given the impact a teaching and/or educational philosophy can have on a job search and subsequent teaching, beginning with syllabus creation, you are strongly urged to write one; one that you regularly revisit and revise as appropriate.

But why, you may be asking, would you want to incorporate such a thing into a syllabus? And how does this help the syllabus function as a learning tool? To begin with, the fact that you likely had to think about your philosophy and then, potentially, write it down, means that it has already served as a learning tool for you – whether you are a novice or seasoned instructor. Beyond writing it, which requires reflection and an examination of your teaching approaches, from delivery methods to assessment techniques, it then asks you to consider whether your current activities (lectures, formative and summative assessments, lab work, and the like) align with your educational philosophy. If they do align, then you have learned something important. If they do not, or they partially do not, you have also learned something, and it should motivate you to ensure your courses are updated to reflect your newfound understanding.

From the students' perspective, at least for those who choose to read it, understanding your approach to education can be eye opening. It helps them prepare for classes because they will better understand your expectations. If you are positivist in your approach then students will be better able to determine if they do or do not need to be present for in-person sessions; they will understand how much reading they need to do ahead of time, and, in conjunction with their experiences in your class, will be better able to allocate their in-person and study time outside the classroom.

Section 3: Creating an Effective Syllabus

The next section will cover different approaches to creating effective syllabi. Spoiler alert: there are several ways to do this, so these are just suggestions. Take what applies to you and use it. But above all, be open to the idea that a syllabus can be an effective learning and teaching tool on a number of levels; once you accept this (rather than feeling frustrated with and/or resigned to), writing and creating your syllabus may become a little less tedious moving forward.

Part 1: Diversity, Equity, and Inclusion (DEI) in the Classroom

Diversity, equity, and inclusion (DEI) is not a new issue, but it has certainly moved to the forefront in the U.S. recently due to the many social, political, and generational changes that have occurred. Healthcare professions, in general, have been traditionally White and male dominated, though that has already changed in veterinary medicine, where according to the American Veterinary Medical Association (AVMA), women made up the majority of the profession for the first time in 2009 and continue to make up the majority of those accepted to veterinary medical programs, with some recent classes being 100% female. While gender equity has tipped in the favor of females within veterinary medicine and is rapidly reaching parity within human medical programs as well (nursing program notwithstanding, as those have, and continue to be, primarily female), it is still predominated by White females of middle to upper socioeconomic status (SeS). Thus, DEI in all its forms still remains a challenge within the profession – meaning that people of color, those with other sexual and gender orientations, varying religious backgrounds, physical and learning disabilities, and others are still underrepresented in veterinary medicine.

There are numerous programs beginning to recognize the value of and need for DEI training during the formal educational process. The Accreditation Council for Graduate Medical Education (ACGME), for example, has "enacted several Common Program Requirements addressing issues of diversity, equity, and inclusion" (ACGME, n.d.). These requirements cover recruitment, safe training environments, and board certification rates beyond first-time passes. For undergraduate medical education, the Liaison Committee on Medical Education (LCME), the accrediting body for medical schools, states in its 12 standards that student diversity and antidiscrimination policies and procedures are required for accreditation (standards 3.3 and 3.4), although it falls short of extending that reach into faculty resources (Liaison Committee on Medical Education [LCME] 2021). The American Psychological Association (APA) has issued accreditation guidelines for both undergraduate (2013) and graduate programs that explicitly require "diversity and. . .the development of cultural competence" (Fuentes et al. 2020, p. 69). In fact, the diversity commitment is addressed in several standards for graduate education, including standards 1 through 4, covering the learning and support environment (standard 1); individual and cultural diversity (standard 2); long-term plans for recruitment and retention of diverse faculty and students, and assessment of those efforts (standards 3 and 4).

In veterinary medicine, there is a movement to incorporate DEI into the accreditation standards. AVMA, the accrediting body for veterinary schools within the U.S. and, in many cases, globally, formed a DEI working group to "address the incorporation of diversity and inclusion language into the Standards of Accreditation" (AVMA.org, accessed 17 Feburary 2022). Although changes were adopted in March 2017 after a period of public comment, the issue has reemerged and was opened for public comment once again in late 2020 through early 2021. This occurred in response to concerns about the nonspecific nature of the new DEI guidelines, which were incorporated into several existing standards rather than inserted as a standalone standard (AVMA.org 2022). At the time of this writing, the process was ongoing.

It is clear then, that DEI is no longer a fad or passing thought; it has permeated the very structures that determine, at least in the United States, the legitimacy of the learning experience. Thus it is imperative that we all expand our ideas of how to infuse this into our teaching, wherever that may take place. And, while comprehensive DEI efforts require full-scale attention and resources, there are myriad steps we can take as individual veterinarians, whether in the classroom, laboratory, clinic, or on the job. Ensuring that students, staff, clients, and the public view us as welcoming and inclusive is not challenging but does require commitment; commitment that starts with understanding and a willingness to recognize that the White female/male society we have grown up in is changing rapidly. A full discussion of DEI efforts within the veterinary profession is not addressed here, but we can discuss one important way that classrooms and teaching labs can promote DEI efforts: through the syllabus.

Part 2: What Makes a Syllabus Inclusive

Inclusive syllabi ideally use universal design for learning (UDL) principles, which is an entire approach to creating classrooms – from syllabi to teaching techniques – with inclusivity in mind. The inclusivity in this instance is that of those with disabilities, however, which is important to keep in mind, as those with disabilities (physical, mental, and/or emotional) are not always the first underserved group to be considered when the concept of DEI is brought up.

UDL originated from CAST, which was first created as the Center for Applied Special Technology but is now known solely by the acronym. Founded in 1984, its purpose is to ensure everyone has appropriate access to learning, and following their beginnings, in 1988 they formally identified a need to fix exclusive curricula rather than focusing on individual student needs. Thus, the idea of UDL was born and was initially defined as "the design of products and built environments that are usable by all people, to the greatest extent possible, without the need for adaptation of specialized design" (Mace 1988). What is good for those with disabilities is also good for everyone else; we see this in everyday technologies that have made all our lives easier, from cutouts in sidewalks to elevators in multistory buildings; yet we have not been able to universally incorporate similar innovations into our everyday curricula. This is where UDL comes in.

There are five principles for designing an inclusive syllabus, according to Helmer (2018). An inclusive syllabus should:

1) be learner centered, focusing on *what* and *how* students will learn;
2) contain inclusive course policies, explaining *what will help* students' learning;
3) have supportive and inclusive rhetoric;
4) incorporate effective visuals and images that are redundant across modes;
5) apply UDL standards to ensure full readability and accessibility.

The full checklist can be accessed through the link in the "additional resources" section of this chapter. That section also includes a link to a podcast interview with Dr. Kirsten Helmer, the creator of this checklist, as well as the UDL on-campus website, where you can go to get some more information and help with creating a syllabus following UDL principles.

For those not sitting at a computer as you read, below are some excerpts from a syllabus that incorporates several of the inclusive syllabus principles. As you are reading through the example, however, what elements are missing based on the UDL information contained in the section just previous to this one?

Course and Program-Specific Information

Course Description

This course provides the building blocks of understanding for applications of educational philosophy and theories to the veterinary school classroom. It examines various learning theorists and their theories of learning, the history of learning and learning theories, the current research in education, and evidence-based practices of classroom and clinical instruction.

Course Goals and Objectives:

Goals: To provide students a solid foundation in educational theory that encourages them to reflect upon their own learning experiences, how they may wish to approach their teaching, and why it is important to understand and apply educational theory in the professional school classroom.

Course Objectives: At the conclusion of this course, students should be able to:

- Describe a variety of learning philosophies and theories, particularly those that resonate with your preferred approach to learning and teaching
- Effectively deliver appropriate lessons about selected educational philosophies and theories
- Demonstrate understanding of personal teaching philosophy using knowledge obtained in the course.

Later in the same syllabus, you will see that *how* the learning of this content will be assessed is addressed through a listing of the assessments (assignments, exams, and quizzes) the students will be required to complete:

For this course, the following assignments and their values include:

Personal introduction	5
Student-led sessions	40
Critical review of book:	10
Educational philosophy:	15
Journals:	10
Open assessments (student assigned): total of 20 points	

Take notice that the information above is then expanded to include a more detailed description of each assessment, as in the example below:

Student-Led Sessions

During this course you will be provided the opportunity to select several theorists and philosophers whose work resonates with you; from there you will create your own content and lessons to be delivered to your classmates – you will become the expert and teacher! You will have two sessions to deliver information and receive feedback from your mentor without a score being attached; your final session will earn your final grade for this assignment. This assignment will evolve throughout the course, as we all get to know each other and work to ensure you gain the content and the skills you desire before moving into your second semester of study. It will be a collaborative effort, however, so no surprises.

In reading the course and learning objectives, and the description of the assignment, consider the language used within each narrative. Is it stiff and autocratic, neutral, or warm and inviting? According to Harnish and Bridges (2011), a warmer-toned syllabus invites students into the classroom, encourages participation, provides students a glimpse of your teaching style and personality, and may improve students' perceptions of your teaching before the course begins (Galardi 2021). In other words, your syllabus is the first impression students have of you and it has the potential to influence how they feel about you and the course before they even meet you.

Now that you understand the power of the language you select for your syllabus, it is important to consider the resources you have selected and must make available to students. Incorporating an "information literacy and technological resources" section within the syllabus helps students understand what learning resources are needed and what resources are available to them. This is part of ensuring students know what will help them learn. Other aspects of this piece of the syllabus include a statement describing where, when, and how office hours will be held; how much time outside the classroom students should anticipate needing to commit to the course; any resources available for students wanting or needing extra help; required and recommend materials, supplies, and/or textbooks; and the like.

Content is another important aspect of the syllabus; it tells the students what they will be learning and how it fits into their overall program of study. It can also shape the students' ideas and perspectives on the topics delivered, so it is important to include information about and from diverse scholars within the field. Working to expand students' understanding of the types of people who work within the field demonstrates and encourages inclusivity; it also provides role models for students from underserved populations. The course from which the syllabus excerpts are taken includes the study of female, male, Black, Latinx, and White scholars within the field. In veterinary medicine, it might be worthwhile to include discoveries made by or influential professionals who are disabled, known to be neurodiverse, are members of the LGBTQIA community, and/or are racial and ethnically diverse, for example.

For added readability and accessibility, include photographs of the required materials along with their title and a brief description, or at least include links to photos of the materials if they are available so that students can click a hyperlink to view the information visually (Yarosh 2021). If there are opportunities to use materials that provide audio recordings and/or accompaniments, incorporate those as well. Consider using a 12- or 14-point font and 1.5 spacing throughout to make the syllabus easier to read and, if possible, use a standardized template for all courses with information provided in the same sequence. Just as we like all our chain stores to be laid out generally the same way so that we can more easily navigate it regardless of which location we shop, if syllabi are set up the same way it reduces the need for students to search through each syllabus to find the information they need to be successful.

Assessments, which include assignments, exams, and quizzes, are another important part of a good and inclusive syllabus. In the example provided, there are a variety of assignments, each with a different purpose but all related to the course goals and objectives. There are no exams for this particular course; it is a graduate-level education course and the instructors felt objective assessments were counter to the learning process and intent of the course. However, for those needing to incorporate exams and/or quizzes, it is appropriate to spell out how such exams will be delivered and at what point during the course they are planned.

Providing a schedule of topics that includes when assignments are due and when exams and quizzes – unless they are pop quizzes – will occur helps students plan accordingly. While a syllabus schedule is not set in concrete, if changes need to be made those should be provided to students in writing and with enough time before the change occurs for them to be able to adjust accordingly. Changing the date of an exam, for instance, should be done rarely and only with at least several weeks' notice to allow students the opportunity to rearrange study schedules as needed.

While UDL provides a great outline for ensuring our students with disabilities are included and supported, there are other ways we can and should show support for students from other underrepresented backgrounds. Chico State University provides some great examples of inclusive statements that could be included in a syllabus, as well as a variety of syllabi that could be adapted for use in your classroom or lab – you can find their website in the additional resources section of this chapter.

In summary, creating a good syllabus can be a challenge the first time around, but once a good one is produced it can be reproduced relatively easily because the template has already been formed. A good syllabus should, by definition, also be an inclusive one. By following the five principles of an inclusive syllabus and providing students a strong roadmap for what, how, when, and why they will learn the content addressed, as well as how their learning will be assessed, your syllabus can help create a positive learning experience for your students before you ever meet them in the classroom, lab, or clinic.

Section 4: The Syllabus as a Tool to Document Scholarship in Teaching and Learning

Before we leave the topic of the syllabus, it is important to discuss the value of a good syllabus for the creator, beyond the benefits already discussed in the previous section.

The syllabus is often viewed as a document intended for students: to be used as a contract, a learning tool, and a permanent record of the content they have learned. While the first and last are also inherently important for the instructor, the second is often viewed solely for the student. Albers (2003), argues that this should not be the case. Before exploring her argument, however, it is important to summarize the beginnings of how scholarship in teaching and learning within the academy came about.

Ernest Boyer is widely regarded as the person who introduced academia to the idea of the *second profession* of teaching, arguing in 1990 that the term *scholarship* should be expanded to "include four distinct, yet overlapping, functions: discovery, application, integration, and teaching" (Fogelberg 2014, p. 28). A decade later, Lee S. Shulman addressed the American Association for Higher Education (AAHE) conference focusing on the idea of the *scholarship of teaching and learning*, or SoTL, as it has come to be widely known as and referred to (Fogelberg 2014). Shulman, in fact, has spent most of his career doing his best to combat George Bernard Shaw's now infamous 1905 line from the stage play *Man and Superman* that "Those who can do, do; those who can't, teach." And while his efforts are laudable and appear to be taking some hold in the academy, the progress has been slow at best.

However, there is some change occurring. In support of her premise, Albers (2003), documents an analysis of Sociology faculty positions available in 2001 and points out that of the 199 open jobs, 14 specifically required course syllabi as part of the application process and asked for teaching portfolios, which are assumed to include syllabi. Another 14 postings required "evidence of teaching ability" and 20 others requested specific "evidence of teaching effectiveness" (Albers 2003, p. 62). A few years later, Vadiya and Urias (2008), noted that there appeared to be a trend in academia toward asking candidates for faculty teaching positions about their prior experiences with and views of education. These papers focused primarily on undergraduate positions, but the same might be noted of professional programs currently, as human and veterinary medical programs are increasingly working to improve the quality of teaching as they come into alignment with the literature that clearly recognizes the effects of quality teaching are significant when it comes to student learning (Ferguson 1999; Hightower et al. 2011; Liston et al. 2008; McCaffrey et al. 2003; Rhoton and Stiles 2002; Rivkin et al. 2000; Rowan et al. 2002; Wright et al. 1997). Human medicine has explicitly recognized the value of high-quality teaching through creation of numerous teaching academies, and at the time of this writing veterinary medicine has successfully started an organization, the Academy of Veterinary Educators (AVE), whose mission includes creation of a rigorous and formal credentialing process to recognize expert veterinary educators within academia and across the profession broadly. It is evident, then, that the idea of teaching being something "anyone can do if they have the content knowledge" is increasingly falling by the wayside.

How one goes about demonstrating their teaching skill is still not fully agreed upon and is a topic for another time, but one aspect of teaching is the syllabus. And while the uses and purposes of the syllabus are still somewhat up for debate, this can be viewed as a good thing – for it allows new ideas to come about and potentially make a positive impact. This is where Albers' (2003) view that the syllabus can be used as a way to document an instructor's scholarship in teaching and learning is pertinent; in her article, she summarizes the purposes of a syllabus as defined by Parkes and Harris (2002) and discussed in previous sections on this chapter. However, Albers (2003), goes on to make the case that the syllabus may also be used as a tool to evaluate teaching effectiveness and has the potential to be used as a way to document scholarship in teaching and learning.

At the heart of Albers' argument that syllabi should be viewed as vehicles for documenting an instructor's scholarly contributions, and in support of this she cites the views and work of Boyer and Shulman. She summarizes three criteria set forth by Boyer in 1990 in his elaboration on the scholarship of teaching. (i) The scholarship of teaching starts with the teacher's knowledge and as such, teachers must be well-read and intellectually connected to their content. (ii) Teaching requires instructors to be able to bridge the gap between their own understanding and the student's learning. (iii) The teaching process includes delivering, transforming, and *extending* knowledge – the last is emphasized to highlight a characteristic consistent with research efforts according to Albers; this author also argues that transforming knowledge is another characteristic of research.

Shulman's contributions to the idea that using syllabi is a way to demonstrate scholarship come in the form of his schemas for understanding and communicating scholarship in teaching. The first is that teaching should be approached as a scholarly argument, which makes the assumption that "effective teaching requires the ability to pose problems, test hypotheses, measure outcomes, explain unexpected discoveries and create knowledge – in short, the same skills that apply to. . .research" (Albers 2003, p. 67). Her assertions are supported by the AAHE's efforts that provided guidelines for evaluating scholarship contained within a syllabus and suggested a variety of scholarly questions to be answered during the evaluation process. For example,

if you think of your course as a scholarly argument, how does it begin and why does it begin there? What are the thesis and key points of your argument? What evidence are you presenting to support your argument? How does your course end, and what do you want to persuade students to know and/or do? (Albers 2003). There are many more questions included in this guide, but this at least provides a solid grounding to help elucidate the types of questions that can be applied to both evaluating the syllabus as evidence of scholarship in teaching and be used to help prepare a syllabus that demonstrates scholarship in teaching.

The second schema of Shulman is that there should be reflection on the curricular content and pedagogical knowledge used in teaching; this "helps to identify key elements in the teaching and learning process" (Albers 2003, p. 68). Curricular content is the basis of the course goals. Therefore, the syllabus should be used to emphasize the importance of the content, how the content or course fits into the educational goals of the university, and to demonstrate the instructor's conviction that the information being delivered is important. Having pedagogical content knowledge – that is, knowledge of how you take what you know about teaching and relate that to what about the content you are teaching – is an imperative in helping your students figure out how to take in new, often challenging, and sometimes abstract, information and absorb it in a way that moves it from short- to long-term memory. If you are well-versed in different teaching techniques and approaches, you can demonstrate this in your syllabus through incorporation of a variety of learning activities that encourage students to be engaged and active learners. Your approaches to teaching can (ideally) help or (suboptimally) hinder students' growth as thinkers and will certainly impact their tendencies with respect to pursuit of lifelong learning versus viewing education as a means to an end. To be fully effective as an educator, then, you must have both content expertise and pedagogical expertise – and be able to connect them to each other. One way you can demonstrate these two types of expertise is through an explicit and well-crafted syllabus.

It should be noted that the syllabus is not the only way to demonstrate scholarship in teaching and learning, nor should it be viewed as such. However, it is an often overlooked piece when educators are looking to support their scholarship in teaching, which is a separate entity from the content-related research we so often reach for and refer to when demonstrating scholarship in higher education. Albers (2003) also cautions that viewing the syllabus as a tool for demonstrating scholarship may result in a more teacher-centered and static presentation of the course and the professor. This can be avoided by using many of the suggestions provided in the "Creating and Effective Syllabus" section in this chapter; it may not be possible to use them all, but selecting those that work for you and your particular area of content expertise is a great start to ensuring your syllabus is welcoming, clear, and supportive of your students' learning while demonstrating your commitment to scholarship in teaching and learning.

Summary

The syllabus has a somewhat fuzzy history but appears to be here to stay. It is an important tool in the classroom because it provides a roadmap of the course that allows the students and the instructor to be on the same page throughout a class. It serves many purposes, including acting as a contract between the students and the instructor; providing a permanent record of the course and its content; and being a learning tool for the students at a minimum. There are some who argue that the syllabus should also be used to demonstrate an instructor's scholarship in teaching; understanding how this can be done may be helpful to both the educator and the students. When viewed as a scholarly effort, teaching can become more engaging for all stakeholders involved and support career progression for educators.

Creating an effective syllabus requires time and attention to the language used, the types of activities planned, and the use of appropriate UDL principles. Syllabi should be inclusive, accessible, clear, and complete. There are a few approaches to creating syllabi, including fully instructor created, fully cocreated by instructor and students, and created by instructor with student input. The way a syllabus is created is up to the instructor and may be influenced by the type of course being delivered, the content of the course, the pedagogical content knowledge of the instructor, the level of the student, the number of students in the course, and the comfort level of the instructor in delivering the course content, among other things.

Overall, while many instructors view syllabi as work that students generally ignore, they are quite important to the smooth delivery and execution of a course. Despite their somewhat obscure beginnings, they have become a centerpiece of higher education and should be viewed as tools in the classroom that guide and support the students, the instructors, and the institutions within which they are created.

References

Accreditation Council for Graduate Medical Education (n.d.). Diversity, equity, and inclusion: overview. https://www.acgme.org/initiatives/diversity-equity-and-inclusion/ (accessed 18 Octoboer 2022).

Albers, C. (2003). Using the syllabus to document the scholarship of teaching. *Teaching Sociology* 31 (1): 60–72.

Bowers-Campbell, J. (2015). Investigating the syllabus as a defining document. *Journal of College Reading and Learning* 45: 106–122. https://doi.org/10.1080/10790195.2015.1030240.

Cooper, P. and Cuseo, G. (1989). The course syllabus. *Teaching Newsletter* 2 (4): 1–4.

Das, J. (2013). Role of syllabus in higher education: a critical study. *Global Research Methodology Journal* 0I–II (7): 1–6.

Eberly, M.B., Newton, S.E., and Wiggins, R.A. (2001). The syllabus as a tool for student-centered learning. *The Journal of General Education* 50 (1): 56–74. https://doi.org/10.1353/jge.2001.0003.

Ferguson, R.F. (1999). Paying for public education: new evidence on how and why money matters. *Harvard Journal on Legislation* 28 (2): 465–498.

Fogelberg, K. (2014). Attitudes and beliefs of university science professors toward the discipline of education. Dissertation.

Fuentes, M.A., Zelaya, D.G., and Madsen, J.W. (2020). Rethinking the course syllabus: Consideration for promoting equity, diversity, and inclusion. *Teaching of Psychology* https://doi.org/10.1177/0098628320959979.

Galardi, N.R. (2021). Syllabus tone, more than mental health statements, influence intentions to seek help. *Teaching of Psychology* 49 (3): 218–223. https://doi.org/10.1177/0098628321994632.

Habanek, D.V. (2005). An examination of the integrity of the syllabus. *College Teaching* 53 (2): 62–64.

Harnish, R.J. and Bridges, K.R. (2011). Effect of syllabus tone: students' perceptions of instructor and course. *Social Psychology of Education: An international Journal* 14 (3): 319–330. https://doi.org/10.1007/s11218-011-9152-4.

Helmer, K. (2018). Six principles of an inclusive syllabus. https://www.mtholyoke.edu/sites/default/fles/TLI-TEFD-Checklist-Inclusive-Syllabus-20180613.pd (accessed 22 November 2023).

Hightower, A.M., Delgado, R.C., Lloyd, S.C. et al. (2011). Improving student learning by supporting quality teaching: key issues, effective strategies. Bethesda, MD: Editorial Projects in Education, Inc. https://www.edweek.org/research-center/research-center-reports/improving-student-learning-by-supporting-quality-teaching-key-issues-effective-strategies (accessed 6 June 2022).

Hudd, S.S. (2003). Syllabus under construction: Involving students in the creation of class assignments. *Teaching Sociology* 31 (20): 195–2002.

Liaison Committee on Medical Education (LCME) (2021). *Functions and Structure of a Medical School: Standards for Accreditation of Medical Education Programs Leading to the MD Degree*. Association of American Medical Colleges https://lcme.org/publications/ (accessed 9 November 2022).

Liston, D., Borko, H., and Whitcomb, J. (2008). The teacher educator's role in enhancing teacher quality. *Journal of Teacher Education* 59 (2): 111–116. https://doi.org/10.1177/0022487108315581.

Lowther, M.A., Stark, J.S., and Martens, G.G. (1989). *Preparing Course Syllabi for Improved Communication*. Ann Arbor: University of Michigan, National Center for Research to Improve Post-secondary Teaching and Learning.

Ludy, M.-J., Brackenbury, T., Folkins, J.W. et al. (2016). Student impressions of syllabus design: Engaging versus contractual syllabus. *International Journal for the Scholarship of Teaching and Learning* 10 (2): 1–23. https://doi.org/10.20429/ijsotl.2016.100206.

Mace, R. (1988). *Universal Design: Housing for the Lifespan of All People. The Center for Universal Design, North Carolina State University* https://disabilityandmultimodality.wordpress.ncsu.edu/universal-design-ud/#:~:text=What%20is%20Universal%20Design%3F,for%20adaptation%20or%20specialized%20design%E2%80%9D (accessed 22 November 2022).

Matejka, K. and Kurke, L.B. (1994). Desiging a great syllabus. *College Teaching* 42 (3): 115–117.

McCaffrey, J. R., Lockwood, D. F., Koretz, D. M., and Hamilton, L. S. (2003). Evaluating value added models for teacher accountability [Monograph]. Santa Monica, CA: RAND Corporation. http://www.rand.org/pubs/monographs/2004/RAND_MG158.pdf (accessed 10 June 2022).

McDevitt, B. (2004). Negotiating the syllabus: a win-win situation? *ELT Journal* 58 (1): 3–9. https://doi.org/10.1093/elt/58.1.3.

Parkes, J. and Harris, M.B. (2002). The purposes of a syllabus. *College Teaching* 50 (2): 55–60.

Rhoton, J. and Stiles, K.E. (2002). Exploring the professional development design process: bringing an abstract framework into practice. *Science Educator* 11 (1): 1–8.

Rivkin, S.G., Hanushek, E.A., and Kain, J.F. (2000). *Teachers, Schools, and Academic Achievement (Working Paper W6691)*. Cambridge, MA: National Bureau of Economic Research.

Rowan, B., Correnti, R., and Miller, R.J. (2002). What large-scale survey research tells us about teacher effects on student achievement: insights from the Prospects study of elementary schools. *Teachers College Record* 104: 1525–1567.

Thompson, B. (2007). The syllabus as a communication document: constructing and presenting the syllabus. *Communication Education* 56 (1): 54–71. https://doi.org/10.1080/03634520601011575.

Vadiya, S. and Urias, D. (2008). Foundation of college teaching – a course for doctoral students: reflections on a case study in college teaching. *International Journal for the Scholarship of Teaching and Learning* 2 (1): 23. https://doi.org/10.20429/ijsotl.2008.020123.

Vaidya, S. and Urias, D. (2008). Foundations of college teaching – a course for doctoral students: reflections on a case study in college teaching. *International Journal for the Scholarship of Teaching and Learning* 2 (1): 1–8.

Wright, S.P., Horn, S.P., and Sanders, W.L. (1997). Teachers and classroom context effects on student achievement: implications for teacher evaluation. *Journal of Personnel Evaluation in Education* 11: 57–67.

Yarosh, J.H. (2021). The syllabus reconstructed: an analysis of traditional and visual syllabi for information retention and inclusiveness. *Teaching Sociology*, 49(2):173–183. https://doi.org/10.1177/0092055X21996784.

Additional Resources

University of Virginia's Center for Teaching Excellence. https://cte.virginia.edu/course-design-institute/sample-syllabi.

University of South Carolina's Center for Teaching Excellence site. https://sc.edu/about/offices_and_divisions/cte/teaching_resources/syllabus_templates/.

Link to full checklist for designing a fully UDL syllabus. https://www.google.com/url?sa=t&rct=j&q=&esrc=s&source=web&cd=&ved=2ahUKEwjay-LFhvP0AhV5l2oFHbk1AD4QFnoECB4QAQ&url=https%3A%2F%2Fwww.mtholyoke.edu%2Fsites%2Fdefault%2Ffiles%2FTLI-TEFD-Checklist-Inclusive-Syllabus-20180613.pdf&usg=AOvVaw0DlEnuylV-X2Nqs1Nhg2ik.

Podcast with Dr. Kiersten Helmer. https://thinkudl.org/episodes/inclusive-syllabus-design-with-kirsten-helmer.

UDL on campus website. http://udloncampus.cast.org/page/planning_syllabus.

Chico State University website for example inclusive syllabus statements. https://www.csuchico.edu/diversity/resources/teaching/syllabi-examples.shtml.

9

Assignments and Rubrics

Jo R. Smith, MA, VetMB, PhD, Post Graduate Diploma in Veterinary Education (PGDipVetEd), DACVIM – SA
University of Georgia College of Veterinary Medicine, Athens, GA, USA

Section 1: Assignments

Part 1: Introduction

Backwards course design starts with the educator defining the student's learning outcomes – what knowledge, skills, and attitudes students will be able to demonstrate at the conclusion of their learning experience (Wiggins and McTighe 2005). Constructive alignment is used to develop appropriate assessments to evaluate the student's performance. Analogous to problem-oriented medicine, the diagnostic tests one selects to progress a patient's case should reflect the specific patient's problem list. Finally, the learning activities and content are created (Biggs 1996). Assessments of learning typically encompass assignments, quizzes, and exams.

Formative assessments are **for** student learning and occur during the course. Ideally, formative assessment should reinforce the skills, knowledge, and attitudes required for the summative assessment, and specific feedback should be provided on the different aspects evaluated in the assignment. Provision of feedback may be time-consuming; however, feedback on formative assessments is often more effective than feedback provided for summative assessments since the student may not have another opportunity to implement the recommendations. Ways to decrease the time spent on providing individual feedback on formative assignments include:

- Providing examples or key answers, either before or after the submission deadline
- Auditing a portion of the assignments rather than reading all of them and providing "group" feedback on frequently encountered issues. In subsequent years, this feedback can be shared with the learners in advance before the formative assignments are submitted, with the aim of enhancing the quality of formative assignments
- Using group assignments to decrease the overall number of assignments
- Providing a rubric and asking for a self-evaluation
- Providing a rubric and implementing peer evaluations

Summative assessments are **of** the learner's competency and typically occur at the midpoint and/or near the conclusion of a course. These often determine the learner's progression within the professional degree – advancement, formal remediation, or dismissal.

Self-regulated learning uses assessment **as** learning. Students can reflect on their learning, self-evaluate their own performance, their strengths and weaknesses, and set personal goals. This gives the students an opportunity to practice metacognition and self-management.

The results of student assessments can also provide educators with feedback on the effectiveness of instructional design. Kirkpatrick's evaluation of training framework proposes different levels of evidence from various educational assessments (Kirkpatrick and Kirkpatrick 2016; Table 9.1).

Miller's prism of clinical competence, or "Miller's pyramid," partially reflects Fitzpatrick's framework as learners progress through *knowing, knowing how, showing how*, and *doing* in the realms of knowledge, skills, and attitudes, or cognitive, psychomotor, and affective domains. It has been suggested that Miller's pyramid be amended to include a fifth level *is*, to reflect professional identity formation and move beyond demonstration of professional behaviors (Cruess et al. 2016; Irby and Hamstra 2016). Different assessment methods have been proposed for each level of clinical competency (Figure 9.1).

Educational Principles and Practice in Veterinary Medicine, First Edition. Edited by Katherine Fogelberg.
© 2024 John Wiley & Sons, Inc. Published 2024 by John Wiley & Sons, Inc.

Table 9.1 Kirkpatrick's training evaluation framework.

Level	Focus	Description
1	Reaction	Assesses the learners' engagement, satisfaction, and their evaluation of relevance, e.g., student teaching evaluations
2	Learning	Assesses the learner's knowledge, skills, attitude, confidence, and commitment
3	Behavior	Performance and workplace assessments evaluate how well the learner applies what they have learned in an authentic environment
4	Results	Outcome assessments evaluate which targeted outcomes occur because of the training. In the preclinical setting, these are often required for accreditation purposes; in the clinical setting, these may include improved patient outcomes

Source: Adapted from Kirkpatrick and Kirkpatrick (2016).

Questions to Consider When Choosing a Learning Assessment Technique or Assignment

- What is your purpose for assessing student learning? Is it a formative, summative, or outcome assessment? This may influence the data output required.
- What learning outcomes are you reinforcing/evaluating?
- How can the assignment best reflect an appropriate degree of realism or authenticity?
- What kind of product do you want the learners to produce? The product should be aligned with, and relevant to, the learning outcome(s) and allow students to demonstrate their learning.
- How complex is the assignment going to be? Will this be mandatory? Will this be graded? What component of the final grade will this assignment constitute?

- What is the instructional context in which you teach – large or small group, onsite, "flipped," online?
- Does the assignment design comply with the Universal Design for Learning Guidelines (CAST 2018)?

Part 2: Learning Outcomes, Activities, and Assignments

As previously stated, development of constructively aligned assessment depends on the learning outcome(s) being evaluated. Well-written learning outcomes are specific, relevant, and measurable (Schoenfeld-Tacher and Sims 2013). Different frameworks have been used to create learning outcomes and can thus form the basis for selecting an apt assignment. Bloom and colleagues created three taxonomies (cognitive, affective, and psychomotor) to reflect the domains of what students should know, feel, and do. However, Bloom's taxonomy is typically used to refer to six levels of knowledge arranged in a hierarchical sequence – *knowledge, comprehension, application, analysis, synthesis, and evaluation* (Bloom and Krathwohl 1956). Lower-order thinking skills are considered foundational for the higher-order thinking skills, although this is not absolute. Learning outcomes that require *analysis* or *evaluation* may be no less complex than those that require *creation*. Airasian et al. (2001) redefined Bloom's cognitive domain as the intersection of the knowledge dimension and a slightly revised order of the cognitive process dimension (Table 9.2).

Specific learning outcomes for what students should know can be created by combining aspects of these two dimensions (Table 9.3).

To convert learning outcomes into learning activities, each learning outcome can be preceded with "Students

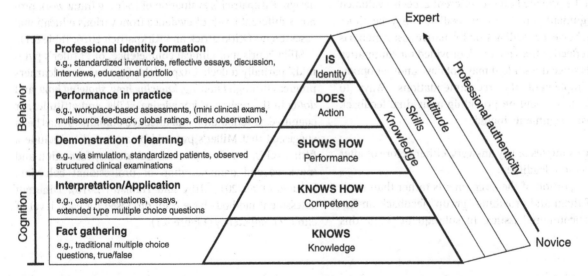

Figure 9.1 Miller's prism of clinical competence. *Source:* Adapted from Mehay and Burns (2012) and Cruess et al. (2016).

Table 9.2 The knowledge dimension of Bloom's taxonomy: the four types of knowledge that the learner is expected to acquire or construct.

Concrete knowledge			Abstract knowledge
Factual	**Conceptual**	**Procedural**	**Metacognitive**
The basic elements to be acquainted with a discipline or solve problems within it • Terminology • Specific details and elements	The interrelationships between basic elements within a larger structure that enable them to function together • Classifications and categories • Principles and generalizations • Theories, models, and structures	How to do something, methods of inquiry, and criteria for using skills, algorithms, techniques, and methods • Subjective-specific skills and algorithms • Techniques and methods • Criteria for determining when to use appropriate procedures	Knowledge of cognition in general as well as awareness of one's own cognition • Strategic knowledge • Knowledge about cognitive tasks including appropriate contextual and conditional knowledge • Self-knowledge

Source: Adapted from Airasian et al. (2001).

will be able to . . ." Learning activities ideally involve lower and higher-order thinking skills and a mix of concrete and abstract knowledge. Well-designed assessments are constructively aligned to evaluate these learning outcomes appropriately.

Tables 9.4 and 9.5 list verbs for learning objectives, learning activities, and suggested assignments organized for the different levels of the cognitive and affective domains of Bloom's taxonomy. Table 9.6 lists the different levels of the psychomotor domain of Bloom's taxonomy, synonyms because the terminology may be obscure, and verbs for learning objectives. Broad learning activities and assessments for technical and nontechnical competencies are suggested – see Chapters 10, 11, and 12 for more detail. Lists of specific day-one competencies or clinical skills that could comprise specific assignments can be found elsewhere (Royal Veterinary College 2007; Coombes and Silva-Fletcher 2018; Read et al. 2021).

Fink (2003) developed an alternate taxonomy of "significant learning" to capture aspects he felt were inadequately described in Bloom's taxonomy. Many of these missing components encompassed "professional skills" and humanism, and this framework provides an alternate basis for the selection of appropriate assignments (Table 9.7).

Similar competencies are also described in the American Association of Veterinary Colleges (AAVMC) Competency-Based Veterinary Education Framework (AAVMC Working Group on Competency-Based Veterinary Education et al. 2018a). See Table 9.8 for a list of suggested assignments for clinical veterinary medicine. These assignments can be integrated to create Entrustable Professional Activities (EPAs; AAVMC Working Group on Competency-Based Veterinary Education et al. 2018b). Rubrics to evaluate veterinary student competency in the EPAs are also available (AAVMC Working Group on Competency-Based Veterinary Education et al. 2019) (Table 9.8).

Part 3: Conclusion

Well-designed assignments should be aligned with, and relevant to, specific learning outcome(s). They should allow students to demonstrate the knowledge, skills, and/or attitudes they have learned. Assignments can be sequenced or scaffolded to support and evaluate progressively more complex learning outcomes, and integrate aspects from cognitive, affective, and psychomotor learning domains. Assignments that are realistic and mimic the competencies required of veterinary graduates will better engage students and reinforce their learning. The students' performance can also provide feedback to educators on the effectiveness of their teaching and indicate areas that may require improvement.

Section 2: Rubrics

Part 1: Introduction and Definition

A rubric is a scoring guide or grading schema that lists specific components evaluated in an assignment. Rubrics permit criterion-referenced assessment, where the measurement of a learner's knowledge or skills against a predetermined standard is not impacted by the performance of the learner's peers. Thus, they are particularly suited to a competency-based education framework, where learners must achieve certain milestones to progress through a curriculum (Education et al. 2019).

Table 9.3 Examples of stratified learning outcomes for the cognitive domain of Bloom's revised taxonomy.

Knowledge dimension	Cognitive process dimension					
	Remember Retrieve relevant knowledge from long-term memory	**Understand** Construct meaning from instructional messages, including oral, written, and graphic communication	**Apply** Carry out or use a procedure in a situation	**Analyze** Break material into constituent parts and determine how parts relate to one another and to an overall structure or purpose	**Evaluate** Make judgments based on criteria and standards	**Create** Put elements together to form a coherent whole; reorganize into a new pattern or structure
Factual The basic elements students must know to be acquainted with a discipline or solve problems within it	**List** *primary and secondary diseases*	**Summarize** *features of a new product*	**Respond** *to frequently asked questions*	**Select** *the most complete list of activities*	**Check** *for consistency among sources*	**Generate** *a log of daily activities*
Conceptual The interrelationships between basic elements within a larger structure that enable them to function together	**Recognize** *symptoms of a specific disease*	**Classify** *substances by toxicity*	**Provide** *advice to novices*	**Differentiate** between *high and low culture*	**Determine** *relevance of results*	**Assemble** *a team of experts*
Procedural How to do something, methods of inquiry, and criteria for using skills, algorithms, techniques, and methods	**Recall** *how to perform a specific technique*	**Clarify** *assemble instructions*	**Perform** *tests on samples*	**Integrate** *compliance with regulations*	**Judge** *efficiency of sampling techniques*	**Design** *an efficient project workflow*
Metacognitive Knowledge of cognition in general as well as awareness of one's own cognition	**Identify** *strategies for retaining information*	**Predict** *one response to culture shock*	**Use** *techniques that match one's strengths*	**Deconstruct** *one's biases*	**Reflect** *on one's progress*	**Create** *an innovative learning portfolio*

Each cell of the table has a **bolded verb** describing the **cognitive** process, and the *italicized text* describes the *knowledge* that the learner is expected to acquire or construct.
Source: Adapted from Airasian et al. (2001) and Heer (n.d.).

Table 9.4 The cognitive domain from Bloom's taxonomy: the intellectual skills and abilities required for learning, thinking critically, and problem-solving.

Learning outcome verbs			Learning activities	Assignments	

1) Remember – retain, recall, and recognize

Acquire	Identify	Recognize	Flashcards	Question-and-answer	Clicker questions	Match
Arrange	Label	Record	Highlight key word	Reading materials	Fill in the blanks	Multiple-choice
Cite	List	Relate	Lecture	Self-awareness	Label	questions
Collect	Match	Repeat	List	inventory		True false
Define	Memorize	Reproduce	Memory activities	Small group discussion		questions
Distinguish	Name	State	Peer teaching	Watching presentation		
Duplicate	Recall		Presentation	Watching video		
				Web-based learning		

2) Understand – translate and interpret

Abstract	Explain	Recognize	Case study	Group discussion	Concept map	Matrix activity
Appreciate	Express	Report	Concept map	Mind map	Create a summary	Multiple choice
Categorize	Extrapolate	Represent	Demonstration	Matrix activity	Essay	questions
Classify	Identify	Restate	• video	Roleplay	Diagrams	One-minute paper
Convert	Indicate	Select	• live	Summarize	Infographics	Presentation
Describe	Locate	Summarize	Diagrams	Think-pair-share	Flow chart	Provide examples
Discuss	Paraphrase		Flowcharts			Short answers
			Gamification			

3) Apply – knowledge to different situations

Apply	Illustrate	Schedule	Calculate	Guided practice with	Create a study	One-minute paper
Calculate	Implement	Show	Case studies	feedback	guide	Presentation
Choose	Interview	Sketch	Concept map	Group work	Discussion board	Problem-solving
Compute	Operate	Solve	Creating example	Lab experiment	post	tasks
Demonstrate	Organize	Translate	Demonstration	Map	E-portfolio	Short answers
Dramatize	Perform	Use	Direct patient contact	Peer teaching	Extended	Tests
Employ	Practice	Write	Flipped classroom	Problem-solving task	matching	
Execute	Restructure		Gamification	Roleplay	questions	
Exhibit	Relate		Guided practice with	Short answer	Lab reports	
			feedback	Simulation		

4) Analyze – break down information to look at relationships

Analyze	Differentiate	Interpret	Brainstorming	Flowchart	Analysis paper	Muddiest point
Arrange	Discriminate	Inventory	Case studies	Graph	Annotated	One-minute paper
Categorize	Distinguish	Investigate	Compare and contrast	Group investigation	bibliography	Research paper
Classify	Examine	Probe	• chart, table	Mind map	Case studies	Review paper
Compare	Experiment	Question	• Venn diagram	Question-and-answer	Deconstruct a	
Contrast	Group	Scrutinize	Concept map	Questionnaire	medical error	
Criticize	Inquire	Survey	Debates	Report/survey	Evaluation criteria	
Diagram	Inspect	Test	Discussions	Think-pair-share	Critique	
Detect				Troubleshooting	hypothesis	
					Critique	
					procedures	

5) Evaluate – make judgments based on evidence found

Appraise	Defend	Rate	Compare and contrast	Direct patient contact	Persuasive essay	
Argue	Determine	Recommend	• charts, tables	Journal	Debates	
Assess	Estimate	Revise	• Venn diagrams	• audio, video, written	Discussions	
Choose	Evaluate	Score	Concept map	Pros and cons list	Presentation	
Compare	Infer	Solve	Debates	Mind map		
Conclude	Judge	Select		Review paper		
Criticize	Justify	Support				
Decide	Measure	Validate				
Deduce	Predict	Value				

(Continued)

Table 9.4 (Continued)

Learning outcome verbs			Learning activities		Assignments
6) Create – compile information to generate new solutions					
Argue	Develop	Plan	Brainstorming	Direct patient contact	Design a
Arrange	Discuss	Predict	Case study	Performance	• Checklist to promote patient safety
Assemble	Formulate	Prepare	Critical review	Presentations	• Instruction manual
Combine	Generalize	Produce	Decision-making	Reflective writing	• Poster
Compose	Hypothesize	Propose	tasks	Research projects	• Rubric
Construct	Imagine	Question	Develop plans	Written assignments	• Standard operating procedure
Create	Incorporate	Summarize	Describe new		• Survey
Design	Integrate	Synthesize	solutions		• Webpage
Invent	Originate	Write			Develop criteria to evaluate product or solution
					Develop exam questions
					Grant proposal
					Outline alternate solutions
					Research proposal or paper

Source: Adapted from Airasian et al. (2001) and Schoenfeld-Tacher and Sims (2013).

Table 9.5 The affective domain from Bloom's taxonomy: the emotional response concerning one's attitudes, values, and appreciation for motivation in learning.

Learning outcome verbs			Learning activities	Assignments
1) Receiving – being willing to listen and being aware to receive knowledge				
Acknowledge	Describe	Listen	Attend focus groups	Feedback forms
Ask	Follow	Name	Listen as an audience to a presentation	Fill-in-the-blanks
Attend	Give	Reply	Read articles/papers/textbooks	Knowledge survey
Choose	Identify	Select	Watch a video	List
				Match
				Memory tests
				One-minute paper
				Qualitative interviews
				Test activities (recall and verbalize reactions)
				Write summary of key points of the presentation
2) Responding – actively participating and engaging to transfer knowledge				
Agree to	Communicate	Indicate	Active participation in classroom activities	Answer questions
Answer	Contribute	Inquire		Ability to follow procedures
Ask	Cooperate	Participate	Brainstorm ideas	Critical questioning
Assist	Discuss	Question	Group discussions	Feedback and peer evaluation
Clarify	Help		Present in front of audience	One-minute paper
			Problem-solving activities	Questionnaires
			Role-play	Willingness to participate
			Written assignments (essays, reports, etc.)	
3) Valuing – finds value and worth in one's learning and is motivated to continue				
Accept	Debate	Identify	Debates	Attendance
Approve	Demonstrate	Initiate	Opinionated writing piece	Accuracy and appearance of submitted work
Complete	Differentiate	Justify	Reflection paper	Meet deadlines
Choose	Explain	Prepare	Self-report	Proposals for new plans
Commit	Establish	Refute		Questionnaires
Describe				Rating scale or rubric
				Reflection paper
				Report on extra-curricular activities
				Ungraded paper

Table 9.5 (Continued)

Learning outcome verbs			Learning activities	Assignments
4) Organization – integrating and comparing values and ordering them according to priorities				
Adapt	Defend	Integrate	Analyze and contrast	Develop realistic aspirations
Arrange	Explain	Modify	● Charts, tables, Venn diagrams	Discuss ethical dilemmas
Categorize	Establish	Order	Concept map	Prioritize time to achieve goals (meet deadlines)
Classify	Formulate	Prepare	● Formal or informal experiences, identify skills	
Compare	Generate	Rank		Focus groups
Complete	Identify	Relate		Questionnaires
				Solve new problems or case studies
5) Characterization – value that will control the outcome and behavior				
Act	Function	Practice	Critical reflection	Criteria for group projects
Arrange	Incorporate	Preserve	Group projects	Self-evaluation
Behave	Influence	Perform	Self-report goals (personally and academically)	SMART goals
Characterize	Justify	Propose		
Defend	Listen	Question		
Display	Maintain	Revise		
Exemplify	Modify			

Source: Adapted from Krathwohl et al. (1964).

Table 9.6 The psychomotor domain from Bloom's taxonomy: the ability to use motor skills that includes physical movement, reflex, nd coordination to develop techniques in execution, accuracy, and efficiency.

Dimension, synonym, and definition				Learning activities	Assignments
1) Set: Prepared – how ready one is to act physically, mentally, and emotionally				**Technical**	**Formative**
				Laboratories	Performance videoed by student
Arrange	Display	Prepare	Respond	● Sample handling	Self-evaluation using a rubric
Begin	Explain	Proceed	Show	● Skills and techniques	Peer-evaluation using a rubric
Demonstrate	Move	React	State		
2) Guided response: Beginner – learns through trial and error and by practicing				Simulations	**Summative**
				● Low fidelity models	Observed structured clinical examination
Assemble	Copy	React	Trace	● High fidelity models	
Attempt	Follow	Reproduce	Try		
Build	Imitate			Live animal laboratories	
3) Mechanism: Intermediate – develops some confidence and proficiency and action becomes habitual				● Physical examination	
				● Handling and restraint	
Assemble	Display	Measure	Organize	● Procedures	
Construct	Fasten	Mend	Sketch		
Dismantle	Fix	Mix			
4) Complex overt response: Expert – high proficiency and performs with accuracy				**Nontechnical**	
				e.g., Verbal communication in simulated scenarios	
Assemble	Display	Measure	Organize	● Peers	
Build	Fasten	Mix	Perform	● Simulated clients	
Construct	Fix	Operate	Sketch		
Dismantle	Heat				
5) Adaption: Flexible – skills are strongly developed and can be modified to different situations					
Adapt	Change	Rearrange	Revise		
Alter	Modify	Reorganize	Vary		
6) Origination: Creative – creates new procedures and solutions to approach various situations					
Arrange	Construct	Formulate	Modify		
Build	Create	Initiate	Originate		
Combine	Design	Make	Redesign		
Compose					

A synonym and definition are provided for each dimension.
Source: Adapted from Clark (1999) and Simpson (1966).

Table 9.7 Fink's taxonomy of significant learning with examples of learning objective verbs and learning activities for each learning dimension.

Dimension	Learning outcome verbs				Topics	Learning activities
1) Foundational knowledge – what key information, ideas, and perspectives are important for learners to know?						
Understanding and remembering developing a full understanding of the concepts associated with a subject to a degree that allows explanations, predictions, etc.	Associate, Compare, Contrast, Define, Describe	Explain, Give example, Identify, Illustrate, Indicate	Recognize, Repeat, Restate, Tell		Concepts, Conclusions, Facts, Models, Organizations, Perspectives, Plans, Problems, Proposals, Purposes, Relationships, Results, Structures, Theories	Gamification, Identify learning issues, Independent study, Large group discussion, Lecture, Presentation, Question-and-answer, Review session, Small group discussion, Peer teaching, Web-based instruction
2) Application – what kinds of thinking, complex projects, and skills are important for learners to be able to do/manage?						
Critical thinking analyzing and critiquing issues and situations	Analyze, Assess, Audit, Catalog, Categorize, Classify, Compare	Contrast, Decipher, Deduce, Derive, Determine, Diagram, Differentiate	Dissect, Distinguish, Examine, Formulate, Hypothesize, Infer, Interpret	Label, Locate, Measure, Organize, Query, Separate, Trace	Assumptions, Conclusions, Ideas, Issues, Processes, Proposals, Results, Situations, Theories	Action plan, Brainstorming, Case study, Clinical rotations, Club, Critical review, Developing research questions, Direct patient contact, Guided practice with feedback
Practical thinking developing problem-solving and decision-making capabilities	Advise, Answer, Apply, Calculate, Certify, Choose	Consult, Debate, Decide, Determine, Diagnose, Evaluate	Give evidence, Judge, Justify, Predict, Prescribe, Propose	Prove, Rank, Select, Solve, Suggest, Test	Conundrums, Issues, Problems	Hands-on procedure, Journal, Laboratory, Live demonstration, Peer teaching, Problem-solving, Question-and-answer
Creative thinking creating new ideas, products, and perspectives	Abstract, Adapt, Amend, Author, Compose, Construct	Convert, Create, Design, Develop, Devise, Discover	Draw, Envision, Experiment, Fabricate, Imagine, Improve	Refine, Reform, Sketch, Theorize, Transform, Write	Ideas, Models, Objects, Plans, Premises, Perspectives, Products, Theories	Role-play, Simulation, Theory and model building, Project, Troubleshooting, Video demonstration

2) Application – what kinds of thinking, complex projects, and skills are important for learners to be able to do/manage?

Description						Examples
Managing complex projects being able to coordinate and sequence multiple tasks in a single project/case and/or multiple projects/cases	Administer Assign Coach Communicate Complete Conduct	Coordinate Delegate Develop Evaluate Facilitate Follow Up	Guide Implement Manage Organize Plan Prioritize	Strategize Supervise Summarize Teach Timeline Train	Cases Projects Tasks Timelines	*See above*
Performance Skills developing capabilities in carrying out psychomotor activities	Conduct Demonstrate Do	Employ Execute Exhibit	Operate Perform Produce	Conduct Demonstrate Do	Interviews Maneuvers Procedures Processes Routines	*See above*

3) Integration – what connections should learners be able to recognize and make within and beyond this learning experience?

Description						Examples
Interdisciplinary learning connecting ideas, disciplines, perspectives, and contexts **Learning communities** connecting people **Learning and living/Working** connecting different realms of life	Associate Combine Compare	Concept map Connect Contrast	Correlate Differentiate Integrate	Link Relate Synthesize	Contexts Disciplines Domains Ideas People Perspectives Realms	Compare and contrast, Concept mapping Cross-disciplinary cases Cross-disciplinary teams Integrated curriculum Multiple examples within and across contexts Theory and model building What if . . .

4) Human dimension – what should learners learn about themselves and about interacting with others?

Description						Examples
Interpersonal relationships with peers, supervisors, patients, and others **Self-authorship** learning to create and take responsibility for one's own life **Leadership** becoming an effective leader **Ethics, character building** living by ethical principles **Multicultural education** being culturally sensitive in interactions with others **Working as a member of a team** knowing how to contribute to a team **Citizenship** of one's profession, community, nation-state, or other political entity **Environmental ethics** having ethical principles in relation to nonhuman world	Acquire Advise Advocate Balance Be aware of Behave Collaborate Communicate Comply Cooperate Critically reflect Decide to Demonstrate Describe	Educate Embody Empathize Express Feel confident Give feedback Help Influence Initiate Inspire Interact with Involve Lead Mediate	Mobilize Motivate Negotiate Nurture Offer Promote Protect Reconcile Reform Resolve conflict Respect Respond sensitively	See oneself as Serve as role model Settle Share Show Suggest Support Suspend judgment Sustain Take responsibility Unite	Ethics Morality Principles Attitudes Values Beliefs Premises Conflicts and implications • Personal • Social • Cultural • Environmental	Authentic project Case study Debate Direct patient contact, Assigned leadership role Group project Journal club, e.g., using ethics articles Patient presentations, Working in diverse teams Simulated patients

(Continued)

Table 9.7 (Continued)

Dimension	Learning outcome verbs				Topics	Learning activities
5) Caring – what changes in learners' feelings, interests, and values are important?						
Wanting to be a good learner wanting to master and achieve high standards **Becoming excited about a particular activity/subject** developing a keen interest **Developing a commitment to live right** deciding to take care of one's wellbeing and living by a certain code	Agree to Be ready to Commit to Decide to Demonstrate	Develop Discover Explore Express Get excited about	Identify Pledge Recognize value of Renew interest	Revitalize Share State Take time to value	Attitudes Beliefs Feelings Interests Opinions Values	Authentic project Debate Reflective writing Role modeling Self-inventory
6) Learning how to learn – what should learners learn about learning, engaging in inquiry, and becoming self-directed?						
How to be a better learner engaging in self-regulated learning or deep learning **How to inquire and construct knowledge** how to engage in the scientific method, historical method, and other forms of inquiry **How to pursue self-directed or intentional learning** developing a learning agenda and plan, becoming an intentional learner, being a reflective practitioner	Construct knowledge about Describe how to Develop a learning plan Frame useful questions Generalize knowledge Identify sources and resources Identify your learning style and barriers Identify what you need to know Inquire	Predict performance Reflect Research Self-assess Self-regulate Self-monitor Set a learning agenda Take responsibility for Transfer knowledge			Accountability Acquisition of knowledge Acquisition of skills Self-improvement Learning Self-direction	Formative assessment Peer teaching Peer feedback Reflective writing Self-assessment Self-awareness exercise Self-awareness inventory Self-feedback

Source: Adapted from the University of New Mexico School of Medicine (2005) and Fink (2003).

Table 9.8 Suggested assignments for various clinical veterinary medicine competencies.

Communication – verbal

Clients

- History
- Relationship-centered care/Case management discussion
- Financial discussion
- Patient updates
- Discharge instruction

Colleagues

- Case presentation using problem-oriented medicine
- Feedback
- Patient handover
- Teamwork

Communication – written

Clients

- History
- Physical examination, including system-specific, e.g., neurologic, ophthalmic, reproductive
- Discharge instructions for a client
- Communication log with a client or referring veterinarian
- Referral letter to a veterinarian

Colleagues

- Consult form for a specialist
- Patient SOAP, i.e., a case summary with a patient/herd assessment that explains clinical rationale and justifies diagnostic, therapeutic, monitoring, and communication plans
- Patient handover
- Patient treatment sheet
- Prescription
- Reports, discipline-specific
  - Anesthesia
  - Health certificate
  - Necropsy
  - Prepurchase examination
  - Procedural – endoscopy, surgery
  - Radiology
- Requisition forms
  - Histopathology submission form
  - Radiology request, etc.

Communication – written

Other

- Brochure or pamphlet, e.g., client handout
- Case report of an individual patient or herd scenario
- Critically appraised topic to demonstrate evidence-based practice or scientific literacy
- Medical error debriefing and development of a checklist or standard operating procedure to minimize recurrence
- Social media posts, e.g., to promote clinic

Career-focused

- Cover letter
- Resume or curriculum vita
- Digital professional network profile

Rounds

- Case-based
- Biomedical topic
- Humanistic and/or professional skills
  - Difficult communication scenarios
  - Ethical dilemmas
  - Wellbeing

Using the concept of backwards course design, rubrics are part of the assessment strategy and should be based on learning objectives. Ideally, the rubric should be created before designing the assignment, learning activities, and content (Biggs 1996). When planning a road trip, we would expect to locate our destination first and then plan the most appropriate route to get there. If teaching involves taking learners on a journey, then our learning outcomes are the destination, and the assignment standards should help learners map their route to achieve them (Chae et al. 2016; Suskie 2009). Irrespective of the type of format used, different rubrics share common advantages and disadvantages.

Advantages of Rubrics for Learners

These assume students are made aware of the rubric prior to instruction and assessment, and the rubric scoring is shared with students after the assignment is evaluated.

- *Clarify expectations.* Permit the learner to understand what criteria or aspects of the assignment are important. This may assist them in knowing where to focus their efforts and how to structure their assignment. Different criteria may be weighted to emphasize key components. If students are involved in the rubric's construction or iterative improvement, then the assignment may become more meaningful to them.
- *Clarify grading decisions.* Rubrics make the basis of grading an assignment transparent by making the grading criteria explicit and more objective. This may increase student satisfaction with the grading process.
- *Inspire better performance.* Students can use the rubric to self-evaluate their own work prior to submission. This may motivate them to revise their assignment and improve its quality. This metacognitive activity can be further extended if rubrics are used for peer evaluation of assignments.
- *Encourage feedback and reflection.* Rubrics can provide specific feedback on the different aspects evaluated in the assignment. This may help learners reflect on how to improve their performance and may be particularly beneficial if the same rubric is used for formative and summative assessments. It may also help to improve the accuracy of the learner's self-evaluation.

Advantages of Rubrics for Educators

- *Save time grading assignments.* Rubrics reduce the uncertainty and subjective nature of grading decisions. The descriptions of different performance levels also provide some feedback and decrease the need for repetitive written comments. Some learning management systems permit additional automated comments depending on the performance level achieved by the student for each criterion, e.g., on how to improve performance.
- *Provide consistency and decrease bias.* All assignments are evaluated using the same criteria, so grading is more transparent and fair. This can be particularly beneficial if multiple graders are evaluating the assignment, provided they have undergone some training. This enhances the defensibility of assigned grades and may reduce student grade appeals. This transparency and reliability may also help with accreditation.
- *Improve teaching.* Involving multiple educators in the rubric's development should enhance its quality. Deconstruction of different components of the knowledge, concepts, or skills may lead to better teaching methodology and more consistent teaching on shared learning objectives.
- *Improve feedback on teaching effectiveness.* Poor student performance on any specific criterion may highlight the need to refine how this aspect is taught (Uhl et al. 2021). If the same rubric is used in subsequent assignments, the impact of this change can be evaluated and documented, and this information can be included in an educator's teaching portfolio.

Disadvantages of Rubrics for Educators

- *Time commitment.* For rubric development, educator training, piloting, and refinement.
- *Reductionist.* Describing more complex competencies with different behaviorally-anchored criteria may be considered derivative, e.g., observable professional behaviors may not capture all aspects of learner professionalism and professional identity formation.

Part 2: Types of Rubrics

Ultimately, the type of rubric that is selected should be aligned with, and reflect, the purpose of the assessment.

Holistic Rubric

- *Description.* A holistic rubric does not have a list of criteria to evaluate assignments; instead, it has a short narrative description of assignment characteristics at different performance levels.
- *Advantages.* These emphasize what the learner can do, rather than what they cannot do. They also acknowledge that performance on an assessment is sometimes more than the sum of its parts. The number of decisions is also minimized, and so these rubrics are typically used for summative assessments that require a rapid turnaround.
- *Disadvantages.* An inability to weight criteria and a lack of specific feedback on learner's strengths or weaknesses. Inconsistent grading may result when the assignment is at varying levels for different criteria, so it may be difficult to select a single best description. Furthermore,

the limited descriptions mean judgments may be relatively subjective, although reliability can be increased by training raters (Table 9.9).

Checklist
- *Description.* These are task-specific and evaluate the presence or absence of each criterion or step. Using

Table 9.9 A holistic rubric for critical thinking.

4 Strong	**Consistently does all or almost all of the following:** Accurately interprets evidence, statements, graphics, questions, etc. Identifies the most important arguments (reasons and claims) pros and cons. Thoughtfully analyzes and evaluates major alternative points of view. Draws warranted, judicious, and non-fallacious conclusions. Justifies key results and procedures and explains assumptions and reasons. Fair-mindedly follows where evidence and reasons lead
3 Acceptable	**Does most or many of the following:** Accurately interprets evidence, statements, graphics, questions, etc. Identifies relevant arguments (reasons and claims) pros and cons. Offers analyses and evaluations of obvious alternative points of view. Draws warranted, non-fallacious conclusions. Justifies some results or procedures and explains reasons. Fair-mindedly follows where evidence and reasons lead
2 Unacceptable	**Does most or many of the following:** Misinterprets evidence, statements, graphics, questions, etc. Fails to identify strong, relevant counterarguments. Ignores or superficially evaluates obvious alternative points of view. Draws unwarranted or fallacious conclusions. Justifies few results or procedures and seldom explains reasons. Regardless of the evidence or reasons, maintain or defend views based on self-interest or preconceptions
1 Significantly Weak	**Consistently does all or almost all the following:** Offers biased interpretations of evidence, statements, graphics, questions, information, or the points of view of others. Fails to identify or hastily dismisses strong, relevant counterarguments. Ignores or superficially evaluates obvious alternative points of view. Argue using fallacious or irrelevant reasons and unwarranted claims. Does not justify results or procedures, nor explain reasons. Regardless of the evidence or reasons, maintain or defend views based on self-interest or preconceptions. Exhibits close-mindedness or hostility to reason

Source: Adapted from Facione and Facione (1994).

multipliers or weighting of specific steps can address the potential issue of a lack of emphasis on key components.
- *Advantages.* The dichotomous decision-making means multiple components of an assignment or skill can be evaluated without resulting in grader fatigue – so they can provide detailed feedback. This rubric format is easy for novice raters to use.
- *Disadvantages.* Performance criteria that are difficult to operationalize will also be difficult to convert into a checklist. Checklists have been considered unsuitable for evaluating increasing competence because the dichotomous grading scale limits nuanced differentiation across the spectrum of performance (Hodges et al. 1999). However, this assumption has been challenged more recently (Ilgen et al. 2015; Wood and Pugh 2020). Checklists can be modified to identify qualities of advanced learners. For example, a checklist could include identification of clinically discriminating items or key features of disease for a simulated patient encounter.
- *Suggested use.* The detailed feedback and ease of use make them suitable for formative assignments, including those that use learner self-and peer-evaluation (Tables 9.10a and 9.10b).

Rating Scale/Global Rating Scale
- *Description.* These are checklist rubrics with a rating scale added to indicate a more qualitative component of each criterion being assessed. The levels of performance may be indicated by a descriptive term, or a Likert-type scale (typically 4–6 points).
- *Advantages.* They are relatively quick and easy to create and use. The multiple levels of performance do allow more discrimination between learners of differing abilities and quantification of competence.
- *Disadvantages.* The major drawback of rating scales is that performance levels are often not clearly described. This can lead to inconsistent grading by different educators and a lack of specific feedback to learners e.g., a checkbox or Likert value does not convey how to improve in any specific criterion.
- *Suggested use.* The ability to discriminate between learners means they are suited to summative assessments, although concerns about reliability mean these are typically "minor" assignments (Tables 9.11 and 9.12).

Operative Component Rating Scale
- *Description.* This type of rubric was initially developed to evaluate surgical residents' operative skills (Kim et al. 2009; Larson et al. 2005; Martin et al. 1997).
- *Advantages.* These can differentiate between learners of differing abilities and provide some feedback on areas of strength or areas in need of improvement. If used by

Table 9.10a Checklist used in scoring performance on the thoracentesis simulator for veterinary students.

	Item	Not done/done incorrectly	Done correctly
1	Assembles butterfly catheter, three-way stopcock, and syringe	0	1
2	Does not contaminate sterile items	0	1
3	Selects a site at the cranial aspect of the rib	0	1
4	Selects a site in the seventh to eighth intercostal spaces	0	1
5	Selects a site between one-third and two-thirds of the way down the chest	0	1
6	Handles butterfly catheter by the plastic wings during insertion	0	1
7	Rests hand on chest wall while advancing butterfly catheter	0	1
8	Inserts needle slowly perpendicular to the chest wall	0	1
9	Place gentle suction (1–4 mm on a 20 ml syringe) on the syringe during insertion	0	1
10	Faces bevel of the needle to sit parallel to the chest wall	0	1
11	Releases butterfly catheter's plastic wings	0	1
12	Performs aspiration gently (no excessive suction)	0	1
13	Avoids sharp movement of the needle	0	1
14	Fills sample tubes with fluid without introducing contamination	0	1
15	Drains effusion without introducing air into the pleural space	0	1
16	Remove needle parallel to the chest wall, avoiding caudal aspect of the rib	0	1

Source: Adapted from Williamson (2014).

experts, they are more reliable and valid than checklists (Regehr et al. 1998).

- *Disadvantages.* They provide less specific feedback to students since they contain fewer criteria (Table 9.13).

Table 9.10b Part of a task-specific checklist to control the hemorrhage and repair a damaged blood vessel for surgical residents.

	Item	Not done/done incorrectly	Done correctly
Control of hemorrhage			
1	Applies pressure to stop bleeding **first**	0	1
2	Asks assistant to suction field	0	1
3	Inspects injury by carefully releasing the damaged blood vessel	0	1
4	Ensures all equipment needed for repair is at hand before starting	0	1
5	Control of bleeding point (use deBakey forceps/ Stainsky clamp, or proximal/ distal pressure)	0	1
Repair			
6	Selects appropriate suture (4.0/5.0/6.0 polypropylene)	0	1
7	Selects appropriate needle driver (vascular)	0	1
8	Selects appropriate forceps (deBakey)	0	1
9	Needle loaded 1/2–1/3 from tip 90% of time	0	1

Source: Adapted from Martin et al. (1997).

Analytic/Descriptive Rubric

- *Description.* An analytic rubric resembles a grid with the different criteria for a learner assignment listed in the leftmost column and with levels of performance listed across the top row, often using numbers and/or descriptive anchors. The AAC&U VALUE rubrics are analytic rubrics developed for 16 essential learning outcomes (Association of American Colleges and Universities 2009). The rubrics include a definition, framing language, and glossary, as well as the grid of criteria and levels of performance (see Tables 9.14a and 9.14b). The wording of item anchors can impact assessors and pass/fail decisions. It is recommended to use descriptors rather than percentage achievement to avoid raters "compensating" for poor scores, across different criteria or items. The cells in the center contain descriptions of behavior across a continuum of performance, although some cells or entire columns may be left blank. The anchor terminology can also impact students perceptions of their performance. For instance, compare the impact of being "labeled" as *Unsatisfactory* or *Failing*, with *Does not meet expectations*, or *Not practice ready*.

Table 9.11 Part of a rating scale rubric used for scoring a simulated ovariohysterectomy for veterinary students.

Making the incision		3 Excellent	2 Good	1 Borderline	0 Unsatisfactory
1	Makes smooth incision through skin (using proper fingertip grip)				
2	Proper sharp dissection to locate body wall – avoids creating dead space				
3	Makes safe abdominal approach – rests hand on patient while using reverse stab with scalpel; tents sufficiently to avoid injury to patient				
4	Extends the incision safely – keeps straight incision, and does not go too deep				

Performing the ovariohysterectomy		3 Excellent	2 Good	1 Borderline	0 Unsatisfactory
5	Proper ligament is identified and grasped with hemostat				
6	Applies correct three-clamp technique proximal to ovary				
7	Places secure circumferential ligation in the groove created by the most proximal clamp using a hand tie				
8	Places a second secure circumferential ligation immediately distal to the first ligature using an instrument tie, demonstrating clamp flashing while tightening				
9	Transects pedicle between two clamps and demonstrates checking pedicles for bleeding before returning to abdomen gently				
10	Locate second ovary and uterine horn using safe efficient technique				
11	Proper ligament is identified and grasped with hemostat, OR first clamp of three-way clamp technique is placed distal to ovary				
12	Applies modified three-clamp technique				
13	Places a secure miller's ligature in the groove created by the most proximal clamp				
14	Transects pedicle between two clamps and demonstrates checking the pedicle for bleeding before returning to abdomen gently				
15	Cranial to the cervix but caudal to the uterine bifurcation; laces three clamps using proper technique				
16	Places secure circumferential ligation at location where hemostat closest to cervix has crushed the tissue				
17	Places a secure trans-fixation ligature immediately distal to the first ligature, demonstrating clamp flashing while tightening				
18	Transects pedicle between two clamps and demonstrates checking the pedicle for bleeding before returning to abdomen gently				

(Continued)

Table 9.11 (Continued)

Collective marks	3 Excellent	2 Good	1 Borderline	0 Unsatisfactory
31 Gentle tissue handling				
32 Good adherence to aseptic technique				
33 Good suture handling, including suture gathering				
34 Good instrument handling; uses appropriate instruments for tasks				

Source: Adapted from Williamson et al. (2019).

Table 9.12 Global rating scale used in scoring performance on the thoracentesis simulator.

	5	4	3	2	1
Procedural performance	Very proficient; smooth technique without much lapse	Proficient; good technique but may have had a minor lapse	Competent; acceptable technique with some lapses noted	Poor performance; multiple or significant lapses in technique	Very poor performance; proper technique is generally absent
Tissue handling	Handled tissues consistently without damage; showed all appropriate safeguards against trauma	Good tissue handling	Handled tissues carefully and showed safeguards, but occasionally caused accidental damage	Unsatisfactory tissue handling	Used excessive force, did not show appropriate safeguards, or repeatedly caused damage
Efficiency	Achieved economy of movement and maximum efficiency	Good efficiency	Acceptable efficiency but made some unnecessary movements	Significant inefficiency	Performed many unnecessary movements
Equipment handling	Fluid handling of equipment	Good handling of equipment	Competent use of equipment, although it appeared awkward at time	Equipment use is stiff or awkward most of the time	Consistently stiff or awkward movements with equipment
Procedural knowledge and flow	Demonstrated familiarity with all aspects of the procedure; procedural flow was effortless	Good procedural knowledge and flow	Knew all important aspects of procedure; steady progression of procedure	Unsatisfactory procedural knowledge and flow	Inadequate knowledge of the procedure; frequently stopped to consider the next step

Source: Adapted from Williamson (2014).

- *Advantages*. Each criterion receives a separate score, and so these types of rubrics can provide useful feedback on learners' strengths and weaknesses. Criterion can be weighted to emphasize the relative importance of each dimension. This typically only impacts borderline learners, so rather than develop weighted rubrics, the time may be more effectively spent on other test development efforts, e.g., rater training or rubric refinement (Homer et al. 2020).
- *Disadvantages*. Analytic rubrics take longer to create and use. Some educators argue they promote a reductionist approach to assignments and may stifle creativity. A possible solution is to combine components from different rubrics. For example, in a simulated client consultation, different communication skills are often treated as distinct constructs and graded using an analytical rubric. However, the separate items are often interrelated and have mutually affecting dynamics (Han et al. 2022). A global rating score can be assigned to the learner's thoroughness and flow or overall efficacy to establish relationship-centered care – whether the client is willing to follow the recommendations or be willing to return for another healthcare visit (Table 9.15).

Table 9.13 Operative component rating scale for open inguinal herniorraphy for surgical residents.

1) Ilioinguinal nerve

1	2	3	4	5
Poor knowledge of nerve anatomy and poor technique in protecting nerve from injury		Aware of potential nerve injury but with inconsistent efforts to protect nerve during procedure		Aware of potential nerve injury; carefully protected nerve during dissection and closure

2) Search for indirect hernia

1	2	3	4	5
Poor technique was used to search for indirect hernia		Moderate efficiency in search for indirect hernia		Careful and meticulous search for indirect hernia proximally; understands need for high ligation

3) Mesh insertion

1	2	3	4	5
Demonstrated inconsistency in accurate placement of mesh sutures		Good placement of mesh sutures to secure mesh with only occasional inaccurate bites		Excellent securing of mesh with consistently appropriate tissue bites

4) Knowledge of anatomy

1	2	3	4	5
Gaps in knowledge of anatomy prevented smooth flow of operation		Basic understanding of anatomy allowed smooth progression of procedure		Excellent understanding of anatomy allowed rapid progression from one step to the next step

5) Femoral vein injury

1	2	3	4	5
Unaware of location of femora vein and potential injury		Aware of potential vein injury but unable to describe management of injury		Understood femoral vein anatomy and described appropriate management of needle injury

6) Prevention of complications (recurrence, cord hematoma, nerve entrapment, elevated testicle)

1	2	3	4	5
Poor knowledge of critical steps to avoid complications		Aware of several critical steps to avoid complications		Aware of most of critical steps to avoid complications

7) Respect for tissue

1	2	3	4	5
Frequently used unnecessary force on tissue or caused damage by inappropriate use of instruments		Careful handling of tissue but occasionally caused inadvertent damage		Consistently handled tissue appropriately with minimal damage to the tissue

8) Time and motion

1	2	3	4	5
Many unnecessary moves		Efficient time/motion but some unnecessary moves		Clear economy of movement and maximum efficiency

9) Flow of operation

1	2	3	4	5
Frequently stopped and seemed unsure of next move		Demonstrated some forward planning with reasonable progression of procedure		Obviously planned course of operation with effortless flow from one move to the next

10) Overall Performance

1	2	3	4	5
Very poor		Competent		Clearly superior

Source: Adapted from Larson et al. (2005).

Table 9.14a Association of American Colleges and Universities (2009).

	Capstone 4	Milestones 3	Milestones 2	Benchmark 1
Knowledge *Cultural self-awareness*	Articulates insights into own cultural rules and biases (e.g., seeking complexity; aware of how her/his experiences have shaped these rules, and how to recognize and respond to cultural biases, resulting in a shift in self-description)	Recognizes new perspectives about own cultural rules and biases (e.g., not looking for sameness; comfortable with the complexities that new perspectives offer)	Identifies own cultural rules and biases (e.g., with a strong preference for those rules shared with own cultural group and seeks the same in others)	Shows minimal awareness of own cultural rules and biases (even those shared with own cultural group[s]) (e.g., uncomfortable with identifying possible cultural differences with others)
Knowledge *Knowledge of cultural worldview frameworks*	Demonstrates sophisticated understanding of the complexity of elements important to members of another culture in relation to its history, values, politics, communication styles, economy, or beliefs and practices	Demonstrates adequate understanding of the complexity of elements important to members of another culture in relation to its history, values, politics, communication styles, economy, or beliefs and practices	Demonstrates partial understanding of the complexity of elements important to members of another culture in relation to its history, values, politics, communication styles, economy, or beliefs and practices	Demonstrates surface understanding of the complexity of elements important to members of another culture in relation to its history, values, politics, communication styles, economy, or beliefs and practices
Skills *Empathy*	Interprets intercultural experience from the perspectives of own and more than one worldview and demonstrates ability to act in a supportive manner that recognizes the feelings of another cultural group	Recognizes intellectual and emotional dimensions of more than one worldview and sometimes uses more than one worldview in interactions	Identifies components of other cultural perspectives but responds in all situations with own worldview	Views the experience of others but does so through own cultural worldview
Skills *Verbal and nonverbal communication*	Articulates a complex understanding of cultural differences in verbal and nonverbal communication (e.g., demonstrates understanding of the degree to which people use physical contact while communicating in different cultures or use direct/indirect and explicit/implicit meanings) and is able to skillfully negotiate a shared understanding based on those differences	Recognizes and participates in cultural differences in verbal and nonverbal communication and begins to negotiate a shared understanding based on those differences	Identifies some cultural differences in verbal and nonverbal communication and is aware that misunderstandings can occur based on those differences, but is still unable to negotiate a shared understanding	Has a minimal level of understanding of cultural differences in verbal and nonverbal communication and is unable to negotiate a shared understanding
Attitudes *Curiosity*	Asks complex questions about other cultures, seeks out and articulates answers to these questions that reflect multiple cultural perspectives	Asks deeper questions about other cultures and seeks out answers to these questions	Asks simple or surface questions about other cultures	States minimal interest in learning more about other cultures
Attitudes *Openness*	Initiates and develops interactions with culturally different others. Suspends judgment in valuing her/his interactions with culturally different others	Begins to initiate and develop interactions with culturally different others. Begins to suspend judgment in valuing her/his interactions with culturally different others	Expresses openness to most, if not all, interactions with culturally different others. Has difficulty suspending any judgment in her/his interactions with culturally different others and is aware of own judgment and expresses a willingness to change	Receptive to interacting with culturally different others. Has difficulty suspending any judgment in her/his interactions with culturally different others but is unaware of own judgment

Source: Intercultural knowledge and competence VALUE rubric. https://www.aacu.org/initiatives/value-initiative/value-rubrics/value-rubrics-intercultural-knowledge-and-competence.

Table 9.14b Association of American Colleges and Universities (2009).

	Capstone	Milestones		Benchmark
	4	**3**	**2**	**1**
Define problem	Demonstrates the ability to construct a clear and insightful problem statement with evidence of all relevant contextual factors	Demonstrates the ability to construct a problem statement with evidence of most relevant contextual factors, and problem statement is adequately detailed	Begins to demonstrate the ability to construct a problem statement with evidence of the most relevant contextual factors, but problem statement is superficial	Demonstrates a limited ability in identifying a problem statement or related contextual factors
Identify strategies	Identifies multiple approaches for solving the problem that apply within a specific context	Identifies multiple approaches for solving the problem, only some of which apply within a specific context	Identifies only a single approach for solving the problem that does apply within a specific context	Identifies one or more approaches for solving the problem that do not apply within a specific context
Propose solutions/ hypotheses	Proposes one or more solutions/hypotheses that indicate a deep comprehension of the problem. Solution/ hypotheses are sensitive to contextual factors as well as all of the following: ethical, logical, and cultural dimensions of the problem	Proposes one or more solutions/hypotheses that indicate comprehension of the problem. Solutions/ hypotheses are sensitive to contextual factors as well as the one of the following: ethical, logical, or cultural dimensions of the problem	Proposes one solution/hypothesis that is "off the shelf" rather than individually designed to address the specific contextual factors of the problem	Proposes a solution/ hypothesis that is difficult to evaluate because it is vague or only indirectly addresses the problem statement
Evaluate potential solutions	Evaluation of solutions is deep and elegant (for example, contains thorough and insightful explanation) and includes, deeply and thoroughly, all of the following: considers history of problem, reviews logic/reasoning, examines feasibility of solution, and weighs impacts of solution	Evaluation of solutions is adequate (for example, contains thorough explanation) and includes the following: considers history of problem, reviews logic/ reasoning, examines feasibility of solution, and weighs impacts of solution	Evaluation of solutions is brief (for example, explanation lacks depth) and includes the following: considers history of problem, reviews logic/ reasoning, examines feasibility of solution, and weighs impacts of solution	Evaluation of solutions is superficial (for example, contains cursory, surface-level explanation) and includes the following: considers history of problem, reviews logic/ reasoning, examines feasibility of solution, and weighs impacts of solution
Implement solution	Implements the solution in a manner that addresses thoroughly and deeply multiple contextual factors of the problem	Implements the solution in a manner that addresses multiple contextual factors of the problem in a surface manner	Implements the solution in a manner that addresses the problem statement but ignores relevant contextual factors	Implements the solution in a manner that does not directly address the problem statement
Evaluate outcomes	Reviews results relative to the problem defined with thorough, specific considerations of need for further work	Reviews results relative to the problem defined with some consideration of need for further work	Reviews results in terms of the problem defined with little, if any, consideration of need for further work	Reviews results superficially in terms of the problem defined with no consideration of need for further work

Source: Problem solving VALUE rubric. https://www.aacu.org/initiatives/value-initiative/value-rubrics/value-rubrics-problem-solving.

Table 9.15 Descriptive anchors for a 4 point-scale of different performance levels.

Poor	Borderline	Good	Excellent
Novice	Advanced beginner	Competent	Proficient
Does not meet expectations	Marginally meets expectations	Meets expectations	Exceeds expectations
Critically deficient	Developing	Ready	Exemplary
Beginning – significant improvement is needed	Progressing – opportunities for growth	Competent – performed correctly	Accomplished – proficient performance

Part 3: Creating Effective Rubrics

Rubrics are better when created by multiple educators. Reaching a consensus may be achieved using one of two methods. Using cognitive task analysis, subject matter experts describe how to complete the task (Clark et al. 2012; Militello and Hutton 1998). It typically involves observation and interviews to elicit both explicit and implicit knowledge about a task, since experts unintentionally omit knowledge when describing a procedure during free recall (Sullivan et al. 2014). This information is then combined to map the task, and key decision points are highlighted. Alternatively, the Delphi technique uses several rounds of questionnaires distributed to a panel of experts; the results are shared after each round; and the responses undergo iterative improvement after each round (Parratt et al. 2016; St-Louis et al. 2020; Tappan et al. 2020). Students can also be involved in the development of rubrics as a means of promoting metacognition, similar to being asked to write exam questions. Alternatively, learners can provide feedback or refine an existing rubric.

As previously mentioned, having multiple educators involved in developing a rubric can increase its quality and also promote more consistent teaching on the shared learning objectives.

The process for developing, e.g., an effective analytic or descriptive rubric includes these steps:

- Define the learning objectives
- Clearly define the learning task – it should be relevant to the learning objectives
- Define the different criteria or items, usually at least 4. These should focus on important aspects of the skill performance, and the traits should be directly demonstrable (knowledge) or observable (skill)
- Create a scoring system, e.g., a 3–6 point scale per item
- Specify the standards of performance across the continuum
- Pilot the rubric – to capture unforeseen events and important critical errors

This will also allow you to determine if the correct amount of time has been allocated to time-bound assignments and whether the test situation reflects the appropriate degree of realism.

Assignment Raters

Raters, or those who are responsible for grading assignments, should be qualified to assess the task being evaluated and ideally be recruited based on their subject expertise. Training is best done with all raters in one group to facilitate consensus and cross-calibration. It should include an introduction to the specific task, a full explanation of the rubric, and frame of reference training (Newman et al. 2016). Raters practice using the rubric with quality control samples of written assessments or videoed performances that span the continuum of performance and receive feedback on their accuracy.

Challenges to Rubric Validity and Reliability

There are multiple ways that the validity of an assessment and accompanying rubric can be invalidated:

- *Face validity*. The assessment is not realistic enough, or it does not represent a task that is relevant
- *Content validity*. The assessment does not sample adequately from the domains of interest
- *Construct validity*. Novices, intermediates, and experts achieve the same scores
- *Predictive validity*. Performance on the assessment does not correlate with the real-world task performance
- *Having poor reliability*

The major cause of poor reliability is rater biases or errors leading to rater inconsistency. A rater bias is the tendency to rate in ways that vary systematically from the scoring rubric (Feldman et al. 2012; Paniagua et al. 2020). There are several types of rater biases (Iramaneerat and Yudkowsky 2007; Royal and Hecker 2016):

- *Central tendency/Restriction of range*. Tendency to score most learners in central performance categories.
- *Drift*. Ratings become more harsh or lenient over time.
- *Fatigue*. Scores are affected by tiredness, which can be exacerbated by rubric complexity.
- *Favoritism*. A well-liked learner is graded more leniently.
- *First impression*. A learner is rated on initial impression and subsequent information is ignored.

- *Gestalt phenomenon.* A learner is judged on an overall impression when implementing an analytical rubric rather than specific aspects of performance.
- *Halo effect.* A learner is rated on characteristics other than the trait being measured, e.g., vocabulary expertise may influence the score in a grammar category, even if it is not explicitly stated as part of the rubric.
- *Leniency/Severity.* Rater tends to score excessively leniently or severely, so-called "doves" and "hawks."
- *Primacy.* A learner is scored in comparison to peers and not the specified rubric, e.g., the rater reviews a cohort of excellent performances and then grades a moderate performance lower than the rubric demands because of scoring relative to the peers rather than the rubric.
- *Skimming.* A learner is judged on a limited section of their performance.
- *Trait.* There is too much focus on one particular aspect of the performance.

Having multiple independent raters score the same assessments may limit the impact of the leniency/severity bias since the "hawks" and "doves" may mitigate each other's impact. Alternatively, training raters for a specific aspect or criterion of the assessment may allow them to evaluate this aspect across all test-takers rather than evaluate multiple aspects of a single test-taker. Allowing for adequate time to evaluate assessments can mitigate against fatigue and repeated training about rater biases may also help. Additional strategies include tracking rater performance and comparing it to their peers to look for evidence of bias, encouraging discussions to allow shared mental models to develop amongst raters, and revising rubrics to refine descriptions and incorporate unanticipated learner responses (Royal and Hecker 2016).

References

AAVMC Working Group on Competency-Based Veterinary Education, A.W.G. on C.-B.V., Molgaard, L.K., Hodgson, J.L., et al. (2019). Competency-Based Veterinary Education: Part 3 – Milestones. https://cbve.org/milestones (accessed 25 November 2022).

AAVMC Working Group on Competency-Based Veterinary Education, Molgaard, L.K., Hodgson, J.L., et al. (2018a). Competency-Based Veterinary Education: Part 1 – CBVE Framework. https://www.aavmc.org/wp-content/uploads/2020/10/CBVE-Publication-1-Framework.pdf (accessed ccessed 25 November 2022).

AAVMC Working Group on Competency-Based Veterinary Education, A.W.G. on C.-B.V., Molgaard, L.K., Hodgson, J.L., et al. (2018b) Competency-Based Veterinary Education: Part 2 – Entrustable Professional Activities Washington, DC.

Part 4: Conclusion

Well-designed rubrics have several advantages for students – they should signpost and inspire better performance, clarify expectations and grading decisions, provide feedback, and encourage self-reflection. Although rubric development, piloting, and refinement all require time, rubrics can enhance teaching by clarifying expectations in team-taught courses, as well as save time grading assignments, enhance grading consistency, and decrease bias. As a means of grading assignments, they can also provide specific feedback to the educator on which teaching areas require improvement and provide a means of demonstrating longitudinal effectiveness if used to compare students' performance over time.

Summary

This chapter has covered different types of assignments that may be used to help students demonstrate their knowledge, as well as provides some background information on how such assignments may be created and delivered depending upon what you desire the students to get out of the assignment. Similarly, the value of rubrics and an explanation of the different types of rubrics are covered. A number of figures and tables within this chapter provide you with some visual aids to use as you consider how you might adjust your own assignments, if needed, and to measure your current assignments if you are interested in assessing your approach to using assignments in general. Overall, this chapter is both quickly applicable and useful as a self-reflection tool for you regarding your use of assessments, where those might be changed for the better, or as an affirmation that what you are already doing is solidly based on the literature.

Airasian, P.W., Cruikshank, K.A., Mayer, R.E. et al. (2001). Chapter 5. The cognitive process dimension. In: *A Taxonomy for Learning, Teaching, and Assessing: A Revision of Bloom's Taxonomy of Educational Objectives*, Completee (ed. L.W. Anderson and D.R. Krathwohl), 63–92. New York: Longman.

Association of American Colleges and Universities (2009). Valid Assessment of Learning in Undergraduate Education (VALUE) rubrics. https://www.aacu.org/initiatives/value-initiative/value-rubrics (accessed 25 November 2022).

Bachelor of Veterinary Medicine Day One Skills (2007). Royal Veterinary College, University of London. www.live.ac.uk/Media/LIVE/PDFs/day_one_handbook.pdf (accessed 25 November 2022).

Biggs, J.B. (1996). Enhancing teaching through constructive alignment. *Higher Education* 32: 1–18.

Bloom, B.S. and Krathwohl, D.R. (1956). *Taxonomy of Educational Objectives: The Classification of Educational Goals by a Committee of College and University Examiners. Handbook I: Cognitive Domain.* New York, NY: Longmans, Green.

CAST (2018). Universal Design for Learning Guidelines version 2.2. https://udlguidelines.cast.org (accessed 25 November 2022).

Chae, S.J., Kim, M., and Chang, K.H. (2016). Can disclosure of scoring rubric for basic clinical skills improve objective structured clinical examination? *Korean Journal of Medical Education* 28 (2): 179–183. https://doi.org/10.3946/kjme.2016.28.

Clark, D.R. (1999). Bloom's Taxonomy: The Psychomotor Domain. http://www.nwlink.com/~donclark/hrd/Bloom/psychomotor_domain.html (accessed 25 November 2022).

Clark, R.E., Pugh, C.M., Yates, K.A. et al. (2012). The use of cognitive task analysis to improve instructional descriptions of procedures. *Journal of Surgical Research* 173 (1): e37–e42. https://doi.org/10.1016/j.jss.2011.09.003.

Coombes, N. and Silva-Fletcher, A. (ed.) (2018). *Veterinary Clinical Skills Manual*, 1e. Wallingford, UK: CABI.

Cruess, R.L., Cruess, S.R., and Steinert, Y. (2016). Amending Miller's pyramid to include professional identity formation. *Academic Medicine* 91 (2): 180–185. https://doi.org/10.1097/ACM.0000000000000913.

Education, A.W.G. on C.-B.V., Molgaard, L.K., Hodgson, J.L., et al. (2019). Competency-Based Veterinary Education: Part 3 – Milestones. https://cbve.org/milestones (accessed 25 November 2022).

Effective use of performance objectives for learning and assessment (for use with Fink's and Bloom's taxonomies). (2005). Teacher & Educational Development, University of New Mexico School of Medicine. https://wit.edu/sites/default/files/2020-10/Effective-Use-of-Learning-Objectives-University-of-New-Mexico.pdf (accessed 25 November 2022).

Facione, P.A. and Facione, N.C. (1994). The holistic critical thinking scoring rubric: a tool for developing and evaluating critical thinking. https://www.insightassessment.com/wp-content/uploads/HCTSR-2014-Insight-Assessment.pdf (accessed 25 November 2022).

Feldman, M., Lazzara, E.H., Vanderbilt, A.A., and DiazGranados, D. (2012). Rater training to support high-stakes simulation-based assessments. *Journal of Continuing Education in the Health Professions* 32 (4): 279–286. https://doi.org/10.1002/chp.21156.

Fink, L.D. (2003). *Creating Significant Learning Experiences.* San Franscico: Jossey-Bass.

Han, H., Hingle, S.T., Koschmann, T. et al. (2022). Analyzing expert criteria for authentic resident communication skills. *Teaching and Learning in Medicine* 34 (1): 33–42. https://doi.org/10.1080/10401334.2021.1977134.

Heer, R. (n.d.). A Model of Learning Objectives–based on A Taxonomy for Learning, Teaching, and Assessing: A Revision of Bloom's Taxonomy of Educational Objectives. Center for Excellence in Learning and Teaching. https://www.celt.iastate.edu/wp-content/uploads/2015/09/RevisedBloomsHandout-1.pdf (accessed 25 November 2022).

Hodges, B., Regehr, G., McNaughton, N. et al. (1999). OSCE checklists do not capture increasing levels of expertise. *Academic Medicine* 74 (10): 1129–1134.

Homer, M., Fuller, R., Hallam, J., and Pell, G. (2020). Shining a spotlight on scoring in the OSCE: checklists and item weighting. *Medical Teacher* 42 (9): 1037–1042. https://doi.org/10.1080/0142159X.2020.1781072.

Ilgen, J.S., Ma, I.W.Y., Hatala, R., and Cook, D.A. (2015). A systematic review of validity evidence for checklists versus global rating scales in simulation-based assessment. *Medical Education* 49 (2): 161–173. https://doi.org/10.1111/medu.12621.

Iramaneerat, C. and Yudkowsky, R. (2007). Rater errors in a clinical. *Evaluation and the Health Professions* 266–283.

Irby, D.M. and Hamstra, S.J. (2016). Parting the clouds: three professionalism frameworks in medical education. *Academic Medicine* 91 (12): 1606–1611. https://doi.org/10.1097/ACM.0000000000001190.

Kim, M.J., Williams, R.G., Boehler, M.L. et al. (2009). Refining the evaluation of operating room performance. *Journal of Surgical Education* 66 (6): 352–356. https://doi.org/10.1016/j.jsurg.2009.09.005.

Kirkpatrick, J.D. and Kayser Kirkpatrick, W. (2016). *Kirkpatrick's Four Levels of Training Evaluation.* Alexandria, VA: ATD Press.

Krathwohl, D.R., Bloom, B.S., and Masia, B.B. (1964). *Taxonomy of Educational Objectives: The Classification of Educational Goals. Handbook II: Affective Domain,* 1e. New York, NY: David McKay Company Inc.

Larson, J.L., Williams, R.G., Ketchum, J. et al. (2005). Feasibility, reliability and validity of an operative performance rating system for evaluating surgery residents. *Surgery* 138 (4): 640–649. https://doi.org/10.1016/j.surg.2005.07.017.

Martin, J.A., Regehr, G., Reznick, R. et al. (1997). Objective structured assessment of technical skill (OSATS) for surgical residents. *British Journal of Surgery* 84 (2): 273–278. https://doi.org/10.1002/bjs.1800840237.

Mehay, R. and Burns, R. (2012). Chapter 29: Assessment and competence. In: *The Essential Handbook for GP Training and Education*, 1e (ed. R. Mehay), 414. http://www.essentialgptrainingbook.com/chapter-29.php.

Militello, L.G. and Hutton, R.J.B. (1998). Applied cognitive task analysis (ACTA): a practitioner's toolkit for understanding cognitive task demands. *Ergonomics* 41 (11): 1618–1641. https://doi.org/10.1080/001401398186108.

Newman, L.R., Brodsky, D., Jones, R.N. et al. (2016). Frame-of-reference training: establishing reliable assessment of teaching effectiveness. *Journal of Continuing Education in the Health Professions* 36 (3): 206–210. https://doi.org/10.1097/CEH.0000000000000086.

Paniagua, M., Swygert, K.A., and Downing, S.M. (2020). Written tests: writing high quality constructed-response and selected response items. In: *Assessement in Healthcare Professions Education*, 2e (ed. R. Yudowsky, Y.S. Park, and S.M. Downing), 109–126. New York, NY: Routledge.

Parratt, J.A., Fahy, K.M., Hutchinson, M. et al. (2016). Expert validation of a teamwork assessment rubric: a modified Delphi study. *Nurse Education Today* 36: 77–85. https://doi.org/10.1016/j.nedt.2015.07.023.

Read, E.K., Read, M., and R., & Baillie, S. (ed.) (2021). *Veterinary Clinical Skills*, 1e. Hoboken, NJ: Wiley-Blackwell.

Regehr, G., MacRae, H., Reznick, R.K., and Szalay, D. (1998). Comparing the psychometric properties of checklists and global rating scales for assessing performance on an OSCE-format examination. *Academic Medicine* 73 (9): 993–997.

Royal, K.D. and Hecker, K.G. (2016). Rater errors in clinical performance assessments. *Journal of Veterinary Medical Education* 43 (1): 5–8. https://doi.org/10.3138/jvme.0715-112R.

Schoenfeld-Tacher, R. and Sims, M.H. (2013). Course goals, competencies, and instructional objectives. *Journal of Veterinary Medical Education* 40 (2): 139–144. https://doi.org/10.3138/jvme.0411-047R.

Simpson, E.J. (1966). *The Classifications of Educational Objectives, Psychomotor Domain*, 1e. Urbana, IL: University of Illinois.

St-Louis, E., Shaheen, M., Mukhtar, F. et al. (2020). Towards development of an open surgery competency assessment for residents (OSCAR) tool – a systematic review of the literature and Delphi consensus. *Journal of Surgical Education* 77 (2): 438–453. https://doi.org/10.1016/j.jsurg.2019.10.006.

Sullivan, M.E., Yates, K.A., Inaba, K. et al. (2014). The use of cognitive task analysis to reveal the instructional limitations of experts in the teaching of procedural skills. *Academic Medicine* 89 (5): 811–816. https://doi.org/10.1097/ACM.0000000000000224.

Suskie, L. (2009). Using a scoring guide or rubric to plan or evaluate an assignment. In: *Assessing Student Learning*, 2e, 137–154. San Fransico: Jossey-Bass.

Tappan, R.S., Hedman, L.D., López-Rosado, R., and Roth, H.R. (2020). Checklist-style rubric development for practical examination of clinical skills in entry-level physical therapist education. *Journal of Allied Health* 49 (3): 202–211.

Uhl, J.D., Sripathi, K.N., Saldanha, J.N. et al. (2021). Introductory biology undergraduate students' mixed ideas about genetic information flow. *Biochemistry and Molecular Biology Education* 49 (3): 372–382. https://doi.org/10.1002/bmb.21483.

Wiggins, G. and McTighe, J. (2005). *Understanding By Design*. Alexandria, VA: Association for Supervision & Curriculum Development.

Williamson, J.A. (2014). Construct validation of a small-animal Thoracocentesis simulator. *Journal of Veterinary Medical Education* 41 (4): 384–389. https://doi.org/10.3138/jvme.0314-037R.

Williamson, J.A., Johnson, J.T., Anderson, S. et al. (2019). A randomizedtrial comparing freely moving and zonal instruction ofveterinary surgical skills using ovariohysterectomy models. *Journal of Veterinary Medical Education* 46 (2): 195–204. https://doi.org/10.3138/jvme.0817-009r.

Wood, T.J. and Pugh, D. (2020). Are rating scales really better than checklists for measuring increasing levels of expertise? *Medical Teacher* 42 (1): 46–51. https://doi.org/10.1080/0142159X.2019.1652260.

10

Assessing Student Learning: Exams, Quizzes, and Remediation

Kimberly S. Cook, Ed.D. MBA
Texas Christian University, Fort Worth, TX, USA

Katherine Fogelberg, DVM, PhD (Science Education), MA (Educational Leadership)
Virginia-Maryland College of Veterinary Medicine, Blacksburg, VA, USA

Patricia Butterbrodt, PhD, MEd
Richard A. Gillespie College of Veterinary Medicine, Lincoln Memorial University, Harrogate, TN, USA

Katrina Jolley, MEd (Educational Leadership)
Richard A. Gillespie College of Veterinary Medicine, Lincoln Memorial University, Harrogate, TN, USA

Malathi Raghavan, DVM, MS, PhD
Purdue University College of Veterinary Medicine, West Lafayette, IN, USA

Jo R. Smith, MA, VetMB, PhD, Post Graduate Diploma in Veterinary Education (PGDipVetEd), DACVIM – SA
University of Georgia College of Veterinary Medicine, Athens, GA, USA

Section 1: Formative Versus Summative Assessments and the Role of Evaluations

Kimberly S. Cook and Katherine Fogelberg

Part 1: Introduction

As someone involved in education, or just life, you have likely seen many programs or classes developed by well-meaning individuals that failed to meet their potential. The scenario is familiar; in fact, you might have even unknowingly played a role. Someone sees a gap in skills, knowledge, or ability that seems important to bridge or fill. That person marshals the resources, plans activities, schedules the dates, opens registrations, and initiates a program. Sometimes, it all goes smoothly, the programs are well received, and the course evaluations are glowing. Often though, we find that what was good could have been better, what was bad caught us by surprise, and the content that seemed fantastic in the idea phase ended up being mediocre in the delivery phase.

So, what happened? Most often, good intentions are not enough to deliver the results we desire. Even with great organization and planning, our intended outcomes are not realized because we failed to incorporate outcomes and evaluations in the planning phase of our education programs. Though we tend to think of evaluation as the final step in a program or class that ultimately "grades" our performance or our participants' performances, embedding evaluation from the outset leads us to have higher impact practices, better data about program outcomes, and a richer understanding of what happens during our classes and programs.

Part 2: Evaluation Overview

When it comes to evaluations, we do them daily, often unconsciously. Additionally, there are many activities that fit under the evaluation umbrella. Merriam-Webster defines evaluation as "determination of the value, nature, character, or quality of something or someone" (Evaluation n.d., n.p.). We make evaluations based on criteria that are either understood, preferred, or specified. Examples of these might include:

- Doggy day care is louder than a library.
- Local coffee shops are better than national chains.
- An 80-lb Beagle is overweight.

Regarding classes and programs, many steps that we already take are evaluative and reflective in nature, even if we don't consider them as such. These can include:

- Examining test data to analyze the difficulty of exam or comprehension of course content.
- Monitoring student engagement to determine the efficacy of a class activity.
- Asking follow-up questions to student responses to ascertain the amount of class preparation and understanding.

Part 3: Evaluation Versus Assessment

Evaluation and assessment are often used interchangeably. According to the Oxford Languages Dictionary, assessment is "the evaluation or estimation of the nature, quality, or ability of someone or something" (accessed 23 September 2022, n.p.). As you can see here, evaluation and assessment essentially *are* interchangeable, although in the educational sense, assessments are broadly encompassing all types of assignments and exams that may be either *formative* or *summative*, where evaluations are primarily focused on exams or more *summative* evaluations.

A *formative assessment* is used when an educator wishes to provide opportunities for students to demonstrate where they are in their learning of new materials, and/or when an educator desires students to learn from mistakes made on an assignment or exam. Such assessments may occur in the form of formal or informal feedback.

Formal feedback may be a low-stakes quiz, for example, such as an in-class, anonymous, online quiz for which students simply earn points for participating rather than for answering correctly. This allows students to gain insights into content they may need to study further or already have a good grasp of. Formal feedback may also be administered through written comments in response to performance during a clinical case as part of the veterinary student's clinical rotations; used formatively, this provides the same learning opportunities as a low-stakes in-class quiz but in the clinical setting.

Informal feedback is provided on a pretty on-going basis; it comes in the form of immediate verbal feedback about a case that went well or not so well; in class when student questions are asked and answered; and during labs when students are performing tasks where instructors have the opportunity to correct their mistakes and affirm their good work in the moment. This type of feedback is generally delivered verbally, but may also be in the form of written feedback if reviewing drafts of assignments or providing mid-block comments to students during clinical rotations, for example.

A *summative assessment* is used to determine whether students have "learned," or at least retained well enough to perform on an exam, the information the instructor intended to deliver and has indicated the student should

take away from a course through their learning objectives. Summative assessments are those we are generally most familiar with, often referred to as mid-terms and finals. They are also often of the "high stakes" variety, meaning that some large consequence may result if a student fails the exam. In K-12 programs, end-of-year assessments that determine whether a student will pass to the next grade is an example; in veterinary medicine, the North American Veterinary Licensing Exam (NAVLE), which determines whether a new graduate will be eligible for a license to practice in the United States, is another.

Summative assessments take many forms, including multiple-choice exams (MCQs), essay exams, objective structured clinical exams (OSCEs), and others that will be explored and discussed later in this chapter and later in this textbook. The important thing, for now, is that there are two basic types of exams used to determine knowledge and skills: formative and summative. Both of these are, of course, evaluations, too, albeit on the individual level. The following sections will cover more specifics of evaluation when taken as a whole, from the individual to the program.

Part 4: Components of Evaluation

Evaluation in an educational or programmatic context can be defined as a method of assessing merit and worth of an evaluand or program by comparison to a standard or desired outcome. Thus, evaluation is the process by which we intentionally compare an element with its ideal or other criteria to determine if it meets that standard, surpasses it, or falls short. The component parts of evaluation, specifically in educational contexts, are as follows:

Evaluand. "The person, program, idea, policy, product, object, performance, or any other entity that you are evaluating" (Mertens and Wilson 2019, p. 5).

Merit. "The absolute or relative quality of the evaluand, either intrinsically or in regard to a particular criterion" (Mertens and Wilson 2019, p. 5).

Outcome. The change that occurs, either intended or unintended, resulting from a program.

Program. An intervention or collection of activities intended to produce change in the participant.

Standard. A target, used implicitly or explicitly, that marks the ideal state and is used to judge merit or worth (Giancola 2021, p. 5).

Worth. "The evaluand's value in a particular context" (Mertens and Wilson 2019, p. 5).

Part 5: Evaluation Purpose

The purposes of evaluation are myriad and complex. Depending on the size and scope of the evaluand or program, they can range from assessing learning outcomes for a particular class session to a final evaluation report for a multi-year grant. Rossi et al. (2019) list a variety of evaluation purposes that include program improvement, accountability, knowledge, and personal agendas. Understanding the purpose of the evaluation is critical to informing the design and scope of the evaluation.

Are you trying to assess the comprehension of a component in a chapter? Then the evaluation may be a test question. Are you trying to evaluate student abilities to synthesize and apply course information? Then possibly you are interested in a case study. Are you attempting to determine the knowledge that each student has acquired after an entire multi-year course of study? Then the evaluation may be a comprehensive examination. Finally, do you want to determine whether your program has effectively prepared students that have graduated for success in a professional capacity? Then an outcome evaluation may be the solution. Each of these is a form of evaluation that differs in complexity and purpose. Identifying what you need to know (evaluation purpose) helps you understand what type of evaluation you need. Also, knowing how the results of your evaluation activities will be used helps ensure that you are evaluating the correct criteria.

Part 6: Program Evaluation

While there are many types of evaluations in educational settings, program evaluation is a type of evaluation that leverages research methods to systematically investigate the structure, efficacy, and processes of programs. Often done in conjunction with grants or other types of funded activities, program evaluation is a domain of applied research that is systematic, focuses on operations and outcomes, is standards-centric, and is concerned with improving programs and policies (Giancola 2021). Rossi et al. define program evaluation as "the application of social research methods to systematically investigate the effectiveness of social intervention programs in ways that are adapted to their political and organizational environments and are designed to inform social action to improve social conditions" (2019, p. 6).

Part 7: Domains of Evaluations

Due to the frequency and utility of evaluations, there are numerous methods of classification and categorization. Rossi et al. (2019) define five primary domains of evaluation and provide corresponding questions that can be used to structure and plan evaluations.

a) *Needs assessments.* **Needs assessments** are an initial evaluation of a gap in services that is demonstrated by the persistence of a problem. Needs assessments should be done in advance of creating a program to understand the nature and magnitude of the problem, the characteristics of the population in need, desirable outcomes, and barriers to intervention. Needs assessments are guided by questions about the social conditions a program is designed to address, the need for the program, feasibility of the program, and an environmental scan to identify resources related to or in competition with the proposed program.

b) *Assessment of program theory and design.* Program theory assessment evaluates the assumptions and design of the program which are in place to bring about the desired change. **Program theory** is the theory of change and action that combine within the program design to elicit changes in the participants. Program theory assessments are guided by questions that focus on the nature of the activities, how the program is structured, and if that structure will bring about the desired change.

c) *Assessment of program process.* Program process assessments investigate how the program or element is delivered by personnel and experienced by participants. Process evaluations are often formative evaluations. **Formative evaluations** are conducted during program operations, and the results are used to make improvements and changes to the existing cycle or next cycle of the program. Process evaluations can also take the form of program monitoring or outcome monitoring to provide evidence of participant progress. Process evaluations are the most common type of program evaluation and are led by questions about program operations, implementation, and participant perceptions (Rossi et al. 2019).

d) *Effectiveness of the program.* Effectiveness evaluations are typically summative in nature. **Summative evaluations** assess the effectiveness and impact of the program and are often utilized to make decisions about continuation or termination of a program. **Outcome evaluations** specifically analyze if and to what extent program outcomes were realized. Impact evaluations take a larger view and investigate intended and unintended outcomes of the program (Giancola 2021). Questions that lead to effectiveness evaluations investigate the amount of change measured in participants in relation to intended program outcomes and the level at which the program contributed to that change.

e) *Cost analysis and efficiency assessment.* Efficiency assessments focus on a cost-benefit calculation to determine the cost of the program per participant in comparison to the benefits produced, and whether similar effects can be produced at a lower cost. Cost analyses and efficiency assessments include a careful accounting of all expenditures and consideration of cost-effectiveness of the program components and delivery.

Part 8: Evaluation in the Classroom

Educational evaluations are not always in the form of a large-scale program evaluation. Obviously, instructors evaluate students in the classroom on an ongoing basis and smaller scale. A variety of evaluation methods are discussed later in this textbook. However, let's consider the purposes for which we evaluate within a classroom setting.

f) *Learning outcomes.* **Learning outcomes** are the enduring concepts that instructors want students to understand at the conclusion of the course. These are typically included in the syllabus and represent the learning goals that the instructor has for the class. Learning outcomes are often phrased according to the level of thinking that is expected to occur during the class. Bloom's Taxonomy (Figure 10.1) provides a framework that is useful for developing learning outcomes. Using Bloom's Taxonomy to construct learning helps both instructors and students understand and clarify the purpose of the course. Additionally, learning outcomes help instructors plan and deliver content, design appropriate evaluations, and ensure that content and evaluation are in alignment with the objectives (Armstrong 2010).

g) *Curricular assessment.* Assessment in a curriculum involves documenting information about a student's learning. This includes many approaches to verify what the student "knows, understands, and can do with their knowledge and skills" (Rhode Island Department of Education 2022). Curricular assessment helps ensure that the curriculum, both at the institutional and classroom level, results in student learning. AAC&U's Teaching-Learning-Assessment framework is one of many examples of a systematic approach to assess teaching and learning in higher education (see link in Additional Resources section of this chapter). Embedding curriculum assessment in the regular planning and implementation of higher education is an important formative evaluation approach to improve student learning outcomes

h) *Action research.* Action research is a methodology developed by practitioners to provide empirical evidence regarding what is occurring within their operational context. **Action research** is any systematic inquiry conducted by educators to gather data on teaching, learning, and operation within a particular educational context (Mertler 2020). Data gathered in this process allows for insight, the development of reflective practice, effecting positive environmental and process change, and improving student learning (Mills 2018). Mertler (2020) indicates that, among others, action research is typified by the following characteristics:

- A focus on process improvement
- Collaboration involving educators/practitioners
- Participation and initiation by the practitioners
- Serving as a bridge between theory and practice
- Occurring in smaller contexts – often classrooms or workgroups
- Being conducted as a cyclical process of planning, acting, developing, and reflecting
- Involving critical reflection about one's own teaching practices

Action research allows educators an opportunity to conduct relevant, systematic inquiry to inform teaching practices in the future.

Part 9: Integrated Evaluation Planning

As mentioned in the introduction, embedding evaluative processes during planning helps ensure that evaluation results are being properly utilized to help improve the program and lead to desired program outcomes. Instructional design and program development should include evaluation planning during the initial phases.

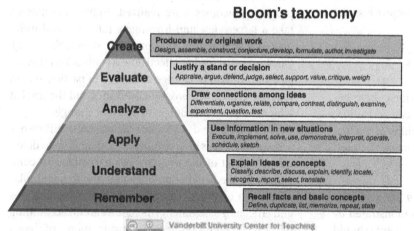

Figure 10.1 Bloom's taxonomy, Vanderbilt University Center for Teaching. *Source:* https://cft.vanderbilt.edu/guides-sub-pages/blooms-taxonomy/

i) *Backward design.* Instructors tend to design courses in a forward manner by planning activities, then assessments, then linking these to the course learning outcomes. Conversely, a backward design approach (Figure 10.2) starts with consideration of desired learning outcomes first, then assessment approaches, prior to planning activities (Bowen 2017). Jay McTighe, author of *Understanding by Design*, provides backward design templates and other resources for educators (https://jaymctighe.com/resources/).

j) *Integrated evaluation planning.* An integrated approach to evaluation in the classroom or learning environment helps increase the quality of data, the efficacy of evaluation efforts, the utility of the information, and ultimately the accomplishment of program goals or learning outcomes. Integrated evaluation incorporates multiple types and instances of evaluations, backward instructional design, and continual process improvement through the flow of evaluation data as depicted in Figure 10.3.

- *Phase 1.* Integrated evaluation begins with a needs assessment to confirm the existence of the knowledge gap, scan the environment for competing service, and assess the feasibility of the idea.
- *Phase 2.* The planning phase involves programmatic, instructional design, and evaluation planning integrating elements of backward design. Stage 1

consists of codifying the desired outcomes of the program. Stage 2 plans for the evidence necessary to demonstrate the desired outcomes. Stage 3 identifies the tactical activities that can viably produce the evidence needed for Stage 2.

- *Phase 3.* The implementation phase is where the program or lesson is implemented. Activity, process, and short and mid-term evaluations are integrated within program activities to provide formative information that is fed back into the planning processes to improve future cycles. At the conclusion of the program activities, summative evaluations are conducted with data from previous formative evaluations to determine program continuity or the need for substantive change.

Part 10: Conclusion

Evaluation in the classroom or other educational context is a critical component of assessment, accountability, and accreditation efforts within higher education. Understanding the types, utility, and process of evaluation helps ensure that your teaching efforts are not wasted and will allow you to gather the evidence needed to demonstrate the learning that is occurring in your program or classroom. Taking an integrated approach will help you and your team incorporate evaluation activities in a manner that is intuitive and not burdensome. We are already conducting many types of evaluations in our programs and classes, so intentionally planning those activities during the program design phase can help maximize time, effort, and quality within our programs.

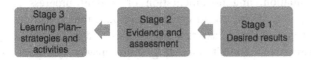

Figure 10.2 The three stages of backward design.

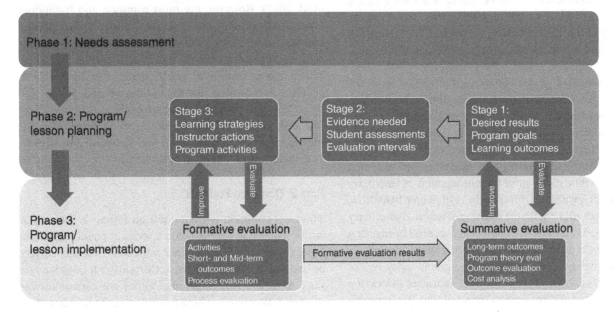

Figure 10.3 Integrating backwards design for program and evaluation planning.

Section 2: Writing Good Exam Questions

Patricia Butterbrodt

Part 1: Introduction

Assessing student knowledge is a daunting task, especially in such a vast pool of information required to be a competent veterinarian. Veterinary schools have affirmed at commencement ceremonies that students have sufficient knowledge to enter the profession for over a hundred years, conferring veterinary medical degrees on thousands of graduates. Yet common sense and practicality clearly indicate there is no possible manner in which the full body of knowledge needed to serve in a medical capacity even to one species, much less multiple species, can be assessed. Therefore, veterinary schools use a wide variety of assessment methods to verify that students are ready to step into the world of veterinary practice. One of the most common methods of assessing knowledge in any educational setting is the written exam, more recently replaced by the digital (computer-based) exam.

While there has been controversy about whether to assess veterinary knowledge by written exam, the fact remains that most veterinary schools still use exams as part of the student assessment in many courses. In this and most situations, the term "written exam" or "written assessment" includes computer-based online testing, where students are asked a question and must either select or write/type in the best answer for the question.

Before the nineteenth century, with the increase in population and therefore number of livestock, there was also an increase in animal plagues, including rabies, influenza, blackleg, Texas fever, and more. There was such a strong need for medical treatment of animals that "that from the founding of the first veterinary school in 1761 to the early part of the nineteenth century practically all of the countries of Europe had their veterinary schools." (Bierer 1940/2014, p. 66) The concept of animal medicine moved to the Americas in the late eighteenth century, when George Washington ordered copies of books on treating animal ailments, which became popular throughout the colonies. However, America continued to have "self-styled animal doctors and farriers (with their empirical and often destructive remedies)" until the introduction of veterinary medicine at Iowa State University in 1879 (Bierer 1940/2014, p. 70; Larkin 2011). With the opening of a formal veterinary school, assessments of learning became central to ensuring students were no longer those self-styled animal doctors.

Unfortunately, many veterinary programs today accept large (100+) cohorts of students, who often learn in lockstep for the first two or three years of their training. It is impractical and unrealistic to expect a veterinary school to assess student knowledge without some kind of evaluation, very often in the form of a written exam, although other assessments can and should be used, including carefully designed activity exams, such as an objective structured clinical exam (OSCE), and/or group projects. However, assessment of preclinical student knowledge now generally happens in a large group setting, with the individual student results being documented and used to move students through the training program and assuring they have the minimum knowledge and skills necessary to practice in the field.

> Assessment is used to measure student achievement of learning outcomes, rank students, maintain academic standards, direct student learning, provide feedback to students and staff, and to prepare students for life. Constructively aligned learning and assessment tasks ensure learners spend the focused time required to sequentially develop programme outcomes. Assessment by staff, peers, and other stakeholders certifies achievement of intended outcomes. Effective assessment also empowers students to define and achieve their own learning outcomes, so they develop the habits of autonomous life-long learning. Evaluation of the quality and consistency of achieved outcomes informs ongoing programme improvement. (Taylor 2009, p. 783)

Several types of assessments can be used for student evaluation, and documentation of student progress is required for successful matriculation into the profession. Several options of assessment are discussed in the CBVE Assessment Toolkit, including short answer questions, essays, direct observation of procedures (DOPs), OSCEs, and clinical evaluation exercises (CEXs) (Foreman et al. 2022). However, the most common and traditional type of assessment, especially in lecture- and lab-based courses, is the written exam. There are several aspects of writing exam questions. We will address format, including MCQs, choose all that apply (CATA), fill-in-the-blank (FITB), short answer, essay, and image-based. For MCQs, by far the most common format, we will also address clear and assessable stem writing, key selection, writing plausible distractors, and using post-exam statistical data to evaluate the effectiveness of an exam item.

Part 2: Question Formats

The most common written question format is a MCQ, in which a question is posed with a series of possible answers listed (distractors). The learner must select the one correct or best answer to the question. Currently, all questions on the NAVLE are MCQs and have either one correct answer or one answer that is a better solution to the problem than the other answers. The art of creating questions in the MCQ format is discussed at length in the next section.

Choose All That Apply (CATA)

A variation on the MCQ is the CATA or Select All That Apply format (CATA). In this case, a question is asked that has many correct answers, and the student must select all that are correct while not selecting answers that are incorrect. There may be two, three, or as many correct answers as are applicable, but this format may lead to guessing and, therefore, credit on a question when a student does not know the content. For example, if there are five choices, and three are correct, then if the student selects three or more choices, credit will be given for one or more correct answer. The item writer needs to have at least twice as many distractors as there are correct answers.

CATAs may be used by instructors as "trick questions," which sets up an unfair testing situation. When students see the prompt to "CATA," the natural implication is that more than one answer is correct. If the writer uses this format but only has one answer, the student by nature will want to select at minimum two answers, as the implied instructions indicate that is the case. In the same manner, using a CATA format and having all of the answers correct is basically writing an "All of the Above" question, and again, goes against the natural understanding of "CATA" as a process. Because of these issues, the CATA format should only be used when it is the only clear way to measure student understanding for a specific content. In these cases, it should be written carefully and fairly to avoid any "trick question" situations. For example, a question may ask what drug would be used to treat a certain condition. If there are three acceptable drugs for the condition, and the objective being assessed is "students will identify specific pharmaceuticals to treat specific conditions," then the CATA format could be appropriate to select those drugs. This is an excellent question option for faculty wanting to use the "not" question, asking "which of these drugs would NOT be used to treat the condition" and list the three plus one incorrect answer, as the "not" question is considered poor MCQ writing. Thus, the best measure of whether the students know the three drugs, if asked as a MCQ, would be to use the CATA format and provide six or more choices, with the three correct being among the choices. Although there is little to no literature covering the CATA format, in this author's experience, it has fairly strong results when used to replace poorly worded or otherwise poorly constructed MCQs.

Fill in the Blank (FITB)

For FITB, the question is asked and the student must come up with the answer, one word, number, or short phrase, on their own. In most exams with FITB, the student will write or type the answer and the faculty must then read through the answers and individually mark them. In the case of a computer-based testing program, there are usually options for a FITB question to be answered by artificial intelligence (AI), where the correct answer is entered into the program and students who type that answer are marked correct.

A FITB question requires more on the part of the student, as they must pull the answer from their own knowledge rather than recognize the answer from the choices. However, there is the time investment by the faculty that is necessary to grade a FITB question. It is nearly impossible to enter all possible versions of a correct answer into a computer program. For example, if the question asks about a species and the answer is "dog," the general expectation would be to enter "dog" as the answer. However, the answers given by the students could include not only other words (e.g., a dog, the dog, canine, a canine, and the canine) but most computer programs identify capitalization, in which case you now must include "dog, Dog, DOG, a dog, the dog, A dog, A Dog, A DOG, canine, Canine. . ." and so on. There is also punctuation that could be included, which now adds "dog. A dog. The dog. It's a dog. The answer is dog. Canine. A canine. . . ." and more to the list of correct answers. Therefore, if faculty choose to use FITB in their exams, they must be willing to put in the time needed to go through each answer and mark it correct or incorrect, as the testing program is limited in its preset correct answer choices. Much time could be saved by indicating in the stem whether the answer should be one word, a short phrase, a number (to how many decimals? Do they write the unit in the answer?), and any other hints on giving the answer that could lead the student to give the answer listed in the testing software.

Short Answer Questions

The short answer question is another format where students provide an answer in written form. Still student generated, it usually requires higher-level thinking than the basic FITB and requires more than one word or number to answer correctly. For a more involved answer, such as a short phrase or set of words, there will be far fewer "correct answers" in the computer program and much more time needed to read through the "incorrect" answers to find those that are correct but were not in the program. If the faculty is willing to put in the time for grading, short answer questions can be highly effective in showing student knowledge and understanding. According to Mujeeb et al. (2010), short answer questions "allow students more flexibility in their response and reflect their individuality of approach in which interpretative skills are developed" (p. 123). Their study demonstrated that multiple-choice scores were significantly higher than short answer scores in all groups – high achieving, low achieving, and those middle performers. In other words, students were better able to recognize a correct answer in a set of choices than they were able to provide the correct answer from their own knowledge. A study by Jonick et al. (2017) found an extreme disparity between the MCQ distractor and the incorrect answers provided in short answer formats. They felt this "indicated that the distracters often did not successfully anticipate how students would be reasoning when they answered incorrectly" (pp. 308–309) and suggested further review by faculty of these incorrect answers as a way to see how the students are free-thinking, which is "stifled when students are limited to only four options" (p. 309). At the Imperial College in London, the very short answer question is used, as they have found that "where MCQs may reward students for a superficial knowledge, VSAs demand a deeper understanding of concepts" (Kalkat et al. 2017, p. 411).

Essay Questions

Essay questions are much more involved than FITB or short answer questions when it comes to grading. Essay questions involve the student understanding the question being asked, then having to think through both any information provided in the stem and their learned knowledge. The student must then write out not only their answer but some kind of justification for that answer. While these are the easiest questions to write for an exam, they are the most difficult to grade; therefore, it is important to determine whether your time is best served by creating well-written questions that are easily and quickly graded beforehand or by reading through and grading each individual essay afterward. The essay is, in fact, the best way for the faculty to assess the student's application and evaluation processes. However, these questions must be very carefully created to avoid ambiguity and misunderstanding. In a study by Shilo (2015), 1500 exam questions were reviewed for flaws and were found to have such problems as leading questions, inaccurate use of action verbs, poorly formulated questions, and unclear questions due to lack of direction or instruction. The study found many essay questions that should be presented as several shorter and clearer questions rather than one long complex question. Her conclusion is that "we must ask questions that are clearly understood from every aspect and detail exactly what the examiner expects" (p. 27).

While an essay could be a good indicator of student knowledge and understanding, grading essay questions is a very delicate process; one that requires a well-designed, clear, detailed rubric to avoid accusations of being unfair, subjective, or showing favoritism. Once again, the biggest challenge for faculty is the time involved in creating a strong rubric and grading the essays. With most veterinary schools having classes of 100 or more students, grading one essay question could take several hours, if not days.

Image-Based Questions

One format that has come into the realm of computer-based testing within the past decade is the image-based or "hot spot" question. This is where the student is asked to identify and click on something on an image such as a bone, artery, muscle, or even a toxic plant in the field. In many computer-based testing programs, one can upload an image and indicate with a circle, square, or rectangle where the correct answer is in the image. The student moves the cursor over their answer and clicks, and the program indicates whether the click was within the indicated area (correct) or not in the answer area (incorrect). This can be a useful question format for simple recall questions such as identification in anatomy, surgery, or pathology, as it only requires the student to know how the correct answer "looks" as opposed to writing a descriptive paragraph. Image identification questions can save time on exams both on the part of the faculty writing the question and the student answering it.

However, the drawback to this type of question is the limit of the shape to be considered correct. For example, if the image is of cells seen on a microscope, and the cell in question is oval and near or overlapping others, the square box indicating the correct cell could include pieces of other cells. If the student is to identify a toxic leaf in a picture of a field, unless the box indicating the correct answer has the same shape as the leaf, it is impossible to limit the correct area to that leaf alone. This can be mitigated by specific instructions, such as "click on the center of the leaf that is toxic to a horse."

Conclusion

Each of the formats listed here can be used on an assessment to effectively determine the results of learning outcomes. Some information being assessed may lend itself more toward one format or another, but with thought and practice, you can become familiar with which format is more appropriate to assess student learning of the information you are responsible for delivering. Ultimately, the most commonly used format is the MCQ, because this is the most efficient for assessing large groups of students quickly and it is the question type found on the NAVLE. It is important to keep in mind that while multiple-choice exams are the most efficient, they are not necessarily the easiest for faculty to execute well, as you will learn in the next section.

Part 3: The Multiple-Choice Exam

Some believe exams in a veterinary program should mirror the layout of the NAVLE, others argue that real life is not multiple-choice, as in practice there are no questions presented in this format. Additionally, students are not limited to what they know, as they have access to almost unlimited information via the Internet, textbooks, and colleagues. While there is a basic body of knowledge a veterinarian should know ("walk around knowledge"), veterinarians are also regularly presented with unusual or uncommon situations, whether that is an unusual disease or a species they are not as familiar with.

It is impossible for anyone to hold in their mind every bit of information presented in every lecture and lab during any program, and this is magnified in professional programs such as veterinary school. However, while in their program, students must be assessed on course content. Thus, the selection of content to be assessed must be carefully considered. For this reason, faculty should present as much applicable content as possible during lectures and labs, but in deciding what questions to use on a test, only content that is expected of a recent graduate and applies going into general practice should be assessed.

The learning objectives presented at the start of a lecture or lab should indicate the most important content from that session and for assessing such learning objectives, the MCQ is an appropriate option. However, creating an effective MCQ, one that measures mastery of a learning objective, involves time and effort as well as training on the part of the instructor. The upside is that a set of well-designed questions, once used and demonstrated to be reliable and valid, can be the basis for a question bank from which the instructor can pick and choose in the future.

When the National Board of Veterinary Medical Education (NBVME) was created in 1948, it was to provide a veterinary-focused mirror to the National Board of Medical Education (NBME), founded in 1915, to develop and manage licensing exams for those entering the human medical field. The NBVME devoted its efforts to develop and manage licensing exams for those entering the multi-species veterinary medical field and based much of its foundation and information on what was already known through the NBME. The NBVME actively collaborated with the NBME and continues to do so today.

The NBME continually updates its Item Writing Guide, which is in its sixth edition as of 2021. When creating exam items for testing, the NBME bases its guidelines on both peer-reviewed research publications and on their own research results, having been involved in years of reviewing countless MCQs, working with hundreds of item writing committees, and providing training for hundreds of individual item writers. In their guide, they state "we can personally attest that each committee and workshop attendee has helped us examine our methods, rethink our arguments, and better frame our thoughts regarding how to write high-quality test items" (NBME, p. 5). The NBME continues to research the most effective practices in testing, both written and now online, to provide the most accurate and effective representation of student knowledge. When creating new versions of the medical exams used by the NBME, item writers must first complete extensive training in how to write effective MCQs. It is the cumulation of the research and the training guide of the NBME that is also used by the NBVME to create the NAVLE, and these guidelines are available to any faculty at a medical education institution for use in creating their own assessment items. The stated purpose of the manual is "to help faculty members across health professions improve the quality of the multiple-choice items they write" (NBME 2021, p. 5).

Research has shown that well-meaning faculty have long been using MCQs for student evaluation, only to later discover these questions are inherently faulty. Caldwell and Pate (2013) showed that questions that deviate from specific item-writing guidelines "can result in poorer student performance on questions with no increased benefit if differentiating higher- from lower-performing students" (p. 71). In two research studies by Tarrant and Ware (2008) and Cook et al. (2020), it was found that the questions used in assessments had issues that either kept students from being able to select the best answer or were presented in a manner that allowed students who did not know the content to answer the question correctly. Tarrant and Ware's (2008) study of high-stakes nursing assessments found that 48% of the questions were identified as having testing flaws. Additionally, "the trend toward discipline-specific higher education in nursing and other health science disciplines means that few academics today have had any formal preparation in educational assessment methods such as item construction" (p. 202). And in a study of assessments in veterinary medicine, Cook et al. (2020) demonstrated that more than 30% of the questions reviewed were flawed, with 43% being identified as flawed by one or more of the reviewers. They found "that instructors at this veterinary school may benefit from information regarding optimal question construction and training in the identification of common flaws in questionings" (p. 502). The authors of each of these studies encourage faculty to learn more about writing effective assessment items.

A test-taker's probability of answering an item correctly should be determined by his or her amount of expertise on the topic being assessed; ideally, that probability will not decrease due to a poorly written item and will not increase due to test-taking strategies (NBME 2021). Research studies showed that the high achievers will continue to perform at a high level, and the low achieving students will continue to perform at a low level, but it is the borderline students who benefit from flawed items, with a greater proportion passing than would have if flawed items were removed. At the same time, it is more often the high achievers whose results are lowered due to poorly written exam items (Tarrant and Ware 2008). Research also shows that item-writing flaws may increase an item's difficulty while decreasing the same item's discriminatory ability (Ali and Ruit 2015). "This means that some MCQs may be unnecessarily difficult due to factors unrelated to the content tested" (Biblier et al. 2017, p. 793).

Faculty can learn to write MCQs that effectively assess student knowledge. Research and experience have shown some clear issues in item writing and studies have identified best practices for faculty to use. By applying the following guidelines, MCQ assessments can be created that are accurate and effective measures of student learning.

Part 4: Writing Effective Multiple-Choice Questions (MCQs)

The Stem

The stem of a question is the piece that includes any background information and data and has the actual question being asked. While the stem could be one sentence or a paragraph with charts and images, the actual question should be asked as an interrogative ending with a question mark. The following are a few issues in the stem that may cause a question not to accurately measure student knowledge.

The Question Is Unanswerable Without Choices

An MCQ has a set of choices from which to select a correct answer, but the student should be able to answer the question without having a list. To truly assess content knowledge, questions should be assessing a specific learning objective, and the question should have one best or one correct answer. It is unfair to the student and a poor indication of the objective to have a question with multiple correct answers or a question for which the student must read through all of the answers and decide, one at a time, if this is true or false, and if another answer is better or "more true" than the one first read. These types of questions are not assessing a single objective, and if the student does not select the correct answer, does not indicate the level of knowledge in the other objectives listed.

For example, the question "Which of the following is true in a ferret?" has infinite answers, and one must read through all of the choices and basically answer "true or false" for each of them. The student does not know what objective is being assessed, and therefore cannot use their knowledge to process their thinking while looking through the answers. Likewise, the question "Which of the following is an NSAID?" has multiple answers, and rather than have one answer in mind that the student is searching for, the student must read through all answers to find which of the many NSAIDs is listed in this item. It takes time, it could be misleading, and it is a flawed question. Be sure exam items can be answered with the desired answer without having to read the choices.

Use of a Negative Stem

Most professionals have seen or written the negative stem. These questions do not ask the student to identify a correct answer but rather to identify the answer that is incorrect. When asking "which of the following is NOT . . ." one is actually requiring the student to answer true/false questions for each of the options. Unfortunately, it is much easier to create a negative question than to find a way to ask a question that shows mastery of the content in many cases. However, the research continues to show that a negative stem is inherently flawed, often overlooked by the nervous test taker, and can make the questions more difficult (NBME 2021; Rush et al. 2016; Tarrant and Ware 2008).

The only time a negative stem could be considered appropriate is in the case of a specific and unusual situation, such as giving a cat acetaminophen. In this case, the word "contraindicated" should be used, rather than a negative such as "NOT" or "NO" in the sentence. Other than such unique and rare medical situations, the question being asked should look for the correct answer, not an incorrect one.

Asking More Than One Question At a Time

When presenting content, it is a common practice to group information. For example, a parasite, its commonly transmitted conditions, its habitat, the species it affects, and how to eliminate it. When creating exam items for this content, you might be tempted to ask "What is this parasite and where does it live?" or "What disease does this parasite transmit and how do you treat cattle for this parasite?" The flaw in this question is that it is assessing two (or more) objectives. Are you assessing parasite identification? Are you assessing how cows get a certain disease? Or are you assessing which parasites are responsible for zoonotic diseases?

Each question should assess one and only one objective. This decreases the cognitive load for the student, increases its validity and reliability, and helps you if several students miss the question because you can identify a weakness in the instruction of that objective. Otherwise, depending on how the choices are written, the results do not show specifically which of the objectives the student knows and which they do not know.

Superfluous Information Is Included

This guideline is somewhat flexible, depending on the objective being assessed and the educational level of the student. For a first-year veterinary student in physiology, a straightforward question about the function of a vessel should be short and clear. However, for a third-year veterinary student in surgery, a question discussing a condition and possible surgery in the area of the vessel might also be asking if the student understands what the function of the vessel is. In an early case study, the history and clinical signs of a problem could be included in the stem. Later in the curriculum, a case study could include a complete history, the results of multiple diagnostic tests, and possible treatments. Near the end of their curriculum, students need to be able to sort through more complex information and identify what is relevant to the question being asked.

In general, however, there are times that information in the stem is unnecessary, takes time for the student to read, and could actually mislead or distract the student from the important information. For example, regardless of placement in the curriculum, a case study regarding a dog that was shot with buckshot does not need to include details about the little boy who saw the event and how mean the neighbor is. Only present the information needed to diagnose and treat the animal.

The Answer Choices Are Longer Than the Stem

Put as much information as possible in the stem. Give the student all the information and any relevant data in the stem, leaving only the answer to the question as the choices. Once the stem is read, the student should have an idea of what the correct answer is and should be able to quickly find the correct answer among the choices. If too much information is in the choices, students may forget what the question was or veer away from the focus of the question. As a result, they may answer incorrectly because their mind was trying to take in all the information in each of the choices rather than because they did not know the content. Identify the objective that is to be assessed, create a question that asks about that objective, and present succinct logical choices from which to choose an answer.

The Distractors

When writing an MCQ, there is one correct answer and a selection of incorrect answers. The correct answer is known as the key and the incorrect answers are called distractors. For a well-written exam item, the most difficult task is creating the distractors. Some people are very test-savvy and able to answer MCQs correctly even without content knowledge, based on subtle (or not so subtle) clues in the way a question is written. Sometimes the distractors will give away the correct answer without having to read the stem. Knowing these clues and writing distractors to avoid them takes time and energy, but results in better exams.

The purpose of the distractors is to appear as tempting solutions to the problem; plausible competitors of the answer for students who do not achieve the objective measured by the test item (Torres et al. 2011). Taking the time to write good distractors will result in assessments that accurately show student mastery of the objectives with questions that are valid and reliable. Distractors should match in length, logic, and syntax and represent realistic incorrect decision-making on the part of the students. There are a few guidelines to follow in writing effective distractors.

Have a Reasonable Number of Distractors

MCQs can come with any number of possible answers. Only having two to choose from does not serve well psychometrically, as students have a 50–50 chance of guessing the answer; this is one of many reasons why a true-false question is not considered an ideal question type for sound assessment. On the other hand, having too many choices usually include what are called nonfunctioning distractors, or those seldom chosen by testers, and therefore only serve as causing time to be lost in reading through and eliminating them (Tarrant and Ware 2008; Ali and Ruit 2015; Haladyna et al. 2019).

Research has been done on how many distractors provide the optimum presentation of true student knowledge. In a review of 20 years of research on MCQs, the team of Haladyna et al. (2019) found results that varied on how many distractors provided the best difficulty, discrimination, and reliability for questions. While some of the evaluations were contradictory, they all had a common theme – distractors must be plausible to be included on an exam to ensure results are an accurate reflection of student knowledge.

Effective distractors create more discriminating exams, but truly plausible distractors are difficult to create. The research does support that as few as two plausible distractors, along with a key, provides reliable valid assessment results (Ali and Ruit 2015). There is little difference between having three, four, or five choices for an MCQ, and if distractors are being added simply to reach a minimum number, it is more academically sound to leave off implausible answers. "The effort of developing that fourth option (the third plausible distractor) is probably not worth it. If the use of four options is preferred, empirical research has established that it is very unlikely that item writers can write three distractors that have item response patterns consistent with the idea of plausibility" (Haladyna et al. 2002, p. 318). The practice of using four options on an MCQ is generally based more on tradition than evidence. According to one research study, "Usually teachers use four option distractors either because it is the traditional practice which they have been accustomed to, or it is the practice adopted by their college, or they feel it covers a large amount of content in the curriculum. There is no doubt that more distractors, if well designed, will add to the reliability of the test" (Rahma et al. 2017, p. 290). But if the distractors are not well designed, are obviously incorrect, or are there as an attempt at humor or frivolity, the distractor adds nothing to the exam, is eliminated quickly, and has served no purpose. In short, it is better to have three choices – two plausible distractors along with the key – than to include a fourth option that has no relevance and students will likely ignore.

Save Humor for the Lectures

First and foremost, distractors must be logical and possible answer to the question. It is tempting to include a nonsense or humorous answer as a distractor to help students relax and give them a chuckle as they test. However, this can backfire. An implausible distractor will rarely or never be chosen and only serves to waste the valuable testing time of the student (NBME 2021).

As an example that actually occurred, a food animal class had a lab away from campus to handle sheep on a certain farm. One student was not able to attend this event but watched the videos and thought she understood what was being experienced. On the exam covering this material, a question was asked about the location of certain plants toxic to sheep. One of the distractors was "Old MacDonald's Farm" and the student was very flustered because she thought that might have been the name of the farm they visited, that the plant had been found there, and it was pointed out to the class on the visit. She selected that response because to her it made more sense than to have a silly children's song on an exam.

Humor absolutely has a place in education; any faculty who has spent time with students knows not to take themselves too seriously and to show students that being a veterinarian has its fun moments and moments so bizarre they can only be handled with a laugh. An exam is not the place for this humor, however; with the pressure on veterinary students to know so much and such varied content, an exam presents enough stress and anxiety on its own without having to decide if someone was trying to be funny or if the student missed something that could lead to this answer. Use humor in lectures and labs – just keep the assessments as realistic and reasonable as possible.

Match Distractors in Length and Logic

One of the most common test-taking clues is to select the answer that is longest or shortest. This is a common but natural mistake that item writers make. For example, in creating distractors and correct responses, you might give more than just a single-word answer, such as "ibuprofen to reduce the swelling," but then not do the same with the other potential responses. If the key has a medication and its action, then the distractors should do the same. For example, "(A) acetaminophen to reduce the fever, (B) amoxicillin to kill the bacteria."

Other common mistakes include:

- the key having a second part, such as a cause or an action, while the distractors do not
- the key having a letter and a number, while the distractors have either a letter or a number.
- the key being rounded to the two decimals and the distractors being rounded to one decimal.

If there are not enough plausible options to make three or four that all match, then the suggestion is to have four choices, with two matching and the other two matching. There could be two antibiotics and two NSAIDs, or two results from a blood test and two results from a urine test.

If the question is for treatment and the key is a drug with a dosage, be sure the other drugs have a dosage with them. As long as two are visually similar and the other two are visually similar, the question can still be effective. If the question asks for a location on the body, and two answers are left ear and right ear, the other two might be right shoulder and left shoulder, but again, they should match in length and logic.

The important point is not to have one answer that is obviously different from the others. Some students will select the different answer simply because it is different. Other students will avoid that answer, again simply because it is different. Students should be selecting an answer by their knowledge of the objective being assessed, not by a visual clue they think is in a set of answers. By avoiding this unmatched outlier, effective item writers are actually helping students show their mastery of the content rather than their prowess as a test taker (NBME 2021).

Specificity in Numbers

If a question is asking for a numerical answer, avoid overlapping numbers. Even if a lecture clearly states a range (kittens become playful between three and five weeks), overlapping times could be argued as correct because part of the time is in the correct range. If the answer is 3–5, do not use 2–4 as a distractor, because it can be argued that 3 and 4 are in both sets of ranges and are correct.

If asking students to calculate an answer (e.g., a drug dosage), be specific about the calculation being requested. The distractors for calculations need to be logical and plausible values that could be calculated with the given information. For example, if the numbers given in the stem are 10, 4, and 3, then plausible answers could include 120 (10*4*3); 17 (10 + 4 + 3), 22 (3*4 + 10), 34 (10*3 + 4), 43 (10*4 + 3), 18 ((10 − 4)*3), and more. But it is not plausible for the numbers 10, 4, and 3 to produce the number 15. Use the numbers in the formula and do it incorrectly to come up with plausible distractors.

When creating numerical distractors, do not create "trick" distractors, such as 3.1, 3.14, and 3.14159 – which are actually the same value, rounded to different decimals. In summary, make your distractors obviously different from the key but plausible enough that someone who is not sure of the content might consider a correct answer.

Avoid Using All or None of the Above as Possible Responses

Psychometric research on all of the above (AOTA) and none of the above (NOTA) questions has shown that these types of questions are not strong indicators for assessing student knowledge (Rush et al. 2016; NBME 2021). In the case of AOTA, the student does not need to know if all the choices are true, they need only know that at least two are true, so the other distractors become irrelevant. In addition, most AOTA questions are asking about multiple objectives and are therefore already flawed.

None of the above questions are flawed for the opposite reason. Students must determine if one of the questions is correct, but if more than one is incorrect, the other distractors become irrelevant, as with AOTA. Additionally, if NOTA is the key, students are not demonstrating what they know, they are simply demonstrating that they know those answers are incorrect. Therefore, if one of the choices is the correct answer, then the distractor "none of the above" is not needed. Ultimately, then, these questions are not assessing the objectives. In fact, research has demonstrated negative psychometric results from these types of questions, supporting that AOTA and NOTA questions are not psychometrically sound (Pachai et al. 2015; Odegard and Koen 2007).

Avoid K-Type Questions

For a while, these K-type questions were popular because there was a belief that they made the test taker think harder about the question. A K-type question has three or four answer options for answers with possible responses being "A Only," "B Only," "A and B Only," "B and C Only," "A and C Only," and so on. Research on this type of question has shown them to be time-intensive because students will read and reread through the options several times, deciding for each one if it is true or not. K-type questions can also cause confusion because they insinuate that a question could have more than one answer, which could be better addressed as a CATA type question. The K-type question is confusing, raises stress in the test taker, and should not be used (NBME 2021).

Part 5: An Alternative Idea – Students Writing Multiple-Choice Questions

It has been mentioned several times that creating a good MCQ involves time and effort. One must not only know the correct answer to a question but must know enough about the content to be able to identify two or three incorrect answers that are plausible. This depth of knowledge is required and expected of the faculty. But using this same expectation on the part of students could be a valuable tool for formative assessment and student learning.

An alternative to the faculty creating the questions is to allow the students to create multiple choice questions on the content. This practice has become more popular in the past decade, as faculty recognize the implications of item writing. The creator of a question must have a strong understanding of the content, as well as be able to recognize what parts of the lecture or lab are important enough to include on an assessment. This would, of course, depend on the student learning objectives identified in the lecture or lab, but while faculty may think that is quite obvious, many are surprised at what the students' interpretation of the objective actually is.

Having students create their own MCQs allows students to "study" (i.e., reinforce learning) with a direct application of the information that was presented, while giving them the freedom of creating their own set of distractors. This one task alone shows the faculty the level of understanding. In a study by Grainger, it was found that "Student-generated questions can also highlight when students have a flawed understanding of the course material more effectively than students' answers to MCQs, and thus provide a formative opportunity to address misconceptions" (Grainger et al. 2018, p. 2). His study required the students not only to write the question with distractors, but to give the justification for why each distractor was plausible but incorrect. He found that "although students did not enjoy the challenging MCQ-generating process, the quality of the question repository and reported problem-solving strategies may indicate engagement with the course material." (Grainger et al. 2018, pp. 6–7).

A literature review on student-generated questions was conducted by a team of medical school instructors. Their findings support the value of having students create the questions. "MCQs-generation exercise broadly improved students' grades. Some studies reported that low performers benefited more from the process of writing MCQs, concordantly with the findings of other studies which indicate that activities promoting active learning advantage lower-performing students more than higher-performing ones. Also, guiding students to write MCQs makes it possible to test higher-order skills as application and analysis besides recall and comprehension" (Touissi et al. 2021, p. 10).

It may seem to some as a tempting way for an instructor to avoid having to create MCQs, but in reality the practice does have educational value, helps reinforce the content for the students who write the questions, and gives the instructor a good indication of the depth of understanding of the students. The findings of employing higher-order skills as application combined with improving lower-performing students' learning give a strong validation for this activity. At the same time, for those well-written questions, it is a way to increase the question bank for use in future classes.

Part 6: The Final Check for a Good Question

Professional program students have traditionally been rewarded for high grades, which are usually determined by test performance. No matter how much we work to get students to be less concerned with grades, they have been conditioned this way for many years and, when they feel they have not earned the grade they felt they should, will often request, sometimes forcefully, that their incorrect answer be considered for at least partial credit.

The best way to prepare for such student pushback is to be able to defend the correct answer while having a clear and specific explanation for why each of the distractors is not the best answer. As each distractor is written, try to verbally express why this answer is incorrect and attempt to understand how a student might be drawn to it as the correct one. This process can help faculty avoid what students term "trick questions" that rely on trivial knowledge or content. Students are looking at your learning objectives; to defend a distractor as being incorrect, your explanation should rely on those clear objectives.

Conclusion

Veterinary instructors want students to succeed and become competent professionals; this involves presenting content and assessing student mastery of that content. Therefore, it should be the goal of veterinary instructors to create valid, reliable, and effective questions to use on exams that will both accurately assess student knowledge and prepare students to pass the NAVLE prior to graduation.

Research has shown that multiple-choice exam questions can be accurate measures of student mastery of objectives (Xu et al. 2016; Biblier et al. 2017; Jonick et al. 2017; NBME 2021). Research has also given examples of specific guidelines for writing questions that are effective, fair, and high-performing (NBME 2021). By taking the time to write good exam items, caring faculty can be assured that students have the knowledge needed to move forward in their academics toward their professional career goals.

Section 3: Exams and Quizzes: Determining Validity and Reliability

Katrina Jolley

Part 1: Introduction

Creating high-quality written exams and quizzes starts with creating a blueprint of both the specific lecture or lab content to be assessed and the types of questions that will be used in the assessment. A course exam may use a combination of multiple-choice and open-response questions to assess student learning from a series of lectures on the cardiovascular system while a quiz may use a small set of FITB questions to assess a student's ability to calculate anesthetic drug dosages. Each serves a different purpose, and the student results from those assessments may have different expectations.

Once the questions have been written and the exam has been given, the next step is to process the results and determine how well the assessment performed. Did the students answer the questions correctly? Did the exam or quiz measure the student learning that was intended? What are the next steps if the exam did not go as planned? Those questions seem very simple on the surface, but they can be quite daunting when it comes time to review the assessment outcomes data.

Exam validity is used to measure how well the exam material assessed what it was intended to assess. This is influenced heavily by both how the questions were written and how well the questions link to the learning objectives. The validity of each item on the exam or quiz contributes to the overall exam validity; the individual components combine to form the whole (Ryans 1939; Flanagan 1939). Reliability refers to how stable an item or exam's results are over time (Phelan and Wren 2006; Bannigan and Watson 2009). The validity and reliability of a set of exam questions are used together to create high-quality assessments.

Validity

Bannigan and Watson (2009) define validity as "the degree to which a scale measures what it is intended to measure" (p. 3238). Validity can be determined qualitatively through faculty review of the exam questions and overall assessment structure. Quantitatively validity can be measured through the "product-moment correlation coefficient" (Flanagan 1939, p. 677). Content validity (face validity), criterion validity (concurrent and predictive validity), and construct validity (convergent, divergent, factorial, and discriminant validity) are the primary types of validity that Bannigan and Watson (2009) use to review and analyze assessments.

Content validity is dependent on content experts (namely, faculty) to determine if the questions are appropriate for the exam or quiz. This includes ensuring that the assessment "has included all the relevant and excluded irrelevant issues in terms of its content" (Bannigan and Watson 2009, p. 3240). Face validity refers to how the questions or assessment as a whole appear on the surface level. It is "the requirement that examinations appear to measure what is popularly understood from the title" (Flanagan 1939, p. 677). Both those who are taking the exam and those who will use the results rely on face validity to ensure that the exam is assessing what it claims to assess (Walsh and Betz 2001). For the purposes of written exams and quizzes in an academic setting, content validity and face validity can be used interchangeably because written assessments should have a great deal of transparency.

Content validity for an assessment can be determined with the help of a carefully defined exam blueprint. Walsh and Betz (2001) recommend including very specific details about what is and is not included in the assessment. Checking that each test question properly links to the learning objectives is a clear and straightforward way to make sure that the assessment as a whole has both content validity and face validity. It is better to check that all exam and quiz questions have a high degree of content validity before the exam is given than it is to wait until the results are back to find out that a large portion of questions did not assess the content that was intended (Bannigan and Watson 2009).

Criterion validity is used to compare a new assessment with an assessment that "has been established as valid" (Bannigan and Watson 2009, p. 3241). Walsh and Betz (2001) described two types of criterion validity: predictive validity and concurrent validity. Predictive validity is used to make determinations on how current performance on a test predicts future performance in the criteria. Concurrent validity measures the relationship between current performance on the test and current performance in the criteria. Placement tests at the beginning of a semester use predictive validity to make assumptions about future performance in an academic area based on current performance on the placement test. When reviewing criterion validity of an assessment, if the correlation between the test and the criterion is "zero or in a direction other than that predicted, the criterion-related validity of our test is cast in doubt" (Walsh and Betz 2001, p. 59).

Construct validity measures the relationship between the assessment under development and the concept it is intended to assess. Carmines and Zeller (1979) describe construct validity as a way to compare an assessment in development with an assessment that has already been determined to be valid. Construct validity includes convergent, divergent, factorial, and discriminant validity (Bannigan and Watson 2009). Discriminant validity is the most applicable type of construct validity to written exams and quizzes because it is used to measure the difference between groups of students. By measuring the difference in assessment performance of upper and lower groups of students, "the more definitely can it be concluded that an item is valid by finding that the upper group is more successful in passing it than the lower group" (Kelley 1939, p. 17). Written assessments should be constructed with questions that are able to discriminate between high-performing and low-performing students.

Reliability

Phelan and Wren (2006) define reliability as "the degree to which an assessment tool produces stable and consistent results" (n.p.). Reliability is measured in how well an assessment "will give the same results on separate occasions" (Bannigan and Watson 2009, p. 3238). Reliability can be measured by giving the same assessment multiple times to different groups of students or by measuring the results between two tests that assess the same content with different questions (ExamSoft 2021b, Validity and Reliability). Carmines and Zeller (1979) found that "the more consistent the results given by repeated measurements, the higher the reliability of the measuring

procedure; conversely the less consistent the results, the lower the reliability" (p. 12).

Test-retest reliability involves administering the same test to the same group of students at two different times. In the field of psychology, test-retest is used to measure the reliability of participant responses. In the field of education, test-retest can be used to measure student growth before and after a unit of study or to confirm student retention of the material assessed. Bannigan and Watson (2009) found that when retesting with the same groups of participants, test-retest reliability can be influenced by participant memory of the first administration. They cautioned that "subjects may not be as careful when using a scale a second time" (p. 3239).

Inter-item reliability is used to measure the internal consistency of an assessment. There are a variety of procedures and mathematical formulas for "measuring the internal consistency including the 'split-half technique', 'Chronbach's alpha' (or 'coefficient alpha') and the 'Kuder-Richardson formula 20' (KR-20)" (Bannigan and Watson 2009, p. 3239). Richardson and Kuder (1939) found that the reliability of the split-half technique was directly related to the way the test was split. Because the standard deviations of the two halves were often unequal, the results were "rather unsatisfactory in practice" (p. 681). Walsh and Betz (2001) cautioned that if the split-half technique were to be used to determine reliability, the split should be made in a way that creates equivalent halves such as "to assign the odd-numbered items to one half and the even-numbered items to the other half" (pp. 51–52). As a means to rectify the inconsistencies in the split-half technique in the 1930s, Richardson and Kuder developed the formula known as KR-20 to measure reliability of dichotomously scored items such multiple-choice and true/false items (items that are right or wrong, yes or no). Determining the reliability of items that are rated on a scale or continuum (such as "strongly agree" to "strongly disagree") is best calculated by using Cronbach's alpha (Walsh and Betz 2001). For more information on how Cronbach's alpha is calculated, see *Statistics for People Who Think They Hate Statistics* by Salkind (2013).

Interrater reliability is used when the same grading scale will be used by multiple content experts at the same time to grade the assessment (Bannigan and Watson 2009). Assessment of hands-on clinical skills and interpersonal professional skills depend on interrater reliability to make sure that the students' skills are being appropriately assessed by the faculty graders and that no one person is grading more harshly than another when using the same grading scale. Determining interrater reliability can also be applied to high-stakes essays, papers, and oral exams if there will be more than one faculty member assessing the students' work.

For exams with a single grader, reliability can also be determined by using alternate forms of the same assessment. Alternate forms reliability is measured by comparing the difference in results from two sets of questions that cover the same learning objectives, administered to two groups of students (Walsh and Betz 2001). Walsh and Betz (2001) cautioned assessment creators to take care when selecting the items for the two forms. "The two forms should contain the same number and type of items and, in tests of ability or achievement, should be approximately equal in difficulty" (p. 51).

Purpose of Validity and Reliability

When used together validity and reliability ensure that the exam or quiz measures what was intended. This can be achieved by making sure that the questions are well written, do not contain any structural flaws, and align with the learning objectives. Thorndike (1982) recommends creating a detailed list of what material should and should not be included in the test with an emphasis on the amount of content covert for each portion of the overall material. Defining the list of learning objectives that will be assessed in the exam or quiz helps the faculty make sure that the questions used adequately cover the content intended. This exam blueprint is further strengthened when "those objectives are themselves clearly and explicitly defined" (Thorndike 1982, p. 185).

For written exam and quiz questions, item validity can be established before item reliability because reliability is dependent on item validity. Newly written questions should have content validity before they are used in an assessment. Reused questions should also have a measure of discriminant validity to make sure that the questions are able to discriminate between higher and lower-performing students. Thorndike (1982) found that a question's ability to discriminate between higher and lower-performing students was especially important when using test questions to place students in remediation or honors courses. Walsh and Betz (2001) cautioned that "if a test does not yield a range of scores, it does not provide us with information about individual differences in the attribute or trait of interest" (p. 73).

The inter-item reliability of the exam questions can be established once the questions have been retested over the course of several administrations of the assessment. Individual exam questions that consistently produce the same results when used on tests that assess the same set of lectures from year to year can be considered to have a high degree of reliability. Inconsistent results may indicate either a problem with the question or with the way the material was presented (e.g., content sequence shifted so that there was less cross-discipline overlap in content, or a course that historically used homework and quizzes before an exam no longer including those formative assignments).

Test-retest reliability in the academic setting is measured when administering the same test containing the same set of questions on a repeated basis. This typically occurs when a faculty member uses the same questions year after year to assess a particular set of lectures. Unfortunately, the reliability of such exams can be misleading as students may come to predict which questions will be asked on the exams when the same questions are used year after year. It is better to use alternate forms of the test or quiz and introduce new questions each time the material is assessed.

Part 2: Using Assessment Data to Measure Validity and Reliability

Most learning management systems (LMS) and testing software platforms provide psychometrics on how the exam or quiz performed. Psychometrics are "essential statistical measures that provide exam writers and administrators with an industry-standard set of data to validate exam reliability, consistency, and quality" (ExamSoft How to Measure Test Validity and Reliability 2021b, n.p.). These are calculated based on how each student performed on each question in the assessment, and they should be used to determine if the exam or quiz performed as expected (ExamSoft Guide to the Statistics 2021a). The assessment's item analysis report shows a breakdown of each question on the assessment and the overall class performance. Some of the most common psychometrics shown on the item analysis are the difficulty (percent correct), discrimination index, point biserial, and the KR-20. These, along with the exam's mean, median, minimum, and maximum scores, can be used to identify questions that may have been confusing or misleading to students.

The item's difficulty or p value is the proportion of students who answered the question correctly. The p value is written in decimal form and can be interpreted as the question's average percent correct. A question with a p value of 0.5 means that 50% of the students answered the question correctly. Walsh and Betz (2001) found that items with a p value of 1.0 are likely too easy for the group, and items with a p value approaching 0.0 are likely too difficult for the group. Tests with too many easy items are not able to "discriminate individuals at the upper end of the distribution," and tests with too many very difficult items do "a very poor job of distinguishing individuals at the lower end of the score distribution" (p. 73). The ideal item difficulty depends on the purpose of that question. For content that all students must master, a higher p value is the target, while content that is more general in nature may have an ideal p value closer to 0.7.

The item's discrimination index is calculated based on the difference in the overall performance between high-performing and low-performing groups of students on an exam on a scale from −1.00 to 1.00 (ExamSoft Guide to the Statistics 2021a). Kelly (1939) found through the use of various formulas that a threshold of the upper and lower 25–27% was ideal in calculating how well an item discriminated in groups of students. Flanagan (1939) confirmed that the differentiation between upper and lower groups was "a maximum when the two tails of the normal distribution each contain 27% of the cases" (p. 677). Thorndike (1982) recommends using the top 27% and bottom 27% of exam takers' overall scores to calculate the biserial according to the "Flanagan *r*" chart published in 1939 in the *Journal of Education Psychology* (p. 678).

Flanagan's (1939) chart assumes a normal distribution of scores following a normal standard deviation. To account for exams that do not have a normal score distribution, a point biserial can be used to determine item validity. A point biserial calculates how well all students performed on each question relative to the whole exam. Walsh and Betz (2001) refer to this type of analysis as "the extent to which people's responses to a given item measuring a construct are related to their scores on the measure as a whole" (p. 74). Because all student results are included in the formula for point biserial calculation, a normal score distribution is not assumed.

Kuder and Richardson developed the KR-20 formula in 1939 as a way to address the inconsistencies of the split-half technique of determining inter-item assessment reliability. The KR-20 measures an exam's reliability and ability to predict the stability and replicability of its results on a scale from 0.0 to 1.0. A higher KR-20 score indicates that the assessment is more likely to produce the same results when administered again, and a lower KR-20 score indicates that the assessment is not as likely to produce the same results in subsequent administrations (ExamSoft Guide to the Statistics 2021a). The best use for a KR-20 score is for exams that are given consistently over the course of several years by reposting the same questions in the same order without altering the assessment blueprint. For exam question security, it is recommended to pull from a wider bank of exam questions and rotate in new questions each time the assessment is given.

Part 3: What to Do When Statistics Are Not Available

From time-to-time students may be assessed outside of a computer-based testing platform or LMS (i.e., paper exam). For certain open response question types, the testing software may not automatically calculate the percent correct, point biserial, or discrimination index. In those instances, it is still possible to determine the validity and reliability of the assessment with a small amount of data entry. Thorndike (1982) described this as "making the practical value of a test explicit [by displaying] the full bivariate table of test score versus criterion scores" (p. 223).

The first step in the process is to create a spreadsheet of the students' exam results by question plus the overall scores. The students' names should be listed vertically on the left-hand side of the spreadsheet with the names beginning in cell A2 (column A, row 2). The question numbers should be listed horizontally beginning in cell B1 (column B, row 1). When practical, create columns for both the question answer and point value (Q1 answer, Q1 points). The total point value and percentage correct for the assessment should be listed to the right of the question columns.

Once the student responses and points earned for each question have been entered into the spreadsheet, the total points earned, item difficulty (p value), and point biserial for each question can be calculated. The total points earned will be a sum of the points earned for each question, and the percent correct will be the points earned divided by the points possible, displayed as a percent. The p value is calculated as the number of students who answered correctly divided by the total number of students. The point biserial is calculated using a combination of the p value, standard deviation for the question, and the overall exam average (ExamSoft Guide to the Statistics 2021a). If the idea of calculating a point biserial in a spreadsheet sounds daunting, keep in mind that even a bare minimum of the p value for each item can help begin to answer the question of item validity.

Part 4: How to Handle Poor Assessment Statistics

Thorndike (1982) found that there are two considerations that should be made when selecting which items to use for a test: item content and item statistics. While this information is helpful in creating the test, the same information should be scrutinized when considering how to handle poor question statistics such as a low p value or negative point biserial. Poor question performance can be caused by a number of factors, including clerical errors when constructing the test questions, conflicting sources of information, and misunderstanding of the material. Walsh and Betz (2001) also point out that poor performance can be caused by a misrepresentation in the amount of course material covered. This can happen when an exam's blueprint does not match the students' expectations of the content to be tested. Phelan and Wren (2006) recommend using a panel of experts to review the assessment blueprint to avoid bias from the exam maker when selecting which content to assess.

When the exam or quiz questions do not perform as expected on the item analysis, particularly the p value and either discrimination index or point biserial, it is considered best practice to make appropriate scoring changes. If the majority of the class chose the same incorrect answer, first check to see that the answer marked for the question is supposed to be marked correct. This kind of error reduces the item's content validity and can cause the test to be scored improperly (Walsh and Betz 2001). When the question is rekeyed and scored correctly, the validity of the question is increased.

If the question performed very poorly and the results are evenly spread across multiple answer choices, deleting the question is the best route to go. Evenly distributed incorrect responses indicate that the students who did not know the answer simply guessed at the question. Deleting the question does not give credit to those who answered correctly, and it removes the point value from the exam (zero points earned and zero points possible for that question).

A question may perform poorly but have a single second answer that a significant portion of the students chose. If this second answer could be considered correct either through the way the question was written or through a supporting source such as a textbook or journal article, it is best to double key the item. This gives credit to students who chose either answer (one point if either answer was chosen and one point possible for the question). If more than two answers need to be counted as correct (triple or quadruple key), it is better to delete the question due to item validity issues.

There are two types of scoring changes that should be used with extreme caution since they have a higher potential to skew an exam question's validity and reliability. It may be theoretically possible to give full credit to all students for a question or to bonus a question, but these are not best practices for high-quality assessments. Giving full credit to all students is best suited to open response question types such as FITB and hot spot where the students provide the answer rather than selecting from a list. This scoring change should only be performed when all responses are very close to the correct answer and could be considered correct.

Bonusing questions is not recommended since this gives credit only to those who answer correctly but does not penalize those who do not answer correctly (one point earned but zero points possible for the question). This makes it mathematically possible to earn more than 100% correct on a quiz or exam. It is better to delete the question from the exam even if there are no students scoring above 100% correct with the item bonused. As accrediting bodies and university administration continue to scrutinize professional schools on their assessment methods and documentation, it is imperative that programs provide high-quality assessments that are both valid and reliable (Hundley and Kahn 2019).

Section 4: Remediation

Malathi Raghavan and Jo R. Smith

Part 1: What Is Remediation?

Remediation may be defined as an interventional pedagogic policy and process facilitating a correction in the learning processes of students to help them achieve the required competencies in which they are struggling. In medical education, remediation has been defined as "the act of facilitating a correction for trainees who started out on the journey toward becoming a physician but have moved off course" (Kalet and Chou 2014, p. xvii).

Accreditation standards for veterinary degrees stipulate that remediation processes must be in place for students who do not meet the required competencies. Accrediting bodies typically do not stipulate the exact structure of remediation, nor do they proscribe how or when students are identified as needing remediation. At a minimum, the process of remediation involves recognizing the deficit in knowledge or skills; developing additional training to overcome the deficit; and determining through reassessment whether learner has successfully met the remediation goals.

Part 2: Factors That May Predispose Students to Needing Remediation

There is a societal contract to deliver trustworthy veterinary professionals and protect patient safety. Concerns have been raised about faculty's "failure to fail" underperforming trainees in healthcare professions and reasons have been identified (Lane and Bogue 2010; Yepes-Rios et al. 2016). However, even previously successful learners may stumble with the volume and pace of veterinary curricula, or when the training requires them to reassess and adjust their learning methods. Veterinary students can struggle because of issues with cognition – knowledge; clinical reasoning; study or testing-taking skills or learning difficulties. They may require more time or more personalized attention to navigate student learning bottlenecks (Middendorf and Shopkow 2017).

Struggling students may also have a bias in their perceptions of what is causing problems (Patel et al. 2015). Poor appreciation of task demands and blame for inaccurate causal attributions (e.g., fixed personal factors or external uncontrollable factors) can lead to ineffective use of learning strategies and maladaptive motivational beliefs (Foong et al. 2022). Thus, these students may be unaware of or reluctant to self-refer to remediation interventions or support. Alternatively, psychosocial stressors in the student's personal life, such as health; family/spouse stressors; finances; emotional issues; cultural adaptation; and social life may by a factor. Biopsychosocial contributors (e.g., stress and anxiety) and affective factors such as personal, interpersonal, and professional attitudes are also some of the descriptors thought to contribute to poor performance ultimately requiring remediation (Lacasse et al. 2019; Mills et al. 2021).

Part 3: Identifying Students to be Remediated

Ideally, students would be detected early in the supportive or corrective phase before remediation is required. Learning analytics have the potential to predict student academic performance and identify at-risk students at an early stage (Weng et al. 2021).

Part 4: Role of Faculty and Administration in Remediating Students

For remediation goals to be achieved, the right attitudes are essential on the part of the faculty and administration offering remediation as well as the students required to undergo remediation. Compassion and a potential change in mindset about delays in academic milestones and failures are needed for struggling students. There may be many reasons why students struggle with a competency achievement, including getting through a student learning bottleneck; going through life struggles; or recognizing an evident mismatch between their earlier preparation for a rigorous program of study and the learning environment encountered (Cleland et al. 2018). Any impressions that students are struggling because they are under-qualified or lacking motivation, responsibility, accountability, or self-efficacy are best dispelled because students have gone through a rigorous and competitive admissions process as instituted by the college and based on its vision and articulated mission. Such impressions and attitudes are also counterproductive as they negatively impact the goals of remediation, which should be thought of as a vital and necessary step in health professional education.

Educators and administrators should understand that emotion and cognition are not separate domains. Emotion plays a large role in learning because of its impact on metacognition and motivation and effecting a gap between the two is rarely helpful to the learner (Posner and Rothbart 2005). There is a small (but growing) body of literature that supports that learning (in the domain of cognition) can be facilitated by building positive, supportive learner-educator relationships (Curtis et al. 2021).

The study of teachers in successfully remediating struggling medical students has identified five core roles as facilitator, nurturing mentor, disciplinarian, diagnostician, and modeler of desired skills, attitudes, and behaviors. Blending these various roles is a complex performance where context and practical wisdom are incorporated through the unique support of an expert teacher (Winston et al. 2012). Teachers who were encouraging, motivating, approachable, and honest with their feedback were appreciated for the support they provided to at-risk medical students. Students also found it important and crucial that teachers challenged their learning and held them accountable for details (Winston et al. 2012).

Faculty training in remediation principles and practice, facilitation skills, and how to provide emotional support should be part of an institutional remediation strategy (Chou et al. 2019). Faculty should be provided opportunities to come together to know about newer, supportive learner-educator theories through seminars and learning commons.

Part 5: How Educational Programs Should Remediate Struggling Students and the Process by Which We Remediate Students

The minimum that is being offered in a remediation intervention is the opportunity to retake subject-specific assessments after a mandatory independent study period. This minimal approach has its merits as a minority of students may just need the extra time to fill gaps in knowledge or to learn clinical skills that were missed due to unexpected circumstances during the academic year. However, remediation is not merely extended time, repetition, or reassessment of learning. Remediation should not just focus on assessment coaching to pass a course if there are additional underlying factors. When required, remediation interventions should also support the development of long-term learning with effective lifelong or learning skills (Cleland et al. 2018).

Self-determination theory comprises three basic psychological needs that promote intrinsic motivation and autonomous self-regulation: competence, autonomy, and relatedness (Ten Cate et al. 2011). Formal remediation may challenge these exact needs that underpin intrinsic motivation. Remediation, by definition, indicates a lack of adequate competence; autonomy is often lost because the learner must follow a mandatory remediation plan and/or change their habits; and relatedness is often lost because of the need to observe confidentiality and the potential stigma associated with remediation can isolate students (Krzyzaniak et al. 2017, 2021). Several evidence-based recommended best practices of healthcare remediation also include the logistics of redressing these specific needs (Bennion et al. 2018; Chou et al. 2019; Kalet et al. 2016). For general recommendations to optimize remediation programs, see Table 10.1. Reprinted with permission.

Long-term competency can be enhanced by combining the learning of content and process and fostering development of students' affective, cognitive, and metacognitive practices, i.e., self-regulated learning (Kirtchuk et al. 2021). Self-regulation is a distinguishing characteristic between high and low academically achieving college students, hence the rationale for including it in remediation interventions (Patel et al. 2015).

To overcome the lack of perceived autonomy, it is recommended that the student is included in devising their remediation plan. Relatedness, or the need for connection to others, can also be addressed by the use of a mentor or learner advocate who can provide additional support (Price et al. 2021). Although self-regulated learning promotes individual agency and internal metacognitive processes, remediation interventions more closely resemble co-regulated learning. There is a shared control of learning and colleagues with more expertise scaffold novices' metacognitive engagement and promote their development of self-regulated learning ability (Rich 2017).

Table 10.1 Summary of guidelines for remediation in medical education.

Systems level, Dos

- Do advertise to the entire medical community that learners commonly need remediation, which is resources and available to all learners
- Do develop a robust feedback culture that impels learner improvement
- Do align selection and assessment systems with desired outcomes and graduate qualities
- Do construct strategies aimed at averting the need for remediation
- Do deliver remediation as highly individualized processes while recognizing common patterns across struggling learners
- Do "feed forward" remediation, with an abundance of caution
- Do provide faculty development and tangible support for frontline educators in early identification of, effective interventions for, and appropriate referral of struggling learners
- Do separate the individual conducting the remediation process from those who determine the outcome of remediation
- Do ensure due process, balancing empathy for individual students' struggles with the medical profession's responsibility to society
- Do create compassionate alternative pathways for those who do not choose to or cannot complete medical training

Remediation process, Dos

- Do aim to detect a need for remediation early
- Do collect relevant information from multiple sources across case content
- Do explore multiple causes of learner struggle beyond educational or workplace issues
- Do intervene proactively with struggling learners – do not rely on their initiative
- Do have trainees in remediation undergo intensive, longitudinal tutoring with emphasis on study skills, collaboratively designed plans, frequent high-quality feedback, and individualized assessment
- Do assess for and improve skills in learning self-regulation
- Do remediate knowledge and skills in small group with expert facilitators
- Do follow up with learners, even after the presumed end of the remediation period

Dont's

- Don't rely solely on traditional academic markers of performance
- Don't merely give more time, repeat the learner experience, give general or vague advice, or just "teach to the test" without additional support

---

Source: Adapted from Chou et al. (2019).

Regular feedback is an essential component of remediation interventions, and provision of this could be viewed as a form of *academic coaching*. Athletic coaches and music teachers perform detailed analyses of recent performances, identify relative strengths and weaknesses, and devise target exercises to enhance performance – dedicating time to improve weaker skills, and developing and practicing strategies for key performances. The process for remediating healthcare students essentially follows the same pattern. The medical analogy is often used in healthcare remediation; we are encouraged to *diagnose* the learner *deficit(s)*. Using coaching language moves away from an implied pathology or dysfunctionality and acknowledges there are likely to be complex factors impacting performance and that students are above-average learners, operating in very demanding environment (Bennion et al. 2018).

A healthcare remediation model has been defined based on five zones of practice: the "normal" curriculum, corrective action, remediation, probation, and exclusion (Ellaway et al. 2018). This may make it easier to normalize both the correction and remediation phases by situating them within a continuous zone of practice and thus decrease the perception of punishment and associated stigma (Kalet et al. 2017). This approach enables educators to plan for remediation as an inevitable aspect of training, "not a failure of an individual" (Kalet et al. 2017, p. 423).

Ideally, remediation programs are not isolated, stand-alone aspects of educational programs, but are embedded in a curricular context with clear learning objectives, competencies, milestones, and performance assessments (Cooke et al. 2010). The most effective remediation is one in which the process is highly individualized for individual learners and their specific challenges, including causes of learner struggle beyond educational issues and issues with self-regulation. The "establishment of appropriate, achievable intervention or learning plan that directly addresses deficiencies" is essential (Chou et al. 2019, p. 328). Following early detection of need to remediate, ideally through multi-source feedback, it is strongly recommended that remediating learners "undergo intensive, longitudinal tutoring with emphasis on study skills, collaboratively designed plans, frequent high-quality feedback, and individualized assessment" alongside content development. A key mode in which to remediate cognitive skills is for expert facilitators to skillfully facilitate small-group learning (Chou et al. 2019).

How specific remediation is accomplished is dependent on the type of deficit (i.e., whether the identified challenge(s) is cognitive or with a technical or nontechnical competency); the timing of failure to make curricular progress and meet academic standards; the extent to which the competency is structured within a program; and the resources available (Guerrasio 2017; Kalet and Chou 2014). Institutions may also have different academic policies on the type and number of remediations that can be attempted over the course of an individual learner's progress in the program.

Part 6: Typical Timing for Remediation

Major resource limitations to offering a well-designed remediation program are faculty time and scheduling of trainees' time for remediation activities. For example, in semester-based programs in the United States, remediation of failures in preclinical didactic courses or specific skills-based courses may need to occur in summer between academic years. Unfortunately, summer remediation may be problematic if the course is failed early in the academic year and serves as foundation for subsequent courses in the same academic year. For these reasons, most colleges may require that students redo the failed courses in their entirety in the following year along with the next class of students. The downside to this is that academic progress may be delayed for the individual learners involved – they may have to wait a whole year to repeat the course and/or they may be unable to register for another course without successfully remediating the original course.

In comparison, remediation of failed clinical rotations may be accomplished in a relatively timely manner if they are offered throughout the year – provided there is the capacity to add an extra learner or two. When deficits in specific clinical skills are required to be remediated, OSCEs or prevailing assessment methods may be used when possible, without relying on the summer months.

Part 7: Remediation of Professionalism

Academic remediation in the first two years of medical school is not related to patient complaints or subsequent disciplinary action by a state board; however, professionalism lapses have been shown to be a significant predictor of subsequent probation or state board complaints (Papadakis et al. 2005). Subsequently, a 3-phase model for how medical educators attend to professionalism lapses has been proposed (Mak-Van Der Vossen et al. 2019). In phase 1, educators are concerned with teachers who explore the lapse from the student's perspective. In phase 2, they coach supportively, providing feedback on professionalism values, improving skills, and promoting reflectiveness. In phase 3, if the student does not demonstrate reflectiveness and improvement, and particularly if patient care was potentially compromised, educators assumed an opposite role: gatekeeper of the profession.

Analysis of client complaints against veterinarians reported that failures of professional behavior included lack of trustworthiness, honesty, good quality care, and acceptable communication with the client (Gordon et al. 2019). Similarly, professional competencies that enhance the veterinarian-client interaction include accountability and integrity; effective communication skills; personal well-being; and quality of care (Gordon et al. 2021). Both of these

studies demonstrate that some *professional skills* may be conflated with *professionalism* (Mossop and Cobb 2013).

The development of medical professionalism has been described in three frameworks: virtue-based professionalism, behavior-based professionalism, and professional identity formation (Irby and Hamstra 2016). Virtue-based professionalism relied heavily on role models and implicit learning. This was impacted by negative role models and the hidden curriculum (Brater 2007).

The behavior-based competency movement focused on performance outcomes and developed in response to frustrations with the subjective measures of character and apparent failures of clinicians to apply moral reasoning to their actions. Identity formation arose from the perceived reductionist and prescriptive behavioral approach to competencies and milestones. Rather than consider professionalism as a trait (character or behavior), professionalization is the process of becoming a member of the profession and includes the processes of socialization and identity formation. It represents the interaction between personal values, professional behavior, and the workplace, and has been proposed as the fifth level of Miller's pyramid of assessment – "is" – when a learner can "think, act, and feel" like a clinician (Cruess et al. 2016, p. 181).

However, without explicitly defining features of veterinary professionalism it is difficult to teach, assess, and remediate professional identity formation (Mossop and Cobb 2013). Educators may perceive their judgment to be more subjective than assessing students' medical knowledge or procedural skills (Ghasemi et al. 2022). Lack of evaluation tools includes the concept that professional behavior occurs along a spectrum, and the point of professionalism incompetency is not clearly defined (Guerrasio et al. 2014; Hafferty and Castellani 2010). The short timeframes of some clinical placements can also compound these difficulties since, ideally, assessment should be longitudinal to emphasize that professional identity formation is a process.

Pedagogic strategies for professional identity formation have been proposed, including direct instruction, role models, case studies, reflective writing, guided discussions, appreciative inquiry, and white coat ceremonies (Armitage-Chan and May 2018; Irby and Hamstra 2016; Mak-van der Vossen et al. 2020). Constructively aligned assessment methods include self-administered rating scales, reflections, educational portfolios, observations and multisource feedback, and critical incident reports on lapses (Cruess et al. 2019; Smith et al. 2021).

Deficits in self-regulated learning and reduced reflective abilities also play a significant role in professional lapses (Brennan et al. 2020; Hoffman et al. 2016). These deficits may also make remediation challenging since insight into one's own behavior and correct attribution is often required for persistent change to occur (Roberts and Stark 2008; Stern et al. 2005). Remediation programs are more effective when a doctor's insight and motivation are developed and behavior change reinforced. Insight can be developed by using advocacy to develop trust in the remediation process and framing feedback sensitively. A sense of control can be created by involving the remediating doctor in remediation planning. Change can be motivated by correcting causal attribution, goal-setting, destigmatizing remediation, and sustained change can be achieved by practicing new behaviors and skills and through guided reflection (Price et al. 2021).

The most common remediation strategies used in medical schools across the United States and Canada were mandated mental health evaluation, remediation assignments, and professionalism mentoring (Ziring et al. 2015). While it has been reported that a paucity of research evidence exists to guide best practices in the remediation of professionalism lapses in medical students, "most interventions were multifaceted and addressed professionalism issues concomitantly with clinical skills, some . . . on specific areas" (Brennan et al. 2020, p. 196).

A framework for assessing veterinary professionalism in clinical rotations has been developed by a cohort of clinical faculty (Armitage-Chan 2016). Categories of behavior and skills include client and colleague interactions, respect and trust, recognition of limitations, and understanding of different professional identities. It details specific teaching and learning activities and assessment criteria centered on reflection and group discussion.

Part 8: Conclusion

Remediation is a "complex, context-dependent process" wherein all elements of the learning environment including students, teachers, curriculum, and educational program interact (Winston et al. 2010, p. e733). What faculty and administration learn from remediating learners could ultimately inform curricular and pedagogical improvements for all learners. Educators will benefit by learning to appreciate the advantages of using diverse teaching tools and learning methods.

References

Ali, S. and Ruit, K. (2015). The impact of item flaws, testing at low cognitive level, and low distractor functioning on multiple-choice question quality. *Perspectives on Medical Education* 4 (5): 244–251. https://doi.org/10.1007/s41137-015-0212-x.

Armitage-Chan, E. (2016). Assessing professionalism: a theoretical framework for defining clinical rotation

Summary

This chapter has covered several distinct, but intimately interrelated, topics. Starting with the broad terms of *assessment* and *evaluation*, a discussion briefly covering formative and summative assessments provided you with a general understanding of the purposes of each and how they differ. A more in-depth discussion of how evaluation can be confused with assessment depending upon how it is used was followed by an opportunity to learn about the components of a good evaluation and how that applies to programs, rather than individual students. In Section 2, you were provided specific information about a variety of different question formats that are suitable for use – in various situations – within the veterinary curriculum, with a focus on MCQs and some pointers for how to write these well.

After learning about the variety of question types that can be used on exams, Section 3 provided you insights into how each question should be approached to determine its validity and reliability – or the proof that you are testing students over the information you think you are testing them over and whether those questions do so over time and with different students. The chapter ends with remediation – what it is, why and when we do it, and the roles of the instructor(s) and administrator(s) in the process.

Assessment and evaluation are things we all know are important but most of us are not particularly fond of. It is also something that many educators have little understanding of – regardless of how long they have been teaching – and often believe they do pretty well in spite of information to the contrary. Although we primarily use MCQs for efficiency, there are also many who may believe they are "easy" to write – then find themselves sadly mistaken as their questions demonstrate poor statistical performance and discrimination. Thus, while we address the issue of remediation for our students explicitly in this chapter, we do not discuss the concept of remediation for faculty when it comes to our educational skills and knowledge. Perhaps we should explore this further – but we will leave that to another time.

assessment criteria. *Journal of Veterinary Medical Education* 43 (4): 364–371. https://doi.org/10.3138/jvme.1215-194R.

Armitage-Chan, E. and May, S.A. (2018). Developing a professional studies curriculum to support veterinary professional identity formation. *Journal of Veterinary Medical Education* 45 (4): 489–501. https://doi.org/10.3138/jvme.1216-192r1.

Armstrong, P. (2010). Bloom's taxonomy. Vanderbilt University Center for Teaching: https://cft.vanderbilt.edu/guides-sub-pages/blooms-taxonomy/ (accessed 15 March 2022).

Bannigan, K. and Watson, R. (2009). Reliability and validity in a nutshell. *Journal of Clinical Nursing* 18: 3237–3243. Blackwell Publishing Ltd. https://www.google.com/url?sa=t&rct=j&q=&esrc=s&source=web&cd=&cad=rja&uact=8&ved=2ahUKEwjyseikpLT2AhWqmeAKHXfYAX8QFnoECBwQAQ&url=https%3A%2F%2Fmy.enmu.edu%2Fc%2Fdocument_library%2Fget_file%3Fuuid%3D299fd446-72fa-4e09-9681-51825a0cb1b7%26groupId%3D4153058%26filename%3Dsbbannigan-nur502.pdf&usg=AOvVaw15os-QLDl8AjJdc2Rl3i0e.

Bennion, L., Durning, S.J., LaRochelle, J. et al. (2018). Untying the Gordian knot: remediation problems in medical schools that need remediation. *BMC Medical Education* 18: 120.

Biblier Zaidi, N., Monrad, S., Grob, K. et al. (2017). Building an exam through rigorous exam quality improvement. *Medical Science Educator* 27: 793–798. https://link.springer.com/article/10.1007/s40670-017-0469-2.

Bierer, B. (1940/2014). Before the nineteenth century. 1940. *Veterinary Heritage* 37 (2): 65–71.

Bowen, R. S. (2017). Understanding by design. Vanderbilt University Center For Teaching: https://cft.vanderbilt.edu/guides-sub-pages/understanding-by-design/ (accessed 15 March 2022).

Brater, D.C. (2007). Viewpoint: infusing professionalism into a School of Medicine: perspectives from the dean. *Academic Medicine* 82 (11): 1094–1097. https://doi.org/10.1097/ACM.0b013e3181575f89.

Brennan, N., Price, T., Archer, J., and Brett, J. (2020). Remediating professionalism lapses in medical students and doctors: a systematic review. *Medical Education* 54 (3): 196–204. https://doi.org/10.1111/medu.14016.

Caldwell, D. and Pate, A. (2013). Effects of question formats on student and item performance. *American Journal of Pharmaceutical Education* 77 (4): 71. https://doi.org/10.5688/ajpe77471.

Carmines, E. and Zeller, R. (1979). *Reliability and Validity Assessment, Quantitative Applications in the Social Sciences*, vol. 17. Thousand Oaks, CA: Sage Publications.

Chou, C.L., Kalet, A., Costa, M.J. et al. (2019). Guidelines: the dos, don'ts and don't knows of remediation in medical education. *Perspectives on Medical Education* 8 (6): 322–338. https://doi.org/10.1007/s40037-019-00544-5.

Cleland, J., Cilliers, F., and van Schalkwyk, S. (2018). The learning environment in remediation: a review. *Clinical Teacher* 15 (1): 13–18. https://doi.org/10.1111/tct.12739.

Cook, A., Lidbury, J., Creevy, K. et al. (2020). Multiple-choice questions in small animal medicine: an analysis of cognitive level and structural reliability, and the impact of these characteristics on student performance. *Journal of Veterinary Medical Education* 47 (4): 497–505.

Cooke, M., Irby, D.M., and O'Brien, B.C. (2010). *Educating Physicians: A Call for Reform of Medical School and Residency*. San Francisco, CA: Jossey-Bass.

Cruess, R.L., Cruess, S.R., and Steinert, Y. (2016). Amending Miller's pyramid to include professional identity formation. *Academic Medicine* 91 (2): 180–185. https://doi.org/10.1097/ACM.0000000000000913.

Cruess, S.R., Cruess, R.L., and Steinert, Y. (2019). Supporting the development of a professional identity: general principles. *Medical Teacher* 41 (6): 641–649. https://doi.org/10.1080/0142159X.2018.1536260.

Curtis, S., Mozley, H., Langford, C. et al. (2021). Challenging the deficit discourse in medical schools through reverse mentoring – Using discourse analysis to explore staff perceptions of under-represented medical students. *BMJ Open* 11 (12): 1–8. https://doi.org/10.1136/bmjopen-2021-054890.

Ellaway, R.H., Chou, C.L., and Kalet, A.L. (2018). Situating remediation: accommodating success and failure in medical education systems. *Academic Medicine* 93 (3): 391–398. https://doi.org/10.1097/ACM.0000000000001855.

Merriam-Webster (n.d.). Evaluation. merriam-webster.com. https://www.merriam-webster.com/dictionary/evaluation (accessed 5 March 2022).

ExamSoft. (2021a). A Guide to the statistics (legacy and enterprise portal). https://community.examsoft.com/s/article/A-Guide-to-the-Statistics-Legacy-and-EnterprisePortal (accessed 15 March 2022).

ExamSoft. (2021b). How to measure test validity and reliability. https://examsoft.com/resources/how-to-measure-test-validity-reliability/

Flanagan, J.C. (1939). General considerations in the selection of test items and a short method of estimating the product-moment coefficient from the data at the tails of the distribution. *Journal of Education Psychology* 30 (9): 674–680.

Foong, C.C., Bashir Ghouse, N.L., Lye, A.J. et al. (2022). Differences between high- and low-achieving pre-clinical medical students: a qualitative instrumental case study from a theory of action perspective. *Annals of Medicine* 54 (1): 195–210. https://doi.org/10.1080/07853890.2021.1967440.

Foreman, J., Read, E., Coleman, M. et al. (2022). *Competency Based Veterinary Education (CBVE) Assessment Toolkit*. AAVMC https://cbve.org/assessment-toolkit.

Ghasemi, A., Gartrell, C.L., and Graves, T. (2022). A qualitative study of how on-campus faculty and off-campus preceptors evaluate veterinary students' professionalism. *Journal of Veterinary Medical Education* https://doi.org/10.3138/jvme-2021-0122.

Giancola, S.P. (2021). *Program Evaluation: Embedding Evaluation into Program Design and Development.* SAGE.

Gordon, S.J.G., Gardner, D.H., Weston, J.F. et al. (2019). Quantitative and thematic analysis of complaints by clients against clinical veterinary practitioners in New Zealand. *New Zealand Veterinary Journal* 67 (3): 117–125. https://doi.org/10.1080/00480169.2019.1585300.

Gordon, S.J.G., Gardner, D.H., Weston, J.F. et al. (2021). Using the critical incident technique to determine veterinary professional competencies important for enhancing the veterinarian-client interaction. *Veterinary Record* 190 (6): 1–9. https://doi.org/10.1002/vetr.943.

Grainger, R., Dai, W., Osborne, E., and Kenwright, D. (2018). Medical students create multiple-choice questions for learning in pathology education: a pilot study. *BMC Medical Education* 18 (2018): https://www.proquest.com/docview/2108916521?accountid=12101.

Guerrasio, J. (2017). *Remediation of the Struggling Medical Learner.* Irwin, PA: Association for Hospital Medical Education.

Guerrasio, J., Garrity, M.J., and Aagaard, E.M. (2014). Learner deficits and academic outcomes of medical students, residents, fellows, and attending physicians referred to a remediation program, 2006–2012. *Academic Medicine* 89 (2): 352–358. https://doi.org/10.1097/ACM.0000000000000122.

Hafferty, F.W. and Castellani, B. (2010). The increasing complexities of professionalism. *Academic Medicine* 85 (2): 288–301. https://doi.org/10.1097/ACM.0b013e3181c85b43.

Haladyna, T., Downing, S., and Rodriguez, M. (2002). A review of multiple-choice item-writing guidelines for classroom assessment. *Applied Measurement in Education* 15 (3): 309–334. http://site.ufvjm.edu.br/fammuc/files/2016/05/item-writing-guidelines.pdf.

Haladyna, T., Rodriguez, M., and Stevens, C. (2019). Are multiple-choice items too fat? *Applied Measurement in Education* 32 (4): 350–364. https://doi.org/10.1080/08957347.2019.1660348.

Hoffman, L.A., Shew, R.L., Vu, T.R. et al. (2016). Is reflective ability associated with professionalism lapses during medical school? *Academic Medicine* 91 (6): 853–857. https://doi.org/10.1097/ACM.0000000000001094.

Hundley, S. and Kahn, S. (2019). *Trends in Assessment: Ideas, Opportunities, and Issues for Higher Education*, Special Institute Edition. Steerling, VA: Stylus Publishing, LLC.

Irby, D.M. and Hamstra, S.J. (2016). Parting the clouds: three professionalism frameworks in medical education. *Academic Medicine* 91 (12): 1606–1611. https://doi.org/10.1097/ACM.0000000000001190.

Jonick, C., Schneider, J., and Boylan, D. (2017). The effect of accounting question response formats on student performance. *Accounting Education* 26 (4): 291–315. https://doi.org/10.1080/09639284.2017.1292464.

Kalet, A. and Chou, C.L. (2014). *Remediation in Medical Education: A Mid-Course Correction.* New York, NY: Springer.

Kalet, A., Guerrasio, J., and Chou, C.L. (2016). Twelve tips for developing and maintaining a remediation program in medical education. *Medical Teacher* 38 (8): 787–792. https://doi.org/10.3109/0142159X.2016.1150983.

Kalet, A., Chou, C.L., and Ellaway, R.H. (2017). To fail is human: remediating remediation in medical education. *Perspectives on Medical Education* 6 (6): 418–424. https://doi.org/10.1007/s40037-017-0385-6.

Kalkat, H., Sonagara, V., and Santhirakumaran, S. (2017). The use of distractors in multiple-choice questions: a medical student perspective. *Advances in Medical Education and Practice* 8 (2017): 411–412. https://doi.org/10.2147/AMEP.S141505.

Kelley, T. (1939). The selection of upper and lower groups for the validation of test items. *Journal of Education Psychology* 30: 17–24.

Kirtchuk, D., Wells, G., Levett, T. et al. (2021). Understanding the impact of academic difficulties among medical students: A scoping review. *Medical Education* (August): 1–8. https://doi.org/10.1111/medu.14624.

Krzyzaniak, S.M., Wolf, S.J., Byyny, R. et al. (2017). A qualitative study of medical educators' perspectives on remediation: adopting a holistic approach to struggling residents. *Medical Teacher* 39 (9): 967–974. https://doi.org/10.1080/0142159X.2017.1332362.

Krzyzaniak, S.M., Kaplan, B., Lucas, D. et al. (2021). Unheard voices: a qualitative study of resident perspectives on remediation. *J Grad Med Educ* 13 (4): 507–514. https://doi.org/10.4300/JGME-D-20-01481.1.

Lacasse, M., Audétat, M.C., Boileau, É. et al. (2019). Interventions for undergraduate and postgraduate medical learners with academic difficulties: a BEME systematic review: BEME Guide No. 56. *Medical Teacher* 41 (9): 981–1001. https://doi.org/10.1080/0142159X.2019.1596239.

Lane, I.F. and Bogue, E.G. (2010). Perspectives in Professional Education and place of nontechnical competencies. *Journal of the American Veterinary Medical Association* 237: 53–64.

Larkin, M. (2011). Pioneering a profession, the birth of veterinary education in the age of enlightenment. *Journal of the American Veterinary Medical Association* 01: 2011. https://www.avma.org/javma-news/2011-01-01/pioneering-profession.

Mak-Van Der Vossen, M.C., De La Croix, A., Teherani, A. et al. (2019). A road map for attending to medical students' professionalism lapses. *Academic Medicine* 94 (4): 570–578. https://doi.org/10.1097/ACM.0000000000002537.

Mak-van der Vossen, M., Teherani, A., van Mook, W. et al. (2020). How to identify, address and report students' unprofessional behaviour in medical school.

Medical Teacher 42 (4): 372–379. https://doi.org/10.1080/0142159X.2019.1692130.

Mertens, D.M. and Wilson, A.T. (2019). *In Program Evaluation Theory and Practice A Comprehensive Guide*, 2e, 5. New York: The Gulliford Press.

Mertler, C.A. (2020). *Action Research: Improving Schools and Empowering Educators*, 6e. Thousand Oaks: Sage.

Middendorf, J. and Shopkow, L. (2017). *Overcoming Student Learning Bottlenecks: Decode the Critical Thinking of Your Discipline*, 1e. Sterling, VA: Stylus Publishing.

Mills, G.E. (2018). *Action Research: A Guide for the Teacher Researcher*, 6e. New York: Pearson.

Mills, L.M., Boscardin, C., Joyce, E.A. et al. (2021). Emotion in remediation: a scoping review of the medical education literature. *Medical Education* January: 1–13. https://doi.org/10.1111/medu.14605.

Mossop, L.H. and Cobb, K. (2013). Teaching and assessing veterinary professionalism. *Journal of Veterinary Medical Education* 40 (3): 223–232. https://doi.org/10.3138/jvme.0113-016R.

Mujeeb, A., Pardeshi, M., and Ghongane, B. (2010). *Comparative assessment of multiple choice questions versus short essay questions in pharmacology. Indian Journal of Medical Sciences* 64 (3): 118–124. https://doi-org.lmunet.idm.oclc.org/10.4103/0019-5359.95934.

National Board of Medical Examiners (2021). NBME item-writing guide: constructing written test questions for the health sciences, Sixth Edition. February 2021. https://www.nbme.org/item-writing-guide (accessed 16 November 2022).

Odegard, T.N. and Koen, J.D. (2007). "None of the above" as a correct and incorrect alternative on a multiple-choice test: implications for the testing effect. *Memory* 15 (8): 873–885. https://web.s.ebscohost.com/ehost/pdfviewer/pdfviewer?vid=2&sid=506bb666-3061-4ccc-9a42-cab29ae5826d%40redis.

Pachai, M., DiBattista, D., and Kim, J. (2015). A systematic assessment of 'none of the above' on multiple choice tests in a first year psychology classroom. *The Canadian Journal for the Scholarship of Teaching and Learning* 6 (3): 1–17. https://doaj.org/article/ad6dbe54394c47a185687a2fbad9291d.

Papadakis, M., Teherani, A., and Banach, M. (2005). Disciplinary action by medical boards and prior behavior in medical school. *New England Journal of Medicine* 353: 2673–2682.

Patel, R., Tarrant, C., Bonas, S. et al. (2015). The struggling student: a thematic analysis from the self-regulated learning perspective. *Medical Education* 49 (4): 417–426. https://doi.org/10.1111/medu.12651.

Phelan, C. and Wren, J. (2006). Exploring reliability in academic assessment. *Created for University of Northern Iowa's Office of Academic Assessment.* https://chfasoa.uni.edu/reliabilityandvalidity.htm.

Posner, M.I. and Rothbart, M.K. (2005). Influencing brain networks: implications for education. *Trends in Cognitive Sciences* 9 (3 SPEC. ISS): 99–103. https://doi.org/10.1016/j.tics.2005.01.007.

Price, T., Wong, G., Withers, L. et al. (2021). Optimising the delivery of remediation programmes for doctors: a realist review. *Medical Education* 55 (9): 995–1010. https://doi.org/10.1111/medu.14528.

Rahma, N., Shamad, M., Idris, M.E.A. et al. (2017). Comparison in the quality of distractors in three and four options type of multiple choice questions. *Advances in Medical Education and Practice* 8 (2017): 287–291. https://doi.org/10.2147/AMEP.S128318.

Rhode Island Department of Education. (2022). Curriculum definition. RIDE: https://www.ride.ri.gov/Instruction Assessment/Curriculum/CurriculumDefinition.aspx (accessed 1 March 2022).

Rich, J. (2017). Proposing a model of co-regulated learning for graduate medical education. *Academic Medicine* 92: 1100–1104.

Richardson, M.W. and Kuder, G.F. (1939). The calculation of test reliability coefficients based on the method of rational equivalence. *Journal of Education Psychology* 30 (9): 681–687.

Roberts, C. and Stark, P. (2008). Readiness for self-directed change in professional behaviours: factorial validation of the self-reflection and insight scale. *Medical Education* 42 (11): 1054–1063. https://doi.org/10.1111/j.1365-2923.2008.03156.x.

Rossi, P.H., Lipsey, M.W., and Henry, G.T. (2019). *Evaluation A Systematic Approach.* SAGE.

Rush, B.R., Rankin, D.C., and White, B.J. (2016). The impact of item-writing flaws and item complexity on examination item difficulty and discrimination value. *BMC Medical Education* 16 (250): 1–10. https://doi-org.lmunet.idm.oclc.org/10.1186/s12909-016-0773-3.

Ryans, D. (1939). A note on methods of test validation. *Journal of Education Psychology* 30: 315–319.

Salkind, N. (2013). *Statistics for People Who (Think They) Hate Statistics*, 3e. Thousand Oaks, CA: Sage Publications.

Shilo, G. (2015). Formulating good open-ended questions in assessment. *Educational Research Quarterly* 38 (4): 3–30. Retrieved from http://lmunet.idm.oclc.org/login?url= https://www.proquest.com/scholarly-journals/formulatinggood-open-ended-questions-assessment/docview/1692023116/se-2.

Smith, K.J., Farland, M.Z., Edwards, M. et al. (2021). Assessing professionalism in health profession degree programs: a scoping review. *Currents in Pharmacy Teaching and Learning* 13 (8): 1078–1098. https://doi.org/10.1016/j.cptl.2021.06.006.

Stern, D.T., Frohna, A.Z., and Gruppen, L.D. (2005). The prediction of professional behaviour. *Medical Education*

39 (1): 75–82. https://doi.org/10.1111/j.1365-2929.2004.02035.x.

Tarrant, M. and Ware, J. (2008). Impact of item-writing flaws in multiple-choice questions on student achievement in high-stakes nursing assessments. *Medical Education* 42 (2): 198–206. https://doi.org/10.1111/j.1365-2923.2007.02957.x.

Taylor, R.M. (2009). Defining, constructing and assessing learning outcomes. *Revue scientifique et technique (International Office of Epizootics)* 28 (2): 779–788. https://web.s.ebscohost.com/ehost/detail/detail?vid=1&sid=11c2dc08-4dd2-4132-9253-a245cc71e683%40redis&bdata=JnNpdGU9ZWhvc3QtbGl2ZSZzY29wZT1zaXRl#AN=20128490&db=mdc.

Ten Cate, O., Kusurkar, R., and Williams, G. (2011). How self-determination theory can assist our understanding of the teaching and learning processes in medical education. AMEE Guide No. 59. *Medical Teacher* 33: 961–973.

Thorndike, R. (1982). *Applied Psychometrics*. Boston, MA: Houghton Mifflin.

Torres, C., Lopes, A., Babo, L., and Azevedo, J. (2011). Improving multiple-choice questions. *US-China Education Review B* 1 (2011): 1–11. https://eric.ed.gov/?id=ED522219.

Touissi, Y., Hjiej, G., Hajjiuoi, A. et al. (2021). Does developing multiple-choice questions improve medical students' learning?. A systematic review. *Medical Education* 27 (1): https://www.tandfonline.com/doi/full/10.1080/10872981.2021.2005505.

Walsh, W. and Betz, N. (2001). *Tests and Assessment*, 4e. Upper Saddle River, NJ: Prentice Hall.

Weng, W., Ritter, N.L., Cornell, K., and Gonzales, M. (2021). Adopting learning analytics in a first-year veterinarian professional program: what we could know in advance about student learning progress. *Journal of Veterinary Medical Education* 48 (6): 720–728. https://doi.org/10.3138/jvme-2020-0045.

Winston, K.A., van der Vleuten, C.P.M., and Scherpbier, A.J.J.A. (2010). At-risk medical students: implications of students' voice for the theory and practice of remediation. *Medical Education* 44 (10): 1038–1047. https://doi.org/10.1111/j.1365-2923.2010.03759.x.

Winston, K.A., Van Der Vleuten, C.P.M., and Scherpbier, A.J.J.A. (2012). The role of the teacher in remediating at-risk medical students. *Medical Teacher* 34 (11): https://doi.org/10.3109/0142159X.2012.689447.

Xu, X., Kauer, S., and Tupy, S. (2016). Multiple-choice questions: Tips for optimizing assessment in-seat and online. *Scholarship of Teaching and Learning in Psychology* 2 (2): 147–158. https://doi.org/10.1037/stl0000062.

Yepes-Rios, M., Dudek, N., Duboyce, R. et al. (2016). Thefailure to fail underperforming trainees in health professions education: a BEME systematic review: BEME Guide No. 42. *Medical Teacher* 38 (11): https://doi.org/10.1080/0142159X.2016.1215414.

Ziring, D., Danoff, D., Grosseman, S. et al. (2015). How do medical schools identify and remediate professionalism lapses in medical students? A Study of U.S. and Canadian Medical Schools. *Academic Medicine* 90 (7): 913–920. https://doi.org/10.1097/ACM.0000000000000737.

Additional Resources

AAC&U's Teaching-Learning-Assessment framework: https://www.aacu.org/initiatives/tla-framework

Gyll, S. and Ragland, S. (2018). Improving the validity of objective assessment in higher education: steps for building a best-in-class competency-based assessment program. *The Journal of Competency-Based Education* 3 (1). 2018. Published 23 February 2018. https://onlinelibrary.wiley.com/doi/full/10.1002/cbe2.1058.

Jandaghi, G. and Shaterian, F. (2008). Validity, reliability, and difficulty indices for instructor-built exam questions. *Journal of Applied Quantitative Methods* 3 (2): 2008 151–155. https://www.google.com/url?sa=t&rct=j&q=&esrc=s&source=web&cd=&cad=rja&uact=8&ved=2ahUKEwi5-bPnpbT2AhWvc98KHSm_AEIQFnoECDkQAQ&url=https%3A%2F%2Ffiles.eric.ed.gov%2Ffulltext%2FEJ803060.pdf&usg=AOvVaw2mtjjbjqWRvNnQp0metMai.

Price, P., Jhangiani, R., and Chiang, I. (2015). Chapter 5: Psychological measurement. In: *Research Methods in Psychology*, 2nd Canadiane. Victoria, BC: Bccampus

https://opentextbc.ca/researchmethods/chapter/reliability-and-validity-of-measurement/.

The Center on Standards and Assessment Implementation (CSAI). (2018). Valid and reliable assessments. *CSAI Update* March 2018. https://www.google.com/url?sa=t&rct=j&q=&esrc=s&source=web&cd=&cad=rja&uact=8&ved=2ahUKEwjRgd7ApLT2AhWhd98KHde2BwkQFnoECCQQAQ&url=https%3A%2F%2Ffiles.eric.ed.gov%2Ffulltext%2FED588476.pdf&usg=AOvVaw1fYpMHoYJQaPrMm4kvlf64.

University of North Texas, Center for Learning Experimentation, Application, and Research (2022). Why reliability and validity are important to learning assessment. https://teachingcommons.unt.edu/teaching-essentials/assessment/why-reliability-and-validity-are-important-learning-assessment

Votaw, D. and Danforth, L. (1939). The effect of method of response upon the validity of multiple-choice tests. *Journal of Education Psychology* 30: 624–627.

11

Assessing Clinical Skills

Stephanie L. Shaver, DVM, DACVM (Small Animal), MS (Health Professions Education)

University of Arizona College of Veterinary Medicine, Oro Valley, AZ, USA

Section 1: Introduction

Assessment in medical education has historically focused on the determination of whether a student is competent or incompetent (Schuwirth and van der Vleuten 2020). In recent years, assessment has evolved from this specific aim to a more inclusive process in which feedback is useful for both student and program, and assessment both *of* learning and *for* learning are of great import (Danielson 2021; Naeem et al. 2012). This change regarding the process of assessment is particularly relevant when it comes to clinical skills training. The term "clinical skills" encompasses a broad array of behaviors, from procedural accuracy to comprehensive patient care decisions. Evaluation of these skills can guide the efforts of a student who will enter clinical practice and provides information for a training program regarding whether the student is competent to do so. Effective assessment of these higher-order behaviors and skills is essential for the development of competent veterinary clinicians.

Miller's (1990) pyramid of clinical competence (Figure 11.1) captures different levels of learning and their expression. Written examinations are well suited to documenting whether a student "knows" or "knows how," but clinical skills are evaluated by assessing a student who "shows how" and "does." Emphasis on action has led to a focus on psychomotor knowledge when discussing clinical skills; however, affective knowledge, as demonstrated through attributes such as professionalism and communication, also comprises essential clinical skills. Furthermore, many clinical skills and their assessment replicate or approximate the reality of practicing veterinary medicine, and as such, involve the confluence of procedural knowledge, basic science knowledge, and clinical reasoning (Michels et al. 2012).

Competency-based veterinary medical education reinforces the necessity of clinical skills assessment, as a principle underpinning of competency-based medical education is programmatic assessment. Programmatic assessment is integrated throughout the system, involves numerous occasions and methods of assessment, and provides regular, timely feedback to the learner. As veterinary medical education has turned toward a competency-based approach, the assessment of clinical skills situated within a program-wide framework is increasingly necessary (Bok et al. 2018; Danielson 2021). Although clinical skills assessments are often emphasized in later years of training, instituting more holistic and higher-level assessment processes earlier in curricular sequencing is a part of moving toward integrated, competency-based education in veterinary medicine (Hecker et al. 2010, 2012a).

Presently, clinical skills assessment is largely accomplished through *performance assessment*, in which students are assessed in situations designed to mimic an authentic setting, and *workplace-based assessment,* in which students are evaluated on encounters in an actual clinical environment. This chapter will discuss the current use of performance and workplace-based assessment in health professions and veterinary education, with essential areas of focus for improving training and providing increasingly valid and constructive clinical skills assessment.

Section 2: Performance Assessment

Performance assessment is an opportunity for students to practice and be assessed on clinical skills in a lower-stakes environment compared to the functioning clinic or hospital. In contrast to clinical experiences, the use of models, simulations, and animals in a situation designed for

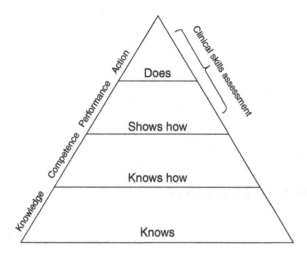

Figure 11.1 Pyramid of clinical competence. *Source:* Modified from Miller (1990).

learning provides a chance to design assessment that is relatively uniform for all students and occurs in a more controlled environment. Clinical work may be driven by available opportunities, while performance assessment is more readily standardized and homogenous. Despite these advantages, performance assessments lack the situational accuracy of a workplace-based experience. Many performance assessments are also resource-intense with material costs and significant time invested on the part of the assessor. Basic clinical skills simulations, however, have been described as a strategy for resource-limited veterinary education programs (Seddon et al. 2020).

An advantage of performance assessments is potential mitigation of the anxiety and stress associated with assessment. The student novice may begin with simple models and short encounters, and progress to more intensive simulations and live animal experiences as increased competence and comfort are demonstrated. Use of models to practice skills prior to live animal encounters has been shown in multiple, disparate settings to increase comfort and self-confidence and reduce stress in veterinary students (da Silva et al. 2021; Goldschmidt and Root Kustritz 2021; Langebæk et al. 2012). This is particularly useful given that some of the skills evaluated via performance assessments are tied to experiences, such as live animal surgery and client interactions, that are sources of apprehension (Kedrowicz 2016; Langebæk et al. 2012).

Competencies that can be assessed with performance tests include those that are not easily evaluated with a written examination; that involve interaction with a client or patient; or include aspects of psychomotor and affective knowledge, such as procedural steps, communication, and interpersonal skills. Three broad categories of performance assessment have been described: artificial, analogue, and actual. Actual performance assessments occur in the setting in which they would ordinarily take place; for instance, a spay/neuter laboratory, which has real consequences and requires a high level of student competence. Analogue performance assessments are those in which a re-creation of the scenario where a task would take place is presented to the student. This is best exemplified in veterinary medicine by communication simulations, in which a standardized client interacts with a student as though an actual clinical encounter were occurring. Artificial performance assessments have the least consistency with a real-life setting, and require the student to mentally create the scenario posed by the assessment and demonstrate problem-solving skills (Reynolds et al. 2006). Performance assessments, particularly artificial assessments, may be distinguished from written evaluations of skill as they involve assessment of multiple criteria and do not focus solely on a single area of student competency. This more inclusive approach to documentation of student proficiency is another way that performance assessment operates at the "shows how" or "does" level of Miller's pyramid.

Table 11.1 demonstrates that simulated learning with models has increased exponentially in veterinary medicine education in recent years (Hunt et al. 2021b). Models have been developed for tasks including abdominal palpation, gonadectomy, intubation, joint injections, nerve blocks, dental cleanings, and rectal palpation, among many others. The fidelity of some models is very basic, in which *psychological fidelity*, the process necessary to complete the task, is the focus. In other cases, a high degree of realism, known as *engineering fidelity* may also be present (Hunt et al. 2021b). This is exemplified by the variety of models described for the canine ovariohysterectomy, which encompass models constructed with materials such as balloons, rubber bands, and gloves that provide an opportunity for students to complete procedural steps, in contrast to highly realistic models that feature vascularized anatomy and controllable blood pressure and heart rate (Au Yong et al. 2019; Langebæk et al. 2015). Despite the disparate experiences and costs associated with these models, psychological fidelity, present in both models, seems to be most important for deliberate practice and student learning (Hamstra et al. 2014; Hunt et al. 2021b). Less lifelike models may be beneficial to allow students to focus on the task without additional stressful stimuli; however, greater realism may improve the focus of more advanced students and allow for additional complexities in the simulated task.

Use of models and simulations has been shown to positively impact veterinary student learning, improving both knowledge and clinical skills (Noyes et al. 2021). Not only are models a chance to advance from abstract to more concrete demonstration of knowledge, but students have

Table 11.1 Various models and simulations described in veterinary medical education, 2020–2021.

Castration-bovine
- Bovine: Anderson et al. (2021)
- Canine: Hunt et al. (2020a)
- Equine: Sheats et al. (2021)

Cerebrospinal fluid collection
- Langebæk et al. (2021)

Clinical reasoning
- Vinten et al. (2020)

Communication
- McCool and Kedrowicz (2020)

Dental cleanings-small animal
- Goldschmidt and Root Kustritz (2021)
- Hunt et al. (2021a)

Endoscopy
- McCool et al. (2020)

Fine needle aspiration
- Luís Pires et al. (2021)
- Stowe et al. (2021)

Fundic examination
- Banse et al. (2021)

Intravenous catheter placement- feline
- Silva et al. (2021)

Intubation- canine
- Canine: Cosford et al. (2020)
- Feline: Clausse et al. (2020)

Ophthalmoscopy
- Dos Santos Martins et al. (2021)

Ovariohysterectomy- canine
- Annandale et al. (2020)
- MacArthur et al. (2021)

Simple interrupted suture
- Baillie et al. (2020)

Ultrasound
- Wichtel et al. (2021)

Venipuncture
- Canine: da Silva et al. (2021)
- Feline: Hunt et al. (2020b)

---

an opportunity for deliberate practice, which has been shown to meaningfully impact the development of skills. Deliberate practice, in which one consciously completes an exercise with an eye toward improvement, receives feedback, and repeats the experience to hone a skill, was originally conceived of for applications in sports, games, and music, but has been shown to apply equally well to the development of expert performance in medicine

(Compton et al. 2019; Ericsson 2008; Sadideen and Kneebone 2012). In deliberate practice, the learner persists in the cognitive-associative phase of learning to consciously develop skill; in this situation, continued experience contributes to developing expert performance, rather than a situation in which behaviors become automatic and experience no longer leads to improvement (Ericsson 2004, 2008). The use of simulated clinical environments and tasks allows the learner to focus on a specific task, receive expert feedback, and repeat and refine their performance. Assessment provided in this context provides external motivation for deliberate practice that meaningfully impacts skill development.

Clinical skills laboratories have been adopted at an increasing number of veterinary education programs as both elective and core features of curriculum (Carroll et al. 2016; Dilly et al. 2017; Morin et al. 2020). These serve the purpose of providing a chance for deliberate practice as well as a place in which formative assessment is routinely provided. Formative assessment is designed to provide feedback to the learner, and is characterized by relative informality, increased frequency, and a nonjudgmental approach. This type of assessment provides students with detailed, ongoing feedback, promotes self-direction, and enhances student engagement (Swanwick 2018). Formative assessment has been shown to promote retention of skills beyond simple practice alone (Sennhenn-Kirchner et al. 2018). Clinical skills laboratories vary considerably in size, scope, and staffing, but typically include low-engineering-fidelity models. Depending on the laboratory, there may be high-fidelity models, cadavers, live animals, and standardized client experiences; it may also be used for training in animal handling, basic psychomotor skills (venipuncture and suturing), clinical skills (communication and history taking), and more advanced technical procedures, such as provision of anesthesia, surgery, and obtaining diagnostic imaging (Hodgson and Pelzer 2017).

In medical education, performance assessments are often occupied with a discussion of the "standardized patient," who is trained to realistically portray a clinical encounter. This type of simulation allows a health professions student to practice and demonstrate communication, history-taking, and clinical reasoning skills. In veterinary medicine, the "standardized client" has been utilized to much the same purpose and has been shown to be a reliable and valid way of assessing communication and clinical reasoning skills in veterinary medicine (Artemiou et al. 2014; Englar 2019a; Vinten et al. 2020). Crucial to the use of a standardized client for assessment is a well-developed script that contains characteristics of the client, history and medical information regarding the patient, and questions or desired responses to particular student behaviors (Yudkowsky et al. 2019). Having a thoroughly developed script along with a well-trained standardized client ensures reliable assessment practices across student encounters. Numerous specific scripts or client vignettes have been described in the veterinary literature in recent years, covering communication topics ranging from accidental death to service dogs to wellness visits (Englar 2019a,b; McCool and Kedrowicz 2020). Additional studies have also evaluated the use of standardized clients as student assessors, and the use of veterinary students as standardized clients and peer-evaluators with promising results (Artemiou et al. 2014; Strand et al. 2013).

Scoring performance assessments is relatively difficult compared to a written examination that is designed to have an objectively correct answer. Performance assessments are inherently subjective and assess multifaceted skills. The two most common means of scoring performance assessments are checklists and rating scales. Checklists require a yes/no assessment on separate behaviors that comprise a skill (Table 11.2). Checklists are advantageous in that they present the assessor with discrete, observable behaviors to grade, and well-trained lay persons can accurately complete a checklist (Artemiou et al. 2014; Bergus et al. 2009). Despite the dichotomous nature of grading a checklist, this does not necessarily result in a more valid

Table 11.2 Checklist for placement of an intravenous catheter in a canine model.

Canine intravenous catheter (IVC) placement checklist	Yes	No
1) Gathers necessary items for catheter placement: 1) catheter 2) T-port 3) 3 cc syringe with needle 4) white tape 5) scrub		
2) Fills 3cc syringe with sterile flush.		
3) Precut tape strips appropriately (3).		
4) Flushes catheter.		
5) Flushes T-port.		
6) Scrubs IVC site and wipes with saline prior to placement.		
7) Wears exam gloves for IVC placement.		
8) Successfully places IVC in vein.		
9) Secures IVC and T-port in place using two strips around catheter and one strip around T-port.		
10) Flushes IVC following placement to confirm patency.		

assessment of student ability, particularly for complex tasks. Rating scales require expert judgment to complete but allow for nuanced evaluation of clinical skills performance. Although subjective, interrater reliability may be enhanced by scale anchors, which include Likert scale items that use task-independent terms (e.g., strongly disagree/disagree/neither agree nor disagree/agree/strongly agree) or linear scale items, in which an adjective is assigned to the valuation (e.g., Not efficient/somewhat efficient/efficient/very efficient). A third type of rating scale item that is particularly effective for improving reliability is a behaviorally anchored rating scale, in which a behavioral description is provided to help an assessor determine how to grade a student, as in the surgical skills assessment shown in Table 11.3 (Schnabel et al. 2013).

Minimizing errors in scoring performance assessments can be accomplished by using validated and reliable checklists and rating scales. At a minimum, multiple colleagues should evaluate a scoring rubric for consistency, clarity, and surface validity. It is critical to ensure that the criteria being evaluated are observable, specific, and that the task is the most direct way of evaluating the pertinent objective. A rating scale or checklist should allow for discrimination between novice, intermediate, and advanced students, and the appropriate grading procedure (checklist or rating scale) should be selected. Training assessors is also critical to reach a uniform consensus about the use of checklists and rating scales; it can also help assessors remain aware of leniency, severity, and central tendency bias, wherein some evaluators tend to give either good, poor, or intermediate scores, respectively, regardless of performance (Reynolds et al. 2006). Ideally, all raters should be trained in a group so that agreement regarding item scoring can be achieved. The exam purpose and items should be explained, and during training, the raters should score at least one performance individually, although scoring performances at different competency levels can be useful. Following individual scoring, raters should discuss each item and reach a consensus regarding scoring on the assessment (Yudkowsky et al. 2019).

The most well-known and widely used performance assessment in health professions education is the Objective Structured Clinical Examination (OSCE). An OSCE comprise a series of performance assessments, or stations, that students complete in sequence. Stations are typically of the same duration for ease of administration, and all students rotate through all stations. The number of stations may vary, but typically range from 10 to 20, with 5–15 minutes allowed per station. The content of an OSCE may be similar, such as multiple communication simulations, or vary and include disparate or unrelated skills such as suturing, venipuncture, or interpretation of diagnostic tests.

Table 11.3 Excerpt, "Veterinary surgical skills assessment form."

Use of forceps on tissue		
1 Holds incorrectly, awkward or inappropriate use	2 3 Holds correctly some of the time, occasional awkward use	4 5 Holds correctly consistently, uses forceps with precision
Needle handling with needle holder		
1 Repeatedly handles and loads needle incorrectly, i.e., not perpendicular to driver and/or not 2/3 up needle shaft	2 3 Mostly acceptable handling and loading, occasional incorrect use	4 5 Consistently smooth handling, loads needle properly, clamps driver onto needle
Needle handling when suturing		
1 Incorrect use and placement of needle, does not follow curve of needle	2 3 Mostly acceptable use and placement, occasionally does not follow curve of needle	4 5 Consistently correct orientation and distance from incision, follows curve of needle
Quality of finished sutures		
1 Poor quality (not square) knots, incorrect knot tension, asymmetric	2 3 Most knots correct, tension sometimes incorrect, partially symmetric	4 5 Square knots, appropriate tension, symmetric

Source: Adapted from Schnabel et al. (2013).

An OSCE may be used formatively in early clinical training to provide the learner information about their skills, or summatively at the end of a semester or unit of clinical skills training, with high-stakes consequences for failure of a station or the examination in its entirety.

The advantages of the OSCE are an increase in standardization and reliability of testing. All students complete the same practical assessments, delivered in the same fashion with the same information and time/environmental constraints. The multi-station nature of the OSCE minimizes testing errors associated with too small a sample size and allows students a greater opportunity to demonstrate the breadth of their clinical skills. Disadvantages are primarily related to the artificial nature of the stations and the extensive resource commitment necessary to successfully hold an OSCE. The large number of stations and lengthy testing periods require significant commitments in examination design, evaluator training, and the time of experts and standardized clients in delivering and scoring the examination.

Scoring of an OSCE is accomplished through checklist or rating scale use. Experienced assessors have greater inter-rater reliability compared to inexperienced assessors, emphasizing the importance of training prior to the examination (Hecker et al. 2012a; Read et al. 2015). Some authors have recommended the use of a global rating scale to capture the student's overall performance in addition to the use of a checklist. This is typically not considered toward the student's final score and is of use in determining a passing standard for the examination; however,

assessor performance has been shown not to meaningfully differ between global rating scale and checklist scores (Read et al. 2015).

Global rating scales require that an expert assessor subjectively rate the overall proficiency of the student on the task. Use of a checklist with a global rating scale is helpful to guide assessors on criteria to consider when making their global assessment, and though global rating scales are associated with a decrease in inter-rater reliability, they have been shown to capture greater interstation reliability. A documented increase in the validity of global rating scales is likely due to checklists failing to capture factors such as efficiency or confidence that an expert assessor will incorporate in a judgment. This is a useful example of the concept that objectivity does not always imply validity of an assessment, and that subjective evaluation by an expert can meaningfully contribute to assessment practices (van der Vleuten et al. 2010).

Global rating scales are of use for setting a passing standard on an OSCE station via borderline group or borderline regression methods. In these approaches, once the OSCE is completed, the checklist scores of students who are borderline or marginally acceptable on the rating scale are used to determine the passing standard. The mean or a linear regression analysis using borderline scores for the group or regression methods, respectively, is performed, allowing a passing standard to be set for each station and for the overall test. A disadvantage of the borderline approach to standard setting is that the pass mark can only be determined after the test has been administered. In contrast, the modified Angoff method uses experts prior to the test who state what items they would expect a borderline test-taker to complete correctly or incorrectly and, as a result, establishes a standard prior to delivery of the examination (Dwyer et al. 2016).

Section 3: Workplace-Based Assessment

Workplace-based assessment encompasses a broad array of assessment strategies taking place as learners encounter clinical practice in a mentored environment. This level of assessment takes place at the highest level of Miller's pyramid, in which the learner *does* by actively taking part in the practice of veterinary medicine. The high fidelity between assessment in this setting and real-world practice ideally allows for assessment based on the premise that what a learner does in workplace-based assessment will mirror what they will do when in practice postgraduation.

Situated learning is a key feature of workplace-based assessment, in that both learning and assessment are taking place in an authentic environment for clinical practice. Situated learning is critical for the establishment of professional identity and learning that takes place within the sociocultural context of the profession (Sadideen and Kneebone 2012). Although it provides challenges for assessment, the importance of professional identity development that takes place in workplace-based learning is such that authors in human medical education have proposed another assessment category that sits above *does* for the apex of Miller's triangle: *Is*. This tier emphasizes that not only does the learner demonstrate behaviors consistent with being a trained healthcare worker, but also that they demonstrate the expected values and attitudes as an individual with an established professional identity (Cruess et al. 2016). Workplace-based assessment focuses on experiences that are inseparable from the setting in which they take place, allowing the learner to demonstrate capabilities and embody attributes required in an actual working clinic.

Workplace-based assessment is closely linked to the evolving focus on competency-based veterinary education (CBVE) and, particularly, entrustable professional activities (EPAs). The EPA was developed to represent a unit of skills, behaviors, or activities essential to practice that the learner can be entrusted to perform independently once deemed competent (Englander et al. 2017). Bridging the gap between defined competencies and clinical practice, the EPA is an observable clinical occurrence that contains a multitude of skills and encompasses areas such as medical knowledge, patient care, and professionalism, which occur confluently in an authentic clinical scenario

(ten Cate and Scheele 2007). Among the conditions of EPAs are that these activities are essential; require a minimum threshold of knowledge, skill, and attitude; have recognized output; and are observable and measurable (ten Cate and Scheele 2007). Entrustment decision-making requires careful assessment of clinical skills, as the assessor must deem the learner's level of capability in performing the activity independently. Furthermore, the assessor must determine that the learner has the necessary ability to handle both current and future situations, requiring a summative assessment of both the efficacy of the learner and their ability to manage risk, ask for help, and adapt to shifting clinical scenarios. The importance of the judgment is such that authors have proposed yet another alternate fifth level to Miller's pyramid: *Trusted* (ten Cate et al. 2021). Medical knowledge and procedural skills must be accounted for, as must trust conditions, such as integrity, reliability, and humility, when making an assessment for the clinical transition to independence (ten Cate 2016).

The provision of feedback to the learner is an important aspect of workplace-based assessment, and nearly all of this type of assessment is in some way formative. Feedback should be delivered in an actionable way that allows the learner to make graduated progress toward clinical independence. To provide assessment that is centered on the learner and provides useful information regarding their proficiency, much workplace-based assessment feedback is delivered in narrative rather than numerical form. There is no single test for clinical ability, and variation among expert evaluators is to be expected as there is no correct answer to many clinical experiences; additionally, assessors may have differing expectations and preferences regarding clinical skills, which underscores the need to provide the learner with specific examples of how to improve performance. Developing a strategy for delivery of feedback that is positive, task-centered, timely, and specific is essential for meaningful workplace-based assessment. The ideal feedback mechanism should be integrated into the workplace, drive learning, and be well understood by the learner (van der Vleuten et al. 2010). A disconnect between assessor and learner can result in the assessment feeling arbitrary or intimidating. It is important to clearly establish the expectations regarding assessment impact (high or low stakes), process (ad hoc or structured), and purpose (formative or summative) to alleviate learner concerns. Ideally, impactful feedback provided in an effective manner is conducive to an environment where assessment drives learning and is not an end in and of itself (Kinnear et al. 2021).

Limitations of workplace-based assessment include that the dynamic hospital or clinical environment precludes uniformity of experience among students. This type of assessment is opportunity-driven, thus not all learners will be able to experience a similar cohort of cases during their education and may encounter significant variation in case numbers, content, severity, and complexity. Likewise, the hospital or clinic is driven by patient care as a priority, and there must be a balance between management of cases and the opportunity for assessment, which can be time-consuming and challenging in specific clinical contexts.

An additional obstacle associated with workplace-based assessment is related to the need for multiple sources of feedback and observations of clinical performance in order to reach a valid conclusion about clinical fitness. Numerous evaluations of performance and workplace-based assessment have found that performance in one clinical scenario does not reliably predict performance in another, a concept referred to as "content specificity" (van der Vleuten et al. 2010). Therefore, it is essential that numerous observations are used to generate any summative or high-stakes evaluation of a learner. The validity of the evaluation process can be further strengthened by incorporating feedback both from multiple occasions and multiple sources.

Subjectivity of the assessor has historically also been perceived as a threat to validity of workplace-based assessments. As noted in the discussion of OSCE scoring, however, objectivity is not necessarily synonymous with validity, and subjective clinical assessments are still a meaningful way of assessing a learner. As with content specificity, multiple assessments, by different qualified, expert assessors, mediate the variability of clinician opinions about treatment options and professional behaviors inherent to clinical practice.

Numerous approaches have been identified for workplace-based assessment. These can be grouped into two categories: those based on direct observation of the learner versus those derived from a compilation of different clinical metrics. Some of the most common direct observation modalities include the mini-clinical evaluation exercise (mini-CEX), direct observation of procedural skills (DOPS), and multi-source feedback (MSF), though other approaches, such as case-based discussion and in-training evaluation reports (ITERs), have also been described (Weijs et al. 2015; Wilkinson et al. 2008). Aggregate assessment information may include data such as case logs, case metrics, procedures, or complication rates, or for a more holistic approach, portfolio development.

The mini-CEX provides assessment while the learner is providing direct patient care. A qualified assessor watches the interaction and then provides the learner with feedback on specific aspects of their practice. This approach was originally developed in human medicine for internal medicine residency assessment; however, the tool has spread widely and been employed in a variety of settings.

Ideally, the mini-CEX is used formatively and serves to identify any student who is performing markedly below expectations while providing feedback to all learners that leads to improved performance. While formative assessment is most common, the mini-CEX has also been used summatively, although the validity of single-instance mini-CEX encounters is a drawback. The mini-CEX may be used to evaluate history taking, physical examination skills, communication, clinical judgment, professionalism, and efficiency, though not all attributes may be able to be evaluated in all settings (Swanwick 2018). Evaluation forms typically allow for characterization of the encounter (clinical setting, severity, new, or follow-up appointment), a Likert scale for whether the learner meets expectations in different domains, and free-text boxes for positive feedback and suggestions for improvement.

The mini-CEX has been shown to correlate with other measures of clinical skill (Swanwick 2018). Educational impact, validity, and reliability have generally be shown to be good; however, the primary limitation is the number of encounters required to achieve the necessary level of reliability (Mortaz Hejri et al. 2020). Frequency of assessment has varied in the human medical literature from one encounter per week to one encounter every two months, depending on setting and rotation duration. In veterinary medicine, the mini-CEX has been described for use in a primary care environment. Hecker et al. (2012b) discuss the use of the mini-CEX and similar evaluation instruments at the Ontario Veterinary College (OVC) and the University of Calgary, providing an example of the OVC's modified mini-CEX evaluation form. This form focuses on six domains: history taking and relationship building, physical exam skills, explaining and planning, clinical judgment, professionalism, and organization/efficiency. There is also an assessment of overall clinical skills and overall communication skills. The form builds on the classic document by adding an area for a development plan and action steps, as well as characterizing the time commitment spent in both evaluating the learner and providing feedback (Hecker et al. 2012b). An additional publication from the OVC describes implementation of workplace-based assessment in a primary care rotation through qualitative feedback from students and instructors (Weijs et al. 2015). In this instance, the mini-CEX was performed twice during a three-week rotation. Both students and instructors found the mini-CEX feasible and worthwhile, though time-intensive, and commented on the assessment as a useful means of facilitating specific, timely feedback.

The DOPS assessment is a modification of the mini-CEX, designed to evaluate procedural skills. As with the mini-CEX, the learner is observed with a real patient in a clinical setting and the instructor provides written and verbal feedback immediately following the observation. DOPS has been used in human medicine to assess short skills such as intubation and arterial blood gas sampling. The learner is assessed on all aspects of the procedure, including clinical understanding, safety, patient comfort, and communication (Swanwick 2018). The limitations of the DOPS are similar to that of the mini-CEX: time required of the instructor and learner, and content specificity requiring multiple DOPS to achieve validity. In veterinary medicine, a study comparing DOPS to multiple choice questions (MCQ) found that students employed deeper learning when preparing for DOPS than MCQ. Students were driven to prepare for DOPS due to a desire to understand the material, whereas they were motivated to study for MCQ due to a fear of failure (Cobb et al. 2013). These differences are likely at least partially due to major structural differences between the two assessment methods; the DOPS is designed for formative assessment of procedural skills whereas MCQ are used for summative assessment of factual knowledge. Despite this, the difference in student motivation is illustrative of the concept of learning driving assessment (or vice versa). DOPS was also evaluated in the small animal primary care setting, where two DOPS were performed (one surgical and one diagnostic) in a three-week rotation. Students and instructors found the DOPS helpful, particularly when time allowed repeated assessments on the same skill, which allowed a learner to evaluate growth and plan future development (Weijs et al. 2015).

ITER or in-training assessments are commonly used during clinical rotations. ITERs provide formative evaluation of the learner at the end of a multi-week period of clinical training. This is usually provided via Likert-scale evaluation of rotation competencies with additional narrative feedback. The evaluation summarizes the learner's demonstrated skills and abilities over the duration of the rotation. However, this assessment method has been criticized for a lack of accuracy and reliability. Assessors demonstrate a low ability to discriminate between learners, either based on a surface-level appreciation of skill or a tendency to give generous ratings regardless of obvious differences in ability. Validity is limited by an inability to address issues of content specificity with a summary method of evaluation. Low correlation between ITER and other assessment methods also raises concerns about accuracy and validity (Govaerts et al. 2007). In a study in veterinary medicine, ITERs were compared to entrustment scales with results demonstrating that scores on entrustment scales increased over time, while ITER scores did not (Read et al. 2021). The narrative feedback provided on entrustment scales was also longer, more specific, and utilized a coaching voice relative to feedback provided on

ITERs. In an another veterinary study, students expressed that nonspecific feedback provided via ITER was not useful, and instructors found it burdensome, repetitive, and time-intensive (Weijs et al. 2015). Suggestions for improving the usefulness of ITERs include making them more context-specific, engaging assessors in evaluation report design and discussion of underlying assessment theory, and modifying prompts for narrative feedback to elicit more specific, actionable, and robust commentary (Govaerts et al. 2007; Hatala et al. 2017).

MSF (also known as 360° feedback) is an approach to assessment that captures the viewpoints of a variety of stakeholders, such as peers, clients, technical staff, and house officers, in addition to faculty instructors. Self-assessment is also often used in MSF. This approach varies in whether the learner chooses who provides feedback, whether the feedback is anonymous, and how the feedback is delivered to the learner (van der Vleuten et al. 2010). MSF also differs from mini-CEX and DOPS in that assessors provide an overall judgment about a learner's skill set, rather than a specific assessment of a single encounter. Learners may be assessed in categories such as clinical care, effective practice (efficiency and technical skills), teaching/training, patient/client relationships, and colleague interactions. The mini-PAT (peer assessment tool) has been used in human medicine for peer evaluations. This instrument features Likert scale ratings for subcompetencies within the larger categories noted above, an overall rating, and area in which the assessor may state any concerns regarding the learner (Swanwick 2018). As with the mini-CEX and DOPS, forms are modified as applicable to the specific setting and evaluator. Using MSF to assess attributes such as professionalism and collegiality has good validity, though multiple assessors are required, and allowing learners to choose evaluators may skew feedback (Magnier et al. 2012; Mossop and Cobb 2013). Drawbacks of MSF are that distributing, collecting, and organizing feedback for the learner can be difficult and time-consuming.

An additional type of evaluation is that which is oriented around case discussions, versions of which have been described in human medical education literature as "case-based discussion" or "chart-stimulated recall." These assessments are focused on the idea of reviewing a learner's reasoning behind case decisions. A case the learner was involved in with regard to time management and medical record documentation is selected by either the assessor or learner; the learner may select two to three cases the assessor subsequently chooses between. The assessor then questions the learner to probe the clinical reasoning behind case management choices. Questions may include focus on areas such as differential list development, diagnostic choices, communication, and treatment/management

Table 11.4 Chart-Stimulated review sample questions.

- Discuss your diagnostic decision-making for this patient. What features of the patient's presentation led you to your top two diagnoses? Was there ambiguity or uncertainty? If yes, how did you deal with it?
- Did you order any labs or tests? What was your rationale? Were there other tests that you thought of but decided against? Why?
- Did you inquire about the patient's (client's) experience of his or her illness and care (feelings, ideas, effect on function, and expectations)? What did you learn?
- Describe your management and treatment decisions. What did you decide was appropriate for follow-up? What factors influenced your decisions?

Source: Adapted from Philibert (2018).

decisions (Philibert 2018). Representative questions from Philibert (2018) may be found in Table 11.4. The learner is asked to discuss the case to articulate their strategy in case management, revealing both an understanding of the medical condition or presenting complaint in question, but also a broader understanding of case management and critical thinking in a clinical setting. Feedback may be provided in written and/or verbal forms; authors have described both the use of a standard and clinical milestones-based rating scale (Reddy et al. 2018).

Aggregate methods of assessment are those that encompass a greater period of time than MSF, DOPS, or mini-CEX. These may span the entire duration of veterinary school or be limited to the clinical year. Case or procedure logs are one of the more commonly employed approaches to aggregate assessment of clinical skills. (Rush et al. 2011) describe a web-based logbook for clinical students to document technical skills over the course of the year. Students were required to complete a minimum number of skills overall from specific subsections and submit these skills for feedback to an assessor (technician, house officer, or faculty member). Students were also asked to self-assess their performance with a scale that identified if they required additional coaching, were competent but inefficient, or competent and efficient. Assessors were asked to correspondingly evaluate the student's performance on the task as not yet competent, competent, or excellent (Rush et al. 2011). Although not commonly framed this way, logbooks are a type of portfolio that focus almost exclusively on student monitoring (van der Vleuten et al. 2010).

Portfolios are described extensively in health professions education as a compilation of learner achievement and feedback (and are covered in detail in Chapter 12 of this textbook). This accumulation of material differs from MSF in that it is broader, spans a greater period of time, and is compiled by the learner from different sources. A number of different models for portfolio construction exist; in one

source, they are colorfully described as the shopping trolley, toast rack, spinal column, and cake mix (Endacott et al. 2004). These descriptions illustrate some of the varying forms possible for a portfolio to take: the shopping trolley, which includes anything the learner deems relevant to their development; toast rack, which indicates a number of required slots that must be filled for a portfolio to be completed; spinal column, wherein a learner gathers material to satisfy a list of elements; and cake mix, which mixes components of the portfolio to create a greater whole with written reflection. Portfolios can also differ in their focus on outcomes of assessing, coaching, or monitoring, with relative emphases on the portfolio containing evidence, reflection, or overviews of the learner's experience (van Tartwijk and Driessen 2009).

Portfolios are capable of serving as multipurpose instruments and are ideally specific enough to provide the learner with objectives but allow a great degree of flexibility in how this is manifested. They should additionally incorporate periodic student reflections that demonstrate to the assessor growth and maturation over the time period designated (van Tartwijk and Driessen 2009). Drawbacks of the portfolio are the time-consuming nature of creation/compilation for the learner, the time required of a mentor/assessor to provide feedback and assess, and the lack of validity and reliability.

The use of e-portfolios, which minimize physical materials and includes user-friendly hyperlinks and easy indexing, facilitates compilation and material review (Tochel et al. 2009; van Tartwijk and Driessen 2009). Portfolios may also differ in whether they are focused on a single objective or competency or are program-wide and all-encompassing (van der Vleuten et al. 2010). Depending on the use for which the portfolio is intended, they may also vary in whether they are formative, summative, or both assessment types concurrently. Reliability is difficult to measure given the wide variety of ways in which portfolio use has been implemented for medical training; use of multiple assessors is helpful in improving reliability. However, a review of portfolio use among different health professions identified increased engagement and personal responsibility for learning, and enhanced professional development associated with well-implemented portfolio use (Tochel et al. 2009).

Section 4: Essential Concepts in Clinical Skills Assessment

In considering the body of knowledge around clinical skills assessment in the health professions, and specifically veterinary medicine, several critical themes emerge:

Part 1: Assessment Both Documents and Drives Learning

At the higher levels of Miller's pyramid, both *shows how* and *does,* assessment methods are authentic and context-rich, providing deeper meaning to knowledge that is acquired. The learner is an integral part of any assessment and as they transition from student to health professional, should be encouraged to embrace ownership of the learning process and drive their own assessment. Many of the assessment methods discussed in this chapter lend themselves to self-directed learning and varying degrees of autonomy with regard to assessment, such as clinical skills labs, simulation use, clinical encounters for mini-CEX and DOPS that the learner selects for evaluation, and self-reflection in MSF and portfolios. The concept of assessment *for* learning, associated with a progressive and humanistic educational framework, is essential to encouraging the development of independence, professional identity, and doctors who can be entrusted with the practice of veterinary medicine.

Although learner-centered and formative assessment processes comprise the main body of assessments used to evaluate clinical skills, there is a countervailing imperative to have documentation *of* learning prior to certification of students as independent professionals. Stakeholders within the institution, the profession, and the public require assurance that education programs are producing competent, proficient, and safe healthcare providers. Summative assessment is achieved through OSCEs, when properly delivered with accurate methods to develop a passing standard, and through clinical work in which students must acceptably demonstrate performance to expert evaluators, as in skills logbooks, or mini-CEX and DOPS, which provide more nuanced feedback. Portfolios provide a holistic assessment of a learner's overall body of work, allowing a program to assess a student's readiness for practice in a wide variety of areas. It is critical for veterinary training programs to select assessment practices that both encourage learner development and ensure integrity of the profession and safety and competence of those allowed to practice.

Part 2: Assessment Purposes Are Made Clear

Andragogy, or the process of teaching adult learners, has several basic tenets pioneered by Malcolm Knowles that are relevant to clinical skills assessment. Adult learners differ from children in their desire for applicable and meaningful knowledge, their store of prior experience, and the need to direct their own learning. Implications of these concepts suggest that where possible, the adult learner should be involved in mutual planning of learning and assessment and have choice in how to carry out learning and assessment plans. Clear communication about the rationale for various assessment practices allows the learner to derive practical knowledge and contextualized meaning from these events rather than seeing them as an obstacle devoid of purpose. Providing autonomy where possible, for instance in the selection of cases for review with an assessor, timing of a clinical evaluation, or the ability to practice a skill in a laboratory with formative assessment prior to higher stakes testing are all examples of applying the framework of andragogy in order to make assessment purposeful, meaningful, and useful to adult learners.

A positive climate for assessment should be established that promotes the learner's physical and emotional safety. Although assessment is inherently stressful to most learners, creating clear expectations about the purposes for and consequences of an assessment can mitigate anxiety. A focus on frequent, ongoing formative assessments also engages learners in the process of their professional growth and acclimatizes them to the process of self-evaluation and receiving structured feedback.

Appropriate assessment selection and design are also critical. While much of clinical skills assessment can be holistic and evaluate both technical proficiency and humanistic attributes, there should still be clear learning objectives for each assessment. Competency-based education and EPAs can be used to facilitate development of learning objectives and outcomes. The level of assessment (*shows how/does/is/trusted*) should be identified and articulated, and more specifically, the desired functions of assessment should be identified. Is the assessment meant to provide a grade, indicate learner readiness, direct student learning, review material, provide quality assurance, or some combination of these elements?

Part 3: The Assessor Is as Important as the Assessment

Feedback is the means through which assessment can be used to generate a change in performance. Effective feedback is a collaboration between teacher and learner that allows the learner to understand gaps between their performance and learning objectives, develop goals, and create a plan to reach them. Many veterinary students are used to didactic courses that rely heavily on summative assessment; performance in these situations is defined by success or failure, rather than a process of gradual, progressive improvement over time. Feedback must be explained to students so that formative assessments are understood as motivational and part of a natural progression of growth, rather than a manifestation of inadequacy.

Characteristics of good feedback are that it is timely, specific, actionable, and task-oriented. Feedback should be

Table 11.5 Seven principles of good feedback practice.

1) Helps clarify what good performance is (goals, criteria, expected standards)
2) Facilitates the development of self-assessment (reflection) in learning
3) Delivers high-quality information to students about their learning
4) Encourages teacher and peer dialogue around learning
5) Encourages positive motivational beliefs and self-esteem
6) Provides opportunities to close the gap between current and desired performance
7) Provides information to teachers that can be used to help shape teaching

Source: Adapted from Nicol and Macfarlane-Dick (2006).

delivered in a safe environment and be related to previously defined learning objectives. Table 11.5 outlines other principles of delivering feedback effectively. Action plans should be developed using the SMART construct, which is an acronym for Specific, Measurable, Attainable, Relevant, and Time-bound (Lee and Chiu 2021). Learners are likely to disregard feedback that they perceive is not constructive, is not delivered from a credible source, or threatens their self-worth (Watling and Ginsburg 2019). Feedback that is poorly delivered can be demotivational to the learner and create the opposite of the desired effect (Swanwick 2018).

An essential aspect of meaningful assessment and worthwhile feedback is that assessors must be well-trained. This is an often-overlooked aspect of assessment delivery; in busy educational institutions, the assessors selected are determined by who is available and who is responsible, with little thought given to individual capability as an assessor (Lockyer et al. 2017). The ability to assess effectively is a learned skill that is unrelated to the content expertise of the assessor. Training is rarely provided for assessment or occurs as an isolated event; however, for all the attention given to assessment instruments, they can only be as effective as the assessors who use them (van der Vleuten et al. 2010).

Various specific training programs have been developed to promote effective assessment practices, such as behavioral observation training, performance dimension training, and frame of reference training, which may add to an assessor's abilities generally (Lockyer et al. 2017). Training on specific instrument use is also critical so that an assessor clearly understands the criteria by which a learner is being evaluated and can distinguish reliably between levels of performance. Sources of bias such as the halo effect (bias due to preexisting information about a learner), a tendency of the assessor toward harsh or permissive evaluation (severity and leniency bias; sometimes referred to as hawk/dove assessors), or personal factors of the assessor, can confound assessment (Magnier et al. 2012). Although bias is unlikely

to ever be eliminated entirely, training and awareness can mitigate its effects. Assessor training should be an ongoing part of delivery of assessment and faculty development at all veterinary education programs. With instruction, staff and faculty can improve their skill with regard to assessment, learning to mitigate bias, understand assessment goals, instruments, and expected outcomes, and developing the ability to provide constructive and useful feedback.

Part 4: Programmatic Assessment Is Essential

Programmatic assessment, in which multiple direct observations over time are used to make judgments about a learner's competency, is an essential assumption of the use of competency-based education in veterinary medicine (Danielson 2021). Both competency-based medical education and clinical skills evaluation rely on formative assessment methods that are designed to assist the learner in progressing further along a continuum of knowledge and skill (Lee and Chiu 2021). The shift away from relatively infrequent assessment that provides summative decisions about a learner's readiness and toward assessment that is ongoing, dynamic, and integrated into the process of learning requires an overall restructuring of how we conceptualize assessment and evaluation in veterinary medicine.

Formative assessment relies on multiple, diverse points of assessment to render a complete picture of a learner upon which summative decisions can be made. Single assessments are prone to a lack of validity due to content specificity and bias; whereas a larger aggregation of assessment material allows for information to be averaged, thus mitigating the noise around the true signal of a learner's competence. Despite concerns about validity and reliability associated with qualitative data, it is clear that content experts who are trained assessors provide valuable information and that subjectivity is not synonymous with bias.

Summary

Assessments should ideally be valid, reliable, feasible, acceptable, defensible, and have educational impact; however, no single assessment type is without limitations, and evaluations from different sources, different methodologies, and different time points all contribute to creating a more comprehensive and accurate assessment picture (Magnier et al. 2012; van der Vleuten 1996). Clinical skills assessment in veterinary medicine will continue to evolve with a persistent focus on learner-centric assessment, constructive feedback that empowers ownership, and self-direction, and is driven by the ultimate goal of creating competent and capable veterinary clinicians.

References

Anderson, S.L., Miller, L., Gibbons, P. et al. (2021). Development and validation of a bovine castration model and rubric. *Journal of Veterinary Medical Education* 48 (1): 96–104. https://doi.org/10.3138/jvme.2018-0016.

Annandale, A., Scheepers, E., and Fosgate, G.T. (2020). The effect of an ovariohysterectomy model practice on surgical times for final-year veterinary students' first live-animal ovariohysterectomies. *Journal of Veterinary Medical Education* 47 (1): 44–55. https://doi.org/10.3138/jvme.1217-181r1.

Artemiou, E., Adams, C.L., Hecker, K.G. et al. (2014). Standardised clients as assessors in a veterinary communication OSCE: a reliability and validity study. *Veterinary Record* 175 (20): 509. https://doi.org/10.1136/vr.102633.

Au Yong, J.A., Case, J.B., Kim, S.E. et al. (2019). Survey of instructor and student impressions of a high-fidelity model in canine ovariohysterectomy surgical training. *Veterinary Surgery* 48 (6): 975–984. https://doi.org/10.1111/vsu.13218.

Baillie, S., Christopher, R., Catterall, A.J. et al. (2020). Comparison of a silicon skin pad and a tea towel as models for learning a simple interrupted suture. *Journal of Veterinary Medical Education* 47 (4): 516–522. https://doi.org/10.3138/jvme.2018-0001.

Banse, H.E., McMillan, C.J., Warren, A.L. et al. (2021). Development of and validity evidence for a canine ocular model for training novice veterinary students to perform a fundic examination. *Journal of Veterinary Medical Education* 48 (5): 620–628. https://doi.org/10.3138/jvme-2020-0035.

Bergus, G.R., Woodhead, J.C., and Kreiter, C.D. (2009). Trained lay observers can reliably assess medical students' communication skills. *Medical Education* 43 (7): 688–694. https://doi.org/10.1111/j.1365-2923.2009.03396.x.

Bok, H.G.J., de Jong, L.H., O'Neill, T. et al. (2018). Validity evidence for programmatic assessment in competency-based education. *Perspectives on Medical Education* 7 (6): 362–372. https://doi.org/10.1007/s40037-018-0481-2.

Carroll, H.S., Lucia, T.A., Farnsworth, C.H. et al. (2016). Development of an optional clinical skills laboratory for surgical skills training of veterinary students. *Journal of the American Veterinary Medical Association* 248 (6): 624–628. https://doi.org/10.2460/javma.248.6.624.

ten Cate, O. (2016). Entrustment as assessment: recognizing the ability, the right, and the duty to act. *Journal of Graduate Medical Education* 8 (2): 261–262. https://doi.org/10.4300/jgme-d-16-00097.1.

ten Cate, O. and Scheele, F. (2007). Competency-based postgraduate training: can we bridge the gap between theory and clinical practice? *Academic Medicine* 82 (6): 542–547. https://doi.org/10.1097/ACM.0b013e31805559c7.

ten Cate, O., Carraccio, C., Damodaran, A. et al. (2021). Entrustment decision making: extending Miller's pyramid. *Academic Medicine* 96 (2): 199–204. https://doi.org/10.1097/acm.0000000000003800.

Clausse, M., Nejamkin, P., Bulant, C.A. et al. (2020). A low-cost portable simulator of a domestic cat larynx for teaching endotracheal intubation. *Veterinary Anaesthesia and Analgesia* 47 (5): 676–680. https://doi.org/10.1016/j.vaa.2020.05.006.

Cobb, K.A., Brown, G., Jaarsma, D.A., and Hammond, R.A. (2013). The educational impact of assessment: a comparison of DOPS and MCQs. *Medical Teacher* 35 (11): e1598–e1607. https://doi.org/10.3109/0142159x.2013.803061.

Compton, N.J., Cary, J.A., Wenz, J.R. et al. (2019). Evaluation of peer teaching and deliberate practice to teach veterinary surgery. *Veterinary Surgery* 48 (2): 199–208. https://doi.org/10.1111/vsu.13117.

Cosford, K., Briere, J., Ambros, B. et al. (2020). Effect of instructional format on veterinary students' task performance and emotional state during a simulation-based canine endotracheal intubation laboratory: handout versus video. *Journal of Veterinary Medical Education* 47 (2): 239–247. https://doi.org/10.3138/jvme.0618-077r1.

Cruess, R.L., Cruess, S.R., and Steinert, Y. (2016). Amending Miller's pyramid to include professional identity formation. *Academic Medicine* 91 (2): 180–185. https://doi.org/10.1097/acm.0000000000000913.

Danielson, J.A. (2021). Key assumptions underlying a competency-based approach to medical sciences education, and their applicability to veterinary medical education. *Frontiers in Veterinary Science* 8: 688457. https://doi.org/10.3389/fvets.2021.688457.

Dilly, M., Read, E.K., and Baillie, S. (2017). A survey of established veterinary clinical skills laboratories from Europe and North America: present practices and recent developments. *Journal of Veterinary Medical Education* 44 (4): 580–589. https://doi.org/10.3138/jvme.0216-030R1.

Dos Santos Martins, T.G., Schor, P., Stuchi, J.A., and Fowler, S.B. (2021). New direct and indirect ophthalmoscopy teaching methodology for veterinary doctors: teaching tip. *Journal of Veterinary Medical Education*, e20200089. https://doi.org/10.3138/jvme-2020-0089.

Dwyer, T., Wright, S., Kulasegaram, K.M. et al. (2016). How to set the bar in competency-based medical education: standard setting after an Objective Structured Clinical Examination (OSCE). *BMC Medical Education* 16: 1. https://doi.org/10.1186/s12909-015-0506-z.

Endacott, R., Gray, M.A., Jasper, M.A. et al. (2004). Using portfolios in the assessment of learning and competence: the impact of four models. *Nurse Education in Practice* 4 (4): 250–257. https://doi.org/10.1016/j.nepr.2004.01.003.

Englander, R., Frank, J.R., Carraccio, C. et al. (2017). Toward a shared language for competency-based medical education. *Medical Teacher* 39 (6): 582–587. https://doi.org/10.1080/0142159x.2017.1315066.

Englar, R.E. (2019a). Tracking veterinary students' acquisition of communication skills and clinical communication confidence by comparing student performance in the first and twenty-seventh standardized client encounters. *Journal of Veterinary Medical Education* 46 (2): 235–257. https://doi.org/10.3138/jvme.0917-117r1.

Englar, R.E. (2019b). Using a standardized client encounter to practice death notification after the unexpected death of a feline patient following routine ovariohysterectomy. *Journal of Veterinary Medical Education* 46 (4): 489–505. https://doi.org/10.3138/jvme.0817-111r1.

Ericsson, K.A. (2004). Deliberate practice and the acquisition and maintenance of expert performance in medicine and related domains. *Academic Medicine* 79 (10 Suppl): S70–S81.

Ericsson, K.A. (2008). Deliberate practice and acquisition of expert performance: a general overview. *Academic Emergency Medicine* 15 (11): 988–994. https://doi.org/10.1111/j.1553-2712.2008.00227.x.

Goldschmidt, S.L. and Root Kustritz, M.V. (2021). Pilot study evaluating the use of typodonts (dental models) for teaching veterinary dentistry as part of the Core veterinary curriculum. *Journal of Veterinary Medical Education*, e20200113. https://doi.org/10.3138/jvme-2020-0113.

Govaerts, M.J., van der Vleuten, C.P., Schuwirth, L.W., and Muijtjens, A.M. (2007). Broadening perspectives on clinical performance assessment: rethinking the nature of in-training assessment. *Advances in Health Sciences Education: Theory and Practice* 12 (2): 239–260. https://doi.org/10.1007/s10459-006-9043-1.

Hamstra, S.J., Brydges, R., Hatala, R. et al. (2014). Reconsidering fidelity in simulation-based training. *Academic Medicine* 89 (3): 387–392. https://doi.org/10.1097/acm.0000000000000130.

Hatala, R., Sawatsky, A.P., Dudek, N. et al. (2017). Using In-Training Evaluation Report (ITER) qualitative comments to assess medical students and residents: a systematic review. *Academic Medicine* 92 (6): 868–879. https://doi.org/10.1097/acm.0000000000001506.

Hecker, K., Read, E.K., Vallevand, A. et al. (2010). Assessment of first-year veterinary students' clinical skills using objective structured clinical examinations. *Journal of Veterinary Medical Education* 37 (4): 395–402. https://doi.org/10.3138/jvme.37.4.395.

Hecker, K.G., Adams, C.L., and Coe, J.B. (2012a). Assessment of first-year veterinary students' communication skills using an objective structured clinical examination: the importance of context. *Journal of Veterinary Medical Education* 39 (3): 304–310. https://doi.org/10.3138/jvme.0312.022R.

Hecker, K.G., Norris, J., and Coe, J.B. (2012b). Workplace-based assessment in a primary-care setting. *Journal of Veterinary Medical Education* 39 (3): 229–240. https://doi.org/10.3138/jvme.0612.054R.

Hodgson, J.L. and Pelzer, J.M. (2017). *Veterinary Medical Education: A Practical Guide*. Wiley.

Hunt, J.A., Heydenburg, M., Kelly, C.K. et al. (2020a). Development and validation of a canine castration model and rubric. *Journal of Veterinary Medical Education* 47 (1): 78–90. https://doi.org/10.3138/jvme.1117-158r1.

Hunt, J.A., Hughes, C., Asciutto, M., and Johnson, J.T. (2020b). Development and validation of a feline medial saphenous venipuncture model and rubric. *Journal of Veterinary Medical Education* 47 (3): 333–341. https://doi.org/10.3138/jvme.0718-085.

Hunt, J.A., Schmidt, P., Perkins, J. et al. (2021a). Comparison of three canine models for teaching veterinary dental cleaning. *Journal of Veterinary Medical Education* 48 (5): 573–583. https://doi.org/10.3138/jvme-2020-0001.

Hunt, J.A., Simons, M.C., and Anderson, S.L. (2021b). If you build it, they will learn: a review of models in veterinary surgical education. *Veterinary Surgery* https://doi.org/10.1111/vsu.13683.

Kedrowicz, A.A. (2016). The impact of a group communication course on veterinary medical students' perceptions of communication competence and communication apprehension. *Journal of Veterinary Medical Education* 43 (2): 135–142. https://doi.org/10.3138/jvme.0615-100R1.

Kinnear, B., Warm, E.J., Caretta-Weyer, H. et al. (2021). Entrustment unpacked: aligning purposes, stakes, and processes to enhance learner assessment. *Academic Medicine* 96 (7s): S56–s63. https://doi.org/10.1097/acm.0000000000004108.

Langebæk, R., Eika, B., Jensen, A.L. et al. (2012). Anxiety in veterinary surgical students: a quantitative study. *Journal of Veterinary Medical Education* 39 (4): 331–340. https://doi.org/10.3138/jvme.1111-111R1.

Langebæk, R., Toft, N., and Eriksen, T. (2015). The SimSpay-student perceptions of a low-cost build-it-yourself model for novice training of surgical skills in canine ovariohysterectomy. *Journal of Veterinary Medical Education* 42 (2): 166–171. https://doi.org/10.3138/jvme.1014-105.

Langebæk, R., Berendt, M., Tipold, A. et al. (2021). Evaluation of the impact of using a simulator for teaching veterinary students cerebrospinal fluid collection: a mixed-methods study. *Journal of Veterinary Medical Education* 48 (2): 217–227. https://doi.org/10.3138/jvme.2019-0006.

Lee, G.B. and Chiu, A.M. (2021). Assessment and feedback methods in competency-based medical education. *Annals of Allergy, Asthma & Immunology* https://doi.org/10.1016/j.anai.2021.12.010.

Lockyer, J., Carraccio, C., Chan, M.K. et al. (2017). Core principles of assessment in competency-based medical education. *Medical Teacher* 39 (6): 609–616. https://doi.org/10.1080/0142159x.2017.1315082.

Luís Pires, J., Payo, P., and Marcos, R. (2021). The use of simulators for teaching fine needle aspiration cytology in veterinary medicine. *Journal of Veterinary Medical Education*, e20200036. https://doi.org/10.3138/jvme-2020-0036.

MacArthur, S.L., Johnson, M.D., and Colee, J.C. (2021). Effect of a Spay simulator on student competence and anxiety. *Journal of Veterinary Medical Education* 48 (1): 115–128. https://doi.org/10.3138/jvme.0818-089r3.

Magnier, K.M., Dale, V.H., and Pead, M.J. (2012). Workplace-based assessment instruments in the health sciences. *Journal of Veterinary Medical Education* 39 (4): 389–395. https://doi.org/10.3138/jvme.1211-118R.

McCool, K.E. and Kedrowicz, A.A. (2020). Evaluation of veterinary students' communication skills with a service dog handler in a simulated client scenario. *Journal of Veterinary Medical Education*, e20190140. https://doi.org/10.3138/jvme-2019-0140.

McCool, K.E., Bissett, S.A., Hill, T.L. et al. (2020). Evaluation of a human virtual-reality endoscopy trainer for teaching early endoscopy skills to veterinarians. *Journal of Veterinary Medical Education* 47 (1): 106–116. https://doi.org/10.3138/jvme.0418-037r.

Michels, M.E., Evans, D.E., and Blok, G.A. (2012). What is a clinical skill? Searching for order in chaos through a modified Delphi process. *Medical Teacher* 34 (8): e573–e581. https://doi.org/10.3109/0142159x.2012.669218.

Miller, G.E. (1990). The assessment of clinical skills/competence/performance. *Academic Medicine* 65 (9 Suppl): S63–S67. https://doi.org/10.1097/00001888-199009000-00045.

Morin, D.E., Arnold, C.J., Hale-Mitchell, L.K. et al. (2020). Development and evolution of the clinical skills learning center as an integral component of the Illinois veterinary professional curriculum. *Journal of Veterinary Medical Education* 47 (3): 307–320. https://doi.org/10.3138/jvme.1217-186r1.

Mortaz Hejri, S., Jalili, M., Masoomi, R. et al. (2020). The utility of mini-Clinical Evaluation Exercise in undergraduate and postgraduate medical education: a

BEME review: BEME Guide No. 59. *Medical Teacher* 42 (2): 125–142. https://doi.org/10.1080/0142159x.2019.1652732.

Mossop, L.H. and Cobb, K. (2013). Teaching and assessing veterinary professionalism. *Journal of Veterinary Medical Education* 40 (3): 223–232. https://doi.org/10.3138/jvme.0113-016R.

Naeem, N., van der Vleuten, C., and Alfaris, E.A. (2012). Faculty development on item writing substantially improves item quality. *Advances in Health Sciences Education: Theory and Practice* 17 (3): 369–376. https://doi.org/10.1007/s10459-011-9315-2.

Nicol, D.J. and Macfarlane-Dick, D. (2006). Formative assessment and self-regulated learning: a model and seven principles of good feedback practice. *Studies in Higher Education* 31 (2): 199–218. https://doi.org/10.1080/03075070600572090.

Noyes, J.A., Carbonneau, K.J., and Matthew, S.M. (2021). Comparative effectiveness of training with simulators versus traditional instruction in veterinary education: meta-analysis and systematic review. *Journal of veterinary Medical Education*, e20200026. https://doi.org/10.3138/jvme-2020-0026.

Philibert, I. (2018). Using chart review and chart-stimulated recall for resident assessment. *Journal of Graduate Medical Education* 10 (1): 95–96. https://doi.org/10.4300/jgme-d-17-01010.1.

Read, E.K., Bell, C., Rhind, S., and Hecker, K.G. (2015). The use of global rating scales for OSCEs in veterinary medicine. *PLoS One* 10 (3): e0121000. https://doi.org/10.1371/journal.pone.0121000.

Read, E.K., Brown, A., Maxey, C., and Hecker, K.G. (2021). Comparing entrustment and competence: an exploratory look at performance-relevant information in the final year of a veterinary program. *Journal of Veterinary Medical Education* 48 (5): 562–572. https://doi.org/10.3138/jvme-2019-0128.

Reddy, S.T., Tekian, A., Durning, S.J. et al. (2018). Preliminary validity evidence for a milestones-based rating scale for chart-stimulated recall. *Journal of Graduate Medical Education* 10 (3): 269–275. https://doi.org/10.4300/jgme-d-17-00435.1.

Reynolds, R.C., Livingston, B.R., and Wilson, V. (2006). *Measurement and Assessment in Education*. Pearson/Allyn & Bacon.

Rush, B.R., Biller, D.S., Davis, E.G. et al. (2011). Web-based documentation of clinical skills to assess the competency of veterinary students. *Journal of Veterinary Medical Education* 38 (3): 242–250. https://doi.org/10.3138/jvme.38.3.242.

Sadideen, H. and Kneebone, R. (2012). Practical skills teaching in contemporary surgical education: how can educational theory be applied to promote effective learning? *The American Journal of Surgery* 204 (3): 396–401. https://doi.org/10.1016/j.amjsurg.2011.12.020.

Schnabel, L.V., Maza, P.S., Williams, K.M. et al. (2013). Use of a formal assessment instrument for evaluation of veterinary student surgical skills. *Veterinary Surgery* 42 (4): 488–496. https://doi.org/10.1111/j.1532-950X.2013.12006.x.

Schuwirth, L.W.T. and van der Vleuten, C.P.M. (2020). A history of assessment in medical education. *Advances in Health Sciences Education: Theory and Practice* 25 (5): 1045–1056. https://doi.org/10.1007/s10459-020-10003-0.

Seddon, J.M., Vo, A.T.T., Kempster, S.R. et al. (2020). Simulated clinical skills for veterinary students supplement limited animal and clinical resources in developing countries. *Journal of Veterinary Medical Education* 47 (s1): 92–98. https://doi.org/10.3138/jvme-2019-0112.

Sennhenn-Kirchner, S., Goerlich, Y., Kirchner, B. et al. (2018). The effect of repeated testing vs repeated practice on skills learning in undergraduate dental education. *European Journal of Dental Education* 22 (1): e42–e47. https://doi.org/10.1111/eje.12254.

Sheats, M.K., Burke, M.J., Robertson, J.B. et al. (2021). Development and formative evaluation of a low-Fidelity equine castration model for veterinary education. *Frontiers in Veterinary Science* 8: 689243. https://doi.org/10.3389/fvets.2021.689243.

da Silva, D.A.F., Fernandes, A.A., Ventrone, A.E. et al. (2021). The influence of low-fidelity simulator training on canine peripheral venous puncture procedure. *Veterinary World* 14 (2): 410–418. https://doi.org/10.14202/vetworld.2021.410-418.

Silva, L.J., Cordeiro, C.T., Cruz, M.B., and Oliveira, S.T. (2021). Design and validation of a simulator for feline cephalic vein cannulation – a pilot study. *Journal of Veterinary Medical Education* 48 (3): 276–280. https://doi.org/10.3138/jvme.2019-0028.

Stowe, D.M., Fiebrandt, K.E., Druley, G.E., and Taylor, A.J. (2021). Implementation of a fine needle aspirate simulation model. *Journal of Veterinary Medical Education*, e20200157. https://doi.org/10.3138/jvme-2020-0157.

Strand, E.B., Johnson, B., and Thompson, J. (2013). Peer-assisted communication training: veterinary students as simulated clients and communication skills trainers. *Journal of Veterinary Medical Education* 40 (3): 233–241. https://doi.org/10.3138/jvme.0113-021R.

Swanwick, T. (2018). Understanding medical education. In: *Understanding Medical Education: Evidence, Theory, and Practice* (ed. T. Swanwick), 1–6. Wiley-Blackwell.

van Tartwijk, J. and Driessen, E.W. (2009). Portfolios for assessment and learning: AMEE Guide No. 45. *Medical Teacher* 31 (9): 790–801. https://doi.org/10.1080/01421590903139201.

Tochel, C., Haig, A., Hesketh, A. et al. (2009). The effectiveness of portfolios for post-graduate assessment and education: BEME Guide No 12. *Medical Teacher* 31 (4): 299–318. https://doi.org/10.1080/01421590902883056.

Vinten, C.E.K., Cobb, K.A., and Mossop, L.H. (2020). The use of contextualized standardized client simulation to develop clinical reasoning in final-year veterinary students. *Journal of Veterinary Medical Education* 47 (1): 56–68. https://doi.org/10.3138/jvme.0917-132r1.

van der Vleuten, C.P. (1996). The assessment of professional competence: developments, research and practical implications. *Advances in Health Sciences Education: Theory and Practice* 1 (1): 41–67. https://doi.org/10.1007/bf00596229.

van der Vleuten, C.P., Schuwirth, L.W., Scheele, F. et al. (2010). The assessment of professional competence: building blocks for theory development. *Best Practice & Research: Clinical Obstetrics & Gynaecology* 24 (6): 703–719. https://doi.org/10.1016/j.bpobgyn.2010.04.001.

Watling, C.J. and Ginsburg, S. (2019). Assessment, feedback and the alchemy of learning. *Medical Education* 53 (1): 76–85. https://doi.org/10.1111/medu.13645.

Weijs, C.A., Coe, J.B., and Hecker, K.G. (2015). Final-year students' and clinical instructors' experience of workplace-based assessments used in a small-animal primary-veterinary-care clinical rotation. *Journal of Veterinary Medical Education* 42 (4): 382–392. https://doi.org/10.3138/jvme.1214-123R1.

Wichtel, J., Zur Linden, A., Khosa, D. et al. (2021). Validation of a novel ultrasound simulation model for teaching foundation-level ultrasonography skills to veterinary students. *Journal of Veterinary Medical Education*, e20200123. https://doi.org/10.3138/jvme-2020-0123.

Wilkinson, J.R., Crossley, J.G., Wragg, A. et al. (2008). Implementing workplace-based assessment across the medical specialties in the United Kingdom. *Medical Education* 42 (4): 364–373. https://doi.org/10.1111/j.1365-2923.2008.03010.x.

Yudkowsky, R., Park, Y.S., and Downing, S.M. (2019). *Assessment in Health Professions Education*. Routledge.

12

Different Approaches to Assessment

Erik H. Hofmeister, DVM, DACVAA, DECVAA, MA, MS
College of Veterinary Medicine, Auburn University, Auburn, AL, USA

Section 1: Introduction and Approaches

Assessments are an essential component for effective education. Students need feedback on their performance (i.e., formative assessments) to improve. Competency-based veterinary education (CBVE) has four levels of competency: novice, advanced beginner, competent, and proficient. Assessing a student's level of competency (i.e., summative assessment) is essential to determine if they are qualified to be a veterinarian. On a fundamental level, assessments drive teaching. Using backward design, the teacher should begin with what they want the students to feel, know, or do, then develop assessments to measure the student's performance, and, finally, design learning activities to meet those outcomes. Without effective assessment design, there is a disconnect between learning activities and student outcomes.

In veterinary medicine, the expectation is that students will achieve the higher levels of Bloom's Taxonomy. For example, students are expected to create a diagnostic plan, evaluate test results, analyze different treatment options, and present the information effectively to an owner. Although it is possible to write multiple choice questions (MCQ) that assess higher levels of Bloom's Taxonomy, without adequate training and analysis, such questions tend to assess lower levels of Bloom's Taxonomy, such as knowledge and comprehension. Other traditional assessment approaches, such as essay questions and matching, may variably assess higher levels of Bloom's Taxonomy, but may not always accurately represent a student's abilities. Additionally, some assessments may not be authentic, meaning that students are not applying their knowledge to real-world problems.

Summative assessments, particularly those leading to a grade, pose a particular challenge in veterinary medicine. Students applying to veterinary school have pushed themselves to earn high grades throughout their undergraduate curriculum, and often have an expectation of earning high grades in veterinary school. However, CBVE is based on competence, not earning a grade. This can create a disconnect, where clinicians want the students to reason through a problem and apply clinical decision-making, while students are focused on earning a high grade. These two goals may often be at odds with each other in a traditional (A-F) grading scheme. Therefore, alternatives to traditional grading and assessments other than MCQ-based exams are worthy of consideration for the veterinary educator.

This chapter presents a variety of different assignments with assessments often considered less traditional or typical. Script concordance questions, extended matching, oral exams, blogging, reflections, readiness assessment tests, image creation, exam question creation, role-playing (RP), presentations (group, individual, and video), podcasts, and portfolios will be presented. Each will also have an example from the author's work to allow the reader to adopt or use as a model for their own use. Alternative grading schemes, including pass/fail, contract grading, specifications (spec) grading, competency-based grading, labor grading, and ungrading will also be presented.

Part 1: Script Concordance Test

One of the challenges for assessment of knowledge related to clinical decision-making is that many clinical scenarios are not clear. That is, the decision to pursue a particular diagnostic or therapeutic path is not obvious. Therefore, some ambiguity in answering a question about a clinical scenario for an assessment may mimic clinical reality more accurately. The script concordance test (SCT) is one attempt to assess clinical reasoning that relies on subjective interpretations of data. Whereas MCQs rely largely on recall of information, the SCT requires students to apply their knowledge (Cobb et al. 2015).

In the SCT, the question presents a clinical scenario and the stem is broken into two parts. The first provides a piece of information and the second asks for a likelihood. An example stem is, "If you knew the heartworm test was positive, that would make a diagnosis of DCM. . ." Then there are five answer options: much less likely, less likely, neither more or less likely, more likely, and much more likely. The question may be scored such that students who get the exact right answer earn full credit, and students who get the adjacent answer(s) earn partial credit. For example, if the correct answer is "much more likely," but "more likely" is plausible, students may earn two points for selecting "much more likely" and one point for selecting "more likely." Alternatively, it can be scored so that students only earn credit for the exact right answer.

The answer choices, and weighting for partial credit, are ideally generated by a panel of experts who answer the questions the same way the students would. This creates an array of answers given by the experts. Although a pool of 10–20 experts is recommended, a panel with nine individuals may be acceptable (Tayce and Saunders 2021). For a single instructor writing questions for a lecture-based class, assembling a pool of experts may be challenging, and they may need to use their own judgment to assign correct answers.

SCTs have been documented to be valuable for testing clinical reasoning skills in veterinary students (Cobb et al. 2015; Tayce and Saunders 2021) as well as veterinary practitioners (Dufour et al. 2012). While 5-point Likert scales (i.e., from "much less likely" to "much more likely") are generally preferred, 3-point Likert scales (i.e., "less likely," "neither more or less likely," and "more likely") have also been used in formative assessments (Tayce and Saunders 2021). Students are unfamiliar with this type of assessment, and so numerous practice opportunities should be provided before including SCT in summative assessments. Guidance on how the instructor approaches creating and answering questions may help students understand the SCT and adapt to it more quickly. In the author's experience, some students express interest in the SCT and like that it mimics real-world clinical scenarios, whereas others express significant displeasure because the answers represent an opinion rather than a quantifiable fact as with an MCQ.

To build an SCT, first consider a diagnostic or therapeutic scenario about which there is uncertainty. Next, build a short clinical scenario with sufficient information for the student to understand the case. This does not need to be extensive; it only needs to include the information relevant to answering the question. Next, create the question stem, giving the student a relevant piece of information and asking them to provide a likelihood on a 5-point Likert scale. The information can be a radiographic image, ECG image, diagnostic test, or similar to recreate a more realistic scenario. For example, instead of phrasing the question, "If the patient had a basketball-shaped cardiac silhouette on radiographs, that would make a diagnosis of pericardial effusion. . ." the question could supply the image: "If the patient had the following radiograph, that would make a diagnosis of pericardial effusion . . ." Additional examples of SCT are in Table 12.1.

Table 12.1 Examples of script concordance questions.

Bruiser, a 9-year-old intact male boxer, has been having episodes of collapse and fainting. If you found his ECG to show a heart rate of 275 bpm, with wide, bizarre QRS complexes, that would make a diagnosis of ventricular tachycardia:

a) Much less likely
b) Less likely
c) Neither more or less likely
d) More likely
e) Much more likely

Boomer, an 11-year-old male castrated toy poodle presents to you with lethargy and dyspnea. The owner complains to you that Boomer has coughing episodes when he lays down at night and when he gets up in the morning. On thoracic auscultation, you note rales indicating moderate pulmonary congestion. A normal cardiac auscultation would make a diagnosis of MMVD:

a) Much less likely
b) Less likely
c) Neither more or less likely
d) More likely
e) Much more likely

You have an 8-year-old female/spayed Golden Retriever mix named Layla. The client is concerned that she has shown reduced activity over the past few months. On presentation, Layla has lost 13 lbs. over the last 5 months. If you knew Layla had not been on heartworm preventative, that would make a diagnosis of weight loss due to right-sided heart failure:

a) Much less likely
b) Less likely
c) Neither more or less likely
d) More likely
e) Much more likely

You have a 2-year-old male goat who presents for depression. On physical exam, he is notably bradycardic. If you knew he had been vomiting, that would make a diagnosis of azalea toxicity:

a) Much less likely
b) Less likely
c) Neither more or less likely
d) More likely
e) Much more likely

Providing students an opportunity to give their rationalization for an answer may help the instructor to gain valuable insight into the student's thought processes (Tayce and Saunders 2021). From the author's experience, it may also help students feel better because they want to be able to explain their rationale if they choose an incorrect answer. SCTs help assess decision-making in a more realistic "gray" clinical decision-making scenario, as opposed to MCQ's "black-and-white" knowledge. Creating valid, reliable SCTs may be challenging for a single instructor. Preparing the students with practice questions and explaining the instructor's rationale for answers is essential, and some students may resent the opinion-based nature of the answers.

Part 2: Extended Matching Questions

Another attempt at assessing clinical decision-making uses extended matching questions (EMQs). Since development of clinical reasoning occurs through compilation of knowledge and integrates with practitioner experience, a method of assessment that evaluates propositional reasoning, rather than yes/no processes, is valuable.

EMQs provide a list of possible diagnostic steps, interventions, or diagnoses, and then give a series of cases. The student can choose any one of the possible answers, which may be the correct answer once, multiple times, or not at all. Common stems include, "For each case described below, choose the single most likely diagnosis from the above list of options," "For each case described below, choose the single most appropriate diagnostic step from the above list of options," and "For each case described below, choose the single most appropriate treatment from the above list of options," each of which would be followed by the brief case description and a list of possible responses.

A complete EMQ might look like the following.

For each case described below, choose the single most likely diagnosis from the provided list of options:

Mitral regurgitation
Tricuspid regurgitation
Pulmonic stenosis
Aortic regurgitation
Tetralogy of Fallot
Physiological/innocent flow murmur
Ventricular septal defect
Physiological PDA
True congenital (pathological) PDA

You are performing a prepurchase exam on a 15-year-old Quarter horse gelding that will be used for weekend trail rides. You identify a grade III/VI diastolic murmur, point of maximal intensity left heart base. The gelding is in excellent body condition (BCS 6/9), has normal peripheral pulses, rebreathing examination is normal, and his heart rate is 32 beats per minute with a regular rhythm. The rest of the prepurchase exam is unremarkable.

Additional scenarios would follow and, in each case, the student would select the best choice from the list of provided options related to that case.

EMQs can be graded electronically, have high reliability, have reduced cueing effects, and have been shown to have good discrimination compared with MCQs (Tomlin et al. 2008a). Veterinary students believe EMQs test clinical decision-making better than other methods and that their clinical experiences prepared them well for such assessments (Tomlin et al. 2008a). However, they may take more time than MCQs, so fewer questions or a longer exam period may be necessary (Tomlin et al. 2008a). Faculty also expressed concern about the EMQ taking longer for students to answer because of the lengthy text associated with case descriptions (Tomlin et al. 2008b). Although one supposed benefit of EMQs is that they are easier to write, one study of veterinary faculty found that only 18% believe they were easier to write than MCQs (Tomlin et al. 2008b). Veterinary faculty generally believed that EMQs are good for assessing clinical reasoning (Tomlin et al. 2008b).

Building an EMQ starts with a clearly defined area of content (e.g., diagnostic options for certain types of presentations and diagnoses for certain case descriptions). Case descriptions are then created for the stems, with enough detail that the questions can be reasonably answered by a student. The actual answers are then added to a list of possible answers, along with other plausible answers. The instructor needs to be careful that more than one answer cannot reasonably apply to the case. Each case is then scored separately, earning full credit only if the correct answer is chosen (no partial credit is granted).

When properly constructed, EMQs can assess knowledge similar to that needed for clinical decision-making. Because they are relatively intuitive for students, significant training and experience for them is unnecessary, although instructors do require training on effective EMQ writing. Fortunately, a large number of case scenarios may be built relatively quickly, using the same bank of answers, thus alleviating the need to create numerous new distractors for each question.

Part 3: Individual Readiness Assessment Tests

Preparing students to learn new material is supported when students engage in pre-reading. Effective integration of new information depends on repeat exposure to and recall of that information. If a student is presented with material in a lecture, recalls it once during study, and recalls it again during an examination, it is less effective than if a student reviews material before a lecture and then continuously recalls the new information. As such, more opportunities for recall and priming are advantageous to learning. A simple technique to support this is the individual readiness assessment test (IRAT).

The IRAT is not intended to test clinical reasoning or higher levels of Bloom's taxonomy; rather, it is a series of short, simple MCQs the students must complete prior to a class session. The questions should ask for simple recall of basic knowledge, aiming at the bottom of Bloom's taxonomy, since their purpose is to ensure the student opened the slides for the lecture and is familiar with foundational concepts.

The IRAT should be part of the course requirement for credit. For example, a low-stakes quiz or a certain number needed to complete to earn a certain grade. IRATs are commonly used in problem-based learning and flipped classroom settings (Kek et al. 2019), and are an integral part of team-based learning (Hopper 2018), but they can be used in any educational setting. IRATs can also be used to reinforce important elements of the syllabus or to determine if students are aware of important parts of the syllabus (e.g., assignments due dates, number or type of assignments, and percentages of class credit for assignments).

In an introductory physics and an intermediate biology course, quizzes given on material to be read before class, constituting 2% and 5% of the grade for each respective course, resulted in 98% of students completing the reading every week or most weeks (Heiner et al. 2014). Students reported that the quizzes forced them to complete the reading, which enhanced their comprehension of material presented during class. In an upper-level genetics class, quizzes on the material prior to class helped to motivate students prepare for the class (Cameron 2003). In an undergraduate exercise physiology course, an online quiz open 48 hours prior to class improved students' engagement and summative assessment scores (Dobson 2008). In the author's experience, students expressed appreciation for the IRATs in a required cardiovascular systems course.

To build an IRAT, the instructor should review the materials they want the students to read prior to the lecture. This may be written materials such as books, journal articles, or, in large lecture classes, simply the PowerPoint slides. Information aiming at the "knowledge" or "understanding" levels of Bloom's taxonomy should be identified and should be understood by the student reading the given material; that is, they should not have to go to sources beyond the reading/slides to answer the questions. An online quiz is then built that is open prior to the lecture covered, 24 or 48 hours being a reasonable window, as a longer window may lead to students completing the quiz far before the session and not retaining the information for use during the

Table 12.2 Examples of Individual Readiness Assessment Test questions.

What causes myocyte depolarization?

1) Opening of potassium channels
2) Opening of sodium channels
3) Opening of calcium channels
4) Closing of chloride channels

Which of the following assignments requires a rough draft submitted to the course coordinator?

1) Exam Questions
2) Reflections
3) Peer Review
4) VetView Case

Which of these pathologic lesions is associated with right-sided heart failure?

1) Nutmeg liver
2) Pulmonary artery hypertrophy
3) Heart failure cells
4) Pulmonary edema

What is a typical cutoff value for systolic arterial pressure to diagnose hypertension in dogs and cats?

1) 190 mmHg
2) 120 mmHg
3) 160 mmHg
4) 220 mmHg

lecture. The quiz should be composed of simple and fact-based recall MCQs, preferably an odd number, so it can be scored full credit if the majority of questions are answered correctly. Each question may be counted for credit separately, although this tends to lessen the formative aspect of the quiz. Examples are provided in Table 12.2.

The IRAT is an easy-to-use tool to help students prepare for learning during class. It moves learning factual information, which is at the bottom of Bloom's taxonomy, out of class time, allowing more in-person time to be used for elaborating on information and teaching higher levels of Bloom's taxonomy. It is not time-consuming for the student, is generally well accepted, is easy for the instructor to build, and improves learning.

Part 4: Blogging/Handout

Effective written communication is considered an essential skill and core competency for veterinarians (Haldane et al. 2017; AAVMC Working Group on Competency-based Veterinary Education et al. 2018). Being able to make a simple illustration, write discharge instructions, and create a summary of a case for referral are all frequently used skills for veterinarians. With a handful of exceptions (e.g., writing radiology descriptions), the opportunity for conducting writing assessments in the preclinical curriculum is often limited. During clinical rotations, students largely write in the medical record and create discharges, which are often more detailed than necessary for the client (Burrows 2008), and it has been documented that students' email responses to clients composed as a course assignment showed that their use of examples, analogies, and images could be improved (Kedrowicz et al. 2017). Creating a client handout or writing a blog are useful ways for students to practice communicating with lay people through writing.

A client handout is a printed, or possibly digital, handout. Often trifold, it is provided to clients to give them additional general information about a condition, treatment, medication, etc. (Dorman et al. 2013). A blog (derived from "web log") is an informational article available on a website consisting of discrete entries. Many businesses build blogs with information aimed at their target consumer to drive traffic to their website; according to DVM360, veterinary clinics can leverage this same approach. In both cases, the goal is to provide clients with useful information in a concise, easy-to-understand format.

Clients have expressed a desire to have written information in various forms, such handouts and information packets (Coe et al. 2008), and medical students and house officers on clinical rotations completing a voluntary blog writing exercise reported a positive learning experience (Manian and Hsu 2019). In an undergraduate biochemistry course, a required blog exercise was well-received by students who indicated that their interest in biochemistry increased and that it was a valuable learning opportunity (Cubas Rolim et al. 2017). Students in a medical microbiology course indicated the exercise was fun and they appreciated the importance of the subject and recommended it for future courses (Lloyd 2021). Toxicology experts, as well as members of the public, found student-generated brochures accurate and valuable (Dorman et al. 2013).

Creating a client information blog or handout assignment is relatively straightforward for the instructor. Student choice is important in this assignment, and was one of the key components that students enjoyed about the assignment in one study (Lloyd 2021). Each student should choose a single topic that is substantially different from anything available online to minimize plagiarism, and images that support the text should be required. Blog posts should have a word count minimum (e.g., 2000 words) and be organized into sections (e.g., similar to a WebMD blog post). The client information assignment can be graded complete/incomplete, or a rubric can be designed to allow a point grade.

Blog posts and handouts help students practice written communication to a lay audience. Blog posts are common and students are likely to encounter them in their daily internet use, so they should be familiar to most students. The assignment is easy to design and encourages students to apply concepts they have learned and have a need to explain.

Part 5: Reflections/Journals

Students completing their veterinary education are not completed professionals. As medical knowledge continues to advance, they will need to learn and adapt their practice over time (Freeman et al. 2022). They will routinely encounter problems their training did not adequately prepare them to solve (Schon 1983). Being able to reflect on the problem in the moment (reflection-in-action) as well as to learn from cases (reflection-on-action) are essential skills for the veterinary practitioner (Dale et al. 2008). Furthermore, reflection can be a powerful learning tool for veterinary students during their training.

Reflections and journals during the veterinary program, which may be written or verbal, are opportunities for students to practice reflecting on knowledge they have learned or experiences they have had. Written assignments are often completed for reflection-on-action about an experience or content the student has learned. Verbal reflections may be done in the moment (a talk-out-loud method) for reflection-in-action or can be after an experience, such as during rounds at the end of a day. Reflection skills progress from no reflection (description only) to surface reflection (general concepts) to developing reflection (including feelings and rationales) to deep reflection (specific, tied to prior experiences; Adams et al. 2006).

Reflective practices and activities are associated with improved learning outcomes (Mann et al. 2009), and have been linked with improved student outcomes, including interactions with standardized patients (Bernard et al. 2012). When feedback is given to medical students, supportive, validating statements, questions to enhance reflection, and focus on the primary concern in the reflection were all valued (Rozental et al. 2021). Students given vague or unspecific instructions for reflection may produce relatively superficial reflections (Adams et al. 2006).

Assignments asking students to reflect require specific, detailed instructions for the production of a high-quality product. Describing the purpose of the reflection and giving the conceptual framework for reflection to the students may be helpful. Once an appropriate mindset has been created for the student, specific guiding questions can be provided. Some questions may be required, or students may be able to choose a certain number of questions from a list.

Requiring a positive, constructive approach to reflection may also encourage students to engage with the assignment in a meaningful way. Evaluating the reflection can be a simple, "meets expectations/does not meet expectations" assessment. This may facilitate student engagement and growth of students' reflective skills (Bernard et al. 2012). The assessment should focus on the process, rather than the content, and feedback should also focus on the process, such as how the student changed or what they learned about themselves (Bernard et al. 2012). Grading rubrics, including some well-validated rubrics, can be used if a point grade is desired (Sandars 2009). An example of a reflection assignment is given in Table 12.3.

Reflecting effectively is a skill and students may not be able to reflect or may only have surface reflection when confronted with an initial reflection assignment (Adams et al. 2006). Having students reflect on professional knowledge or experiences – rather than personal ones – may be better received in the context of an assignment (Duret et al. 2022).

Part 6: Image Creation

Integrating information from numerous sources and applying it is a complex cognitive process. Students who encounter a single piece of information one time are unlikely to commit that information to memory and successfully incorporate it into their knowledge base for future clinical decision-making. Exercises requiring students to integrate knowledge in different ways improve learning.

Image creation is simply making a graphical representation (drawing) of a concept or actual structure (anatomic, histologic, etc.). Students may use pen-and-paper or drawing tools on their tablet or computer. When drawing, students have to make meaning of the content, integrate it into a mental model, and then incorporate verbal and non-verbal representations. These processes all encourage retrieval practice, elaboration, and dual-coding, which are known to be effective tools for learning (Weinstein et al. 2018).

Most evidence for the value of image creation comes from anatomy and histology, but it could be applied in any discipline. One study concluded that students who drew epithelium and heart cells had improved retention of knowledge compared to students not in the drawing group (Balemans et al. 2016). In another study of college students, those told to summarize a chapter using pictorial representations scored better than students told to read the material twice or those who summarized the chapter by writing about it (Alesandrini 1981). And most students in another study considered art to be a useful tool for learning histology (Cracolici et al. 2019).

An image creation assignment can be completed during class or outside of class. During class, it can be a useful starting point for discussion for areas of confusion, particularly if students can anonymously submit images, which can be accomplished via a learning management system (Kotzé and Mole 2015). Wide latitude should be given for the quality of the image; as long as the concepts are well represented, the student should get credit. Image creation may seem more obvious in some disciplines, such as anatomy, histology, surgery, and radiology, but it can be used in all disciplines. For example, in anesthesia, students could be asked to draw the pathway a pain signal takes from the periphery and indicate where various analgesic drugs exert their effects. Students might also be asked to draw a decision flowchart for various clinical problems (e.g., hypotension, PU/PD, and hyporexia), or a setup for a procedure such as catheter placement.

Assessment can be done on a complete/did not complete basis. If an image creation is graded, a rubric with specific requirements should be created and shared with students prior to the assignment.

Drawing can be a powerful learning tool, thus image creation assignments can be used in a wide variety of disciplines to reinforce learning. While the time to complete the assignments may be longer than some students want to invest (Balemans et al. 2016), creating and evaluating the assignment is usually straightforward for the instructor.

Part 7: Exam Question Creation

One of the goals of veterinary medical education is to have students create, which is one of the highest steps of the updated version of Bloom's Taxonomy. Given that veterinarians must create treatment plans, diagnostic plans, anesthetic protocols, etc., traditional assessments, such as multiple choice questions, are rarely elaborate enough to have students participate in the act of creation. Furthermore, students are often frustrated by exam questions and do not understand the difficulty in creating quality exam questions. Writing high-quality exam questions is a distinct skill, and veterinary faculty do not always write high-quality multiple choice questions (Shaver et al. 2020). Having students, some of whom may one day become faculty members, practice writing questions can be beneficial for their future careers.

When students are asked to write exam questions, they have to integrate information. If the exam questions may be used in an actual exam, this changes the students' studying behavior and increases their confidence (Baerheim and Meland 2003). Exam questions may be multiple choice questions, short-answer, or any other format the instructor

Table 12.3 Written reflection assignment example description and assessment.

Purpose: To practice reflective assessment for the student's own development.

Reflection is:

- A form of personal response to experiences, situations, events, or new information.
- A "processing" phase where thinking and learning take place.

There is neither a right nor a wrong way of reflective thinking, there are just questions to explore.

Doing this involves revisiting your prior experience and knowledge of the topic you are exploring. It also involves considering how and why you think the way you do. The examination of your beliefs, values, attitudes, and assumptions forms the foundation of your understanding.

Reflective thinking demands that you recognize that you bring valuable knowledge to every experience. It helps you therefore to recognize and clarify the important connections between what you already know and what you are learning. It is a way of helping you to become an active, aware, and critical learner.

Use this resource to work through your writing if you need help:

https://www.ed.ac.uk/reflection/reflectors-toolkit/reflecting-on-experience/gibbs-reflective-cycle

Reflective writing is:

- Documenting your response to experiences, opinions, events, or new information
- Communicating your response to thoughts and feelings
- A way of exploring your learning
- An opportunity to gain self-knowledge
- A way to achieve clarity and better understanding of what you are learning
- A chance to develop and reinforce writing skills
- A way of making meaning out of what you study

Reflective writing is not:

- Just conveying information, instruction, or argument
- Pure description, though there may be descriptive elements
- Straightforward decision or judgment, e.g., about whether something is right or wrong, good or bad
- Simple problem-solving
- A summary of course notes
- A standard university essay.

Pathology Reflection

Write a reflection about your experience in the gross pathology lab associated with this course. Answer five of the following questions. You may answer additional questions of your own making if you like. Be constructive.

- What did you like about the experience?
- What did you learn?
- Why does it matter?
- How did your involvement and participation in this fit into your broader goals for developing yourself?
- What would you change?
- What is the most important thing I personally learned?
- How will I use what I've learned in the future?

Criteria for success/Assessment (Meets Expectations/Does Not Meet Expectations)

- Meet deadline for submission
- Answered five questions.
- Maintained a constructive, positive approach to reflection.
- Clearly identified what the student has learned as part of the process.
- Statements are accurate and nonjudgmental.
- Ideas are expressed clearly, using relevant examples when necessary.
- Appropriate grammar, spelling, and organization.

---

feels is valuable for students to practice writing and answering. Exam questions generated by the students can be shared with each other to create a built-in practice quiz as part of the assessment.

A meta-analysis of student question writing found a positive learning effect of students writing exam questions (Touissi et al. 2022). Students generally enjoyed making questions, although there was some resistance on the basis of the time to reward efficiency (Touissi et al. 2022). Encouraging students to write high-quality questions, rather than questions requiring recall and comprehension, enhance the quality of the educational experience (Touissi et al. 2022). In veterinary medicine, students who answered more peer-generated questions performed better in a course, increased their depth and breadth of understanding, and provided a valuable resource for studying (Rhind and Pettigrew 2012).

Supporting students to create high-quality questions that target higher levels of Bloom's Taxonomy is important for this assignment. Students should be given clear directions on how to write quality exam questions, such as the best practices used by the National Board of Medical Examiners. Faculty should review questions before allowing them to be posted to a peer practice quiz format to ensure accuracy of the information and correctness of the answer choices (Rhind and Pettigrew 2012). It is suggested that as much choice as possible be built into the assignment, allowing students to select the topic and type of question, although encouraging students to choose topics with which they struggle is recommended.

Students need to tie a learning objective from the course to the question, and must provide the correct answer. In the case of a short-answer question, the student should create a simple rubric for scoring (Table 12.4). An exam question template may help students include all components of the assignment. Assessment can be done by simple pass/fail, or students may be given feedback if they have designed a question poorly (for example, the student used "all of the following except" format and that is brought to their attention) and allowed to resubmit the question. Alternatively, it may be graded on the basis of an established rubric.

Creating exam questions requires students to integrate information and achieve a high level of Bloom's Taxonomy. It also requires effort from the instructor to educate students on how to write high-quality questions. However, assessment can be relatively simple, such as the rubric given in Table 12.5. Students may resent the time required or not understand or appreciate the applicability of the exercise to their learning, though research demonstrates that this assessment practice improves student learning (Rhind and Pettigrew 2012).

Table 12.4 Example scoring rubric for a student-submitted short answer question.

Learning Objective: Diagnose common canine arrhythmias.

Max, a 13-year-old male neutered DSH, is presented at your clinic for ADR. Your technician performs thoracic radiographs and an ECG. Before you even have a chance to look at the tracing, your technician states she expects that Max has a second-degree AV block.

Discuss how you think the ECG tracing will appear given the technician's prediction. How will this differ from a normal sinus rhythm?

Rubric

+1 – P-waves with no corresponding QRS

+1 – Normal QRS

+1 – Normal sinus rhythm regular ventricular contractions; 2nd-degree AV block sometimes absent ventricular contractions

Table 12.5 Example scoring rubric for a student-generated question.

Questions will be marked according to the following key. Any marking besides "Meets expectations" indicates that the question will need to be revised.

Meets expectations	Earned the Meets expectations mark for this question
LO	No Learning Objective listed
Rubric	No rubric provided for a short answer
N	Negatively worded question stem (e.g., "Which one of the following is NOT. . ." or "which of the following is false")
OBA	One Best Answer. Do not use "all of the above," "none of the above," "A and B," etc.
Long	Correct answer is notably longer than distractors
TMI	Too Much Information. Shorten answers to be more concise/cut extraneous information
B	Binary choice in answers (i.e., the answer could be reduced to 2 possible instead of 4 possible because of binary answer choices).
	A: Abnormal – Sinus Arrhythmia
	B: Abnormal – Second Degree AV Block
	C: Normal – Second Degree AV Block
	D: Normal – Third Degree AV Block

Part 8: Role-Playing

Some skills are challenging or impossible to fully learn merely by reading, studying, and doing assessments. For example, nontechnical skills like communication can be learned by reading and studying, but application of communication principles is difficult without practice. Affective learning objectives, such as empathy, may be difficult for students to learn by traditional means. Moral reasoning, appropriate use of clinical autonomy, and recognition of limitations are other skills veterinarians must learn that are difficult to assess. Furthermore, in extreme situations such as the COVID-19 pandemic, students may not have the opportunities to practice professional skills such as communication.

RP involves a student taking on the role of another, such as a client, a veterinarian, or even another student. The student is asked to imagine the thoughts and feelings of such a person and then to act as though they were a person with those thoughts and feelings. Students are given a situation to immerse themselves in, one that should mimic a real clinical scenario or challenge. RP requires few resources or equipment and may not require much instructor involvement, depending on how it is used.

RP has been used extensively in simulations and communication skills training. Veterinary students believe that RP is an effective way to teach communication, even while they are anxious about doing RP exercises because of inexperience with that teaching modality (Brandt and Bateman 2006). In a workshop with veterinary educators, high-order learning outcomes were generated by an RP exercise, and RP allowed creation of complex learning outcomes that are hard to define but that students need for clinical practice (Armitage-Chan and Whiting 2016). Veterinary students participating in an RP simulation of a case reported positive perceptions of the experience, and felt RP was an important part of the learning process (Baillie et al. 2010). Empathy has been taught using RP in pharmacy students, where an RP experience significantly increased their physician empathy scale scores (Chen et al. 2008). During the COVID-19 pandemic, teaching experiences where students created cases and then role-played as the client or veterinarian were positively received in part because of positive engagement, student-centered learning, and peer-to-peer interaction (Alvarez et al. 2023).

An RP assignment should provide as much flexibility as possible. For example, students should be able to work with whomever they like, on their own schedule, and/or on a topic of their choosing. However, RP can happen in more structured settings, as well, such as communication courses. The specific goals of the assignment should be clearly articulated, and students should be advised of what role they are going to inhabit. Specific prompts, such as reflecting on what the person in that role may be thinking or feeling, may be helpful. Students may record themselves on video or audio but this is not always necessary.

RP may take place over an online video or audio platform in the event students cannot physically be together (e.g., during the COVID-19 pandemic). RP assignments may be graded pass/fail, or a rubric may be created to ensure students complete essential parts of the assignment with a high degree of quality. Valid assessment tools, such as the Liverpool Undergraduate Communication Assessment Scale, are available for application if a detailed rubric is desired (Huntley et al. 2012).

A reflection is an important component of an RP assignment. Merely participating in the RP activity is not sufficient for achieving the learning objectives of RP. Many of the goals of RP, such as enhancing empathy, benefit from structured reflection-on-action. Some specific prompts for reflection of RP are listed in Table 12.6. Reflections on RP should be a required part of completion of the assignment and can be graded similar to other reflections (pass-fail or by a rubric). If points are awarded for RP, the reflection should comprise a substantial portion of the point (e.g., 50% of the assignment).

RP may be one of the few ways that veterinary educators can elicit evolution of students in affective domains such as ethics, communication, and knowing their own limitations. Students need to be given clear instructions, and the flexibility of the assignment encourages its use in a variety of settings. Communications training currently relies heavily on RP at many institutions.

Part 9: Presentations

Public speaking skills are valuable for veterinarians. They may present continuing education to peers, present to the public about disease conditions, explain to stakeholders the importance of various interventions, report research findings, or otherwise be called upon to speak in front of a large group of people. Students report that the most important reason they do not participate in discussions during classes is because of an aversion to speaking in public (Moffett et al. 2014). Organizing one's thoughts and presenting them in a coherent fashion is an important skill and one that takes time and practice to develop. Providing students with opportunities to practice presentations is one way to develop those skills.

A public speaking assignment is when a student verbally presents information to one or more audience members. The audience may be peers, instructors, clients, or a mixture. Presentations to small groups happen daily during

Table 12.6   Role-playing assignment example description and assessment.

Communication Lab

You will role-play with your chosen partner in person or via video chat. Each of you will play the role of the veterinarian and the role of the client. You will do two interactions, with a different case for each interaction. For the first, one of you will be the veterinarian and the other will be the client. For the second interaction, flip roles.

For the role of the client, choose from among these approaches/attitudes. Do not share your approach/attitude with your partner playing the veterinarian.

- Upset
- Frustrated
- Cost-conscious
- Happy
- Confused
- Internet-Knowledgeable (I looked it up on the Google before coming in!)
- Breeder (supposedly knows more about their breed than the vet)
- Rock (not communicative, answers in single-word responses)
- Eager
- Easy going

For each interaction, choose a different case from the list below, or create your own case.

- 9-year-old F/S Shih Tzu presents for wellness visit, and grade II/VI left apical systolic heart murmur is auscultated.
- 4-year-old M/I Boxer dog presents for fainting on numerous occasions when playing fetch with client.
- 3-month-old F/I mixed breed dog presents for puppy vaccinations and a grade IV/VI continuous murmur is auscultated.
- 5-year-old M/C miniature schnauzer presents for lethargy of 3 months duration.
- 11-year-old M/C Labrador presenting for acute collapse.

In each case, begin by welcoming the client, collecting a history, and discuss your diagnostic plan. Continue through getting diagnostic test results and discussing a diagnosis, treatment plan, and prognosis.

Use the information presented in the communication class period such as:

- Build rapport
- Ask open-ended questions
- Reflective listening
- Express empathy
- Nonverbal communication
- Organization
- Eliciting client's perspective
- Asking permission
- Signposting
- Using easy-to-understand language
- Chunk and check
- Assessing client's knowledge
- Offering partnership
- Summarizing
- Contracting for next steps
- Final check

Write a reflection about your experience in the communication lab associated with this course. Answer the following questions. You may answer additional questions of your own making if you like. Be constructive.

- What did you like about the experience?
- What did you learn?
- Why does it matter?
- How did your involvement and participation in this fit into your broader goals for developing yourself?
- What would you change?
- What is the most important thing I personally learned?
- How will I use what I've learned in the future?

Criteria for success/Assessment (Meets Expectations/Does Not Meet Expectations)

- Meet deadline for submission
- Completed Communication Reflection
- Clearly identified what the student has learned as part of the process.
- Statements are accurate and nonjudgmental.
- Ideas are expressed clearly, using relevant examples when necessary.
- Appropriate grammar, spelling, and organization.

rounds for students on clinical rotations, and presentations to larger groups might include events like grand rounds, group summaries to the class on a specified topic, or at functions such as a veterinary school open house.

The assignment may be performed individually, or as a member of a group where different students present different parts of a topic. Students may even present some of the actual content of a course, if presented during regularly scheduled class time.

There is little evidence that there are efforts to develop public speaking skills in veterinary medicine, even though it has been identified as a critical skill for veterinarians for over 20 years (Humble 2001). Public speaking skills, such as eye contact, pacing, and a logical progression of ideas can be applied to many other communication contexts in which veterinarians participate, such as counseling a client. A leadership program for incoming veterinary students included public speaking as a component, but evaluated public speaking as a component of communication rather than as a separate skill (Moore and Klingborg 2006). In one teaching certificate program for veterinary students, which included a module aimed at client education, students felt more confident in public speaking (Hughes et al. 2022). Public speaking per se has not been evaluated as a separate skill from general communication or outside the context of broader training programs. This lack of evidence is similar to the situation in human medicine, where developing public speaking skills is acknowledged as important, but there is scant literature supporting the development of those skills (Nie et al. 2020).

To build a presentation assignment, the instructor should be explicit about the skills they want students to display and the way they want content delivered (e.g., PowerPoint slides, extemporaneous verbal delivery, rehearsed or scripted verbal delivery, and use of images). The assignment should also help the student understand the value of such assignments, as public speaking has been found to develop the ability to improvise, deliver information well, and use frameworks (Nie et al. 2020). In addition, providing guidance regarding use of the SEED method public speaking (statement, evidence, emotion, and demonstration), facilitates students having a go-to model for how to present information, particularly when speaking to clients (Nie et al. 2020). Students must organize their information, potentially design presentation slides, and orally deliver pieces of or entire presentations. Assessment can be pass/fail, or a rubric can be designed to evaluate the key components of the presentation, as described to the students in the assignment.

Presentations are common in clinical rotations but are not often presented as formal assignments with meaningful assessments and feedback for veterinary students. Providing students more opportunities for public speaking with effective feedback will enhance their presentation skills.

Part 10: Oral Exams

Ultimately, the goal of the veterinary educator is to produce a clinician who can make appropriate clinical judgments about a patient. This is a complex process and assessing the ability of a student to manage a case is challenging. Students must progress from knowing, to knowing how, to showing how, to actually doing a task. An oral exam may be the best way to test clinical decision-making in a complex way without using individual patients. Two types of assessments that often and easily incorporate oral responses are the objective structured clinical exams (OSCEs) and Mini-Clinical Evaluation Exercises for trainees (Mini-CEX); they also provide opportunities to assess students on *showing how* and *actually doing* a task (for more detailed information about these types of assessments, see the competency-based veterinary education assessment toolkit at www.cbve.org).

Oral exams have a long history; they consist of an instructor asking a question to a student or group of students and receiving a verbal answer. This can be done formally or informally, as any individual interactions between instructors and students are a form of oral exam. In a clinical setting, oral exams happen routinely, but are usually considered conversations between the instructor and the student and are not graded directly. The format of an oral exam can be highly structured (specific questions are always asked) to highly flexible (questions are asked as the instructor thinks of them).

Oral exams are often used in veterinary education outside of the United States (Hewson et al. 2005), often show poor relationship with subjective performance of medical students during clinical rotations (Saberi et al. 2021), and have been found to correlate less strongly with overall GPA than portfolios (Isbej et al. 2022). These findings suggest that oral exams, as well as clinic performance scores, are both subject to significant bias and variability.

To construct an oral exam in a classroom setting, using standardized questions is recommended to reduce bias. Exams may be scored pass/fail, where the student clearly demonstrates sufficient understanding of a concept or is not able to articulate their knowledge sufficiently. Alternatively, a rubric may be designed to score specific points the student must bring up during the specific questions. It is also important to keep in mind that oral exams are likely to induce significant anxiety, similar to giving a presentation (Huxham et al. 2012).

Oral exams are time-consuming to deliver, but may be effective to probe the limits of a student's knowledge. Scoring oral exams is highly subjective, and performance may not correlate with student ability. However, for students with disabilities related to reading, for example, such exams may provide them an opportunity to more fully demonstrate their learning (Huxham et al. 2012).

Part 11: Portfolios

Student learning may occur in isolation in the curriculum, and there is often no mechanism to document progression of learning as students advance through it. Students may not return to content or material taught in previous courses, causing them to silo knowledge rather than integrate it.

Portfolios are a collection of evidence that document student learning; they are composed of artifacts, such as documents and pictures, and may even include physical objects such as a suture board. They encourage reflective learning and iterative improvement, which complements CBVE. They also serve as an alternative to traditional methods of assessment and are able to document performance in a holistic fashion. Ideally, the content within the portfolio was created by the student (i.e., many of the assessments described in this chapter) rather than performance on exams in a course (i.e., percentage scores on summative assessments).

Portfolios have been associated with positive student perceptions and improved student knowledge in medical education (Buckley et al. 2009). They also encourage students to take ownership of their learning (Mossop and Senior 2008). However, both staff and students may be resistant to portfolios, as they represent a new and dramatic paradigm shift in assessment (Mossop and Senior 2008), and those that are high-stakes summative assessments may be difficult for judges to evaluate reliably (Bok et al. 2013; Favier et al. 2019). For this reason, portfolios may serve better as formative assessments than summative assessments.

Portfolios may be presented in a single course, across all courses in a semester, across an academic year, or across multiple years, with longer time spans providing the best evidence for student learning over time. They may be used in the preclinical or clinical curriculum; may be voluntary or compulsory; may be formative, summative, or both; and the content may be assigned or chosen by the student.

Voluntary portfolios tend to be started but not completed by students (Buckley et al. 2009), while required portfolios with more autonomy in completing assignments tend to increase student motivation, thus allowing students to choose the content is recommended. Students should also be given opportunities to create assignments that can be included in a portfolio (e.g., RP, reflection, and blog posts). Separate reflections on the students' learning over multiple courses, semesters, or years, is strongly recommended. A summary for the portfolio should be included, drawing together the concepts and knowledge gained in the assignments that are included.

In short, portfolios can be a powerful tool for growth and learning for students, as well as provide a great jump start to a student's career because they are tangible documentation of a student's learning, growth, and skills over time. Opportunities to create artifacts that can be included in the portfolio need to be identified in classes. Although using a portfolio as a summative high-stakes assessment may be challenging, given significant inter-rater reliability issues, using them formatively can be highly effective and rewarding.

Part 12: Audio and Video Options

Since students often have an aversion to speaking and presenting in public (Moffett et al. 2014), an alternative that achieves cognitive learning objectives without having to navigate the psychological anxiety of public speaking may be valuable. Allowing students to record their assignments gives them more flexibility as to when they complete the assignment (i.e., it doesn't have to occur during class time). Similarly, having a recording allows the faculty to assess the assignment on a flexible schedule. Audio or video recordings may be done for any assignment in lieu of written or presented material. For example, a student may record a vlog (video log) instead of performing a written reflection (Gajria et al. 2022). Students performing a RP experience may video record the interaction to submit the assignment. A blog, handout, or client communication could be audio recorded as an interview, question, and answer, or a discussion among speakers about a topic. Adding an audio or video component can be a required part of any other assignment or can be made optional, to allow for more student choice.

Section 2: Implementing New Assignments

Veterinary students are most familiar with standardized exams, often including multiple choice questions, matching, and similar objective question types that can be more efficiently graded. As a result, introducing novel assignments to assess learning in different ways may be challenging for them (Hofmeister et al. 2023a). For this reason, some care is necessary when introducing different approaches to assessment.

As with any educational intervention, the instructor should start with the end in mind. What do they want the student to be able to do at the end of the course? Knowing this, learning objectives can be constructed that can serve as the basis for building teaching activities and assessments that achieve those learning objectives.

Specific types of assessments are best for certain learning objectives. For example, SCT questions and EMQs are most useful for testing clinical decision-making. IRAT prepare students for engaging in active learning during class. Presentations, reflections, and RP are valuable for developing communication and empathy. Blogging, image creation, and exam question creation can be used to assess students' integration of information. An example of learning objectives matched with the different assignments is included in Table 12.7.

Individual assignments may be added to an existing course or may supplant existing assessments. Although a complete course redesign allows the instructor significant flexibility in how to structure assignments, updating is generally less time-consuming. If assignments are added, the

Table 12.7 Assessments that can be used to demonstrate achievement of example learning objectives.

Script concordance test	Interpret diagnostic test results leading to a diagnosis
Extended matching question	Interpret diagnostic test results leading to a diagnosis
	Create a treatment plan for commonly encountered diseases
Individual readiness assessment test	Compare diagnostic and treatment plans during class for given cases
Blogging/handouts	Explain the need for diagnostics and treatments and provide a prognosis to a client
Reflections/ journals	Express empathy with a client in a difficult situation
Image creation	Create a treatment plan for commonly encountered diseases
Exam question creation	Compare diagnostic and treatment plans during class for given cases
Role-playing	Explain the need for diagnostics and treatments and provide a prognosis to a client
Presentations	Explain the need for diagnostics and treatments and provide a prognosis to a client
Oral exams	Create a diagnostic plan, interpret results, and create a treatment plan for commonly encountered cardiovascular diseases of dogs, cats, horses, and food animals
Portfolios	Demonstrate progress of learning throughout the course

instructor should be careful not to use the assignments to get "more material" into the course or otherwise overload the students. For example, an inappropriate use of IRATs would be to add them but continue to use class time for lectures rather than active learning. Traditional examinations may be removed to allow students more time to complete assignments such as blogging or presentations. Some assignments may be optional, such as allowing students to complete a reflection to resubmit an assessment they did not perform well on. Class content may be cut away to allow students to give presentations during class time.

Regardless of the instructor's intention, clear communication is essential. A detailed explanation of the assessment should be created. This should include the purpose of the assignment (what the student will learn and why it matters), associated learning objectives, detailed instructions for completing the assignment, criteria for success, whether the student must complete it alone or may solicit peer feedback, due date, and method for submission. Students should always be given as much choice as possible when completing an assignment, and assignments tied to future applications (e.g., what they need to do as a veterinarian) are recommended. A video tutorial for some assignments may be helpful. Providing exemplar assignments, such as from past years' students, is extremely helpful to give students a clear idea of what an exceptional final product looks like.

Section 3: Novel Grading Schemes

Historically, grades are a relatively recent invention, dating only to the 1700s. During the 1800s, grades became more standardized with the A-F system originating in the late 1800s. However, even as early as the 1970s, only two-thirds of primary and secondary schools were using letter grades (Schinske and Tanner 2014).

Grades take the complexity of teaching and learning and reduce them to a single score. Grading is often at odds with institutional missions and can be very subjective, potentially propagating systemic biases like racism, classism, and sexism (Malouff and Thorsteinsson 2016). Grades may also be at odds with a growth mindset, which has recently been touted as a desirable characteristic in veterinary professionals (Routh et al. 2022). Essentially, grades are designed to sort and rank students, rather than facilitate education.

There are other approaches to grading. According to Nilson (2015), the ideal grading system should have 15 characteristics: upholds high academic standards; reflects student learning outcomes; motivates students to learn; motivates students to excel; discourages cheating; reduces student stress; makes students feel responsible for their own grades; minimizes conflict between faculty members and students; saves faculty members' time; gives students useful feedback; makes expectations clear; fosters higher-order cognitive development and creativity; has authentic assessment; has high inter-rater agreement; and is simple. Traditional A-F grading schemes suffer from numerous deficiencies in these ideal characteristics. For example, compared with feedback alone, when both grades and feedback are both given, students focus on the grades rather than the (more useful for their development) feedback (Butler and Nisan 1986). Numerous strategies have been created to manage these deficiencies, most focused on changing the way students are assessed and graded. While an ideal grading system has not yet been designed, alternatives to traditional grading schemes provide veterinary educators with tools to minimize the flaws of an A-F grading paradigm.

Part 1: Contract Grading

In contract grading, the instructor makes an agreement with each student about the amount and type of work that students will do to demonstrate learning and earn a certain grade (the contract). This agreement is individualized to each student and focuses on what that student needs to be successful. There is a list of assignments from which students may select to demonstrate their learning. Students also create their own consequences for failing to meet deadlines, which they establish, or failing to fulfill the other elements of the contract, such as quality of work. Typically, students who submit assignments that are below expectations receive feedback and can resubmit the assignment.

The student and the instructor both sign the contract. At the end of the semester, the student earns the grade they contracted for at the beginning of the course, unless the contract stipulates otherwise. Nursing students had generally positive responses to contract grading in one study, but studies in human or veterinary medical students have not been published (Kruse and Barger 1982). Contract grading achieves numerous goals of the ideal grading system, but it does not save faculty time and is not simple because of the individualized nature of creating each contract.

Part 2: Specifications Grading

Spec grading is a variation on contract grading. With this approach, the instructor creates a bundle of assignments for each grade for all students in the class, rather than entering into contracts on an individual basis. Once the instructor creates assignments, they designate how many of the assignments must be completed to meet baseline expectations (i.e., a grade of "C"). From there, additional assignments represent greater demonstration of learning the content and therefore represent higher grades of "B" and "A." If students do not meet the minimum criteria but do some assignments, a grade of "D" may be assigned. And if students do not meet the absolute minimum, they earn an "F." Each assignment is assessed as meeting expectations, typically consistent with a "B" level of performance, or not meeting expectations. If the assignment does not meet expectations, students may resubmit the assignment with some associated cost (e.g., a limited number of resubmits per semester or having to write a reflection as part of the resubmission).

Although spec grading theoretically meets all of the ideal requirements described by Nilson in 2015, in practice this is not completely true. The amount of work done by the instructor can be substantial, depending on how they give feedback for assignments (Hofmeister et al. 2023b). It may also paradoxically increase student stress, since it is a new system and students may not adapt well to change (Hofmeister et al. 2023a).

Part 3: Labor Grading

Labor grading resembles spec grading, except students' work is not evaluated for the quality of the product. Instead, only the amount of labor students spend on the task gets credit. This may be quantified as time on task, number of words written, and/or number of words read. The premise is that all learning requires labor and is the most fundamental task we expect of students. In traditional grading systems, students labor to acquire grades, which are given by the instructor. It is not for the student, but rather as a system of exchange. Labor grading is primarily used in writing classes, and examples could not be found in the medical literature. Since it does not necessarily meet the goal of reflecting student learning outcomes, discouraging cheating, fostering higher-order cognitive development, or being authentic, labor grading probably has limited applicability in veterinary education.

Part 4: Competency-Based Grading

In competency-based grading, students are evaluated and graded on their ability to conduct a specific task or entrustable professional activity (EPA). Ultimately, students need to be competent clinicians. Grading them on the basis of their competence aligns assessment with effort. That is, students will spend effort to achieve the stated assessment goals. Ultimately, students achieve a grade that is aligned with their ability to perform a task. Competency-based grading is currently in its infancy, and clear guidelines for developing this grading system are still being built.

Part 5: Pass/Fail Grading

With pass/fail grading, students receive a single grade at the end of a course, either a pass or a fail. The assignments given during the course may be scored traditionally (i.e., by points) or also on a pass/fail basis. Determination of the final grade could be earned through successful completion of a certain number of assignments, could be based on reaching or not reaching a certain average percentage on exams, or a combination of both.

Pass/fail grading has been the focus of a substantial amount of research, and the majority of medical schools have transitioned to a pass/fail system for preclinical courses. Pass/fail grading has been shown to reduce student anxiety and resulted in equitable student performance during residency with those training in a traditional grading system (Bloodgood et al. 2009; Wang et al. 2021). Pass/fail grading most closely approximates reality, where clinicians are faced with situations in which a decision must be made, prevents grade inflation, which is a known and growing problem (Rush et al. 2009), and achieves most of Nilson's characteristics of an ideal grading system.

Part 6: Ungrading

It has been noted that grades generally inhibit learning (Schinske and Tanner 2014). Research has also demonstrated grades tend to diminish students' interest in what they are learning and decrease intrinsic motivation (Kohn 2018). Therefore, in ungrading, assignments are not graded in any way, and only feedback is presented to the students. Assignments with self-assessment and reflections are completed by the students, and exams are formative in nature and are often open-book and self-graded. Students also conduct regular reflections on their learning throughout the class, then assign themselves a grade at the end of the course. Ungrading moves the power in the classroom from the instructor to the students. It achieves most of the goals of an ideal grading system, with the arguable exception of upholding high academic standards, reflecting student learning outcomes, or saving faculty time. Since feedback and having a dialogue with students is an important component of upgrading, performing it in a large classroom may be prohibitive from a time standpoint.

Section 4: Implementing Novel Grading Schemes

Before starting a course with a novel grading scheme, the instructor should discuss it with their direct supervisor and any administrators who play a significant role in shaping and maintaining the curriculum. As these novel schemes may cause distress in veterinary students, it is essential to ensure administration is aware of the instructor's efforts, reasons for pursuing the novel scheme, and plans to manage challenges along the way (Hofmeister et al. 2023a). Numerous excellent blogs are available about spec grading and upgrading, which should serve as inspiration. The instructor implementing pass/fail grading may be concerned that students will shift focus to graded courses but, at one institution where some classes were pass/fail and others were graded in the same semester, this did not occur (Sprunger, personal communication 2022).

The instructor should write a detailed syllabus, providing all the information about the new grading scheme. During the first class period, the rationale for using the new grading scheme should be presented to the students, along with a detailed explanation of how the new scheme will be implemented in the course. A video tutorial that students can refer to is also recommended. The instructor should check in with the students regularly, make sure they are on track, and provide feedback on their performance. A midcourse anonymous survey to students may help elicit problems and confusion while allowing enough time to correct before the course ends. The instructor should be prepared for a variety of student feedback on course evaluations, as some students may appreciate the efforts while others will revile the instructor for doing something different (Hofmeister et al. 2023a).

Summary

Assessments and grading are an integral part of the current higher education paradigm. Assessments help determine a student's level of knowledge and competence, while grades are a summative way to rank and evaluate students. Alternatives to both allow the instructor to have greater flexibility, achieve different learning objectives, and facilitate student growth. Veterinary education is expanding and keeping to "tried and true" may be doing a disservice to our students. Expanding our horizons with regard to educational approaches may help shepherd our students into a new era and help maintain a more sustainable future for our profession.

References

AAVMC Working Group on Competency-Based Veterinary Education, Molgaard, L.K., Hodgson, J.L., Bok, H.G.J. et al. (2018). *Competency-Based Veterinary Education: Part 1 – CBVE Framework*. Washington, DC: Association of American Veterinary Medical Colleges.

Adams, C.L., Nestel, D., and Wolf, P. (2006). Reflection: a critical proficiency essential to the effective development of a high competence in communication. *Journal of Veterinary Medical Education* 33 (1): 58–64. https://doi.org/10.3138/jvme.33.1.58. PMID: 16767639.

Alesandrini, K.L. (1981). Pictorial–verbal and analytic–holistic learning strategies in science learning. *Journal of Educational Psychology* 73 (3): 358–368. https://doi.org/10.1037/0022-0663.73.3.358.

Alvarez, E., Nichelason, A., Lygo-Baker, S. et al. (2023). Virtual clinics: a student-led, problem-based learning approach to supplement veterinary clinical experiences. *Journal of Veterinary Medical Education* 50 (2): 147–161. https://doi.org/10.3138/jvme-2021-0144. PMID: 35500194.

Armitage-Chan, E. and Whiting, M. (2016). Teaching professionalism: using role-play simulations to generate professionalism learning outcomes. *Journal of Veterinary Medical Education* 43 (4): 359–363. https://doi.org/10.3138/jvme.1115-179R. PMID: 27404549.

Baerheim, A. and Meland, E. (2003). Medical students proposing questions for their own written final examination: evaluation of an educational project. *Medical Education* 37 (8): 734–738. https://doi.org/10.1046/j.1365-2923.2003.01578.x. PMID: 12895254.

Baillie, S., Pierce, S.E., and May, S.A. (2010). Fostering integrated learning and clinical professionalism using contextualized simulation in a small-group role-play. *Journal of Veterinary Medical Education* 37 (3): 248–253. https://doi.org/10.3138/jvme.37.3.248. PMID: 20847333.

Balemans, M.C., Kooloos, J.G., Donders, A.R., and Van der Zee, C.E. (2016). Actual drawing of histological images improves knowledge retention. *Anatomical Sciences Education* 9 (1): 60–70. https://doi.org/10.1002/ase.1545. PMID: 26033842.

Bernard, A.W., Gorgas, D., Greenberger, S. et al. (2012). The use of reflection in emergency medicine education. *Academic Emergency Medicine* 19 (8): 978–982. https://doi.org/10.1111/j.1553-2712.2012.01407.x. PMID: 22818356.

Bloodgood, R.A., Short, J.G., Jackson, J.M., and Martindale, J.R. (2009). A change to pass/fail grading in the first two years at one medical school results in improved psychological well-being. *Academic Medicine* 84 (5): 655–662. https://doi.org/10.1097/ACM.0b013e31819f6d78. PMID: 19704204.

Bok, H.G., Teunissen, P.W., Favier, R.P. et al. (2013). Programmatic assessment of competency-based workplace learning: when theory meets practice. *BMC Medical Education* 11 (13): 123. https://doi.org/10.1186/1472-6920-13-123. PMID: 24020944; PMCID: PMC3851012.

Brandt, J.C. and Bateman, S.W. (2006). Senior veterinary students' perceptions of using role play to learn communication skills. *Journal of Veterinary Medical Education* 33 (1): 76–80. https://doi.org/10.3138/jvme.33.1.76. PMID: 16767642.

Buckley, S., Coleman, J., Davison, I. et al. (2009). The educational effects of portfolios on undergraduate student learning: a Best Evidence Medical Education (BEME) systematic review. BEME Guide No. 11. *Medical Teacher* 31 (4): 282–298. https://doi.org/10.1080/01421590902889897. PMID: 19404891.

Burrows, C.F. (2008). Meeting the expectations of referring veterinarians. *Journal of Veterinary Medical Education* 35 (1): 20–25. https://doi.org/10.3138/jvme.35.1.020. PMID: 18339951.

Butler, R. and Nisan, M. (1986). Effects of no feedback, task-related comments, and grades on intrinsic motivation and performance. *Journal of Educational Psychology* 78 (3): 210–216. https://doi.org/10.1037/0022-0663.78.3.210.

Cameron, V.L. (2003). Teaching advanced genetics without lectures. *Genetics* 165 (3): 945–950. https://doi.org/10.1093/genetics/165.3.945. PMID: 14668355; PMCID: PMC1462828.

Chen, J.T., LaLopa, J., and Dang, D.K. (2008). Impact of Patient Empathy Modeling on pharmacy students caring for the underserved. *American Journal of Pharmaceutical Education* 72 (2): 40. https://doi.org/10.5688/aj720240. PMID: 18483606; PMCID: PMC2384215.

Cobb, K.A., Brown, G., Hammond, R., and Mossop, L.H. (2015). Students' perceptions of the Script Concordance Test and its impact on their learning behavior: a mixed methods study. *Journal of Veterinary Medical Education* 42 (1): 45–52. https://doi.org/10.3138/jvme.0514-057R1. PMID: 25526762.

Coe, J.B., Adams, C.L., and Bonnett, B.N. (2008). A focus group study of veterinarians' and pet owners' perceptions of veterinarian-client communication in companion animal practice. *Journal of the American Veterinary Medical Association* 233 (7): 1072–1080. https://doi.org/10.2460/javma.233.7.1072. PMID: 18828715.

Cracolici, V., Judd, R., Golden, D., and Cipriani, N.A. (2019). Art as a learning tool: medical student perspectives on implementing visual art into histology education. *Cureus* 11 (7): e5207. https://doi.org/10.7759/cureus.5207. PMID: 31565612; PMCID: PMC6758967.

Dale, V.H., Sullivan, M., and May, S.A. (2008). Adult learning in veterinary education: theory to practice. *Journal of Veterinary Medical Education* 35 (4): 581–588. https://doi.org/10.3138/jvme.35.4.581. PMID: 19228912.

Dobson, J.L. (2008). The use of formative online quizzes to enhance class preparation and scores on summative exams. *Advances in Physiology Education* 32 (4): 297–302. https://doi.org/10.1152/advan.90162.2008. PMID: 19047506.

Dorman, D.C., Alpi, K.M., and Chappell, K.H. (2013). Subject matter expert and public evaluations of a veterinary toxicology course brochure-writing assignment. *Journal of Veterinary Medical Education* 40 (1): 19–28. https://doi.org/10.3138/jvme.0912.082R. PMID: 23475408.

Dufour, S., Latour, S., Chicoine, Y. et al. (2012). Use of the script concordance approach to evaluate clinical reasoning in food-ruminant practitioners. *Journal of Veterinary Medical Education* 39 (3): 267–275. https://doi.org/10.3138/jvme.0112-13R. PMID: 22951462.

Duret, D., Terron-Canedo, N., Hannigan, M. et al. (2022). Identifying the barriers to incorporating reflective practice into a veterinary curriculum. *Journal of Veterinary Medical Education* 49 (4): 454–461. https://doi.org/10.3138/jvme-2020-0040. PMID: 34097581.

Favier, R.P., Vernooij, J.C.M., Jonker, F.H., and Bok, H.G.J. (2019). Inter-rater reliability of grading undergraduate portfolios in veterinary medical education. *Journal of Veterinary Medical Education* 46 (4): 415–422. https://doi.org/10.3138/jvme.0917-128r1. PMID: 30920333.

Freeman, D., Hodgson, K., and Darling, M. (2022). Mentoring new veterinary graduates for transition to practice and lifelong learning. *Journal of Veterinary Medical Education* 49 (4): 409–413. https://doi.org/10.3138/jvme-2021-0036. PMID: 34342545.

Gajria, C., Gunning, E., Horsburgh, J., and Kumar, S. (2022). Using vlogging to facilitate medical student reflection. *Education for Primary Care* 33 (4): 244–247. https://doi.org/10.1080/14739879.2022.2070868. PMID: 35638935.

Haldane, S., Hinchcliff, K., Mansell, P., and Baik, C. (2017). Expectations of graduate communication skills in professional veterinary practice. *Journal of Veterinary Medical Education* 44 (2): 268–279. https://doi.org/10.3138/jvme.1215-193R. PMID: 27689946.

Heiner, C.E., Banet, A.I., and Wieman, C. (2014). Preparing students for class: how to get 80% of students reading the textbook before class. *American Journal of Physics* 82 (10): 989–996.

Hewson, C.J., Baranyiová, E., Broom, D.M. et al. (2005). Approaches to teaching animal welfare at 13 veterinary schools worldwide. *Journal of Veterinary Medical Education* 32 (4): 422–437. https://doi.org/10.3138/jvme.32.4.422. PMID: 16421823.

Hofmeister, E., Fogelberg, K., Conner, B.J., and Gibbons, P. (2023a). Specifications grading in a cardiovascular systems course: student and course coordinator perspectives on the impacts on student achievement. *Journal of Veterinary Medical Education* 50 (2): 172–182. https://doi.org/10.3138/jvme-2021-0115.

Hofmeister, E., Gibbons, P., Fogelberg, K., and Conner, B.J. (2023b). Specifications grading for veterinary medicine. *Journal of Veterinary Medical Education* 50 (1): 15–18. https://doi.org/10.3138/jvme-2021-0116.

Hopper, M.K. (2018). Alphabet Soup of Active Learning: Comparison of PBL, CBL, and TBL. *HAPS Educator* 22 (2): 144–149. https://doi.org/10.21692/haps.2018.019.

Hughes, K., Hudson, N., Bell, C. et al. (2022). Exploring student experiences of an undergraduate certificate in veterinary medical education. *Journal of Veterinary Medical Education*: e20210098. https://doi.org/10.3138/jvme-2021-0098. PMID: 35588307.

Humble, J.A. (2001). Critical skills for future veterinarians. *Journal of Veterinary Medical Education* 28 (2): 50–53. https://doi.org/10.3138/jvme.28.2.50. PMID: 11553869.

Huntley, C.D., Salmon, P., Fisher, P.L. et al. (2012). LUCAS: a theoretically informed instrument to assess clinical communication in objective structured clinical examinations. *Medical Education* 46 (3): 267–276. https://doi.org/10.1111/j.1365-2923.2011.04162.x. PMID: 22324526.

Huxham, M., Campbell, F., and Westwood, J. (2012). Oral versus written assessments: a test of student performance and attitudes. *Assessment & Evaluation in Higher Education* 37 (1): 125–136. https://doi.org/10.1080/02602938.2010.515012.

Isbej, L., Cantarutti, C., Fuentes-Cimma, J. et al. (2022). The best mirror of the students' longitudinal performance: portfolio or structured oral exam assessment at clerkship? *Journal of Dental Education* 86 (4): 383–392. https://doi.org/10.1002/jdd.12823. PMID: 34811760.

Kedrowicz, A.A., Hammond, S., and Dorman, D.C. (2017). Teaching tip: improving students' email communication through an integrated writing assignment in a Third-Year Toxicology Course. *Journal of Veterinary Medical Education* 44 (2): 280–289. https://doi.org/10.3138/jvme.0816-124R2. PMID: 28375070.

Kek, B., Buchanan, J., and Adisesh, A. (2019). An introduction to occupational medicine using a team-based learning methodology. *Journal of Occupational and Environmental Medicine* 61 (2): 132–135. https://doi.org/10.1097/JOM.0000000000001499. PMID: 30475307.

Kohn, A. (2018). *Punished by Rewards*, 1e. San Francisco: Harper One.

Kotzé, S.H. and Mole, C.G. (2015). Making large class basic histology lectures more interactive: the use of draw-along mapping techniques and associated educational activities. *Anatomical Sciences Education* 8 (5): 463–470. https://doi.org/10.1002/ase.1514. PMID: 25650015.

Kruse, L.C. and Barger, D.M. (1982). Development and implementation of a contract grading system. *The Journal of Nursing Education* 21 (5): 31–37. https://doi.org/10.3928/0148-4834-19820501-07. PMID: 6286572.

Lloyd, C. (2021). Blogging as a tool for real-time learning in medical microbiology. *Frontiers in Microbiology* 12: 576145. https://doi.org/10.3389/fmicb.2021.576145. PMID: 33746910; PMCID: PMC7970246.

Malouff, J. and Thorsteinsson, E. (2016). Bias in grading: a meta-analysis of experimental research findings. *Australian Journal of Education* 60. https://doi.org/10.1177/0004944116664618.

Manian, F.A. and Hsu, F. (2019). Writing to learn on the wards: scholarly blog posts by medical students and housestaff at a teaching hospital. *Medical Education Online* 24 (1): 1565044. https://doi.org/10.1080/10872981.2018.1565044. PMID: 30693840; PMCID: PMC6352928.

Mann, K., Gordon, J., and MacLeod, A. (2009). Reflection and reflective practice in health professions education: a systematic review. *Advances in Health Sciences Education: Theory and Practice* 14 (4): 595–621. https://doi.org/10.1007/s10459-007-9090-2. PMID: 18034364.

Moffett, J., Berezowski, J., Spencer, D., and Lanning, S. (2014). An investigation into the factors that encourage learner participation in a large group medical classroom. *Advances in Medical Education and Practice* 5: 65–71. https://doi.org/10.2147/AMEP.S55323. PMID: 24648783; PMCID: PMC3956477.

Moore, D.A. and Klingborg, D.J. (2006). The University of California Veterinary Student Leadership Program: comparison of a five-day with a three-day course. *Journal of Veterinary Medical Education* 33 (2): 284–293. https://doi.org/10.3138/jvme.33.2.284. PMID: 16849312.

Mossop, L.H. and Senior, A. (2008). I'll show you mine if you show me yours! Portfolio design in two UK veterinary schools. *Journal of Veterinary Medical Education* 35 (4): 599–606. https://doi.org/10.3138/jvme.35.4.599. PMID: 19228915.

Nie, J., Torabi, S., Peck, C. et al. (2020). Teaching public speaking to medical students. *The Clinical Teacher* 17 (6): 606–611. https://doi.org/10.1111/tct.13153. PMID: 32202383.

Nilson, L.B. (2015). *Specifications Grading*, 1e. Oxfordshire: Routledge.

Rhind, S.M. and Pettigrew, G.W. (2012). Peer generation of multiple-choice questions: student engagement and experiences. *Journal of Veterinary Medical Education* 39 (4): 375–379. https://doi.org/10.3138/jvme.0512-043R. PMID: 23187030.

Cubas Rolim, E., Martins de Oliveira, J., Dalvi, L.T. et al. (2017). Blog construction as an effective tool in biochemistry active learning. *Biochemistry and Molecular Biology Education* 45 (3): 205–215. https://doi.org/10.1002/bmb.21028. PMID: 27862849.

Routh, J., Paramasivam, S.J., Cockcroft, P. et al. (2022). Stakeholder perspectives on veterinary student preparedness for workplace clinical training – a qualitative study. *BMC Veterinary Research* 18 (1): 340. https://doi.org/10.1186/s12917-022-03439-6. PMID: 36085152; PMCID: PMC9461096.

Rozental, L., Meitar, D., and Karnieli-Miller, O. (2021). Medical students' experiences and needs from written reflective journal feedback. *Medical Education* 55 (4): 505–517. https://doi.org/10.1111/medu.14406. PMID: 33141960.

Rush, B.R., Elmore, R.G., and Sanderson, M.W. (2009). Grade inflation at a north american college of veterinary medicine: 1985–2006. *Journal of Veterinary Medical Education* 36 (1): 107–113. https://doi.org/10.3138/jvme.36.1.107. PMID: 19435997.

Saberi, R.A., Kronenfeld, J.P., Hui, V.W. et al. (2021). Surgical clerkship: do examination scores correlate with clinical performance? *American Journal of Surgery* 222 (6): 1163–1166. https://doi.org/10.1016/j.amjsurg.2021.09.016. PMID: 34602278.

Sandars, J. (2009). The use of reflection in medical education: AMEE Guide No. 44. *Medical Teacher* 31 (8): 685–695. https://doi.org/10.1080/01421590903050374. PMID: 19811204.

Schinske, J. and Tanner, K. (2014). Teaching more by grading less (or differently). *CBE Life Sciences Education* 13 (2): 159–166. https://doi.org/10.1187/cbe.cbe-14-03-0054. PMID: 26086649; PMCID: PMC4041495.

Schon, D.A. (1983). The Reflective Practitioner: How Professionals Think in Action. Basic Books, New York.

Shaver, S.L., Patterson, C.C., Robbins, E.A., and Hofmeister, E.H. (2020). Faculty perspectives regarding day one-ready examination items. *Journal of Veterinary Medical Education* 47 (6): 695–699. https://doi.org/10.3138/jvme.0718-087r2. Epub 2019 Nov 15. PMID: 31738681.

Tayce, J.D. and Saunders, A.B. (2021). The use of a modified script concordance test in clinical rounds to foster and assess clinical reasoning skills. *Journal of Veterinary Medical Education* 16: e20210090. https://doi.org/10.3138/jvme-2021-0090. PMID: 34784257.

Tomlin, J.L., Pead, M.J., and May, S.A. (2008a). Veterinary students' attitudes toward the assessment of clinical reasoning using extended matching questions. *Journal of Veterinary Medical Education* 35 (4): 612–621. https://doi.org/10.3138/jvme.35.4.612. PMID: 19228917.

Tomlin, J.L., Pead, M.J., and May, S.A. (2008b). Attitudes of veterinary faculty to the assessment of clinical reasoning using extended matching questions. *Journal of Veterinary Medical Education* 35 (4): 622–630. https://doi.org/10.3138/jvme.35.4.622. PMID: 19228918.

Touissi, Y., Hjiej, G., Hajjioui, A. et al. (2022). Does developing multiple-choice questions improve medical students' learning? a systematic review. *Medical Education Online* 27 (1): 2005505. https://doi.org/10.1080/1087298 1.2021.2005505. PMID: 34969352; PMCID: PMC8725700.

Wang, A., Karunungan, K.L., Shlobin, N.A. et al. (2021). Residency program director perceptions of resident performance between graduates of medical schools with pass/fail versus tiered grading system for clinical clerkships: a meta-analysis. *Academic Medicine* 96 (11S): S216–S217. https://doi.org/10.1097/ACM.0000000000004321. PMID: 34705719.

Weinstein, Y., Sumeracki, M., and Caviglioli, O. (2018). *Understanding How We Learn: A Visual Guide*, 1e. London: Routledge.

Additional Resources

Helpful Blogs About Alternative Grading Schemes

https://rtalbert.org/
https://www.jessestommel.com/ungrading-an-faq/
https://composingpossibilities.com/
http://oudigitools.blogspot.com/
https://vetducator.com/specifications-grading-my-experience/

13

Program Outcomes

Patricia Butterbrodt, PhD, MEd
Richard A. Gillespie College of Veterinary Medicine, Lincoln Memorial University, Harrogate, TN, USA

Katrina Jolley, Med (Educational Leadership)
Richard A. Gillespie College of Veterinary Medicine, Lincoln Memorial University, Harrogate, TN, USA

Introduction

Katherine Fogelberg

When administering any program, it is important to consider how you will determine whether you are teaching what you intend to teach, where topics are being taught within the program, and if the students are achieving the goals set forth by the program. Program outcomes are generally set by the individual accrediting bodies and their expectations, which should be based on stakeholder information and a deep understanding of the needs of the profession.

In Chapter 10, the student aspect was covered with regards to formative and summative exams, as well as several different types of traditional exams that could be used to determine student performance. There was also a brief section covering program evaluation in that same chapter. This chapter provides deeper discussion covering ways to track what students are supposed to be learning (curriculum mapping), how to work toward ensuring students *are* learning, and methods for tracking outcomes at the individual, cohort, and clinical levels.

Section 1: Curriculum Mapping

Patricia Butterbrodt

There are several different purposes for which you may desire a geographical map. To travel from one city to another, you need a map showing roads, directions, and landmarks. A map can identify specific locations in a city, such as Italian restaurants or shoe stores, and a map can locate the desired location for the reader. If you are planning an extended hike and camping trip, a topographical map could show where the rises and falls along the path will come and how steep they are, so you could plan the steepest parts as downhill hikes rather than uphill climbs. There are maps showing political tendencies, population densities, land use, or just about any information needed about a location. You can even log into a live interactive map that shows traffic information as it is happening. The concept of a map indicates the user is searching for some information and has gone to the map to provide the information needed, with targeted layers of information available in maps with different foci.

Just as a map is useful for a variety of purposes, so can a map be used to identify information about a curriculum. There are a variety of curriculum maps that each have a specific purpose. Some maps show detailed pathways and links from assessment items through course objectives to professional competencies. Others show individual competencies and where they are introduced, reinforced, and assessed. Still, others show the content in courses being taught simultaneously or consecutively to look for content flow, lapses, and surplus. Depending on what information is being sought, a curriculum map in one form or another can give a picture of what is being taught when, where, and even how.

Part 1: Why Map the Curriculum?

A map provides a picture of what is being done in the curriculum. There are several uses of the various configurations of a curriculum map based on the needs of the people seeking information about the curriculum. In their curriculum design process at Texas A&M University CVM, the curriculum designers, including mapping as an important part of the process, stating that it "provides information regarding the relative contact time currently allocated to teaching and assessing each NGO (New Graduate Outcome) to enable the identification of gaps, redundancies, and misalignment in the curriculum" (Chaney et al. 2017, p. 556). As Al-Eyd and his colleagues found when they created a curriculum map for a new College of Medicine, curriculum mapping "made the curriculum transparent and communicable; it identified content gaps and redundancies and strengthened the content integration" (2018, p. 7). Rackard and Cashman (2019) used curriculum mapping at the School of Veterinary Medicine in Dublin as the method by which to gather data in preparation for their accreditation review by the AVMA. They actually created several different versions of a map to use in their various analyses of the curriculum and found that "mapping to stage outcomes and showing how they align to Day One Competencies could enhance the validity of data gathered on curriculum coherence" (2019, p. 286).

Likewise, when the world animal health organization (OIE) released a set of Day 1 Competencies necessary for veterinary graduates to be recognized, schools responsible for training veterinarians globally were now held responsible for producing graduates who have mastered these competencies. In Tanzania, the only professional veterinary degree program in the country, the College of Veterinary Medicine and Biomedical Sciences (CVMBS) found itself required to provide opportunities for students to demonstrate competence in these areas. With the OIE guidelines as the framework, the CVMBS looked to mapping to show its compliance. "The curriculum mapping process is key to developing a successful outcome-based curriculum, as it provides a means to examine the extent to which these outcomes are being addressed and assessed in the curriculum" (Komba et al. 2020, p. 21).

Curriculum mapping is not limited just to the curriculum of a single educational institution. In 2017, the pharmaceutical profession published a new set of Core Entrustable Professional Activities (EPAs) for pharmacy graduates, made up of six domains with 15 EPAs identified for new graduates to master to demonstrate competency in the pharmacists' responsibilities. The pharmaceutical common core task force was charged with mapping these EPAs to the pharmacy education guidance documents, of which there are five. This task force, made up of nine members, went through an extended three-phase process to map these EPAs to the competencies identified in each of the educational guidance documents. Their work resulted in identifying gaps in the competencies that were addressed in the EPAs and the reverse. More importantly, it created a comprehensive document encompassing the competencies from all of the various education guidance documents, showing "the necessary connections among the

educational guidance documents so that the EPAs may better serve as a foundation for schools and colleges of pharmacy to use in curricular development and assessment" (Kanmaz et al. 2020, p. 1538). Mapping the new graduate EPAs of the pharmaceutical profession to the educational competencies of the professional education institutions resulted in a clearer understanding of the profession, its various responsibilities, and the expectations of the profession on the educational institutions.

The basic purpose of a map is to provide a visual representation of the curriculum. The curriculum map is made up of a set of data about instruction that occurs, what is being taught, where and when it is being taught, and why it is being taught. According to Komenda and colleagues, "curriculum mapping is about spatially representing the different components of the curriculum so that the whole picture and the relationships and connections between the parts of the map are easily seen" (2015, p. 3). A curriculum map, then, takes the details of what occurs in a program of instruction and presents that data in a visual construct that allows the audience to understand the curriculum for the purposes of identifying what is occurring and using that information to improve the educational program.

Part 2: The Two-Level Curriculum Map

Many programs use a two-level curriculum map to show that required objectives are being taught. A simplified example of this could be for a college-level general studies mathematics curriculum as shown in Figure 13.1. The courses are listed along the top axis, and the required math content is on the left axis. An "X" indicates that the course includes that content in its curriculum. While simple in its design, this map provides a clear overview of what content is offered in which course(s) in this program.

These two-level curriculum maps serve a very important purpose. They show the reader in which courses certain student learning objectives are presented and show how often the content is addressed. They are simple to understand and give a concise view of the information. Two-level maps generally give information on one variable, such as timing of content presentation, overlaps of content, forms or timing of assessment, or other single variables for review.

The two-level map can be more detailed, with the level of coverage for the content being identified. For example, a map may show where content is introduced, where it is reinforced, at which point mastery is expected and assessed, and where it is applied to further content. Consider this map of a music theory curriculum in a Bachelor of Arts in music degree (Figure 13.2).

By indicating in which courses the objective is introduced, reinforced, mastered, and then used in application. This map shows the levels at which the students are

Student learning objectives	College algebra	Trig	Calculus 1	Calculus 2	Discrete structures	Differential equations	Linear algebra
Reasoning/Problem solving	X		X	X		X	
Set theory	X						
Functions	X	X	X				X
Identities		X	X				X
Matrices	X				X		X
Sequences	X				X		
Integrals			X	X			
Parametric curves		X		X			
Ordinary Diff Eq						X	
Eigenvectors							X
Boolean algebra	X				X		

Disclaimer: This is not meant to be an accurate summary of a mathematics degree; it is simply an example of a 2-level map.

Figure 13.1   Sample of simple two-level map.

I = introduction, R = Reinforcement; M = mastery (assessment); A = Application of the objective

Music theory curriculum	Sem 1	Sem 2	Sem 3	Sem 3	Sem 4	Sem 4	Sem 5
Student learning objectives	Intro to theory	Theory I	Theory II	Composition I	Theory III	Composition II	Adv theory and comp
Notation – treble/bass clefs	I	R	M	R	A	A	A
Other clef notation			I		R	R	M
Major/minor scales	I	R	R	R	M	A	A
Other modal scales			I		R	R	M
Time Signatures and Note values	I	R	R	R	M	M	A
Chords and Chordal Progression	I	R	R	R	M	A	A
Phrasing		I	R	R	M	M	A
Tempo and Dynamics	I	R	R	R		M	A
Musical Forms		I	R	R	R	R	M
Voicing – Vocal		I	R	R	R	M	A
Voicing – Instrumental			I	I	R	R	M

Disclaimer: This is not meant to be an accurate summary of a music degree; it is simply an example of a 2-level map.

Figure 13.2   Sample of mastery-based two level map.

expected to perform for each objective. Once mastered, the objective is then applied to meet the objectives for other strains of the curriculum, in this case possibly the performance or composition parts of the music curriculum.

In a veterinary curriculum, a two-level curriculum map could be used to identify where a concept is introduced, how many times it is reinforced through different courses, and at what point the concept is expected to be mastered and will be formally assessed. This may be especially helpful in mapping clinical skills, which are more difficult to follow than a lecture-based course. If there is a skill that several students are struggling to master, a curriculum map can show where and when it is introduced, where and when it is reinforced, and possibly help identify lapses in the curriculum. If drawing blood from a dog is introduced in semester two and reinforced in semester three, but then not seen again until semester six, perhaps this skill needs a reinforcement review in either semester four or five. Likewise, if tying knots is introduced in semester one, reinforced in semesters two and three, and mastered and assessed in semester four, it does not necessarily need to be assessed again in semesters five or six. At that point, knot tying can be applied to skills and procedures that are more advanced, such as surgical objectives.

A two-level map can also be used to set a schedule for content. Consider a vet tech program in which five instructors each have students for whom they are instructing in the lab techniques of a complete physical exam. To keep the course uniform, a curriculum map can show a schedule of when each topic is to be covered for each species. This would act very similar to a calendar, but with the species across the top axis, the procedure along the left, and showing the date of the lesson in the body of the map. This does not restrict the faculty in HOW they teach the content but does set a common structure to show WHEN they are expected to cover specific content for specific species.

A more recent type of two-dimensional curriculum map is the heat map, as explained by Clark and his team at the University of Glasgow. Their curriculum heat map was "developed as a way to visualize where and when topics are taught, in an easier-to-understand format" (Clark et al. 2021, p. 1). They used two variables – what area of biomedical science is being taught and whether that area is within the Intended Learning Outcomes (ILO) for their program. This project produced a two-dimensional curriculum map that showed the week-by-week coverage of each ILO across the entire curriculum. The darker the shading on the map, the more times that ILO was included in that week's instruction in all included courses. If there was no color under an ILO, then it was not present in the content that week. Then by collapsing the chart down to just the ILOs, the curriculum could be presented in a single

document, showing the absolute number of sessions covering any specific topic on the map. This curriculum heat map made it easier to interpret for staff and students. In particular, they found that "this tool can (1) highlight stranding of key topics within a curriculum and (2) provide a way for leads to easily identify sessions which cover their topic so that they may review those together to see how a student's knowledge is built as the course progresses" (Clark et al. 2021, p. 7).

The two-level curriculum map is a tool that can be used to report student learning objective coverage information to an outside entity, such as a committee, a board, or an accrediting body. It is a straightforward and minimal way to present a two-dimensional structure of the learning that will be obtained through the course of a program. For many schools and many programs, the two-dimensional map is all that is required, as several versions of the map can represent several perspectives of the curriculum. A set of two-dimensional maps can give information clearly on only those variables in question for each individual situation or audience. But internally, while each of these two-level maps does give a snapshot of one particular variable or set of variables, a more detailed curriculum map can have many more intricate uses. Sometimes more detail may be needed, and then a multi-level map could be used to provide more information on the curriculum.

Part 3: The Multi-Level Curriculum Map

Ideally, the best road trip plan comes from a combination of several various versions of street maps: a digital map search, perhaps a topographical map, and even a globe. Depending on the information needed, a map can show how to navigate to or from a location, give alternative routes if a detour is desired, identify whether the roads are interstate, state highways, or two-lane roads, show the layout of the land and any mountains or canyons in the path, show the size of a town or city being traversed, tell what amenities are available at any location, and even show in real time where there are construction delays or traffic incidents. An entire trip can be planned with the combined use of maps on paper and through digital sources.

A multi-level curriculum map, then, also has many uses. Depending on the information included, the viewer can use the map to see how a course was designed last semester or how the previous professor laid out the content. Faculty can use the map to explore other courses and plan horizontally with their peers to have cooperative lessons that cross course disciplines and look vertically at courses prior to their own to discover whether certain content has already been presented to students in other courses or formats. They can also view courses that come after their own to see if their content is reintroduced and followed up on by other faculty.

Faculty and administration can review the curriculum map for content redundancies as well as for missing content. Should students show a lack of mastery of an outcome or objective as they move toward graduation, faculty can use the curriculum map to discover where that objective was first introduced, where it was followed up on, and how often it was formally assessed. The map can then be used to redesign the curriculum to cover the required objective more effectively. The accrediting body might use a multi-level curriculum map to assure all required objectives are being taught, see at what level they are being taught, determine how they are assessed, and decide if the content meets the academic requirements put forth in their accreditation guidelines. In other words, the map can and should be used by multiple entities as, according to Komba et al. (2020), "curricular gap analysis has been considered a benchmark for educational transformation" (p. 25), and the map is the best place to do this analysis.

A curriculum map is a place to get answers to questions about the curriculum. Whether the map encompasses one-degree program, one general education department, or the entire curriculum offered across a campus, a map is a one-stop shopping place for information. A multi-level curriculum map can be used to answer questions such as:

- Where is this taught? What semester and what class?
- Why are we teaching this? How does it address any of our student learning outcomes? Can we eliminate it from the curriculum or make it an elective?
- Where are we teaching this? Our graduates get jobs and then seem unable to do this activity. Do we need to include this in our curriculum or increase where and how often we present and reinforce the content?
- How is this assessed? Is there a written exam, a project, or an activity to complete?
- Is this content approached from several different perspectives in several different courses? Do we need to adjust where it is covered?
- Are these two courses similar enough to combine into one course?
- Is this course overloaded with content so much that we need to break it into two courses?
- Could the content of this five-credit course be taught in a three-credit format?
- Dr. Smith won the lottery, resigned, and moved to Jamaica. Could you step in where he left off and take over his classes for the rest of this semester?
- Scientists have just discovered another process to do this marvelous thing and we need to add it to our content. Where would it best fit into our curriculum?

- These students are struggling to get the physiology of this muscle set. Where were they taught that before or is this the first time they are seeing it? Should it be taught before my course?
- How can every student have an A in this course? Is the assessment truly measuring mastery of the objectives? (Butterbrodt 2020, p. 4).

This list could go on with many more curriculum-related questions. By studying the completed curriculum map, decisions about adjusting and improving the curriculum can be made. The curriculum redesign team at Texas A&M University found that "Curriculum mapping is also an important component in the evaluation of the current curriculum and a method of establishing a baseline for the redesign effort" they undertook in rebuilding their College of Veterinary Medicine (Chaney et al. 2017, p 557). The curriculum map should be the go-to place for answers about the content of the educational program being mapped.

Part 4: Time and Human Resources Needed

Before getting into the actual design of a multi-level map, it needs to be stressed that creating a curriculum map, especially from scratch, is not an overnight task. Depending on the size of the educational program(s) being mapped, the stability and history of the curriculum, and the participation from the faculty, it could take several months or even a couple of years to finally have a meaningful and usable map. If several staff members are involved in data entry, the task moves quicker. It is also imperative to have qualified and knowledgeable faculty involved in the linking of the levels of the map. Staff can type objectives and assessment items but are not necessarily qualified to determine what question content from a lecture should be linked to which course and/or competency.

Once it has been decided that a curriculum map is needed, desired, and often required, it is necessary to get the buy-in of all stakeholders. Most importantly, the program director, the dean of the college, the president of the university, or the chairman of the board must be passionate about the project. If it is not supported from the top, the efforts to complete the curriculum map will be greatly challenged. When the administration demonstrates the many varied and useful benefits of having a curriculum map and keeping it updated, the faculty learn their own uses for the information in the map and how important it is for them to both follow the direction in which the map points and to keep the map accurate from term to term. Having support for the map from the top down increases its perceived value and encourages participation at the faculty level.

Participation from the faculty in creating the map must be strongly encouraged, and with some effort, could be a positive and creative process. While very few educators consider mapping to be "fun," they do appreciate what the end result gives them. It is important to have at least a few "cheerleaders" among the faculty who will not only complete their piece of the map but use it actively and share with others how having the map has helped them. The faculty of the veterinary school in Tanzania found that mapping enhanced faculty members' relationships and initiated conversation among the participants. "At times, discussions and debates among faculty teaching different courses led to identification of overlapping contents between courses, especially in the delivered curriculum" (Komba et al. 2020, p 27). When people see their peers finding value in a product or service, they ask about it, they watch their peers use it, and they start to see themselves getting the same benefits.

There needs to be a team who will input the actual data into the map. These detail-oriented personnel will enter the objectives at each level of the map, and according to the information provided by the faculty, identify the links. They are also responsible for inputting keywords, the key to making a map user-friendly and searchable. These data-inputting staff are the worker bees who create the map and should be adequately acknowledged and appreciated.

If you have ever traveled extensively by car in the United States, you know that at any given time there is construction on the interstates, construction in the cities, destruction of old roads, and construction of new roads. The map used must continually be updated to reflect these changes to accurately present directions to the destination. The same is true of an educational curriculum. As may be expected, the curriculum goes through small – and sometimes large – modifications each semester. A new faculty member comes on board. Courses are moved from one semester to another. New information in the content area must be included somewhere in the content. Thus, the data entry for the curriculum map does not end; it is a living document that changes with the curriculum of the program, and it is the responsibility of all involved in these changes to see that the information gets to the curriculum map for regular updates.

Finally, there needs to be a single person (or at most two) who is ultimately responsible for regularly using current information to update the map and make sure it is easily accessible to all concerned parties. This person or persons will make sure the map is updated at regular intervals, is available to faculty and administration to use, and is able to speak to the map at all levels and links. This master of the map will be the heart of the value of the curriculum map, the one person with the big picture who can find the answer to all of those questions asked on the map. Whether answering internal content or assessment questions, working with committees to identify gaps or redundancies in the curriculum, or helping with co-curricular experiences with another school, the map master will be a great asset in the continual improvement of any educational system.

Part 5: Levels of the Map

How many levels a curriculum map has depends on how deep into the curriculum the institution wants to map. That, in turn, depends on the desired function of the map. Do you need a map of a city, a state, a country, or the world? Will the curriculum map only show one department's curriculum? Or is the map of a full degree program? Are you mapping an entire undergraduate curriculum offering at a university, or is this a map of a certificate program? Or is it a map of the timing of content presentation in a single course?

There is no correct answer to the number of levels on a curriculum map. Many function very well with a set of two-level maps, some use three or four levels, while some administrations prefer all the details available and will have as many as six levels or more. These multi-level maps are huge documents and very complex in their design and creation. For the sake of example, we will look at one of these six-level maps.

In this hypothetical example, we will look at a curriculum map of a professional veterinary school program – the curriculum required at Horseshoe State University CVM (HSU-CVM) to obtain a DVM degree – Doctor of Veterinary Medicine. The purpose of the map is to document everything that is taught during the program at every level.

This map has six levels, each with its own set of objectives, goals, competencies, or educational expectations. At each level, the individual objectives are listed and linked up to the higher level and down to the lower level. Thus, by selecting any objective at any level, one can identify why it is being taught and the ultimate goal of the content.

Level 1 holds the university's strategic goals. Each university has a set of goals, values, or priorities listed in its mission statement.

Level 2 has the mission statement and goals of the College of Veterinary Medicine. Each of these leads directly back to one of the Level 1 goals of the university.

Level 3 is the list of professional veterinary competencies as outlined by the American Veterinary Medical Association (AVMA) or the Association of American Veterinary Medical Colleges (AAVMC). These competencies are shared by nearly all colleges of veterinary medicine, and this map can be linked to the college goals in Level 2.

Level 4 contains the courses included in the curriculum. Each course has a set of course learning objectives, and those objectives tie directly to one or more of the Level 3 professional competencies.

Level 5 is a listing of each and every lecture, lab, and curricular activity that takes place in every course during the four-year program toward the DVM. This is an extensive level, and each lecture or lab objective is tied directly back to one of the course objectives. This level is the heart of the curriculum and holds the details of exactly what is being taught where and when and by whom. This is the level where the keywords live, although they occasionally can be found in other levels as well.

Level 6 has its own separate document. Level 6 holds the assessment information for every lecture and lab presented – it shows exactly how student learning is assessed and how mastery of the competencies is measured. Level 6 is also a very high-security document, as it has the actual exam questions, quiz items, OSCE stations, project rubrics, and grading mechanisms for every quiz, test, project, and graded assignment used for student assessment. Each item is linked back to the lecture or lab objective that it is assessing and can be identified with keywords usually found in the stem of the question or project (Figure 13.3).

The professional program outlined in the example above chose to begin the curriculum map with the mission statement of the university at the highest or "top" level, followed by the college mission at level two. Many curriculum maps would not include the top two levels. Some only map to the professional competencies, while others may not

Figure 13.3 Map levels identified.

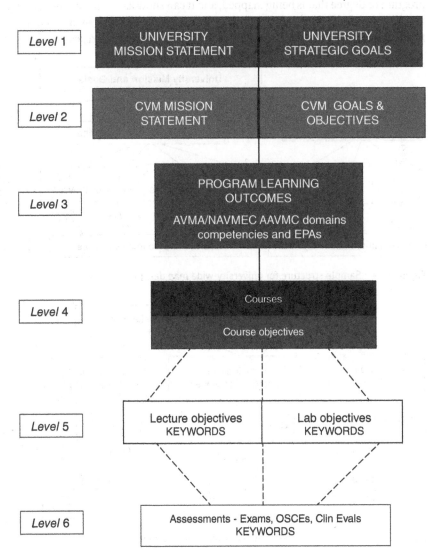

Sample CVM curriculum map

include the individual exam questions as part of the curriculum map. To give another view of the extent of a multi-level map, consider the volume of data in each level of a map designed for a medical school in the Czech Republic. They begin with four major sections, which are then mapped down through 44 medical disciplines into 144 courses, and within those, they map 1347 learning units with a total of 6974 learning objectives. Each learning objective can then be mapped back to one of the original four major sections, giving a complete picture of the curriculum of this school (Komenda et al. 2015, p. 11).

Selecting what the map is going to be designed to show and how many levels the map will need is the first step in creating the complete curriculum map. Within a department, there may only be three or four levels. For an entire university map or undergraduate program map, there may be 8 or 10 branches at a level, one for each department or one for each degree offered. The beauty of a curriculum map is that it can be designed and customized to match the program or degree that is being mapped, and it can show as much or as little detail of the curriculum as is needed to fulfill the desired function. A map of a full university program might externally show four levels, from the course objectives to the university goals, for the Board of Directors and program accreditors, as shown in the figure below (Figure 13.4).

As an example, consider the structure of a veterinary school. If the organization is divided into departments for instruction, then these departments could represent a level on the map, with the individual course's learning objectives as the sub-level, and the veterinary competencies as the professional goals at the top of the curriculum map. This three-level map covers the objectives from each course as they link to the individual department's specific goals, which then link to the veterinary competencies (Figure 13.5).

Or the veterinary school could map the courses by professional skill competencies, such as basic sciences, diagnosis, medical treatment, and surgical treatment. Here again, the same course objectives are being mapped to the competencies, but through skills categories rather than departments (Figure 13.6).

A map could use any organizational setup as a level, or basically any set of objectives that link to another set of

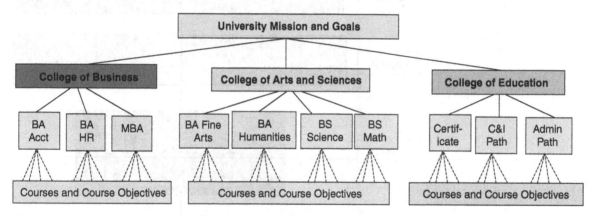

Figure 13.4 Sample structure for university-wide map design.

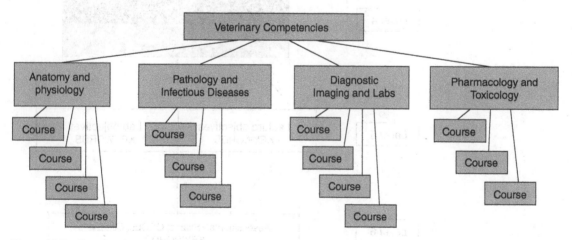

Figure 13.5 Sample of veterinary map design by department.

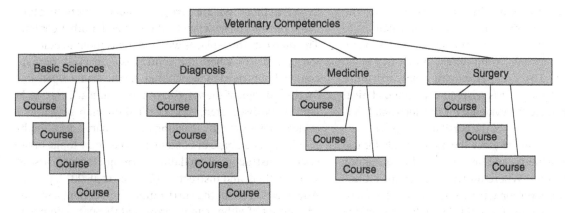

Figure 13.6   Sample of veterinary map design by skill areas.

objectives that link to the competencies. However, the organization of the school is set up, and the curriculum map can be designed to match the levels of that system. The map would then be a true reflection of the educational program, easily recognized by those involved, and easily explained to those who are searching for information on the map.

Part 6: Software for a Curriculum Map

There are many educational software programs in existence that have the capability to create a curriculum map. Several common learning management systems (LMS) have a curriculum mapping feature. Some export information directly into the map, while with others, the user has to input information into the mapping section of the software. If a school is using a two-dimensional curriculum map, whether showing the basic content of the courses or showing the introduction, reinforcement, mastery, and application of the content, there are several software programs, testing and assessment programs, and LMS already in existence that will automatically populate the map based on other data input, such as assessment items or lecture or lab objectives. These programs have various options as to their design and reporting and are very helpful for an educational program to have regular reporting capability on the instructional content of the professional objectives. If a school has the option, it is well worth the time and effort to include a review of the mapping capabilities of software before selecting what will be used for the institutional program.

Many curriculum mapping programs come with a preset mapping format and the map matches what the programmers decided it should look like. Others can be customized and may or may not show relationships from level to level. Still others do not have the capability to hold the detailed information required in an extended multi-level map. Some institutions find curriculum mapping software to fit their needs and that certainly makes the initial creation and subsequent maintenance of the map much easier than doing it from scratch. For the previous example of the HSU-CVM program, the institution did not find a program whose mapping software fit what they were trying to do. In such a situation, general programs such as spreadsheets or databases can be used to create a curriculum map to the specific organizational designs desired by the institution. This, of course, requires a map master who is thoroughly familiar and comfortable with the software and willing and able to do the work needed to design the map in a way that can be easily understood and manipulated by the stakeholders. In many cases, a readily available program already in place at an institution, such as Microsoft Excel® or Access®, is chosen as the software for mapping.

A spreadsheet program such as Excel may be chosen largely due to the capability for searching the entire document for a word or term. It is this ability to search quickly and easily that makes a curriculum map most useful in the day-to-day educational business of a school. Any software program chosen for the curriculum mapping of an educational program needs to have the capability to be searched thoroughly to identify all related information. Ideally, a database would be preferable to a spreadsheet for a map, as a change in one area will automatically transfer to other areas where that objective is used. Creating a spreadsheet with such referential operations would be comparable to learning to use a database. If an institution has a chance to have a database programmed for its curriculum map and is large enough to handle the data, the capabilities of that program to cross-reference the information on the different levels of the map would make it much more user-friendly than a spreadsheet.

Part 7: Searchability – Keywords and Codes

Keywords are the heart of the multi-level map. If you relate a curriculum map to a road map, the keywords are the roads that used to get from place to place, from city to city, or from house to restaurant. In a curriculum map, the keywords are the "roads" that connect one course to another, a lecture objective to an exam question, or a course objective to a professional competency. As Al-Eyd et al. (2018) discovered, "The results of searching the Curriculum Map database using keywords related to basic and clinical sciences demonstrated the evidence for the horizontal, vertical, and spiral integration of the curriculum" (p. 4).

Once the keywords are in place the map is ready for use by faculty administrators and anyone who has questions about the curriculum. Where do we teach about rabies? Search the lecture level for rabies. Why do we teach students to estimate the size of a marble? Search estimate size and follow the links up to the competency that requires estimating the size of a tumor in an organ or the progression of a pregnancy. Does the first semester expose students to research citations? Search for citations and see which courses use that concept. Do the accreditors want to know how competency two is assessed? Go to competency two and follow the links down to level 6 Assessments. Everything that links up to competency two is an assessment of that competency.

If there are a set of specific goals, competencies, or student learning objectives that are the heart of the program, such as standardized testing competencies, specific nursing competencies, or competencies required for a degree, these can be abbreviated with an alphanumeric code to make searching and data input much easier. In the HSU-CVM map example, the code for an objective may look like this: 3.25 (level 3 – professional competencies, competency #25) or like this 5.710.44.3 (level 5 – lecture objectives, course 710 – Anatomy, lecture #44, objective #3) so the map master can search by code rather than typing in an entire sentence or paragraph. By looking for 3.25, the entire map can be searched to see which objectives link to competency 25. These codes for the objectives would be created by the map maker and have a logical set of parameters clearly outlined so those seeking information can not only find what they seek but understand what they find.

Part 8: Summary of Curriculum Mapping

A curriculum map is very useful tool for understanding what is being taught, where, and how. It is a picture of the intended design of the curriculum and can be used to answer questions about the curriculum. Inclusion of keywords makes a curriculum map searchable and allows flexibility in identification of objectives at all levels of the map. When a curriculum is under review, the map allows for a complete and transparent view of the current design of the curriculum. It also shows objectives that are not reinforced as well as those that are covered so much content that they could possibly be lessened to allow room for other content. The map can show places where there is room to add content and places where the content is so packed, perhaps contact hours need to be required. As the team responsible for the redesign of the veterinary curriculum at Texas A&M University discovered, "the curriculum map serves as a critical tool for faculty teaching in veterinary education by providing a database of content searchable by topic, organ system, instructional modality, learning outcome, assessment method, and instructor" (Chaney et al. 2017, p. 557). Any question about the curriculum of a program, a school, or a subset of either can be answered through a complete and accurate curriculum map.

Section 2: Accountability in Assessment Outcomes

Katrina Jolley

Tracking student outcomes allows colleges and universities to ensure that their students are meeting or exceeding the standards set forth by the institution and its programs of study. The most recognizable ways to track outcomes are through the use of course grades and grade point averages. Institutions also use outcomes on standardized assessments, licensing exams, and graduation rates to measure outcomes between cohorts of students and convey program performance over time. In veterinary medicine, the end result is to be able to prove that graduates have the skills needed to enter the field they have been training for and for the school to use those outcomes to identify ways for continued curricular improvement.

Graduate and professional programs are under an increased amount of scrutiny of student outcomes "because of the additional debt students accrue when they pursue advanced degrees" (Hundley and Kahn 2019, p. 112). Expectations for outcomes assessment in veterinary education are also held to a high standard due to concerns about patient safety and practice readiness (Hundley and Kahn 2019, p. 112; AVMA 2022 section 7.11). Additionally,

> Recognizing that assessment must be conducted to meet requirements imposed by accreditors or government, and also may be frequently requested by other stakeholders, many higher education institutions have embraced the accountability process as a strategic opportunity to quantify and qualify institutional efficiency and effectiveness, and to analyze learning outcomes to improve educational quality through strategic change (Hernon et al. 2006, p. 103).

Rather than becoming overwhelmed by the seemingly daunting task of documenting student outcomes, it is best to see this necessary task as a means to evaluate the strengths and weaknesses of the veterinary curriculum being implemented.

The goal of accountability is to make sure the institution is achieving its own goals for student learning outcomes no matter who is looking at the data (Henning et al. 2022). The records should be kept up to date and easy to reference for accreditors, external stakeholders (such as boards of trustees), and internal institutional reporting. Hernon et al. (2006) recommend keeping accountability documentation simple and manageable, because by having continuous access to the right assessment data, all necessary parties can stay up to date on how each student and cohort are performing throughout the semester as well as identify "what kinds of emerging or persistent challenges need to be addressed to enable students to equitably progress" through the curriculum (Henning et al. 2022, p. 297). This allows for continuous improvement in multiple areas, from individual courses all the way to institutional-level outcomes, as required by the AVMA-COE (Henning et al. 2022, p. 8; AVMA 2022 standard 7.11).

Proper documentation is key to accountability for both internal and external stakeholders because both record the results (e.g., course grades), show where the results came from, and demonstrate how they lead to the outcomes assessment reports (Brun 2016). Brun (2016) recommends documenting all outcomes "as if someone might conduct an audit of the entire evaluation process. Such thorough and comprehensive documentation will provide evidence and support of the decisions made along the way" (p. 330). When student assessment results are supported by documentation, this protects faculty from accusations of arbitrary grade discrimination and justifies the grades for any issues that move forward to academic council review (i.e., student in danger of dismissal for poor academic performance).

Most of the course documentation will come from faculty who "have the primary responsibility in assessing student academic performance and assigning grades to students" (Hu 2005, p. 12). This documentation should come in a combination of assignment grades, test scores, and grading rubrics for projects. These should be tracked for each student using some form of student identification number or other unique identifier so that individual student outcomes can be tracked over the course of the academic program. Other forms of documentation may include student feedback on end-of-course surveys, clinical outcomes, and data from standardized assessments such as the NAVLE and the veterinary educational assessment (VEA®).

While in the early years of higher education students were assessed to ensure teacher effectiveness, assessment now is used "to measure levels of mastery, provide feedback to students, account to important stakeholders, and improve programs and services" (Miller 2007, p. 32). But to drive improvement, the learning outcomes tracked must "reflect the values of all stakeholders" (Henning et al. 2022, p. 101). However, often those responsible just make a list of the expected values, without providing support for their inclusion (Brun 2016). This can create confusion when the reason why certain data is being tracked is not made clear. Students and faculty are more likely to provide appropriate input when they know how their information and input are being used to drive improvement.

One of the ways colleges can remain accountable to both internal and external stakeholders is through the use of comparative analysis and benchmarking. Within a single veterinary school, for example, cohorts can be compared against each other to measure outcomes for part or all of the veterinary curriculum. And when a comparison is made between two or more schools, this analysis lets "stakeholders know how an institution stacks up against its peers," especially those that it is trying to emulate (Terkla 2008, p. 21). External stakeholders may choose to focus on retention and graduation rates as targets for learning outcomes, while program administrators likely take a more comprehensive and detailed look at outcomes (Hernon et al. 2006). Hernon et al. (2006) further state that "the commitment to student learning outcomes should be evident in how the institution goes about developing its set of intended student learning outcomes" and implements them in the classroom (p. 11).

Section 3: Ensuring Students Meet Benchmarks for Student Learning

Katrina Jolley

Clear criteria and standards are critical to ensuring that grading measures the desired outcomes (Barkley et al. 2014). Dufour and Marzano (2011) recommend the use of "SMART goals that are (1) strategically aligned with school and district goals, (2) measurable, (3) attainable, (4) results-oriented (that is, requiring evidence of higher levels of student learning on order to be achieved), and (5) time bound" (p. 24). While this concept is generally geared toward K-12 education, it is transferable to professional-level programs. The benchmarks for veterinary education should be strategically aligned with both the AVMA and institutional goals, measurable through the use of outcomes assessment, attainable by resulting in the DVM degree, results oriented by developing practice-ready veterinarians, and time-bound in that there is a specified progression toward degree completion. The end result of setting up SMART goals is a series of benchmarks along the way that can be measured through assessment to determine whether students are learning what is intended (Terkla 2008).

The curriculum map can be a great place to start when deciding on the benchmarks for the veterinary curriculum. The benchmarks should identify the key concepts, or the knowledge, skills, behaviors, and attitudes that students are expected to learn and master at the learning unit (lecture series), course, and program level (Terkla 2008; Hernon et al. 2006). Creating benchmarks for specific content that must be taught in specific courses, regardless of who is coordinating or instructing the content, ensures the curriculum is sufficient to cover the necessary concepts and makes sure that "there is enough instructional time available to actually teach the content identified as important" (Dufour and Marzano 2011, p. 91). This process helps to identify what should be measured for tracking and improvement purposes and highlights any areas of overlap or gaps in the curriculum (Alstete 1995).

One of the components to consider when setting benchmarks is the level of mastery or competence the students are expected to achieve with each benchmark. Ambrose et al. (2010) found that "for students to achieve mastery within a domain, whether narrowly or broadly conceived, they need to develop a set of key component skills, practice them to a point where they can be combined fluently and used with a fair degree of automaticity, and know when and where to apply them appropriately" (p. 95). Just as the veterinary curriculum builds on itself, so should the benchmarks build upon themselves as students are expected to combine components of tasks together into more complex skills and knowledge foundations.

As students progress through the curriculum, they are expected to fluently combine knowledge from multiple content areas and component skills into more complex procedures (e.g., leading up to live surgery or creating a treatment plan for a real patient). It is crucial that students learn to see these procedures as one skill rather than a series of tasks; for mastery to occur they must undergo less multitasking, as this risks degrading their overall performance. If students are continually viewing complex tasks as a series of individual tasks, their cognitive load is more easily exceeded, which leaves them "with insufficient attention and other cognitive resources to complete the task effectively" (Ambrose et al. 2010, p. 103).

Another approach that can be taken for setting benchmarks is to begin with the end in mind: graduate veterinarians who are ready to enter the field from day one (AVMA 2022, section 7.11). What skills are necessary for students to meet this goal? Brun (2016) recommends

looking at the professional organizations' standards for "the principles and behaviors expected of all members of that organization" (p. 62). "Dating back to the creation of the Council on Medical Education (CME) in 1904, governing bodies in medicine were among the first to require programs to meet specific standards and benchmarks of quality and effectiveness" (Hundley and Kahn 2019, p. 108). The AVMA Council on Education (AVMA-COE) requires schools to document that students are observed and assessed on nine different competencies:

1) comprehensive patient diagnosis (problem-solving skills), appropriate use of diagnostic testing, and record management
2) comprehensive treatment planning including patient referral when indicated
3) anesthesia and pain management, patient welfare
4) basic surgery skills and case management
5) basic medicine skills and case management
6) emergency and intensive care case management
7) understanding of health promotion, biosecurity, prevention, and control of disease including zoonoses and principles of food safety
8) ethical and professional conduct; communication skills including those that demonstrate an understanding and sensitivity to how clients' diversity and individual circumstances can impact healthcare
9) critical analysis of new information and research findings relevant to veterinary medicine (AVMA 2022 section 7.11).

These nine competencies are intended to give students the necessary skills and foundation for entering the veterinary field. Keep in mind, there are numerous frameworks for beginning with the end in mind. These include the AAVMC's Competency-Based Veterinary Education (CBVE); the Royal Veterinary College's (RVC) Day One competencies, the World Organization for Animal Health's (OIE) Day 1 graduates' competencies, and the Ontario Veterinary College's "Essential Skills and Abilities" to name a few; all are readily accessible via the internet.

The final assessment of a student's content knowledge and career readiness comes from the North American Veterinary Licensing Exam (NAVLE). Because the NAVLE is standardized and designed to assess all students' full knowledge of the curriculum, it is frequently used to show how well a program is doing on its own and compared to others (Hundley and Kahn 2019, p. 111). The AVMA-COE "expects that 80% or more of each college's graduating senior students sitting for the NAVLE will have passed at the time of graduation" (AVMA 2022, section 7.11); this benchmark is required to be met each year to maintain a veterinary college's accreditation through the AVMA-COE. It is therefore recommended that schools shape their learning targets to help students pass the NAVLE and prepare for clinical practice and other veterinary careers. In other words, begin with the NAVLE in mind.

When working by backward design, the benchmarks are broken down and nested together. There should be benchmarks set for each semester and course that lead to the end goal. With this approach, it is helpful to establish the benchmarks for the final courses in the curriculum then determine what benchmarks are needed in the prerequisite courses and finally the foundational courses. Within each course, there should be goals for students to direct and focus their learning and monitor their progress (Ambrose et al. 2010). These goals should be "stated in terms of something students do, which automatically leads to more concrete specifications that students can more easily interpret correctly" (Ambrose et al. 2010, p. 129). If needed, the course content can be further subdivided into benchmarks for specific learning units. This is especially helpful for courses where the content builds upon itself such as anatomy, physiology, pathology, and skill-based courses.

Once the benchmarks for a course or set of courses have been created, the next step is to identify the key concepts, projects, and tasks that students must achieve minimum proficiency in in order to advance in the curriculum. "Rather than trying to assess every desired outcome, an institution should assess those that are most critical and would provide the most information for analysis and reporting" (Hernon et al. 2006, p. 106). Neufeld and Norman (1985) suggest avoiding rarely used skills and primarily assessing commonly used skills; if necessary, the "common components of several complex procedures" can be assessed rather than the whole procedure (p. 259). Monitoring and measuring these goals allows students to track their progress and faculty to provide feedback "to help students refine their performance or learning" (Ambrose et al. 2010, p. 129). Brown et al. (2014) also recommend having low-stakes quizzes and practice exercises count toward at least a small portion of the course grade because "students in classes where practice exercises carry consequences for the course grade learn better than those in classes where the exercises are the same but carry no consequences" (p. 227).

Section 4: Tracking Student Outcomes

Katrina Jolley

Part 1: Individual

The primary way to track individual student outcomes is through the use of course and assignment grades. The grading plan should reflect the benchmarks set for the course and sufficiently document the results in a timely manner (Moss and Brookhart 2012; AVMA 2022). It is recommended that the assessment director create a master gradebook so that key administrators (i.e., those in academic support and student affairs) can see individual student progress throughout the curriculum. While grade reports for individual courses can be pulled and compiled into longitudinal reports as needed, it is much less frustrating to already have the information in a secure, centralized location. This allows for a complete picture of a student's academic record to identify areas in need of improvement (Terkla 2008).

To create a cohesive picture, the final course grades need to be reported on the same scale (typically as a percent correct). This allows administrators to see the big picture with minimal confusion. For transparency of student grades, it is good practice to document both the original points or rubric scores as well as the percentage score on each assignment so that grades can be compared and analyzed on the same scale (Moss and Brookhart 2012). Dufour and Marzano (2011) advise that these assessment scores should be seen as "snapshots taken at a point in time of students' progress toward a specific goal" (p. 119). Group projects should be graded as a combination of individual and group scores. "In this model, the combination of individual and group grades is weighted as appropriate for the assignment (e.g., 75% individual grade, 25% group grade for high-stakes assignments, and percentages reversed for low-stakes assignments)" (Barkley et al. 2014, p. 114). This gives a more complete picture of how an individual student's performance aligns with the group as a whole.

When assessments and assignments are aligned with curricular benchmarks, course grades become a form of tracking document to show student learning throughout the curriculum (Moss and Brookhart 2012). To further track student learning throughout a course, assessment scores can be reported with subsection scores when the assessment is comprised of more than one-course content area (i.e., multiple learning units or multiple body systems). While this type of score reporting is not critical for keeping track of student grades, Dufour and Marzano (2011) advise providing this level of feedback to students so they can focus on mastering the content rather than calculating what score they will need to pass the class. If a course's assessments are given through testing software or the LMS, it is usually possible to create a category report from a single assessment or range of assessments to provide students with more detailed data on how they are performing in different areas of the curriculum (e.g., species, system, and content area).

Scores from summative and formative assessments can be used in conjunction with student perceptions of their own performance. This metacognition allows students to reflect on their level of understanding about a topic and identify areas for self-improvement (Brown et al. 2014; Angelo and Cross 1993). This provides an opportunity for the faculty to "compare the students' assessments with his or her own assessment of their competence" as well as the students' level of preparation on the content (Angelo and Cross 1993, p. 284).

Moss and Brookhart (2012) report that "good self-assessment requires students to have a clear concept of the learning goals and criteria for success, to be able to recognize these characteristics in their own work, and to be able to translate their self-assessments into action plans for improvement" (p. 80). Individuals who have an inaccurate self-analysis of their skills and knowledge are unable to improve because they cannot identify their areas of weakness and may have trouble completing the curriculum (Brown et al. 2014; Davis and Murrell 1993). "The upshot is that even the most diligent students are often hobbled by two liabilities: a failure to know the areas where their learning is weak – that is, where they need to do more work to bring up their knowledge – and a preference for study methods that create a false sense of mastery" (Brown et al. 2014, p. 17). Therefore, it is important that in the first year of veterinary school students be taught to accurately assess their own skills and knowledge base so they can maximize their learning and improvement in the curriculum.

Part 2: Tracking Student Outcomes

Cohort

Comparing outcomes between cohorts of students can highlight the strengths and weaknesses of the veterinary curriculum. Cohort analysis with groups of veterinary students works well because each cohort is made of similar populations of students, the same points of comparison are used, and there is little movement between cohorts (i.e., relative attrition; Glenn 2005). The most basic cohort comparison is to compare the class averages from one cohort to another (i.e., this year's class average in Anatomy compared to last year's). Assessment category performance (e.g., species or system), professional standards outcomes, NAVLE pass rates, and benchmark performance each provide additional opportunities to track and compare cohort outcomes. If using end-of-course surveys to track cohort outcomes, it is important that both the questions asked and the response choices stay the same for all groups. "What seem to be minor differences in question wording can produce substantial differences in responses, as can differences in the order in which response alternatives are presented" (Glenn 2005, p. 44).

Viewing the results of multiple cohorts over time is even more useful and can help identify areas of the curriculum that students tend to do well in or struggle with consistently (Glenn 2005). As curricular changes are implemented, cohort analysis provides a means to show how those changes impact student outcomes. Alstete (1995) identified three types of performance gaps or trends in educational outcomes: negative, parity, and positive. When comparing outcomes for different cohorts, a negative trend indicates a need to change and analyze "why the differences exist and determine the specific contributing factors or enablers" (p. 75). The process is likely to result in some sort of curricular revision within specific courses. Unless the results are consistently very low, outcomes that are at parity, (have little difference) or have a positive trend are generally acceptable when tracking outcomes for cohorts across time. The goal is to maintain a high-quality curriculum and ensure that students and cohorts are meeting benchmarks.

Part 3: Tracking Outcomes

Clinical

Tracking outcomes in the clinical setting can be a bit more involved than tracking outcomes in the classroom setting. Rather than using assignment scores or exam scores, clinical outcomes tend to lean more toward individual student portfolios and evaluations of skills as measures of student performance. Global rating scales and rubrics can be used to measure students' clinical skills that are hard to evaluate using traditional written exams (Neufeld and Norman 1985). The global rating scale used by The Royal College of Physicians and Surgeons (RCPS) of Canada functions as a scoring rubric to assess a student's ability in fundamental skills, professional attitudes, technical skills, and knowledge, with an optional section to add additional criteria to be measured. When written in clear and concise terms, the global rating scale can allow the student to see "exactly which areas need improvement and may facilitate discussion with the faculty about these deficiencies" (RCPS, pp. 123–124). The scale should be divided for each item into only as many parts as are necessary for the raters to "discriminate among levels of performance in different areas" (RCPS, p. 137). Some items may have more rating points than others because the skill being rated has more variance from the low end of the spectrum to the high end.

Case logging can be used for students to track the skills performed each day while on rotations. This method should only be considered a formative part of the students' performance because "there is no way of determining from the log which activities constitute good or competent behavior, and which are poor, and which activities fall in the mid-range" (Neufeld and Norman 1985, p. 22). What case logs can show are the frequency that a student has performed a skill within a given time frame. This can be analyzed to identify any gaps in the clinical skills where a student may need an opportunity to practice. For example, if a student has not logged any limb bandaging over three rotations, the student may need an opportunity to demonstrate that skill.

Case logs and medical records should be reviewed by an attending veterinarian or clinical preceptor to assess for clinical competence (Neufeld and Norman 1985). This review can be used as both formative and summative assessments. The attending clinician is uniquely positioned to provide feedback on the student because they work closely with the student and can provide feedback from first-hand observation of the student's skills. Neufeld and Norman (1985) also point out that this provides an opportunity for the student to participate in the goal setting and "to review and think through the evidence for what constitutes competent care" (p. 167).

The result of the clinical year should be that soon-to-be graduates are able to complete a number of EPAs. These are "tasks that can be entrusted to a trainee once sufficient competence is attained to ensure that the tasks can be carried out in unsupervised settings" (Hundley and Kahn 2019, p. 112). EPAs go one step further than clinical competencies by creating "combinations of competencies (knowledge, skills, and attitudes) that students achieve progressively" (Hundley and Kahn 2019, p. 112). In other words, EPAs are the basic skills and tasks that students should be able to perform on their own by the time they graduate as veterinarians.

Part 4: Tracking Outcomes

Program

Program-level outcomes tend to focus on performance over time for both cohorts and courses. In veterinary education, the predominant focus of program outcomes is the school's overall NAVLE pass rate. While the AVMA requires schools to achieve an 80% minimum NAVLE pass rate (AVMA 2022), other outcomes "such as professionalism, collaboration, and ethical decision-making, which are less easily assessed by traditional means," are also being used to assess program health and stability (Hundley and Kahn 2019, p. 107). End-of-course evaluations, alumni surveys, job placement rates, attrition rates, and category performance over time can all be used to assess program health (Miller 2007; Hernon et al. 2006; Terkla 2008). While it is easy to fixate on one measure of student learning as an indicator of program outcomes, it is better to consider multiple types of cohort data to get a complete picture to determine both program and institutional effectiveness (Hernon et al. 2006).

When curricular changes are implemented, cohort comparisons can be used to show how those changes affected the program outcomes (Hernon et al. 2006). "Institutions oftentimes deploy a systematic, hierarchical framework with horizontal and vertical levels to plan, gather, analyze, and report information, and to make changes to institutional and educational outcomes and objectives, as part of their effort to demonstrate accountability through assessment" (Hernon et al. 2006). Outcomes are mapped and reported from the institutional level (mission statement) to the colleges, departments, disciplines, and courses, as detailed earlier in this chapter. Reporting then maps back up to the top and is sent out to the external stakeholders for accountability (Hernon et al. 2006). When test questions are linked to the curriculum map, outcomes data can be tracked hierarchically and considered as a measure of student learning and overall program health (Terkla 2008).

Part 5: Legal Implications for Tracking Outcomes

For tracking individual student results throughout their education, the gradebooks should include the student ID number in addition to first and last name so student data can be tracked consistently as legal names may change over time. Keeping record of students' grades by course, term, and cohort is necessary in case the records are ever challenged in court.

> When a student alleges that a grade has been awarded improperly or that credits or a degree have been denied unfairly, the court must determine whether the defendant's action reflected the application of academic judgment or an arbitrary or unfair application of institutional policy. If the court is satisfied that the decision involved the evenhanded application of academic judgment, the court will typically defer to the institution's decision. But if the student can demonstrate arbitrary, discriminatory, or bad faith actions on the part of the faculty or administrators, then the court will scrutinize the decision and may not defer to the institution's decision. (Kaplin et al. 2020, p. 546)

Ensuring that faculty are following the grading scheme laid out in the course syllabus closes a potential loophole that students can use to successfully argue for a change of grade. For example, if a course's grading scheme includes 10% for case studies and the faculty never assign any case studies, the student can successfully argue that their otherwise course grade of 68% would have been one letter grade higher had the case studies been given and graded; for programs where this is considered a failing score, the student would have failed the course because they were counting on all parts of the grading scheme listed in the syllabus to be included in the final course grade, but one or more grading categories were not given. The onus is on the student to show "either that the institution did not follow its own policies and procedures or that the policies and procedures themselves were unfair" (Kaplin et al. 2020, p. 618).

As with disciplinary issues, schools are expected to follow due process when addressing academic issues. "Although courts have not required public institutions to provide the type of procedural due process required for disciplinary sanctions to sanctions based upon academic performance, institutions must still provide reasons for their decisions and an opportunity for the student to respond (at least where a liberty or property interest is at stake)" (Kaplin et al. 2020, p. 614). Tracking student outcomes through grade records, performance evaluations, and established benchmarks gives the institution the documentation needed to justify academic decisions. If a student chooses to challenge an academic outcome, those records will be necessary to demonstrate that the student received the appropriate course credit and/or academic decision (e.g., remediation, recession, or dismissal).

While the number of disputes of performance evaluations in the clinical setting have increased, they are rarely successful (Kaplin et al. 2020). "The leading case on the subject of judicial review of academic judgments is *Board of Curators of the University of Missouri v. Horowitz*, 435 U.S. 78 (1978)" (Kaplin et al. 2020, p. 614). Horowitz's academic dismissal from medical school was based on her poor clinical performance, poor interpersonal relations, and lack of personal hygiene during clinical rotations. The student was "allowed to take a special set of oral and practical exams, administered by practicing physicians in the area, as a means of appealing the council's determination" (Kaplin et al. 2020, p. 614). The Supreme Court determined that the school went above and beyond the constitutionally required due process in allowing the student to be assessed by area physicians to determine that grading of the student's skill was accurate.

In *Lekutis v. University of Osteopathic Medicine*, 254 N.W.2d (Iowa 1994), the Supreme Court of Iowa upheld the university's decision to dismiss a medical student for his inappropriate behavior in the clinical setting (Kaplin et al. 2020). While the student "had completed his coursework with the highest grades in his class and had scored in the 99th percentile on standardized tests," Lekutis also had "serious psychological problems" that resulted in hospitalization multiple times during his academic studies, resulting in dismissal from medical school because "during several clinical rotations, his professors found his behavior bizarre, inappropriate, and unprofessional and gave him failing grades" (Kaplin et al. 2020, p. 619). When the dismissal was ultimately challenged in court, the Supreme Court of Iowa found "that the staff did not treat the student in an unfair or biased way and that there was considerable evidence of his inability to interact appropriately with patients and fellow medical staff" (Kaplin et al. 2020, p. 619).

Part 6: Grading Issues

Course, assignment, and examination grades serve as numerical representations of a student's mastery of course content. However, the representation may be skewed if the numerical grade is inflated or does not accurately portray the student's level of content mastery. Hu (2005) performed a study of 22,792 self-reported grades from the mid-1980s to the mid-1990s at 124 four-year schools, and they found that there was an increase in college grades over time resulting from "a complex combination of students' changing background, changing grade-awarding, and in some cases, artificial inflation of grades in colleges and universities" (p. 33). Grade inflation refers to "the increase of grades over a specified period of time with higher grades being awarded for the same quality of work" (Hu 2005, p. 15). This can result from changes in faculty characteristics, institutional policies, or shifting academic cultures (Hu 2005). Adjunct and nontenured faculty tend to give higher grades than tenured faculty, partly in an effort to receive positive student evaluations (Hu 2005). When this issue is spread across multiple courses, particularly multiple sections of the same course, inflated grades can lead to inflated student GPAs as students choose the course section they feel will give them the higher grade (Hu 2005).

Kamber and Biggs (2002) argue that "the problem is not only that most institutions have accepted grading practices that persistently blur the distinction between good and outstanding performance, while they award passing grades for showing up and turning in work – even when that work is poor. It is also that students and faculty members, administrators and trustees, accrediting bodies, and higher-education associations have been united for more than 25 years in their willingness to ignore, excuse, or compromise with grade inflation rather than fight it" (p. B14). To maintain fairness and equity in grading, "students with similar performances [should be] awarded similar grades" and "student with different performances [should] receive different grades. The higher the student performance, the higher the grade" (Hu 2005, p. 24). Using a standardized grading rubric for key assignments can help prevent some of the grading disparity that can lead to inflated grades.

When grade inflation reaches the extreme, a new issue arises as the numerical score no longer delineates the quality of student performance and the grades are no longer a reliable measure of student learning (Hu 2005). The grading system essentially becomes pass/fail when the majority of students receive an A, and in this system "students are less motivated to learn, feel that they learn less, and show lower achievement in pass/fail courses than in regular courses" (Hu 2005). "On the other end of the scale, great damage has also been done by the metamorphosis of F from an academic grade for 'failing to do acceptable college-level work' into a disciplinary category for 'failing to come to class' or 'failing to submit assignments'" (Kamber and Biggs 2002, p. B14). A side effect of inflated and ambiguous grades being so widespread is that students have conditioned themselves to believe that high grades are so necessary that they argue for more lenient grading policies and policies for dropping or retaking courses to replace unwanted low grades (Kamber and Biggs 2002).

Faculty members should not be deterred from accurately assessing student work, and "accreditors must recognize that giving low grades for low performance – even if this causes students to transfer, drop out, or fail – is not only a legitimate college function but is essential to the fulfillment of the academic mission in society" (Kamber and Biggs 2002, p. B14). It may take a shift in the institution's culture to counteract the overall grade inflation. Additional training is needed to teach faculty effective grading practices and "to increase faculty awareness and willingness to grade students fairly and vigorously" (Hu 2005, pp. 67–68). Faulty may also find it helpful to have examples of key assignments that represent various qualities of work to use alongside the scoring rubric to use as a grading reference (e.g., examples of outstanding, good, mediocre, and poor).

Part 7: Conclusion

The starting point for tracking outcomes and ensuring students meet benchmarks is to provide transparency to all stakeholders about what data is being collected and how that information is being used. The learning benchmarks should be made available to the students so they can track their own progress through the curriculum and see how their content knowledge is helping them reach the goal of becoming practice-ready veterinarians. Faculty and administrators need to be informed of how outcomes tracking can show overall program health and lead to curricular change when areas for improvement are identified.

Additional training on the best practices for grading should be offered to the faculty periodically. The timing and frequency of this training will vary based on the needs of the instructors, and it should be offered to new faculty members as part of their first academic year experience. Best practices must include keeping appropriate records and should include methods to prevent grading bias and grader fatigue. By paying attention to the details, individual, cohort, and program outcomes can be accurately tracked to ensure that students are meeting benchmarks for learning and that the program is delivering a guaranteed and viable curriculum.

Summary

Educational programs are being increasingly scrutinized due to rising tuition costs and societal pressures to tangibly demonstrate what students and parents are "getting for their money." A professional education is one of the biggest investments a person will make in their lifetime, and understandably whoever endeavors to go through such a program desires proof that what they are learning will provide them the skills and knowledge necessary to be successful in their field. This chapter has provided an in-depth look at the ways such "proof" can be produced and tracked, so that at any given time during a program all stakeholders involved – from those who work within the program to students and their families, from potential employees to accrediting bodies, from licensing boards to administrators – can accurately determine whether students are achieving the goals set forth by the program, the college or university, and the profession.

References

Al-Eyd, G., Achike, F., Agarwal, M. et al. (2018). Curriculum mapping as a tool to facilitate curriculum development: a new school of medicine experience. *BMC Medical Education* 18: https://doi-org.lmunet.idm.oclc.org/10.1186/s12909-018-1289-9.

Alstete, J. (1995). Benchmarking in higher education: adapting best practices to improve quality. *ASHE-ERIC Higher Education Reports, No. 5 1995*. Washington, DC: The George Washington University, School of Education and Human Development.

Ambrose, S., Bridges, M., DiPietro, M. et al. (2010). *How Learning Works: 7 Research-Based Principles for Smart Teaching*. San Francisco, CA: Wiley.

American Veterinary Medical Association (2022). COE Accreditation Policies and Procedures: Requirements. July 2021. https://www.avma.org/education/accreditation-policies-and-procedures-avma-council-education-coe/coe-accreditation-policies-and-procedures-requirements (accessed 19 November 2022).

Angelo, T. and Cross, K.P. (1993). *Classroom Assessment Techniques: A Handbook for College Teachers*, 2e. San Francisco, CA: Wiley.

Barkley, E., Major, C., and Cross, K.P. (2014). *Collaborative Learning Techniques: A Handbook for College Faculty*, 2e. San Francisco, CA: Wiley.

Brown, P., Roediger, H., and McDaniel, M. (2014). *Make It Stick: The Science of Successful Learning*. Cambridge, MA: The Belknap Press of Harvard University Press.

Brun, C. (2016). *A Practical Guide to Evaluation*, 2e. New York, NY: Oxford University Press.

Butterbrodt, P. (2020). *The Curriculum Mapping Process from Lincoln Memorial University*. Urbana, IL: University of Illinois and Indiana University, National Institute for Learning Outcomes Assessment.

Chaney, K., Macik, M., Turner, J.S. et al. (2017). Curriculum redesign in veterinary Medicine: Part I. *Journal of Veterinary Medical Education* 44 (3): 552–559. https://doi.org/10.3138/jvme.0316-065R1.

Clark, R., Bell, S., Roccisana, J. et al. (2021). Creation of a novel simple heat mapping method for curriculum mapping, using pathology teaching as the exemplar. *BMC Medical Education* 21 (371): https://doi.org/10.1186/s12909-021-02808-3.

Davis, T. and Hillman Murrell, P. (1993). Turning teaching into learning: the role of student responsibility in the collegiate experience. *ASHE-ERIC Higher Education Reports, No. 8 1993*. Washington, DC: The George Washington University, School of Education and Human Development.

Dufour, R. and Marzano, R. (2011). *Leaders of Learning: How District, School, and Classroom Leaders Improve Student Achievement*. Bloomington, IN: Solution Tree Press.

Glenn, N. (2005). Cohort analysis. In: *Quantitative Applications in the Social Sciences*, 2e, vol. 5 (ed. T.F. Liao, L.C. Shaw, and C.A. Hoffman). Thousand Oaks, CA: Sage Publications.

Henning, G., Baker, G., Jankowski, N. et al. (2022). *Reframing Assessment to Center Equity: Theories, Models, and Practices*. Steerline, VA: Stylus Publishing, LLC.

Hernon, P., Dugan, R., and Schwartz, C. (2006). *Revisiting Outcomes Assessment in Higher Education*. Westport, CT: Libraries Unlimited.

Hu, S. (2005). Beyond grade inflation: grading problems in higher education. *ASHE Higher Education Report, Vol. 30, No. 6*. Hoboken, NJ: Wiley Periodicals.

Hundley, S. and Kahn, S. (2019). *Trends in Assessment: Ideas, Opportunities, and Issues for Higher Education*. Special Institute Edition. Steerling, VA: Stylus Publishing, LLC.

Kamber, R., and Biggs, M. (2002). Grade conflation: a question of credibility. *Chronicle of Higher Education* (12 April), Vol 48(31). B14. http://lmunet.idm.oclc.org/login?url=https://www.proquest.com/trade-journals/grade-conflation-question-credibility/docview/214698457/se-2

Kanmaz, T., Culhane, N.S., Berenbrok, L.A. et al. (2020). A curriculum crosswalk of the core entrustable professional activities for new pharmacy graduates. *American Journal of Pharmaceutical Education* 84 (11): 1532–1538. https://doi.org/10.5688/ajpe8077.

Kaplin, W., Lee, B., Hutchens, N., and Rooksby, J. (2020). *The Law of Higher Education*, 6e. Student Version. Hoboken, NJ: Jossey-Bass.

Komba, E., Kipanyula, M.J., Muhairwa, A.P. et al. (2020). Evaluation of the Bachelor of Veterinary Medicine (BVM) Curriculum at Sokoine University of Agriculture in Tanzania: Mapping to OIE Veterinary Graduate 'Day 1 Competencies'. *Journal of Veterinary Medical Education* 47 (s1): 20–29. https://doi.org/10.3138/jvme-2019-0120.

Komenda, M., Víta, M., Vaitsis, C. et al. (2015). Curriculum mapping with academic analytics in medical and healthcare education. *PLoS One* 10 (12): e0143748. https://doi.org/10.1371/journal.pone.0143748.

Miller, B. (2007). *Assessing Organizational Performance in Higher Education*. San Francisco, CA: Wiley.

Moss, C. and Brookhart, S. (2012). *Learning Targets: Helping Students Aim for Understanding in Today's Lesson*. Alexandria, VA: ASCD.

Neufeld, V. and Norman, G. (1985). *Assessing Clinical Competence*, Springer Series on Medical Education, vol. 7. New York, NY: Springer Publishing Company.

Rackard, S. and Cashman, D. (2019). Curriculum mapping as a tool for review of the professional veterinary medicine curriculum at University College Dublin – strategic organizational considerations. *Journal of Veterinary Medical Education* 46 (3): 278–288. https://doi.org/10.3138/JVME.0617-084rl. Retrieved from: https://web-s-ebscohost-com.lmunet.idm.oclc.org/ehost/detail/detail?vid=1&sid=2025bac9-d5e9-4963-8666-9aca97ac4891%40redis&bdata=JnNpdGU9ZWhvc3QtbGl2ZSZzY29wZT1zaXRl#AN=31460845&db=mdc. (accessed 20 September 2022).

Terkla, D. (2008). Institutional research: more than just data. *New Directions for Higher Education, Number 141, Spring 2008*. San Francisco, CA: Wiley Subscription Services, Inc.

14

Mentoring Students

Micha C. Simons, VMD, MVEd
Virginia-Maryland College of Veterinary Medicine, Blacksburg, VA, USA

Stephanie Thomovsky, DVM, DACVM (Small Animal), MS (Health Professions Education)
Purdue College of Veterinary Medicine, West Lafayette, IN, USA

Julie A. Hunt, DVM, MS
Richard A. Gillespie College of Veterinary Medicine, Lincoln Memorial University, Harrogate, TN, USA

Katrina Jolley, MEd (Educational Leadership)
Richard A. Gillespie College of Veterinary Medicine, Lincoln Memorial University, Harrogate, TN, USA

Section 1: Veterinary Student Mentorship

Micha C. Simons and Stephanie Thomovsky

Part 1: Introduction

Mentoring in education is an effective and impactful way to develop and build lifelong relationships with future colleagues. Along with excellent teaching, it may be one of the most important and impactful roles a faculty member can undertake (Johnson 2016). Mentors can occupy a variety of roles, including educator, sponsor, collaborator, evaluator, role model, encourager, counselor, and friend (Ambrosetti and Dekkers 2010; Etzkorn and Braddock 2020). However, the success of any mentorship relationship is contingent on the development of a thoughtful and goal-orientated mentoring program. Forced mentoring relationships or poor mentor–mentee selection can often be more damaging than the absence of a mentoring program (Collins 2005; Johnson 2016).

Part 2: Definitions

A *mentorship* is a reciprocal relationship where personal and professional knowledge and/or experiences are shared. A *mentor* is defined as a more experienced and/or knowledgeable person who actively helps guide a less experienced and/or knowledgeable person, also called the *mentee* (Elce 2021). One goal of mentorship is to help the mentee grow personally and professionally, all while developing their own identity (Elce 2021). Contrast this interaction with an *advisor* who is an individual providing advice in a single area or field based on their expertise (Elce 2021).

Mentorship can occur in many forms, both through formal and informal means. *Formal* programs are designed by the institution, or a department, and outline specific roles, expectations, and duties for the mentor. The mentor is then assigned to a mentee either randomly or through a matching process. The program will also make recommendations for the frequency of meetings and objectives for the relationship. Contrast this with an *informal* program, where the participants initiate and establish the relationships without official guidelines. These are often mentee initiated and driven.

Discussed here are some broad categories that encompass the majority of mentor-mentee relationships (Elce 2021). *Peer-to-peer mentoring* is a supportive relationship built within the same social group. The mentor is selected from a higher academic level, and in some cases, may be older. *Group mentoring* is defined by having multiple mentors, each bringing their unique characteristics and goals to support the mentee. Group mentoring provides a well-rounded approach and allows for mentor-mentee relationships to develop and dissolve as the mentee progresses through their training or career. Lastly, and somewhat related, is *mosaic mentoring* which is a form of group mentorship focused on life and career progression.

As with any relationship, establishing the primary goal is critical to the success of the mentorship. For veterinary students, the goal is typically two-fold (i) learning how to successfully negotiate the preclinical and clinical years of their veterinary education, and (ii) career-related. These goals fit well within Kram's concept of mentorship function (Kram 1983). Mentoring, at its best, should be a balanced and democratic relationship, based on support, transparency, and sincerity (Collins 2005).

Part 3: Common Mentorships in Veterinary Education

Some common forms of these mentorships within veterinary education include (Collins 2005):

Faculty-to-student mentorship – often designed to help with the transition into veterinary school and to help with academic success and/or challenges. There are often formal and preassigned relationships, however as students become more comfortable and have increased interactions with faculty members, they may self-select a mentor who is more aligned with their goals and long-term career interests.

Peer-to-peer mentorship – these relationships were defined earlier in this section. In veterinary medicine these typically include the relationship between a senior student and junior student; students can offer advice and support on joining the veterinary student community, course-related questions, or other areas specific to the individual (e.g., location or culture-specific challenges). These relationships can develop formally, assigned by the college or faculty, or they can be more organic or informal in nature.

Clinician-to-student mentorship – created to aid in the development of professional and clinical skills. These relationships can occur during the clinical year or may be longstanding connections formed during the pre-veterinary experiences and/or extracurricular activities. These relationships will often transition to an *experienced practitioner's mentor to house officer or new graduate mentorship* where support is offered in the context of a professional role.

Mentorship is of the utmost importance for everyone at all stages of their educational and professional career. Certain time points wherein exposure to mentorship has been identified as extremely important include (Collins 2005):

1) Pre-veterinary
2) Immediately post-matriculation/enrollment
3) Clinical Year
4) Upon entering the workforce (and any other career change)

Part 4: A Faculty Clinician's Insight into Veterinary Student Mentorship in the Clinical Year

Veterinary school is difficult. In the North American system students work hard for three years learning physiology and basic medicine, all with the goal of applying what they have learned to clinical practice in their fourth year, as they rotate through clinics. Nevertheless, this application and integration of knowledge is not the only stress placed on students during the clinical year of study it is during the clinical year that career decisions also have to be made. Many students enter the clinical year of study unsure of exactly in what direction they want to take their career. This means that the final year is also used to solidify their goals and aspirations. For all of these major decisions, mentorship is necessary.

Being a mentor for these clinical students is critical; they rely on those with experience to guide them through this decision-making process and act as a sounding board often dispensing advice. Mentors should help students consider what subjects or topics interest them and what courses are preferred, and help students consider some of the important information that should be taken into account when finalizing career decisions. This can be done throughout the clinical year as it progresses, with the mentor encouraging students to take into account which rotations interested them most. Other important considerations include: which blocks challenged them, which blocks interested them, which blocks they missed most and which blocks made them yearn for more! Ultimately, with appropriate mentorship, after four years of veterinary training students must determine which type of veterinarian they want to be.

Just a mere four months into the beginning of the clinical year (for most), students must determine whether they want to pursue a rotating internship and potential residency, or whether they want to pursue general practice. Both avenues of study are commendable and both require a good deal of work. The Veterinary Internship and Match Program (VIRMP) is the program through which those who want to pursue veterinary rotating internships (and many residency programs) in North America must enroll.

The pros and cons of internship must be considered. A rotating internship is required as a precursor to many specialty internships and residency positions, although not a requirment, the same internship can also be considered if a student wishes to gain additional experience prior to becoming a general practitioner. An internship is a considerable commitment, so mentors should point out the positive and the negative aspects of pursuing a rotating internship. Advantages include: (i) structured learning, (ii) an extra year of training in an environment focused on rotating through a myriad of veterinary specialties, (iii) an environment in which instructors are expected (and paid) to teach, (iv) an extra year focused on learning rather than making money for a clinic/making commission. Disadvantages include: (i) less compensation for your work, (ii) another year of deferred student loans, and (iii) your living location is, in many cases, selected for you.

If a student decides to pursue an internship, it is the job of his or her mentor to help them consider and weigh what type of internship is best for them, the choices generally being academic or private practice. There are advantages and disadvantages to both opportunities. Academic internships, as a general rule, are focused on lecture-based learning (e.g., rounds and journal clubs) in addition to case learning – often ideal locations for those who learn better when given time to think rather than those who learn better by seeing a multitude of cases. The private sector, on the other hand, allows for increased caseload and can be ideal for learners who do best through seeing and doing. Academic internships are those in which instructors are paid to teach, private practices typically are focused on case workup, often allowing less time for more lecture-based teaching. Opportunities to teach are more abundant for the intern in academic internships as students are always present in some capacity; while students can rotate through private practices, they are not typically always present. For those considering academic internships. Teaching may also be viewed as a disadvantage to some so early in their career, as student teaching can be intimidating, especially for a recent veterinary graduate with little to no training in how to do so.

Once a clinical year student has made the decision to pursue an internship, it is the mentor's responsibility to guide them through the ranking process. Going through each program and what is offered and giving insight into the upside and downside to each available internship opportunity, is important. It would behoove the mentor to share any "intel" he or she has on a specific internship. For example, perhaps the mentor knows a former student who completed an internship at a specific location, or maybe the mentor knows that his or her clinical year student, based on personality, would excel at one location over another.

Regardless of whether a student goes forward to complete an internship or decides to forgo the internship year and delve right into general practice work, an interview is often one of the next steps. It is less common for those who pursue internships to be required to interview, but at some clinics a virtual or in-person interview may be required. Meanwhile, for those who go into general practice an interview is always required. Sometimes this interview may be in the form of a "working interview" during an externship in the clinical year. Alternatively, it may be a more traditional job interview involving a series of questions, a binder, a ballpoint pen, and a business suit. Regardless of the type of interview, it is prudent for the student to have an updated curriculum vitae (CV), and he or she should show up prepared physically, academically, and emotionally. The mentor can help with this preparation by guiding the student to ensure he or she is familiar with the veterinary practice and the different members of its staff, for example. Familiarity with the clinic at which one is interviewing is critical to interview success. Making oneself memorable in a good way is something the mentor can help the student with prior to the student's interview. Setting up mock interviews with commonly asked questions, ensuring students have high-quality questions of their own, and reminding the student that they are interviewing the practice as much as the practice is interviewing them, all help set the mentee up for success.

Representing oneself well during the interview process is critical, and it is equally important during the negotiation process once a job offer has been made. Those pursuing work in general practice will be presented with a contract and, for many, this may be the first contract experience in their lives. If comfortable, the mentor can help the student navigate the contract, making sure to guide them as they negotiate salary, commission, healthcare, desired equipment, moving expenses, vacation time, funding for continuing education, liability insurance, association memberships, state and drug enforcement agency licensure fees and nursing staff hires. The mentor can also make sure the student understands the nuances of a noncompete clause. Though the mentor should look at the contract and weigh in on what is missing and unfair, ultimately consulting with a lawyer versed in contract law is necessary to ensure that the student gets a fair contract. Most importantly, veterinarians are a needed commodity; the student should be empowered to take his or her time in considering the job offer and contract.

Part 5: Successful Mentorship

Formal mentor programs tend to be effective and successful when the institutional culture demonstrates value in the process of mentorship. This value is contingent on both administrator and faculty buy-in, and making sure necessary time and resources are provided (Etzkorn and Braddock 2020). Additionally, success is directly related to the effort put into the relationship from both parties and the connection that is developed.

Research validating formal evaluation of mentoring programs and their effects in veterinary education is lacking. Additionally, the veterinary profession is facing many challenges related to well-being, diversity, and inclusion, as well as recruitment and retention, and successful mentorship programs and mentor opportunities have been cited as strategies to minimize these issues (Barbur et al. 2011; Jelinski et al. 2009; Niehoff et al. 2005). Thus, it is in the profession's best interest to provide as many mentorship opportunities for students and veterinarians as possible, regardless of their experience level and/or career path.

Section 2: Mentoring Students in Educational Research

Julie A. Hunt

Part 1: Why Veterinary Educational Research?

Veterinary medical research has driven gains in animal and human health that have occurred in the past several decades, resulting in longer lifespans for companion animals, a safer food supply for humans, and a better understanding of how zoonotic diseases move through populations. Veterinary research has also contributed significantly to human medical advancements (National Research Council Committee on the National Needs for Research in Veterinary Science 2005). One specific type of veterinary research is veterinary educational research (VER), which is focused on evaluating educational methods, assessments, and factors impacting veterinary student success. The rapidly growing field of VER is essential for the continued improvement of veterinary education.

Recognizing the importance of veterinary students having an understanding of research, accrediting bodies, including the American Veterinary Medical Association Council on Education (AVMA CoE) and the Royal College of Veterinary Surgeons (RCVS) require that veterinary colleges run substantial, high-quality research programs and that interested students have the opportunity to participate in research (AVMA CoE 2021; RCVS 2017). As a result, veterinary schools have focused on providing their students with access to high-quality veterinary research projects and numerous veterinary faculty members internationally have chosen to perform educational research as a means of meeting the accrediting bodies' requirements.

Being a part of a research project early in a veterinary student's career can be a defining experience, especially when coupled with good-quality mentorship and counseling on graduate training options (McGregor and Fraser 2006). Students who play an active part in the research process are thought to be more likely to enter research-based careers or careers in academic medicine (Frei et al. 2010). Mentoring veterinary students in research is important to meeting the demand for veterinarians working in research-based careers and in academic medicine. Students who do not choose these careers but instead enter clinical practice still benefit long-term from their participation in research; these students have an improved understanding of the research process and an enhanced ability to critically evaluate veterinary research studies they may encounter during their careers.

Part 2: How to Involve Students in Research

There are numerous ways for students to become involved in research at a veterinary college, including working as a student research assistant, enrolling in a dual-degree program, or taking an elective research course within the veterinary curriculum. Some veterinary schools also have required coursework in research to expose all students to important research principles.

Veterinary educators who are willing to mentor students with an interest in research can let students know this from the beginning of their veterinary school education. For example, faculty members who are willing to be research mentors can introduce themselves at veterinary school orientation or during the first laboratory or lecture session they teach, providing information about their research interests, current projects, and willingness to involve and mentor interested students. Faculty members can provide quality mentorship that helps to guide students through the research process, veterinary school, advanced training, and into their careers. In return, enthusiastic and productive students can, once trained, help to drive a faculty member's research projects forward. However, the primary aim of a research university is not merely to complete projects but to inspire students and teach them how to perform research (Gonzalez 2001), so this should remain the focus.

Part 3: Reasons Students Choose to Participate in Research

Veterinary students choose to pursue research opportunities for a variety of reasons, and understanding a student's motivation for participating in research can assist a faculty member in providing the best possible experience and mentorship. Some students may participate in research because they are interested in exploring or pursuing a research-based career, although these students are the minority (AVMA 2005). Other students may pursue research opportunities to advance the breadth of their professional qualifications, both in research generally but also in the specific research topic. For example, students planning to work in academic veterinary medicine may choose to participate in an educational research project specifically. Finally, some students may participate in paid research positions to support their tuition costs or living expenses during veterinary school. Although the latter group of students appears superficially to be motivated by income, the author's experience suggests that they often also have nonmonetary goals they hope to achieve during their participation in research.

When starting a mentorship relationship, it is important to understand a student's motivation for participating in research, the goals they wish to reach through their participation, and their ultimate career aims. For students who do not plan to pursue a research-based or academic career, there are still benefits from participating in research projects; students who plan for a clinical or general practice career may be more interested in research with immediate, practical implications for animal care, such as case studies or clinical trials. A good research mentor will assist a student in finding a study that matches the student's personal and career goals, whether that project is led by the mentor or by another researcher at their institution.

Part 4: Selecting a Good Student Research Assistant

Choosing a capable and dedicated student research assistant is important to the success of the mentoring relationship and the research project. Key qualities to look for include an interest in research and a willingness to commit the required time to the project (Morrison-Beedy et al. 2000). Experience or competence in the area of the research project may be helpful but generally is not necessary as long as a student is willing to commit the time and effort to learning. While grade point average (GPA) may indicate how successful a student is in their coursework, it is unlikely to indicate their performance as a research student. However, by setting a minimum GPA requirement, faculty may avoid having a student's participation in research jeopardize their performance in the academic curriculum (Leong and Austin 1996). Some researchers have suggested that students be required to commit to at least two semesters of work so there is adequate time for them to work on the research project after completing the necessary training and introduction to the project (Leong and Austin 1996).

Part 5: The Initial Meeting

When a faculty member and a student interested in research initially meet, they should review the student's motivation for participating in research, their career goals, and their goals for participating in research. If the student's interest is not a good fit for the faculty member's project(s), the faculty member can refer the student to other colleagues whose research projects may be better aligned with the student's interests. If the student's interest appears to be a good fit for the faculty member's research project(s), then the conversation can continue. Students may be under the false impression that an educational research project will be easier to complete than a biomedical or clinical research project (Fogelberg et al. 2021); faculty mentors can kindly correct this misconception and ensure that the student is still interested.

The faculty member can discuss their project(s), the aims or research questions that those project(s) hope to answer, and what role the faculty member sees a student playing in the project. This can spark a dialogue about the project and gives both parties the ability to see whether the student's interests, aims, and existing skills are a good match for the project. This discussion also begins to set expectations between the mentor and student, which help to prevent misunderstandings that can negatively impact the project. For example, the faculty member should discuss the number of hours and schedule that will be worked, whether there is any flexibility in scheduling, how much and when the student would be paid, how much supervision the student would have on a daily basis, what type of tasks the student would be asked to perform, and whether there are institutional expectations placed on the student, such as completing institutional training or giving a presentation at the college's research day. The faculty member should also discuss the importance of confidentiality and protection of research subjects during the study, particularly if the student will have access to data with identifiers.

A discussion of the student's anticipated role, if any, in the dissemination of research outputs is also a good idea. Will the student be expected or permitted to participate in writing or editing a manuscript for publication? If so, the mentor should state what the expectations would be for the student to achieve authorship, if offered. Will the student be expected or permitted to present the results of the research at a conference? If so, the mentor should again state their expectations regarding this opportunity. Having these discussions at an early stage allows students who are interested in pursuing publication or presentation as a qualification builder to gauge the likelihood that these aims could be achieved. It also allows a student to state what they prefer not to do (e.g., write, present results in front of a group), which is equally helpful information.

Part 6: Expected Roles of the Research Mentor and Student

A research mentor is responsible for ongoing supervision of the project, assistance with the student's personal growth, encouragement of the student, and help in building a professional network. Increasingly, research students want a personal connection with their research mentors, and time should be scheduled for regular check-ins. The mentoring relationship should be designed to assist the student in achieving personal and professional growth. Mentored students benefit the most from faculty who are committed to providing mentorship, willing to share their knowledge and skills, and show a personal interest in students' professional advancement (Hayes 2000).

A research student's role is to work in a focused manner on the project, ask questions as they arise, attend project meetings as scheduled, and accept constructive criticism. A mentorship relationship will be most fruitful if both the research mentor and the student continually assess the mentorship relationship and feel empowered to discuss issues or potential areas for improvement.

When a faculty member mentors multiple students, it creates a multidimensional team where each team member brings their own strengths, experiences, and ideas to the project. This type of team can handle diverse tasks more effectively and efficiently. If a faculty member mentors multiple students and retains some students over a multiyear period, the more experienced students can assist with training less experienced students and can serve as role models for engagement in a research project. Faculty members who leverage the participation of research students are likely to see an increase in their own overall research productivity (Morrison-Beedy et al. 2001), which can come into consideration on promotion and tenure decisions.

Part 7: Good Practices Once the Student Joins the Project

Once a student has agreed to join a project, there are four key steps that are essential for good quality research mentoring (Morrison-Beedy et al. 2001). The first is to set clear goals for the project; these should have been succinctly communicated at the initial meeting between student and mentor. The elaboration of these goals should include how the study will gather and disseminate valid, meaningful data. Throughout the project, should these goals change or evolve, this should also be conveyed to the student.

The second step is to define expectations for the student. These should be shared in a broad sense at the initial meeting with the student; after the student joins the project, expectations can be further elaborated. Faculty who mentor multiple students may wish to write these expectations down so that they are certain to provide consistent and complete instructions to each student. These expectations may also need to be revisited as the project progresses, as the student's interests may change, and the needs of the project may also evolve.

The third step is to establish and maintain good quality communication among the entire research team. Busy faculty researchers are often drawn in multiple directions, and research at times may be deprioritized as compared with other tasks. However, remaining committed to projects that students are working on is very important to ensure

that students have a positive experience with research. When discussing the project, faculty members should offer students the opportunity to bring forward suggestions or concerns about the project. If miscommunication occurs, the faculty researcher is responsible for restoring open communication so that research can continue unhindered.

The final step is for the researcher to share their values and opinions of veterinary research and the profession of veterinary medicine. Students are in the process of developing their professional identity, and sharing these values and opinions can assist students in developing their own values and professional identity. Sharing the theories and/ or frameworks that underpin the research can also assist students in having a deeper understanding of the research being performed.

Some students may express an interest in pursuing graduate studies in a topic related to the research. These students should be guided to the strongest programs available, programs where important research questions are asked and answered, where science is practiced at a high level, and where the student will graduate in a position to be competitive for employment (McGregor and Fraser 2006). For students performing educational research who are interested in pursuing graduate programs in education, the options include programs specific to veterinary education, more general programs in medical or healthcare professions education, and finally, broad degrees (e.g., a Master of Education) that cover all of higher education, or even education in general (e.g., K-12 and higher education).

Part 8: Conclusions

Mentoring veterinary students in research is beneficial for both the student and the faculty mentor. Students have the opportunity to participate in research and learn about theoretical frameworks and the research process, as well as about the topic of the specific research project they are working on. With a good mentor, students will be guided on their career path according to their interests and may be provided with opportunities to publish, present, and network with other researchers.

Faculty mentors benefit from research students' unique perspectives, experiences, and their labor toward completing the project. Research mentors can set their students up for success by setting and communicating clear goals for the project, defining their expectations for students' participation in the project, maintaining good communication among the research team members, and sharing their views and values on the research being performed.

Section 3: Cheating and Other Unethical Student Behavior

Katrina Jolley

Part 1: Introduction and Overview

The American Veterinary Medical Association (AVMA) set forth a foundation of appropriate behaviors and expectations for the veterinary community in its Principles of Veterinary Medical Ethics, and these standards are expected to be upheld by all veterinarians (AVMA 2019). Principle 3 states that "a veterinarian shall uphold the standards of professionalism, be honest in all professional interactions, and report veterinarians who are deficient in character or competence to the appropriate entities" (AVMA 2019, n.p.). Annotations 1, 3, and 9 further detail the expectations about the reporting of violations, teaching ethics to veterinary students, and addressing impaired cognitive function:

> *1. Complaints about behavior that may violate the Principles should be addressed in an appropriate and timely manner.*
>
> *3. Veterinary Medical educators should stress the teaching of ethical issues as part of the professional veterinary curriculum for all veterinary students. Concomitantly, veterinary medical examiners are encouraged to prepare and include questions regarding professional ethics on examinations.*
>
> *9. Veterinarians who are impaired must not act in the capacity of a veterinarian and shall seek assistance from qualified organizations or individuals. Colleagues of impaired veterinarians should encourage those individuals to seek assistance and to overcome their impairment.*

The AVMA Council on Education further stipulates in Standard 9, Curriculum, that veterinary colleges must provide "opportunities throughout the curriculum for students to gain an understanding of professional ethical, legal, economic, and regulatory principles related to the delivery of veterinary medical services, personal and business finance, and management skills" (AVMA 2022, n.p.).

Despite an obligation by the governing body to instill ethical behavior in students, one of the unfortunate realities of education is that where there is a will to cheat, the student (or students) will find a way. Skshidlevsky (2022a) defines cheating as "using various types of materials, information, or devices that are not allowed when completing an academic task" (n.p.). This can also include "communicating with other test-takers without the consent of the proctor" and accessing electronic resources on a phone or other electronic device without permission (Skshidlevsky 2022a, n.p.). The rapid advances in technology have only furthered the availability to find information, including copies of exam questions and class assignments (Skshidlevsky 2022b).

Part 2: History of Cheating

Students in the Antebellum Period (1760–1860) were held to a high standard of academic integrity and behavior. Any student found cheating or misbehaving faced dismissal or lowering of academic rank (Gallant 2008). While these penalties were steep enough to deter many from misconduct, this was "likely mitigated by the ease with which removed students could purchase degrees from one of the many diploma mills that emerged during this time in history" (Gallant 2008, p. 14). To avoid facing dismissal from a university or failure of a class, a student in the Antebellum Period could cite the honor code "to justify his cheating, especially if his honor was being threatened by failure in a course or public humiliation by his teacher" (Gallant 2008, p. 15).

During the Research University Period (1869–1945), access to advanced copies of examinations was easily obtained from friends, from which they could fill in their self-provided examination booklets prior to the scheduled exams (Gallant 2008). It was also common practice for students to use cheat sheets on exams during this period. This practice, known as "cribbing," was used "on oral, recitation, and standard examinations" (Gallant 2008, p. 18). Unfortunately, the practice of cribbing has stood the test of time and is still in use by students today.

According to Gallant (2008), the Mass Education Period (1945–1975) brought about increased scrutiny and public interest in academic ethics. The current code of ethics in research, including regulations for research using human subjects, is a result of the "litigations and scandals involving academic scientists" (p. 21). There were also some broadly publicized student cheating scandals that occurred at the Air Force Academy, the University of Florida, and the University of Wisconsin between 1964 and 1975, which caused the public to question the ability of colleges and universities to effectively monitor and control their student bodies and to ask whether honor codes were all that effective (Gallant 2008). In addition, the practice of obtaining exam questions and course materials carried over from the Research University Period and was a continued source of concern. It was a well-known practice for faculty to reuse the same exam questions and assignments from year to year, and students were able to access previously graded papers and exams from previous semesters through fraternity and sorority friends (Gallant 2008).

Public concern about academic integrity grew to such a level that in the 1960s that it formed a movement within the higher education system to crack down on students who were cheating on examinations, which occurred at the same time that such institutions were beginning to address academic integrity through legislation of en masse policies and procedures (Gallant 2008). While this may have been in response to a public perception of the publicized cheating scandals, it is more likely that institutions were putting measures in place to uphold constitutional due process for violations of ethics and honor codes. "To avoid turning academic discipline over to the courts, colleges, and universities began to uniformly institute university-administered discipline and due process procedures to back up student-run honor codes" (Gallant 2008, p. 24).

A good, recent example of the application of such policies and procedures is when The Ohio State University – College of Veterinary Medicine followed its own due process procedures in 2016. In this instance, a group of 85 veterinary students "were found to have shared answers on online take-home tests, which is prohibited under the college's honor code" (Larkin 2016). The college's Student Judiciary Committee determined that the honor code was breached by those students, and the case was then reviewed by the group of faculty and administrators on the college's Executive Committee (Larkin 2016). While the outcomes of the individuals involved were not publicized, "sanctions in the college's honor code for unauthorized collaboration range from warnings to dismissal and include grade penalties, which could mean receiving a score of zero on the assessment" (Larkin 2016). The college has since implemented changes to how faculty assess students outside of the classroom and provided additional training to both faculty and students on academic integrity issues (Larkin 2016; Dey 2021).

Part 3: Statistics and Driving Factors

Exact statistics of academic dishonesty are somewhat difficult to pinpoint despite a variety of studies seeking students to self-report that information. Annual studies by the Educational Testing Service (1999) have found that anywhere from 75–98% of college students report that they have cheated in high school. This is a stark difference from the 1940s when roughly 20% of college students reported the same academic dishonesty (Educational Testing Service 1999). According to the 1998 findings from the "29th *Who's Who Among American High School Students Poll* (of 3,123 high-achieving 16- to 18-year-olds – that is, students with A or B averages who plan to attend college after graduation). . .80% of the country's best students

cheated to get to the top of their class" (Educational Testing Service 1999).

Dr. Donald McCabe and the International Center for Academic Integrity have been researching academic integrity since 1990 for a variety of student populations. Through surveys of over 70,000 high school students, they found that "64% of students admitted to cheating on a test, 58% admitted to plagiarism, and 95% said they participated in some form of cheating, whether it was on a test, plagiarism, or copying homework" (International Center for Academic Integrity 2022, n.p.). McCabe's research on academic integrity shows that "more than 60 percent of university students freely admit to cheating in some form" (n.p.). Of the students who admitted to cheating in college, the Educational Testing Service and the Ad Council found that 75–98% of those students began cheating in high school, and the trend for "academic dishonesty is showing up among even younger students, meaning that it is starting to take place not only in high school, but also in elementary school" (Skshidlevsky 2022a, n.p.).

The most common reasons college students have given for cheating center around stress and anxiety, a fear of failure, a general culture of cheating, and poor time management (Skshidlevsky 2022a, 2022b). McCabe et al. (1999) found that a large portion of the cheating that does occur is due to the pressure to succeed students face, and some students "even justified their cheating by noting the need to maintain a minimum GPA to retain their financial aid awards" (p. 231). The Educational Testing Service (1999) also noted that a lack of honor code, no severe penalties for being caught, and low faculty support of what policies may be in place were also top reasons given by students for academic dishonesty. The incidence rate for cheating was also "higher at larger, less selective institutions" (Educational Testing Service 1999, n.p.). While larger class sizes may not be a driving factor in the incidence rate of cheating, a course that uses the same essays, case studies, or exam questions provides ample opportunity for academic dishonesty as students will pass down the assignments and answers from year to year (Gallant 2008).

Part 4: Prevention Techniques

One way that colleges and universities are trying to prevent academic misconduct issues is through educating students and faculty on ethics and academic integrity. Schools such as the University of Georgia and The Ohio State University are setting clear guidelines that define what academic misconduct is, the ways violations can be identified and should be managed at the classroom level and beyond, and providing resources to faculty so they can better understand the processes (Dey 2021).

Ethics education is used in conjunction with school honor codes and ethics committees are often appointed, so that when ethics violations occur, they are available to review any allegations (Gallant 2008). And in spite of the public's questioning of the effectiveness of honor codes in the middle part of the century, research by McCabe et al. (1999) found that honor codes helped to "shape the ethics, values, character, attitudes, and behaviors that students carry forward from their collegiate experiences" (p. 216). The hope is that by teaching students what constitutes academic dishonesty, the number and severity of cases of violations can be minimized.

The other component to ethics education that should be addressed is acknowledging the pressures placed on students to perform well academically and providing the resources for support to help students who may be struggling academically, socially, or emotionally. Using this approach, sanctions for infractions then focus on ways to develop the student's "ethical reasoning and moral judgment" (Gallant 2008, p. 40). In other words, coming at cheating from this perspective is less about convincing them to stop the behavior and more about fostering an environment where learning is interesting and motivates students to engage with the material in a way that promotes learning and decreases emphasis on grades (Gallant 2008). Gallant (2008) also recommends using a combination of clearly communicated learning objectives, assignments, and discussions that require higher-order thinking, and modeling expected learning behavior.

Skshidlevsky (2022b) reports that one of the more common reasons students choose to cheat is a lack of time to complete the assignments or study for the tests. One way to mitigate this issue is to analyze course content to determine whether the delivered content is still relevant and if there is too much repetition on assessments within the course or program (Skshidlevsky 2022b). Faculty should only give assignments and tests that are relevant to the course content and ensure that they clearly link assessments to learning outcomes. This information should also be clearly relayed to students, so they understand from the beginning how interconnected the learning objectives and assessments work together to build their knowledge and skills (Gallant 2008).

The Center for Innovation in Teaching and Learning at the University of Illinois (2022) recommends that faculty pay careful attention to how their assessments are constructed and administered in an effort to minimize cheating. Faculty should create fair tests with clear instructions that cover the material the students were told it would cover, and there should be plenty of time for students to complete the exam (Center for Innovation in Teaching and Learning 2022). When setting the time limit for remote assessments, it should be carefully considered so that students who are not prepared do not have an unlimited amount of time to look up the answers. This is important, because setting a time limit impacts unprepared students the most, as they may spend their time going over a small handful of items, thus decreasing the likelihood that they will have enough time left to complete the exam (Northern Illinois University Center for Innovative Teaching and Learning 2022).

Test construction is one area within the faculty member's control that can minimize the opportunities for students to cheat on an exam. When possible, new exam questions should be rotated in every semester so that students are less likely to predict which questions will be used based on past students' experience (Center for Innovation in Teaching and Learning 2022). This need not be an overly onerous task; making the new questions can be as simple as flipping the question stem and answer choices or asking for a treatment instead of a differential diagnosis on a case.

The use of alternate formats or test question pools can further enhance exam security and minimize the opportunity for academic misconduct (Northern Illinois University Center for Innovative Teaching and Learning 2022; Skshidlevsky 2022b; Center for Innovation in Teaching and Learning 2022). Alternate formats do not have to be completely new questions; they can include the same questions in a different order and/or have the answer choices scrambled (Skshidlevsky 2022b). The Center for Innovation in Teaching and Learning (2022) further recommends using different mathematical values across alternate formats of the exam. For example, version A of the exam may ask the students to find the value of x if $15 = 2x + 3$, and version B of the exam may ask for the value of x if $25 = 6x - 5$. Both versions of the question assess the same learning objective by asking students to solve the same type of equation. In veterinary medicine, alternate lab values, patient signalment, or species can serve the same purpose when creating alternate versions of exam questions.

Test question pools can be used, when possible, for a testing software to select a specific number of items from the pool rather than providing the same questions to all students. This is most appropriate when the pools are made of questions that cover the same "topic, subject matter, question type or difficulty of question" (Northern Illinois University Center for Innovative Teaching and Learning 2022, n.p.).

Setting the testing software to scramble the test questions and answer choices can help enhance exam security for both in-person and remotely delivered assessments. This results in a very small likelihood that two students sitting next to each other will be answering the same question at the same time (Northern Illinois University Center for

Innovative Teaching and Learning 2022). Using answer choices of similar length (or pairs of answers with similar length) makes the choices look visually similar from a distance in the event that a student can see another's exam. Open-response questions can both enhance exam integrity and "help students to develop problem-solving skills and critical thinking" (Skshidlevsky 2022b). By not having a set list of answers to choose from, a student must create their own response based on the knowledge they have learned.

The last piece of exam security that faculty can use to help mitigate cheating is determining how much feedback to give to the students after the exam and determining the number of attempts the students have before that feedback is released. When using testing software or testing through a learning management system, there are settings that can be put in place to show the correct answer to each question when the student submits the exam or quiz file. The Northern Illinois University Center for Innovative Teaching and Learning (2022) cautions that providing the correct answers to students for take-home or remote tests provides an opportunity for students to share answers with their classmates. They can also correctly guess the right answer through a process of elimination if they are allowed to take the test multiple times. When using testing software to deliver in-person exams to a group of students, one possibility is to allow an immediate review of only the questions the student misses. Because all students are testing at the same time, the opportunity to share answers is minimized; this has been successful in decreasing student cheating in this author's experience.

For quizzes taken at home, where students are not testing at the same time, faculty might consider releasing the correct answers after the deadline for submission has passed. This is how several of the faculty at LMU-CVM choose to balance quiz security with the opportunity for students to learn from what they missed, which helps them study for upcoming exams. Allowing the students to see what questions were missed on a quiz or exam provides them a valuable opportunity to identify strengths and weaknesses in their performance and help direct their study of the content for future use (Northern Illinois University Center for Innovative Teaching and Learning 2022). If strategically timed well, the results of a formative quiz can help the students prepare for a summative exam on the same content.

Part 5: Proctoring Student Exams

When students are completing an exam, one of the most effective ways to monitor for cheating is to proctor the exam. By watching the students take the exam, the faculty and/or proctors can ensure that the students are staying focused on their own work and set a tone of exam integrity. A sufficient number of proctors is especially important in larger classes where the incidence rate of cheating is higher (Educational Testing Service 1999; Skshidlevsky 2022b). The Center for Innovation in Teaching and Learning at the University of Illinois (2022) recommends a minimum of one proctor for every 40 students, and the proctor should never leave the exam room unattended.

Proctors should pay close attention to the students, remain focused on the exam environment, and periodically walk around the exam room. "They should not be reading or involved in unnecessary conversation with other proctors" (Center for Innovation in Teaching and Learning 2022). While not directly tied to suspicious student behavior, any noise from the proctors can disrupt the testing environment, causing the proctors to be a distraction to the student's testing. Reading and other activities that draw the proctor's attention away from the exam create an opportunity for students to cheat. A student who is waiting for an opportunity to cheat sees that their behavior is likely to go unnoticed because the proctor's focus is on another activity.

Proctors should be on the lookout for students glancing at neighboring students' computer screens or exam papers. Students who are frequently looking down may have a cell phone or notes in their lap that they may be using to access answers or communicate with other exam takers. In Spring 2020, California State University, Los Angeles, investigated a large cheating incident "after one student alleged that her peers were sharing exam answers through a GroupMe chat" (Dey 2021; Loeb 2021). It is recommended to limit the items that students are allowed to have access to while they are testing.

For exam security reasons, students should store bags, backpacks, jackets, notes, and extra devices away from the testing area. Ideally, these items should not be brought into the exam room at all, but that may not be practical depending on the testing schedule, campus layout, or other factors. Drinks, if allowed, should be in a clear or solid color container without writing, labels, or stickers and with a reasonably spill-proof lid, as there have been reports of students replacing such labels with homemade ones that contain potential exam answers (Hayes et al. 2006). Watches, fitness trackers, cellphones, headphones, earbuds, and extra electronic devices should be turned off and stored away from the testing area. If these items are accessed during the exam, the proctor should confiscate the device if they are spotted (Skshidlevsky 2022b).

Computer-based exams should be password protected to help prevent unauthorized access to the exam questions before the exam begins. Scratch paper, when used, should be handed out after the exam password is given to lessen the chance of students copying their notes down before beginning the exam, and the paper should be collected before the students leave the exam room to make sure no copies of the test questions are smuggled out. Using a different color of paper for each exam administration further reduces the odds that a student will provide their own cheat sheet for the exam. Privacy screens are recommended in conjunction with dimming a device's brightness level to assist in exam security. When the privacy screen fully covers the testing device's screen, it is much more challenging for a student to see what his or her neighbor's answers are when viewed from the side or at an angle; these devices are required for students at Lincoln Memorial University's Richard A. Gillespie College of Veterinary Medicine (LMU-CVM) and have proven to be effective in reducing students' ability to intentionally or unintentionally view a classmate's screen during an exam.

When possible, the testing room should be cleared of students while the proctors set up the testing environment. This gives the proctors the opportunity to check for any paper notes that may be stashed in the seating area. Using assigned seating with randomized seating charts is recommended no matter the class size as cheating is more prevalent when students are allowed to select their own seats. "It should be no surprise that cheaters choose to sit near each other" (Center for Innovation in Teaching and Learning 2022, n.p.). If the exam is being given on paper, another option is to number the tests and seats and have students sit in the seat assigned to their test number. This method can easily allow faculty and/or proctors to hand out multiple forms of the test, "taking into account students sitting laterally as well as those sitting in front and back of each other" (Center for Innovation in Teaching and Learning 2022, n.p.).

Part 6: Proctoring Remote Exams

Sometimes the need arises for students to take exams remotely or in a virtual setting. Ensuring that the exams remain secure and the students are practicing academic integrity becomes a bit more challenging when students are testing outside of the classroom. Where in-person exams rely on proctors to monitor multiple students simultaneously and circulate the room frequently, remote exams are proctored using video capture through the student's testing device. Proctoring services such as ProctorU, Examity, Respondus, Proctorio, and ExamSoft's ExamMonitor use a combination of software features such as screen capture and video recording to monitor exams electronically (Loeb 2021). The exam footage is reviewed through a computer algorithm and any suspicious behavior is flagged by an artificial intelligence system. A human

proctor must then review any flags generated by the software to determine if the behavior was a confirmed case of cheating or not.

The proctoring software is tracking the students' eye movements to look for any off-screen gazing, listening for any noise that may indicate cheating, and watching for any objects to be brought in view of the camera (Loeb 2021; Dey 2021). As with in-person exams, students may attempt to keep a cell phone or notes hidden from view of the proctor in an attempt to cheat. One student at Middle Tennessee State University was even caught using his "smart speaker to find answers during an exam, according to Michael Baily, the school's director of academic integrity" (Dey 2021, n.p.). It is recommended that students perform a security sweep of their testing room by panning the camera slowly to show a 360° view of the room, followed by the ceiling, desk/table, and floor around the desk/table to show the virtual proctor that there are no resources in the testing area.

Faculty must balance the benefit of students being able to write down calculations or diagrams for their course's content with the need for exam security when deciding to allow scratch paper on remotely given exams. If scratch paper is allowed for remote exams, the students should show the front and back of the blank paper at the beginning of the exam and the front and back of the completed paper at the end. While the scratch paper will likely be flagged by the monitoring software, this allows the human proctor to confirm that exam questions were not written down (creating a potential for them to be shared).

Through the use of Examity, Middle Tennessee State University saw an increase in reports of cheating "jump by more than 79% from fall of 2019 to spring of 2021" when the university made a large shift to remote testing due to the COVID-19 pandemic (Dey 2021, n.p.). During the 2020–2021 school year, the University of Georgia saw more than double the amount of academic misconduct reports compared to the previous academic year, and Virginia Commonwealth University saw more than triple the number of academic misconduct reports (Dey 2021). The increase in reported cases is likely due to a combination of more instances of students cheating and a higher number of cheating incidents being caught and confirmed.

Concern has been raised by students that the use of monitoring software is an invasion of privacy since the students are video recorded in their personal space (Dey 2021). "Ken Leopold, a chemistry professor at the University of Minnesota, says he and other faculty must balance privacy concerns with the need to guard against cheating" (Dey 2021, n.p.). Other concerns brought up by Miami University (Ohio) students say that the monitoring service Proctorio discriminates against students who consistently fidget or glance away under normal circumstances due to

ADHD and similar conditions. The students also suggested that Proctorio discriminated against students with darker skin tones because they believed the software was unable to accurately recognize and track their movements (Dey 2021). For this reason, final determinations on what constitutes unethical behavior in a remote assessment should always be made by a person in your institution rather than a computer or person at the remote monitoring software company. The faculty and staff at your institution can more easily determine what is normal behavior for the student testing versus what is academic dishonesty.

Part 7: Plagiarism and Other Unethical Behavior

According to Title 17 Chapter 1 Section 102 of the United States Code, "copyright protection subsists, in accordance with this title, in original works of authorship fixed in any tangible medium of expression, now known or later developed, from which they can be perceived, reproduced, or otherwise communicated, either directly or with the aid of a machine or device" (US Copyright Office 2021, p. 8). Using an author's work in whole or in part without their consent violates this legal code and constitutes plagiarism. Plagiarism is commonly performed through the copy/paste feature of computer software (such as Microsoft Word), whereby students find a previously written work by one or more authors, copy all or portions of that work, and paste it into their own paper without appropriately citing the original in an attempt to pass it off as their own (Skshidlevsky 2022a). In such cases, if the original author of the work discovers that their material has been used without permission, the student(s) who plagiarized the work may be sued for copyright infringement (Skshidlevsky 2022b). Many colleges and universities use plagiarism monitoring software such as SafeAssign or TurnItIn to detect "matches between students' submitted assignments and existing works by others. These works are found on a number of databases including ProQuest ABI/Inform, Institutional document archives, the Global Reference Database, as well as a comprehensive index of documents available for public access on the internet" (Northern Illinois University Center for Innovative Teaching and Learning 2022, n.p.). It should be noted that plagiarism monitoring tools can also serve as a teaching aid to help instruct students on proper citations for direct quotes and paraphrasing (Northern Illinois University Center for Innovative Teaching and Learning 2022).

On occasion, a student or group of students may infringe on the copyright of a faculty member's lecture materials by distributing course content to others outside of the class (such as future students). In the 1969 case of *Williams v. Weisser*, the courts ruled in favor of a UCLA professor who "sued a company, Class Notes, to prevent the dissemination of his lectures and to seek monetary damages" (Sun and Baez 2009, p. 24). Sun and Baez (2009) note that there is some debate on whether the copyright of the course content lies with the faculty or the institution (p. 23). Regardless of who owns the copyright, the student(s) can be charged with academic misconduct for disseminating course materials without permission.

Unprofessional conduct can also extend beyond the classroom into activities that occur off-campus or online. Educational institutions can enforce guidelines for appropriate student conduct outside the classroom "particularly if the misconduct also violates criminal law and the institution can demonstrate that the restrictions are directly related to its educational mission or the campus community's welfare" (Kaplin et al. 2020, p. 624). Honor codes are one way that schools can establish the expected conduct of their students and how it relates to the students' education.

Part 8: Honor Codes and Codes of Conduct

Honor codes are policies that include a combination of elements centering around academic integrity. Honor codes typically include "a written pledge in which students affirm that their work will be or has been done honestly" (McCabe et al. 1999, p. 213), and they may further define academic misconduct to include "plagiarism, cheating, forgery, or alteration of institutional records" (Kaplin et al. 2020, p. 623). Student codes of conduct expand the honor code to include social misconduct in addition to academic misconduct, regardless of whether the misconduct violates state or federal civil or criminal laws (Kaplin et al. 2020). Both Gallant (2008) and Skshidlevsky (2022b) stress the importance of educating students about ethical behavior and academic integrity to "ensure that students (and faculty) understand how they can fulfill all their roles and responsibilities" (Gallant 2008, p. 108). McCabe et al. (1999) echo this sentiment in saying that "honor codes seem to be successful when the vast majority of the student community understands that each student plays a vital role in the success of the code" (p. 232). Their research into academic integrity between schools with an honor code and those without found that while students who sign and/or are asked to adhere to honor codes experience the same societal pressures as students not asked to do so, they are far less likely to rationalize or justify their own cheating by citing such pressures (McCabe et al. 1999).

When writing codes of conduct, administration should be mindful of the way the codes are written and what is stipulated in them. Codes of conduct should include what conduct the code addresses, how reported violations of the code will be handled, and what consequences may be imposed for those found to have violated the code, with such consequences ranging in severity and being assigned proportionately according to the significance of the infraction (Kaplin et al. 2020). For example, students caught cheating on exams risk failing the assignment or failing the class, whereas in an extreme case, a student might be dismissed if they were found to have "flagrantly violated the rules of academic integrity" (Skshidlevsky 2022b, n.p.). Importantly, there must also be clear definitions of appropriate behavior so that claims of due process violations can be minimized, (Kaplin et al. 2020).

Part 9: Reporting Procedures

The procedure for reporting academic dishonesty partially depends on the situation. If a student is suspected of cheating during an exam, the Center for Innovation in Teaching and Learning recommends allowing them to finish testing in case it is later found that the student was not cheating (2022). The proctor should move closer to the student exhibiting suspicious behavior and carefully monitor the student to confirm that any cheating is taking place and verify how for documentation. All confirmed cases of cheating must be documented in writing immediately after the incident takes place. The campus procedures for violations of the student code of conduct and/or honor code will then be set in motion (Center for Innovation in Teaching and Learning 2022). Documentation must include a complete description of what happened, who was involved, when the incident occurred, and what specific policy was violated (Kaplin et al. 2020). Similar documentation is expected for infractions of student codes of conduct. The incident must be reported following the school's protocols for such behaviors. In some states reporting inappropriate conduct, such as hazing, is mandated by state law, and failure to report can "result in a fine or imprisonment" (Kaplin et al. 2020, p. 625 in reference to Tex. Educ. Code Ann. § 37.152).

Proper documentation and following of procedures are necessary in the event that a code of conduct issue is brought to court. Committees at the institution that review misconduct violations, whether academic, ethical, or behavioral, must specify in writing "the membership of judicial bodies, the procedures they use, the extent to which their proceedings are open to the academic community, the sanctions they may impose, the methods by which they may initiate proceedings against students, and provisions for appealing their decisions" (Kaplin et al. 2020, p. 629). If such procedures are not established or are established but not followed, if a case goes to court, the student's appeal is less likely to succeed if such procedures are established and followed (Kaplin et al. 2020). The Center for Innovation in Teaching and Learning (2022) advises faculty to be prepared to experience some uneasy feelings when reporting academic dishonesty or violations of student conduct; "these are common and do not mean that you have made a mistake or are being unreasonable" (n.p.).

Part 10: Due Process

The constitutional right to due process also extends to college and university-level misconduct hearings. Students have the right to receive written notice of the charges being brought against them and the specific policy or policies that were violated (Kaplin et al. 2020), and they have the right to appeal any decision made by the committee reviewing the case (Center for Innovation in Teaching and Learning 2022). Any student wishing to claim a violation of due process "must demonstrate that they have been deprived of a liberty or property interest that is considered 'fundamental,' or (if the interest is not fundamental) that the action depriving them of a liberty or property interest was arbitrary and capricious" (Kaplin et al. 2020, p. 604). In *Byrnes v. Johnson County Community College,* 2011 WL 166715 (D. Kan. 2011), a nursing student was able to successfully prove a violation of due process after being suspended from nursing school without a hearing for posting a photo with three other students and a patient's placenta on Facebook because the "college had not established that the students' action was a clear violation of professional conduct" and the student was under the impression that they "had their instructor's permission to post the photo" (Kaplin et al. 2020, p. 600). Even though the actions of the student were a clear violation of professional and ethical conduct, the court reinstated the student's enrollment because the college had failed to properly document the issue and follow its own procedures for code of conduction violations (Kaplin et al. 2020).

When reviewing cases of due process violations, courts will generally side with the school if the charges made to the student(s) are specific, clearly linked to the policies violated, and the procedures for reviewing the charges were followed. Charges of off-campus misconduct should also include the relationship between how the conduct affects the "well-being of the college community," particularly if off-campus conduct is included as part of the student code of conduct (Kaplin et al. 2020, p. 629). Institutions are expected by the courts to follow their own rules when it comes to disciplinary hearings with three exceptions.

> *First, an institution may be excused from following its own procedures if the student knowingly and freely waives his or her right to them, as in Yench v. Stockmar, 483 F.2d 820 (10th Cir. 1973), where the student neither requested that the published procedures be*

followed nor objected when they were not. Second, deviations from established procedures may be excused when they do not disadvantage the student, as in Winnick v. Manning, 460 F.2d 545 (2d Cir.1972), where the student contested the school's use of a panel other than that required by the rules, but the court held that the "deviations were minor ones and did not affect the fundamental fairness of the hearing" (see also Barsoumian v. Williams, 29 F. Supp. 3d 303 (W.D.N.Y. 2014), affirmed sub nom. Barsoumian v. University at Buffalo, 594 F. App'x 41 (2d Cir. 2015)). And third, if an institution provides more elaborate protections than constitutionally required, failure to provide nonrequired protections may not imply constitutional violations (Kaplin et al. 2020, p. 641–642).

Students may waive their right to follow the procedures laid out for code of conduct violations, and schools may go above and beyond what is required by the constitution for protections of due process. When dealing with cheating and other unethical behavior the best practice is to document everything in writing, provide notice to the student, and follow the procedures established by the college or university. This way, if a student appeals a decision for academic, ethical, or behavioral misconduct, it will be clear that due process was upheld by the institution.

Summary

The bottom line is that students who want to cheat will find a way to do so. Academic dishonesty has been around in one form or another for centuries and will continue to exist as long as there are students. It is our job as educational professionals to take the steps necessary to minimize instances of cheating and academic dishonesty. Proctoring exams, writing a few new questions for each exam, creating new written assignments, and using plagiarism monitoring software can all be used to deter unethical academic behavior from students. Being mindful of student stressors and providing resources to support academically struggling students can help minimize the "need" to cheat by addressing the most common reasons cited for academic dishonesty.

When a student or group of students is suspected of cheating, it is imperative that the incident be documented immediately. Any suspicion of academic dishonesty must then be followed up with an investigation to confirm that an incident of cheating has taken place. During a proctored exam setting, this is as simple as the proctor moving closer to the student(s) and confirming that the student's behavior is indeed suspicious. For instances that require administrative investigation, the suspicion must be documented so that the administration or investigative committee can follow up and confirm that any academic dishonesty has taken place. The school's procedures for handling ethics and honor code violations will then be followed.

Proper documentation is key when handling academic integrity issues. The student must receive written notice of the specific policy that was violated and the specific behaviors that resulted in that violation. Due process must be followed as required by the constitution. If a student accused of violating a school's ethics and honor code chooses to take the issue to court, the court will be looking for the institution to have provided proper documentation of the violation and to have followed due process for its own policies.

References

Ambrosetti, A. and Dekkers, J. (2010). The interconnectedness of the roles of mentors and mentees in pre-service teacher education mentoring relationships. *Australian Journal of Teacher Education* 35 (6): 42–55.

American Veterinary Medical Association (2005). *AVMA Membership Directory and Resource Manual*. Schaumburg, IL: American Veterinary Medical Association.

American Veterinary Medical Association (2019). Principles of veterinary medical ethics of the AVMA. https://www.avma.org/resources-tools/avma-policies/principles-veterinary-medical-ethics-avma (accessed 28 October 2022).

American Veterinary Medical Association Council on Education (2021). COE accreditation policies and procedures: requirements. https://www.avma.org/education/accreditation-policies-and-procedures-avma-council-education-coe/coe-accreditation-policies-and-procedures-requirements (accessed 03 November 2022).

American Veterinary Medical Association (2022). COE accreditation policies and procedures: requirements. July 2021. https://www.avma.org/education/accreditation-policies-and-procedures-avma-council-education-coe/coe-accreditation-policies-and-procedures-requirements (accessed 03 November 2022).

Barbur, L., Shuman, C., Sanderson, M.W., and Grauer, G.F. (2011). Factors that influence the decision to pursue an internship: the importance of mentoring. *Journal of Veterinary Medical Education* 38 (3): 278–287.

Center for Innovation in Teaching and Learning (2022). Teaching and learning: dealing with cheating. https://citl.illinois.edu/citl-101/teaching-learning/

resources/classroom-environment/dealing-with-cheating (accessed 30 October 2022).

Collins, H. (2005). Mentoring veterinary students. *Journal of Veterinary Medical Education* 32 (3): 285–289.

Dey, S. (2021). Reports of cheating at colleges soar during the pandemic. https://www.npr.org/2021/08/27/1031255390/reports-of-cheating-at-colleges-soar-during-the-pandemic (accessed 29 October 2022).

Educational Testing Service. (1999). Cheating is a personal foul: The Educational Testing Service/Ad Council campaign to discourage academic cheating. http://www.glass-castle.com/clients/www-nocheating-org/adcouncil/research/cheatingfactsheet.html and http://www.glass-castle.com/clients/www-nocheating-org/adcouncil/research/cheatingbackgrounder.html (accessed 30 October 2022).

Elce, Y. (2021). The mentor-mentee relationship, addressing challenges in veterinary medicine together. *The Veterinary Clinics of North America. Small Animal Practice* 51 (5): 1099–1109.

Etzkorn, K.B. and Braddock, A. (2020). Are you my mentor? A study of faculty mentoring relationships in US higher education and the implications for tenure. [Faculty mentoring in US higher education]. *International Journal of Mentoring and Coaching in Education* 9 (3): 221–237. https://doi.org/10.1108/IJMCE-08-2019-0083.

Fogelberg, K., Hunt, J., and Baillie, S. (2021). Young and evolving: a narrative of veterinary educational research from early leaders. *Education in the Health Professions* 4 (3): 124–133.

Frei, E., Stamm, M., and Buddeberg-Fischer, B. (2010). Mentoring programs for medical students – a review of the PubMed literature 2000–2008. *BMC Medical Education* 10 (1): 1–14.

Gallant, T. (2008). Academic integrity in the twenty-first century: a teaching and learning imperative. *ASHE Higher Education Report* 33 (5). San Francisco, CA: Wiley Periodicals: 1–114.

Gonzalez, C. (2001). Undergraduate research, graduate mentoring, and the university's mission. *Science* 293 (5535): 1624–1626.

Hayes, E. (2000). The preceptor/student relationship: implications for practicuum evaluation. *The Nurse Practitioner* 25 (5): 118–124.

Hayes, D., Hurtt, K., and Bee, S. (2006). The war on fraud: reducing cheating in the classroom. *Journal of College Teaching & Learning* 3 (2): 1–12.

International Center for Academic Integrity (2022). Facts and statistics. https://academicintegrity.org/resources/facts-and-statistics (accessed 04 November 2022).

Jelinski, M.D., Campbell, J.R., MacGregor, M.W., and Watts, J.M. (2009). Factors associated with veterinarians' career path choices in the early postgraduate period. *The Canadian Veterinary Journal = La revue veterinaire canadienne* 50 (9): 943–948.

Johnson, B. (2016). *On Being a Mentor: A Guide for Higher Education Faculty*, 2e. New York, NY: Routledge.

Kaplin, W., Lee, B., Hutchens, N., and Rooksby, J. (2020). *The Law of Higher Education*, 6e. Student Version. Hoboken, NJ: Jossey-Bass.

Kram, K.E. (1983). Phases of the mentor relationship. *Academy of Management Journal* 26: 608–625.

Larkin, M. (2016). Ohio State disciplines veterinary students for cheating. JAVMA News. August 01, 2016 Issue. https://www.avma.org/javma-news/2016-08-01/ohio-state-disciplines-veterinary-students-cheating (accessed 30 October 2022).

Leong, F. and Austin, J. (1996). *The Psychology Research Handbook: A Guide for Graduate Students and Research Assistants*. Sage Publications.

Loeb, L. (March 31, 2021). Cal State LA was caught in a large-scale cheating scandal, but it's not alone. *Golden Gate Express*. https://goldengatexpress.org/97004/campus/cal-state-la-was-caught-in-a-large-scale-cheating-scandal-but-its-not-alone/ (accessed 04 November 2022).

McCabe, D.L., Trevino, L.K., and Butterfield, K.D. (1999). Academic integrity in honor code and non-honor code environments: a qualitative investigation. *The Journal of Higher Education* 70 (2): 211–234. https://doi.org/10.2307/2649128.

McGregor, D. and Fraser, D. (2006). Counseling veterinary students who aspire to careers in science. *Journal of the American Veterinary Medical Association* 229 (5): 668–671.

Morrison-Beedy, D., Aronowitz, T., Dyne, J., and Mkandawire, L. (2001). Mentoring students and junior faculty in faculty research: a win-win scenario. *Journal of Professional Nursing* 17 (6): 291–296.

Morrison-Beedy, D., Beeber, L., and Hahn, E. (2000). Progressive involvement of baccalaureate nursing students in research. *Nurse Educator* 25 (4): 155–156.

National Research Council (US) Committee on the National Needs for Research in Veterinary Science (2005). The role of veterinary research in human society. In: *Critical Needs for Research in Veterinary Science*, 13–19. National Academies Press.

Niehoff, B.P., Chenoweth, P., and Rutti, R. (2005). Mentoring within the veterinary medical profession: veterinarians' experiences as proteges in mentoring relationships. *Journal of Veterinary Medical Education* 32 (2): 264–271.

Northern Illinois University Center for Innovative Teaching and Learning (2022). Tips for preventing cheating. https://www.niu.edu/blackboard/guides/tips-for-preventing-cheating.shtml (accessed 05 November 2022).

Royal College of Veterinary Surgeons (2017). RCVS standards and procedures for the accreditation of veterinary degrees.

https://www.rcvs.org.uk/document-library/rcvsaccreditation standards/ (accessed 05 November 2022).

Skshidlevsky, A. (2022a). Academic dishonesty statistics. https://proctoredu.com/blog/tpost/5dk67zrns1-academic-dishonesty-statistics (accessed 05 November 2022).

Skshidlevsky, A. (2022b). Preventing cheating in college. https://proctoredu.com/blog/tpost/3tih8y7or1-prevent-cheating-in-college (accessed 05 November 2022).

Sun, J. and Baez, B. (2009). Intellectual property in the information age: knowledge as commodity and its legal implications for higher education. *ASH Education Report* 34 (4): 13–30. San Francisco, CA: Wiley Periodicals.

U.S. Copyright Office. (May 2021). Copyright law of the United States and related laws contained in Title 17 of the United States code. Circular 92. https://www.copyright.gov/title17/title17.pdf (accessed 05 November 2022).

Additional Resources

Larkin, M. (2016). Ohio State disciplines veterinary students for cheating. JAVMA News. August 01, 2016 Issue. https://www.avma.org/javma-news/2016-08-01/ohio-state-disciplines-veterinary-students-cheating (accessed 30 October 2022).

National Board of Medical Examiners (2021). NBME Item Writing Guide: constructing written test questions for the health sciences. https://www.nbme.org/item-writing-guide (accessed 30 October 2022).

15

Educational Development

Jesse Watson, Ed.S (Education Specialist), MS
North Carolina State University College of Veterinary Medicine, Raleigh, NC, USA

Sherry A. Clouser, Ed.D
University of Georgia College of Veterinary Medicine, Athens, GA, USA

Section 1: Introduction

Part 1: Educational Development in Veterinary Education

This chapter discusses the history of faculty development in veterinary education and makes a case for creating educational development programs oriented around support for individual educators, instructional teams, and organizational growth. It begins with establishing the need for educational development in Colleges of Veterinary Medicine (CVMs) to best meet the challenges of a changing field. Next comes a brief look into the history of educational development in medical education over the last 30 years. The following section explores the variety of labels given to such programs and the implied understandings, then segues into breaking down the three common types of educational development models found in our field. The later pages break down key decision points for building a program in line with an organization's mission and vision for education. We have sprinkled one-page callouts outlining different existing programs in veterinary medical education for example. Many thanks go to the folks from each program who helped us write them.

Part 2: History

More than 80 years ago, the 1948 President's Commission on Higher Education concluded "that college teaching is the only major learned profession that does not have a program to develop the skills essential for its practitioners" (Zook (1948), p. 16). Forty years later, at the World Conference on Medical Education, conference attendees released a list of improvements in medical education, including a recommendation to the World Health Organization to "train teachers as educators, not content experts alone, and reward excellence in this field as fully as excellence in biomedical research or clinical practice" (World Federation for Medical Education 1988, p. 2). Even today, university-level educators in most disciplines, including veterinary medicine, receive little to no training in teaching and learning before being hired as teaching professionals (Gordon-Ross et al., 2020).

So, if veterinary educators are not hired with training in teaching and learning, what has their on-the-job training looked like? Gaff and Simpson (1994) provide a timeline of events in the United States in the 1960s and 1970s, including student protests that "attacked irrelevant courses and uninspired teaching" (p. 168), an influx of nontraditional students demanding innovation, and research demonstrating the complex nature of teaching and learning. These events led to the creation of programming for supporting college faculty with their teaching roles, including programs focused on the faculty themselves, instructional design and delivery, and organizational structures that encouraged good teaching. The 1980s brought the establishment of central units responsible for developing and implementing those programs, which in the 1990s would include opportunities for graduate students to add training in college teaching to their preparation for professorial roles. In 2005, the Royal Veterinary College, University of London, received funding to establish the first such unit specific to veterinary education (Pirkelbauer et al. 2008) (Box 15.1).

In the field of medical education, interest groups gained formality and stature at some institutions with the formation of institutional academies of educators. According to Irby et al. (2004), these academies were established to

---

Box 15.1   Royal Veterinary College

Mission: The RVC provides a three-phase MSc in Veterinary Education, whose overall mission is, through pedagogical support, scholarly inquiry, and education research, to enhance the quality of worldwide veterinary education, specifically in producing graduates who will be lifelong independent learners. The Postgraduate Certificate specifically aims to enhance the professional development of educators in the veterinary and para-veterinary sectors to (i) facilitate the development of staff that have a substantial role in all areas of teaching and learning; (ii) develop skills and knowledge in all areas of teaching and assessment; (iii) maintain evidence-based education practice; and (iv) develop reflective practitioners, who have a commitment to being engaged in the UK Higher Education Professional Standards Framework (UKPSF).

Primary Model: Training

Leadership: The MSc, Postgraduate Diploma, and Certificate in Veterinary Education are led by the LIVE Team at the Royal Veterinary College. This is a Centre for Excellence in Teaching and Learning, which has a dual role in both education teaching and research. The team and the Veterinary Education programs are led by the LIVE Centre Director, who is a Professor of Higher Education, assisted by the individual phase leads: two Senior Lecturers (Associate Professors) in Veterinary Education, a Lecturer (Assistant Professor) in Veterinary Education, and a Senior Teaching Fellow. Three additional Lecturers in Education support the teaching.

Membership: Open to all who contribute to teaching students of veterinary medicine and the allied veterinary professions. Participants are from a diverse educational background. Some are already curriculum leaders within their own institutions, with tertiary (doctorate level) degrees and specialist qualifications. Others are in nonacademic primary care or specialist veterinary practices (as veterinarians or veterinary nurses/technicians), and some have no prior undergraduate degree. Participants originate from the UK as well as North and South America, the Caribbean, Asia, Europe, and Australasia. The membership is diverse in profession, job role, international region, and prior education background, and we are particularly proud of our success in contributing to veterinary education leadership across this diversity of members.

Activities: Certificate and Degree-granting courses; Learning cohorts with defined social spaces and network building

Awards: Postgraduate Certificate in Veterinary Education, which qualifies them to progress to a Postgraduate Diploma and MSc, if desired. They also become Fellows of the UK Higher Education Academy, an internationally recognized body for teaching excellence.

Founding: LIVE was established as a Centre for Excellence in Teaching and Learning in 2005, and its formal educational programs were launched in September 2009.

Thanks to Dr. Liz Armitage-Chan and Dr. Stephen May for this!

"advance school-wide missions of education" (p. 729). Academies have since been established at many institutions of medical and veterinary education, and though their structures vary widely, some common characteristics include:

- A mission that advances and supports educators, provides faculty development, promotes curriculum improvement, advances educational scholarship, and offers protected faculty time for education;
- A membership composed of distinguished educators who are selected through a rigorous peer review process that assesses contributions to teaching, mentoring, curriculum development and leadership, and educational scholarship;
- A formal school-wide organizational structure with designated leadership; and
- Dedicated resources that fund mission-related initiatives (p. 730).

How might the case be made to establish such an academy?

Part 3: The Case for Educational Development

Council on Education (COE) accreditation standards require that we "provide a basis for a variety of career activities including clinical patient care, research, and other nonclinical options relevant to animal and human health. These fundamentals should be the basis for a lifetime of learning and professional development" (American Veterinary Medical Association 2021, p. 9). More personally as educators, we want to give our students the best veterinary education experience possible. To this end, CVMs guide students in learning the core fundamentals of veterinary care using the best information, practices, and educators to deliver purpose-built curricula. Student learning is our metric for success in this endeavor, and good learning comes from good teaching and a supportive learning environment.

However, definitions of "core" fundamentals and "best" information or practices are in a state of constant evolution spurred by changes in our understanding of the medical and learning sciences. Today's best solution may fall below tomorrow's standards. Much as a surgeon is expected to stay up on recent research into best techniques for patient safety, so should an educator follow developments in teaching and learning.

Staying up to date further assumes that educators have attained satisfactory knowledge and skills in the first place. Most veterinary educators enter their first teaching roles with little to no teaching experience and even less training. They do their best, but rarely do they have the time and support to sufficiently develop their ability to teach while also juggling service and research expectations. The result is generation after generation of veterinary educators carrying forward teaching strategies not because they are supported by research, but because these are the methods they already know.

Various groups work both inter- and intra-institutionally to resist educational stagnation and drive development. The American Veterinary Medical Association (AVMA) accreditation standards require that faculty and staff have time and support for professional development (American Veterinary Medical Association 2021). The Association of American Veterinary Medical Colleges (AAVMC) produced a competency-based veterinary education (CBVE) framework for guiding conversations around setting universally agreed-upon benchmarks for defining practice-ready veterinarians (Competency Based Veterinary Education Working Group 2018). At the regional level in the United States, consortia have formed to coordinate resource sharing between colleges in the West Region, Northeast, and Southeast. Recent years have seen an upswell in programs focused on developing veterinary education and education research within CVMs, such as the Center for Innovation in Veterinary Education and Technology (CIVET) at Lincoln Memorial University CVM, the Teaching Commons at the University of Georgia CVM, and the Academy of Educators at NC State University CVM, to name but a few.

The belief that we can and should be making systematic efforts to improve the quality of veterinary education is central to all this. Providing the best possible education in the face of changing needs requires resources and adaptability on the part of educators, support teams, college leadership, and the institution itself. This is "lifelong learning" at an organizational level. It is also modeling the very practices of self-reflection and self-development we seek to instill in our students. Alas, systematically supported cultures of learning and growth that are explicitly and implicitly developed at all levels of the curriculum and institution do not simply spring into existence. Focused leadership working to stay up to date on evidence-based teaching, instructional, and curricular design practices are needed. Systems for communicating the relevance and meaning of education research to veterinary educators are needed. Time, space, and resources for growing as educators are needed. In a nutshell, educational and educator development programs are needed (Box 15.2).

Box 15.2 Teaching Academy of the Consortium of West Region CVMs

Mission: The mission of the Regional Teaching Academy is to ensure that the members of the (West Region) consortium collaborate to develop, implement, and sustain the best practices in veterinary medical and biomedical education in our colleges, and to establish veterinary medical educator/biomedical educator as a valued career track. Through these efforts, we hope to meet the needs of society and the profession.

The Consortium includes: Colorado State University, Midwestern University, Oregon State University, University of Arizona, University of California – Davis, Washington State University, and Western University of Health Sciences.

Primary Model: Academy of Excellence

Leadership: The Academy has a chairperson who leads a steering committee with two representatives from each of the seven schools. Positions are limited in duration, chosen by the deans of their respective colleges.

Membership: There are 76 members as of March 2022. Academy members are faculty who "play a significant role in the teaching mission" as determined by a nomination process and requiring notable achievement in two of the following categories: teaching effectiveness, innovation in teaching, development of enduring educational materials, effective and creative uses of evidence-based teaching methods, educational scholarship, and educational leadership. Members are expected to participate through committees, producing educational resources and white papers, delivering academy courses, and mentoring junior faculty.

Activities: Members engage with faculty development through modules, peer observations of teaching, and external peer reviews of teaching using a portfolio system designed by the Teaching Academy.

Activity Timing: Variable, often according to individual members

Major Events: Biennial academy meeting

Founding: 2011

https://teachingacademy.westregioncvm.org/

Section 2: Educator Development

Part 1: From "Faculty Development" to "Educator Development"

Programs focused on the development of teaching skills in higher education contexts have many names that are sometimes conflated and other times conflicting. More than simple monikers, these labels indicate philosophical approaches and models for developing educational quality that brings with them certain strengths and gaps. Pulling from multiple fields of literature and our own experience, we recommend veterinary education turn its energies away from *faculty development* toward *educational development* and *educator development* as guiding mindsets for improving educational quality.

Veterinary education literature regularly describes the development of medical educators as *faculty development* (e.g., Barr et al. 2020; Lane et al. 2020), an umbrella term housing many ideas. According to Steinert (2014):

> Faculty development will refer to all activities health professionals pursue to improve their knowledge, skills, and behaviors as teachers and educators, leaders and managers, and researchers and scholars, in both individual and group settings (p. 4).

Faculty development in modern veterinary medical education seeks to support growth as academics and content experts. It can also recognize the critical training gap: that so very few veterinary educators receive sufficient training on how to actually teach the content with which they have achieved expertise. The field has largely moved past assumptions that grasp of the content or strong scholarship alone makes one a capable teacher (e.g., Figlio and Schapiro 2017), and accepted that we should treat teaching skills development as a core professional practice for faculty (World Federation for Medical Education 1988; Irby and O'Sullivan 2018). To this end, many faculty development programs seek to nurture the faculty member's growth as an educator. Developing a novice educator into an expert is an exercise in scaffolding rather similar conceptually to taking DVM aspirants from day-one students to day-one doctors. In this case, novice educators are provided skills and knowledge training with targeted outcomes in terms of educational capability.

Staff development is often used interchangeably with faculty development. This broader term theoretically opens doors to equitably support veterinary technicians and other nonfaculty educators in their growth (Steinert 2014; Steinert et al. 2016). Nonetheless, confusion remains as to the extent to which veterinary technicians and other nonfaculty educators are supported by "staff" development programs that often remain faculty focused in their content. Faculty development and staff development are conceptually broad constructs with aspects that have received significant attention in their own right.

Professional development, another common term in the medical education literature, typically refers to career and/or scholarly development and is most often concerned with faculty (Centra 1978). Topics include the leadership, management, research, and scholarship aspects of faculty development. Programs employing academy of excellence models in particular have a tendency to lean heavily into this aspect of development through public recognition. Membership itself is often a prestigious reward for those who have demonstrated a minimum level of capability in the realm of education (e.g., Barr et al. 2020; Buja et al. 2013; Dewey et al. 2005).

Where professional development focuses on the educator's success outside of the learning environment, *instructional development* concerns itself with the improvement of course design and student learning support within classroom, lab, and clinical contexts (Stes et al. 2010; Centra 1978). That is, it develops the educator's instructional strategies to improve student learning. It is important for program developers to distinguish between instructional development – focused on growth – and *instructional support* services provided to assist educators in the delivery of content instruction. Though it is entirely possible to serve up both "development" and "support" in the same moment, to assume that one inherently includes the other without intentional design creates an environment ripe for error and missed opportunities.

Professional development and instructional development equally, if differentially, describe programs targeting faculty, staff, and others, and are aspects of holistic faculty or staff development programs (Marschner et al. 2021; Irby and O'Sullivan 2018; Taylor and Rege Colet 2010). Whether training educators singly or in groups, the drive of such programs has traditionally been to support individual educators' growth, even when considering that individual as a member of a group. The expectation is that student-learning outcomes will improve when educators are "trained up" through workshops, seminars, and courses focused on educator growth.

A truly broad and holistic perspective on development to improve teaching and learning must consider not just the educators (Faculty Development, Staff Development), but also the organizational context in which teaching and learning occur. To this end, *organizational development* "is about maximizing an institution's resources to meet organizational objectives and to achieve broad institutional missions," (Taylor and Rege Colet 2010, p. 142). Leadership support, messaging, funding, institutional culture, time allowed for development activities, expectations for promotion ... there are a multitude of organizational and institutional factors influencing successful development of educators at the individual or group level (Marschner et al. 2021; Irby and O'Sullivan 2018). For a community of educators to grow effectively requires an alignment of their learning needs and the support provided. This alignment must further be adaptable to shifting trends as educators, learners, content, and learning environments change over time. Essentially, the organization must evolve and grow along with its educators and the context in which they teach (Gordon-Ross et al. 2020; Mallette and Rykert 2018; Irby 2014).

In summation, faculty development – the most common term in veterinary education – is too broad a concept for our purposes, as it includes ideas unrelated to teaching and learning. Yet it is not broad enough, as the name itself excludes nonfaculty educators and does not describe critical organizational elements for individual and programmatic success. Therefore, the authors recommend the veterinary education field embrace "educator development" and "educational development" for the purpose of improving student learning outcomes.

Educator development as used here refers to programming intended to develop the skills, knowledge, and behaviors of faculty, staff, residents, and anyone else who works with students – regardless of institutional rank or experience – for the purpose of supporting student learning and growth. The educator is identified as having membership in a group of professional learners responsible for building their individual capacities and collaborating with peers to construct a positive learning environment for students.

As a case example: in North Carolina State University's Academy of Educators, the original charter described a program to serve faculty growth. However, early reflection brought about an awareness that many aspects of faculty development were covered by other units in the college (specifically the office of Continuing Education), and that the community responsible for educational quality extended beyond the faculty. This led to a reenvisioning of the Academy as one that served all educators in the college, to better meet the mission of the program. Activities are now designed to meet the needs of various groups and encourage meaningful interactions between educators with shared goals.

Educational development, as borrowed from the Academic Development literature, is itself a term that has been stretched to cover many concepts over the decades. For the purposes of this chapter, we choose a conception of educational development that is inclusive of educator development practices and extends further to consider the organizational or institutional context in which teaching and learning at both the educator and student levels occur. It is not a fixed construct, and the educational development programming of one school may differ notably from the next. According to Gibbs (2013), "Educational development is defined within an institution by the subset of change mechanisms in use that they are responsible for" (p. 5).

Gibbs (2013, p. 6) provides a detailed list of common areas for development, including:

- Teachers' practice, motivation, thinking, and ability to "self-improve"
- Communities of practice and leadership of teaching
- Learning environments
- Institutional growth in the form of
  - facilities that support teaching
  - educational policies, learning and teaching strategies, pedagogy
  - aligning components within the teaching and learning strategy
- Influencing the external environment
- Identifying emergent change and spreading "best practice"
- Student study skills, self-efficacy, and meta-cognitive awareness
- Quality assurance systems
- Developing the credibility of teaching improvement efforts
- Educational evaluation
- Educational research and scholarship support

Consider educational development programs as intentionally designed systems or strategic plans for improving educational practices at the organizational, group, and individual (educator) levels. Educator development is a critical component for targeting educational development at the individual instructor level. That is, educator development exists within the context of an educational development plan at the organizational level. The best programs deploy both educator and educational development processes in tandem. At the Virginia–Maryland CVM, for example, educators participating in curriculum redesign were encouraged to engage with related programming offered by the campus teaching center as well.

Part 2: Educator Development Models in Medical Education

Educator development is a process that progresses across the career span (Schor et al. 2011). Early career programming may include community building, mentoring relationships, and practical strategies for getting started in teaching environments. While these types of activities may continue into mid-career, educators at this stage are often more prepared to explore learning theory and develop curricula using innovative, evidence-based teaching practices. Our most experienced educators often learn from serving as mentors to newer colleagues and reflecting on their experiences of what works and what doesn't in various teaching contexts. Such mentoring relationships are not a one-way street, as new educators may help experienced educators to view teaching, learning, and learners from modern perspectives (Clarke et al. 2019).

There are several models for framing educator development. One familiar model includes offering training opportunities organized around specific objectives. Activities in the *training model* may be developed to address how to perform common teaching tasks, such as presenting ideas clearly in the classroom or providing effective feedback on the clinic floor (O'Sullivan and Irby 2011; Lane and Strand 2008); to bring attention to context-specific situations such as curriculum renewal or other program changes (Root Kustritz et al. 2017; Warman et al. 2015); and to highlight advancements in evidence-based practice, such as in universal design for learning and inclusive teaching (Jackson et al. 2022). Training may take many forms, including workshops, seminars, and small-group discussions. These may be face-to-face or online, synchronous or asynchronous, stand-alone, or in a series (Steinert 2014).

Another approach is the *academy of excellence model,* which we previously described, where accomplished teachers are recognized with membership in the academy (Barr et al. 2020; Dewey et al. 2005). In this model, members of the academy may be asked to share their expertise with other educators, or they may sponsor special events with outside experts. This approach is focused on expertise and methods for disseminating that expertise.

While training is focused on building expertise and academies are focused on rewarding and disseminating expertise, communities of practice combine the best of both these models. The *community of practice model* shifts the focus from individuals to developing "groups of people who share a concern or a passion for something they do and learn how to do it better as they interact regularly" (Wenger-Trayner and Wenger-Trayer 2015, What are communities of practice?, para. 1). Sometimes referred to as "communities of teachers," these social spaces highlight collaborative interactions among educators with different experiences, skills, and backgrounds to cocreate and share new knowledge. Development activities in this framework aim to grow the group culture as much, or even more, than individuals' skill sets (de Carvalho-Filho et al. 2020; Barab et al. 2002). Communities of practice are increasingly perceived as central to providing high-quality educational programming that supports educator skills, knowledge, and identity development (de Carvalho-Filho et al. 2020; Lane et al. 2020; Steinert et al. 2016) (Box 15.3).

Box 15.3   UTK Master Teaching Program

Mission: Provide the resources, programs, and leadership that support the highest quality of professionalism and instruction within the various educational missions of the college.

Primary Model: "Community of practice with the approach of a teaching academy"

Leadership: Organizing Committee of one DVM, one DVM/educational EdD, one educational EdD, and one educational PhD. Leadership is based on interest rather than administrative appointment, and three members are founding members.

Membership: "Open invitation to all interested college faculty, staff, and students. Attendance at sessions is dependent on participant interest in the topic."

Activities: Monthly one-hour sessions with occasional, additional multi-hour workshops and one-hour brown bag sessions. Topics are both educational theory-driven and applied. Over the years, some of the topics have included providing student feedback, small group facilitation, how people learn, writing effective multiple choice questions, lecture "don'ts," writing student learning outcomes, classroom technology, technicians as teachers, etc. Attendance at monthly sessions in 2021 (all online) averaged 33 people; there were 95 unique attendees throughout the year (some sessions were also open to SEVEC schools).

Activity Timing: Regular sessions are held on the third Thursday of each month at 8:00 a.m. Workshops typically span the lunch hour to continue conversations into that space. Brown bag sessions generally occur during the lunch hour and are in partnership with student clubs or other affinity groups.

Major Events: Annual fundamentals of teaching workshop

Recognition/Awards/enticements: MTP Fundamentals of Classroom Teaching Certificate (Online Self-Paced; eight hours). An annual letter is provided to department heads and supervisors to outline MTP participation of their direct reports. For faculty, participation is included in their effort allocation calculation. Sessions are approved for continuing education credit for college clinicians. Support for travel to veterinary/medical education conferences is available to faculty and staff. Faculty and staff presentation at MTP sessions is also encouraged, and MTP-branded "swag" is often provided to attendees.

Founding: 2008

Thanks to Dr. Misty Bailey for this!

Section 3: Building an Educator Development Program

Part 1: Establish Needs

Educator development is ultimately a change management process (Bell 2013). The requirements of our students and our profession undergo constant evolution driven by economic, generational, cultural, and other forces, not least of which is our growing understanding of veterinary and veterinary educational sciences. CVMs require curricular and instructional agility to keep up with changing needs, lest they fall behind. Laying out a plan for an educator development program has many parallels with the competency-based backward design processes currently gaining traction within the AAVMC (Competency Based Veterinary Education Working Group 2018). Essentially, planners must establish the type and level of teaching competency they wish their veterinary educators to achieve, and work backward in planning how to bring their educators to that point. These needs-based goals are instrumental to establishing the purpose of the program.

Development planners frequently focus on programming to meet specific immediate needs. The sudden transition to online and hybrid learning in the face of COVID-19, for example, spurred a plethora of conversations around how to teach through virtual meeting platforms like Zoom. The purpose of such programming is vital: to resolve pressing issues in content delivery and support faculty during a difficult time. Now, CVMs across the globe must decide what role these new teaching modalities will play in their curricula going forward (Routh et al. 2021), and once again reorient their educator development programming to a more hybridized teaching world.

Planners should regularly ask themselves: Are the needs being met temporary or lasting issues? Will the program being designed summarily answer those needs, or will the issue require more constant vigilance? What needs will the future hold and how can we begin to address them?

There is a natural temptation to focus on emergent issues, and often good reasons to do so! The danger lies in failing to also look beyond the immediate and pressing to future and ongoing needs. In particular, there may be underlying, less obvious issues in your educator community that are root causes for more obvious problems. Consider the conversation in a recent Southeast Veterinary Education Consortium (SEVEC) workshop discussing clinical communication for Safety Culture education, where hierarchical challenges underlying staff and faculty communication norms in learning environments were identified as a root cause of problems. Working on communication skill sets without addressing the power differential issues as a community would be akin to treating the symptom, not the disease.

It is incumbent upon developers to perceive the direction of change necessary to meet both current and future needs and resolve root causes. They are to devise and implement strategic programming initiatives to guide positive change, inspire broad participation and engagement among their educators, and evaluate the effectiveness of their work for future growth (Bell 2013; By 2005). In other words, developers should create a change management plan to scaffold their programming direction and community development.

Such plans begin with determining the needs of the organization and its stakeholders through in-house assessments and metrics, comparison against benchmarks and standards (e.g., AVMA accreditation), education literature research, and a healthy dose of listening to the community members, e.g., students, faculty, staff, employers, alumni, etc. (Oakes 2021). Developers first learn about their own CVM and its educational development needs, then establish where those needs are and are not being met, and explore root causes. Meeting these needs becomes the direction, or purpose, toward which all the program planning will be oriented.

Part 2: Establish Purpose

The purpose of educator development at an institution should be clearly laid out so that (i) planning is driven by a consistent conception of needs and directions, (ii) success in meeting the purpose can be defined and evaluated, and (iii) changes reflecting evolving needs can be made at all levels. Purpose definition often begins with establishing a mission statement, or a "formal expression of an institution's core values" in regard to educational development (Williams 2013, p 371). Mission statements are not consistently formatted across or even within industries and contexts, though all provide a starting point for making programmatic decisions. For example, consider the Teaching Academy of the Consortium of West Region CVM:

> The mission of the Regional Teaching Academy is to ensure that the members of the consortium collaborate to develop, implement, and sustain the best practices in veterinary medical and biomedical education in our colleges, and to establish veterinary medical educator/biomedical educator as a valued career track. Through these efforts, we hope to meet the needs of society and the profession (Teaching Academy n.d.).

No matter the final mission statement design, it is critical to support the idea of growing the skills and capacities of our educators and our educator support programs. First, because as previously established through various reviews (see: Gordon-Ross et al. 2020), too few of our veterinary educators have sufficient training on how to be high-quality educators. Second, because the challenges facing veterinary education are constantly changing in ways that call for an evolving response (e.g., the COVID-19 pandemic). Finally, because the best educational environments support lifelong learning habit development among our students; habits that are best taught through modeling. Essentially, we will never be done learning as a profession, and educator development strategies and programming should reflect that growth.

Mission statement in hand, the next step is to begin planning how to achieve that mission and thereby answer the needs of your organization. This includes blueprinting who will lead and facilitate the program, defining clearly who is served by the program, the best model for shaping the program, what content will be delivered and how.

Part 3: Define Leadership and Membership

Leadership

Educator development programming functions over many years and requires an individual or team to steer design, facilitation, evaluation, and adaptation across that time. While leadership teams need not be permanent positions, key responsibilities should be assigned in a way that preserves the structure of the program through changes in personnel. These are the leaders that carry forth the mission (and perhaps vision) of the organization. Trusting an educator development program to survive without leadership is akin to starting down a trail on a bicycle, then taking your hands off and hoping for the best. It may work for a time, but the first bump likely means disaster.

Leaders can come from many areas of the CVM. A senior faculty member or academic dean chairing a rotating committee of veteran academic decision-makers is a classic model (e.g., Teaching Academy of the Consortium of West Region CVMs). Alternatively, a smaller team of two or three veterinary educators working with an educational specialist can prove more dexterous while increasing individual load (e.g., UTK Master Teaching Program). Funding permitting, part- or full-time hires with the explicit purpose of running the organization can provide consistent and reliable planning. Such leaders could be drawn from veterinary faculty with notable training on education or from non-veterinary backgrounds, such as educational psychology, curriculum and instruction, instructional design, etc.

In many ways, a leader's background matters less than what they are able to do once they are in position. Leaders need to be able to develop or guide development of educational programming to meet the mission of the organization and do so in a way that gives confidence to participants not only that the direction taken is correct, but that it is well planned. This calls for sufficient understanding of educational principles and literature, organizational management skills, and empowerment from administration to act. Choose your leadership thoughtfully and support them appropriately.

Membership

Who has access to the development of programming, and the method by which they gain or maintain that access, is not only a critical element of the program design, but perhaps the clearest enactment of philosophy, mission, and vision. Academy of Excellence models will typically restrict access to those who have demonstrated a minimum level of competence already and by their nature tend toward smaller, more elite, membership group structures. This approach combines well with promotion planning and establishing leadership groups for guiding educational initiatives.

Training and Certification models tend to be more open access for entry, as their intention is to raise the skill level of novice educators to meet the very same minimum standards an Academy of Excellence may require for entry. There is a natural dovetail in combining the two approaches. Though access may be open, programs may also be designed in a way that entails certain costs in terms of time or money that will dissuade potential applicants. Assuming those costs are directly related to providing excellent training, this is less of a failing and more of a balance point to be considered. Lower costs mean more folks can engage in the full program, but also that the program may not be able to provide the level of rigor desired.

Community of Practice models tend to be the easiest to access and engage with and will often maintain the highest volumes of membership as a result. Such approaches are best when the goal is to affect cultural change around how education is thought of within an organization, and to shift the teaching practices of a majority of educators within the college. On the other hand, engagement is naturally more variable in these models than in entry-bound academies or regulated training. The degree of impact on individual educators ranges more widely as a result.

As an example, the NC State Academy of Educators prioritizes the growth and recognition of a community of educators whose efforts intersect to train DVM students. It allows any member of the CVM to join by simply asking to be added and is more in line with community models than an academy of excellence model, despite the name. Instead, to encourage engagement, participation in programming across each academic year is tracked and used for determining "Active Membership." Access to additional resources such as research grants and conference support requires Active Membership status, which in turn requires a minimum degree of engagement. Members who struggle to make meetings (e.g., Second shift technicians) can reach out to the program director to be connected with learning partners via email exchanges and recordings of events. Programming frequently encourages collaboration and discussion as peers to reflect on information provided by experts (Box 15.4).

Part 4: Select a Model

A well-designed educator development program will have an operating model like those previously discussed (Academy of Excellence, Community of Practice, Training, or Certification). The leadership team defines the model early in the development process and manages both the implementation and adaptation of that model over time. As demonstrated by University of Tennessee, it is entirely possible, even to some extent likely, that an educator development program will be best defined as belonging to one model or another at different points in its lifespan (Lane et al. 2020).

Neither is a development program limited to selecting just one model. For example, the NCSU Academy of Educators is primarily defined by its community of practice model while maintaining elements for recognizing excellence through annual awards. In another instance, the Royal Veterinary College Post-Graduate Training Certification for Veterinary Educators, while very much defined by its excellent training focus, also seeks to establish localized communities via cohorts and study groups. To this end, a model is more of a guide than a bounded set of activities, and it is likely that any given program can identify elements of multiple models within its organizational principles. The crucial element is that the leadership understands the nature and intention of their chosen model – amalgam that it likely is. It is the model that guides decision-making toward completion of mission and vision.

Box 15.4   The NC State University CVM Academy of Educators

Mission: To nurture the growth of a skilled, knowledgeable, innovative, and mutually supportive community of veterinary educators.

Primary Model: Community of Practice

Leadership: Director (Educational Specialist) collaborates with a President (Faculty or Staff elected from membership) and working groups formed for major questions or projects.

Membership: 173 members as of March 2022, including faculty, staff, residents, graduate students/postdocs, administration, and a few DVM Students. Interested CVM community members of all levels are invited to participate.

Activities: Combination of workshops, seminars, journal clubs, and community building averaging five events a month. Weekly listserv discussion prompt.

Activity Timing: Varies. One-hour sessions, 8 a.m.~6 p.m., M~F.

Major Events: Education Day in early summer

Recognition/Awards/Enticements: Annual Awards for Excellence in Education, Innovation, and Wellness Allyship. "Active" members have access to research, conference travel, and training registration support. Four members take the RVC PG Certification program annually.

Learning Resources: Recordings of past events, recommended reading lists online and in library, and research consultants.

Founding: 2018

Part 5: Select Content, Learning Objectives/Outcomes

To determine program content, the needs of the college, program, and individuals should all be considered. This can be done in a top-down way, with administrators leading a formal needs analysis to identify gaps between existing and desired knowledge, skills, and attributes, or bottom-up, with the educators themselves identifying areas of interest.

Once the needs are determined, curriculum development may proceed using a strategy similar to backward course design, starting with the learning objectives, moving through assessment strategies, and finally learning activities. Just as CBVE frameworks focus instruction on professional outcomes in veterinary medicine, educational development programs may be focused on professional outcomes for educators. Several such frameworks exist with outcomes for medical educators; however, none have been specifically identified for veterinary educators. For example, Sherbino et al. (2014) suggest seven competency domains for clinician educators: assessment, communication, curriculum development, education theory, leadership, scholarship, and teaching. A community might choose a set of domains like this one including defined competencies, and then develop activities that support development in each domain. Assessments, such as student experience surveys, peer observations of teaching, educator self-reflection, and teaching portfolios, might be implemented to identify levels of competence and further understand the needs of the community members.

At the University of Georgia CVM, staff in the Office of Academic Affairs started with the CORE Values of the College – Compassion, Openness, Respect, and Entrepreneurialism – and developed a mission statement for the UGA CVM Teaching Commons:

> Teaching Commons programs will foster instructors who show compassion for our students and their learning processes; are open to sharing their teaching challenges and successes with others; are respectful

of students' ideas, contributions, and feedback; and forward-thinking in developing and implementing innovative models for teaching. (S.A. Clouser, personal communication, May 8, 2019).

This mission statement provides a foundation for developing programming and resources and keeps the activities focused on what matters to the College. More specifically, the goal of the Teaching Commons "is to support veterinary educators across the College as a community, with a variety of opportunities to participate in conversations and read about teaching and learning" (S.A. Clouser, personal communication, May 8, 2019). The mission statement and the goal of the Teaching Commons are specific enough to ensure direction to programming, yet broad enough to provide flexibility.

Lane and Strand (2008) offer another approach to identifying goals for educator development. They interviewed educators at their institution about the strengths and weaknesses of the clinical setting, and then developed programming incorporating their findings. They reported four themes related to learning in the clinical setting:

> (1) maximizing learning during the initial client-patient encounter, (2) maximizing learning and optimizing use of time related to patient-centered activities, (3) maximizing the educational value of the existing caseload, and (4) maximizing the educational contributions of all members of the medical team (p. 400).

The authors connected these themes, along with "the clinician's time, energy, and level of comfort with teaching in the clinics," and they "recognized that the common thread in clinical teaching is the teacher's skill in giving the learner *feedback*" (Lane and Strand 2008, p. 401). After identifying these concepts that facilitate learning in clinical settings, the authors were able to develop activities that were community-centered and focused on the values and needs of community members (Box 15.5).

Box 15.5   University of Georgia College of Veterinary Medicine Teaching Commons

Mission: The mission for the UGA CVM Teaching Commons is situated in the CORE values of the College (Compassion, Openness, Respect, Entrepreneurialism): Teaching Commons programs will foster instructors who show compassion for our students and their learning processes; are open to sharing their teaching challenges and successes with others; are respectful of students' ideas, contributions, and feedback; and forward-thinking in developing and implementing innovative models for teaching.

Primary Model: Training

Leadership: Director of Instructional and Curricular Innovation (Education Specialist, Non-DVM)

Membership: All faculty, staff, and students at the college have access to most Teaching Commons programs; the Teaching Certificate is limited to faculty and veterinary nurses.

Activities: Workshops, Seminars, Guest lectures, Online resources, Certificate program

Activity Timing: Synchronous events are typically held during the week and recorded for later viewing.

Major Events: Summer Teaching Series, including workshops and guest speakers; Teaching Certificate Program

Learning Resources: Workshop/Seminar recordings; Links to recommended books, articles, and teaching websites; Links to teaching conferences; Information about teaching strategies and curriculum renewal; Blog including posts from Teaching Certificate participants

Recognition/Awards/Enticements: Teaching Certificate recipients are included in annual presentation of all faculty and staff awards

Founding: 2019

Part 6: Select Activities

No matter the model, educator development activities may take a variety of forms. Some programs may be formalized, highly organized, and result in a degree or certificate for the participant. There are several such programs specific to veterinary education, such as the Royal Veterinary College certificate and master's programs and the Lincoln Memorial University Master of Veterinary Education program. Most educational development in veterinary education is workplace-based and not as formal as these programs, though many such activities are deliberately constructed. However, unlike formal activities, they do not result in a formal credential.

Activities such as workshops and journal clubs can be planned for large or small groups to occur synchronously, asynchronously, or in some combination. They may accommodate community and individual needs via sessions that can be stand-alone or in a series; perhaps theme-based or time-based, such as a summer series. Sessions can be prepared and led by more-expert educators or facilitated by peers. At the University of Tennessee, for example, the interview study on clinical teaching resulted in a list of synchronous and asynchronous clinical teaching sessions:

> Feedback: The Nuts and Bolts
> The Teaching Moment
> Teaching During Rounds
> Evaluating Clinical Performance
> Improving Narrative Comments in Clinical Assessments
> Effective Mentoring (Lane and Strand 2008, p. 401)

Each session includes opportunities for participants to reflect on their own experiences and learn strategies for teaching in specific situational contexts. As feedback is important in clinical teaching, the authors also recognize that feedback is important for continuous improvement of these sessions and note how they provide opportunities for

participants to comment on their experience in the program. (Lane and Strand 2008)

Another example of a workplace-based program is the UGA CVM Teaching Certificate, which is one opportunity available to faculty and veterinary nurses through the UGA Teaching Commons. As with all Teaching Commons programs, Teaching Certificate activities are all aligned with the Teaching Commons mission, previously cited. The Certificate program includes a series of six online, self-paced modules including opportunities for asynchronous discussions with colleagues and the Certificate instructors. Learning objectives for the certificate were developed based on a literature search of teaching competencies. Following successful completion of the program, participants should be able to:

- Identify major learning theories and their relevance in veterinary education contexts;
- Apply the principles of integrated course design to select and develop learning activities and assessments;
- Describe techniques for providing effective feedback;
- Evaluate education-related literature; and
- Practice a scholarly and reflective approach to teaching (Office of Academic Affairs 2019).

For each module, participants respond to a reflective prompt, and then instructors direct each participant to readings appropriate for each individual. Instructors also provide a follow-up reflective prompt for the participant to consider following the assignment. Additionally, participants pair up to observe and be observed in one instructional context, such as the classroom or clinic. Pre-observation, in-observation, and post-observation guidelines are provided, as well as suggestions for providing gentle feedback.

A final type of educational development is more spontaneous and happens on the job through workplace conversations, experiences, and observation. We can, and should, capture and build on these learning experiences

---

Box 15.6 Lincoln Memorial University College of Veterinary Medicine Veterinary Educator Training Seminar Series (VETSS)

Mission: This seminar series is designed to provide a brief overview of educational philosophy, psychology, and research supporting a variety of effective teaching practices in the adult classroom and to enhance the teaching skills of current faculty.

Primary Model: Community of Practice

Leadership: Director of the Center for Innovation in Veterinary Education and Technology (CIVET), in coordination and consultation with the other assigned faculty members to CIVET (both veterinarians, both with advanced training in education).

Membership: All faculty, staff, and students interested in the topics who are affiliated with participating schools in the Southeast Veterinary Education Consortium (SEVEC).

Activities: 10, One-hour virtual lectures/workshops, opportunities for peer observation and feedback.

Activity Timing: Monthly at lunchtime, 10 months out of the year (Jan–May, August–December)

Recognition/Awards/Enticements: Participants meeting specific criteria are eligible to earn a certificate of completion and/or a certificate of skilled teaching each year.

Learning Resources: Online repository of all session recordings, PowerPoint slide decks from the speakers, accompanying literature or links to available literature, and quizzes for those wishing to obtain attendance credit.

Founding: 2019

Thanks to Dr. Katherine Fogelberg and Dr. Micha Simons for this!

---

by referring to them in planned activities. Including reflective prompts in a workshop or meeting with a mentor can help educators associate their lived experiences with organizational learning goals and teaching competencies (Box 15.6).

Section 4: Recommendations for Success

We have discussed the philosophies behind educator and educational development programs and made a case for their implementation. We then covered major components and decision points in building a program to meet the needs of your organization, coupled with examples of successful programs in callout boxes. Note from the examples that educator development programs rarely look exactly alike in form, function, and activity from organization to organization. Rather, each should speak to the particular needs, preferences, resources, and quirks of their home organization.

The following are a set of general recommendations to keep in mind as you build your own program. These apply to all educator and educational development programs in some way, though interpretations can vary.

Part 1: Growth is Adaptation and Change

For your program to remain healthy in the long term, it will need the ability to grow. That means adapting plans to meet changing needs, reworking activity structures, revisiting and updating content, and otherwise treating your program as a living thing that may look a bit different from year to year. Resist the temptation to "lock in" set training or activity structures, and keep an eye out for how aspects could benefit from updating or refreshing. Just as you assess the quality and impact of your student programs, reflect on each component of your educator development programs, implement improvements that support current needs, and repeat. This will not only keep your program healthier and more engaging long term, but will model the sort of thinking we expect from our educators and veterinary students.

Part 2: Make the Wheels Fit, Don't Invent New Ones

There is a vast pool of literature on educational skills training and development in medical and other professional contexts that is perfectly applicable to our populations and contexts. We recommend due diligence and searching for answers to your complex questions before inventing new solutions whole cloth. Please do not invent a new learning theory without considerable reading into what exists!

At a localized programming level, this advice also applies to modifying existing structures to fit your needs where possible before adding entirely new and sometimes overlapping programs. When building your program, consider what relevant programming already exists in your organization, and decide whether it might be adopted as is, adapted for your context, absorbed to support a larger population, or perhaps developed further in collaboration with the existing program leaders.

Part 3: Teaching Skills Development is Professionalism

In veterinary medical education, practitioners first develop their professional identities around medical practice. The same is true for PhD scholars and their identities as experts and researchers in their fields of study. They may not consider themselves as educators, or they may not perceive teaching as having the same level of importance as their content expertise and content-specific skill sets. To engage these members of your community in educational growth, you must instill within them the recognition that in their current roles, teaching is not a tack-on duty but rather a key aspect of their professional identity. They are veterinary medical educators, and as such veterinary teaching skills development is a responsibility of professional practice. This messaging should begin with administration and continue through community spaces and across organizations.

Summary

Because most educators in colleges in universities have little to no training in education before they are hired as academics, educational development is imperative to improving the quality of learning that occurs in higher education classrooms. This is particularly true of professional training programs, which encompass veterinary medicine. There are some unique challenges in veterinary medical education, as well, and that includes the various skills and training of the educators who contribute to the veterinarian's education – including veterinary technicians, non-veterinarians (e.g., PhD-trained but not medically trained), and staff (e.g., those trained in business, lawyers). Providing a consistent, high-quality educational development program for all involved in veterinary education is important and is becoming increasingly viewed as being so. This chapter has provided support for the value of creating such programs, laid out a process for doing so, and ends with recommendations to aid programs in ensuring the best possible success in the process.

References

American Veterinary Medical Association (2021). Accreditation policies and procedures of the AVMA Council on Education (COE). https://www.avma.org/education/accreditation-policies-and-procedures-avma-council-education-coe (accesssed 29 April 2022).

Barab, S.A., Barnett, M., and Squire, K. (2002). Developing an empirical account of a community of practice: characterizing the essential tensions. *The Journal of the Learning Sciences* 11 (4): 489–542.

Barr, M.C., Hines, S.A., Sprunger, L.K. et al. (2020). An inter-institutional collaboration to "make teaching matter": The Teaching Academy of the Consortium of west region colleges of veterinary medicine. *Journal of Veterinary Medical Education* 47 (5): 570–578. https://doi.org/10.3138/jvme-2019-0102.

Bell, C.E. (2013). Faculty development in veterinary education: are we doing enough (or publishing enough about it), and do we value it? *Journal of Veterinary Medical Education* 40 (2): 96–101. https://doi.org/10.3138/jvme.0113-022R.

Buja, L.M., Cox, S., Lieberman, S. et al. (2013). A university system's approach to enhancing the educational mission of health science schools and institutions: The University of Texas Academy of Health Science Education. *Medical Education Online* 18 (1). https://doi.org/10.3402/meo.v18i0.20540.

By, R.T. (2005). Organisational change management: a critical review. *Journal of Change Management* 5 (4): 369–380. https://doi.org/10.1080/14697010500359250.

de Carvalho-Filho, M.A., Tio, R.A., and Steinert, Y. (2020). Twelve tips for implementing a community of practice for faculty development. *Medical Teacher* 42 (2): 143–149.

Clarke, A.J., Burgess, A., van Diggele, C., and Mellis, C. (2019). The role of reverse mentoring in medical education: current insights. *Advances in Medical Education and Practice* 10: 693–701. https://doi.org/10.2147/AMEP.S179303.

Competency Based Veterinary Education Working Group (2018). Competency based veterinary education framework. American Association of Veterinary Medical Colleges. https://cbve.org/framework (accessed 28 September 2021).

Centra, J.A. (1978). Types of faculty development programs. *The Journal of Higher Education* 49 (2): 151–162.

Dewey, C.M., Friedland, J.A., Richards, B.F. et al. (2005). The emergence of academies of educational excellence: a survey of US medical schools. *Academic Medicine* 80 (4): 358–365.

Figlio, D.N. and Schapiro, M. (2017). Are great teachers poor scholars? *Evidence Speaks Reports* 2 (6): 1–7.

Gaff, J.G. and Simpson, R.D. (1994). Faculty development in the United States. *Innovative Higher Education* 18 (3): 167–176.

Gibbs, G. (2013). Reflections on the changing nature of educational development. *International Journal for Academic Development* 18 (1): 4–14. https://doi.org/10.1080/1360144X.2013.751691.

Gordon-Ross, P.N., Kovacs, S.J., Halsey, R.L. et al. (2020). Veterinary Educator Teaching and Scholarship (VETS): a case study of a multi-institutional faculty development program to advance teaching and learning. *Journal of Veterinary Medical Education* 47 (5): 632–646. https://doi.org/10.3138/jvme-2019-0089.

Irby, D.M. (2014). Excellence in clinical teaching: knowledge transformation and development required. *Medical Education* 48 (8): 776–784. https://doi.org/10.1111/medu.12507.

Irby, D.M. and O, Sullivan, P.S. (2018). Developing and rewarding teachers as educators and scholars: remarkable progress and daunting challenges. *Medical Education* 52 (1): 58–67. https://doi.org/10.1111/medu.13379.

Irby, D.M., Cooke, M., Lowenstein, D., and Richards, B. (2004). The academy movement: a structural approach to reinvigorating the educational mission. *Academic Medicine* 79 (8): 729–736.

Jackson, M.A., Moon, S., Doherty, J.H., and Wenderoth, M.P. (2022). Which evidence-based teaching practices change over time? Results from a university-wide STEM faculty development program. *International Journal of STEM Education* 9 (22). https://doi.org/10.1186/s40594-022-00340-4.

Lane, I.F. and Strand, E. (2008). Clinical veterinary education: insights from faculty and strategies for professional development in clinical teaching. *Journal of Veterinary Medical Education* 35 (3): 397–406.

Lane, I.F., Sims, M., Howell, N.E., and Bailey, M. (2020). Sustaining a collegewide teaching academy as a community: 10 years of experience with the master teacher program at the University of Tennessee College of Veterinary Medicine. *Journal of Veterinary Medical Education* 47 (4): 384–394. https://doi.org/10.3138/jvme.0918-106r1.

Mallette, C. and Rykert, L. (2018). Promoting positive culture change in nursing faculties: getting to maybe through liberating structures. *Journal of Professional Nursing* 34 (3): 161–166. https://doi.org/10.1016/j.profnurs.2017.08.001.

Marschner, C.B., Dahl, K., and Langebæk, R. (2021). Creating a pedagogical development program for veterinary clinical teachers: a discipline-specific, context-relevant, bottom-up initiative. *Journal of Veterinary Medical Education* 48 (2): 129–135. https://doi.org/10.3138/jvme.2019-0042.

Oakes, K. (2021). *Culture Renovation: 18 Leadership Actions to Build an Unshakeable Company*. McGraw Hill.

O, Sullivan, P.S. and Irby, D.M. (2011). Reframing research on faculty development. *Academic Medicine* 86 (4): 421–428. https://doi.org/10.1097/ACM.0b013e31820dc058.

Pirkelbauer, B., Pead, M., Probyn, P., and May, S.A. (2008). LIVE: the creation of an academy for veterinary education. *Journal of Veterinary Medical Education* 35 (4): 567–572.

Root Kustritz, M.V., Molgaard, L.K., and Malone, E. (2017). Curriculum review and revision at the University of Minnesota College of Veterinary Medicine. *Journal of Veterinary Medical Education* 44 (3): 459–470. https://doi.org/10.3138/jvme.0217-029R.

Routh, J., Paramasivam, S.J., Cockcroft, P. et al. (2021). Veterinary education during COVID-19 and beyond – challenges and mitigating approaches. *Animals* 11 (6): 1818. https://doi.org/10.3390/ani11061818.

Schor, N.F., Guillet, R., and McAnarney, E.R. (2011). Anticipatory guidance as a principle of faculty development: managing transition and change. *Academic Medicine* 86 (10): 1235–1240. https://doi.org/10.1097/ACM.0b013e31822c1317.

Sherbino, J., Frank, J.R., and Snell, L. (2014). Defining the key roles and competencies of the clinician-educator of the 21st century: a national mixed-methods study. *Academic Medicine* 89 (5): 783–789. https://doi.org/10.1097/ACM.0000000000000217.

Steinert, Y. (2014). Faculty development: core concepts and principles. In: *Faculty Development in the Health Professions: Innovation and Change in Professional Education*, vol. 11 (ed. Y. Steinert), 3–25. Dordrecht: Springer. https://doi.org/10.1007/978-94-007-7612-8_1.

Steinert, Y., Mann, K., Anderson, B. et al. (2016). A systematic review of faculty development initiatives designed to enhance teaching effectiveness: a 10-year update: BEME Guide No. 40. *Medical Teacher* 38 (8): 769–786. https://doi.org/10.1080/0142159X.2016.1181851.

Stes, A., Min-Leliveld, M., Gijbels, D., and Van Petegem, O. (2010). The impact of instructional development in higher education: the state-of-the-art of the research. *Educational Research Review* 5 (2010): 25–49. https://doi.org/10.1016/j.edurev.2009.07.001.

Taylor, K.L. and Rege Colet, N. (2010). Making the shift from faculty development to educational development: a conceptual framework grounded in practice. In: *Building Teaching Capacities in Universities: A Comprehensive International Model* (ed. A. Saroyan and M. Frenay), 139–167. Stylus Publishing.

The Teaching Academy of the Consortium of West Region Colleges of Veterinary Medicine (n.d.). Main. https://teachingacademy.westregioncvm.org/ (accessed 28 September 2021).

Warman, S., Pritchard, J., and Baillie, S. (2015). Faculty development for a new curriculum: implementing a strategy for veterinary teachers within the wider university context. *Journal of Veterinary Medical Education* 42 (4): 346–352. https://doi.org/10.3138/jvme.1214-124R1.

Wenger-Trayner, E. and Wenger-Trayner, B. (2015). Introduction to communities of practice: a brief overview of the concept and its uses. https://www.wenger-trayner.com/introduction-to-communities-of-practice/ (accessed 3 April 2022).

Williams, D.A. (2013). Activating the diversity change journey. In: *Strategic Diversity Leadership*, 371. Stylus Publishing, LLC.

World Federation for Medical Education, World Conference on Medical Education (1988). The Edinburgh Declaration. Retrieved from the World Health Organization website: https://apps.who.int/iris/bitstream/handle/10665/163121/EB83_Inf.Doc-3_eng.pdf?sequence=1&isAllowed=y (accessed 28 September 2021).

Zook, G.F. and President's Commission on Higher Education(1948). *Higher Education for American Democracy: A Report of the President's Commission on Higher Education*. Washington, DC: United States Government Printing Office.

16

Documenting Teaching for Career Advancement

Misty R. Bailey, MA, PhD
College of Veterinary Medicine, University of Tennessee, Knoxville, USA

Susan M. Matthew, PhD, BVSc (Hons), BSc (Vet)(Hons), GradCertEd Stud(HigherEd)
Washington State University College of Veterinary Medicine, Pullman, WA, USA

Section 1: Introduction

Effectively documenting teaching for career advancement goes beyond the traditional method of presenting a quantitative list of what was taught, when, where, and with whom. Effectively documenting teaching also requires giving evidence of quality, effectiveness, and impact; and adopting a scholarly approach to educational work (Boyer 2016; Glassick et al. 1997; Gusic et al. 2007, 2014; Hines et al. 2020; Simpson et al. 2007). These criteria apply across all domains of educator activity: teaching, mentoring and advising, learner assessment or outcome assessment, educational research and scholarship, curriculum and program development, and educational leadership and administration (Baldwin et al. 2012; Gusic et al. 2014; Hines et al. 2020; Simpson et al. 2007). Few educators are active in all these domains (Hines et al. 2020; Teaching Academy 2022), and for early career educators, providing evidence of a scholarly approach to teaching, together with quantity, quality, effectiveness, and impact in one or two domains of educator activity, is a more realistic expectation (Hines et al. 2020).

Effective evidence is built on qualitative and quantitative data gathered repeatedly from a range of different perspectives on the educator's efforts: students, peers and colleagues, administrators, and self (Baldwin et al. 2012; Benton and Young 2018; Hoyt and Pallett 1999; Simpson et al. 2007; Theall 2017). The goal is to show evidence of quality and advancement in effectiveness as a teacher and a commitment to ongoing professional development through engagement with the education community (Benton and Young 2018; Hoyt and Pallett 1999; Simpson et al. 2007). In the realm of medical education research, Friesen et al. (2019) recommend using "grey metrics" to capture an educator's influence in the field (p. 956). They suggest that the influence of education research cannot be fully captured with conventional metrics such as impact factor or grant dollars. Instead, Friesen et al. (2019) argue that an educator's meaningful effects on policy, practices, and perspectives should be illustrated with metrics that are better aligned with the purposes of the field. Examples provided are informal and formal consultations, listserv mentions, citations on websites, and slide sharing requests. Additionally, the authors suggest documenting communications that specify appreciation, application or inclusion of developed resources or their use to inform innovative practices (Friesen et al. 2019). Such metrics may be expanded to provide meaningful evidence of impact in all domains of educator activity.

Part 1: The Importance of a Scholarly Approach

Effective teaching and educational leadership are built on a scholarly approach that is informed by relevant education literature and best practices (Baldwin et al. 2012; Boyer 2016; Gusic et al. 2014; Sullivan 2018). This includes systematic planning to achieve educational goals using methods that are based on sound principles and best practices drawn from the literature and other experts (Baldwin et al. 2012). Adopting a scholarly approach is the foundation for engaging in educational scholarship (Simpson et al. 2007). Excellent educational scholarship fulfills six criteria: clear goals, adequate preparation, appropriate methods, significant results, effective presentation of results for review, and reflective critique (Glassick 2000; Glassick et al. 1997). These criteria are aligned with a growth mindset that educational practices such as teaching can be learned and improved rather than being a fixed characteristic of an individual (Benton and Young 2018; Dweck 2006). Such improvement requires engagement with the educator community (Boyer 2016; Shulman 1998; Simpson et al. 2007) and a mastery goal orientation that encompasses openness to experimenting with new practices and receiving feedback on performance, as well as persistence in ongoing learning and improvement through critically reflective practice (Baldwin et al. 2012; Benton and Young 2018; Boud 1985; Svinicki 2017).

Part 2: Showcasing Educator Activities and Outcomes

The teaching component of an educator's curriculum vitae (CV) can be structured using six broadly applicable domains of educator activity to showcase the breadth, effectiveness, and impact of an educator's accomplishments (Hines et al. 2020). A reflective portfolio of showcased activities, known as an educator's reflective document or teaching portfolio, can complement the educator's CV by giving additional evidence of the scholarly approach that underpins how and why particular teaching and educational leadership approaches were used (Academy of Medical Educators 2021; Hines et al. 2020; Shinkai et al. 2018; Simpson et al. 2007). The portfolio may be framed by a position description; an educational philosophy statement, also known as a teaching philosophy, that articulates the principles underlying an educator's approach to teaching and educational leadership; and a statement of five-year goals (Gusic et al. 2007, 2013; Hines et al. 2020; Schönwetter et al. 2002). This is followed by summaries that showcase the scholarly approach, importance, creativity, innovation, and impact of a selection of educational activities (Gusic et al. 2007, 2013; Hines et al. 2020; Shinkai et al. 2018; Simpson et al. 2007). Appendices can be used to provide detailed supporting evidence for activities highlighted in the portfolio entries. Clear and succinct presentation of quantitative and qualitative data using reader-friendly formatting such as tables, figures, graphs, and white space aids subsequent review (Baldwin et al. 2012; Simpson et al. 2007).

Together, the educator's CV, portfolio, and appendices form a professional dossier that can be used to showcase the educator's teaching and educational leadership activities for career advancement decisions (Academy of Medical Educators 2021; Hines et al. 2020; Teaching Academy 2022). Several guidelines, toolboxes, and templates exist for structuring the educator's professional dossier to showcase activities and outcomes (Academy of Medical Educators 2021; Gusic et al. 2013, 2014; Simpson et al. 2007; Teaching Academy 2022). Table 16.1 provides an outline of the components of an educator's professional dossier designed to showcase evidence for teaching and educational leadership activities based on the dossier format from the Regional Teaching Academy of the West Region Consortium of Colleges of Veterinary Medicine (Teaching Academy 2022). Figure 16.1 presents example extracts from an educator's reflective document based on the template from the Regional Teaching Academy (Teaching Academy 2022).

Table 16.1 Components of an Educator's Professional Dossier Designed to Showcase Evidence for Teaching and Educational Leadership Activities.

Typical components of the Educator's Professional Dossier[a]		
Curriculum Vitae	**Portfolio**	**Appendices**
Section: Teaching 1) Teaching 2) Mentoring and advising 3) Learner assessment or outcome assessment 4) Educational research and scholarship 5) Curriculum and program development 6) Educational leadership and administration Other sections of the CV detail achievements in the other areas of the educator's work appointment, e.g., professional education, employment history, research, service, outreach, etc.	1) Position description 2) Educational philosophy statement/ Teaching philosophy 3) Five-year goals 4) Executive summary of achievements highlighted in the portfolio entries 5) Series of portfolio entries that showcase selected teaching and educational leadership activities	Series of appendices that provide detailed supporting evidence for the portfolio entries

Note. Based on the educator's professional dossier from the [a]Academy of Medical Educators at the University of California San Francisco School of Medicine and the Regional Teaching Academy of the West Region Consortium of Colleges of Veterinary Medicine (Academy of Medical Educators 2021; Hines et al. 2020; Teaching Academy 2022).

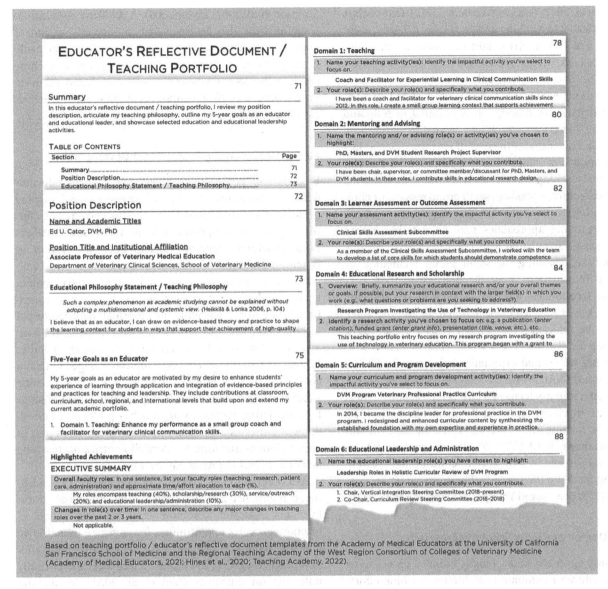

Figure 16.1 Example Extracts from an Educator's Reflective Document.

Part 3: Structure of this Chapter

The sections of this chapter are structured according to the six broadly applicable domains that typically characterize educator effort (Hines et al. 2020):

1) Teaching
2) Mentoring and advising
3) Learner assessment or outcome assessment
4) Educational research and scholarship
5) Curriculum and program development
6) Educational leadership and administration

Each section contains a review of relevant principles and literature, as well as suggestions for how activities might be documented in an educator's professional dossier to demonstrate evidence of not only quantity but also of quality and a scholarly approach.

Section 2: Teaching

Part 1: Describing Teaching

Traditional methods of documenting teaching for career advancement focus on quantifying teaching efforts. This includes lists of courses taught and the teaching hours involved, what years and semesters they were taught, and the numbers and level of learners involved – undergraduate, professional, or postgraduate (American Association of University Professors [AAUP] 1975; Gusic et al. 2007;

Simpson et al. 2007; Teaching Academy 2022). Out-of-class activities related to teaching and professional development seminars and workshops taught to colleagues may also be included (AAUP 1975; Glassick et al. 1997; Gusic et al. 2007). However, quantitative descriptions alone provide little to no evidence of teaching context and strategy. Additional narrative description is required to fully and accurately describe teaching activities (Simpson et al. 2007). This includes the type of teaching, such as lecture, laboratory, or clinical teaching, and a brief description of the teaching format, such as traditional lecture, interactive lecture, workshop, small group session, or clinical precepting (Gusic et al. 2007; Teaching Academy 2022). Specific teaching approaches may be detailed within these, such as team-based learning, case-based learning, problem-based learning, or small group facilitation or coaching. Information about the delivery method, e.g., online or face-to-face, and the location of the teaching audience, e.g., local, regional, national, or international, may also be relevant to document (Gusic et al. 2007). Explaining the alignment of teaching goals and effort with institutional values and expectations can provide further useful context (AAUP 1975; Benton and Young 2018). For example, if a primary focus of a unit is on teaching clinical content to veterinary students, then articulating how an educator's teaching fulfills this aim can enhance a case for career advancement (AAUP 1975; Benton and Young 2018; Theall 2017). In all cases, the specific contribution to teaching being made by the individual educator must be clear (AAUP 1975; Benton and Young 2018; Simpson et al. 2007).

Part 2: Demonstrating a Scholarly Approach

A scholarly approach to teaching is founded on engaging with the educator community to inform teaching efforts through published literature and best practices (Simpson et al. 2007). Engagement is followed by systematically designing and implementing the teaching activity, critically reflecting on the outcomes, and making further changes for ongoing improvement (Simpson et al. 2007; Teaching Academy 2022). The scholarly approaches adopted by an educator in their teaching can be articulated in the educator's portfolio, starting with the educational philosophy statement. A systematic approach to teaching can also be demonstrated through constructive alignment of intended learning outcomes or objectives, student assessment, and teaching activities in the process of "backward design" (Biggs 2003; Wiggins and McTighe 2005). Demonstrating alignment of learning objectives with curriculum goals, graduate attributes, and relevant education frameworks and standards provides additional evidence for a systematic approach to teaching (Baldwin et al. 2012;

Simpson et al. 2007; Taylor 2009). A scholarly approach to teaching may also be evidenced in scholarly design of enduring instructional materials that are used repeatedly or used by others, such as audiovisual resources, teaching cases, textbooks or textbook chapters, and shared test questions (Gusic et al. 2013; Simpson et al. 2004, 2007; Teaching Academy 2022).

Part 3: Documenting Professional Development

Engaging in professional development as an educator demonstrates a commitment to effectiveness and ongoing professional growth (AAUP 1975). This encompasses formal teaching development such as professional certifications, teaching programs, formal peer observation or coaching programs, conferences, workshops, and seminars. It also encompasses informal teaching development such as independent reading and peer review of educational literature, engaging in informal observation of teaching, and creating a personalized professional development plan based on critically reflective practice. Professional development opportunities engaged with and completed may be listed in the educator's CV (Teaching Academy 2022). The educator's portfolio provides scope for articulating a scholarly approach to professional development either as a complete portfolio entry or as part of appropriate preparation for portfolio entries on teaching activities (Teaching Academy 2022).

Peer observation of teaching, also known as peer coaching, can enhance teaching practices for individual educators and educator communities. Peer observation of teaching provides opportunities for engaging in collective dialogue about teaching and learning, experimenting with new practices, giving and receiving feedback, and critically reflecting on outcomes (Bell et al. 2020; Benton and Young 2018; Bernstein et al. 2000; Theall 2017). Though peer observation may be used as part of evaluating teaching, most peer coaching programs in medical schools accredited by the Association of American Medical Colleges are structured to provide formative feedback with the sole purpose of improving teaching (Bell et al. 2020). Observers or coaches may be colleagues or peers who are internal to the educator's teaching unit, department, or college; faculty development specialists; or external reviewers (Benton and Young 2018).

It is important for rigor that a standardized tool and process is used for peer observation, and that observers are trained, rather than observation being casual, one-time, and uncritically positive (Hines et al. 2020). Peer observation of teaching often starts with a review of course materials such as syllabi, teaching goals, test questions, and instructional methods (AAUP 1975; Benton and Young 2018;

Bernstein et al. 2000; Teaching Academy 2022). Collegial discussion with sharing of goals, evidence, and experience may then occur in advance of scheduled teaching observation sessions (Bell et al. 2020; Bernstein et al. 2000; Sullivan et al. 2012). This allows the observation process and feedback to be tailored to the educator's context and goals (Bernstein et al. 2000; Sullivan et al. 2012). This preparatory discussion is followed by direct observation of teaching sessions by one or more observers, followed by feedback and collaborative discussion (Bell et al. 2020; Bernstein et al. 2000; Sullivan et al. 2012; Teaching Academy 2022). Critical reflection on feedback received, further investigation if needed, and setting new goals for teaching performance complete the cycle of reflective practice (Boud 1985; Simpson et al. 2007; Sullivan et al. 2012). Portfolio entries and a summary report of process and outcomes can be used to document engagement with and results of the peer observation process (Simpson et al. 2007; Sullivan et al. 2012).

Documenting reflective practice that is based on self-examination and collegial discussion of data arising from teaching activities as part of professional development can be a useful addition to an educational portfolio (AAUP 1975; Benton and Young 2018; Svinicki 2017). For example, an initial self-analysis of teaching practices and feedback from students and colleagues may identify a need for improvement in knowledge, skill, or performance (Benton and Young 2018). Discussion with and input from colleagues can help to motivate and guide these analyses and balance interpretations arising from them (AAUP 1975; Hoyt and Pallett 1999). The educator can develop a professional development plan with clearly articulated goals and rationale, identify and engage with relevant professional development opportunities, and critically reflect on how their own learning may improve their teaching (Baldwin et al. 2012; Boud 1985; Svinicki 2017). The outcomes considered beneficial can be applied in teaching, assessed, and critically reflected upon as part of a scholarly approach to teaching (Glassick 2000). Focusing on a limited number of teaching components to develop at a time helps to sustain motivation and build teacher self-efficacy (Benton and Young 2018; Hoyt and Pallett 1999). Improvement in performance indicated by progressive student evaluation ratings, peer observation and coaching feedback, and annual performance review evaluations by department heads can be used to document evidence of increasing effectiveness in teaching (Benton and Young 2018; Hoyt and Pallett 1999; Svinicki 2017).

Part 4: Assessing Teaching

First and foremost, educator and administrator buy-in and mutual understanding are required for a successful program for assessing teaching effectiveness. The importance of assessment, evaluation, and measurement at all levels of higher education has increased over the last 25 years, partly because of higher stakeholder expectations of accountability (Chapman and Joines 2017; Estelami 2015; Leveille 2006; Lombardi 2013; Warman 2015). It is important to assure higher education stakeholders – students and their families, administrators, accrediting bodies, governing boards, and legislators – that colleges and universities are fulfilling their duty to educate students and prepare graduates (Chapman and Joines 2017; Estelami 2015; Lombardi 2013; McCarthy 2012). Evaluating teaching is one form of assessment to gauge the success of students' education. Additionally, the American Veterinary Medical Association's (AVMA 2021) Council on Education requires that all accredited veterinary schools collect "sufficient qualitative and quantitative information" to ensure "instructional quality and effectiveness" (p. 27). In this section, several different evaluation methods are described that taken together, comprise a holistic program for assessing teaching. A successful program will likely require stakeholder education on appropriate use of student evaluations of teaching (SETs) combined with additional measures of teaching quality (Addison and Stowell 2012; McKeachie 1969) (Figure 16.2).

Student Evaluations of Teaching (SETs)

SETs in higher education have existed for nearly 100 years (Addison and Stowell 2012), and student feedback is an important part of the evaluation of teaching effectiveness. Originally, SETs were intended as formative assessments to be used by instructors to improve their teaching (Smalzried and Remmers 1943). In the 1950s, the focus began to shift

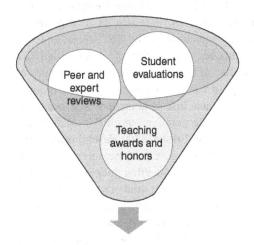

Holistic assessment of teaching

Figure 16.2 Components of a Holistic Assessment of Teaching Program.

toward summative use of SETs (Addison and Stowell 2012), and by 1993, 86% of higher education institutions were using SETs (Hoefer et al. 2012). The summative function of SETs is a source of controversy because administrators now use them to contribute to decisions about faculty career advancement and salary (Algozzine et al. 2004). This summative function has made SETs one of the most researched and debated topics in academia (Beran et al. 2012; Clayson 2009). Still, most SETs have been found to be valid and reliable instruments (Adams 2012; Addison and Stowell 2012; Hativa 2013; McCarthy 2012).

Colleges of veterinary medicine use SETs for evaluating both teaching in a classroom setting and clinical teaching in a hospital or practice setting (Fossum et al. 1993). An SET form typically contains a set of Likert scale-type items that assess how well an instructor establishes a positive learning environment, promotes understanding and retention of information, evaluates learner achievement of desired outcomes, and provides feedback to learners (Rhind and Bell 2017). The quantitative, numeric scale data resulting from these items are summarized as means for a given course or rotation/clerkship and over a given period, such as a semester or clinical year. Qualitative comments are typically also solicited and included in summary reports for the same parameters described above.

Persistent Misconceptions

Despite widespread use of SETs, many instructors perceive SETs as a platform for students to vent frustrations and express anger, at the detriment of educator career advancement (Eckhaus and Davidovitch 2019; Nasser and Fresko 2002). Results from studies on the relationship between grades and SETs are conflicting, but a positive correlation between grades and SET scores has been found to range between 0.14 and 0.47 (Aleamoni 1999; Hativa 2013; Marsh and Roche 1997). In those studies, as expected or actual final grades increased, so did SET scores, and vice versa. Such results beg the question of whether high SET scores are a product of grading leniency or an indicator of student learning. In contrast, other research has brought into question the idea that grading leniency positively affects SET data (Algozzine et al. 2004; Marsh and Roche 1997; Nasser and Fresko 2002). Several researchers have shown that SETs are more than measures of popularity and that students are qualified judges of teaching (Nasser and Fresko 2002). In fact, students have been found to be as effective at evaluating teaching as recent graduates (Hativa 2013; Theall and Franklin 2001). Learners are uniquely situated to consistently evaluate teaching because they are participating in longitudinal evaluation. Peer and administrator perspectives are often cross-sectional, and their content knowledge hinders their ability to fully appreciate the perspective of a novice (Hativa 2013; Theall and Franklin 2001).

When compared to other measures of instructional effectiveness, SETs have generally been found to be valid and reliable, and minimally affected by common biases when used for summative and formative purposes (Adams 2012; Addison and Stowell 2012; Hativa 2013; McCarthy 2012). What has been found to positively affect student ratings includes prior student interest in the subject being taught and, perhaps surprisingly, a more difficult workload (Adams 2012; Marsh and Roche 1997). Researchers exploring gender bias in a veterinary student population looked at retrospective data from 1981 to 1991 and found that women faculty were more highly rated than men for every evaluation parameter (Christopher and Leskosky 1997). Others have found that female instructors are sometimes rated lower by male students and higher by female students, and lower ratings have been seen with young female instructors (Basow and Martin 2012).

Evidence-Based Recommendations and Best Practices for SET Use

Advice for Instructors Instructors seeking to use SETs to improve their teaching might start by reviewing the numeric results for each item and then reviewing written comments in consideration of the numeric results. Some points to keep in mind during this process (I. Lane, personal communication, June 21, 2022):

- Recognize that a 3 on a 5-point scale is the visual average for students.
- While all questions provide input on teaching quality, "global" questions are most valid in reflecting overall teaching effectiveness. These questions usually are phrased as, "This instructor's overall effectiveness is. . ." or something similar and are usually the key numeric measure used in summative reviews, such as educator dossiers.
- Compare current numeric results to previous results. Use a spreadsheet or table to track results over time.
- Identify items with strong numeric results and items with weaker results. Consider these results in relation to primary teaching and course objectives (some items will be less relevant than others).
- Review written comments and look for consistent or repeated comments related to content and rigor of the material, organization of material, delivery or personal style/enthusiasm, and interactions with students. Organizing comments into these four categories better enables seeing and making sense of patterns.
- Avoid focusing on isolated, irrelevant, or unprofessional comments.
- Compare feedback gained from SETs to information gained from peer review of teaching or other sources.

- Determine one or two areas for improvement and determine ways to develop skills in these areas.
- Summarize reflections in written form for use in future career advancement or award application documents.
- Look for trends indicating improvement (or sustained outstanding performance).

Instructors may also use professional teaching consultants, trusted colleagues, and/or mentors to help make meaning of SET results and exercise reflective practice (Beran et al. 2012; Carmack and LeFebvre 2019; Ismail et al. 2012; Marsh and Roche 1997).

Advice for Peer Reviewers, Department Heads, and Promotion and Tenure Committees Those reviewing summaries of SETs should avoid reviewing one set of evaluations in isolation. Instead, focus on individual efforts and compare an instructor's current and past performance, rather than comparing one educator to another. This helps foster a mindset of developing better teaching, instills confidence, treats individuals fairly, and leads to growth and success (I. Lane, personal communication, June 21, 2022).

- Consider results in relation to the instructor's primary teaching and course objectives (some items will be less relevant than others and should bear less weight).
- Compare feedback gained from student evaluations to information gained from peer review of teaching or other sources.
- In collaboration with the instructor, determine one or two areas that provide opportunities for improvement, and determine ways to help the instructor develop materials or skills in these areas.
- Consider SET results in context with other documentation about teaching, such as self-assessment and peer review, to form a more comprehensive basis for evaluation (Addison and Stowell 2012; McKeachie 1969; Nasser and Fresko 2002; Wilson and Ryan 2012).

The scholarly consensus is that SETs should be used as part of a *holistic* framework for assessing teaching quality. Therefore, SETs should not be used in isolation; rather, they should be used to document patterns in an individual's teaching over time. Evaluation of teaching is more reliable when it is based on multiple measures. Lastly, as adult learning scholar Brookfield (2015) notes, instructors need to be "able to teach in creative and purposeful ways with a minimum of external interference. . . [with] a buffer that allows us to try things out. . . without immediate institutional punishment" (p. 253).

Peer and Expert Review
Formal reviews of teaching efforts by educational peers and experts offer another measure of teaching quality and effectiveness as part of a balanced, holistic evaluation system (AAUP 1975; Benton and Young 2018; Simpson et al. 2004). This review may be based on written materials and/or direct observation of teaching, with the results captured using standardized rubrics that may include overall ratings for performance (Benton and Young 2018; Hines et al. 2020; Teaching Academy 2022). Direct observation of teaching by internal or external reviewers gathers observational evidence of teaching performance that may be used to complement SETs (AAUP 1975; Benton and Young 2018). However, reviewers undertaking teaching observations must keep in mind that teachers' performance may be negatively impacted by stress and anxiety associated with being reviewed (Theall 2017). While external observers might be considered more reliable in assessing teaching practices, logistics and resource constraints may preclude their systematic involvement in directly observing face-to-face teaching (AAUP 1975). Instead, external observers may be invited to provide formal reviews of teaching on an individual case basis as warranted (AAUP 1975).

Review of written materials may also be used to assess teaching quantity, quality, effectiveness, and impact. Materials reviewed may include the educator's position description, CV, course materials, SETs, summary letters from peer observations of teaching, educational philosophy statement, and scholarly approaches to teaching detailed in a reflective portfolio (Bell et al. 2020; Glassick et al. 1997; Hines et al. 2020; Simpson et al. 2004). For ease of review, these materials may be collected into an educator's professional dossier based on standardized document formats with sufficient detail to facilitate effective and efficient review, including focused templates to structure and guide teaching portfolio entries (Hines et al. 2020; Shinkai et al. 2018; Teaching Academy 2022). Rigorous assessment of the dossier by members of an independent external review committee that comprises educational peers and experts from other institutions, and that is summarized in a letter of external review, provides internal evaluators, such as departmental colleagues and administrators, with an additional measure of an educator's teaching quality and effectiveness (Hines et al. 2020). Engaging in external reviews is recommended, where available, for educators with significant teaching responsibilities, or those who consider teaching as an essential part of their professional identity (Hines et al. 2020).

Teaching Awards and Honors
Another component in holistic evaluation of teaching is formal recognition of teaching improvement and teaching excellence. Nominations for teaching awards and honors most often originate with students or peers but might also come from administrators or committees (Seppala and

Smith 2020). Opportunities for teaching honors range from the department level to the college or school, university, and national levels. Regardless of their origin or level, teaching awards can be valuable evidence of effective teaching (Huggett et al. 2012; Zhu and Turcic 2018). To be considered for an award, nominees typically submit formal materials that often include a reflection component.

Teaching awards have been shown to motivate and encourage instructors to try new strategies to further enhance student learning (Seppala and Smith 2020), as well as to contribute to career advancement (Huggett et al. 2012; Zhu and Turcic 2018). To maximize the motivation of teaching awards, these honors should be considered in career advancement and performance review criteria (Seppala and Smith 2020; Zhu and Turcic 2018). Awards as evidence of teaching quality are most valuable and useful when their evaluative criteria and standards, from nomination to selection, are clear (Huggett et al. 2012). Many award programs' criteria are vague and do not enable objective differentiation between candidates (Chism 2006). An example of a transparent teaching award is the American Association of Veterinary Medical Colleges (AAVMC) Distinguished Veterinary Teacher Award. The AAVMC shares on its website what materials are submitted, what criteria are considered, and a list of past recipients. When considering teaching awards for career advancement, such information should be compared to the values and expectations of the institution, as well as the instructor's effort allocation, also known as appointment description, and rank (Huggett et al. 2012).

Section 3: Mentoring and Advising

Some schools of veterinary medicine make a distinction between the roles of mentors and advisors. Advisors are usually those who provide guidance toward meeting academic requirements and recommend resources to meet academic and career goals (Frei et al. 2010; Woods et al. 2010). Mentors guide mentees toward their highest potential in personal and professional development (Frei et al. 2010). True advisor/advisee partnerships are usually assigned, whereas mentoring relationships often develop organically based on mutual interests between the learner and mentor. Of course, mentorship can develop from an advising relationship, and one can certainly serve as an advisor and mentor simultaneously. Regardless of how we define these terms, the success of the learner is a measure of the success of the mentor or advisor (Lunsford 2012). Evidence of learner success depends on the type of learner – veterinary professional student, master's or doctoral graduate student, intern, or resident – and the goals and expected learner outcomes of a given program.

The quality of advising and mentoring relationships may be demonstrated in an educator portfolio by sharing mentee/advisee goals, how those goals were realigned over time to meet changing learner needs, and how milestones and goals were ultimately met (Gusic et al. 2013). Quantitative measures are outlined in Table 16.2. Additionally, dissemination and recognition by others of the value of mentoring and advising methods is an indicator of educator impact. For example, have the methods been published or presented (via invitation or otherwise)? Have others adopted the methods? Have the methods been recognized with honors or awards? (Gusic et al. 2013).

Recognizing mentorship and advising as a formal teaching activity that may contribute to educator career advancement helps provide educators with the protected time necessary to make these important connections with learners and rewards educators for their efforts (Frei et al. 2010; Gusic et al. 2013; Woods et al. 2010). In 2019, the mentoring and advising domain was being considered in nearly half of US medical colleges' promotion and tenure decisions (Ryan et al. 2019). Table 16.3 presents a completed example of an educator's portfolio entry for the mentoring and advising domain based on the educator's reflective document/teaching portfolio template from the Regional Teaching Academy of the West Region Consortium of Colleges of Veterinary Medicine (Academy of Medical Educators 2021; Teaching Academy 2022).

Section 4: Learner Assessment or Outcome Assessment

In a survey that explored the types of educational activities used by committees evaluating faculty promotion and tenure, learner assessment was noted as being considered by more medical schools than educational scholarship (Ryan et al. 2019). More broadly, in US veterinary education, the AVMA Council on Education expects student achievement to be included in its accreditation standard for outcomes assessment (AVMA 2021). Although including course syllabi summaries in an educator's dossier will enable a review team to determine the quantity and perhaps the context of assessment methods, more detailed indicators are needed to demonstrate quality and scholarly approach (Gusic et al. 2013).

Again, evidence of development of quality assessment methods begins with backward design (Wiggins and McTighe 2005), which starts with quality intended learning outcomes/objectives or competencies that specify what learners are expected to be able to do at the end of a given experience (laboratory, lecture, course, rotation, clinical program, etc.). The content of exemplar assessments should

Table 16.2 Quantitative Measures of Learner Success in Advising and Mentoring Relationships.

Measure	Student type			
	Professional	Graduate (non-DVM)	Interns	Residents
Merit-based grants, scholarships, and honors	X	X	X	X
Scholarly products, such as publications or presentations	X	X	X	X
Advanced training or job placement	X	X	X	X
Passing the North American Veterinary Licensing Examination (NAVLE)	X			
Student evaluations of teaching		X		X
Time to degree completion		X		
Contribution of mentorship to others		X	X	X
Achievement of milestones			X	
Progression on mock board exams				X
Clinician evaluations of competence				X
Passing board examinations				X

Note: AAVMC 2018; Collins 2005; Fascetti 2008; Gusic et al. 2013; Lunsford 2012; Newkirk et al. 2020.

reflect the learning objectives. Showing the relationship between learning objectives and written assessments may be accomplished with an exam blueprint that maps exam questions or assignment prompts to the desired objectives (Gusic et al. 2013). When using multiple choice questions, item analysis psychometrics will help ensure the validity of the assessment (e.g., discrimination index, point biserial, or Kuder–Richardson Formula 20 [KR-20] values; ExamSoft 2022). When synthesized, such information, taken together with learner and peer feedback, provides guidance to instructors on how to improve exams and exam questions (Gusic et al. 2013). Support for the quality of an assessment will likely also include de-identified, summary comparisons of learner performance over time.

To demonstrate an understanding of how assessment not only measures learning, but also contributes to learning, educators may include in their educator's dossier a suitable range of implemented assessment methods that are supported by literature. Examples of such variety include formative and summative, direct and indirect, written and practical, and low- and high-stakes methods. It is also important to list and describe professional development in assessment activities, such as those aimed at improved question writing, clinical skill assessment, effective test construction, rubric creation, competency-based education, assessment theory, etc. (Gusic et al. 2013; Salisbury and Cornell 2022). Finally, involvement in assessment

activities as part of teaching service for the institution includes training for and participation on teams to create, administer, and/or evaluate objective structured clinical exams (OSCEs), practical exams, simulated skill assessments, rubrics, comprehensive exams, theses, and dissertations. National program leadership roles in assessment consist of such activities as question writing, exam creation, and/or portfolio review for high-stakes exams like the North American Veterinary Licensing Examination (NAVLE) and specialty board certifications.

Section 5: Educational Research and Scholarship

Educational research and scholarship are built on scholarly engagement with the education community and a commitment to teaching quality and effectiveness (AAUP 1975; Gusic et al. 2014; Shulman 1998; Simpson et al. 2007; Sullivan 2018). Educational scholarship produces educational resources that have been publicly disseminated for peer review, critique, and building upon by others (Gusic et al. 2014; Shulman 1998; Simpson et al. 2007; Sullivan 2018). Educational research focuses on advancing knowledge of education and learning processes and may be directed at any of the other five domains of educator activity (American Educational Research Association 2022;

Table 16.3 Example of an Educator's Portfolio Entry for Mentoring and Advising.

Domain 2: Mentoring and Advising[a]

1) Name the mentoring and/or advising role(s) or activity(ies) you have chosen to highlight:

Doctoral, Master's, and DVM Student Research Project Supervisor

2) Your role(s): Describe your role(s) and specifically what you contribute.

I have been chair, supervisor, or committee member for doctoral, master's, and veterinary student research projects. In these roles, I educate and train students in research design, qualitative data analysis, academic writing, time management, and oral presentation skills.

3) Mentees and amount of contact: Describe types, levels, and numbers of mentees; amount of contact you have with them.

Since 2014, I have been chair or committee member for four doctoral students (three current) and four master's students, and primary or co-supervisor for four veterinary student research projects. I meet with students weekly when chair/primary supervisor and as needed when a committee member/co-supervisor.

4) Goals and learning objectives: List goals and learning objectives of program and/or individual mentees. If these are extensive, provide just a few illustrative examples.

My goal for research student advising is to foster student curiosity and creativity, engender commitment to academic rigor, and promote clear and engaging presentation of research processes and outcomes. Program learning objectives are aligned with those of my department's doctoral program:

1) Enable students to develop as successful professionals for highly competitive positions in academia, industry, and government.
2) Prepare students to be effective researchers (clinical, translational, and basic sciences).
3) Enhance the national and international visibility of graduate education and research in the department, college, and university.

5) Methods: Describe the methods used for instruction, how these align with objectives, and rationale for choices.

I adopt a student-centered, conceptual-change approach to my teaching by questioning students about their thoughts, knowledge, skill proficiency, perceptions, and assumptions related to their research content and process (Brew 2001; Ramsden 2003). I provide detailed formative feedback on my students' written work and oral presentations to help them prepare for successful publication of their research in a variety of formats (Hattie and Timperley 2007). I encourage my students to present their work at conferences and publish peer-reviewed journal articles to establish them as independent scholars in the discipline. Through this, I achieve program learning objectives 1–3 above.

I meet with students weekly when chair/primary supervisor to maintain open channels of communication and support during their research journey. During these meetings, I not only help students move their research projects forward by providing guidance on research methods and publication, but also enquire about how they are doing personally. Knowing the challenges my students are facing helps me to modulate my expectations and offer support where needed.

6) Rationale: Describe why and how you chose the mentoring and advising method(s) you use.

My overarching aim in my work is to help members of the veterinary profession achieve success in their chosen career. This goal underpins all my teaching, including mentoring and advising veterinary, master's, and doctoral research students. My goal for all my research students is that they make a unique contribution to the discipline based on thorough knowledge and rigorous research methods. These contributions may be in a variety of formats, including presentations, dissertations, and peer-reviewed research articles. My desire for my doctoral and master's students specifically is that they will develop a unique professional identity that will guide and sustain their professional life and contributions to society during their subsequent career. I apply evidence-based principles and practices for advancing the conceptual and practical skill development of my research students. I have indicated some of these principles in my citations to peer-reviewed literature above. I first learned these principles and practices through experience and training as an undergraduate and postgraduate research student. I have since honed my understanding through formal and informal training in research supervision and processes as a faculty member. Particularly helpful was the Foundations of Research Supervision program that I completed in 2012.

7) Results and impact: Describe evidence of mentee ratings for mentoring, learning outcomes, career trajectories, impact on educational programs, and/or mentoring awards.

In total, my students have submitted 11 peer-reviewed research articles, given 13 conference presentations, and won three awards. Three are now faculty or adjunct faculty at veterinary schools in the USA or internationally.

8) Reflective critique: Describe your reflections, what went well, and plans for improvement.

I am pleased with the outcomes achieved by my research students in their research productivity and career trajectories. The research supervision training programs I have undertaken and my experiences as a faculty member have enabled me to critically reflect on my performance through engaging with the literature, peer and student feedback, and self-reflection (Brookfield 1995). I have recently learned values-based (Kraemer 2011) and affiliative (Goleman et al. 2002) leadership strategies in professional development for my administrative roles. I plan to review and synthesize the resources I have on these strategies and research supervision to identify additional ways in which I can support the personal and professional development of my research students.

9) Dissemination: If applicable, describe how your efforts have been recognized by others externally through peer review, dissemination, use by others, or mentoring awards nationally.

In 2018, I was awarded an Academic Advisor Excellence Award by the Graduate and Professional Student Association in recognition of my skills in and commitment to mentoring and advising.

Note: Portfolio entry is based on the teaching portfolio / educator's reflective document template from the [a] Academy of Medical Educators at the University of California San Francisco School of Medicine and the Regional Teaching Academy of the West Region Consortium of Colleges of Veterinary Medicine (Hines et al. 2020; Teaching Academy 2022).

Simpson et al. 2007). These activities may be listed and/or tabulated in the educator's CV, as well as showcased and expanded upon in the educator's portfolio.

Engagement with the education community through educational research and scholarship may be demonstrated through journal publications, textbooks or textbook chapters, conference presentations, invited talks, consulting for other schools on teaching, peer review work, and editorials (AAUP 1975; Baldwin et al. 2012; Gusic et al. 2013; Simpson et al. 2007; Teaching Academy 2022). Documenting the details of internal and external grants used to support educational research provides additional evidence of quality, impact, and engagement with the education community (Simpson et al. 2007). This includes details of the funding agency, amount, title, and investigators, together with an additional brief description of the focus of the grant and the educator's specific role in delivering the intended outcomes (Teaching Academy 2022).

Evidence for the impact of educational research and scholarship can be provided using both traditional metrics and "grey metrics" (Friesen et al. 2019; Glassick et al. 1997; Simpson et al. 2007). Publication citation rates, journal rankings and impact factors, and social media metrics can be used to indicate the quality and impact of peer-reviewed scholarship and research (Cabrera et al. 2017; Teaching Academy 2022). Adding a description of the readership and practical impact of an educational journal in a specific field can be important if journal impact factors based on article citation rates do not align with these. Noting the specific contribution of the educator to each publication, including if the first author is a mentored student, is also informative. "Grey metrics" may be used to illustrate additional meaningful impact in the field (Friesen et al. 2019). Evidence of engagement with and impact in the educator community can be shown by listing invited talks and conference presentations in the educator's CV, including whether submitted abstracts were peer-reviewed (AAUP 1975; Teaching Academy 2022). Evidence of adoption or adaption by others of the outcomes of educational scholarship provides additional evidence of impact (Gusic et al. 2014; Friesen et al. 2019; Teaching Academy 2022).

Section 6: Curriculum and Program Development

Educator contributions to curriculum and program development are likely to vary widely within and between schools and colleges of veterinary medicine. Curricular responsibilities could entail developing or revising sessions (lectures, laboratories, discussions, etc.), units/modules, courses, rotations/clerkships, semesters or years of a program, or an entire veterinary medical curriculum. Additionally, many of the components of curricular development and revision are intertwined with and closely linked to assessment, teaching practices, and evaluation of teaching. This section of the chapter first describes ways in which educators might contribute to curriculum development and then lists some best practices for documenting involvement in curriculum and program development for career advancement.

Standard 9 of the AVMA Council on Education's accreditation standards requires veterinary schools to review their curriculum as a whole at least every seven years and to use both qualitative and quantitative information in evaluating curricula (AVMA 2021). Therefore, ample opportunities exist for veterinary medical educators to become involved in curricular revision, even if one holds a relatively small teaching appointment. Here, ways to contribute to the curriculum are explored, starting with the session (micro) level and moving to the program (macro) level.

For anyone who teaches, curriculum development or revision begins with establishing or revising student learning objectives – statements of what students will be expected to do at the end of a given learning opportunity (Schoenfeld-Tacher and Sims 2013). As noted previously, this backward design approach is well established in the literature and can be used by everyone from instructors who teach lecture-based sessions to those who lead rounds in a clinical setting. At the micro level, curriculum development might include offering a new lecture, laboratory, elective, or topics rounds series. In contrast, curriculum revision might include revising an inherited lecture, laboratory, or topics rounds series and making decisions about what content to retain and what to replace or discard (O'Connor and Yanni 2013). Such work contributes to the larger curriculum through its contributions to the program's curriculum map, where it is important to identify the written, taught, learned, and assessed curricula (Lam and Tung 2016; Rackard and Cashman 2019).

Course-level development and revision follow the same principles as those at the session level but include the additional task of understanding and incorporating accreditation requirements (O'Connor and Yanni 2013). At this level, the process might also include deciding course content based on an alteration in contact or credit hours or on the availability of teaching staff or infrastructure. Educators might also have responsibility for coordinating or directing a course with various additional instructors, which necessitates sequencing of material for optimal student learning. At both the session and course levels, instructors might be contributing to curricular innovation by incorporating service learning, universal design, and/or inclusivity into a program of study (CAST n.d.; Milstein et al. 2022; Sathy and Hogan n.d.; Van Patten et al. 2021).

At a more macro level, educators might serve on curriculum committees or subcommittees within a veterinary school or the veterinary profession. Most veterinary colleges maintain a formal committee that guides the curriculum, but professional organizations such as the AAVMC also offer opportunities to engage in areas of curricular interest. For example, at the time of this writing, the AAVMC supports groups such as the Primary Care Veterinary Educators (PCVE), the Academic Veterinary Wellbeing Professionals (AVWP), the newly formed Academy of Veterinary Educators (AVE), the Council on Outcomes-based Veterinary Education (COVE), and three working groups in competency-based veterinary education.

Contributions to curriculum development may be quantified by listing time devoted, meetings attended, stakeholders involved, breadth and duration of work, invitations to provide educator development and/or peer review other curricula, and resulting scholarship. Documenting the quality of curriculum development efforts may be accomplished in an educator's portfolio with a narrative describing the application of models found in the literature, reviews from students and peers, evidence of trainee learning or effectiveness of the approach, and adoption by others (Gusic et al. 2013; Teaching Academy 2022). Grey metrics recommended for illustrating the impact of educational research (Friesen et al. 2019) may be expanded to include work in curricular development, revision, and reform to help establish faculty as change agents.

Section 7: Educational Leadership and Administration

Effective educational leadership and administration are vital for the ongoing success and impact of education programs (Boyer 2016; Gusic et al. 2014; Hines et al. 2020). Educational leadership and administration may be at several levels: it may be at the course level, e.g., as a course or rotation director; at a curricular oversight level, e.g., as chair of the curriculum committee; at a program level, e.g., as an associate dean for professional programs or academic affairs; or at a university level (Baldwin et al. 2012). It also encompasses leadership roles in regional, national, or international educational organizations (Gusic et al. 2014). As when documenting teaching practices, it is important to provide evidence of quantity, quality, effectiveness, impact, and a scholarly approach. Quantifying educational leadership and administration efforts includes the number and titles of roles with which an educator is engaged, the hours taken to serve in each of these roles, and the number of

constituents involved (Simpson et al. 2007). Effort and impact are further articulated through qualitative descriptions of the scope of the role, committee, or organization; the educator's specific contributions; individual and collective outcomes; and their impact.

Quantitative details and brief descriptions of educational leadership and administration efforts may be included in an educator's CV and expanded upon in an educator's portfolio. A scholarly approach to educational leadership and administration is demonstrated by evidence that approaches used are founded in the literature and best practices, including the way in which leadership is conceived of and approached within educational institutions (Ramsden 1998; Simpson et al. 2007). Establishing clear goals, engaging in adequate preparation, implementing appropriate methods, gaining significant results that are presented effectively for review by relevant constituents, and reflecting critically on processes and outcomes complete the components of a scholarly approach for assessment by reviewers (Glassick 2000; Glassick et al. 1997). Evidence of alignment with the institution's educational priorities can provide additional context for evaluating the importance and value of educational leadership and administration efforts (AAUP 1975).

Section 8: Institutional and Administrative Support for Teaching for Career Advancement: A Case Study

In 2002 at the University of Tennessee College of Veterinary Medicine, an office was created to emphasize enhancement of the learning environment. The need for the office was first conceived in the mid-1990s with a college curriculum renewal that included plans to integrate problem-based learning. Upon realizing the extensive effort required to implement problem-based learning into the curriculum, the dean of the college supported a proposal to restructure a faculty appointment to devote 50% effort toward the faculty development and direction required to achieve the college's curriculum goals (I. Lane, personal communication, June 21, 2022). In 2006, "strengthen all teaching programs to meet societal needs" was the first goal of a five-year college strategic plan. A group of three faculty members with an interest in veterinary medical education proposed a teaching academy model to help meet the strategic goal. Thereafter, this faculty-driven committee conducted a limited needs assessment, recruited core faculty as charter members, and sought formal recognition, through the college's executive committee, of the newly developed Master Teacher Program (MTP; April 2008). The MTP quickly became institutionalized, and faculty involvement was validated via recognition for participation in formal effort allocation, which serves as the college's de facto currency for faculty review, promotion, and tenure (Lane et al. 2020). The program and the college's devotion to teaching continue to be highlighted in the recruitment of new faculty members, and in 2016, MTP sessions were added to the list of approved continuing education units that faculty and staff may use to maintain their Tennessee veterinary professional licensure. Additionally, financial support has enabled faculty and staff to pursue professional development opportunities in veterinary medical education. In this case, college leadership promoted teaching as an important component in career advancement with their messaging, strategic goals, and budget decisions.

Section 9: Summary

Teaching and educational leadership activities may be grouped into six broad domains: teaching, mentoring and advising, learner assessment or outcome assessment, educational research and scholarship, curriculum and program development, and educational leadership and administration. Though few educators will have activities in all of these domains, the principles for documenting activities are similar across each domain. Evidence of quantity, quality, effectiveness, impact, and a scholarly approach is essential, as is a reader-friendly format that aids evaluation. An educator's professional dossier structured in alignment with these principles can be used to showcase excellence in educator activities and outcomes for career advancement decisions.

References

Academy of Medical Educators (2021). *Educator's Portfolio*. University of California San Francisco School of Medicine Center for Faculty Educators https://meded.ucsf.edu/faculty-educators/educators-portfolio.

Adams, C. (2012). On-line measures of student evaluation of instruction. In: *Effective Evaluation of Teaching: A Guide for Faculty and Administrators* (ed. M.E. Kite), 50–59. Society for the Teaching of Psychology.

Addison, W.E. and Stowell, J.R. (2012). Conducting research on student evaluations of teaching. In: *Effective Evaluation of Teaching: A Guide for Faculty and Administrators* (ed. M.E. Kite), 1–12. Society for the Teaching of Psychology.

Aleamoni, L.M. (1999). Student rating myths versus research facts from 1924 to 1998. *Journal of Personnel Evaluation in Education* 13: 153–166.

Algozzine, B., Beattie, J., Bray, M. et al. (2004). Student evaluation of college teaching: a practice in search of principles. *College Teaching* 52: 134–141. https://doi.org/10.3200/CTCH.52.4.132-141.

American Association of University Professors (1975). Statement on teaching evaluation. https://www.aaup.org/report/statement-teaching-evaluation (accessed 29 July 2023).

American Association of Veterinary Medical Colleges (2018). Veterinary internship guidelines. http://www.aavmc.org/assets/data-new/files/About_AAVMC/AAVMC%20Veterinary%20Internship%20Guidelines%20(ID%2096740)%20(ID%2096741).pdf (accessed 29 July 2023).

American Educational Research Association (2022). *What is education research?* https://www.aera.net/About-AERA/What-is-Education-Research (accessed 29 July 2023).

American Veterinary Medical Association Council on Education (2021, July). COE Accreditation Policies and Procedures: Requirements. https://www.avma.org/education/accreditation-policies-and-procedures-avma-council-education-coe/coe-accreditation-policies-and-procedures-requirements (accessed 29 July 2023).

Baldwin, C., Chandran, L., and Gusic, M. (2012). Educator evaluation guidelines. *MedEdPORTAL* 8: 9072. https://doi.org/10.15766/mep_2374-8265.9072.

Basow, S.A. and Martin, J. (2012). Bias in student evaluations. In: *Effective Evaluation of Teaching: A Guide for Faculty and Administrators* (ed. M.E. Kite), 40–49. Society for the Teaching of Psychology.

Bell, A.E., Meyer, H.S., and Maggio, L.A. (2020). Getting better together: a website review of peer coaching initiatives for medical educators. *Teaching and Learning in Medicine* 32 (1): 53–60. https://doi.org/10.1080/10401334.2019.1614448.

Benton, S.L. and Young, S. (2018). *IDEA Paper #69: Best Practices in the Evaluation of Teaching*. The IDEA Center https://www.ideaedu.org/Portals/0/Uploads/Documents/IDEA%20Papers/IDEA%20Papers/IDEA_Paper_69.pdf (accessed 29 July 2023).

Beran, T.N., Donnon, T., and Hecker, K. (2012). A review of student evaluation of teaching: applications to veterinary medical education. *Journal of Veterinary Medical Education* 39: 71–78. https://doi.org/10.3138/jvme.0311.037R.

Bernstein, D.J., Jonson, J., and Smith, K. (2000). An examination of the implementation of peer review of teaching. *New Directions for Teaching and Learning* 83: 73–86.

Biggs, J. (2003). *Teaching for Quality Learning at University: What the Student Does*, 2e. Open University Press.

Boud, D. (1985). Promoting reflection in learning: a model. In: *Reflection: Turning Experience into Learning* (ed.D. Boud, R. Keogh, and D. Walker), 170. Kogan Page.

Boyer, E.L. (2016). *Scholarship Reconsidered: Priorities of the Professoriate* (expanded ed.). Jossey-Bass.

Brew, A. (2001). Conceptions of research: a phenomenographic study. *Studies in Higher Education* 26:271–285.

Brookfield, S. (1995). *Becoming a Critically Reflective Teacher*. Jossey-Bass.

Brookfield, S.D. (2015). *The Skillful Teacher: On Technique, Trust, and Responsiveness in the Classroom*, 3e. Jossey-Bass.

Cabrera, D., Vartabedian, B.S., Spinner, R.J. et al. (2017). More than likes and tweets: creating social media portfolios for academic promotion and tenure. *Journal of Graduate Medical Education* 9 (4): 421–425. https://doi.org/10.4300/JGME-D-17-00171.1.

Carmack, H.J. and LeFebvre, L.E. (2019). "Walking on eggshells": traversing the emotional and meaning making processes surrounding hurtful course evaluations. *Communication Education* 68: 350–370. https://doi.org/10.1080/03634523.2019.1608366.

CAST (n.d.). UDL in higher ed. http://udloncampus.cast.org/page/udl_landing (accessed 29 July 2023).

Chapman, D.D. and Joines, J.A. (2017). Strategies for increasing response rates for online end-of-course evaluations. *International Journal of Teaching and Learning in Higher Education* 29: 47–60.

Chism, N.V.N. (2006). Teaching awards: what do they award? *The Journal of Higher Education* 77: 589–617.

Christopher, M.M. and Leskosky, L. (1997). Effect of faculty gender on veterinary student teaching evaluations. *Journal of Veterinary Medical Education* 24: 36–42.

Clayson, D.E. (2009). Student evaluations of teaching: are they related to what students learn? A meta-analysis and review of the literature. *Journal of Marketing Education* 31: 16–30.

Collins, H. (2005). Mentoring veterinary students. *Journal of Veterinary Medical Education* 32: 285–289.

Dweck, C.S. (2006). *Mindset: The New Psychology of Success*. Random House.

Eckhaus, E. and Davidovitch, N. (2019). How do academic faculty members perceive the effect of teaching surveys completed by students on appointment and promotion processes at academic institutions? A case study. *International Journal of Higher Education* 8: 171–180.

Estelami, H. (2015). The effects of survey timing on student evaluation of teaching measures obtained using online surveys. *Journal of Marketing Education* 37: 54–64.

ExamSoft (2022). White paper: Exam quality through the use of psychometric analysis. https://examsoft.com/white-papers/exam-quality-use-psychometric-analysis/?submissi onGuid=768db3dc-c679-452f-b7e4-256279a949bf (accessed 29 July 2023).

Fascetti, A.J. (2008). Resident and graduate training in veterinary nutrition. *Journal of Veterinary Medical Education* 35: 292–296.

Fossum, T.W., Ruoff, W.W., Rushton, W.T., and Paprock, K.E. (1993). Patterns of and criteria for evaluating clinical teaching performance: perceptions of a national sample of teaching veterinary clinicians. *Journal of Veterinary Medical Education* 20: 24–27.

Frei, E., Stamm, M., and Buddeberg-Fischer, B. (2010). Mentoring programs for medical students – a review of the PubMed literature 2000–2008. *BMC Medical Education* 10: 32.

Friesen, F., Baker, L.R., Ziegler, C. et al. (2019). Approaching impact meaningfully in medical education research. *Academic Medicine* 94: 955–961.

Glassick, C.E. (2000). Boyer's expanded definitions of scholarship, the standards for assessing scholarship, and the elusiveness of the scholarship of teaching. *Academic Medicine* 75: 877–880.

Glassick, C.E., Huber, M.T., and Maeroff, G.I. (1997). *Scholarship Assessed: Evaluation of the Professoriate*. Jossey-Bass.

Goleman, D., Boyatzis, R., and McKee, A. (2002). *Primal Leadership: Realizing the Power of Emotional Intelligence*. Harvard Business School Press.

Gusic, M.E., Chandran, L., Balmer, D. et al. (2007). Educator portfolio template of the academic pediatric Association's educational scholars program. *MedEdPORTAL* 3: 626. http://doi.org/10.15766/mep_2374-8265.626.

Gusic, M.E., Amiel, J., Baldwin, C.D. et al. (2013). Using the AAMC toolbox for evaluating educators: you be the judge! *MedEdPORTAL* 9: 9313. http://dx.doi.org/10.15766/mep_2374-8265.9313.

Gusic, M.E., Baldwin, C.D., Chandran, L. et al. (2014). Evaluating educators using a novel toolbox: applying rigorous criteria flexibly across institutions. *Academic Medicine* 89: 1006–1011. https://doi.org/10.1097/ACM.0000000000000233.

Hativa, N. (2013). *Student Ratings of Instruction: Recognizing Effective Teaching*. Oron Publications.

Hattie, J. and Timperley, H. (2007). The power of feedback. *Review of Educational Research* 77: 81–112.

Hines, S.A., Barr, M.C., Suchman, E. et al. (2020). An interinstitutional external peer-review process to evaluate educators at schools of veterinary medicine. *Journal of Veterinary Medical Education* 47: 535–545. https://doi.org/10.3138/jvme.2019-0094.

Hoefer, P., Yurkiewicz, J., and Byrne, J.C. (2012). The association between students' evaluation of teaching and grades. *Journal of Innovative Education* 10: 447–459.

Hoyt, D.P. and Pallett, W.H. (1999). *IDEA Paper #36: Appraising Teaching Effectiveness: Beyond Student Ratings.* IDEA Center https://www.ideaedu.org/idea_papers/appraising-teaching-effectiveness-beyond-student-ratings (accessed 29 July 2023).

Huggett, K.N., Greenberg, R.B., Rao, D. et al. (2012). The design and utility of institutional teaching awards: a literature review. *Medical Teacher* 34: 907–919.

Ismail, E.A., Buskist, W., and Groccia, J.E. (2012). *Effective Evaluation of Teaching: A Guide for Faculty and Administrators* (ed. M.E. Kite), 79–91. Society for the Teaching of Psychology.

Lam, B.H. and Tung, K.T. (2016). Curriculum mapping as deliberation–examining the alignment of subject learning outcomes and course curricula. *Studies in Higher Education* 41: 1371–1388.

Lane, I.F., Sims, M., Howell, N.E., and Bailey, M. (2020). Sustaining a collegewide teaching academy as a community: 10 years of experience with the master teacher program at the University of Tennessee College of Veterinary Medicine. *Journal of Veterinary Medical Education* 47: 384–394.

Leveille, D.E. (2006). *Accountability in Higher Education: A Public Agenda for Trust and Cultural Change.* Center for Studies in Higher Education.

Lombardi, J.V. (2013). *How Universities Work.* Johns Hopkins University Press.

Lunsford, A. (2012). Doctoral advising or mentoring? Effects on student outcomes. *Mentoring & Tutoring: Partnership in Learning* 20: 251–270.

Marsh, H.W. and Roche, L.A. (1997). Making students' evaluations of teaching effectiveness effective: the critical issues of validity, bias, and utility. *American Psychologist* 52: 1187–1197.

McCarthy, M.A. (2012). Using student feedback as *one* measure of faculty teaching effectiveness. In: *Effective Evaluation of Teaching: A Guide for Faculty and Administrators* (ed. M.E. Kite), 30–39. Society for the Teaching of Psychology.

McKeachie, W.J. (1969). Student ratings of faculty. *American Association of University Professors Bulletin* 55: 439–444.

Milstein, M.S., Gilbertson, M.L.J., Bernstein, L.A., and Hsue, W. (2022). Integrating the Multicultural Veterinary Medical Association actionables into diversity, equity, and inclusion curricula in United States veterinary colleges. *Journal of the American Veterinary Medical Association* https://doi.org/10.2460/javma.21.10.0459.

Nasser, F. and Fresko, B. (2002). Faculty views of student evaluation of college teaching. *Assessment & Evaluation in Higher Education* 27: 187–198.

Newkirk, K.M., Xiaocun, S., and Bailey, M.R. (2020). Correlation of mock board examination scores during anatomic pathology residency training with performance on the certifying exam. *Journal of Veterinary Medical Education* 47: 39–43.

O'Connor, L.G. and Yanni, C.K. (2013). Promotion and tenure in nursing education: lessons learned. *Journal of Nursing Education and Practice* 3: 78–88.

Rackard, S. and Cashman, D. (2019). Curriculum mapping as a tool for review of the professional veterinary medicine curriculum at University College Dublin–strategic and organizational considerations. *Journal of Veterinary Medical Education* 46: 278–288.

Ramsden, P. (1998). *Learning to Lead in Higher Education.* Routledge.

Ramsden, P. (2003). *Learning to Teach in Higher Education.* Routledge Falmer.

Rhind, S.W. and Bell, C.E. (2017). Assessing teaching effectiveness. In: *Veterinary Medical Education: A Practice Guide* (ed. J.L. Hodgson and J.M. Pelzer), 301–315. Wiley Blackwell.

Ryan, M.S., Tucker, C., DiazGranados, D., and Chandran, L. (2019). How are clinician-educators evaluated for educational excellence? A survey of promotion and tenure committee members in the United States. *Medical Teacher* 41: 927–933.

Salisbury, K. and Cornell, K. (2022). *Coaching in CBVE.* American Association of Veterinary Medical Colleges https://cbve.org/coaching-and-feedback?ss_source=sscampaigns&ss_campaign_id=6228b859c2c7 f60492fcac90&ss_email_id=6246fde5fe3e89546aa5a632&ss_campaign_name=CBVE+Newsletter-March+2022&ss_campaign_sent_date=2022-04-01T13%3A28%3A26Z (accessed 29 July 2023).

Sathy, V. and Hogan, K.A. (n.d.). *How to Make your Teaching more Inclusive: Advice Guide.* The Chronicle of Higher Education https://www.chronicle.com/article/how-to-make-your-teaching-more-inclusive/ (accessed 29 July 2023).

Schoenfeld-Tacher, R. and Sims, M.H. (2013). Course goals, competencies, and instructional objectives. *Journal of Veterinary Medical Education* 40: 139–144.

Schönwetter, D.J., Sokal, L., Friesen, M., and Taylor, K.L. (2002). Teaching philosophies reconsidered: a conceptual model for the development and evaluation of teaching philosophy statements. *The International Journal for Academic Development* 7 (1): 83–97.

Seppala, N. and Smith, C. (2020). Teaching awards in higher education: a qualitative study of motivation and outcomes. *Studies in Higher Education* 45: 1398–1412.

Shinkai, K., Chen, C.A., Schwartz, B.S. et al. (2018). Rethinking the educator portfolio: an innovative criteria-based model. *Academic Medicine* 93: 1024–1028. https://doi.org/10.1097/ACM.0000000000002005.

Shulman, L.S. (1998). Course anatomy: the dissection and analysis of knowledge through teaching. In: *The Course Portfolio: How Faculty Can Examine their Teaching to Advance Practice and Improve Student Learning* (ed. P. Hutchings), 5–12. American Association for Higher Education https://eric.ed.gov/?id=ED441393 (accessed 29 July 2023).

Simpson, D., Hafler, J., Brown, D., and Wilkerson, L. (2004). Documentation systems for educators seeking academic promotion in U.S. medical schools. *Academic Medicine* 79: 783–790.

Simpson, D., Fincher, R.-M.E., Hafler, J.P. et al. (2007). Advancing educators and education by defining the components and evidence associated with educational scholarship. *Medical Education* 41: 1002–1009. https://doi.org/10.1111/j.1365-2923.2007.02844.x.

Smalzried, N.T. and Remmers, H.H. (1943). A factor analysis of the Purdue Rating Scale for Instructors. *The Journal of Educational Psychology* 34: 363–367.

Sullivan, G.M. (2018). A toolkit for medical education scholarship. *Journal of Graduate Medical Education* 10 (1): 1–5. https://doi.org/10.4300/JGME-D-17-00974.1.

Sullivan, P.B., Buckle, A., Gregg, N., and Atkinson, S.H. (2012). Peer observation of teaching as a faculty development tool. *BMC Medical Education* 12 (1): 26–26.

Svinicki, M.D. (2017). From Keller's MVP Model to faculty development practice. *New Directions for Teaching and Learning* 2017 (152): 79–89. https://doi.org/10.1002/tl.20270.

Taylor, R.M. (2009). Defining, constructing and assessing learning outcomes. *Revue Scientifique et Technique (International Office of Epizootics)* 28 (2): 779–788.

Teaching Academy (2022). *Applicant Toolbox*. Regional Teaching Academy of the Consortium of West Region Colleges of Veterinary Medicine https://teachingacademy. westregioncvm.org/initiative-eprt-applicanttoolbox (accessed 29 July 2023).

Kraemer, H.M. (2011). *From Values to Action: The Four Principles of Values-Based Leadership*. Jossey-Bass.

Theall, M. (2017). MVP and faculty evaluation. *New Directions for Teaching and Learning* 2017 (152): 91–98. https://doi.org/10.1002/tl.20271.

Theall, M. and Franklin, J. (2001). Looking for bias in all the wrong places: a search for truth or a witch hunt in student ratings of instruction? *New Directions for Institutional Research* 109: 45–56.

Van Patten, K.M., Chalhoub, S., Baker, T. et al. (2021). What do veterinary students value about service learning: insights from subsidized clinics in an urban environment. *Journal of Veterinary Medical Education* 48: 477–484. https://doi.org/10.3138/jvme-2019-0074.

Warman, S.M. (2015). Challenges and issues in the evaluation of teaching quality: how does it affect teachers' professional practice? A UK perspective. *Journal of Veterinary Medical Education* 42: 245–251.

Wiggins, G. and McTighe, J. (2005). *Understanding by Design*. Association for Supervision and Curriculum Development.

Wilson, J.H. and Ryan, R.G. (2012). Formative teaching evaluations: is student input useful? In: *Effective Evaluation of Teaching: A Guide for Faculty and Administrators* (ed. M.E. Kite), 22–29. Society for the Teaching of Psychology.

Woods, S.K., Burgess, L., Kaminetzky, C. et al. (2010). Defining the roles of advisors and mentors in postgraduate medical education: faculty perceptions, roles, responsibilities, and resource needs. *Journal of Graduate Medical Education* 2: 195–200.

Zhu, E. and Turcic, S.M. II (2018). Teaching awards: do they have any impact? *The Journal of Faculty Development* 32: 7–17.

17

Educational Research

Jill R. D. MacKay, M.Sci, PhD, Senior Fellow of the Higher Education Academy (SFHEA)

The Royal (Dick) School of Veterinary Sciences, University of Edinburgh, Midlothian, Scotland, UK

Shelly Wu, PhD (Science Education)

Peter O'Donnell Jr. School of Public Health, University of Texas Southwestern Medical Center, Dallas, TX, USA

Section 1: Introduction to Educational Research

Jill R. D. MacKay

Veterinary education research (VER) is a form of discipline-based education research (DBER). Education research is concerned principally with the methods and approaches to exploring learning (Nisbet 2008), and DBER utilizes this alongside scholarship of teaching and learning (SoTL) within the domain-specific context of a given discipline (Roxå et al. 2017). As such, VER is necessarily an interdisciplinary field, exploring aspects of medical education, animal welfare, educational psychology, anthropology, and even meta-research. With such a broad scope, it can be useful to think back to basics. What are we trying to achieve when we embark on VER?

When training the next generation of veterinarians, we may have many questions we want answered. How do veterinary students learn? What is the most effective method of teaching? Can we make an improvement that will benefit the whole class? Why do students fail exams? The research process allows us to answer these questions with evidence. By approaching these questions about the world in a standardized manner, we can properly evaluate that evidence and decide whether to act upon it. Education research can be acted upon quickly, with educators able to enact changes for another cohort, and so it is important that we explore the veracity of educational research, or we risk making poor choices (Oancea 2005).

Generally, most veterinary scientists will be familiar with the "hypothetico-deductive" model of research, perhaps more familiar as the observation – hypothesis – prediction – analysis cycle (Figure 17.1). In this approach, the researcher expects to repeatedly make observations about the world and tests the assumptions made to confirm whether a given prediction based on the assumption was correct. These findings are written up and shared with other researchers, most commonly after the process of peer-review, a sort of "sense check" where other researchers evaluate the work for clarity and veracity. If all steps of this process are conducted properly, we should be confident in the results obtained and make the best choices to support the learning for our students.

For many readers, this may be an unquestioned truth of the world, but in fact, the process of research described above is shaped by many underlying biases, assumptions, and certain epistemologies. It is not a process guaranteed to produce unbiased results but is often blind to its own flaws. This approach is a paradigm or a model which guides thinking, and as with all models, it has limitations. Perhaps the most well-known limitation of the hypothetico-deductive paradigm is the flaws surrounding null hypothesis significance testing (NHST), which has been much discussed in the sister field of psychology. By describing educational research methods, this chapter seeks to explore and describe a process which is currently undergoing debate, revision, and contest. It is a chapter that invites and encourages critical response. No research guide committed to text can remain the canonical approach to how research is done, because the research paradigms themselves must always be evaluated in light of new evidence. What this chapter aims to do is to equip the reader with the tools they need to remain responsive to research in the veterinary education world and to enable them to pick up new approaches. In some ways, this chapter is a call for veterinary education researchers to critically evaluate their own practice to improve the research of the field.

Part 1: When Research Goes Wrong

The concept that basic processes of research may be fundamentally flawed can be a distressing idea. After all, research has brought us many great advances and improved our quality of life. How can there be such uncertainty regarding its methods? In fact, there have been many critiques of the findings of educational research, often pointing at poor methodology (Lortie-Forgues and Inglis 2019; Makel et al. 2021; Norman 2003; Oancea 2005). There is less certainty in the world than you may expect. As an example, many educators may have heard of learning styles, which explore how students feel they learn in visual, auditory, written, and kinesthetic spaces. The designer of the system states it is a useful tool for self-reflection, enabling learners to explore what methods of learning they may need to work on (Fleming and Baume 2006). The "VARK" questionnaire, however, is very difficult to validate in any meaningful way; it does not relate to student attainment, nor does adjusting teaching to these styles make measurable impact on student learning (Kirschner 2016). And yet, VARK is commonly used by educators at all levels to inform their teaching, without the evidence base to support its use (Franklin 2006). Much criticism of VARK has been published since the mid-2000s; one author of this chapter has used VARK to influence her teaching as recently as the late 2010s. Is this an example of ignorant teaching? Or the difficulty of disseminating good research?

To understand why unvalidated findings can be so widely disseminated, we can look to the so-called replication crisis as a case study. The replication crisis (sometimes referred to as the reproducibility crisis or repeatability crisis) is a general name for a series of findings, mainly focusing on psychology research, which has prompted changes in the conceptualizing of the research process. The replication crisis is a valuable case study for any chapter on research, not least because it is an indication of what practices to avoid in research, but also because it involves several key concepts that are useful for critically evaluating any piece of research.

Part 2: The Replication Crisis: A Primer

In 2005, Ioannidis made the eye-catching claim that most research findings published were false. How can this be true? First, we must explain what we mean by "false" research findings. In general, these are findings that cannot be independently confirmed or replicated by researchers in other labs. In fundamental biology, this is easy to understand. An agar plate growing the same strain of bacteria treated with the same antibacterial substance should show reduced growth whether the laboratory was in Scotland or South Carolina. How does this manifest in educational research? Let us consider a fictional example.

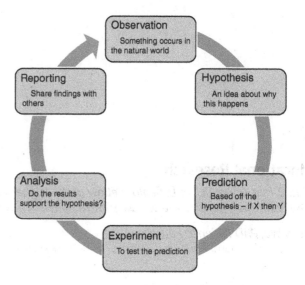

Figure 17.1 A general overview of veterinary science's research process.

A group of education researchers in School A has developed a new tool, Clever Online Open Learning (COOL), which they hope will improve the test scores of veterinary students using the tool. They start with a *hypothesis*.

Hypotheses

Thinking back to Figure 17.1, a hypothesis enables a prediction to be made in a given situation. Hypotheses are potential explanations for the observed effect(s). As predictions are formed from the hypothesis, hypotheses are therefore necessarily tied to study design. In the COOL example, we could test this in multiple ways. The researchers in School A could deploy COOL to a group of 100 students, then ask them in a survey whether they thought the tool improved their learning. In this case, the hypothesis would be: *students using COOL perceive benefits to their learning*.

Alternatively, School A might split the students into two groups of 50. They might give the study group access to COOL, and the control group access to the standard materials. The hypothesis would then be: *students using COOL will achieve higher test scores than students using traditional materials*.

Both hypotheses are valid, and both explore aspects of COOL's validity as an educational tool, but they are only valid in their respective study designs. It would be impossible to test the first hypothesis in the second study setting, and vice versa. This can sometimes lead to confusion when we insist to the novice researcher that they come up with a hypothesis prior to the study design. If a hypothesis cannot be tested in the final study design, it is the hypothesis that must change!

Hypotheses are specific to the experimental design and identify an outcome or response variable and an explanatory variable. For every hypothesis we create, there is also a null hypothesis, which predicts no relationship. These are often written as H_1 and H_0, e.g.:

H_1: students using COOL will achieve higher test scores than students using traditional materials.

H_0: students using COOL will not achieve different scores compared to students using traditional materials.

In these examples, which we will continue to use in this theoretical COOL study, we are specific to our research design, and we have a testable prediction. That is, we are interested in the response (test scores) across the explanatory variable (COOL versus Control). We even know what direction we expect the response to go (we expect it to increase in COOL compared to control). These are all the hallmarks of a good hypothesis. Hypothesis writing is a skill, and one that even practicing researchers can find it useful to review from time to time.

With their H_1 and H_0 formed, the researchers in School A run their class and collect their scores. They use NHST to decide if their hypothesis was "right" or not.

Null Hypothesis Significance Testing

NHST is part of how we test predictions and is the refutation of the null hypothesis. Take our above example, which gave us a specific and testable prediction. School A runs its study and receives a distribution of data as in Figure 17.2.

The school can see that the average of the control group is lower than the average of the COOL group. The mean score for the control group is 73% ± standard deviation 7.8, and the mean of the study group is 77% ± standard deviation 7.1. Is the difference between these groups meaningful? The researchers at School A run a *t*-test to find out, and discover that with a $p = 0.034$, this is just under the typically held cutoff of $p = 0.05$ for significance. They

conclude that there is a significant difference between the COOL and control groups in their assessment scores and that COOL have significantly higher test scores.

There are some subtle considerations about this conclusion that are important to raise here. When making a statement about significance, we are saying that we have either rejected the null hypothesis or failed to reject the null hypothesis. A fundamental underlying concept with NHST is that School A knows they have not tested every single student in the world. They only have a sample of students. They hope that the sample mean is close to the true population mean, and that is why they include a measure of the variation in their sample (standard deviation). Any statistic which calculates a *p* value is a branch of "frequentist" statistics, where probability is treated as a frequency. Frequentist statistics explore whether it is reasonable that the estimates of the true mean for the control and condition samples could overlap. In other words, is it feasible that the difference between these two groups could be 0? The *p* value represents the conditional probability of these findings, that is to say, a significant *p* value of $p < 0.05$ means that we think the observed difference could occur fewer than 1 in 20 times if the null hypothesis (that there is no effect of materials on scores) is true. The condition is that the null hypothesis is true, and the *p* value relates to how often we would expect these findings if that condition was met.

Often *p* values are reported in isolation without the test statistics and confidence intervals. In this imaginary study, if we followed APA reporting guidelines we would say:

Those in the COOL group performed better ($M = 77\%$, $SD = 7.1$) than those in the control group ($M = 73\%$, $SD = 7.8$) and this was significant ($t_{\text{Welch}}(97.01) = -2.15$, $p = 0.034$).

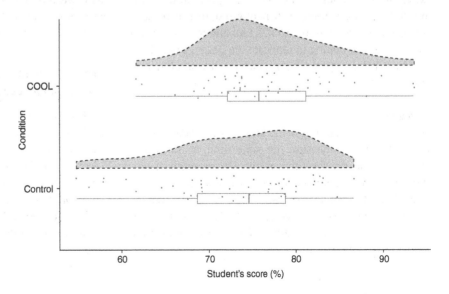

Figure 17.2 Raincloud plot (see Allen et al. 2019) demonstrating distribution of student scores between the control condition, using standard materials, and the study condition, using the COOL tool. The "cloud" density layer shows the distribution, the "rain" dot layer shows individual responses, and the "land" boxplot layer shows the medial and inter-quartile range for each group.

The combination of test statistic ($t = -2.15$) and the degrees of freedom (97.01), give us more information with which to judge the p value. The p value was never intended to be an absolute arbiter of whether a result was interesting, but rather an indication of what relationships should be explored in more detail.

This finding allows School A to reject the H_0, there is a difference between COOL and control groups, but it is only their study design which allows them to accept H_1 as the most likely alternate hypothesis (more on this later). There are many issues with NHST, and these are mostly linked to the conceptual leap that p values are not proof of a hypothesis. Instead, they disprove a null hypothesis. It is critical thinking that helps a researcher decide the correct alternate hypothesis to accept instead.

School A decides to accept their alternate hypothesis, that COOL is responsible for the rise in test scores, and they write up their findings for a respected journal. The journal is an important one, and keen to get a publication, researchers from School A do not entertain the possibility of alternative explanations for their findings. They are at the risk of introducing *errors* into the literature. Their paper is peer-reviewed, without catching this error, and publication ensues. What kind of errors might the researchers from School A have made?

Type I and Type II Errors

Something bound to strike fear into the heart of any researcher or student is being asked to remember the difference between Type I and Type II errors. They are more easily remembered as false positives and false negatives. False positives, or Type I errors, claim there is an effect when there is not one. False negatives, or Type II errors, claim there is no effect when there is one.

At this point, researchers from School B read School A's paper on COOL at their weekly journal club. They are excited to try the same work, and so they set out to repeat the study. They do exactly as School A did, recruit 100 students, and assign 50 to the COOL tool and 50 to a control group. They are hoping to replicate the findings of School A, which brings up two new concepts: *repeatability* and *reproducibility*.

Repeatability

Repeatability in research is the idea that the same person should be able to measure the same thing again, in the same way, and get the same result. For example, if you measure the width of a wardrobe with a tape measure, you would expect to get a very similar measure if you were to measure it again the next day. In the COOL study, if School A repeated its test on the same student populations, they should have similar results.

Reproducibility

Reproducibility in research is the idea that if you measure the same thing in the same way as someone else, you should obtain similar results. For example, if 10 people measure the same wardrobe with 10 different tape measures, we would expect them to get very similar measures. In the COOL study, if School B runs the study on 100 students from the same population as School A, they should both have similar results.

School B runs their study, but they do not find the same results. In fact, they cannot find any evidence of the significant difference between their two groups. They have failed to reject the null hypothesis. The findings of the COOL study have failed to *replicate*.

Replication

Replication is the idea that multiple groups of scientists can use the same process to measure and test a phenomenon in their own research contexts and obtain the same results. The replication crisis is, therefore, a concern that actually very few studies, when replicated, provide the same results. There have been alternative, perhaps more useful definitions of replication, for example, Nosek and Errington (2020) propose that replication is "a study for which any outcome would be considered diagnostic evidence about a claim from prior research," (p. 2) but regardless of this more lenient definition, replication should allow for researchers to be able to provide the same or diagnostically similar results.

What has gone wrong in the fictional COOL study example? Has School B done something wrong, such as not applying COOL correctly? Did School A accept the wrong alternate hypothesis? Should School A has considered the potential errors in their findings more? With the information we have here, we simply cannot tell. And this is why Ioannidis says that most research claims are false. There are many unknowns in research, and by ignoring them, we lose faith in our findings. The replication crisis is, in part, a call to be clearer about the unknowns in research.

Part 3: The Replication Crisis and Open Versus Questionable Research Practices

Replication studies, where a different team uses the same methods to come to the same findings, are surprisingly rare. In education research, one study found less than 0.03% of studies could be replicated by an independent team (Makel and Plucker 2014).

A proposed overarching explanation for the replication crisis is questionable research practices (John et al. 2012; Open Science Collaboration 2015). Questionable research practices are a series of habits and unchallenged assumptions in the hypothetico-deductive model that contribute in different ways to the lack of replication in research. Some of these questionable research practices that have been measured and found to be prevalent (John et al. 2012; Makel et al. 2021) include:

- Within methods, making choices about analysis as a response to findings, e.g.:
  - choosing to collect more or less data after finding a significant result
  - excluding certain data because of their impact on the result
  - choosing not to explore impact of demographics, or ignoring impact of demographics
  - falsifying data
- Within write-ups, questionable research practices mainly surround misleading the reader, e.g.:
  - neglecting to mention all of a study's potential explanatory variable
  - neglecting to report all conditions of a study or even whole studies that do not support the hypothesis
  - generously rounding p values, so $p = 0.051$ becomes $p < 0.05$
  - Hypothesizing After Results Are Known (HARKing, Kerr 1998) or doing so secretly in the introduction (SHARKing, Hollenbeck and Wright 2017) or Critiquing the methods and findings After Results are Known (CARKing)

The reader may have many reactions to this type of list, ranging from "well of course I wouldn't do that" to "I don't see why that is a problem." While falsifying data should, hopefully, raise eyebrows in any coffee room, some of these practices are subtly or actively encouraged. Many anxious research students are advised not to worry during data collection, they can tweak their hypothesis later in the process. Is HARKing such a sin? Surely some surprising findings have to come out after you have found them? There is a distinction between doing this secretly and openly (Hollenbeck and Wright 2017). Openly admitting that you were expecting Result A and subsequently determining an alternative explanation to account for Result B describes clearly why you made certain choices about your research design (Rubin 2017) and is an excellent example of open research practices.

Much of these questionable practices stem from a lack of transparency. It would be hard to falsify data or drop demographic variables from an analysis if the data could be reviewed by others. Similarly, if a study's write-up communicated the researcher's choices clearly, it would be easier for other researchers to understand why they may not have been able to replicate findings. This is hinted at in the description of the COOL study above. When School A wrote up their paper, they did not entertain alternative explanations, and perhaps engaged in more of these questionable research practices. There may be many differences between the studies that School A and School B ran that explain why the work did not replicate, but without changes to the research process, including the publication process, it is impossible to say.

Intuitively, the counterpoint to these questionable research practices is open research practices. Open research practices aim to improve transparency and clarity of research at all stages, with a view to improving the overall replicability of science. A selection of approaches to open research practices is described in Table 17.1.

While there is promising evidence for open research practices and their impact on science (Nosek et al. 2015), we must also be aware of the impact of so-called "bropen science" (Whitaker and Guest 2020), where these tenets are used as a stick to threaten researchers as opposed to the carrot to promote good practice. Minority and vulnerable

Table 17.1 Approaches to open and reproducible science.

Area of research	Approach	Example
Methods	Improving methodological training and understanding	Improved teaching of statistics and methodology
	Independent support of methodology	Including methodologists at earlier stages in research
		Review of methods (pre-registering, registered reports)
	Increased collaboration	Multiple laboratories working on repeating studies
Writing and reporting of results	Promoting pre-registering and registered reports	Utilizing repositories such as Open Science Framework, EdArXiv, PsyArXiv, etc.
	Improving the quality of reports	Using checklists Writing transparently
	Disclosing conflicts of interest	
Peer review	Diversifying peer review	Utilizing pre-prints to make pre-review comparisons more available
		Pre- and post-publication peer review

Source: Adapted from Munafò et al. (2017).

groups can be particularly exposed to this form of "bullying" within academia (Nosek 2017; Pownall et al. 2021). This chapter advocates strongly for open research practices, including the use of clear mission statements to make the performance and communication of research as transparent as possible. Therefore, the rest of this chapter will adopt an open research framework as in Table 17.1 to illustrate good VER. The chapter will highlight what appropriate critiques of research can be presented in this framework, but unequivocally rejects a framing that researchers who are not part of open science are lesser. This chapter aims to evaluate research, not researchers.

Section 2: Designing the Educational Research Study

Jill R. D. MacKay

Research design is a series of choices for the study in question. Each choice will likely have ramifications for the practicalities of running a study, limiting aspects, and potentially opening new possibilities. Some of these choices tend to the mundane: will you have the funding to pay for the person-hours needed to interview 100 people? Some can be more complicated: does your epistemological approach limit your understanding of the field? Navigating this series of choices can feel daunting at first, but it can be useful to return to a guiding question: what am I trying to measure?

Knowing what you want to measure can help identify which choices are most important, and which will have the biggest impact on your research. The following section will detail some of the trade-offs and considerations that are most common in veterinary education studies. There is no "gold standard" for a veterinary education study, other than one that is fully transparent regarding its motivations, biases, approaches, and analysis, and that allows for the critical evaluation of its findings. All studies will have weaknesses, and hopefully some strengths.

Part 1: Ontology, Epistemology, and Reality

It is possible to come some way in veterinary science without encountering ontology or epistemology. Others may have very sophisticated ideas about their ontological stance. Broadly speaking, ontology is the "study of being," (Palermo et al. 2021) or a stance about what is "real" and what is not. For the purposes of this chapter, there are generally two ontological camps, with ontological realists believing that there is an underlying truth to the world, regardless of how we view it. Ontological relativists believe that reality is subjective and only perceived by an individual (Jenkins 2010).

A helpful and greatly simplified analogy may be that of a table. To a realist, a table is inherently a table, regardless of whether a group of children is using it to sit on or as a play-fort. To a relativist, the table ceases to be a table when it is no longer perceived that way by those interacting with it. Epistemology is the "study of knowledge" (Palermo et al. 2021), and is interested in how individuals and societies consider knowledge to be acquired. Similar to the two ontological stances, there are different approaches to epistemology. Objectivist epistemology is similar to a realist ontological stance, believing that there is one truth that can be measured by people, and this measurement could be replicated by others. In contrast, a constructionist epistemology believes that knowledge and facts are grown from a combination of our interactions with our environment, encompassing our languages, our cultures, and our own human bodies. To take the table analogy a step further, an objectivist epistemological approach would suggest the children playing on the table would eventually puzzle out its function (whether that be a table or play-fort), and other children would do the same if they attempted to measure it in the same way. A constructionist epistemological approach might assume that each group of children could come to entirely independent ideas about the use of the table if the children had never interacted or shared their understanding of the measurement.

Ontology and epistemology are philosophical approaches with a wide range of positions beyond these simple examples; however, they have an impact in education. Most scientists are educated in a positivist tradition, which tends to marry a realist ontological approach with objectivist epistemology (Riley 2014; Staller 2012). Many of our discussions regarding the replication crisis are couched in this gentle assumption: the reason results do not replicate must be some flaw in how the work was conducted or described. We have not really considered whether the thing being measured is "real" or "measurable."

A constructionist approach takes a more social approach to learning and considers reality formed by the joint experiences of a group (Alanazi 2016). While discussions around transparency of methods may begin to acknowledge elements of more constructionist approaches, in that we require more collaboration and shared understanding to approximate the same results, there is still an underlying belief that we should achieve the same results if we apply the correct method. In this way, this chapter has already taken an ontological stance of sorts, that there is validity and reason in wanting to find repeatable measures. Critiques of this chapter, and the ideas proposed within it, should incorporate that ontological stance, and consider their own ontological stances. Our ontological and epistemological stances inform our theoretical frameworks,

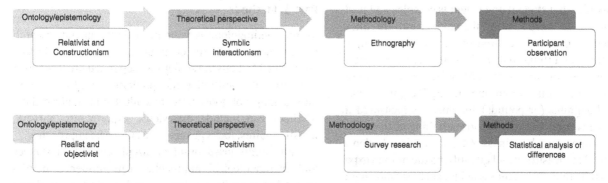

Figure 17.3 Ontological and epistemological impacts on research approaches, per Crotty (1998).

which allow us to identify a methodology, a stance on how our knowledge and theories will be developed, and ultimately a method or an approach to collecting evidence (Crotty 1998). Figure 17.3 demonstrates how different stances can approach a research question in different ways.

Even for those who have not considered their various stances, their methodological and methodical choices reflect underlying biases. It has been argued that being unaware of ones' stance, and the impact on research, limits the researcher's ability to critique research (Braun and Clarke 2006; Twining et al. 2017), although these arguments tend to fall to the qualitative researcher, who often has to make more obvious choices between their theoretical perspective and methodology. There are other, perhaps more esoteric, concerns regarding epistemological influences on research. In many countries, research is competitively funded by government, which often drives institutions to selectively hire researchers who meet certain metrics (Stern 2016). These metrics are often primed to positivist paradigms, with belief in the validity and underlying "realness" of any metric, and so alternative approaches are often ignored in funding strategies (Staller 2012). It is easy to see then how this small disadvantage can be magnified with time. As more positivist-learning researchers obtain funding, and earn the notoriety to sit on panels, they will expect to see research that looks like what they are used to.

If being naïve to our inherent assumptions about ontology and epistemology can bias research, it stands to reason that ignoring the internal and external forces acting on research exposes us to bias, too. Part of the explanation for the replication crisis included pressure to publish papers and biases within journals for positive or interesting results. Perhaps the biases within research funding help maintain a lack of understanding of alternative approaches in education research. Some researchers may be comfortable playing with epistemologies, for example, constructionist realism is an ontological and epistemological approach that broadly considers there to be "real" reality that is only perceived by humans through their own experiences

(Cupchik 2001).[1] For clarity, this is the stance adopted by the author (JM) of this chapter, and so is the stance that influences the advice given therein. Not all researchers may be comfortable with exploring alternative epistemologies, and this is perfectly fine. This chapter does not maintain there is a "correct" philosophy to take, only that there are implications of a researcher's position on how they conduct their research.

Part 2: Methodology

One of the more difficult aspects of educational research is that we are measuring humans. Humans are frustratingly complex and ornery. Often, the "things" we are interested in are constructs as opposed to tangible traits (see this chapter's ontological stance above!). Consider student enjoyment of a course. What kind of data is this? Could we ask students whether they enjoyed the course: yes or no? Does this binary category capture the wealth of different experiences students may have on the course, or allow us to differentiate between smaller changes? So perhaps we use a scale, and ask students to rate themselves, how strongly on a 5-point scale do they agree that they enjoyed the course? But why a 5-point scale; is that enough to detect the vastness of student experience? Would 10 be better (Dawes 2008)? Could we make do with three (Jacoby and Matell 1971)? Do some students "agree" more than others by default, even if their experience was not the same (Krosnick 2018; Lee et al. 2002)? Perhaps we can make use of a nearby laboratory and instead ask the students to donate a sample so we can measure oxytocin levels, although we also know that hormones and behaviors are complex, and no one hormone can scale precisely to enjoyment (Pfaff 2005).

---

1 Chupchik refers in fact to constructivist realism. Constructionists come to their understanding of the world through dialogue with others, constructivists through their own personal experiences, per Rob and Rob (2018).

The issue is that student enjoyment is complex and multifactorial. If we were to grind the student into the finest particulate, we would not find one molecule of "enjoyment." It is not a thing that can be counted. In the veterinary sciences, we are often told as undergraduates to remember the "unit" we are measuring. Weight is measured in kilograms (or pounds) and speed is measured in meters per second, but there is no such thing as the *nanojoy* that can measure happiness. Yet, entire fields of science are devoted to measuring and quantifying the human experience. Traits that we are interested in, such as enjoyment, satisfaction, anxiety, and amount learned, are constructs that encompass different things for different people. Student engagement with learning, for example, is dependent on the student's history, their emotional states, the behaviors they demonstrate, and the mental processes happening within (Fredricks et al. 2004). We call this collection of processes "engagement" and attempt to measure it by proxy.

Proxy measures are very effective and can achieve reproducibility and repeatability that would satisfy any positivistically inclined researcher. This may be why they are often not questioned, and a Likert-like scale asking a student to rate enjoyment is taken as a pure measure of enjoyment. But constructs do not behave normally. For example, in studies of animal personality, it can be debated whether fear and boldness are two independent traits, or two extremes of the same trait (MacKay 2018). Returning to student experience, can a student enjoy a course while finding it stressful? What does the answer to that question imply about a student saying they really did not enjoy a course?

Understanding your own ontological and epistemological stance may help you in answering these questions. Knowing what you want to measure, and how you develop the knowledge on those theories, is part of your *methodology*. Methodology can be thought of as the justification for the method you choose to use. Methodological approaches encompass phenomenology, ethnography, participatory research, action research, grounded theory approaches, and many more forms of research. For example, if your methodology identifies student experience as a complex and unmeasurable thing, you may be led to a qualitative methods approach, which seeks more to describe than to quantify. However, if your methodology identifies a research question such as how student experience differs across groups, you may choose a more quantitative method and use a proxy measure of experience, such as the Likert-like scale. To choose the appropriate methodology, the researcher must understand how they conceive of the traits of interest for that particular study.

Part 3: Methods

Where methodology is your perspective on the research design, methods are the ensuing approaches to collecting your data. Methods are sometimes separated into the broad categories of quantitative and qualitative, but they encompass a range of tools used to collect and analyze data. Methods can include interviews, experiments, surveys, questionnaires, focus groups, and statistical approaches.

While undisclosed ontological/epistemological stances and methodological approaches can influence how a researcher conceives of the research project, undisclosed methods are a far more intuitive explanation for the replication crisis. If one group of researchers uses Software A, which presents p values to three decimal places, and another group of researchers use Software B, which presents p values to six decimal places, the researchers using Software B will always be presenting more granular values, even with exactly the same data. This difference, while small, is very common. Very popular statistical programs do this, and the difference may be completely unknown to many peer reviewers. Methods can also be more deliberately obscured; for example, a questionnaire design may be retained as intellectual property and not published, meaning other researchers might need to pay for access to the same questions and data.

A full description of methods does not have to be the purview of positivist approaches only. Qualitative method descriptions are just as important. In interview research, was the interview structured, semi-structured, or entirely free? Was a codebook (DeCuir-Gunby et al. 2011) used in analysis? How did the researchers decide they had analyzed the data enough (Braun and Clarke 2019)? There are some very good pieces of work producing guidance on how qualitative methods should be described (Twining et al. 2017), including considerations such as:

How did the researchers decide on their sample?
How were participants in the sample approached? Who did not participate and why?
Where might there be gaps in the sample or potential sources of bias?

Within qualitative methods, there should be recognition that often the goal of this research is not replicability, at least not as it is commonly known (although perhaps Nosek and Errington's definition is closer). A key aspect of many positivist forms of research is generalizability, the idea that findings in one cohort should be broadly applicable elsewhere. Qualitative research does not consider generalizability as so key, instead, it views findings more as a model for future work (Noble and Smith 2015; Smith 2018).

Part 4: An Overview of Key Terminology

The jigsaw of pieces that is research design can be overwhelming, and the terminology is often not helpful. With similar words (methodology versus methods) and an abundance of "ologies," Table 17.2 may serve as a useful lookup to ensure the enterprising veterinary education researcher is kept right.

Part 5: Study Design

The prevalence of choices available to researchers may seem daunting, but often a need for pragmatism is a useful way to hone a researcher down to a particular choice. This section will give a broad overview of a range of study design choices and sources of data, including perspectives on practicalities that may sway educational researchers one way or another. For this section, there are two caveats to bear in mind: the design influences the hypothesis and no one design will be able to measure everything.

Caveat One, that design influences the hypothesis (and indeed, the research question), may seem obvious, and yet in teaching research methods we often ask the prospective researcher, "what is your hypothesis?" far too early in the process. From a teaching point of view, this makes sense. It is easy to offer feedback on a hypothesis. Hypotheses are highly structured and a fundamental concept in understanding the process of the hypothetico-deductive model of research. It is much easier for a tutor to give feedback on a hypothesis than on a poorly described experimental design. From the tutor's perspective, a hypothesis can help identify what the prospective researcher thinks the explanatory and response variables are, or how they might think the analysis

is working. In the author's experience, this focus on the hypothesis can often lead the prospective researcher to think they need to come up with the hypothesis first. Instead, hypothesis and design should be developed in tandem. This should become clear in the following examples.

Caveat Two, that no one design is capable of measuring everything, is more subtle. A well-designed study should be very specific about what data it is collecting and what that data are thought to represent (methodology). This seems obvious in what might be thought of as the traditional study, a manipulation study. You change one variable between groups and measure the response variable in each group to establish whether a difference exists. Let us say a new study technique has been shown to have an impact on acquired grade; we still do not know about the study experience, the student's knowledge retention after the fact, or what aspects of the study can be easily generalized. Some prospective researchers may think there are ways to continue refining the study, to add more and more variables perhaps, or to use more sophisticated statistical analyses to answer some of these questions. This is a fool's errand. Ultimately, a study is conducted under highly specific circumstances and in certain time frames. It can never be all things to all people. This is true of all research. There is a very interesting theory on modeling that no research model can maximize the three fundamental components of specificity, generalizability, and precision (Levins 1966). One component must always be sacrificed, or the statistical model will have fully replicated the real world. Similarly, in research design, we have constraints on all approaches. The more complicated the organisms being studied are, the harder it is to minimize all three constraints. These are: bias, confounding variables, and variation.

Table 17.2 An overview of key research terminology.

Considerations	Level	Considerations
Theoretical stance	Ontology Epistemology	How does your theoretical stance influence your approach to data? Is data real and reproducible, or is data constructed by the researcher and approximated through similar methods?
Approach	Methodology	Quantitative approaches Qualitative approaches
	Design	How does it align with your methodology? What are the ethical considerations inherent in the design?
Data	Methods	Your methods should be fully specified before you start (necessary for ethical approval), and practical in the context of your research
	Instruments	Are your tools for collecting data robust? Were there adaptions along the way and how will these be detailed?
	Analysis	Should align with theoretical stance, approach, and methods/instruments used to collect data. Consider alternative explanations for findings and link to the overall relevance of the work

Source: Adapted from Twining et al. (2017).

The constraints on study design are an integral part of the research process. Research publishing, which will be visited later, commonly uses a structure that explicitly sets aside time to critically evaluate the findings of any study. This is the Discussion section (see Section 6: Reporting the Educational Study). Critical evaluation of findings describes the process of considering what potential alternative explanations may exist for your results. All research should be critically evaluated, which involves exploring how a given set of results fits with the surrounding literature, and how the methodology and methods may have weaknesses (Hek 1996; Roever et al. 2016).

The evaluation of a piece of research does not mean that the findings are disputed, or that the study is poorly done. It is, most importantly, not a personal attack on the researchers. Critical analyses of research should be specific, relating to the findings of the research; reasonable, relating to the issue of concern and with a clear impact; and fair, avoiding assumptions regarding intent or motivations of the researchers. Critical evaluation goes beyond merely describing the results of previous research, but instead offers a comparison and contrast, synthesizing new understanding from the analysis. It is often considered as being the "why" questions of research, "why do these findings differ from previous research?," or "have all likely alternative explanations for the findings been covered?" A good report of research will have done much of this work for the reader by highlighting weaknesses in the discussion; however, this is not always guaranteed, and this is the reason it is important to evaluate the literature alongside one's own findings.

Bias, Confounding Variables, and Variation

The three principal critiques of any study (Ruxton and Colegrave 2011) are bias, confounding variables, and variation. These are elements of study design that researchers try to minimize, but they must be cognizant of their intractability. In each study, the prospective researcher will work hard to design all three elements out, and yet they must still address them in their critique. Knowing the weaknesses of a study does not invalidate its findings, but instead helps you understand why it may or may not replicate or generalize in certain circumstances.

Bias

Bias is a systematic error in measurement that introduces inaccuracy to a variable. Measurement inaccuracy is often discussed along with measurement imprecision, and there is an important distinction between them. Inaccuracy is the systematic error (or bias), for example, if a researcher purchased a slightly cheap measuring tape with all the marks slightly too-close together, then all measurements

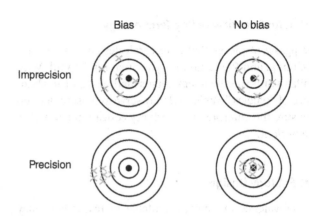

Figure 17.4 Bias, imprecision, and their interactions.

taken by that tape would be an underestimate of the true measurement. This would be an obvious source of error if another researcher was trying to replicate their findings. The error in this measurement is all in a consistent direction and therefore the error in one individual measure is highly associated with the measure of another individual data point. That is to say, they would both be underestimated by a similar amount. When the error between measurements is not associated, or random, we have imprecision in our measurements. Technically, bias is the systematic error or inaccuracy within measurement, but it is worth considering it alongside imprecision as they can both interact, as commonly depicted in Figure 17.4.

Imprecision occurs where there is random error in any measurement. For example, if the researcher measured each data point with a different poorly made tape measure, knowing whether or not data point A was underestimated would not help deciding whether data point B was underestimated or overestimated.

One of the easiest ways to combat bias is through explicit detailing of methods. If you have ever wondered why journals insist on knowing the brand of microscope used in a laboratory, or who made precisely what statistical software that was utilized, it is to try and identify where bias may exist. If, for example, a particular software always reported p values of <0.001 as $p = 0.000$, we know that there may be quite a bit of variation in the p values reported by that software as $p < 0.001$. Explicit detail goes beyond the reporting of specific tools used in the methods and should also carry out to protocol. Ethograms, which many veterinary scientists will be familiar with due to their extensive use in nonhuman animal behavior, are an excellent example of this.

Bias is also an issue for qualitative work. The analysis and interpretation of qualitative findings are highly associated with the researcher. Research in widening participation, the process of ensuring underrepresented groups are represented in education, is a good example of this. There is systematic bias in how different types of universities admit and discriminate against students from disadvantaged backgrounds (Boliver 2015), so, therefore, any research done within a university is necessarily biased by its own population.

The position of the researcher is an important aspect that can introduce bias into the interpretation of results. Researcher position includes the researcher's ontological and epistemological stance (and therefore the previously discussed assumptions within those), and the researcher's methodological approach to the data, e.g., whether they felt they facilitated collection of data that was pure, or whether their own collection of the data influenced the data itself (Grbich 2011). In science, technology, engineering, maths, and medicine (STEMM) fields, stating the position of the researcher can be controversial, perhaps because it makes bias obvious, and positivistic leaning fields place great value on a lack of bias. There have been many calls for education research to make its researcher position more explicit in methodology (Braun and Clarke 2006; Twining 2010) to facilitate more critical evaluation of findings. For example, in a piece on widening participation in education (MacKay et al. 2021b), the researcher position clarifies that the universities sampled in the study were biased and that the researchers themselves had many shared experiences that would likely make them less sensitive to particular aspects of the widening participation student experience, such as being from certain ethnic backgrounds. To evaluate the research, these limitations must be borne in mind just as the brand of microscope or statistical software are. The position of the researcher is a potential source of bias because the researcher themselves are a tool.

To tackle bias in research we must be both aware of it and accepting of it. Ultimately, choices must be made in study design, and as mentioned, no one design is perfect. By acknowledging what biases exist in research, we can identify why other studies may or may not replicate the work.

Confounding Variables

In the hypothetico-deductive model, we are usually interested in "does x affect y?" Confounding variables are when z, which is not accounted for in our measurements, affects y and we draw a false conclusion, either a false positive (Type I error) or false negative (Type II error). Confounding variables are easiest understood in the context of a correlation. Consider a scenario where researchers theorize that studying more will increase grades. Their null hypothesis is that there will be no relationship between time spent in the library and final grades for a certain cohort of students. They record when each student swipes in and out of the library, and then their final grade for the test. When they put their findings together the researchers are surprised to discover their null hypothesis is not refuted by the statistics, and time spent in the library has no clear relationship with attainment. The researchers were unaware that during the study period, time spent in the library was confounded, as the nearby social café was closed for refurbishments and a floor on the library was co-opted for a café space. Time in library was confounded by time in café. These researchers are in danger of accepting a false negative.

Confounding variables can be difficult to track, as unknown unknowns can remain hidden from researchers through no fault of the researcher's own. Some confounding variables are obvious (ice cream sales and homicide rate are highly associated in New York, but it is clear that the link here is weather, as hot weather makes people grumpier and more prone to buying ice cream). More subtle confounding variables can only really be identified through continued study or a bit of fortune on the behalf of the researcher noticing the café had moved.

The difference between bias and confounding variables is sometimes blurred in study design. An easy distinction between them is that bias affects the process of measurement, whereas confounding variables are that the measure itself is not accurate.

Variation

The third and final general critique of study design is that of natural variation. Variation is principally considered in terms of statistics. It is a basic principle of science that the natural world varies. We know intuitively that we cannot simply measure one veterinary student and then consider their measurements as representative of every veterinary student. Let us take the example of final grade for a course. Often in research, we want to make the best "guess" for an individual's measurement that we can. Imagine a course of 100 students, and the only information we have is each student's final grade. If we wanted to describe the performance of any given student but we could not look up their specific grade, our best "guess" at their grade would be the mean grade of the class. The mean is an estimate of a population's central tendency. We expect that most populations are "normal," that is to say the mean is a fair approximation of most individuals within the population. Many populations are not normally distributed, and with these populations, the median or middle values, is a better estimate of the population's central tendency. In the absence of any other information, the central tendency, be it mean, mode, or median, is a guess for any unknown individual's value.

The spread of data around the central tendency is the natural variation in the world, or "noise." When there is

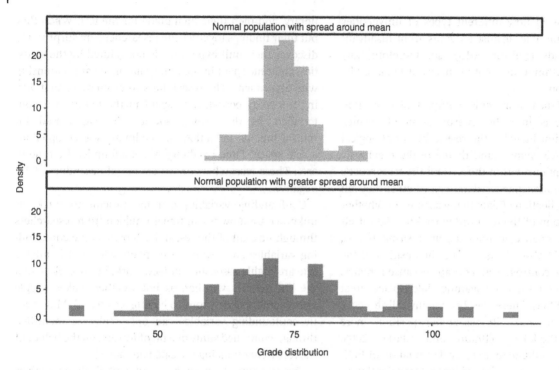

Figure 17.5 Histograms of grade for two student samples, both with a mean of 73, but with different amounts of noise around the mean.

lots of noise or variation around the central tendency, we are less confident that the central tendency is a good measure of the population. Figure 17.5 describes two classes of 100 students, both with a mean of 73 for their final grade. The mean is clearly a better guess of any individual student's grade for the first sample in comparison to the second sample.

If we take the central tendency as a prediction for each individual in the population, the distance between the prediction and the observed result is referred to as the fit, or residual. The wider the spread around the mean, the greater the range of fitted values. In this example, Sample A has a mean of 73 ± 5.2, and the fits range from -14.8 (i.e., the lowest performing student achieved 14.8 marks less than the mean) to 12 (i.e., the highest performing student achieved 12 marks more than the mean). Sample B has the same mean of $73 \pm$ a standard deviation of 15.1. The lowest-performing student scored 41.6 points less than the mean, with the maximum fit being 37.3. It is easy to see here that the mean is a poorer "guess" for any given individual in Sample B. What may be less obvious is the implication for study design.

Increased numbers allow for more certainty in the estimate of the central tendency. This is related to the concept of statistical power, the probability that a significance test will detect a deviation from the null hypothesis if a deviation exists. In this example, we have calculated the mean of both populations as 73, but is it statistically different from a historical mean grade of 74? For Sample A, we can say that the mean grade (73 ± 5.2) was significantly smaller than the historical average of 74 in a one-sample t-test ($t_{(99)} = -2.39$, $p = 0.019$). For Sample B, which remember has the exact same arithmetic mean as Sample A, we can say that the mean grade (73 ± 15.1) is not different from the historical average of 74 in a one-sample t-test ($t_{(99)} = -1.02$, $p = 0.310$). The increased variation in Sample B makes the estimate of central tendency more unreliable, and so a t-test cannot reject the possibility that the true mean could be 73. If we had a thousand students in Sample B we could say that the same mean grade (73 ± 15.1) was significantly lower than the historical average of 74 in a one-sample t-test ($t_{(19999)} = 108.85$, $p < 0.001$). Although the mean and the standard deviation are the same, having more individuals allows us more confidence in our estimate. An implication of this is that with enough individuals a significant p value can be found for any test (Sullivan and Feinn 2012). A statistician may say that a p value is simply a test of sample size and should always advise the use of effect size estimates (see Frequentist Analyses). For now, it is enough to recognize that we need to account for the variation in the natural world in designing our studies to ensure we have captured enough variation to describe the population while also ensuring we understand our sample size.

There is one more issue with variation, however. The need to have more than one observation in a (quantitative) study is often referred to as replicating an observation. Each individual student in our samples above was a replicate, that is to say, each student was independent of one another, and knowing one particular student's grade would give us no information on the next student. The assumption of independent observations is a vital assumption in frequentist statistics. We need independent replicates to find the patterns in our data when we ask the question "does x affect y?" Pseudoreplication is similar to confounding variables or bias where there is an underlying pattern in the data of which the statistical analysis is unaware. One hundred observations on the same student are a clear example of pseudoreplication, but what if the final grade was allocated by a project where students had to work in pairs? In this case, we would have 50, rather than 100 replicates, in our samples, as each pair would have associated grades. Pseudoreplication can be very tricky, and it depends on what your observation is intended to be. In our grades example, if we think that we have taught the class exactly the same way, we can compare our 100 students to the historical average, but if we are concerned that the way we have taught the classes has changed and we want to compare the performance of the teaching over time, our 100 students are simply one observation of the teaching and learning of the class. This is particularly true if you adhere to a constructivist epistemology, where the teaching and learning in the class is co-constructed by all the class participants, i.e., that each student was influencing one another and influencing the teaching received. Common environments, common influences, and social relatedness are common sources of pseudoreplication in research (Ruxton and Colegrave 2011). Some pseudoreplication is inevitable; for example, we will always have the shared environment of Earth to contend with, but study design should do its best to be aware of and mitigate pseudoreplication where possible. Pseudoreplication is very similar to confounding variables but specifically relates to the assumptions of statistics and the independence of observations from one another.

Quantitative, Qualitative, and Mixed Methods Study Designs

The dichotomy between qualitative and quantitative research paradigms is a fundamental aspect of methodology, and yet it refers more to the approach to the data (see Table 17.2) than necessarily aspects of the design. For example, if a researcher wanted to explore students' responses to a new form of teaching, this may be set up as a manipulation study (with half receiving the new intervention and half not) or as an observational study (exploring students' perspectives about the new intervention). In both scenarios, the approach taken could be quantitative or qualitative. Quantitative and qualitative study designs differ in the measures recorded and the approaches taken to the data, but these can be applied across different types of studies.

One of the fundamental differences between qualitative and quantitative approaches is the outcome. With quantitative research, we often aim to produce a definitive answer to a question posed by a hypothesis: has the prediction proved true? With qualitative research, we are often aiming to generate a new theory consolidating information to propose a new explanation for why a phenomenon exists in the natural world, promoting understanding of what is "behind" the numbers. Generally, quantitative studies are better for making comparisons across populations or time points, and qualitative studies are better for characterizing processes, populations, or events. However, there can be exceptions to this, and often a "mixed-methods" approach is used to collect both types of data to enable methodological triangulation on a research question (Burke Johnson et al. 2007).

The level of integration between these methodological and method approaches is sometimes debatable and is a topic of consternation when attempting to define the approach. A typology of mixed designs (Leech and Onwuegbuzie 2009) describes a research design in terms of how mixed the methods are, either fully or partially, with the data collected either concurrently or sequentially. The emphasis placed on one type of data, either both approaches being considered equal, or one dominant, provides the final dimension. For example, a fully mixed concurrent equal status design would integrate both quantitative and qualitative research paradigms throughout the study design, including within epistemological approach, etc., collect all qualitative and quantitative data together, and place equal value on the findings from each type of data collection. A partially mixed sequential (quantitative) dominant status design might have a study design based predominantly on quantitative epistemologies and approaches, with all quantitative data collected first, and then qualitative data being collected afterward to elaborate on certain findings, but to be considered only in light of the quantitative findings. It is not always common for mixed methods study designs to identify their structure in this typology; however, it can be a useful approach, particularly when trying to establish where ones' epistemological approach fits into the different data types in a mixed methods design. More informed use of this typology may support better understanding and dissemination of these mixed methods designs.

Given that the thrust of mixed methods allows for triangulation on the research question, it is important that the integration of the methods is an integral part of the study design. Do you expect the findings from the different methods to converge, complement, or provide a dissonant finding (O'Cathain et al. 2010)? For example, your study design may be a mixed methods approach into how students utilize virtual learning environments (VLE) prior to exams. Quantitative data may come in the form of analytics, while follow-up semi-structured interviews with a subset of participants may provide the qualitative data. A convergent approach would expect to see a pattern of behavior in the analytics, borne out by the participant's reasoning, e.g., student visits to the VLE increasing before exams and interview data revealing students want to visit the VLE. A complementary approach may show student visits to the VLE increasing, and interviews revealing that students preferred to start their literature searches through the VLE as it provided a list of resources, explaining and elaborating on the observed behavior. A dissonant finding might be that visits to the VLE increase, but in interviews, students talk about the VLE being a poor place to start their studies. The potential reasons for this dissonance in findings might reveal some new understanding to advance our knowledge. Perhaps the VLE learning analytics are not measuring what we really think they are, or perhaps those students who are accessing the VLE are getting frustrated by a lack of resources. Pursuing any of these lines may help to further develop the finding and integrate the data in a mixed methods study. The sequence may be reversed or altered depending on your mixed design typology, and no one specific sequence is applicable for all research questions. When evaluating a mixed methods design, the key questions of bias, confounding variables, and variation can still be considered, particularly for the quantitative work. The qualitative work must also be interrogated on its merits, and there also are specific evaluation points that can be used for mixed methods designs, see Leech et al. (2010).

Manipulation Studies

Manipulation studies are probably the most familiar type of study to a veterinary scientist, as they are the "proto example" of research used to teach the subject. Manipulation studies, or experimental studies, are often considered to be the only type of study design that can provide unequivocal evidence that your explanatory variable has an effect on your response variable (Ruxton and Colegrave 2011), although this of course depends on the study's design.

In a manipulation trial, the researcher identifies the relationship of interest, that old question of does x affect y, and isolates what measurements can be taken of x and y in study design. It then requires x to be artificially changed or adapted by the researcher, so there are discrete levels of x that we would expect to see defined differences in y between them.

Manipulation trials generally treat the explanatory variable as a categorical grouping variable. For example, a study exploring the benefit of models in surgical skill training might have a control group without models and intervention group with models. The explanatory variable may also be an ordered (ordinal) variable. For example, associating provision of resources with final exam score might have a number of ordered categories in the explanatory variable from no supplied resources (control), one supplied resource, two supplied resources, and all supplied resources.

There are ethical implications in choosing the manipulation that may impact the study design. Particularly within education, it may be considered unethical to deprive participants of certain resources. It may also impact recruitment into a study, as participants may be unlikely to opt into a study if it may have an impact on their final grades, for example. The ethical implications of controls will be discussed in later, but for now, it is important to recognize that these choices about study design are not made in a vacuum, but are impacted by ethical and pragmatic considerations.

Balancing and Randomization

Within a manipulation study, one of the most important aspects is how to assign participants to their treatment (also known as intervention) group. There can be balanced or unbalanced designs, and participants can be assigned randomly or with an underlying structure. Balanced designs have the same number of participants in all treatment and control groups. Balanced designs have advantages in terms of statistical analysis, but can often become unbalanced (with uneven numbers) if participants are likely to drop out of a study throughout the process. Designs can be balanced if they are one-way designs, i.e., there is one variable of interest, such as the impact of a new study technique on attainment. A balanced one-way (or one-factor) design would have equal numbers of participants randomly drawn from the population in both the control and treatment groups. Balanced designs can also be two-way (two-factor) or three-way, four-way, etc. For example, if we were interested in both the new study technique and a new study environment in the library, we would need to balance participants across both treatments, i.e., 100 participants would need to be randomly assigned to the Control Study Technique – Control Environment ($n = 25$), Control Study Technique – New Study Environment ($n = 25$), New Study Technique – Control Environment ($n = 25$), and New Study Technique – New Study Environment ($n = 25$). If you wanted a three-way design, if

Table 17.3 A balanced three-way design exploring the effect of a novel study strategy, study environment, and coffee administration on attainment.

Study strategy	Environment	Coffee Intake	*n*
Control	Standard	Control	25
Control	New	Control	25
Control	Standard	Increased	25
Control	New	Increased	25
Novel	Standard	Control	25
Novel	New	Control	25
Novel	Standard	Increased	25
Novel	New	Increased	25

say you were also interested in the administration of coffee to the study environment and wanted to retain 25 participants in each group you would need 200 participants in total (Table 17.3). To have a fully balanced design takes a great deal of work and fervent hoping that all participants remain in the study. It does, however, make the statistical analysis far easier, as assumptions on random sampling, i.e., that any one participant is as likely to be in any one condition as the other, are upheld. As with so many study designs, the choice to balance your design requires effort, time, and resources, often financial.

Blocking

Similar to a multifactorial design, we can also attempt to control for variation within the population that we think will impact our outcome variables. If we felt our new study technique would also be impacted by whether or not a student had a prior degree, a balanced blocked design would have equal numbers of graduates and nongraduates in both the control and novel technique treatment group. Similar to multi-way design, if we wanted to balance on multiple blocked variables, we would need to balance the numbers in each group. In this particular study, if we were also concerned that gender might impact the use of the novel study technique, we would need equal numbers of female graduates, male graduates, female nongraduates, and male nongraduates in both the control and treatment groups to have a fully balanced and blocked design. Of course, this assumes that we only have male and female genders in this study design (and says nothing about assigned sex). Blocking is done when you know that there are underlying structures of variation in your population, and you want to ensure that with your randomization, you do not randomly over-sample some parts of the population. In other words, you can design a multi-way design to test multiple forms of intervention at once. You can create a blocked design to account for structures of variation that are inherent within your population that you suspect will impact your study outcome. Multi-way designs allow you to describe differences between groups, whereas blocking allows you to discard differences due to the variables of concern in your population.

Types of Control

There are many different types of control groups that can exist in manipulation study designs. The typical example of a control group, such as those described above, are negative concurrent controls, in that the different trial groups happen over the same time period and the control is the absence of the manipulation. In pharmaceutical studies, concurrent negative controls are very popular, as often there is an ethical concern of the intervention doing harm. It would be difficult to justify a study design considered harmful for human participants, particularly where the benefits of such a design are for an optional benefit like education. Depriving students of an educational resource in the name of producing a negative concurrent control is hard to defend, and requires considerable thought and ethical justification.

Due in part to the ethical concerns with depriving students of resources, in education it is common to use a positive, rather than negative, control. In this situation, the treatment group has a particular intervention and the control group has another intervention of known quality. With positive controls, it is very important to recognize that these designs require a known quality of intervention. The pharmaceutical example would be a novel drug being compared with a currently used drug, and in education, we might have a novel learning design being compared with the existing learning design. Again, designs can be balanced or unbalanced in a positive concurrent control study, perhaps useful if there is concern regarding a new curriculum.

Finally, controls can be historical. Historical controls, while not ideal, are often a pragmatic study design, especially in human trials. This would be, for example, comparing two years of exam scores before and after a new "how to study" resource is included. Historical controls can avoid the ethical concerns over how to assign participants to a treatment condition considered less advantageous to the student's overall attainment or experience. They can also be more pragmatic in that it is often simply easier to deliver one form of teaching versus multiple forms of teaching, particularly when an intervention may be multimodal, e.g., a combination of new lectures and tutorials.

Historical controls are difficult to disentangle from confounding variables and bias. Having a defined structure of time that defines the sample of the population in one group introduces bias because we cannot be sure that we are truly looking at the difference between the treatment and the time. There may be confounding variables we are unaware of that are related to the time point. Historical controls are perhaps a necessary evil in study design when there are real-world constraints that keep us from utilizing a concurrent control. Note that while a historical control is sometimes the only option, a future control is unacceptable. Historical controls accept the trade-off of bias and confounding variables for the benefit of being able to enact a treatment on a full sample population. A future control does not save any effort of running the treatment on a full sample population, as the same group must be deprived of something, and as a future control is not concurrent it introduces bias and confounding variables. Future controls are one of the few examples in this chapter of a design choice that cannot be defended. If a control group is going to be run at all, it should be done concurrently.

Randomized Controlled Trials

Earlier in this section, we said there was no such thing as a gold standard. Some readers may have frowned at this and argued that the gold standard for any study is a randomized controlled trial (RCT). As the name implies, RCTs take the form of a manipulation study where there is a concurrent control group, which may be a negative or a positive control. Each individual within the study is randomly assigned to their treatment group, and there may be multi-way or blocking elements to the design. They are usually balanced, or at least set out to be balanced at their conception. RCTs aim to allow for direct comparison of the treatment with the control group, making the best use of the existing variation in the population and minimizing bias, often through techniques such as blinding, and confounding variables, through techniques such as blocking.

Blinding

In a pharmaceutical RCT, we would expect the patients and experimenters to both be blinded (a double-blinded trial, or double-blind label trial). Neither the prescribing physician nor the patient would not know if they were administering the active ingredient or the placebo. This has obvious advantages in terms of bias. If a patient knew they were not receiving the active ingredient, they may feel that other measures were pointless, and not continue healthy behaviors. Alternatively, they may feel more motivated to seek out additional treatments or perform healthy behaviors to an increased intensity in an attempt to compensate for not receiving the drug. Likewise, if the physician knew, any recordings of outcome variables they made may be questionable. Their motivation to have a "successful" study would bias them, even with the best of intentions to remain impartial. Blinding, specifically double

blinding, where participant and experimenter are both unaware of the experimental condition the participant is in, is an excellent way to reduce some forms of bias, but it has weaknesses.

Pragmatically, one of the first weaknesses of blinding is that is very hard to blind participants in an educational study to the condition they are in. In an educational study, it is hard to hide whether or not the participant has received the educational intervention. In these cases, often the experimenter or examiner is blinded to the experimental condition. For example, one study explored whether healthy-eating interventions for children under five years of age improved health-related behaviors in families (Iaia et al. 2017). In this trial, nurseries were randomly allocated to an intervention group, where the staff was trained in educating healthy eating and a series of activities were planned, and a control group, where the routine curriculum was in place and individual families were sent a leaflet on diet guidelines. Obviously, the families would be aware of what intervention they were receiving, even if they were not sure what other nurseries were receiving. The behaviors of the children were assessed by assessors who were blind to what nursery (and thus which experimental group) each participant was in. In this semi-blind design, there is still some potential for bias to creep in. Behaviors were recorded via a family diet and activity diary, but there is still the chance of these being influenced by the intervention without reflecting an underlying behavioral change. Additionally, as children were assigned into their experimental groups via their nursery, some confounding effect(s) with nurseries influencing how the diaries are written is still possible. There is some attempt to control for this statistically; for example, the mother's education level was accounted for in the models, which we might expect has an impact on the diaried behaviors, but this reflects our questions regarding whether one study can measure everything. It would have been wonderful to observe these behaviors directly instead of using diaries, but how were the researchers supposed to observe this without accidentally uncovering from excited five-year-old participants what they learned in nursery today? It is important to note here that these questions do not imply this is a poor design or a flawed study! Instead, they serve to highlight the great difficulty in blinding in educational studies.

Another weakness of blinding is the extent to which it is possible. In the well-designed and preregistered study on feedback, Fyfe et al. (2021) explored the impact of feedback being immediate or delayed in 38 classes of consisting of over 2000 total students. Each student received both treatments, with the order randomized (i.e., some students received immediate feedback first and some students received delayed feedback first). This makes sense as the student must consent to be in the study and will be aware of when they received their feedback. They cannot be blind to their own experiences. As a note, this study was preregistered, allowing for comment and critique ahead of its being conducted, which given its scale is a very sensible investment. For those interested, delayed feedback appeared to have no impact on the student's attainment. Blinding is a valuable tool in study design, but it is not always achievable, and it is not always as fully blind as it may be purported. Recognizing where bias and confounding variables may impact the study can help determine how important it is to blind aspects of a given design.

Critiques of Randomized Control Trials

With all of this work to minimize bias, account for confounding variables, and take the variation of the population into account, why might RCTs not be considered the gold standard? They are, after all, a tenet of evidence-based medicine; should they not also be a hallmark of evidence-based education (Davies 1999)? Unfortunately, RCTs are expensive, both in terms of labor and financial cost. Furthermore, they are very good for answering certain kinds of questions, but for exploring more holistic questions, such as "why do students like X?," they are less useful. An RCT allows for a statement like "x is the most likely cause of y" or "studying increases student attainment in standard exams" but it does not explain why Student 1 did not engage with study sessions, or why Student 2 found them so stressful. One might argue these are different research questions, and that different RCTs would allow for their disentanglement. This is questionable. As mentioned above, education research rarely has an easy placebo and so fully blinded RCTs are rare. Furthermore, engaging enough students to account for the huge variation in human experience to make an RCT statistically powerful enough to detect a difference is often predicated on other forms of motivation and education levels (Wrigley 2018), immediately introducing confounding variables. RCTs also have an ethical implication, as they require evidence prior to change to justify the use of controls. Surely this is good? Would it not be unethical to impose an untested treatment on a population, or blindly try a new form of education?

Recent global events have offered a very interesting counter to this argument. Intervention must be considered on risks and harms case-by-case approach. Early in the SARS-COV-19 (COVID-19) global pandemic, there were severe lockdowns that restricted human behavior and commerce, and hospitals were overloaded with severe COVID-19 cases with little knowledge on how best to treat them. The use of face masks emerged as a potential measure to potentially mitigate the spread and protect societies.

This led to fierce debate. On the one hand, masks had not been subject to an RCT to explore the extent to which they prevented the spread of COVID-19 (Marasinghe 2020). There were also concerns that the public would use masks inexpertly, choosing substandard masks, improperly applying them, or being more tempted to touch their face while using them (Mantzari et al. 2020). In other words, there were risks of potential harm from mask use. On the other hand, countries with mask use had been observed to have lower rates of COVID-19, and the risks of improper mask usage were arguably very small and potentially misleading to the public (Mantzari et al. 2020). The precautionary principle dictated that as a small, majority-harmless intervention, the risk of wearing masks was so dwarfed by the risk of catching COVID-19 that it made sense to advocate for their usage in the absence of gold-standard RCT evidence (Greenhalgh et al. 2020; Javid et al. 2020). This has been contested, with other researchers suggesting that the harms of masks, such as their impact on communication and the potential for contaminating oneself with COVID-19 through touching masks, and thus their use cannot be recommended (Lazzarino et al. 2020). Without "evidence" that we can all be convinced of, how can this argument be resolved?

Many large public health interventions are so complicated and multifaceted that they will never lend themselves to an RCT (Greenhalgh 2020). To be effective, RCTs need to be highly specific and constrained. Historically this has led to whole populations being quietly ignored in studies. RCTs in acute coronary disease have historically under-represented women (Lee et al. 2001). A common explanation for this bias is that there are sex differences that make the study harder to control; for example, female body temperature varies significantly with the menstrual cycle, and so measures of temperature are confounded by an underlying variable for women, one that most women are likely not aware of (ovulation). The systematic under investigation and underreporting of certain populations are historic and has been critiqued as being part of Western Science's colonial approaches (Henrich et al. 2010). Sadly, we know that being aware of these issues and indeed legislating against them does not significantly improve the problem; women are still underrepresented in clinical RCTs (Geller et al. 2018). It is unlikely that all these scientists are deliberately setting out to disenfranchise groups, or that they are trying to introduce systemic bias in the literature. Instead, they may well simply be trying to produce the best RCT they can, one which aims to act ethically (such as not recruiting women who may be pregnant to trial a potentially dangerous drug), and yet considering only one type of evidence as "gold standard" results in a gap in our data.

Observational Studies

A large proportion of veterinary educational studies are likely observational studies. Observational studies have many advantages over manipulation studies but also have their own disadvantages. They may be common in education for many of the pragmatic issues highlighted in the overview of manipulation studies. The biggest advantage of manipulation studies is that great efforts can be made to minimize sources of bias and account for confounding variables. With appropriate design and prior information on the distribution of traits, it is also possible to account for the natural variation of the world by ensuring you sample enough of the population to make reasonable inferences to the rest of the population. Observational studies are often criticized on all three points. In an observational study, you are limited in how and what you can measure and may have restrictions on recruitment, e.g., access to data, which impacts your ability to ensure you have accounted for the natural variation in a population. These are all reasonable critiques of any study, but by bearing these critiques in mind, one can design an observational study of great value to the field.

Observational studies involve identifying the variables of interest and how best to measure them within the study environment. Observational studies are not necessarily free of intervention; for example, a researcher may administer a personality test to a sample of students and then look for associations between the outcomes of the test and educational outcomes. While the test was administered as part of the study, no manipulation of the study participants happened, i.e., the researchers did not neatly divide the sample population into two personality groups by artificially manipulating the personalities of the participants. This is a double-edged sword. Observational studies often have less statistical power with which to detect differences as one cannot artificially ensure there is representation across the explanatory variable of interest; by contrast, they allow for exploration of the relationship between traits where there is little preexisting evidence.

The hypothetico-deductive model clearly states the process of scientific investigation begins with observation, and so observational studies can be thought of as a formalization of this initial step. Through observational studies, researchers can collect prior information regarding the distribution of a trait. For example, if a robust observational study showed there was some convincing evidence that personality and educational outcome might be associated, a manipulation-type study could be set up recruiting into specific groups individuals of certain personalities, controlling and balancing for all other variables. To justify the expense and labor of such a trial, we would expect the observational study to have shown very convincing evidence, perhaps demonstrating it had controlled statistically for all other confounding variables on a large sample of the population to account for natural variation, with a highly robust "gold standard" personality test to account for potential biases in the measurement of the explanatory variable, and a highly robust assessment which could account for potential biases in the measurement of the response variable. A common refrain around observational studies is that correlation does not equal causation. Not all observational studies must be analyzed through correlations, but this dismissal of correlations negates the fact that a correlation is necessary for causation. Where no correlations exist, it is unlikely that any further manipulation trial will be more successful at finding a relationship between two variables. Observational studies should have a very important place in the hypothetico-deductive model, allowing researchers to refine and target their research questions and potential analyses prior to conducting a potentially costly larger manipulation trial.

Observational studies also have value outside of this narrow interpretation of the hypothetico-deductive model. Often, observational studies may be the only practical approach to studying a phenomenon, such as when ethical or practical concerns make a manipulation study impossible. No one would wish to induce hardship on students to study how interventions can support students in need, and so we may instead try to identify when these situations arise so we can record how our current interventions work. Additionally, where useful historical data has been identified, that data often will often not be structured in an intervention, and so an observational study must be used.

Retrospective Versus Prospective Studies

Across both manipulation and observation studies, data can be collected retrospectively or prospectively. Historical data sources, or retrospective studies, can be an economic use of data. The obvious drawback is that there is no ability to modify the study protocol in light of new information. A good retrospective study will have access to a great deal of information regarding the data collection protocol to make informed judgments about what measurement biases may exist. Anyone who has attempted to standardize historical clinical records will be well aware of the shifts in trends that can influence how someone records data. To minimize measurement bias, strict criteria are often required for data cleaning. Wherever possible, data cleaning should adhere to principles of repeatability, with explicit outlines of each step (Kitzes et al. 2018). This is not outside the realms of possibility and can be achieved even in large textual datasets with the right tools (MacKay 2021a). Researchers on retrospective trials are also at the mercy of what data were historically thought to be useful to account for their confounding variables and, depending on access to data, may need to seek out more data to contextualize their variables. Finally, retrospective studies must also be concerned with data use aspects, not all available data are available for the use of researchers. This is of particular note in studies making use of data from online sources, which are often mistakenly thought to be a "free-for-use" source of data (Zimmer 2010). Prospective studies can avoid these concerns through the careful designing out of measurement bias, accounting for confounding variables, and ensuring proper ethical consent is obtained for all data. Unsurprisingly this comes with financial and labor costs.

Section 3: Collecting Data

Jill R. D. MacKay

While some aspects of study design are impacted by philosophical positions on the nature of reality, the practical implications of running a study, and the funding available to the researcher, another key aspect of design is how to collect the data itself. There are myriad data sources available to the education researcher, and many of them can be utilized in a variety of study designs. In this section, we will cover what types of data can be collected where, some of the most obvious biases that can impact these measurements, and some typical use cases. However, there is a veritable smorgasbord of data sources in the world, and exploring new ways of utilizing data can bring great insights into any research question. It should also be noted that the collection of data should be considered concurrently with the analytical methods chosen. In this chapter, they are presented sequentially, but in practice, the data recording method cannot truly be separated from the data analysis method.

Data collection methods can be utilized in a variety of different designs. A survey, for example, may be used in a manipulation trial to collect data from the control and treatment groups, or in an observational trial to explore events happening in the natural world.

Part 1: Research Surveys

One of the most common tools in the educational researcher's arsenal is the research survey. For those starting out in education or interdisciplinary research, surveys are often referred to as, or outright dismissed as, qualitative data collection. This is inaccurate and potentially misleading information. There is a range of different data types that can be collected via a survey, and purely qualitative surveys require exceptional consideration to design and

administer, so much as to merit their own subheading in this chapter. Examples of different types of data and forms of questions are given in Table 17.4.

Surveys allow for standardized collection of data from participants as each participant receives the questions in the same format, attempting to minimize the impact of bias or poor measurements. This means that the design and consideration of the questions is a crucial aspects of ensuring surveys are fit for purpose. There are many common challenges or pitfalls in the design of survey questions that can introduce aspects of bias or confounding variables into the data.

An Overview of Question Types

Generally, questions in a survey can be "fixed response" or "open response." A fixed response question provides a list of potential answers and forces the participant to choose one of the options. Fixed responses can be multiple responses (sometimes referred to as "check box"), i.e., the participant can indicate as many answer options as they feel is appropriate to them; or single response (sometimes referred to as "radio button"), i.e., the participant must choose the single most appropriate answer from the list. Open response questions allow the participant to answer the question in their own words. Open response questions can have limitations, such as a word limit, and are valuable because they minimize limitations on the participant's ability to respond. In cases where there is little information regarding how participants might respond it can be useful to provide an open response question to collect and summarize this data. They are also essential for qualitative surveys.

For all question types, the manner of asking the question has the potential to influence the answer. A question can be poorly written and difficult for the participant to parse. This can be because of jargon or regional dialects. For example:

Have you ever clapped a pig?

Would be very clear to someone from Scotland, but would require elaboration to someone from the rest of the United Kingdom (and other English-speaking countries).

Have you ever clapped (sometimes called stroking or petting) a pig?

By providing elaboration, we ensure that regardless of where the participant is from, they infer the same meaning from the question. Questions can commonly be made confusing by attempting to assess too many things at once. For example:

Were the induction and orientation sessions useful?

Table 17.4 Example questions and their corresponding data types utilized in research surveys.

Data type	Example question	Example data
Numerical The data is provided as a number, and the interval between each number is consistent.	What is your age to the nearest year?	18, 19, 20 . . . 100
	To the nearest hour, how many hours would you say you studied in the average week?	2,3,4. . .168
Ordinal There is a rank order to the data, which may often be coded as numerical data for analysis, but the interval between each number is not consistent	Does the following statement describe you well or poorly?	Describes me very poorly Describes me poorly Describes me neither well nor poorly Describes me well Describes me very well
	How frequently do you study in the average week?	At least daily At least every two days At least twice a week At least once a week Less often than once a week
Categorical There is no implicit order to the data	How would you describe your gender?	As a man As a woman In another way
	Which of the following study methods have you used? Please tick all that apply.	Cover-and-recall method Reading and rewriting notes Pomodorino method

This question will result in conflation between the sessions in the data, and if one session was good while the other was poor, how does a participant respond? Two separate questions will provide less biased data.

Was the induction session useful?
Was the orientation session useful?

There is an important distinction between fixed multiple response questions and fixed single response questions from a data analysis point of view that is often overlooked. The naïve or unwary researcher may see little difference between the following two questions:

Which one of the following statements best describes your reaction to this chapter (select only one)?
I found this chapter useful
I found this chapter engaging
I found this chapter frustrating

And

Which of the following statements describes your reaction to this chapter (select as many as apply):
I found this chapter useful
I found this chapter engaging
I found this chapter frustrating

In your final data, the first option provides one column of categorical data with three levels (useful/engaging/frustrating). The second option provides three columns of categorical data each with two levels (useful yes/no; engaging yes/no; and frustrating yes/no). This can surprise researchers who expect that they have only asked one question when they realize they have in fact asked three and need to analyze all three separately.

Item Anchors

In many types of fixed response questions, we use set item "anchors," or descriptions of the scale to standardize responses. Along with the question, the answer scale can also impact how participants answer the question. It is common for scales to be numbered to save on space and formatting issues. Potentially, as the researcher intends to analyze the responses by coding the values to numerical, numbering the scale may also feel less biased to the researcher.

How strongly do you agree or disagree that this course was useful?

1) Strongly disagree
2)
3)
4)
5) Strongly agree

In fact, numerical and partially labeled response items create more ambiguity for the participant, and thus introduce more bias into the data (Krosnick 2018). Instead, all options should be labeled verbally only, which is the most descriptive and unambiguous form of labeling and requires the participant to do less work in interpretation.

Furthermore, agreement anchors, often called Likert scales, are subject to biases, where some people will be more likely to agree than disagree. Instead, anchors should be Likert-like, and explicitly phrase the construct of interest in the question (Artino et al. 2014; Dillman et al. 2009; Krosnick 2018).How useful was this course?

Not at all useful
Not useful
Neither useful nor not useful
Useful
Very useful

From an analysis point of view, these scales are often converted into numbers, but fundamentally these data are about the relationship between observations (participants). This will be discussed further later. What is important to recognize is that we cannot rely on all participants agreeing on the points of the numerical scale, and by providing explicitly labeled anchors, we reduce some of the variation in participants' responses (Christian et al. 2009). Arguments that numbers might be more objective miss an underlying point: there is no fundamental unit of usefulness. A course cannot double in usefulness; treating the scale as ratio data can convey false meaning.Item anchors can also be worded in unipolar fashion, where the important concept within the description, often a word, is repeated, e.g.:

Was the induction helpful?
  Not at all helpful
  Not helpful
  A little helpful
  Helpful
  Very helpful

Whereas a bipolar scale provides two concepts and encourages the participant to choose between them, e.g.:

Was the induction helpful?
  Completely unhelpful
  Unhelpful
  Neither helpful nor unhelpful
  Helpful
  Very helpful

There is some evidence to suggest that unipolar scales often have a moderate middle item, whereas bipolar scales are interpreted as having a neutral middle item (Menold 2021; O'Muircheartaigh et al. 1995) and that in practice, we tend to see bipolar scales as showing more agreement than unipolar scales (Höhne et al. 2020). Further research on the impact of unipolar versus bipolar scales is necessary, particularly as these assessments of response bias are often conducted using questions with agreement items, which as previously discussed may be prone to agreement bias in certain cultures and contexts (J. W. Lee et al. 2002; Schaeffer and Dykema 2020). Potentially this agreement bias is in fact a bipolar bias given it is phrased as strongly disagree to strongly agree; it is difficult to know for sure at this stage.

The final element of item anchors to consider is how many anchors are required. Odd scales, such as 3 items, 5 items, or 7 items, often lend themselves to a neutral middle point, in bipolar scales at least. Even scales, such as 2, 4, or 6 items more often omit a middle point, forcing the participant to make a choice one way or the other. While forcing participants to avoid the middle is often attractive, studies into how people respond to questions suggest this negatively impacts the quality of data (Wang and Krosnick 2020). Often people simply feel neutrally about a question, particularly where it has little relevance to them. One argument for scales with more anchor points is that central point tendency theorem allows for parametric statistics to be used on larger scales, but it is also contested that parametric statistics can be used on shorter scales if desired (Norman 2010). There is some evidence to suggest that larger scales produce less extreme responses, but are comparable (Dawes 2008). On the other hand, a simple 3-item scale can also be considered reliable and valid when used as agree, uncertain, or disagree in certain situations (Jacoby and Matell 1971).

As with so much in research design, "best practice" in question writing is about being aware of the potential ways your methods can be biased because there is no perfect question that can completely minimize bias. Instead, continually evaluating how we ask questions is the best way we have of considering the replicability of our findings.

Survey Delivery Mode

Surveys can be administered in a variety of ways. Surveys can be verbal (also known as a structured interview), where the researcher asks each question in a standardized fashion and records the answer through face-to-face, telephone, or video call meetings. Verbal surveys have great advantages when accessibility may be an issue for participants, where literacy levels are known to be poor, or for younger participants. Historically they were thought to have better response rates than paper surveys (Hox and De Leeuw 1994), although the ever-changing impact of the Internet on society encourages researchers to utilize verbal surveys more when there are accessibility reasons for doing so rather than to ensure high response rates.

Surveys can also be administered through writing, whether through print or the Internet. Response rates generally favor Internet surveys in comparisons of the two (Boyer et al. 2002), but there are elements of design that impact this. Participants are more likely to complete shorter surveys and surveys without progress bars (when online, Liu and Wronski 2017). Often paper-based surveys will have more options in terms of design than the "off the shelf" online survey tools, such as being able to visually differentiate between non-applicable answer options (which can be useful for data quality, see Dillman et al. 2009). However, online survey tools have more ability to quality control data, such as ensuring participants select only one option in a fixed response single item question, or tracking participants through emails.

Ultimately the delivery mode will reflect more about your own pragmatic design considerations. Offering incentives can improve reach into underrepresented demographics (Dykema et al. 2013), and can be a useful tool alongside multimodal survey distribution where there are concerns that certain demographics will be missed.

Instruments

It is important to distinguish between research surveys and research instruments. A survey aims to ask a series of questions in a standardized fashion. A research instrument aims to use a standardized and validated set of questions to measure an underlying construct of variation. As previously mentioned, constructs are otherwise hard-to-measure traits thought to impact multiple behaviors or affective states. Designing an instrument requires considerably more work than a survey, and the time investment means that they are often considered proprietary by the researcher, limiting their ability to be used by other researchers in the field.

Artino et al. (2014) recommend a 7-step process in instrument design (which they call a survey scale):

1) Conduct a literature review to align the survey's purpose with prior research
2) Conduct interviews and/or focus groups to formalize the process
3) Synthesize your construct of interest from participant data and literature review
4) Develop the items thought to be affected by the construct
5) Conduct expert validation of items to ensure they relate to construct
6) Conduct interviews with potential participants to ensure the items relate to the construct
7) Conduct pilot testing of the items in their proposed form to establish construct validity such as through Crohnbach's alpha.

The design and validation of a survey instrument would greatly benefit from the inclusion of psychology researchers and statisticians, alongside the considerable investment in the preliminary stages incorporating stakeholders in assessing the validity of the proposed construct.

Qualitative Surveys

Recently, qualitative surveys have garnered attention for their own utility (Braun et al. 2020). Qualitative surveys feature open-ended questions and share many similarities with interviews (see below). When designing a qualitative survey in comparison to a research interview, the researcher needs to ensure they provide enough opportunity for the participant to provide the same depth of response that is possible in an interview where the participant can be prompted by the researcher. However, qualitative surveys can be administered widely and are more highly economic in terms of data collection time. The ability for the participant to choose when they respond can also be of benefit to them. This makes qualitative surveys particularly good for exploring the early stages of an analysis where there may be limited information in the literature regarding how an issue is perceived by a certain demographic, for example. Qualitative surveys require the same consideration as to question wording, etc., if not more since the researcher cannot clarify as they would in an interview, and there is guidance on their design in the literature (Braun et al. 2020; Terry and Braun 2017). One advantage of qualitative surveys that is of particular interest to education research is their ability to be piped into more automated textual analyses, which can have great benefits for research over long periods of time, such as course evaluations (MacKay 2019, 2021a).

Piloting Surveys

Given the many varied ways that surveys can be asked, the piloting and testing of surveys ahead of time is an important element of their design. No instrument should be developed without a rigorous and theory-led approach, but research surveys should also be developed in conjunction with participants and ideally with interviews/focus groups to ensure the questions are being interpreted properly. Most commonly, surveys are piloted in a family and friends test of the researcher, checking for spelling errors and, in the case of online surveys, errors in data quality control measures. Again, proper piloting takes time and resources, which are often hard to come by in education. Papers rarely feature clear and honest descriptions of exactly how piloting was conducted. To better improve our understanding of the biases inherent in any survey, it would be beneficial to have a clearer, more accurate understanding of what piloting was done, even when that was simply a family and friends test, as opposed to construct validity assessments. We must remember that publication is highly incentivized, and by accepting the honest limitations of a research piece we may improve replicability more generally.

Part 2: Research Interviews

The research interview is a powerful tool for collecting data. It is most suited for qualitative data collection, although in some limited cases, they can also collect quantitative data (see structured interviews). Interviews feature a researcher and participant sharing a space (physical or virtual) and having a conversation, meaning that research interviews mainly collect a form of data related to naturally occurring talk (Silverman 2014, p. 316). A conversation is conducted by both agents, and so this form of data collection allows both the participant and researcher to direct the conversation, seek out clarification on meaning, and jointly ensure meaning is reached (Byrne 2016). As conversation is a tool used daily by most people, there is very little training or skill acquisition that a researcher needs to do to interview appropriately (Rapley 2011).

The nature of interviews seems to lend them to a constructionist epistemology, where the researcher and participant jointly negotiate the understanding of the data, but Silverman (2014, p. 173) describes how they can also be used in positivist epistemologies, with questions designed to uncover standardized "facts" (much like a survey), and sampling considerations around this. Finally, they can come from naturalist epistemologies, which focus on describing the authentic experience of the participant, with less concern as to the previous assumptions of the researcher. These three approaches are broadly suited to three types of research interviews: structured, semi-structured, and unstructured.

Structured Interviews

Structured interviews and verbal surveys are highly related. They both suit more positivist approaches to data, seeking standardized questions that should not be altered after the study begins. In practice, this means that participants are not able to provide elaboration or clarify their position. Imagine a scenario where a researcher has a question in their structured interview: Do you find this textbook useful? Please answer yes or no. In a sample of 10 participants, the first five answered quickly, but the sixth seems uncertain. They elaborate "Yes, it was useful, because I used it to prop up my laptop when working from home." The researcher may be tempted to amend the interview question for the seventh participant and specify "useful for your research?" within the question, but this does not fit with a positivist approach to data. As the first five participants did

not have access to that question, changing the question splits the dataset. The tool for data collection has changed, meaning there are now two smaller datasets. Alternatively, retaining a question that is now known to be inaccurate prompts considerable discussion as we cannot be confident in the findings.

As with surveys, proper piloting hopes to minimize these risks. The financial and other resources of a researcher and participant sitting through a structured interview are significant. Consider as well that the data from the interview must be inputted. The cost investment of a structured interview when it does not offer the advantage of a full conversation makes it an unusual choice, except in cases where there may be identifiable accessibility risks to written surveys.

Semi-structured Interviews

The semi-structured interview may be a "best of both worlds" approach to interview data. In a semi-structured interview, the researcher has an outline of questions they want to address in the given time. These questions are open-ended and aim to explore the participant's feelings and experiences. Semi-structured interviews are valuable for exploring these unquantifiable phenomena and, importantly, allow the researcher to adapt to the discussion from the participants, following new avenues of inquiry as they arise (Adams 2015). A short schedule for a semi-structured interview can also feature prompts that can help to elaborate on a question where participants are slow to engage. Not all prompts will be used for all participants, indeed not all questions may be needed for all participants. After all, if a participant naturally answers question two in the course of responding to question one, it would not be a particularly natural conversation to then go back and repeat the question!

For the positivist, this may evoke a shiver down the spine. How can consistency between participants be achieved with such a flexible approach? This is a key point: the aim is not consistency; the aim is joint understanding. The researcher wants to describe the participant's feelings on a set of events or phenomena and is not necessarily trying to imply those feelings are representative of a larger sample. Indeed, interviews are sometimes at their most useful in understanding the experiences of atypical participants. Generally, interviews aim to collect data about experiences and feelings, then characterizing what can be observed from such interactions.

Semi-structured interviews work best with how, what, and why questions, so the data collected often lends itself to analyses such as reflexive thematic analysis or constructionist grounded theory, which condense and summarize information to propose explanations for phenomena in education. As semi-structured interviews do require the prior planning of questions, they require identification of the analytical method and research framework ahead of time. Sometimes researchers will collect interview data when they are unsure what they intend to do with the data, believing that qualitative methods are flexible enough to apply to a variety of scenarios. There is some truth to this, particularly in how qualitative analytical methods can be applied to naturally occurring data, but semi-structured interviews still have the researcher developing the data during its collection. This is an opportunity for bias to be introduced, and therefore identifying the analytical methods is a useful step in the design of the research study. Remember that bias is ever-present within research and must be acknowledged where it cannot be minimized.

Unstructured Interviews

The unstructured interview is an odd beast. As the name implies, there are no fixed questions that should be addressed in each interview; instead, the researcher and participant generate data together around the research topic and may go in any direction that is of interest to either party. Unstructured interviews follow a naturalist approach to data and analysis (Silverman 2014). If this is naturally occurring data, such as those found in unstructured documents (see below), then there are implications for analysis. One perspective is that this kind of data can fit multiple analytical methods, as the data itself is so "pure" that it cannot be biased by underlying flaws in the data collection, which Silverman terms a maximalist approach, as participants are not expected to conceptualize aspects of their lived experience to fit a research agenda. Alternatively, this naively discounts the impact of the researcher and overly simplifies the data collection and analysis process (Potter and Hepburn 2005), which Silverman terms a minimalist approach. Ultimately the researcher's own perspectives and research approach will influence the researcher to one or other of these views. The unstructured interview can be a way of collecting natural data, but this should not be used to avoid making choices regarding the analysis of data unless this is a specific aspect of the researcher's position, and as such should be made explicit in the design of the study from the beginning.

Part 3: Focus Groups

One of the great limitations of interviews is that each interview captures only the self-reported and subjective experience of an individual. While this can be valuable, it falls to the researcher in the analysis stage to explore how findings can be transferred to other contexts. Focus groups aim to combat this at the data collection stage by drawing from the collective experience of participants, giving them the opportunity to review and comment on the experiences of others. Focus groups often work much like semi-structured interviews, with a schedule of questions and prompts. These can sometimes take the form of statements intended to provoke the participants into discussion, such as "this course is in need of radical reform, what do we think about this?" (Conradson 2005). Focus groups are facilitated by either a trained facilitator or the researcher acting as the facilitator. The facilitator's role is there to ensure that ground rules regarding respect and shared participation are followed, and one of their most important roles is to keep discussion and interaction between participants flowing (Kitzinger 1995). The great advantage of focus groups is that participants can share experiences, build consensus, and highlight areas where consensus does not exist (Kitzinger 1994). The interaction between participants is the most important aspect of a focus group, and it can be particularly valuable in situations where there is a power discrepancy between the researcher and participants, such as for marginalized groups (MacKay et al. 2021b; Wilkinson 1999), but this is also very useful in education research where often the participants are in a student–educator relationship with the researchers. The "strength in numbers" aspect of focus groups allows participants to contradict the facilitator's expectations. This of course depends on many factors, including appropriate sampling, to ensure the composition of the group is representative of the desired experiences (Bloor et al. 2002) and appropriate facilitation to ensure certain voices do not become dominant (Smithson 2000).

Part 4: Recording Behavior

Asking people via surveys or interviews what they do can provide self-reported data on behavior and activities. Self-reports are vulnerable to the participant's unintentional incorrect assumptions about what they do and their intentionally misleading answers. These are common phenomena in public health. For example, participants often under-report weight and over-report height (Elgar and Stewart 2008), which may be both an unintentional mistake (after all, who does not get a surprise on the scales sometimes), or an intentional one (it can be embarrassing to reveal the true number). Self-reports with behavior can be similarly error-prone. There can be alternative methods of collecting data on behavior that suit a more positivist epistemology.

Ethograms

Ethograms can be a suitable approach to recording human behavior. They use literature and prior observations to create agreed upon definitions of behavior and sampling protocols that allow for replicable recordings of behavior (Martin and Bateson 1993). This form of behavior recording is commonly used in classroom taxonomy protocols (Eddy et al. 2015; Lund et al. 2015; Wood et al. 2016), although these tools have been criticized for not explicitly adopting ethogram approaches and designing them with replicability in mind (Kinnear et al. 2021).

Think-Alouds

The form of behavior recorded by ethograms is best suited for describing what happens during a session. It is not always clear why a behavior occurs (indeed, good ethogram development discourages the researcher from assuming motive behind behaviors). Think-aloud sessions can be thought of as a halfway house between ethogram and interview. Think-alouds involve the researcher watching the participant's behavior, perhaps making objective notes regarding what is happening, but couples that with standardized interruptions to ask questions about why a behavior is occurring (Cooke 2010). Think-alouds require the participant to verbalize aspects of the process and so can require some gentle facilitating and leading, much like an interview (Willis and Artino 2013). Think-alouds are common in user experience design research and can be a good fit for exploring how students utilize technology in particular (such as studying with lecture recordings; MacKay et al. 2021a).

Part 5: Secondary Data

The majority of data collection methods discussed so far have been methods where the researcher sets out to collect specific data prospectively. In our increasingly digitized world, there are more and more opportunities to use naturally occurring data, either prospectively or, where ethically appropriate, retrospectively.

While not all data that are accessible to researchers should be considered available for research (Zimmer 2010), with due ethical concern and consideration there can be many opportunities for utilizing data sources from elsewhere in the world. These might be considered more natural forms of data for those who are particularly concerned about how the researcher's practice might impact the data. There are many forms of secondary data in the world, some of which lend themselves to positivist approaches (such as learning analytics or grades) and some of which may be more constructionist (such as blogs or social media). These are only tendencies and should not be treated as absolute rules.

Secondary data may often fall under the purview of "data mining," particularly when looking at retrospective sources of data. Data mining is defined as the automated or convenient extraction of data from a wide variety of databases that are not explicitly designed for analysis from the outset (Calders and Custers 2013). Data mining can provide vast quantities of data relatively cheaply and can be a very

tempting resource; however, there are many specific data management, ethics, and statistical considerations to data mining (Hand 1998) which cannot be fully elaborated upon here. Suffice it to say data mining, while powerful, is not easy, and collaboration with methodologists will be advantageous to most researchers embarking on a data mining project.

Learning Analytics

Learning analytics are a topic of increasing interest in the education research literature, in terms of how they can support educational outcomes and how they might also support institutions to develop their own strategies (Tsai et al. 2018). Learning analytics are commonly gathered from the Learning Management System and can include a variety of measures, such as the number of times a resource has been viewed, the times resources have been accessed, the number of discussions or flags raised on a piece of content, the duration of time a piece of content has been viewed (particularly in video resources) and the types of resources accessed (Dietz-Uhler and Hurn 2013; Paterson et al. 2019). There can also be synthesized measures from analytics, such as active class sizes (MacKay et al. 2016) and identifying resources with unusual access patterns, e.g., those videos that were watched more than one standard deviation beyond the average video (MacKay et al. 2021a).

Grades are a particular form of learning analytics that are readily accessed and compared across years and groups. Previous chapters have already discussed the many biases and concerns within assessment, and so most readers should already be aware of the limitations of grades as a direct comparison between students. While they can be a useful source of data and one with obvious relevance to educational research questions, they cannot be assumed to be pure indications of learning.

The use of learning analytics requires consideration of potential bias within the measures, e.g., when might the analytics not truly reflect what we think it does. Massive open online courses (MOOCs) commonly use "retention" as a metric of success, with student retention rates between 5% and 10% being considered successful (Daniel 2012). However, retention can not only be calculated in different ways, such as active class size, but these metrics may offer very narrow glimpses into whether a MOOC was successful for any given individual student who may fairly have engaged with a MOOC for a limited purpose and been successful in this need (MacKay et al. 2018). What "success" is within the learning context requires careful consideration and can rarely be considered as simple as a single number derived from the interactions with the digital environment. However, large analyses can be surprisingly informative of general patterns of behavior and can be useful in informing policy decisions (Tsai and Gasevic 2017). While we may yet be some way away from highly personalized learning environments based on learning analytics usage, they can be a useful and economic source of data for evaluation when appropriate critiques are borne in mind.

Unstructured Documents

A final source of data that may be commonly forgotten is unstructured documents, which most commonly now probably fit into the online space. Unstructured documents can include a wide range of materials, such as images, blog posts, diaries, social media posts, emails, etc. While these documents will often have some form of structure (i.e., there are often unwritten formatting rules regarding social media posts; Kietzmann et al. 2011), the creator of the document has a great deal of choice regarding what and how they will present their data.

This data is commonly found online, so it is vital that researchers intending to utilize data sources such as this consider the ethical implications of their research. The Association of Internet Researchers has important guidance regarding how such documents can be explored in an appropriate manner (Markham and Buchanan 2012). At the very least, participants providing documents, such as discussion board posts, etc., should be aware that their data may be used for research, or better yet, actively give consent for specific research. It is possible to utilize these data sources prospectively, e.g., to ask participants to reflectively blog for the express purpose of understanding their thought processes over a period of time (Chinnery et al. 2021). Where there may be ethical concerns regarding participants' experiences in the online environment, it can also be possible to create mock online environments, such as showing an example of an artificial social media post and inviting participants in a study to respond as though it were real (Riddle and MacKay 2020).

Given the broad and varied nature of these documents, the researcher's position and analytical methods chosen will impact how they can be used. For example, if using blogs as your data source, sampling the blogs will depend on whether the researcher is aiming to characterize a representative cross-section of the population or is exploring a specific phenomenon (Hookway 2008).

Section 4: Analyzing Data

Jill R. D. MacKay

There are many approaches to analyzing data, which may typically be split into quantitative and qualitative forms of analysis. Readers of this chapter will now be able to predict the overarching theme at all points of choice in research methodology, and that is that choices made about data analysis reflect the researcher's position and epistemology (Gelman and Hennig 2017). There are broadly some differences between quantitative and qualitative analyses. Generally, quantitative analyses are interested in predicting responses for others, with data being generalized from one context to another. Qualitative analyses are less interested in generalizing, but may be interested in producing a theory to model future quantitative research around. Qualitative analysis also often centers the researcher's bias, making those assumptions explicit, and this should be likewise encouraged in quantitative analyses. Analyses are not separate from research design and the sensible researcher generally has an idea as to how they will analyze data prior to collecting it. This is a requirement in preregistrations, part of a suite of strategies to tackle the replication crisis, and this holds true for qualitative analyses too (Haven and Van Grootel 2019). Wherever possible, it is best to seek out the experience of someone familiar with the type of analysis you are doing during the design stage of research to help point out the pitfalls of any particular approach. Test analyses, either on randomly generated data or on data similar in structure to your own, are an excellent approach to explore the suitability of a given pairing of data and analysis. Particularly within statistical analyses, researchers should not shy away from generating fake data to explore potential methods (DeBruine and Barr 2021). If this alarms the reader – after all, what is to stop a researcher from using that fake data if their own data does not prove as useful? – then this is even more incentive to share data where appropriate and to highlight the methodological choices being made.

Part 1: The Purpose of Research Analysis

At this point, it is worthwhile revisiting the purpose of research, particularly in light of how choices made in the data analysis stage can impact the uses of research. At the top of the chapter, we discussed how research could be used to make improvements through the application of findings to similar contexts. This is frequently considered "generalizability," something we have discussed at great length in the design of quantitative studies. In qualitative research, "generalizability" is more complicated.

There are a number of related terms that are commonly used interchangeably, perhaps even within this chapter. Generalizability can be considered a description of the internal and external validity of a study and the researcher's informed opinion as to whether the findings have relevance for another setting (Kukull and Ganguli 2012). In this definition, a researcher may be very concerned regarding elements of study design more suited to quantitative design, such as the relationship of the sample to the population. In qualitative research we sometimes discuss the transferability of findings, e.g., does the researcher have enough confidence in the appropriateness of the design and analysis to allow them to transfer the findings to another setting (Kuper et al. 2008)? In many of the discussions surrounding the integration of qualitative research into historically more quantitative fields, the term "rigor" is used to capture methodological validity (Tong et al. 2007) which can then be used to inform the researcher as to the utility of the findings for their own context.

For all three terms, generalizability, transferability, and rigor, there is a key similarity. The researcher must judge whether the findings are applicable in other contexts. This can only be done through the considered evaluation of methods with the aim of understanding whether the choices made throughout the research process were appropriate. If so, and if the study is relevant to one's own context, then something of the findings should be of use. The purpose of research is to support making better decisions, and if a piece of research is conducted well, it has utility in future decision-making, regardless of its method.

Part 2: Quantitative Analyses

Frequentist Analyses

For most researchers, quantitative analyses are synonymous with p values. p values, however, are the domain of a particular type of quantitative analysis called frequentist statistics. Frequentist statistics have had a great deal of impact on study design. Indeed, the RCT is often how frequentist statistics are explained. We explore the frequency of a given event in a sample of interest compared to a population, e.g., a treatment and control group. The p value is a calculation of the strength of evidence against a given null hypothesis (Grafen and Hails 2002), i.e., it tells us the probability of obtaining the observed results by chance alone if the null hypothesis was true. There are many assumptions and philosophical stances within this statement. For example, you may have been told in the past that data that is not normally distributed should be analyzed via nonparametric forms of statistics, but in fact, most modern approaches to frequentist analysis recognize that it is the normality of the residuals (the difference of the predicted value from the observed value) that is important (Grafen and Hails 2002, p. 159) to frequentist assumptions, not the observed values themselves. In fact, some would argue that even non-ratio data such as Likert-like scales can be analyzed as parametric data (Norman 2010), although that may seem shocking to researchers from highly positivist backgrounds.

The ins-and-outs of frequentist analyses are outside the scope of this chapter (the author recommends Grafen and Hails for an excellent introduction to frequentist model building), but for our purposes, we must recognize an important element of the frequentist approach, and that is that the p value is not a particularly useful criterion. The p value, as defined, is a test of evidence strength, not a test of whether the evidence itself is good. Large sample sizes, for example, provide more strength of evidence and therefore are able to provide significant differences between groups, even though the quality of the evidence is poor. For this reason, it is critical that educational researchers adopting frequentist analyses recognize the value of reporting effect sizes and confidence intervals. These are far more valuable to the reader than simply a p value.

When we discussed NHST as being part of the problem with the replication crisis, we used a fictional example where a control group received standardized materials and the treatment group received COOL materials for study (back in Figure 17.2). The difference in grades between the two groups was found to be significant. Ideally, when we were reporting that study, we should have also reported the effect size and confidence interval around that effect size, as below:

> Those in the COOL group performed better ($\mu = 77\%$, SD $= 7.1$) than those in the control group ($\mu = 73\%$, SD $= 7.8$) and this was significant ($t_{Welch}(97.01) = -2.15$, $p = 0.034$). The effect size ($g_{Hedges} = -0.43$, 95% CI [-0.82, -0.03]) was medium.

Reporting effect size allows us to compare this finding with other findings in different papers. We also see that the confidence interval around this effect size is broad, and it is plausible the effect size could be as small as -0.03 or as high as -0.82. In essence, there is not a lot of confidence around this estimate. The difference of 4% marks between the average grades of the two groups may not be considered very meaningful, and it may be much less. However, the effect size could feasibly be greater than we have calculated, and so it is clear that we are not terribly confident in our estimate. This is more informative than simply saying "significant at the level of $p < 0.05$."

Bayesian Analyses

Where frequentist approaches philosophically can only explore the evidence against a null hypothesis, Bayesian approaches allow us to describe evidence for and against a hypothesis (Kruschke 2014). Bayesian approaches are becoming more popular as the computing power required to adopt them becomes cheaper and more accessible (Kruschke 2013). Instead of comparing only against a null hypothesis, Bayesian approaches compare the distributions of populations (called the prior distribution) to calculate the likelihood of a difference between the population (Perkins and Wang 2004). Philosophically, a Bayesian approach considers probability to be a degree of belief in the unknown, versus the Frequentist consideration of probability, the *p* value, as being a threshold at which we would consider something unusual if the null hypothesis was true. Neither approach is necessarily "correct," but Bayesian approaches can be more useful in cases of small data, in cases where frequentist assumptions may not be met, and in cases of very large data where *p* values would be expected to be significant purely due to sample size (Bayarri and Berger 2004). An excellent example of this is the exploration of "grade inflation" in the United Kingdom using Bayesian models, which was able to highlight that only some of the increase in grades awarded from 2010 to 2019 was unexplained by other factors, such as improvements to teaching (Jephcote et al. 2020).

With the same COOL study, we can explore a few measures from Bayesian analyses that can inform our understanding of the data. We might report the following measures: the region of practical equivalence (ROPE), the probability of effect direction, and the Bayes Factor (Makowski et al. 2019). The ROPE, which we can define based on our own beliefs about the data, is a range of data values that are practically equivalent to a null effect (Kruschke 2014, Ch 12). Bayesian analyses calculate highest density interval (HDI), which can be thought of as similar to the frequentist confidence interval. The HDI is the range of values of the parameter that are credible, and just to confuse people further we often use 89% credible intervals for HDI as opposed to the 95% confidence intervals in frequentist statistics. The ROPE looks to see how much of the HDI (the most likely values of the data) falls within this predefined range of values that are considered equivalent. In other words, is this effect likely to be of interest or not? Finally, we can also look at the Bayes Factor, which is a calculation of how much the data favor the null hypothesis versus the alternate hypothesis (Kruschke 2013). We could then report the same data for the COOL experiment with the following Bayesian analysis.

> In a Bayesian linear model, the COOL condition was found to have a 3.2% (95% CI [0.31, 6.18% points]) point increase in median grade. The probability of a positive effect of the COOL treatment was 98.5%, and 0% of the parameter fell within the ROPE. The Bayes Factor was 0.48 which, per Raftery (1995), is weak evidence against the null hypothesis.

This is a very uninformed usage of the Bayesian approach; for example, we have simply used default criteria to set the ROPE. We may have decided that we were only interested in differences larger or smaller than 5% points, which may have reasonably pushed some students over a grade boundary, and could have explicitly set this in

our calculations. Regardless, one advantage the Bayesian approach has over the Frequentist approach is that while we have good evidence of a positive effect (the probability of direction was 98.5% positive), we have only weak evidence against the null hypothesis. We can explore the evidence for both hypotheses. Regardless, both Bayesian and Frequentist approaches to this data have not provided convincing evidence regarding the impact of the COOL resources. Our decision to continue their use should be based on whether we think there are critiques of the study design that weaken our findings and the value of the small percentage point increase to this group, not an arbitrary *p* value cutoff.

Full Bayesian reporting guidelines can be found alongside Bayesian tutorials with open-source software (Kruschke 2014; van Doorn et al. 2020). These analyses were run using the "easystats" package in R (Makowski et al. 2020).

Text Mining

Another form of quantitative data analysis that may be very useful to the educational researcher is text mining. Text mining covers a range of approaches and involves processing a corpus of text, which may be a single document or a collection of multiple documents, most often with computer processing. Text mining can produce a range of measures, such as most common words or "tokens" (which may be strings of words or root words), most unique words, and sentiment analyses (Greaves et al. 2013; Silge and Robinson 2018). Text mining requires a context-informed approach to support research, i.e., simple descriptions of the most common word in a corpus are not likely to reveal much of interest unless there is underlying knowledge on the part of the researcher regarding what may be expected within this context (Liberman 2018; MacKay 2021a). For most purposes, text mining allows the classification of words into categories that can then be used to explore differences across groups or times. There are many advantages to text mining, especially when done with reproducible considerations in mind. In particular, it can be applied to make better use of the types of secondary data often collected in standard course evaluation questionnaires that are routinely administered in many educational institutions.

Part 3: Qualitative Analyses

Content Analysis

The range of potential qualitative analytical methods available to the researcher is just as varied as the range of quantitative methods. Much as quantitative methods seek to summarize and condense large amounts of numerical data into something that can be understood by someone unfamiliar with the data, qualitative methods seek to summarize and condense large amounts of qualitative data. Content analysis is a form of classification, i.e., reading through text and finding parts of the text that can be systematically characterized to a certain category (Smith 2000). Often content analyses will make use of a codebook (DeCuir-Gunby et al. 2011; Fonteyn et al. 2008), which describes how a reader might recognize aspects of a category within the text, and thus enable multiple researchers to "code" the same piece of text with relative accuracy as within (MacKay et al. 2022). Content analyses can therefore support quite positivist approaches to qualitative data, allowing for the measurement of agreement between coders, and replicable work across time and context.

Thematic and Reflexive Thematic Analyses

Thematic analysis may be considered as a step beyond content analysis, although it is important to distinguish between thematic analysis and reflexive thematic analysis as first proposed by Braun and Clarke (2006). Thematic analysis is similar to content analysis in that is seeks to identify patterns across data but is less "categorizable" than content. Instead, thematic analysis looks for "themes" or "patterns" (Braun et al. 2019).

Reflexive thematic analysis as described by Braun and Clarke (2019) is intended to formalize (and thus improve the reproducibility of) the process of thematic analysis, while encouraging active identification of the epistemological approach to the data.

Grounded Theory, Constructivist, and Otherwise

Another form of qualitative analysis that may be familiar in passing is Grounded Theory. There are two main brands, classic grounded theory, and constructivist grounded theory. Both aim to characterize the main concern within participant data and develop a theory that explains the data (Breckenridge 2014). In classic grounded theory, this theory should arise from the data abstract from prior knowledge and purely from the data (Glaser 2002). Contra, Constructivist Grounded Theory recognizes the bias and position of the researcher and encourages use of the literature to support and develop the theory alongside the data (Charmaz 2008).

Theory-led Analyses

While there are many, many other approaches to qualitative data (see Silverman 2014; Denzin and Lincoln 2018; Stake 2010) it is worth highlighting a broad arrangement we can term "theory-led analyses." Theory-led analyses start with an existing approach, such as feminist theory, social identity theory, or social capital theory, and apply that to the data through an analysis that may follow reflexive thematic analysis or constructivist grounded theory approaches. The description of a full theory-led analysis is beyond the scope of this chapter, but they can be highly valuable approaches.

Section 5: The Ethics of Educational Research

Shelly Wu

Part 1: Introduction and Overview of Ethics in Educational Research

Thus far, the chapter has provided an overview of how the researcher's theoretical stance influences the study design, including the specific methodological and analytical choices to address the goals of the study. To coincide with the research process, ethical provisions should be made throughout the entirety of the research plan to ensure that the researcher is also protecting the rights and welfare of research participants.

Researcher–Participant Relationship

There is an inherent power difference between the researcher and participant, but this role will vary from a more hierarchical relationship to more co-participatory relationship, depending on the paradigmatic frame of the research (Lincoln et al. 2011; Karnieli-Miller et al. 2009). The researcher should clearly outline the researcher–participant roles throughout the study and identify opportunities where participants can contribute, such as being able to provide feedback to the researcher to build trust (Karnieli-Miller et al. 2009). Instead of treating participants as a means to achieve end goals for the research, using an ethic of care with participants is important for promoting respect with participants and can also enhance the trustworthiness of the research (Rallis and Rossman 2010).

Along with building trust with participants, researchers should be transparent about their role in the research and disclose any conflict of interest (COI) with participants. COI is defined as "Any financial or other interest which conflicts with the service of the individual because it (1) could significantly impair the individual's objectivity or (2) could create an unfair competitive advantage for any person or organization" (The National Academies 2003, p. 4). COI can include financial conflicts such as receiving payment from the sponsor that is funding the study, or non-financial conflicts such as making biased decisions to benefit the outcome of the research. It is recommended that the researcher reports COI to all applicable stakeholders such as the institution and manage their COI to create trust in the research (Hale and Nelson 2022).

Recruitment

The researcher should identify what is the target population of interest in relation to the research topic being investigated by defining the specific inclusion and exclusion criteria (Van den Broeck et al. 2013). The researcher should also consider the planned number of participants to enroll in the study. This is important because the enrollment should be justified in relation to the methodology of the study and be sufficient to address the objective of the study. Enrollment should be reasonable with an appropriate number of participants, such that the researcher is not enrolling too many participants and exposing individuals to unnecessary risk (if applicable) in the study (Brestoff and Van den Broeck 2013). Second, the selection of participants is important to ensure there is equitable selection of subjects in the recruitment process. In other words, participants should not be chosen out of convince to avoid taking advantage of participants (Van den Broeck et al. 2013).

Once the target population is defined, the researcher should consider how the potential research participants will be recruited including the place, timing of communication, nature of communication, and use of recruitment materials. Additional considerations should be taken for recruitment at places where the researcher does not have an association and would like to gain access to the population of interest. For example, if a researcher wants to recruit and conduct research at an organization, school, or institution where they do not have any association, the researcher should obtain appropriate permission in advance to build a positive relationship with personnel at the site, such as school officials (Creswell and Poth 2018; Rice et al. 2007). The researcher can build trust with participants by tailoring the recruitment process with cultural considerations for the participants, such as developing trust with the community, being respectful of the setting, and reducing the power difference such that the researcher is approachable to potential participants (Gyure et al. 2014).

Compensation

Compensation information can be provided during the recruitment and consent process. For example, an advertisement for the research study may indicate the compensation amount being offered for participation, and the consent process may describe the details of compensation further regarding the specific research procedures that need to be completed to receive compensation. The compensation plan should follow applicable institutional guidelines and compensation should be fair for all the participants in relation to what is being asked of their participation for completing research procedures.

Additional considerations should be made such that the compensation does not unduly influence participants to agree to participate against their own best interest (Brown and Largent 2022).

Consent

Consent can be viewed in several ways such as a form that provides information about the study, a process that helps the participant understand the research study, and also a decision that person makes to decide their participation in the study or not (Eyal and Magalhaes 2022). A consent form should provide an adequate overview of information including (but not limited to) the purpose of the study, study procedures, risks and benefits, compensation, alternatives to participating in the study, measures to protect confidentiality, a statement participation is completely voluntary, and contact information. It should meet all regulatory requirements and furthermore, be written in a manner that facilitates participant's level of comprehension to understand the research (Eyal and Magalhaes 2022; Wester 2011).

Prior to obtaining consent, the researcher should be trained on how to obtain informed consent adequately and have a plan for how the consent process will occur such as the use of a consent form, timing of consent, location to protect the potential participant's privacy, documentation of written consent (when applicable), how long participants can decide to participate or not, and measures to minimize coercion (Eyal and Magalhaes 2022; Green and Rosenfeld 2022). Additional considerations should be planned when consenting to vulnerable populations that require further protections. For example, if a study involves children in schools, there should be a plan to obtain both the child's agreement, also known as assent, and parental consent to participate in the research (Nelson and Synder 2022). During the assent and consent process, it should be clear that participation is completely voluntary and their decision to withdraw from the study would not have any impact on their academic performance. The consent process will vary depending on the study, but it is the responsibility of the researcher to be familiar with the regulatory requirements of informed consent, and additionally, ensure that a participant's decision to participate is truly autonomous and ongoing.

Data Collection, Analysis, and Representation

In educational research, data collection methods often include interaction with participants, with examples discussed earlier such as the use of surveys and interviews. When data is being collected, the researcher should consider the provisions in advance to protect privacy and confidentiality. Privacy is defined by the ". . .control over the extent, timing, and circumstances of sharing oneself [physically, behaviorally, or intellectually] or information about oneself, with others" (Buchanan 2022, p. 644). The research plan should include steps to protect participant's privacy, such as conducting interviews in a private room such that others do have access to hearing participant's sensitive information. Confidentiality refers to the processes used to protect information such as only collecting de-identified data, or if identifiable data is collected, assign pseudonyms or a numeric subject ID to each participant. Researchers need to consider how the data collected will be protected such as de-identification, reporting aggregate data, and using secure data storage methods. If there are not enough protections for privacy and confidentiality, data breaches can lead to increased risk to participants. For example, breaches in participant's information such as health status or involvement in illegal activities can lead to increased stigma or job discrimination (Turcotte-Tremblay and Mc Sween-Cadieux 2018). It is important for the researcher to have a clear plan to protect privacy and confidentiality.

During the data analysis stage and reporting process, the researcher should be familiar with the methodological strategies in their paradigmatic framework to ensure the data is being ethically represented. For example, if a qualitative study is reporting participant's perspectives, the researcher might solicit feedback from the participant to confirm that they have not misrepresented their voices, and the results should be comprehensive to not only include positive findings, but also any negative findings. The qualitative researcher should also use reflexivity in their writing to be clear about their theoretical stance, bias, and interpretation of the findings (Creswell and Poth 2018; Karnieli-Miller et al. 2009). Lastly, as a manuscript is finalized for publication, the researcher should follow best practices in their discipline, such as disclosing any COI and listing authorship based on their intellectual contribution to the study (Creswell and Poth 2018).

In summary, the researcher should be intentional about embedding ethics throughout the entirety of the research process from the beginning to the end of the study. Identifying the specific ethical challenges that are contextual to each research study may help a researcher anticipate ethical challenges and address them adequately. Furthermore, it is encouraged to think critically about the research design beyond meeting procedural codes of ethics to intentionally implement actions that will demonstrate respect for the research participants. The research plan should be written into a research protocol and submitted to the appropriate ethics entity for review and approval. The next section describes ethical review of studies involving animal and human subjects research.

Part 2: IACUC Versus IRB

Institutional Animal Care and Use Committee (IACUC)

The exploitation of animals in research has led to the creation of regulatory oversight to promote ethical treatment. In the United States, popular articles in the 1960's exposed how dogs were stolen, abused, and sold for medical research experiments (Rozmiarek 2014). In response, the Laboratory Animal Welfare Act (AWA) was passed in 1966 with regulatory oversight by the US Department of Agriculture (USDA). It was amended several times and led to the formation of the Institutional Animal Care and Use Committee (IACUC) in 1985 (Cardon et al. 2012; Rozmiarek 2014). In the same year, the Health Research Extension Act of 1985 led to the creation of the Public Health Service (PHS) Policy to provide guidance on the ethical use of animals in research (NRC 2009).

IACUC is responsible for providing oversight on research studies with vertebrate animals. The definitions of what animals are covered depend on which regulations are applied, with Animal Welfare Regulations (AWR) having a stricter definition to exclude mice, rats, and birds that are bred for research purposes, for example. This contrasts with PHS policy which has a broader definition of animal to include other vertebrates that are not mammals such as reptiles, amphibians, and fish. For species not covered under the AWA, the PHS policy is applied when institutions receive federal funding from the PHS such as National Institutes of Health (NIH) (NRC 2004). The IACUC's role is to promote the ethical treatment of animals and "ensure that the animals are used in a way that is scientifically meaningful," such as considering the benefits and risks (Mohan and Huneke 2019, p. 43). An important ethical framework for evaluating animal research is The Principles of Humane Experimental Technique (1959), which outlined the 3 Rs for consideration in animal research: (1) reduction, which pertains to reducing the number of animals needed for the research, (2) replacement, which considers alternative procedures to replace the use of animals, such as computer models, and (3) refinement, which is used to enhance research procedures such that they minimize distress to animals (Díaz et al. 2021; Russell and Birch 1959).

Mohan and Foley (2019) described that during IACUC review, the committee is looking for consideration of the 3 Rs to justify the study design and procedures, including nonsurgical and surgical procedures. In addition to rationale for the study procedures, the PHS policy states that IACUC evaluates whether appropriate methods (e.g., anesthesia) are used for painful procedures to minimize stress and, if applicable, euthanasia is practiced in alignment with the American Veterinary Medical Association (AVMA).

The research should also maintain appropriate animal housing and care by qualified personnel (NRC 2011).

Institutional Review Board (IRB)

Several historical events with human experimentation gave rise to the current regulations governing human subjects research. In the 1940's, the Doctor's Trial in Nuremberg, Germany charged Nazi physicians for subjecting prisoners to unethical experiments against their will, such as freezing and poisoning. This led to the ideas created in the Nuremberg Code including but not limited to: voluntary consent to participate in research, the participant's right to leave the research without consequence, and consideration of the risks in relation to the benefits (Annas and Grodin 2018; Rice 2008). Another notable event was the Tuskegee Syphilis Study from 1932 to 1972, in which African American men with and without syphilis were being studied and received free treatment; however, the men did not know they were participating in research, and when penicillin became available, treatment was withheld from many suffering from syphilis and the study was prolonged for years (McCallum et al. 2006; Rice 2008). In response, the National Research Act of 1974 led to the creation of the Institutional Review Board (IRB) (Gordon and Shriver 2022). Around the world, similar committees may be referred to as Independent Ethics Committees (Das and Sil 2017).

The IRB provides oversight on research studies with human subjects. An important ethical document to guide human subjects research is the Belmont Report, which was produced by the National Commission for the Projection of Human Subjects of Biomedical and Behavioral Research in 1979 (Gordon and Shriver 2022). This report underlies three major ethical principles: (1) respect for persons, which is to recognize that individuals have autonomy in decision-making, (2) beneficence to promote good and minimize harm, and (3) justice to "evaluate the appropriate distribution of risks and burdens" on participants (Hurley and Shriver 2022; White 2020, p. 21). In human subjects research, there are several criteria to consider for IRB approval. The IRB will review the following criteria: the risks are minimized, the risks are within reason in relationship to the benefits, there is an fair selection of subjects, the informed consent process follows the elements of informed consent, informed consent is appropriately documented or waived, there is a sufficient plan for protecting privacy and confidentiality, and have a safety monitoring plan (if applicable). The research should also include additional protections for vulnerable participants such as prisoners and children (Pech et al. 2007; Protection of Human Subjects 2018).

Part 3: CITI Training

In 2000, the US Department of Health and Human Services (DHHS) stated that researchers who obtained NIH funding were required to complete human subjects research training (Shalala 2000). To address the need for adequate training, the Collaborative Institutional Training Initiative (CITI Program) was developed in the same year (https://about.citiprogram.org/en/homepage/). Ten participating institutions initially collaborated to create online modules (Braunschweiger and Goodman 2007). Following initial development, the CITI Program has expanded its efforts internationally. For example, Ichikawa and Motojima (2012) stated that because there was no foundation for teaching medical ethics in Japan, the CITI Program was translated and modified for Japan's culture and regulations. Currently, the CITI Program is being used by at least 40 countries (Braunschweiger and Hansen 2010).

The CITI Program's goal is to provide communities with training that addresses their research needs, which "include courses in ethics, research, meeting regulatory requirements, responsible conduct of research, research administration and other topics pertinent of the interests of member organizations, individual learners, and society" (CITI 2022, n.p.). In 2000, the program began with human subjects research training but over the years has created new course offerings in multiple content areas, including but not limited to: clinical research, animal research with IACUC, responsible conduct of research, and biosafety. Furthermore, diverse users include various organizations such as medical centers, universities, government agencies, and industry (Braunschweiger and Hansen 2010; CITI 2022). Compliance training is increasingly important as educational curricula are either already incorporating or suggesting the implementation of the CITI Program to prepare students for research, such as in the nursing and pharmacy disciplines (Lee et al. 2010; Slattery et al. 2016).

If researchers intend to conduct human subjects or animal research, CITI Program training could be required. To fulfill the training requirements, the user should refer to their institution's website to see what module(s) must be completed. If training is required by the institution, there may be an institutional subscription, which covers the individual's cost and allows them to login to the website through their organization. If the researcher has already completed CITI training modules at one institution and moves to another institution, they can affiliate multiple institutions with the same account to avoid redundancy. If there is no institutional subscription, the user can register as an independent learner and pay a fee.

The CITI training requirements may vary depending on two major factors: (1) The nature of the research study, including species of study and the research activities that will occur. For example, if a researcher will focus on animal research, they might complete the *working with IACUC* course on the CITI website as a foundation course. If a researcher will specifically work with mice, the institutional policies might require additional courses, such as *Working with Mice in Research Settings* and *Post-Procedural Care of Mice and Rats in Research*. Similarly, in human subjects research, a researcher may only need to complete the *Human Subjects Protection (HSP)* course on the CITI website if they are conducting minimal risk studies. The user can choose the HSP course with a Biomedical focus, Social–Behavioral–Educational focus, or combined, depending on their area of research. However, if a researcher will be involved in clinical studies, additional modules may be required, such as the *Good Clinical Practice (GCP)* course. (2) Training also varies by the position of the user in relation to research activities. For example, for IACUC courses, there are different courses for researchers, community members, IACUC members, and the IACUC chair. Likewise, there are distinct human subjects research courses for various roles, such as the IRB Chair and the Institutional Official (CITI 2022). It may benefit the user to explore elective modules for their research needs.

CITI Program module formats can vary, such as following the pace of a recorded voice reading the text on the screen, or the user can read the written text and scroll at their own pace, then complete a quiz at the end of the module, which generally requires 80% correct responses to pass. Upon completion of the course, the user will receive a record of their certificate and completion report with quiz scores. Once the training is complete, the researcher should review institutional requirements for how often the training needs to be retaken as continuing education. For example, if the institution requires training every three years, users may complete the refresher courses for the same content previously completed (CITI 2022).

When a researcher submits a research protocol, CITI training needs to be documented, but it might be recorded differently, depending on the institution. For example, in a paper-based IRB protocol, the researcher might include an image of the CITI certificate or completion report in the protocol. In an electronic IRB (eIRB) system, the researcher may have a user profile that lists the dates of completion for the training. The administrative reviewer of the protocol should check that the user's training is current according to institutional requirements and if it has expired, the reviewer may request a stipulation to complete the required training. Depending on the institution, the reviewer may also have administrative access on the CITI website to search for members and review their training records to confirm if they are complete.

While the CITI program is used to complete training requirements, a critique of the CITI program is that broad application of the modules still may not be suitable enough for community-based research (Brown et al. 2017). For example, Kue et al. (2018) aimed to prepare three Southeast Asian research members with limited English and identified challenges with the CITI program, including academic terminology and assumptions of prior knowledge of research; to address this, the team created modified training to prepare their research staff for their cultural context. Similarly, Pearson et al. (2014) developed an alternative training module for American Indian and Alaska Native members; participants either completed a regular CITI module or the modified CITI module with community-based information and found that those who took the latter had overall higher quiz scores and connected with the relevancy of the content better. In moving forward, it is important for researchers to assess the appropriate level of training for their research staff in addition to the CITI Program and prepare accordingly for the specific research context.

Comparison

Fundamentally, both IACUC and IRB function to review animal and human subjects research protocols, respectively within an institution. For researchers to obtain approval for their studies, a research protocol must be submitted. Both IACUC and IRB protocols ask the researcher(s) to describe the background context for the research, the objectives of the research and hypotheses, study design and procedures being conducted, alternative procedures, justification for the research, and evidence of appropriate training from the research team.

Once the protocol is submitted, a pre-review process is completed. The rationale for the pre-review process is to ensure the protocols comply with the regulations and institutional policies and that submissions are complete. If there are issues with the protocol, such as missing information, regulatory issues, or ethical concerns, pre-review comments will be communicated to the research team. Study procedures that involve components requiring additional ancillary committee review (e.g., biosafety) should be initiated. Once the stipulations are addressed, the study can be reviewed by designated review or full-board review, depending on the nature of the study (Prentice et al. 2014).

Committee Meetings

The composition of both IACUC and IRB committees should reflect diverse members that have the appropriate expertise and experience. For example, the IRB committee requires a minimum of five members including at least one scientist, one nonscientist, and one member who has no affiliation with the institution (Protection of Human Subjects 2018). Similarly, PHS policy describes that IACUC requires at least five members with at least one scientist, one doctor of veterinary medicine, a nonscientist, and one member with no affiliation with the institution (NRC 2011). Both IACUC and IRB meetings require *quorum*, meaning that they must have a minimum number of members present for a decision to be made. For IACUC, a quorum consists of "a majority (>50%) of the voting members of the IACUC" (NIH 2002, p. 15). Similarly for IRB, a quorum requires that greater than half of the members are present. If quorum is not maintained, the meeting is stopped until quorum requirements can be met again (Bibeault and Ludwig 2022). During both IACUC and IRB meetings, the chair and the committee members have an agenda of the studies that will be discussed. The primary reviewer (and secondary reviewer, if applicable) present an overview of the study, including any concerns and stipulations they would like to propose for corrections to improve the study. The chair of the committee opens the discussion to the committee for any comments and at the end of each discussion, the committee votes to approve it, approve it with stipulations, defer, or disapprove it (Jones and Waltz 2022; Silverman et al. 2015).

If the research study is approved, there are several considerations for researchers. One consideration for both IRB and IACUC protocols is continuing review and ensure that studies continually comply with regulations. Depending on the policies and procedures, researchers may report information in their continuing review that includes, but is not limited to, the status of the project and ongoing activities, the study's progress towards achieving the objectives of the study, the number of subjects involved in the study, how subjects responded to the research procedures, any adverse events, and unanticipated problems (Coleman and Scott 2022; Oki and Prentice 2014). A second consideration is that if the researchers decide to alter the original approved protocol (e.g., the methodology), an amendment must be approved prior to implementing the changes. A final consideration for researchers is that they should submit reportable events when they occur. Although reportable events will vary for IACUC and IRB, such events may include cases of unexpected and serious harm to subjects that are directly related to the research procedures or incidents of noncompliance, among others.

In summary, both IRB and IACUC function to provide oversight for ethical use and treatment of animals and humans involved in regulated research. As IRB and IACUC have underlying ethical principles and regulatory requirements, researchers should take these into consideration when conceptualizing all aspects of their research design. The study should be justified to demonstrate its valuable contribution to society and minimize unnecessary harm to subjects. It is ultimately the research team's responsibility to be familiar with the regulations, institutional policies, and procedures so they remain in compliance for the duration of the research, from initial submission to study closure.

Section 6: Reporting the Educational Study

Jill R. D. MacKay

After you have done all the hard work of conducting your research to the best possible standards, it would be foolish to keep that work to yourself. Unfortunately, journals have long been criticized for inadvertently discouraging appropriate reporting due to limitations of the peer review process (Bland and Altman 1986). Given the interdisciplinary nature of educational research, it is worth evaluating what should be included within an educational research report. There are many forms of guidance, e.g., on how to report mixed methods studies (Creswell and Tashakkori 2007), how to report various forms of analysis (Twining et al. 2017; van Doorn et al. 2020), and how best to support the peer review process (Aczel et al. 2021; Vaesen and Katzav 2017). As a field, educational research would do well to embrace best reporting guidelines.

Part 1: What Needs to Be Included?

This chapter has hopefully impressed upon the reader the many, many choices available to the researcher in the research process. Every choice in the process of research is a potential source of poor replication. Traditionally, a research report follows the structure of Introduction – Methodology – Results – Discussion, and this is well-suited for describing the choices made in the research process. An Introduction describes the previous knowledge and biases of the researcher, helps contextualize the variation that may be expected, and what confounding variables may exist. It should also unequivocally state research questions and hypotheses, even if these are general, e.g., to characterize a data source. Peer reviewers should be wary of pushing researchers to identify hypotheses/research questions post-hoc, as this is a common problem for replication

(Rubin 2017). The methodology section should allow for full replication of the work, including an understanding of the position of the researchers and other potential sources of bias in measurement, such as sampling, etc. It should also clearly detail what ethical guidelines were followed, if any, and what ethical approvals were granted. Results and Discussion sections can be combined, particularly for some qualitative analyses, which depend upon informed comparisons of findings with the literature, but a Discussion section should always clearly describe how bias, confounding variables, and variation may impact the consideration of findings. It is perfectly acceptable to present null results, or results so specific they cannot be generalized. We must accept that at present, publication is so highly incentivized for researchers that publications will continue to increase in number. It is better that we can clearly identify the findings worth further pursuit.

Part 2: The Role of Preprinting

Preprinting is one aspect of open research practices. Prior to submitting a research article for peer review, an article is hosted on an open-access repository such as EdArXiv.org. This allows for findings to be made more widely available and facilitating open and transparent peer review (Bourne et al. 2017; Ginsparg 2021). When combined with metadata systems such as Open Research and Contributor ID (OrcID) to identify who researchers are even when they move disciplines or change names, etc. (Haak et al. 2012), preprinting can support the researcher at an individual level alongside the societal level by both providing a complete record of how research outputs changed and adapted with peer review and how the researcher themselves adapted to the feedback.

Part 3: Preregistering and Data Sharing

As part of improving the reproducibility of research, preregistered reports and data and analysis sharing can be very useful (Kitzes et al. 2018; MacKay 2021b). Preregistered reports describe what analyses are intended prior to the collection of data (or prior to the exploration of data if the study is retrospective). This should not be a big ask, as most ethical approvals require an understanding of what will be done with the data before being granted, and how can a researcher have made appropriate choices regarding their data collection if they have not thought through the data analysis? Nor does preregistering lock researchers into unproductive paths, as deviations from the preregistration can be clearly highlighted and explained; see Nordmann et al. (2021). The provision of

data, where appropriate, can support reproducibility through making it easier to spot questionable research practices. However, it should be very important that this is used as a carrot, not a stick to beat researchers with. Data sharing can of course be frightening to researchers because who wants to be caught in a mistake? Therefore, we should be accepting and compassionate to those who are open about their science.

Part 4: Questions of Style

There are aspects of academic writing that impact how understandable research is. Traditionally, many scientific manuscripts have been written in the third person, and often in passive voice. It is now more common for first person and active voice to be used, at least in some sections, partly to avoid ambiguity with regards to who did what, and whether a statement is established in previous literature or is author opinion. Consider the following two examples:

Student anxiety had no impact on exam performance in this study. It is considered that students may not be accurate judges of their own performance.

Student anxiety had no impact on exam performance in this study. We consider that this may imply students are not accurate judges of their own performance.

In the second example, it is clearer that it is the author's opinion being proposed as a potential explanation for the finding. Many academics decry the use of first person for being egotistical; however, it is recommended throughout a publication by the APA Style Guide (Lee 2014) as it avoids ambiguity or attesting opinions to others. For example, if one was to use "we often worry about student anxiety" to imply it was a global phenomenon, it confers an opinion on the reader that they may not hold. Instead "many in higher education worry about student anxiety" is a clearer and more specific description of who is worried. The APA Style Guide (7th Edition) has many helpful tips for all aspects of writing and reporting and should be consulted for questions of grammar, format, referencing, results reporting, and many other aspects of research.

Summary

There is no one "right" path to researching education. Educational research is more like a garden, cultivated depending on the type of soil (the research's underlying principles), the choices made by the gardener (the researcher's choice of data and analysis), and is always unique to its own context. No one research approach will ever answer the totality of human experience, and with the wide variety of approaches available to us, clear understanding of the methodology can often require collaboration and support across research groups. Education research is a fundamentally interdisciplinary and collaborative endeavor, which can be a force for enhancing its value, not lessening its ability to answer the questions we face.

References

Aczel, B., Szaszi, B., and Holcombe, A.O. (2021). A billion-dollar donation: estimating the cost of researchers' time spent on peer review. *Research Integrity and Peer Review* 2 (6): 14.

Adams, W.C. (2015). Conducting semi-structured interviews. In: *Handbook of Practical Program Evaluation*, 4e, Issue 1970 (ed. J.S. Wholey, H.P. Hatry, and K.E. Newcomer), 492–505. Wiley. https://www.researchgate.net/publication/301738442_Conducting_Semi-Structured_Interviews.

Alanazi, A. (2016). A critical review of constructivist theory and the emergence of constructionism. *American Research Journal of Humanities and Social Sciences* 2 (March): 1–8. https://doi.org/10.21694/2378-7031.16018.

Allen, M., Poggiali, D., Whitaker, K. et al. (2019). Raincloud plots: a multi-platform tool for robust data visualization. *Wellcome Open Research* 4 (63): 1–40. https://doi.org/10.12688/wellcomeopenres.15191.1.

Annas, G.J. and Grodin, M.A. (2018). Reflections on the 70th anniversary of the Nuremberg doctors' trial. *American Journal of Public Health* 108 (1): 10–12. https://doi.org/10.2105/AJPH.2017.304203.

Artino, A.R., La Rochelle, J.S., Dezee, K.J., and Gehlbach, H. (2014). Developing questionnaires for educational research: AMEE Guide No. 87. *Medical Teacher* 36 (6): 463–474. https://doi.org/10.3109/0142159X.2014.889814.

Bayarri, M.J. and Berger, J.O. (2004). The interplay of Bayesian and frequentist analysis. *Statistical Science* 19 (1): 58–80. https://doi.org/10.1214/088342304000000116.

Bibeault, R.D. and Ludwig, B.M. (2022). Administrative tasks during each IRB meeting. In: *Institutional Review Board Management and Function*, 3e (ed. E.A. Bankert, B.G. Gordon, E.A. Hurley, et al.), 63–68. Jones and Bartlett Learning.

Bloor, M., Frankland, J., Thomas, M., and Robson, K. (2002). Focus groups in social research. In: *Introducing Qualitative Methods*, 1e (ed. D. Silverman). SAGE Publications. https://doi.org/10.4135/9781849209175.

Boliver, V. (2015). Are there distinctive clusters of higher and lower status universities in the UK? *Oxford Review of Education* 41 (5): 608–627. https://doi.org/10.1080/03054985.2015.1082905.

Bourne, P.E., Polka, J.K., Vale, R.D., and Kiley, R. (2017). Ten simple rules to consider regarding preprint submission. *PLoS Computational Biology* 13 (5): 8–13. https://doi.org/10.1371/journal.pcbi.1005473.

Boyer, K.K., Olson, J.R., Calantone, R.J., and Jackson, E.C. (2002). Print versus electronic surveys: a comparison of two data collection methodologies. *Journal of Operations Management* 20 (4): 357–373. https://doi.org/10.1016/S0272-6963(02)00004-9.

Braun, V. and Clarke, V. (2006). Using thematic analysis in psychology. *Qualitative Research in Psychology* 3 (2): 77–101. https://doi.org/10.1191/1478088706qp063oa.

Braun, V. and Clarke, V. (2019). To saturate or not to saturate? Questioning data saturation as a useful concept for thematic analysis and sample-size rationales. *Qualitative Research in Sport, Exercise and Health* 13 (2): 201–216. https://doi.org/10.1080/2159676X.2019.1704846.

Braun, V., Clarke, V., Hayfield, N., and Terry, G. (2019). Thematic analysis. In: *Handbook of Research Methods in Health Social Sciences*, 1e (ed. P. Liamputtong), 843–860. Springer Nature. https://doi.org/10.1007/978-981-10-5251-4_103.

Braun, V., Clarke, V., Boulton, E. et al. (2020). The online survey as a qualitative research tool. *International Journal of Social Research Methodology* 24 (6): 641–654. https://doi.org/10.1080/13645579.2020.1805550.

Braunschweiger, P. and Goodman, K.W. (2007). The CITI program: an international online resource for education in human subjects protection and the responsible conduct of research. *Academic Medicine* 82 (9): 861–864.

Braunschweiger, P. and Hansen, K. (2010). Collaborative institutional training initiative (CITI). *Journal of Clinical Research Best Practices* 6 (4): 1–6.

Breckenridge, C.J. (2014). *Doing Classic Grounded Theory: The Data Analysis Process, SAGE Research Methods Cases*. SAGE Publications Ltd. https://doi.org/10.4135/9781446273050014527673.

Brestoff, J.R. and Van den Broeck, J. (2013). Study size planning. In: *Epidemiology: Principles and Practical Guidelines* (ed. J. Van den Broeck and J.R. Brestoff), 137–155. Springer.

Brown, J.S. and Largent, E.A. (2022). Payment of research subjects. In: *Institutional Review Board Management and*

Function, 3e (ed. E.A. Bankert, B.G. Gordon, E.A. Hurley, et al.), 877–886. Jones and Bartlett Learning.

Brown, E.R., Lu, Y., Beaven, J. et al. (2017). Engagement and quality of life in under–represented older adults: a community–based participatory research project. *Narrative Inquiry In Bioethics* 7 (1): E7–E9.

Buchanan, E.A. (2022). Internet research. In: *Institutional Review Board Management and Function*, 3e (ed. E.A. Bankert, B.G. Gordon, E.A. Hurley, et al.), 635–648. Jones and Bartlett Learning.

Burke Johnson, R., Onquegbuzie, A.J., and Turner, L.A. (2007). Towards a definition of mixed methods research. *Journal of Mixed Methods Research* 1 (2): 112–133. https://doi.org/10.1002/9781119410867.ch12.

Byrne, B. (2016). Qualitative interviewing. In: *Researching Society and Culture*, 4e (ed. C. Seale), 217–236. SAGE Publications Ltd. https://www.research.manchester.ac.uk/portal/en/publications/qualitative-interviewing(f922c775-aa31-4769-a9a4-dbbb0e6746d4)/export.html.

Calders, T. and Custers, B. (2013). What is data mining and how does it work? In: *Discrimination and Privacy in the Information Society. Studies in Applied Philosophy, Epistemology and Rational Ethics*, 1e, vol. 3 (ed. B. Custers, T. Calders, B. Schemer, and T. Zarsky), 27–42. Berlin Heidelberg: Springer. https://doi.org/10.1007/978-3-642-30487-3_2.

Cardon, A.D., Bailey, M.R., and Bennett, B.T. (2012). The Animal Welfare Act: from enactment to enforcement. *Journal of the American Association for Laboratory Animal Science* 51 (3): 301–305.

Charmaz, K. (2008). Constructionism and the grounded theory method. In: *Handbook of Constructionist Research* (Issue September) (ed. A. Holstein and J.F. Gubrium), 397–412. The Guilford Press.

Chinnery, S., MacKay, J.R.D., and Hughes, K. (2021). What'd I miss? A qualitative exploration of student and staff experiences with lecture recording over an academic year. *Journal of Perspectives in Applied Academic Practice* 9 (1): 8–17. https://doi.org/10.14297/jpaap.v9i1.467.

Christian, L.M., Parsons, N.L., and Dillman, D.A. (2009). Sociological methods & for web surveys. *Methods* 37 (3): 393–425.

Coleman, L. and Scott, M. (2022). Continuing review. Historical timeline. In: *Institutional Review Board Management and Function*, 3e (ed. E.A. Bankert, B.G. Gordon, E.A. Hurley, et al.), 359–366. Jones and Bartlett Learning.

Collaborative Institutional Training Initiative: CITI. (n.d.). https://www.citiprogram.org/ (accessed 7 March 2022).

Conradson, D. (2005). Focus groups. In: *Methods in Human Geography. A Guide for Students Doing a Research Project*, 2e (ed. R. Flowerdew and D. Martin), 128–142. Pearson Prentice Hall. https://doi.org/10.2307/j.ctt46nrzt.12.

Cooke, L. (2010). Assessing concurrent think-aloud protocol as a usability test method: a technical communication approach. *IEEE Transactions on Professional Communication* 53 (3): 202–215. https://doi.org/10.1109/TPC.2010.2052859.

Creswell, J.W. and Poth, C.N. (2018). *Qualitative Inquiry and Research Design: Choosing Among Five Approaches*, 4e. SAGE Publications, Inc.

Creswell, J.W. and Tashakkori, A. (2007). Editorial: developing publishable mixed methods manuscripts. *Journal of Mixed Methods Research* 1 (2): 107–111. https://doi.org/10.1177/1558689806298644.

Crotty, M. (1998). Introduction: the research process. In: *The Foundations of Social Research. Meaning and Perspective in the Research Process*, 1–17. SAGE Publications.

Cupchik, G.C. (2001). Constructivist realism: an ontology that encompasses positivist and constructivist approaches to the social sciences. *Forum Qualitative Sozialforschung* 2(1): 1–8. 10.17169/fqs-2.1.968.

Daniel, J. (2012). Making sense of MOOCs: musings in a maze of myth, paradox and possibility. *Journal of Interactive Media in Education* 18: 1–20.

Das, N.K. and Sil, A. (2017). Evolution of ethics in clinical research and ethics committee. *Indian Journal of Dermatology* 62 (4): 373–379. https://doi.org/10.4103/ijd.IJD_271_17.

Davies, P. (1999). What is evidence-based education? *British Journal of Educational Studies* 47 (2): 108–121. https://www.learn.ed.ac.uk/bbcswebdav/pid-3122003-dt-content-rid-4669003_1/courses/ls_PGDE_Secondary_2017/What is Evidence Based Education%281%29.pdf.

Dawes, J. (2008). Do data characteristics change according to the number of scale points used? An experiment using 5 point, 7 point and 10 point scales. *International Journal of Market Research* 50 (1): 1–19.

DeBruine, L.M. and Barr, D.J. (2021). Understanding mixed-effects models through data simulation. *Advances in Methods and Practices in Psychological Science* 4 (1): 1–15. https://doi.org/10.1177/2515245920965119.

DeCuir-Gunby, J.T., Marshall, P.L., and McCulloch, A.W. (2011). Developing and using a codebook for the analysis of interview data: an example from a Professional Development Research Project. *Field Methods* 23 (2): 136–155. https://doi.org/10.1177/1525822X10388468.

Denzin, N.K. and Lincoln, Y.S. (ed.) (2018). *The Sage Handbook of Qualitative Research*, 5e. SAGE Publications Inc.

Díaz, L., Zambrano, E., Flores, M.E. et al. (2021). Ethical considerations in animal research: the principle of 3R's. *Revista de Investigación Clínica* 73 (4): 199–209. https://doi.org/10.24875/ric.20000380.

Dietz-Uhler, B. and Hurn, J. (2013). Using learning analytics to predict (and improve) student success: a faculty perspective. *Journal of Interactive Online Learning* 12 (1): 17–26. http://www.ncolr.org/jiol/issues/pdf/12.1.2.pdf.

Dillman, D.A., Phelps, G., Tortora, R. et al. (2009). Response rate and measurement differences in mixed-mode surveys using mail, telephone, interactive voice response (IVR) and the Internet. *Social Science Research* 38 (1): 1–18. https://doi.org/10.1016/j.ssresearch.2008.03.007.

van Doorn, J., van den Bergh, D., Böhm, U. et al. (2020). The JASP guidelines for conducting and reporting a Bayesian analysis. *Psychonomic Bulletin & Review*. https://doi.org/10.3758/s13423-020-01798-5.

Dykema, J., Stevenson, J., Klein, L. et al. (2013). Effects of e-mailed versus mailed invitations and incentives on response rates, data quality, and costs in a web survey of university faculty. *Social Science Computer Review* 31 (3): 359–370. https://doi.org/10.1177/0894439312465254.

Eddy, S.L., Converse, M., and Wenderoth, M.P. (2015). PORTAAL: a classroom observation tool assessing evidence-based teaching practices for active learning in large science, technology, engineering, and mathematics classes. *CBE Life Sciences Education* 14 (2): 1–16. https://doi.org/10.1187/cbe-14-06-0095.

Elgar, F.J. and Stewart, J.M. (2008). Validity of self-report screening for overweight and obesity: evidence from the Canadian community health survey. *Canadian Journal of Public Health* 99 (5): 423–427. https://doi.org/10.1007/bf03405254.

Eyal, N. and Magalhaes, M. (2022). The functions of informed consent. In: *Institutional Review Board Management and Function*, 3e (ed. E.A. Bankert, B.G. Gordon, E.A. Hurley, et al.), 247–256. Jones and Bartlett Learning.

Fleming, N. and Baume, D. (2006). Learning styles again: VARKing up the right tree! *Educational Developments* 7 (4): 4–7.

Fonteyn, M.E., Vettese, M., Lancaster, D.R., and Bauer-Wu, S. (2008). Developing a codebook to guide content analysis of expressive writing transcripts. *Applied Nursing Research* 21 (3): 165–168. https://doi.org/10.1016/j.apnr.2006.08.005.

Franklin, S. (2006). VAKing out learning styles: why the notion of 'learning styles' is unhelpful to teachers. *Education 3–13* 34 (1): 81–87. https://doi.org/10.1080/03004270500507644.

Fredricks, J.A., Blumenfeld, P.C., and Paris, A.H. (2004). School engagement: potential of the concept, state of the evidence. *Review of Educational Research* 74 (1): 59–109. https://doi.org/10.3102/00346543074001059.

Fyfe, E.R., de Leeuw, J.R., Carvalho, P.F. et al. (2021). Many classes 1: assessing the generalizable effect of immediate feedback versus delayed feedback across many college classes. *Advances in Methods and Practices in Psychological Science* 4 (3): 1–24. https://doi.org/10.1177/25152459211027575.

Geller, S.E., Koch, A.R., Roesch, P. et al. (2018). The more things change, the more the stay same: a study to evaluate compliance with inclusion and assessment of women and minorities in randomised controlled trials. *Academic Medicine* 93 (4): 630–635. https://doi.org/10.1097/ACM.0000000000002027.The.

Gelman, A. and Hennig, C. (2017). Beyond subjective and objective in statistics. *Journal of the Royal Statistical Society: Series A (Statistics in Society)* 180 (4): 967–1033. https://doi.org/10.1111/rssa.12276.

Ginsparg, P. (2021). Lessons from arXic's 30 years of information sharing. *Nature Reviews Physics, 0123456789*. https://doi.org/10.1038/s42254-021-00360-z.

Glaser, B.G. (2002). Constructivist grounded theory. *Forum: Qualitative Social Research* 3 (3): 93–105. https://doi.org/10.1111/j.1741-5446.2002.00409.x.

Gordon, B.G. and Shriver, S.P. (2022). Historical timeline. In: *Institutional Review Board Management and Function*, 3e (ed. E.A. Bankert, B.G. Gordon, E. Hurley, et al.), 17–26. Jones and Bartlett Learning.

Grafen, A. and Hails, R. (2002). *Modern Statistics or the Life Sciences* (First). Oxford University Press.

Grbich, C. (2011). The position of the researcher. In: *New Approaches in Social Research* (ed. C. Grbich), 67–79. SAGE Publications Ltd. https://doi.org/10.4135/9781849209519.n5.

Greaves, F., Ramirez-Cano, D., Millett, C. et al. (2013). Use of sentiment analysis for capturing patient experience from free-text comments posted online. *Journal of Medical Internet Research* 15 (11): 1–9. https://doi.org/10.2196/jmir.2721.

Green, J.M. and Rosenfeld, S. (2022). The functions of informed consent. In: *Institutional Review Board Management and Function*, 3e (ed. E.A. Bankert, B.G. Gordon, E.A. Hurley, et al.), 247–256. Jones and Bartlett Learning.

Greenhalgh, T. (2020). Will COVID-19 be evidence-based medicine's nemesis? *PLoS Medicine* 17 (6): 4–7. https://doi.org/10.1371/journal.pmed.1003266.

Greenhalgh, T., Schmid, M.B., Czypionka, T. et al. (2020). Face masks for the public during the covid-19 crisis. *The BMJ* 369 (April): 1–4. https://doi.org/10.1136/bmj.m1435.

Gyure, M.E., Quillin, J.M., Rodríguez, V.M. et al. (2014). Practical considerations for implementing research recruitment etiquette. *IRB* 36 (6): 7–12.

Haak, L.L., Fenner, M., Paglione, L. et al. (2012). ORCID: a system to uniquely identify researchers. *Learned Publishing* 25 (4): 259–264. https://doi.org/10.1087/20120404.

Hale, K.N. and Nelson, D.K. (2022). Conflicts of interest: researchers. In: *Institutional Review Board Management and Function*, 3e (ed. E.A. Bankert, B.G. Gordon, E.A. Hurley, et al.), 923–934. Jones and Bartlett Learning.

Hand, D.J. (1998). Data mining: statistics and more? *The American Statistician* 52 (2): 112–118. https://doi.org/10.1080/00031305.1998.10480549.

Haven, T.L. and Van Grootel, D.L. (2019). Preregistering qualitative research. *Accountability in Research* 26 (3): 229–244. https://doi.org/10.1080/08989621.2019.1580147.

Hek, G. (1996). Guidelines on conducting a critical research evaluation. *Nursing Standard* 11 (6): 40–43. https://doi.org/10.7748/ns.11.6.40.s48.

Henrich, J., Heine, S.J., and Norenzayan, A. (2010). The weirdest people in the world? *Behavioral and Brain Sciences* 33: 61–135. https://doi.org/10.1017/S0140525X10000725.

Höhne, J.K., Krebs, D., and Kühnel, S.M. (2020). Measuring income (in)equality: comparing survey questions with unipolar and bipolar scales in a probability-based online panel. *Social Science Computer Review* 1–16. https://doi.org/10.1177/0894439320902461.

Hollenbeck, J.R. and Wright, P.M. (2017). Harking, sharking, and tharking: making the case for post hoc analysis of scientific data. *Journal of Management* 43 (1): 5–18. https://doi.org/10.1177/0149206316679487.

Hookway, N. (2008). "Entering the blogosphere": some strategies for using blogs in social research. *Qualitative Research* 8 (1): 91–113. https://doi.org/10.1177/1468794107085298.

Hox, J.J. and De Leeuw, E.D. (1994). A comparison of nonresponse in mail, telephone, and face-to-face surveys – applying multilevel modeling to meta-analysis. *Quality & Quantity* 28 (4): 329–344. https://doi.org/10.1007/BF01097014.

Hurley, E.A. and Shriver, S.P. (2022). Ethical foundations of human research protections. In: *Institutional Review Board Management and Function*, 3e (ed. E. Bankert, B.G. Gordon, E.A. Hurley, et al.), 3–16. Jones and Bartlett Learning.

Iaia, M., Pasini, M., Burnazzi, A. et al. (2017). An educational intervention to promote healthy lifestyles in preschool children: a cluster-RCT. *International Journal of Obesity* 41 (4): 582–590. https://doi.org/10.1038/ijo.2016.239.

Ichikawa, I. and Motojima, M. (2012). Creating the CITI-Japan program for web-based training: where ethics, law and science experts meet. In: *Promoting Research Integrity in a Global Environment* (ed. T. Mayer and N.H. Steneck), 255–261. World Scientific.

Ioannidis, J.P.A. (2005). Why most published research findings are false. *PLoS Medicine* 2 (8): e124. https://doi.org/10.1371/journal.pmed.0020124.

Jacoby, J. and Matell, M.S. (1971). Three-point Likert scales are good enough. *Journal of Marketing Research* 8 (4): 495–500.

Javid, B., Weekes, M.P., and Matheson, N.J. (2020). Covid-19: should the public wear face masks? *The BMJ* 369 (April): 11–12. https://doi.org/10.1136/bmj.m1442.

Jenkins, C.S. (2010). What is ontological realism? *Philosophy Compass* 5 (10): 880–890. https://doi.org/10.1111/j.1747-9991.2010.00332.x.

Jephcote, C., Medland, E., and Lygo-Baker, S. (2020). Grade inflation versus grade improvement: are our students getting more intelligent? *Assessment and Evaluation in Higher Education* 46 (4): 1–25. https://doi.org/10.1080/02602938.2020.1795617.

John, L.K., Loewenstein, G., and Prelec, D. (2012). Measuring the prevalence of questionable research practices with incentives for truth telling. *Psychological Science* 23 (5): 524–532. https://doi.org/10.1177/0956797611430953.

Jones, M.F. and Waltz, A. (2022). Full committee review. In: *Institutional Review Board Management and Function*, 3e (ed. E.A. Bankert, B.G. Gordon, E. Hurley, et al.), 237–243. Jones and Bartlett Learning.

Karnieli-Miller, O., Strier, R., and Pessach, L. (2009). Power relations in qualitative research. *Qualitative Health Research* 19 (2): 279–289. https://doi.org/10.1177/1049732308329306.

Kerr, N.L. (1998). HARKing: hypothesizing after the results are known. *Personality and Social Psychology Review* 2 (3): 196–217. https://doi.org/10.1002/9781118901731.iecrm0112.

Kietzmann, J.H., Hermkens, K., McCarthy, I.P., and Silvestre, B.S. (2011). Social media? Get serious! Understanding the functional building blocks of social media. *Business Horizons* 54 (3): 241–251. https://doi.org/10.1016/j.bushor.2011.01.005.

Kinnear, G., Smith, S., Anderson, R. et al. (2021). Developing the FILL+ tool to reliably classify classroom practices using lecture recordings. *Journal for STEM Education Research.* https://doi.org/10.31219/osf.io/7n6qt.

Kirschner, P.A. (2016). Stop propagating the learning styles myth. *Computers & Education* 106: 166–171. https://doi.org/10.1016/j.compedu.2016.12.006.

Kitzes, J., Turek, D., and Deniz, F. (2018). The basic reproducible workflow template. In: *The Practice of Reproducibility: Case Studies and Lessons from the Data-Intensive Sciences* (ed. J. Kitzes, D. Turek, and F. Deniz). Oakland, CA: University of California Press. http://www.practicereproducibleresearch.org/.

Kitzinger, J. (1994). The methodology of focus groups: the importance of interaction between research participants. *Sociology of Health & Illness* 16 (1): 103–121. https://doi.org/10.1111/1467-9566.ep11347023.

Kitzinger, J. (1995). Qualitative research: introducing focus groups. *BMJ [British Medical Journal]* 311 (7000): 299–302. https://doi.org/10.1136/bmj.311.7000.299.

Krosnick, J.A. (2018). Improving question design to maximize reliability and validity. In: *The Palgrave Handbook of Survey Research* (ed. D.L. Vannette and J.A. Krosnick), 95–101. Cham: Palgrave Macmillan. https://doi.org/10.1007/978-3-319-54395-6_13.

Kruschke, J.K. (2013). Bayesian estimation supersedes the *t* test. *Journal of Experimental Psychology: General* 142 (2): 573–603. https://doi.org/10.1037/a0029146.

Kruschke, J.K. (2014). *Doing Bayesian Data Analysis: A Tutorial with R, JAGS, and Stan*, 2e. https://doi.org/10.1016/B978-0-12-405888-0.09999-2.

Kue, J., Szalacha, L.A., Happ, M.B. et al. (2018). Culturally relevant human subjects protection training: a case study in community-engaged research in the United States. *Journal of Immigrant and Minority Health* 20 (1): 107–114.

Kukull, W.A. and Ganguli, M. (2012). Generalizability: the trees, the forest, and the low-hanging fruit. *Neurology* 78 (23): 1886–1891. https://doi.org/10.1212/WNL.0b013e318258f812. PMID: 22665145; PMCID: PMC3369519.

Kuper, A., Lingard, L., and Levinson, W. (2008). Critically appraising qualitative research. *BMJ* 337. https://doi.org/10.1136/bmj.a1035.

Lazzarino, A.I., Steptoe, A., Hamer, M., and Michie, S. (2020). Covid-19: important potential side effects of wearing face masks that we should bear in mind. *The BMJ* 369 (May): 2020. https://doi.org/10.1136/bmj.m2003.

Lee, C. (2014, May 22). *APA Style 6th Edition Blog: "Me, Me, Me": How to Talk About Yourself in an APA Style Paper*. APA Style Blog. https://blog.apastyle.org/apastyle/2014/05/me-me-me.html. (accessed 01 May 2022).

Lee, P.Y., Alexander, K.P., Hammill, B.G. et al. (2001). Representation of elderly persons and women in published randomized trials of acute coronary syndromes. *Journal of the American Medical Association* 286 (6): 708–713. https://doi.org/10.1001/jama.286.6.708.

Lee, J.W., Jones, P.S., Mineyama, Y., and Zhang, X.E. (2002). Cultural differences in responses to a Likert scale. *Research in Nursing and Health* 25 (4): 295–306. https://doi.org/10.1002/nur.10041.

Lee, M.W., Clay, P.G., Kennedy, W.K. et al. (2010). The essential research curriculum for doctor of pharmacy degree programs. *Pharmacotherapy* 30 (9): 1–12.

Leech, N.L. and Onwuegbuzie, A.J. (2009). A typology of mixed methods research designs. *Quality & Quantity* 43 (2): 265–275. https://doi.org/10.1007/s11135-007-9105-3.

Leech, N.L., Dellinger, A.B., Brannagan, K.B., and Tanaka, H. (2010). Evaluating mixed research studies: a mixed methods approach. *Journal of Mixed Methods Research* 4 (1): 17–31. https://doi.org/10.1177/1558689809345262.

Levins, R. (1966). The strategy of model building in population biology. *American Scientist* 54 (4): 421–431.

Liberman, M. (2018). Applying human language technology in survey research. In: *The Palgrave Handbook of Survey Research* (ed. D.L. Vannette and J.A. Krosnick), 129–133. Cham: Palgrave Macmillan. https://doi.org/10.1007/978-3-319-54395-6_17.

Lincoln, Y.S., Lynham, S.A., and Guba, E.G. (2011). Paradigmatic controversies, contradictions, and emerging confluences, revisited. In: *The SAGE Handbook of Qualitative Research* (ed. N.K. Denzin and Y.S. Lincoln), 199–265. SAGE Publications, Inc.

Liu, M. and Wronski, L. (2017). Examining completion rates in web surveys via over 25,000 real-world surveys. *Social Science Computer Review* 1–9. https://doi.org/10.1177/0894439317695581.

Lortie-Forgues, H. and Inglis, M. (2019). Rigorous large-scale educational RCTs are often uninformative: should we be concerned? *Educational Researcher* 48 (3): 0013189X1983285. https://doi.org/10.3102/0013189X19832850.

Lund, T.J., Pilarz, M., Velasco, J.B. et al. (2015). The best of both worlds: building on the COPUS and RTOP observation protocols to easily and reliably measure various levels of reformed instructional practice. *CBE Life Sciences Education* 14 (2): 1–12. https://doi.org/10.1187/cbe.14-10-0168.

MacKay, J.R.D. (2018). *Animal Personality: The Science Behind Individual Variation*. 5M Publishing Ltd.

MacKay, J.R.D. (2019). On the horizon: making the best use of free text data with shareable text mining analyses. *Journal of Perspectives in Applied Academic Practice* 7 (1): 57–64.

MacKay, J.R.D. (2021a). Freeing the free-text comment: exploring ethical text mining in the higher education sector. In: *Analysing Student Feedback in Higher: Using Text-Mining to Interpret the Student Voice Education*, 1e. Routledge: Taylor & Francis.

MacKay, J.R.D. (2021b). Open science for veterinary education. *Frontiers in Veterinary Science* 8: 745779. https://doi.org/10.3389/fvets.2021.745779 INTRODUCTION.

MacKay, J.R.D., Langford, F., and Waran, N. (2016). Massive open online courses as a tool for global animal welfare education. *Journal of Veterinary Medical Education* 43 (3): 287–301. https://doi.org/10.3138/jvme.0415-054R2.

MacKay, J.R.D., Paterson, J., Sandilands, V. et al. (2018). Lessons learned from teaching multiple massive open online courses in veterinary education. *Journal of Perspectives in Applied Academic Practice* 6 (2): 22–40.

MacKay, J.R.D., Murray, L., and Rhind, S.M. (2021a). The use of lecture recordings as study aids in a professional degree program. *Journal of Veterinary Medical Education*. https://doi.org/10.3138/jvme-2020-0067.

MacKay, J.R.D., Nordmann, E., Murray, L. et al. (2021b). The cost of asking 'say that again?': a social capital theory view into how lecture recording supports widening participation. *Frontiers in Education* 6 (734755). https://doi.org/10.3389/feduc.2021.734755.

MacKay, J.R.D., Bell, C.E., Hughes, K. et al. (2022). Development and evaluation of a faculty based accredited continued professional development route for teaching and learning. *Journal of Veterinary Medical Education* 49 (6): 759–769.

Makel, M.C. and Plucker, J.A. (2014). Facts are more important than novelty: replication in the education sciences. *Educational Researcher* 43 (6): 304–316. https://doi.org/10.3102/0013189X14545513.

Makel, M.C., Hodges, J., Cook, B.G., and Plucker, J.A. (2021). Both questionable and open research practices are prevalent in education research. *Educational Researcher.* https://doi.org/10.3102/0013189X211001356.

Makowski, D., Ben-Shachar, M.S., Chen, S.H.A., and Lüdecke, D. (2019). Indices of effect existence and significance in the Bayesian framework. *Frontiers in Psychology* 10 (December): 1–14. https://doi.org/10.3389/fpsyg.2019.02767.

Makowski, D., Ben-Schachar, M. S., and Lüdecke, D. (2020). *The {easystats} collection of R packages.* GitHub. https://github.com/easystats/easystats (accessed 01 May 2022).

Mantzari, E., Rubin, G.J., and Marteau, T.M. (2020). Is risk compensation threatening public health in the covid-19 pandemic? *BMJ (Clinical Research Ed.)* 370: m2913. https://doi.org/10.1136/bmj.m2913.

Marasinghe, K. M. (2020). A systematic review investigating the effectiveness of face mask use in limiting the spread of COVID-19 among medically not diagnosed individuals: shedding light on current recommendations provided to individuals not medically diagnosed with COVID-19. 1–19. https://doi.org/10.21203/rs.3.rs-16701/v1.

Markham, A. and Buchanan, E. (2012). Ethical decision-making and internet research recommendations from the AoIR Ethics Working Committee. In: *Recommendations from the AoIR Ethics Working Committee (Version 2.0).* www.aoir.org.

Martin, P. and Bateson, P. (1993). *Measuring Behaviour. An Introductory Guide* (Second). Cambridge: University Press.

Martin Bland, J. and Altman, D. (1986). Statistical methods for assessing agreement between two methods of clinical measurement. *The Lancet* 327 (8476): 307–310. https://doi.org/10.1016/S0140-6736(86)90837-8.

McCallum, J.M., Arekere, D.M., Green, B.L. et al. (2006). Awareness and knowledge of the US Public Health Service syphilis study at Tuskegee: implications for biomedical research. *Journal of Health Care for the Poor and Underserved* 17 (4): 716–733. https://doi.org/10.1353/hpu.2006.0130.

Menold, N. (2021). Response bias and reliability in verbal agreement rating scales: does polarity and verbalization of the middle category matter? *Social Science Computer Review* 39 (1): 130–147. https://doi.org/10.1177/0894439319847672.

Mohan, S. and Foley, P.L. (2019). Everything you need to know about satisfying IACUC protocol requirements. *Institute for Laboratory Animal Research Journal* 60 (1): 50–57. https://doi.org/10.1093/ilar/ilz010.

Mohan, S. and Huneke, R. (2019). The role of IACUCs in responsible animal research. *Institute for Laboratory Animal Research Journal* 60 (1): 43–49. https://doi.org/10.1093/ilar/ilz016.

Munafò, M.R., Nosek, B.A., Bishop, D.V.M. et al. (2017). A manifesto for reproducible science. *Nature Publishing Group* 1 (January): 1–9. https://doi.org/10.1038/s41562-016-0021.

National Institutes of Health (2002). *Institutional Animal Care and Use Committee Guidebook.* Office of Laboratory Animal Welfare. https://grants.nih.gov/grants/olaw/guidebook.pdf.

National Research Council (2004). *Science, Medicine, and Animals.* The National Academies Press. https://doi.org/10.17226/10733.

National Research Council (2009). *Scientific and Human Issues in the Use of Random Source Dogs and Cats in Research.* The National Academies Press. https://doi.org/10.17226/12641.

National Research Council (2011). *Guide for the Care and Use of Laboratory Animals*, 8e. The National Academies Press. https://doi.org/10.17226/12910.

Nelson, R.M. and Synder, D.L. (2022). Subpart D research: additional protections for children. In: *Institutional Review Board Management and Function*, 3e (ed. E.A. Bankert, B.G. Gordon, E.A. Hurley, et al.), 515–526. Jones and Bartlett Learning.

Nisbet, J. (2008). What is educational research. In: *An Introduction to the Study of Education* (ed. D. Matheson), 319–333. Routledge. https://books.google.co.uk/books?hl=en&lr=&id=EiOsAgAAQBAJ&oi=fnd&pg=PA319&dq=what+is+educational+research&ots=eIRocjq1sJ&sig=iYFi6tiPRubHNmoYCoI4aCauJQs#v=onepage&q=what is educational research&f=false.

Noble, H. and Smith, J. (2015). Issues of validity and reliability in qualitative research. *Evidence Based Nursing* 18 (2): 34–35. https://doi.org/10.1136/eb-2015-102054.

Nordmann, E., Clark, A., Spaeth, E., and MacKay, J.R.D. (2021). Lights, camera, active! Appreciation of active learning predicts positive attitudes towards lecture capture. *Higher Education.* https://doi.org/10.31234/osf.io/2jgcs.

Norman, G. (2003). RCT = results confounded and trivial: the perils of grand educational experiments. *Medical Education* 37 (7): 582–584. https://doi.org/10.1046/j.1365-2923.2003.01586.x.

Norman, G. (2010). Likert scales, levels of measurement and the "laws" of statistics. *Advances in Health Sciences Education* 15 (5): 625–632. https://doi.org/10.1007/s10459-010-9222-y.

Nosek, B. (2017, May 5). *How can we improve diversity and inclusion in the open science movement?* Center for Open Science Blog. https://www.cos.io/blog/how-can-we-improve-diversity-and-inclusion-open-science-movement.

Nosek, B.A. and Errington, T.M. (2020). What is replication? *PLoS Biology* 18 (3): e3000691. https://doi.org/10.1371/journal.pbio.3000691.

Nosek, B.A., Alter, G., Banks, G.C. et al. (2015). Promoting an open research culture. *Science* 348 (6242): 1422–1425. https://doi.org/10.1126/science.aab2734.

Oancea, A. (2005). Criticisms of educational research: key topics and levels of analysis. *British Educational Research Journal* 31 (2): 157–183. https://doi.org/10.1080/0141192052000340198.

O'Cathain, A., Murphy, E., and Nicholl, J. (2010). Three techniques for integrating data in mixed methods studies. *BMJ (Online)* 341 (c4587). https://doi.org/10.1136/bmj.c4587.

Oki, G.S.F. and Prentice, E.D. (2014). Continuing review of protocols. General concepts of protocol review. In: *The IACUC Handbook*, 3e (ed. J. Silverman, M.A. Suckow, and S. Murthy), 199–210. CRC Press.

O'Muircheartaigh, C., Gaskell, G., and Wright, D.B. (1995). Weighing anchors: verbal and numeric labels for response scales. *Journal of Official Statistics* 11 (3): 295–308.

Open Science Collaboration (2015). PSYCHOLOGY. Estimating the reproducibility of psychological science. *Science (New York, N.Y.)* 349 (6251): aac4716. https://doi.org/10.1126/science.aac4716.

Palermo, C., Reidlinger, D.P., and Rees, C.E. (2021). Internal coherence matters: lessons for nutrition and dietetics research. *Nutrition and Dietetics, February* 252–267. https://doi.org/10.1111/1747-0080.12680.

Paterson, J., Keys, C., Phillips, K. et al. (2019). Peer-led academic support for pre-arrival students of the BVM&S degree. *Journal of Veterinary Medical Education* 46 (4): 481–488. https://doi.org/10.3138/jvme.1017-149r.

Pearson, C.R., Parker, M., Fisher, C.B., and Moreno, C. (2014). Capacity building from the inside out: development and evaluation of a CITI ethics certification training module for American Indian and Alaska Native community researchers. *Journal of Empirical Research on Human Research Ethics* 9 (1): 46–57.

Pech, C., Cob, N., and Cejka, J.T. (2007). Understanding institutional review boards: practical guidance to the IRB review process. *Nutrition in Clinical Practice* 22 (6): 618–628. https://doi.org/10.1177/0115426507022006618.

Perkins, J. and Wang, D. (2004). A comparison of Bayesian and frequentist statistics as applied in a simple repeated measures example. *Journal of Modern Applied Statistical Methods* 3 (1): 227–233. https://doi.org/10.22237/jmasm/1083371040.

Pfaff, D. (2005). Hormone-driven mechanisms in the central nervous system facilitate the analysis of mammalian behaviours. *Journal of Endocrinology* 184 (3): 447–453. https://doi.org/10.1677/joe.1.05897.

Potter, J. and Hepburn, A. (2005). Qualitative interviews in psychology: problems and possibilities. *Qualitative Research in Psychology* 2 (4): 281–307. https://doi.org/10.1191/1478088705qp045oa.

Pownall, M., Talbot, C.V., Henschel, A. et al. (2021). Navigating open science as early career feminist researchers. *Psychology of Women Quarterly* 45 (4): 1–44. https://doi.org/10.1177/03616843211029255.

Prentice, E.D., Oki, G.S.F., and Mann, M.D. (2014). General concepts of protocol review. In: *The IACUC Handbook*, 3e (ed. J. Silverman, M.A. Suckow, and S. Murthy), 139–277. CRC Press.

Protection of Human Subjects, 45 CFR § 46 (2018). https://www.ecfr.gov/on/2018-07-19/title-45/subtitle-A/subchapter-A/part-46 (accessed 8 August 2021).

Raftery, A.E. (1995). Bayesian model selection in social research. *Sociological Methodology* 25: 111–163.

Rallis, S.F. and Rossman, G.B. (2010). Caring reflexivity. *International Journal of Qualitative Studies in Education* 23 (4): 495–499. https://doi.org/10.1080/09518398.2010.492812.

Rapley, T. (2011). Interviews. In: *Qualitative Research Practice* (ed. C. Seale, G. Gobo, J. Gubrium, and D. Silverman), 16–34 (Online Version). SAGE Publications Ltd. https://doi.org/10.4135/9781848608191.

Rice, T.W. (2008). The historical, ethical, and legal background of human-subjects research. *Respiratory Care* 53 (10): 1325–1329.

Rice, M., Bunker, K.D., Kang, D. et al. (2007). Accessing and recruiting children for research in schools. *Western Journal of Nursing Research* 29 (4): 501–514. https://doi.org/10.1177/0193945906296549.

Riddle, E. and MacKay, J.R.D. (2020). Social media contexts moderate perceptions of animals. *Animals* 10 (845): 16. https://doi.org/10.3390/ani10050845.

Riley, D. M. (2014). What's wrong with evidence? Epistemological roots and pedagogical implications of "evidence-based practice" in STEM education. *ASEE Annual Conference and Exposition, Conference Proceedings,* Indianapolis. American Society for Engineering Educaiton.

Rob, M. and Rob, F. (2018). Dilemma between constructivism and constructionism: leading to the development of a teaching-learning framework for student engagement and learning. *Journal of International Education in Business* 11 (2): 273–290. 10.1108/JIEB-01-2018-0002.

Roever, L., Resende, E.S., Diniz, A.L.D. et al. (2016). Critical analysis of clinical research articles: a guide for evaluation. *Evidence Based Medicine and Practice* 2 (e116). https://doi.org/10.4172/2471-9919.1000E116.

Roxå, T., Larsson, M., Price, L., and Mårtensson, K. (2017). Panel: Constructive friction? Charting the boundary between Educational Research and The Scholarship of Teaching and Learning. *International Society for the Scholarship of Teaching and Learning*, Online. https://guidebook.com/guide/113423/event/16623086/.

Rozmiarek, H. (2014). Origins of the IACUC. In: *The IACUC Handbook*, 3e (ed. J. Silverman, M.A. Suckow, and S. Murthy), 1–10. CRC Press.

Rubin, M. (2017). When does HARKing hurt? Identifying when different types of undisclosed post hoc hypothesizing harm scientific progress. *Review of General Psychology* 21 (4): 308–320. https://doi.org/10.1037/gpr0000128.

Russell, W.M.S. and Burch, R.L. (1959). *The Principles of Humane Experimental Technique*. Methuen.

Ruxton, G.D. and Colegrave, N. (2011). *Experimental Design for the Life Sciences*. Oxford University Press.

Schaeffer, N.C. and Dykema, J. (2020). Advances in the science of asking questions. *Annual Review of Sociology* 46: 37–60. https://doi.org/10.1146/annurev-soc-121919-054544.

Shalala, D. (2000). Protecting research subjects – what must be done. *New England Journal of Medicine* 343 (11): 808–810.

Silge, J. and Robinson, D. (2018). *Text Mining with R*. O'Reilly. https://www.tidytextmining.com/.

Silverman, D. (2014). *Interpreting Qualitative Data* (ed. K. Metzler), 5e. SAGE Publications.

Silverman, J., Lidz, C.W., Clayfield, J.C. et al. (2015). Decision making and the IACUC: Part 1—protocol information discussed at full-committee reviews. *Journal of the American Association for Laboratory Animal Science* 54 (4): 389–398.

Slattery, M.J., Logan, B.L., Mudge, B. et al. (2016). An undergraduate research fellowship program to prepare nursing students for future workforce roles. *Journal of Professional Nursing* 32 (6): 412–420.

Smith, C.P. (2000). Content analysis and narrative analysis. In: *Handbook of Research Methods in Social and Personality Psychology*, 313–335. Cambridge University Press. https://doi.org/10.1093/acprof.

Smith, B. (2018). Generalizability in qualitative research: misunderstandings, opportunities and recommendations for the sport and exercise sciences. *Qualitative Research in Sport, Exercise and Health* 10 (1): 137–149. https://doi.org/10.1080/2159676X.2017.1393221.

Smithson, J. (2000). Using and analysing focus groups: limitations and possibilities. *International Journal of Social Research Methodology* 3 (2): 103–119. https://doi.org/10.1080/136455700405172.

Stake, R.E. (2010). *Qualitative Research: Studying How Things Work*. The Guilford Press.

Staller, K.M. (2012). Epistemological boot camp: the politics of science and what every qualitative researcher needs to know to survive in the academy. *Qualitative Social Work* 12 (4): 395–413. https://doi.org/10.1177/1473325012450483.

Stern, N. (2016). *Building on Success and Learning from Experience. An Independent Review of the Research Excellence Framework* (Issue July). Department for Business, Energy & Industrial Strategy, UK Government.

Sullivan, G.M. and Feinn, R. (2012). Using effect size—or why the P value is not enough. *Journal of Graduate Medical Education* 4 (3): 279–282. https://doi.org/10.4300/jgme-d-12-00156.1.

Terry, G. and Braun, V. (2017). Short but often sweet. In: *Collecting Qualitative Data* (ed. V. Braun, V. Clarke, and D. Gray), 13–14. Cambridge University Press. https://doi.org/10.1017/9781107295094.003.

The National Academies (2003). Policy on committee composition and balance and conflict of interest for committees used in the development of reports. http://www.policyscience.net/nas.policies1.pdf (accessed 8 August 2021).

Tong, A., Sainsbury, P., and Craig, J. (2007). Consolidated criteria for reporting qualitative research (COREQ): a 32-item checklist for interviews and focus groups. *International Journal for Quality in Health Care* 19 (6): 349–357. https://doi.org/10.1093/intqhc/mzm042.

Tsai, Y.-S. and Gasevic, D. (2017). Learning analytics in higher education – challenges and policies. *Proceedings of the Seventh International Learning Analytics & Knowledge Conference on – LAK'17*, 233–242. https://doi.org/10.1145/3027385.3027400.

Tsai, Y., Gaševi, D., Whitelock-Wainwright, A., et al. (2018). *SHEILA Supporting Higher Education to Integrate Learning Analytics Research Report* (Issue November). The SHEILA Project ISBN 978-1-912669-02-8.

Turcotte-Tremblay, A. and Mc Sween-Cadieux, E. (2018). A reflection on the challenge of protecting confidentiality of participants while disseminating research results locally. *Ethics and Global Health* 19 (1): 5–11. https://doi.org/10.1186/s12910-018-0279-0.

Twining, P. (2010). Educational information technology research methodology: looking back and moving forward. In: *Researching IT in Education: Theory, Practice and Future Directions*, 1e (ed. A. McDougall, J. Murnane, A. Jones, and N. Reynolds), 153–168. Routledge. https://doi.org/10.4324/9780203863275.

Twining, P., Heller, R.S., Nussbaum, M., and Tsai, C.C. (2017). Some guidance on conducting and reporting qualitative studies. *Computers & Education* 106: A1–A9. https://doi.org/10.1016/j.compedu.2016.12.002.

Vaesen, K. and Katzav, J. (2017). How much would each researcher receive if competitive government research funding were distributed equally among researchers? *PLoS One* 12 (9): 4–6. https://doi.org/10.1371/journal.pone.0183967.

Van den Broeck, J., Sandøy, I.F., and Brestoff, J.R. (2013). The recruitment, sampling, and enrollment plan. In: *Epidemiology: Principles and Practical Guidelines* (ed. J. Van den Broeck and J.R. Brestoff), 171–196. Springer.

Wang, R. and Krosnick, J.A. (2020). Middle alternatives and measurement validity: a recommendation for survey researchers. *International Journal of Social Research Methodology* 23 (2): 169–184. https://doi.org/10.1080/13645579.2019.1645384.

Wester, K.L. (2011). Publishing ethical research: a step-by-step overview. *Journal of Counseling & Development* 89 (3): 301–307. https://doi.org/10.1002/j.1556-6678.2011.tb00093.x.

Whitaker, K. and Guest, O. (2020). #Bropenscience is broken science. *The Psychologist* 33: 34–37. https://doi.org/10.5281/zenodo.4099011.

White, M.G. (2020). Why human subjects research protection is important. *The Ochsner Journal* 20 (1): 16–33.

Wilkinson, S. (1999). Focus groups: a feminist method. *Psychology of Women Quarterly* 23: 221–244.

Willis, G.B. and Artino, A.R. (2013). What do our respondents think we're asking? using cognitive interviewing to improve medical education surveys. *Journal of Graduate Medical Education* 5 (3): 353–356. https://doi.org/10.4300/jgme-d-13-00154.1.

Wood, A.K., Galloway, R.K., Donnelly, R., and Hardy, J. (2016). Characterizing interactive engagement activities in a flipped introductory physics class. *Physical Review Physics Education Research* 12 (1): 1–15. https://doi.org/10.1103/PhysRevPhysEducRes.12.010140.

Wrigley, T. (2018). The power of 'evidence': reliable science or a set of blunt tools? *British Educational Research Journal* 44 (3): 359–376. https://doi.org/10.1002/berj.3338.

Zimmer, M. (2010). "But the data is already public": on the ethics of research in Facebook. *Ethics and Information Technology* 12 (4): 313–325. https://doi.org/10.1007/s10676-010-9227-5.

18

Building Bridges Between Research and Practice

Julie A. Hunt, DVM, MS

Richard A. Gillespie College of Veterinary Medicine, Lincoln Memorial University, Harrogate, TN, USA

Section 1: Introduction

Veterinary educators desire research that guides and supports their instruction and assessment methods. Veterinary educational researchers want to publish impactful studies that will prove useful to educators and will serve as a springboard for further research to understand educational phenomena. However, there can be a disconnect between the two groups, and not all veterinary educational research is useful in informing educational practices. This chapter will discuss how veterinary educational research findings can support, advance, and refine educational practices by looking at the challenges facing modern veterinarians, how adjustments to veterinary education can address these challenges, how educational theory can drive educational research, what struggles educational research faces, the barriers to implementing changes in higher education, and examples of how veterinary educational research findings have been successfully incorporated into educational practices.

Part 1: How Will Veterinary Education Adapt?

> An adequate philosophy of higher education would seek to widen the conceptual landscape by identifying universal and imaginative concepts that can assist not merely in understanding the university or in defending the university, but in changing it. (Barnett 2017, p. 78)

Many challenges facing the field of veterinary medicine can be addressed during students' veterinary education. In 1989, William Pritchard stated in his landmark Pew report:

> Veterinary education is a key leverage point for change in the profession. There are numerous

catalysts for change at work in the profession... A question of paramount importance is: How well will veterinary education structure itself so that it can support the needs of a rapidly developing profession with static or diminishing resources? (Pritchard 1989)

The Pew report identified key changes, including the increasing value of animals to society, the changing status of animals, expectations of high-quality service, a focus on health and not disease, an explosion of available information, advances in healthcare and science, changes in animal agricultural practices, and globalization. The report stated that one result of these societal changes was that an increasing number of veterinarians would seek to limit their professional practice exclusively to a single class of animals or species. The report made 13 recommendations for the modification of veterinary education, including a focus on health instead of disease, teaching students to find and use information rather than recalling facts, and moving toward more collaboration between veterinary colleges. Although the Pew report is now decades old, the trends it recognized are still in place in veterinary medicine.

Twelve years after the Pew report, in 2011, a broad group of veterinary educators, accreditors, and licensing assessors met and established the North American Veterinary Medical Education Consortium (NAVMEC), subsequently publishing a report that defined professional core competencies for veterinarians and identified the highest priority items for veterinary educational research (NAVMEC 2011). In the years following the Pew and NAVMEC reports, veterinary education has encountered additional pressures for change, including:

- As adult learners, students expect more flexibility and accommodation with their learning than ever before, and educators have responded with increased virtual teaching, live streaming, and lecture capture options. However, this flexibility adds to educators' workload and stress, as they navigate a landscape of students in front of them, students watching on livestream, and those who will watch the recording later.

- As public funding for veterinary training has declined, tuition has increased, and new graduate veterinarians' debt-to-income ratio has risen unsustainably.

- The indebtedness of new graduates impacts their career choices and limits their desire to purchase veterinary practices. This has driven many veterinary practices to be sold to corporations.

- Veterinary medicine's struggle with wellness, burnout, and mental health has become more widely researched, understood, and discussed. Research has demonstrated that veterinary students struggle to adapt to clinical practice after graduation, particularly in disciplines like surgery (Routly et al. 2002).

- Medical and surgical advancements continue to be made at an unprecedented rate, and veterinary education, fixed in duration, consists of more educational content crammed into the same amount of educational time. Many veterinary schools are allotting a growing amount of time to professional and life skills training, including topics like communication, collaboration, leadership, and financial literacy; though these topics are critically important to professional success, their inclusion in the curriculum further constricts the time available for traditional content.

- As societies grow more litigious, veterinary programs increasingly feel the need to make their assessments, and the decisions made from those assessments, more legally defensible.

- Clinical training methods are evolving away from academic veterinary teaching hospitals; each of the most recent veterinary schools in the United States features a distributed model of clinical training instead. Distributed models offer students a more realistic view of private and corporate practice than the potentially skewed view of the profession seen in most academic settings. However, distributed programs also engage students in a learning environment that is less supervised by college faculty.

- Veterinary colleges are increasingly called upon by accrediting bodies to provide outcome assessment data on their graduates. Educators seek to gather meaningful data that will allow them to draw meaningful conclusions about outcomes and guide continual improvement of their programs.

How veterinary education adapts to these and other modern forces of change depends on numerous factors. First, the profession must recognize and state the need for change. Second, there must be at least a minimum level of agreement on what adjustments or advancements are needed for this change to take place. The Pew and NAVMEC reports attempted to create consensus on these advancements, although these reports are both over a decade old. Change at the individual college level is perhaps the easiest to effect, although changes to accreditation standards can drive more widespread change on important issues. Finally, there must be retrospective analysis of the changes made and a realistic appraisal of the impact these changes had on veterinary students and new veterinary graduates.

Section 2: Educational Theory's Impact on Veterinary Educational Research

> Knowledge is theory, with the power to account for phenomena and predict beyond the particular. But that only happens when the bond between theory and study is intimate and dynamic, which in education, it rarely is (Norman 2007, p. 2)

Both the Pew and NAVMEC reports recommended that research be afforded a higher priority in veterinary education (NAVMEC 2011; Pritchard 1989). The field of veterinary educational research has grown in recent decades, as demonstrated by the expansion of research reports in the *Journal of Veterinary Medical Education*, the only journal devoted exclusively to veterinary education (Olson 2011; Schoenfeld-Tacher and Alpi 2021). Veterinary educational research has also been published in other veterinary journals, health professions education journals, and higher education journals. The number of conferences devoted to veterinary education has also increased in recent years, including the addition of the International Veterinary Simulation in Teaching (INVEST) conference starting in 2011 and VetEd Down Under beginning in 2018. The profession's opinion of educational research as a valid, meaningful pursuit has also grown, as have inter-disciplinary collaborations with fields like psychology and education (Fogelberg et al. 2021). The dissemination of well-designed educational research, which rests on educational theory, can help to answer the questions and challenges posed by modern society and its shifting requirements for veterinary medicine and its practitioners.

Researchers in health professions education have articulated how they see educational research impacting health professions education. Kevin Eva states:

> Scholarship is about determining how to best adapt the empirical findings present in the literature to

the needs and constraints of one's local context (and engaging in continuous quality improvement exercises to ensure that one's adaptations are meeting their mark). It is not about simply ordering the most effective educational therapy off the formulary. That pill doesn't exist (Eva 2009)

Eva purposefully avoids the term evidence-based teaching, believing that the term evidence-based has evolved to mean proof that something works and that in health professions education, a more accurate view is that the research forms a body of knowledge that is continually being built upon. Angela Brew describes research in higher educational settings as ideally being a community of scholars where free discussion and debate can occur (Brew 2001). Brew goes on to state that ideally, the link between teaching and research should be intimate and symbiotic, where teaching is in harmony with research and student learning aligns with faculty research activities.

Veterinary educational research studying the scholarship of teaching and learning can guide the development and evolution of veterinary education. However, there are limitations to how fully educational theory can inform teaching in a real educational setting. Educational research offers no definitive answers, but it can contribute to a knowledge base that can be used to formulate an answer or adaptation to the concerns facing modern veterinary medicine and veterinary education.

Section 3: How Educational Research Can Increase its Impact on Educational Practice

> Medical education research is not the 'poor relation' of medical research because it is not a relation at all. Instead, it belongs to a different family altogether. (Monrouxe and Rees 2009, p. 198)

The greatest value of educational research is its potential to refine how students are taught. Educational research can increase its influence on educational practice by:

Part 1: Undertaking Studies that Adhere to the Principles of Design-Based Research

The aim of design-based research is to advance theoretical knowledge about learning that can be applied to educational practices. Design-based research has five characteristics (Barab and Squire 2004). First, it involves a continuous cycle of design, evaluation, and redesign. Second, it occurs in real-life learning settings. Third, it aims to test or refine educational theories and advance practice. Fourth, it typically involves mixed methods studies, which allow researchers to determine how different variables influence each other and help to elucidate the how and why of an intervention's outcome (Dolmans and Tigelaar 2012). Finally, design-based research involves a close interaction between designers, researchers, and educators with varying expertise.

Educational theory and its foundations, assumptions, and claims are central to performing design-based research studies. Development studies seek to use existing theories and develop them further, while validation studies aim to test or prove theories (Nieveen et al. 2006). While design-based research studies take place in a local environment, generalization to other settings is based on educational theories grounding the design and on the inclusion of a thorough description of the local setting where the study took place. Good design-based research studies contribute to an understanding of the characteristics that are critical for an intervention to be successful in a specific setting.

Part 2: Changing the Focus of Educational Research from "Did It Work?" to "Why or How Did It Work?"

Educational research is a subset of social science research, not of medical research. As a social science discipline, educational research should seek to fully understand why and how educational phenomena occur, not just measure outcomes as biomedical and clinical research do. Most studies in medical educational research have been justification studies, which seek to answer the question "Did it work?," instead of clarification studies that answer "Why or how did it work?" (Cook et al. 2008). Educational research should seek an imperative of understanding the complexity of an outcome, not simply an imperative of proof of whether or not an intervention works (Cook et al. 2008; Regehr 2010). The value in educational research is generated less by researchers proving that their intervention was successful and more by the researchers' honest and thorough discussion of what they learned over the course of the study about students, processes, assessments, outcomes, and assumptions about learning. These types of discussions contribute to the real value of educational research, which is its contribution toward the building of a body of knowledge and advancement of educational theories (Monrouxe and Rees 2009).

Part 3: Evaluating Educational Interventions by Comparing Them to Existing Educational Methods

Veterinarians are trained as scientists and are thus most adept at biochemical and clinical research methodologies, which include quantitative research methods and the perceived "gold-standard" randomized controlled trial. However, if a veterinarian's career path includes veterinary educational research, the veterinarian must discover qualitative methodologies and recognize that the randomized controlled trial is no longer the best option for educational research. When comparing an educational intervention to a control group that receives no educational intervention, almost any intervention will prove better than nothing. Instead, a more valuable measure is to compare a new educational method to an established or traditional educational method. This allows the researcher to determine whether the new method is inferior, equivalent, or superior to the existing method, which helps educators make choices in designing curricula and learning opportunities. The direct comparison of two or more learning methods also advances educators' understanding of how students learn best and what specific components of an intervention lead to improved educational outcomes.

Part 4: Choosing Meaningful Outcome Measures When Assessing the Effectiveness of an Educational Intervention

Health professions educational research has been criticized for collecting data that is convenient to gather but has limited validity for answering the research question. In 1970, Kirkpatrick published a hierarchy for assessment of educational interventions (Kirkpatrick 1970). The ascending steps in Kirkpatrick's hierarchy are assessment of reaction (the trainee's opinion of the intervention), learning (the trainee's level of knowledge after the intervention), behavior (the trainee's behavior on the job following the intervention), and results (the tangible changes in outcomes attributed to the intervention) (Kirkpatrick 1970).

In 1990, Miller published his pyramid of assessment, which can also be considered when designing studies that assess learning (Miller 1990). The ascending levels in Miller's pyramid are knows (assessment of knowledge), knows how (assessment of application of knowledge or knowledge of a procedure), shows how (assessment of a demonstration of skill in a simulated environment), and does (assessment of workplace-based performance).

In 2009, Moore et al. published an expanded framework for assessing learning outcomes in medical education (Moore et al. 2009). This framework features ascending

Table 18.1 Levels of outcomes measures in medical education: a comparison of Moore et al.'s framework (Moore et al. 2009), Miller's pyramid of assessment (Miller 1990), and Kirkpatrick's hierarchy (Kirkpatrick 1970).

Moore et al.'s framework	Miller's pyramid	Kirkpatrick's hierarchy
Level 1 – Participation		
Level 2 – Satisfaction		Reaction
Level 3A – Learning declarative knowledge	Knows	Learning
Level 3B – Learning procedural knowledge	Knows how	
Level 4 – Competence	Shows how	
Level 5 – Performance on the job	Does	Behavior
Level 6 – Patient health		Results
Level 7 – Community health		

levels of participation, satisfaction, learning declarative or procedural knowledge, competence, performance on the job, patient health, and community health. A comparison of Moore et al.'s levels with Kirkpatrick's and Miller's can be seen in Table 18.1.

Educational researchers should avoid using participation, satisfaction, and reaction as sole measures for evaluating the effectiveness of an educational intervention, as they are subject to numerous biases, including confirmation bias. Learning and competence are better measures that are typically able to be collected. Higher-level measures, such as performance on the job and impact on patient and community health, are also valuable but are generally more difficult to collect and are typically influenced by many more variables than just the educational intervention being studied.

Part 5: Explaining the Local Context that the Research Is Conducted in Thoroughly, So Others Can Judge How the Findings May Apply to Learners in Their Context

Educational research that seeks to understand the problems and issues occurring in the discipline, rather than focusing on a singular solution, requires a thorough description of the problem; explanation of the local context of the study; evaluation of the study's assumptions about learning, competence, and assessment; and thorough description of what did not work in addition to what did work (Regehr 2010). The description of local context, including setting, students and their past educational history, faculty and their training, and how information is delivered and learning assessed, is critical to allowing those reading the research to determine how effectively the same intervention might be incorporated into their local context.

Reflexivity is also important in educational research and particularly necessary in qualitative research. The reader needs to be informed of the researchers' backgrounds, their pre-existing assumptions and expectations, and the lenses through which they designed and conducted the study (Bunniss and Kelly 2010). Reporting these features acknowledges the educational researcher's inherent bias and allows readers to reflect on how to adapt others' educational interventions or solutions for implementation in their local context.

Part 6: Following Coordinated Lines of Inquiry that Over Time Will Advance Veterinary Education Through an Iterative Building of Understanding

Knowledge and truth are not finite items waiting to be discovered; they are constructed by a community of inquirers through iterative study (Rorty 1990). Researchers and educators have observed that medical educational research does not frequently follow a coordinated line of inquiry but instead has often focused on the first step of observation and the final step of testing, while ignoring the important middle steps of model formation, theory building, and prediction, which guide educators in selecting instructional methods and assessments and promote the field's advancement over time (Cook et al. 2008).

Veterinary educational researchers should seek to follow a consistent and coordinated line of inquiry (e.g., what features of small animal surgical skills training models lead to effective learning, or how effectively a diagnostic imaging curriculum can be delivered remotely). Each study in the line of inquiry advances the knowledge of how learning takes place and can contribute to developing or revising educational theory as it applies to that topic. Veterinary educational research projects are frequently opportunistic and too rarely follow a coordinated line of inquiry that could truly advance the collective knowledge of a single area in a meaningful way.

Section 4: Educational Research Challenges

The practice of education cannot be the object of a science (Pring 2000, p. 29)

Educators in the health professions have complained that there is a gap between educational research results and educational practices (Badley 2003). In part, this gap results from educational research that does not build or refine educational theories in a way that could be instructive to educators. Healthcare professions educators have also noted that educational research is frequently repetitive and opportunistic, performed by researchers who demonstrate a limited understanding of educational theory and practice, especially qualitative methods, which are critical to social sciences research (Albert et al. 2007; Norman 2007). When educational researchers fail to link their study's methodology and findings to an educational theory, the study is inherently restricted to a description of findings that are not able to add to the larger conversation or body of knowledge. Theories provide different lenses through which to consider complicated issues, and they broaden our understanding of local situations (Reeves et al. 2008).

Veterinary educational research is also subject to numerous limiting factors that must be understood by those who perform research, implement findings, and create educational policies. Some of these limitations include inflated stakeholder expectations of how educational research should influence practice, the divide between quantitative and qualitative researchers and their methods, and rapidly changing conditions in veterinary education and employment.

Some stakeholders may have falsely inflated expectations of what it can accomplish and how educational research should impact practice. Increasingly, government and regulatory agencies are demanding evidence-based educational research to use to address perceived educational problems. However, the pragmatist approach rejects the notion that educational research can be used to specify educational practices and instead posits that educational research can only provide possible lines of action that can be considered for implementation in the local context (Badley 2003). Martyn Hammersley (2002) agrees that educational research is not able to provide a unified, comprehensive recommendation for educational practice, opining that educational practice cannot be founded on research outputs because practice also draws upon teachers' knowledge, experience, motivation, and other behavioral factors (p. 52). Additionally, school environments are complex, with changing social interactions and life events that daily impact the generalizability of educational research findings, and science is inadequate in explaining and predicting human behavior (Berliner 2002).

Educational research is also plagued by the epistemological and ontological divide that often separates quantitative and qualitative researchers (Pring 2000). Quantitative researchers and scientists generally believe in a single, objective reality that can be measured, while qualitative researchers are typically constructivists who argue that reality is a social construction and therefore can be changeable. As a rule, quantitative researchers believe in the importance of separation between the researcher and the researched, while qualitative researchers blur this distinction by stating that research findings are created rather than discovered and are a matter of consensus among researchers, each of whom brings their own biases to the interpretation of qualitative data.

However, the divide between quantitative and qualitative research methodologies is not insurmountable. Richard Pring (2000) states that the gap between these research methodologies is inappropriate and represents a false dualism; he recommends that educational researchers use both qualitative and quantitative methodologies. Mixed methods studies, or studies including both qualitative and quantitative methodologies, frequently impart a better understanding of the phenomenon being studied than either method used alone.

Incorporating educational research findings into changed educational practices is also limited by time and the degree of change taking place in educational settings and places of employment. The changing social environment in education means that educational research findings may not be valid or useful a decade after the initial research (Berliner 2002). Unfortunately, good-quality educational research takes time to design, perform, analyze, and disseminate; frequently, years may go by between the inception of a study and its dissemination to a broader audience. The changing face of higher education and the dynamic needs of the new veterinary graduate mean that once published, educational research may become outdated relatively soon afterward.

While none of these limitations of veterinary educational research are catastrophic, they must be considered when designing and performing research, or when seeking to incorporate research findings into educational practices. However, they are not the only barriers that exist to implementation. Educational institutions, faculty, and students can also pose significant barriers to changing educational methods that reflect the most recent educational research findings.

Section 5: Barriers to Changing Educational Methods

> It is easier to change the location of a cemetery than to change the school curriculum. Woodrow Wilson (Larkin 2010, p. 474)

Veterinary colleges in North America have been teaching students with little change in methods since the inception of the programs. The current educational model, pioneered by medical educators, is based on a clinical clerkship training model established by William Osler in the late 1800s (Dornan 2005) and modified by recommendations in the Flexner Report, published in 1910 (Flexner 1910). Influenced by physician training methods used in Europe, Flexner recommended additional scientific training of medical doctors in North America; medical schools subsequently established a preclinical phase, where students learn biomedical sciences, followed by a clinical phase of education. This model of training persists today in both medical and veterinary education.

While the overall format of veterinary education has not changed, educational research findings continue to highlight ways in which current practices could be improved and refined. For example, research has demonstrated that students retain less information delivered in lecture format as compared with an active learning format (Freeman et al. 2014). One of the reasons that widespread change toward active learning methods has been implemented slowly in veterinary curricula is because faculty prefer and are more prepared to teach using the familiar lecture-based system that they themselves learned through (Pollock 1985). Veterinary educational researchers have also stressed the importance of developing students' critical thinking skills; however, they also acknowledge that teachers will need to modify their beliefs about knowledge and learning, learn new strategies for teaching and assessment, and practice new classroom habits to assist students' development of critical thinking skills (Paul and Wilson 1993). Several colleges already offer their veterinary faculty additional training in methods of instruction and assessment (Bell 2013; Silva-Fletcher and May 2015), though the majority still lag. If educational theory is to impact veterinary educational methods, faculty development will be necessary to train faculty in new practices.

Veterinary students may also resist a change in teaching methods, particularly if the new methods are not implemented beginning on the first day of veterinary school (Dale et al. 2008). Unfortunately, transformations of veterinary educational methods have often been introduced piecemeal, during the middle or later years of the veterinary curriculum. Changes are more often focused on teaching methods than on changing the format of assessments, which may be determined at a college level. Therefore, for students who are motivated by assessment practices, these isolated teaching innovations have failed to change the overall learning culture because the assessments continue to reward traditional teaching and learning methods (Dale et al. 2008).

The veterinary college at Texas A&M University published an example of the barriers to changing the veterinary curriculum, in this case from a traditional lecture-based curriculum to a problem-based curriculum with more independent learning (Herron et al. 1990). Although students recognized that problem-solving was an important skill and students generally desired more problem-solving in their curriculum, students and faculty noted some barriers, including faculty resistance due to the belief that students' academic success depended on memorizing facts and student resistance to independent self-study in lieu of lectures and laboratories (Herron et al. 1990).

Section 6: How Educational Research Has Changed Veterinary Education Practices

> Change is the end result of all true learning. Change involves three things: first, a dissatisfaction with self – a felt void or need; second, a decision to change – to fill that void or need; and third, a conscious dedication to the process of growth and change – the willful act of making the change, doing something. Leo Buscaglia (Chang 2006, p. 114)

Despite the potential shortcomings of educational research and the resistance of students and faculty toward changing educational methods, some veterinary educational research has impacted how veterinary students are taught and assessed. Examples of a few of these situations are described below.

Part 1: Active Learning

Historically, veterinary colleges have delivered knowledge using a lecture-based curriculum. However, lectures encourage surface learning methods, such as note-taking and memorization, instead of promoting deep learning that comes from reflection and modification of students' existing mental schemas (Biggs 1999). Active learning teaching formats require student engagement, such as for analysis, reflection, problem-solving, and discussion. Active learning methods have demonstrated improved student learning and retention (Freeman et al. 2014).

Numerous veterinary schools have recently incorporated active learning into lecture-based courses (Dooley et al. 2018; Gordon et al. 2022), skills-based courses (Keegan et al. 2012; Moffett and Mill 2014), and into active learning tracks throughout the curriculum (Crowther and Baillie 2016). One common form of active learning is the flipped classroom, where students review materials prior to attending lecture or laboratory and then use their existing knowledge during active learning classroom activities. An international survey study demonstrated that 95% of veterinary educators were familiar with the flipped classroom technique, and 64% had used it in their teaching (Matthew et al. 2019).

Problem-based learning (PBL) is another active learning method used at several veterinary schools (Fletcher et al. 2015). PBL teaches clinical concepts through the completion and study of real and meaningful cases, which are designed to help students develop rich cognitive models of the problems given to them. True PBL curricula are cumulative and require students to take responsibility for their own learning. The problems presented must allow for free inquiry, and collaboration is essential for solving the problems. PBL generally features a closing analysis phase where students share what they have learned about the problem, its concepts, and associated principles. Self- and peer-assessment are typically carried out regularly.

PBL curricula are based on several learning theories (Newman 2005). Social constructivist theory supports the use of small group learning, and theories of self-regulation and metacognition allow students to adopt attitudes and strategies that allow them to be responsible for their learning with the teacher serving as a facilitator. Schema theory supports students' activation of prior knowledge and application of that knowledge in context during their problem-solving process. Finally, motivational theories support students' internal motivation to learn, which is critical in PBL curricula.

Part 2: Competency-Based Veterinary Education

One of the strategic goals identified by the NAVMEC report was to graduate new veterinarians who are career-ready and proficient in an agreed-upon set of core competencies (NAVMEC 2011). Veterinary educators proposed that these competencies must be clearly defined, taught across the entire curriculum, and assessed with valid and reliable measures to be impactful (Hodgson et al. 2013). Multiple attempts have been made to create a competency framework to underpin veterinary curricula because this framework allows educators to design curriculum with outcomes in mind, a concept known as backwards design. Once competencies are established, courses can be built, and assessment methods can be created and validated.

Harold Bok et al. (2011) created a competency framework for veterinary students in Europe through focus group interviews with practicing veterinarians and a Delphi procedure. Along with a group of international educators, Bok went on to assess international veterinarians' perspectives on the created competency framework, including what skills were expected of veterinarians and what should be taught in veterinary school (Bok et al. 2014). In a subsequent study, Bok et al. (2013a) investigated a program of assessment that could be used to evaluate student competencies. In the next two studies, Bok et al. (2013b, 2016) evaluated students' feedback-seeking behavior in the clinical workplace and clinical teachers' perspectives on teaching interactions in the workplace, including teachers' use of the mini-clinical evaluation exercise to provide student feedback. Finally, Teunissen and Bok (2013) used a social cognitive model of motivation about implicit self-theories to explain behaviors that arise when individuals are confronted with challenges such as seeking and providing constructive workplace-based feedback. In this series of six studies, Bok and his team demonstrated how researchers can pursue a single line of inquiry to promote a meaningful change in educational practices and contribute to a more nuanced understanding of an educational phenomenon, in this case feedback-seeking and feedback -giving behaviors.

Bok et al. were not the only ones interested in developing a competency framework. The American Association of Veterinary Medical Colleges (AAVMC) assembled a competency-based veterinary education (CBVE) working group to create and publish a framework describing nine domains of competence (Molgaard et al. 2018a). Not surprisingly, the working group included Bok, no doubt in recognition of his role in creating a veterinary competency framework in Europe. Each of the domains described by the working group contained several competencies that veterinary graduates should be able to perform, with sample sub-competencies listed for illustrative purposes. The working group subsequently published eight entrustable professional activities (EPAs), representing skills that students could be assessed upon, each of which was linked back to several of the nine domains of competence (Molgaard et al. 2018b). Finally, the working group published milestones, which defined the skill level expectations for each competency at a range of levels from novice to proficient (Salisbury et al. 2019). Collectively, the CBVE framework, EPAs, and milestones represent the most substantial pedagogical project that the AAVMC has ever undertaken, and the framework, EPAs, and milestones have begun to be incorporated into veterinary curricula and student skills assessments (Hays et al. 2020). Numerous veterinary schools currently map their curricula to the CBVE competencies, and several schools are utilizing the EPAs to determine students' readiness to graduate during their clinical rotations.

Part 3: Early Clinical Exposure

Medical educators dating back to William Osler in the late 1800s espoused the value of clinical training and allowed students to learn from patients and their diseases while standing bedside (Dornan 2005). Distinct preclinical and clinical phases became the standard in medical education – and veterinary education quickly followed – shortly after the Flexner report's call for an increased emphasis on the biomedical sciences (Dornan 2005; Flexner 1910). However, 73 good-quality educational studies have demonstrated that early clinical exposure can motivate and satisfy health professions students, help them to adapt to clinical environments, impart improved clinical skills, assist them in developing a professional identity, allow them to interact with patients more confidently and with less stress, improve their ability to self-reflect, and strengthen their learning of biomedical sciences (Dornan et al. 2006). These studies of early clinical exposure draw upon multiple educational and social science theories, including situated learning theory, contemporary social and learning theory, and workplace learning theory.

As a result of research supporting early clinical exposure, several veterinary schools have begun to integrate students into the clinical environment during the first half of veterinary school, which traditionally has been spent learning the biomedical sciences. One of these schools, Charles Sturt University in Australia, has veterinary students spend time in rural veterinary practices beginning in the first year of their veterinary education to gain animal handling skills and a better understanding of the veterinary profession, veterinary workplaces, and a veterinarian's role in their community (Abbott 2009). Early clinical experiences also serve as potent motivators for on-campus student learning.

Part 4: Clinical Skills Laboratories

Numerous educators have noted that veterinary students struggle with the transition from classroom to clinical workplace (Jaarsma et al. 2008; Mellanby and Herrtage 2004; Routly et al. 2002). Specifically, clinical-year veterinary students and recent graduates tend to report challenges in learning and practicing clinical skills, including performing surgery. In addition to early clinical exposure as a method of assisting students in the transition between classroom and clinic, many veterinary schools have established clinical skills laboratories, where preclinical students learn to perform clinical skills in a standardized environment on models or cadavers with instructor feedback prior to entering the real clinical environment with client-owned patients (Dilly et al. 2017). A myriad of models and simulators have been developed for use in teaching veterinary students, and the field continues to expand rapidly (Baillie 2007; Hunt et al. 2022; Scalese and Issenberg 2005).

Educators have recognized the value of standardized, focused skills training that takes place outside of the clinical environment; Monkhouse (2010) stated, "Two hours of focused surgical training is worth more than eight hours of chaotic, random educational encounters" (p. 167). Veterinary students have also accepted alternative models for teaching procedures as long as the instructor imparts clinical relevance (Johnson and Farmer 1989). Practicing clinical skills on models and simulators has resulted in equivalent or superior educational outcomes to training on live animals (Olsen et al. 1996) or cadavers (Caston et al. 2016; Griffon et al. 2000) and has resulted in reduced procedural times on subsequent live animal performances (Annandale et al. 2020).

A 2017 survey study of 18 veterinary colleges with established clinical skills laboratories in North America, the Caribbean, and Europe demonstrated that 15 of the colleges (83%) held formal instruction in the laboratory, 14 (78%) allowed students to practice skills in an open access format, and 13 (72%) formally assessed students in the laboratory (Dilly et al. 2017). The number of veterinary clinical skills laboratories, available models, and educational research to support these programs continues to expand rapidly.

Summary

Modern veterinary education faces numerous challenges, including a decline in public funding, increased student debt, improved understanding of students' and educators' mental health concerns, and expansion of disseminated clinical training. Veterinary educational research findings and the further development of educational theories relevant to veterinary medicine will help the profession to answer the questions and challenges posed by modern society, including its shifting expectations of veterinary practitioners.

Veterinary educational researchers seek to perform and publish studies that are relevant to educators and will advance the field's body of knowledge. However, educational research often falls short of being able to provide evidence-based answers; more likely, educational research can build a body of knowledge that with time will improve veterinary educators' ability to answer the questions that arise in their classrooms, laboratories, and clinical training sites. Using the principles of design-based research can help educational researchers to design and perform meaningful studies that contribute to the field's development and refinement of knowledge. Educational research that evaluates meaningful outcome measures, compares new educational interventions to existing evidence-informed practices, describes the local context of all interventions, and contributes to a coordinated line of inquiry is particularly valuable to educators.

The findings of veterinary educational research may be challenging to implement in veterinary colleges. Two main forces against implementation include faculty and student resistance to change. However, there have been numerous examples of successful implementation of educational research-based findings in veterinary education in recent years. The combined efforts of veterinary educators and veterinary educational researchers will continue to shape the future of veterinary education and the veterinary profession as a whole.

References

Abbott, K. (2009). Innovations in veterinary education: the Charles Sturt University programme (Wagga Wagga, Australia). *Revue Scientifique et Technique* 28 (2): 763.

Albert, M., Hodges, B., and Regehr, G. (2007). Research in medical education: balancing service and science. *Advances in Health Sciences Education* 12 (2): 103–115.

Annandale, A., Scheepers, E., and Fosgate, G.T. (2020). The effect of an ovariohysterectomy model practice on surgical times for final-year veterinary students' first live-animal ovariohysterectomies. *Journal of Veterinary Medical Education* 47 (1): 44–55.

Badley, G. (2003). The crisis in educational research: a pragmatic approach. *European Educational Research Journal* 2 (2): 296–308.

Baillie, S. (2007). Utilization of simulators in veterinary training. *Cattle Practice* 15 (3): 224.

Barab, S. and Squire, K. (2004). Design-based research: putting a stake in the ground. *The Journal of the Learning Sciences* 13 (1): 1–14.

Barnett, R. (2017). Towards a social philosophy of higher education. *Educational Philosophy and Theory* 49 (1): 78–88.

Bell, C. (2013). Faculty development in veterinary education: are we doing enough (or publishing enough about it), and do we value it? *Journal of Veterinary Medical Education* 40 (2): 96–101.

Berliner, D. (2002). Educational research: the hardest science of all. *Educational Researcher* 31 (8): 18–20.

Biggs, J. (1999). What the student does: teaching for enhanced learning. *Higher Education Research & Development* 18 (1): 57–75.

Bok, H., Jaarsma, D.A.D.C., Teunissen, P. et al. (2011). Development and validation of a competency framework for veterinarians. *Journal of Veterinary Medical Education* 38 (3): 262–269.

Bok, H., Teunissen, P., Favier, R. et al. (2013a). Programmatic assessment of competency-based workplace learning: when theory meets practice. *BMC Medical Education* 13 (1): 1–9.

Bok, H., Teunissen, P., Spruijt, A. et al. (2013b). Clarifying students' feedback-seeking behaviour within the clinical workplace. *Medical Education* 47 (3): 282–291.

Bok, H., Teunissen, P., Boerboom, T. et al. (2014). International survey of veterinarians to assess the importance of competencies in professional practice and education. *Journal of the American Veterinary Medical Association* 245 (8): 906–913.

Bok, H., Jaarsma, D.A.D.C., Spruijt, A. et al. (2016). Feedback-giving behaviour in performance evaluations during clinical clerkships. *Medical Teacher* 38 (1): 88–95.

Brew, A. (2001). *The Nature of Research: Inquiry in Academic Contexts*. Routledge Falmer.

Bunniss, S. and Kelly, D. (2010). Research paradigms in medical education research. *Medical Education* 44 (6): 358–366.

Caston, S.S., Schleining, J.A., Danielson, J.A. et al. (2016). Efficacy of teaching the Gambee suture pattern using simulated small intestine versus cadaveric small intestine. *Veterinary Surgery* 45 (8): 1019–1024.

Chang, L. (2006). *Wisdom for the Soul: Five Millenia of Prescriptions for Spiritual Healing*. Gnosophia Publishers.

Cook, D., Bordage, G., and Schmidt, H. (2008). Description, justification and clarification: a framework for classifying the purposes of research in medical education. *Medical Education* 42 (2): 128–133.

Crowther, E. and Baillie, S. (2016). A method of developing and introducing case-based learning to a preclinical veterinary curriculum. *Anatomical Sciences Education* 9 (1): 80–89.

Dale, V., Sullivan, M., and May, S. (2008). Adult learning in veterinary education: theory to practice. *Journal of Veterinary Medical Education* 35 (4): 581–588.

Dilly, M., Read, E.K., and Baillie, S. (2017). A survey of established veterinary clinical skills laboratories from Europe and North America: present practices and recent developments. *Journal of Veterinary Medical Education* 44 (4): 580–589.

Dolmans, D. and Tigelaar, D. (2012). Building bridges between theory and practice in medical education using a design-based research approach: AMEE guide no. 60. *Medical Teacher* 34 (1): 1–10.

Dooley, L., Frankland, S., Boller, E., and Tudor, E. (2018). Implementing the flipped classroom in a veterinary pre-clinical science course. *Journal of Veterinary Medical Education* 45 (2): 195–203.

Dornan, T. (2005). Osler, Flexner, apprenticeship, and "the new medical education". *Journal of the Royal Society of Medicine* 98 (3): 91–95.

Dornan, T., Littlewood, S., Margolis, S. et al. (2006). How can experience in clinical and community settings contribute to early medical education? A BEME systematic review. *Medical Teacher* 28 (1): 3–18.

Eva, K. (2009). Broadening the debate about quality in medical education research. *Medical Education* 43 (4): 294–296.

Fletcher, O., Hooper, B., and Schoenfeld-Tacher, R. (2015). Instruction and curriculum in veterinary medical education: a 50-year perspective. *Journal of Veterinary Medical Education* 42 (5): 489–500.

Flexner, A. (1910). *Medical Education in the United States and Canada: A Report to the Carnegie Foundation for the Advancement of Teaching*. Boston: Merrymount Press.

Fogelberg, K., Hunt, J., and Baillie, S. (2021). Young and evolving: a narrative of veterinary educational research from early leaders. *Education in the Health Professions* 4 (3): 124–133.

Freeman, S., Eddy, S.L., McDonough, M. et al. (2014). Active learning increases student performance in science, engineering, and mathematics. *Proceedings of the National Academy of Sciences of the United States of America* 111 (23): 8410–8415.

Gordon, S., Bolwell, C., Raney, J., and Zepke, N. (2022). Transforming a didactic lecture into a student-centered active learning exercise--teaching equine diarrhea to fourth-year veterinary students. *Education Sciences* 12 (2): 68.

Griffon, D.J., Cronin, P., Kirby, B., and Cottrell, D.F. (2000). Evaluation of a hemostasis model for teaching ovariohysterectomy in veterinary surgery. *Veterinary Surgery* 29 (4): 309–316.

Hammersley, M. (2002). *Educational Research, Policymaking and Practice* (ed. P. Chapman). London: Paul Chapman Publishing.

Hays, R., Jennings, B., Gibbs, T. et al. (2020). Impact of the COVID-19 pandemic: the perceptions of health professions educators. *MedEdPublish* https://doi.org/10.15694/mep.2020.000142.1.

Herron, M., Wolf, A., and DiBrito, W. (1990). Faculty and student attitudes toward problem solving and independent learning in the veterinary medical curriculum. *Journal of Veterinary Medical Education* 17 (1): 19–21.

Hodgson, J.L., Pelzer, J.M., and Inzana, K.D. (2013). Beyond NAVMEC: competency-based veterinary education and assessment of the professional competencies. *Journal of Veterinary Medical Education1* 40 (2): 102–118.

Hunt, J., Simons, M., and Anderson, S. (2022). If you build it, they will learn: a review of models in veterinary surgical education. *Veterinary Surgery* 51 (1): 52–61.

Jaarsma, D.A.D.C., Dolmans, D., Scherpbier, A., and Van Beukelen, P. (2008). Preparation for practice by veterinary school: a comparison of the perceptions of alumni from a traditional and an innovative veterinary curriculum. *Journal of Veterinary Medical Education* 35 (3): 431–438.

Johnson, A. and Farmer, J. (1989). Evaluation of traditional and alternative models in psychomotor laboratories for veterinary surgery. *Journal of Veterinary Medical Education* 16 (1): 11–14.

Keegan, R., Brown, G., and Gordon, A. (2012). Use of a simulation of the ventilator-patient interaction as an active learning exercise: comparison with traditional lecture. *Journal of Veterinary Medical Education* 39 (4): 359–367.

Kirkpatrick, D. (1970). Evaluation of training. In: *Evaluation of Short-Term Training in Rehabilitation* (ed. P. Browning), 40–61. University of Oregon.

Larkin, M. (2010). Long road ahead to change veterinary education. *Journal of the American Veterinary Medical Association* 237 (5): 474–478.

Matthew, S., Schoenfeld-Tacher, R., Danielson, J., and Warman, S. (2019). Flipped classroom use in veterinary education: a multinational survey of faculty experiences. *Journal of Veterinary Medical Education* 46 (1): 97–107.

Mellanby, R. and Herrtage, M. (2004). Survey of mistakes made by recent veterinary graduates. *Veterinary Record* 155 (24): 761–765.

Miller, G.E. (1990). The assessment of clinical skills/competence/performance. *Academic Medicine : Journal of the Association of American Medical Colleges* 65: S63–S67.

Moffett, J. and Mill, A. (2014). Evaluation of the flipped classroom approach in a veterinary professional skills course. *Advances in Medical Education and Practice* 5: 415–425.

Molgaard, L., Hodgson, J., Bok, H. et al. (2018a). *Competency-Based Veterinary Education: Part 1 – CBVE Framework*. Association of American Veterinary Medical Colleges.

Molgaard, L., Hodgson, J., Bok, H. et al. (2018b). *Competency-Based Veterinary Education: Part 2 – Entrustable Professional Activities*. Washington, DC: Association of American Veterinary Medical Colleges.

Monkhouse, S. (2010). Learning in the surgical workplace: necessity not luxury. *The Clinical Teacher* 7 (3): 167–170.

Monrouxe, L. and Rees, C. (2009). Picking up the gauntlet: constructing medical education as a social science. *Medical Education* 43 (3): 196–198.

Moore, D., Green, J., and Gallis, H. (2009). Achieving desired results and improved outcomes: integrating planning and assessment throughout learning activities. *Journal of Continuing Education in the Health Professions* 29 (1): 1–15.

NAVMEC Board of Directors (2011). The north American veterinary medical education consortium (NAVMEC) looks to veterinary medical education for the future: "Roadmap for veterinary medical education in the 21st century: responsive, collaborative, flexible". *Journal of Veterinary Medical Education* 38 (4): 320–327.

Newman, M. (2005). Problem based learning: an introduction and overview of the key features of the approach. *Journal of Veterinary Medical Education* 32 (1): 12–20.

Nieveen, N., McKenney, S., and van den Akker, J. (2006). Educational design research: the value of validity. In: *Educational Design Research* (ed. J. van den Akker, K. Gravemeijer, S. McKenney, and N. Nieveen), 151–159. Routledge.

Norman, G. (2007). Editorial – how bad is medical education research anyway? *Advances in Health Sciences Education* 12 (1): 1–5.

Olsen, D., Bauer, M., Seim, H., and Salman, M. (1996). Evaluation of a hemostasis model for teaching basic surgical skills. *Veterinary Surgery* 25 (1): 49–58.

Olson, L. (2011). Content analysis of a stratified random selection of JVME articles: 1974-2004. *Journal of Veterinary Medical Education* 38 (1): 42–51.

Paul, R. and Wilson, R. (1993). Critical thinking: the key to veterinary educational reform. *Journal of Veterinary Medical Education* 20 (2): 34–36.

Pollock, R. (1985). Problem solving cannot be taught. *Journal of Veterinary Medical Education* 12 (1): 9–12.

Pring, R. (2000). *Philosophy of Educational Research*. Continuum.

Pritchard, W. (1989). *Future Directions for Veterinary Medicine*. The Canadian Veterinary Journal.

Reeves, S., Albert, M., Kuper, A., and Hodges, B. (2008). Qualitative research: why use theories in qualitative research? *BMJ* 337 (7670): 631–634.

Regehr, G. (2010). It's not rocket science: rethinking our metaphors for research in health professions education. *Medical Education* 44 (1): 31–39.

Rorty, R. (1990). Introduction: pragmatism as anti-representationalism. In: *Pragmatism from Pierce to Davidson* (ed. J. Murphy), 1–6. Westview Press.

Routly, J., Dobson, H., Taylor, I. et al. (2002). Support needs of veterinary surgeons during the first few years of practice: perceptions of recent graduates and senior partners. *Veterinary Record* 150 (6): 167–171.

Salisbury, S., Caney, K., Ilkiw, J. et al. (2019). *Competency-Based Veterinary Education: Part 3 – Milestones*. Association of American Veterinary Medical Colleges.

Scalese, R.J. and Issenberg, S.B. (2005). Effective use of simulations for the teaching and acquisition of veterinary professional and clinical skills. *Journal of Veterinary Medical Education* 32: 461–467.

Schoenfeld-Tacher, R. and Alpi, K. (2021). A 45-year retrospective content analysis of JVME articles. *Journal of Veterinary Medical Education* https://doi.org/10.3138/jvme-2020-0073.

Silva-Fletcher, A. and May, S. (2015). Developing teachers in veterinary education. *REDU: Revista de Docencia Universitaria* 13 (33–51): 33–51.

Teunissen, P. and Bok, H. (2013). Believing is seeing: how people's beliefs influence goals, emotions, and behaviour. *Medical Education* 47 (11): 1064–1072.

19

History and Purpose of Higher Education

Donald B. Mills, A.B., M.Div., Ed.D
Texas Christian University, Fort Worth, TX, USA

Kimberly S. Cook, Ed.D., MBA
Texas Christian University, Fort Worth, TX, USA

Section 1: Introduction

In 1620, a group of Protestant separatists set sail from Plymouth, England, determined to start a new life and establish a new church in North America. After two stormy months at sea, the Mayflower reached Cape Cod and set about establishing a colony. That group of devout men and women were the first colonists in New England but were soon followed by many others, including a significant number of graduates of Cambridge and Oxford Universities. Perhaps, then, it is not surprising that within two decades of the first colonist's arrival, the provincial government and colony leaders established a college along the banks of the Charles River (Rudolph 1990). That was Harvard College. The year was 1636 and the unwieldy system of higher education in America had its first member.

Unlike the centralized system of higher education found in most countries of the world, the system in the United States is highly decentralized. Although initially based on European models of education, higher education in the United States has evolved into a variety of governance structures. Private not-for-profit institutions, state-sponsored university systems, locally sponsored community college systems, and private for-profit institutions enroll almost all the higher education students in the United States. But these designations do not always provide adequate clarity in describing institutions.

Approximately, 3,700 institutions of higher education enroll nearly 19 million students. Clearly, there is a wide range of enrolled students, from 2 to 3 dozen at Deep Springs College to over 70,000 at Arizona State University. Some trustees (also called regents, or directors) are elected, some appointed by governors, and some boards are self-selecting. Some institutions are sponsored by religious denominations, others are state-affiliated, some are county supported, and some operate on a business profit orientation answerable to shareholders. Yet with all their differences, all (or almost all) receive support from federal, state, and local governments. All (or almost all) use a model that requires students to pay for their education – or at least earn their tuition.

Within these categories, there are a myriad of subcategories, from highly selective admissions to open admissions, from research-intensive to teaching emphasis, from associates degrees to doctorates, and from general education to narrowly focused curricula. Some institutions focus on traditionally aged students (18–23) while others focus on adult students.

In this chapter we will discuss:

- the growth of higher education from a single institution in colonial New England to multiple institutions in every state in the country.
- who attends these institutions.
- the purpose of higher education.

Section 2: Brief History of Higher Education in the United States

Part 1: Colonial Colleges

After the founding of Harvard College in 1636, it was another half century before another college was founded in the colonies. William and Mary opened in 1694 as the nation's second college. By 1771, another seven[1] had joined

---

1 Yale college in 1902, College of New Jersey (now Princeton) in 1747, King's College (now Columbia) in 1754, College of Philadelphia (now University of Pennsylvania) in 1754, Rhode Island College (now Brown) in 1766, Dartmouth College in 1770, and Queen's College (now Rutgers) in 1771.

Educational Principles and Practice in Veterinary Medicine, First Edition. Edited by Katherine Fogelberg.
© 2024 John Wiley & Sons, Inc. Published 2024 by John Wiley & Sons, Inc.

the first two, but total enrollments at all nine were only 721 in 1775. Between 1769 and 1775 only 825 students had graduated and of those 29% were planning a career in ministry. The law was becoming a popular choice, with about 15% of graduates, and medicine was the career choice of about 12% (Geiger 2015). All of the students were white men and for many, college was a chance to achieve status in the new society being created in the new world. For a good portion of graduates, college served its purpose, but undoubtedly many also headed west and became explorers of the frontier.

Religious roots run deep in the early colleges and the curriculum reflected the founder's theology. However, the purpose of the early colleges went well beyond religious training. As Rudolph (1990) points out:

> A college develops a sense of unity where, in a society created from many of the nations of Europe, there might otherwise be aimlessness and uncontrolled diversity. A college advances learning; it combats ignorance and barbarism. A college is a support of the state; it is an instructor in loyalty, in citizenship, in the dictates of conscience and faith. A college is useful: it helps men to learn the things they must know in order to manage the temporal affairs of the world; it trains a legion of teachers. All these things a college was. All these purposes a college served (p. 13).

How well these early institutions succeeded in accomplishing their purposes was mixed. Although nominally founded by religious organizations, the separation of church and government was unclear. Many of the early colleges were creations as much of the local governments as of the denominations they were expected to serve. Whether they were state colleges or church colleges is probably unimportant. Suffice it to say that the leaders of colonial governments viewed higher education as a necessary part of their communities (Rudolph 1990; Dorn 2017).

The American Revolution touched virtually every institution of higher learning, either because of active involvement of students and faculty or because the war itself impacted campuses. (The exception was Dartmouth that was spared being impacted by the war because it was so remote.) Campuses were closed, used to house soldiers, and endowments were destroyed or used in the war effort. The war effort, initially an effort to achieve independence, evolved into an effort to recognize that each man stood as an equal before God. This new way of thinking overtook colleges and college curricula much to the dismay of college leaders who preferred the classical liberal curriculum of the great institutions of Europe. Higher education leaders lamented that Americans seemed more interested in managing their own affairs than having their affairs well-managed. The involvement of higher education institutions in the war effort marked the first of many instances when campuses were central to significant issues facing the country. And not for the last time the effects of war played a significant role in higher education in the United States.

After the war, state legislators recognized that a new relationship was evolving between existing colleges and the state and that citizens were demanding that additional institutions be established to meet the need for advanced education in a changing and diverse country. From Maine in the north to the Carolinas and deep south, there was a clamor for education. In Maine, Bowdoin College was established with an express purpose to promote the common good (Dorn 2017). This was not a unique characteristic among the early American colleges, but rather fostering the practice of civic virtue and commitment to the common good was the norm. While differentiating between public and private institutions is commonplace today, in the late eighteenth and early nineteenth centuries all institutions were referenced as "public" institutions because their focus was the public good.

The first colleges were established in the most heavily populated areas along the Atlantic seaboard. The elite in the more rural southern colonies sent their sons to school in the north. As the country began to grow and expand, so too did state legislatures begin to recognize the need for institutions of higher education. South Carolina was not the first state to charter a college, but it was the first to both issue a charter and provide the funds to support the enterprise. In North Carolina, as was true elsewhere in the fledgling republic, there remained some resistance to education for young men who were not of the elite. The Federalist ideal of a privileged few did not easily bend to the newer populist ideas of the citizen. But in South Carolina the legislature chartered and supported South Carolina College, recognizing that leadership of the state would come from both the coastal elites and the Piedmont settlers. Indeed, South Carolina College later provided the intellectual rationale for states' rights and secession movements. In many ways, South Carolina provided the model that was adopted by other states to establish publicly supported higher education (Geiger 2015).

The movement to establish colleges continued throughout the 1700s. Catholic institutions were established in the mid-Atlantic states with a view to educate students to take their place in promoting the interests of society and to implant virtue. Georgetown University, established in 1789, (at least that is the date celebrated by the institution; the exact date is a little unclear) manifested its purpose in ways that would be indistinguishable from Bowdoin or South Carolina College. The focus was on an ethos of civic-mindedness. Georgetown offered a classical curriculum in the Jesuit tradition of faith and reason being mutually illuminating, and social justice and care for the marginalized were core values. Because Georgetown was not established as an institution for the training of clergy, it recruited students from a wide variety of denominations with a wide variety of interests. Interestingly, a number of international students enrolled during the early national period, enabling the school to have a distinctive international flavor. The mid-Atlantic location was appealing to students from both the north and south, which led to "contentious and sometimes polarizing debates in the years leading up to the civil war" (Geiger 2015, p. 52).

The country was moving west, and new settlements across the west demanded new institutions. The destruction of the revolutionary war slowed the momentum of establishing colleges, but between 1820 and 1860 approximately 180 colleges did emerge, almost all of which were denominationally sponsored. Even though most colleges were denominationally affiliated, there was nothing systematic about the expansion of higher education. Geiger (2015) reports:

> Indeed, local and religious factors intertwined in the hundreds of founding sagas. Localities played three types of roles. In some cases local boosters took the initiative in founding colleges; colleges were also founded by concentrated religious communities to provide local education of the right kind; and, as standard practice, churches solicited offers and placed new colleges in towns that promised the most attractive financial package (p. 195).

Part 2: Expansion

Established by an act of the State of Virginia Assembly in 1780, Transylvania Seminary became the pioneer institution west of the Allegheny Mountains. Located in Danville, Kentucky, the first classes were held in the home of a Presbyterian minister in 1785. In 1793, Transylvania trustees accepted an offer of land to relocate and maintain the institution in Lexington, Ky. In 1799, Transylvania University was established, creating the first law school and medical school in the west. Like many newly established schools, Transylvania looked to the east for leadership. In 1818, Horace Holley was hired as President. Faculty were soon being sent to Europe for training and Transylvania established a reputation for outstanding education, particularly its medical and law schools. So, what happened?

The Transylvania story is echoed throughout higher education and its story is not atypical. The medical school closed in 1859. The Civil War interrupted campus operations. Transportation, particularly the railroad, meant folks could travel farther from home for college. The state of Kentucky established the University of Kentucky as the state's land grant institution and with its establishment went its support and funding. To survive, Transylvania merged with other local institutions, affiliated with the Christian Church (Disciples of Christ) denomination, but could never find the support to be a major force in the national higher education conversation. Today Transylvania is a well-regarded regional liberal arts school with about 1000 students (Geiger 2015).

Small liberal arts institutions are established, face a crisis, survive but are unable to achieve national relevance, and remain regionally important for reasons of economy and civic pride. The number of private, not-for-profit institutions that close their doors is quite small. But the percentage of students who attend these institutions is also quite small, which is fortunate since this process appears to be a common one.

Part 3: Morrill Act

During the height of the Civil War, Congress passed one of the most consequential laws in the history of the US Republic. The Morrill Act established support for higher education institutions in each of the states. The goal was to establish institutions that focused on the practical aspects of education, particularly agriculture. The concept was the brainchild of Vermont Congressman, James Morrill, who believed that what the new country needed was not higher education that simply mirrored the education conducted in Europe, but rather focused on science. The impetus to change the curriculum to meet the demands of an economy moving from agrarian to industrial was taking place throughout the country. But like most things related to higher education, there was no systematic approach until Morrill brought his ideas to Congress (Rudolph 1990; Geiger 2015).

In true American fashion, there was considerable pushback from members of Congress. Some were concerned that education should remain firmly in the hands of the states with no involvement from the federal sphere. Some believed that apprenticeships provided the best training in agriculture and mechanics. Some believed that college was best a symbol of social standing rather than educational attainment. Some felt that creating land grant colleges would destroy the agrarian nature of society (the romantic notion of the family farm), while others believed that a focus on scientific agriculture in land grant colleges would keep talented youth from being tempted to leave the farm for the city. Some advocates of the legislation suggested that land grant colleges would provide education that would induce young people to stay at home and others suggested that more colleges would enable more people to attend college. Of course, to some legislators making education more achievable was not necessarily a desirable outcome!

The Morrill Act was passed in 1862 with little or no fanfare (there was, of course, a war being waged with some significant existential stakes). The Act provided for the sale of federal lands in the states and the proceeds to be used to provide in each state at least one institution where the emphasis would be on learning essential to agriculture and mechanical arts, but not to the exclusion of other learning. The resulting sale of the land would provide financial support for the colleges. Up to 10% of the proceeds could be used to purchase land for a college site or an experimental farm; the remainder was to be placed in a perpetual endowment that would be invested at a return of 5% (Geiger 2015; Dorn 2017).

The Morrill Act did not provide guidelines to the states to determine how to spend the money. Some states established new institutions. Others introduced new programs at existing state-sponsored institutions. Others delegated the responsibility to private institutions already engaged in scientific study. And in all cases, the actual curriculum differed by state because the legislation provided no guidance. Some preferred a strictly vocational approach, eliminating much, if not all, the classical curriculum. Others viewed the purpose of higher education as being to educate a student to take their rightful place in society, not to be equipped for a particular position or job, an argument that continues today.

A second Morrill Act was passed in 1890, which provided two significant additions to the initial act. First, the 1890 legislation provided for annual appropriations for land-grant colleges. Initial opposition present in the states and among farmers had dissipated as a result of the scientific advances that had taken place under the leadership of the colleges. For example, scientists at Cornell discovered a cure for black rot in vineyards. In Texas, faculty found answers to questions about cotton agriculture and fertilizer. And in Washington, professors turned to the study of salmon and salmon reproduction. Seed research resulted in increased harvests and higher income for farmers (Geiger 2015; Rudolph 1990).

The second important aspect of the 1890 legislation was the requirement that states could not receive appropriations under the Morrill Act if students were denied admission based on race unless those states also created separate but equal facilities. Seventeen states had such laws. Many of the Historically Black Colleges and Universities (HBCUs) were established by states in order to continue receiving appropriations under the Morrill Act but without integrating existing campuses. It is clear that higher education did not significantly challenge the efficacy of a separate but equal policy, but rather was complicit in it. It was not until 1954 that the Supreme Court ruled separate but equal was an unconstitutional concept in education and still decades after that when higher education was fully, at least by law, integrated.

Many historians have marked the Morrill Act as the time when higher education in the United States began to truly flourish. States that had been lukewarm toward higher education began to more fully and robustly support the state institutions newly created and funded by the Morrill Act. Prior to 1860, many states had depended on private institutions to provide higher education. States were intertwined with private institutions with both finances and policy. When it became clear that the state-owned institutions would receive annual appropriations from the federal government, then loyalty and support were transferred to the newer forms of state-supported education. Tribal colleges, funded by local tribal monies, were created for Native American students. The first such college, Diné College, was founded by the Navajo Nation in 1968.

The rise of state institutions occurred at least in part because of the sense that education should be made available to all. President Eliot of Harvard spoke to the elitism of higher education near the end of the nineteenth century when he declared that the farmer or laborer should not bear the cost of education for the lawyer's son or the doctor's son. But it was the Jeffersonian ideal of education as a democratizing tool that carried the day. So as the nineteenth century drew to a close and the twentieth century opened to new promises, higher education stood ready to blossom (Rudolph 1990).

Wealth exploded in some quarters and entrepreneurs in the railroad, communication, shipping, finance, and education industries, among others, found themselves with money for philanthropy beyond anything the country had seen before. Rockefeller provided the financial fuel for the University of Chicago; Mr. and Mrs. Leland Stanford established a new university in California to honor their son who died as a youth; and Andrew Carnegie, Cornelius Vanderbilt, and Johns Hopkins all provided financial footing to establish universities that still bear their name (Rudolph 1990). Northern philanthropists were also active in establishing institutions for African American students who were unable to attend some universities, notably in the south (Obas 2018).

Part 4: An Emerging Model

The Johns Hopkins University in Baltimore opened its doors in 1876 with a mission to be the first true research university in North America. It is a model now emulated throughout the world. In his inaugural address, first

President Daniel Gilman (https://www.jhu.edu/about/history/) stated "Our simple aim is to make scholars, strong, bright, useful, and true" (n.d.). The mission he described remains the Johns Hopkins mission, "To educate its students and cultivate their capacity for lifelong learning, to foster independent and original research, and to bring the benefits of discovery to the world." In creating the research university, Gilman found a ready audience among the newly established land grant and state institutions as a means to separate themselves from the traditional liberal arts curricula of the early private institutions. The search for truth would become the purpose, rather than just preparing the elite for their proper role in society. The search for knowledge would have a democratizing effect as it was available to all, not just a few.

Johns Hopkins also differentiated itself from other institutions as it was faculty centric. Institutional focus centered on the work of the faculty, primarily research, and advanced study. The focus was on graduate education. Hopkins PhDs were in high demand by universities across the country. Hopkins developed a new model of graduate fellowships. By the end of the nineteenth century, research had become the primary preoccupation of the most ambitious universities in the country, both new and old (Geiger 2015).

Section 3: Specialized Institutions

As the public education movement spread across the country, the need for teachers became quite evident. Prior to the Civil War, most school teachers were men, many of whom were not college graduates. The expanding economy after the war attracted men to higher-paying positions in industry, leaving the lower-paid teaching posts to be filled by others, in this case, mostly women. Although women in higher education were not a new phenomenon, there was still resistance. But a growing population needed teachers, and many argued that women with their natural maternal instincts were better suited for teaching than men. Undoubtedly, the fact that women could be paid less than men and would not be competing directly with men for jobs made the feminization of the teaching field more palatable to civic leaders. Normal schools were established throughout the country to provide teachers, and many of these schools grew into very large state universities offering a full range of studies. The University of Chicago and the University of Michigan became two of the first institutions to engage in the study of the art and practice of teaching. Some likened the study of education to the study of agriculture to improve the work of the farmer.

The normal school movement provided a means for persons previously unable to receive a college education and an opportunity to continue on to postsecondary education. The students at normal schools were predominantly women, many of them from families with limited economic resources. Normal schools were the vehicle for higher education, even though many of the students chose not to pursue a career in teaching. In this regard, the normal schools were not different from the A&M colleges, where many students did not contemplate a career in agriculture, but the school became the vehicle for higher education. In short, these schools had a democratizing effect (Dorn 2017).

Part 1: Medical Schools

Providing medical education was common from the early days of higher education in America. However, most medical education was provided by autonomous proprietary schools until Harvard moved its separate medical school under the university's umbrella in 1870. Relatively few medical schools followed Harvard's lead, leaving most medical education to proprietary institutions. Discoveries in Europe of the scientific basis of disease made transforming medical education an imperative. The opening of the Johns Hopkins Medical School and Hospital in 1893 raised standards for all medical schools. Hopkins required an undergraduate degree and a four-year course of study in medical school. Some of the most reputable medical schools saw the value of affiliating with universities, but medical education was still uneven at best. The Council on Medical Education did a study of the nation's medical schools in 1904 and found half to be acceptable, 30% could be improved to become acceptable, and 20% were worthless. The Flexner Report in 1910, a study of medical education in the United States and Canada, delivered stunning information. Flexner noted that the ideal medical school should have ample facilities of laboratories, teaching hospitals, and endowments. The practice of medicine needed not only scientific knowledge but also hands-on clinical experience. The Flexner Report provided a roadmap for medical education (Rudolph 1990). Roughly half of all medical schools closed, and those that remained adopted the best practices of medical education, leading the United States to provide what is arguably the best medical education in the world.

Part 2: Law Schools

Legal education grew dramatically at the end of the nineteenth century. Some law schools required high standards for admission and offered rigorous coursework, but many others had low or no admission standards and lower course standards. Many law schools catered to part-time students and were seen as a reliable source for financial resources for schools. A stratification developed among law schools between those that required an undergraduate degree and had high standards and those that adopted a more open, inclusive approach. Ultimately, the law schools continued offering different models of education, but the conflict highlighted issues that affected American higher education throughout the twentieth century and are still evident now – academic meritocracy, selective admissions, and open, part-time learning opportunities (Rudolph 1990).

Part 3: Veterinary Schools

Veterinary medicine originated in Europe but emerged in North America in the population centers of the country. The immediacy of horses, physicians, and medical schools made the profession viable and necessary. Veterinary medicine was largely an equine practice that was challenged and transformed by the arrival of the internal combustion engine (Smith 2013). The history of veterinary medical education shares characteristics of other higher education professional education, primarily having its roots in proprietary schools and the advent of land-grant colleges, significantly altering the educational landscape.

The development of veterinary medical education can be described in three clusters. First are the proprietary schools, which by 1913 numbered 30 schools. The second cluster established veterinary medicine as part of university medical schools. The third cluster of schools was located at institutions established through the Morrill Act. The proprietary schools had generally failed by the time of the Great Depression, although Iowa State University, the first veterinary medical school in the United States, continues today. Only the veterinary medicine college at the University of Pennsylvania survived from the second cluster, and all of those established at land-grant institutions remain.

After World War II, the existing schools could not meet the demand for veterinary education, in large part because of veterans using the G.I. Bill to fund their studies. Eight institutions were established between the mid-1940s and 1960. This brought the total number of veterinary schools to 18. However, only two veterinary colleges remained in urban areas; veterinary education had moved to rural areas. Between 1960 and 1980, an additional nine institutions were established, again virtually all at land-grant institutions. Until the early 2000s, the most recent veterinary school established in the United States was in 1998. Because of the shortage of seats, US students began to seek training in other locales, notably in the Caribbean veterinary schools. However, a recent surge of new veterinary

schools is coming on board, with three new programs emerging in the decade between 2011 and 2020, and another three coming online over the early part of the decade beginning in 2020.

The practice of veterinary medicine has moved primarily from equine, other large animals, and agriculture to public health, small animal, and companion-animal practice. Yet the location of most veterinary schools away from urban population centers and sources of funding being rooted in agriculture production may conflict with the needs of the profession moving forward (Smith 2013).

Section 4: Students

For most of American higher education history, the students were upper-class males. These students were expected to be the keepers of the culture and become the governing elite. In the earliest schools, it was expected that the students would be trained for the ministry, but this was never the sole purpose of the schools. As higher education spread to the frontier of the new country, the students generally remained remarkably the same – the sons of landowners and successful merchants (Horowitz 1987).

By the nineteenth century, the composition of the student body had changed somewhat. A few schools had opened their doors to women and some institutions had established a relationship with a corresponding women's college. High-quality women's institutions[2] were established, but the students were predominantly the daughters of the elite of society. In the east, public education had not taken hold as it had in the west. So, it was the western state universities that used the public schools as feeder institutions and opened their doors to women students in the 1850s and 1860s.[3] Indeed the role of women in the west had a more egalitarian sense than in the east. Life in the west depended on each person working hard and assuming responsibility for the sustainability of the community. The woman in the west was not set apart but a person who demanded respect in her own right (Rudolph 1990). In 2020, women accounted for 58% of bachelor's degrees awarded. Forty years earlier women accounted for 50% of degrees awarded. Not only are more women enrolling in college, but they are also graduating at a higher rate.

Students of color were generally denied education throughout the south until after the Civil War and even then it was limited. In the northern states, higher education

---

2 For example, Wellesley, Bryn Mawr, Mount Holyoke and Vassar.
3 University of Iowa in 1855, University of Wisconsin in1863 followed by Indiana, Missouri, Michigan, and California.

was theoretically available, but few took advantage or had the means to take advantage of the opportunity. The first institutions to provide education to African Americans were in the north.[4] After the Civil War, institutions were developed for African American students. Philanthropists and freed slaves helped establish several institutions throughout the south. Between 1865 and 1869, 22 institutions for African American students opened their doors in southern states (Suggs 2018).

The era of mass education really began after World War II. The G.I. Bill brought education within reach for hundreds of thousands of soldiers from a variety of backgrounds and experiences. Campuses exploded with new students, many of whom had seen the world in the most difficult of circumstances. Snyder reports:

> The 1950s and 1960s marked two major developments. First, large numbers of young people entered college and second, public colleges expanded dramatically to meet the demand. College enrollment rose by 49 percent in the 1950s, partly because of the rise in the enrollment/population ratio from 15 percent to 24 percent. During the 1960s, enrollment rose by 120 percent. By 1969, college enrollment was as large as 35 percent of the 18- to 24-year-old population. About 41 percent of the college students were women. Public institutions accounted for 74 percent of enrollment, and about one-fourth of all students were enrolled at 2-year colleges (1993, p. 66).

In fall 2020, college enrollment totaled 15.85 million undergraduate students nationwide. This represents a decline of 3.3% year over year, the most noteworthy drop since 1951. Graduate students represent 16.5% of students. Hispanic or Latino students have increased 455.9% since 1976 and now represent almost 20% of all students. African American students represent 12.5% of the student population. Female students represent nearly 59% of all college students, an increase of nearly 100% since 1947 (Hanson 2022).

College enrollment statistics indicate that more Americans are forgoing higher education, which may be a reflection of cost and a cost/value calculation by students and their families. The rate of enrollment among new high school graduates declined by 5.3% year over year in 2020. The pandemic undoubtedly played a role in the decline as well, but college enrollment peaked in 2010 and has declined by almost 10% since then.

The data are clear. The era of mass education has continued to the present. The largest institutions exceed 60,000 students. Classes are offered both on campus and online. However, the number of high school graduates is decreasing and the number moving directly to college is also decreasing. Most postsecondary students attend degree-granting four-year public institutions although about a quarter of them attend two-year colleges. Students choose public institutions at a rate of approximately 3 : 1 (Hanson 2022).

Section 5: Purpose

In 1967, California was the envy of the higher education world: tuition to state institutions was covered by the state, there was a seat at a state institution available for each student in California, and the University of California system was considered among the best in the country. But at a press conference in 1967, California Governor Ronald Reagan maintained that taxpayers should not be subsidizing intellectual curiosity. Higher education, he argued, should be teaching workforce entry skills. If universities were not in the business of developing economic opportunities, the cost is too great for the state (Berrett 2016).

This conversation continues. What is the purpose and what is the value of higher education? Nobel laureate Daniel Kahneman in response to that question stated, "Well, I think that's quite obvious. It's to change what you believe." As Pasquerella (2019) explained, what makes liberal education transformative is that it enables individuals to have the facility to consider that one's most fundamental beliefs may not be correct. Thus, education is core to prepping for global citizenship and furthering a sense of well-being and social responsibility.

The value of a liberal education is questioned and challenged at all levels (Pasquerella 2019), as demonstrated by the fact that recent research has shown that students consider the primary purposes of higher education are to get a job or prepare for a career, yet in the future, credentialing for employment may come from many places beyond colleges and universities. Selingo (2020) maintains that higher education leaders have failed to recognize the new reality and continue to assume that the traditional models of higher education will be successful in the future. Today's students may be seeking more flexible models with more immediate, recognizable benefits upon completion.

Higher education is a complex industry with multiple constituencies. That situation alone assures differences of opinion regarding the purpose of higher education. If a constituency is student-focused, it will center on the student experience and determining what students should

---

4 Cheyney University (PA) in 1837, Lincoln University (PA) in 1854, Wilberforce University (OH) in 1856.

learn. A faculty-centric focus might say that the search for truth, through research, is the purpose of higher education. A politician might say that meeting the state's workforce needs should be at the center of the university's activities. Parents also have a particular sense of what the purpose of an institution should be, like employability. Perhaps the true purpose of higher education may be a combination of all the above, resulting in more than how to make a living – perhaps it is also teaching students how to make a life.

Because the United States has no central system and thousands of institutions, the purpose of higher education cannot be determined by edict. Individual colleges or a state system might have a clear understanding of purpose, but it is unlikely that all associated with the institution agree on priorities and/or purpose. This decentralization leads to an interesting web of competing institutions where each exploits its strengths, but decentralization also leads to an ambiguity of purpose. Lack of clarity of purpose may also be a feature of the challenges facing higher education in the future.

Summary

Public confidence in higher education may be waning. Funding for higher education has become a national issue. As campus populations expanded over the past 50 years, so did campus physical plants. Those must still be maintained even though populations of students may decrease. The nation appears to be in a conundrum: philosophically all who want a college education and qualify should be able to get a college of education. It is less clear that there is agreement about the purpose of that education. Is higher education a good value? Who should pay for it? Is a college education a public good or a private privilege? (Moody 2022)

References

Berrett, D. (2016). The day the purpose of college changed: after February 28, 1967, the main reason to go was to get a job. *The Chronicle of Higher Education* 63 (11): 103. https://link.gale.com/apps/doc/A471473976/ITBC?u=txshracd2573&sid=summon&xid=e054aea6.

Dorn, C. (2017). *For the Common Good: A New History of Higher Education in America*. Cornel University Press.

Geiger, R.L. (2015). *The History of American Higher Education: Learning and Culture from the Founding to World War II*. Princeton University Press.

Hanson, M. (2022). *College Enrollment & Student Demographic Statistics*. EducationData.org. https://educationdata.org/college-enrollment-statistics.

Horowitz, H.L. (1987). *Campus Life: Undergraduate Cultures from the End of the Eighteenth Sentury to the Present*. University of Chicago Press.

Moody, J. (2022, June 6). A grab for power. Inside Higher Ed. https://www.insidehighered.com/news/2022/06/06/draft-legislation-shows-desantis-plan-control-higher-ed (accessed 5 October 2022).

Obas, K.H. (2018). The history of Historically Black Colleges and Universities and their association with whites.

International Journal of Education and Human Developments 4 (1): 1–6.

Pasquerella, L. (2019). The purpose of higher education and its future. *Liberal Education* 105 (3): 2–3.

Rudolph, F. (1990). *The American College and University: A History*. University of Georgia Press.

Selingo, J.J. (2020). Colleges need to rethink their market – and maybe their mission: too many institutions are stuck in the last decade. *The Chronicle of Higher Education* 66 (22): B9.

Smith, D.F. (2013). Lessons of history in veterinary medicine. *Journal of Veterinary Medical Education* 40 (1): 2–11. https://doi.org/10.3138/jvme.1112.04.

Snyder, T.D. (ed.) (1993). *120 Years of American Education: A Statistical Portrait*. U.S. Department of Education.

Suggs, E. (2018). HBCUs: Born in the North but most needed in the South. The Atlanta Journal-Constitution. https://www.ajc.com/news/local/hbcus-born-the-north-but-most-needed-the-south/Q7NI3b0Gnnzak6eWX6p3BJ/ (accessed 5 October 2022).

20

Private and Public Institutions

Kimberly S. Cook, EdD, MBA
Texas Christian University, Fort Worth, TX, USA

Donald B. Mills, A.B., M.Div., EdD
Texas Christian University, Fort Worth, TX, USA

Section 1: Introduction

There are many ways to classify or delimit postsecondary educational institutions. Just a few ways include the Carnegie System, levels of enrollment (undergraduate and graduate), typical time to degree (two-year versus four-year), profit motivation (nonprofit versus for-profit), and subject focus (liberal arts versus occupational/technical). However, one of the most common identifiers for colleges is public versus private, which can indicate levels of governmental involvement, funding sources, and cost to attend.

In this chapter, we will consider the structure and function of institutions through the following topics:

- Public and private institutions
- For-profit and nonprofit education
- Funding
- Governance
- Accreditation
- Contemporary issues.

The National Center for Education Statistics (2022c) indicates that for the academic year 2019–2020 there were 5,999 postsecondary institutions in the US serving just over 22.2 million students. This includes 2,017 nondegree granting institutions and 3,982 degree-granting schools. Public institutions comprise 1,933 schools, private nonprofit include 1,774, and private for-profit number 2,292. Approximately 17.2 million students were enrolled at public institutions, while almost 3.4 million were enrolled at private nonprofit colleges, and 1.6 million attended private for-profit institutions.

Section 2: Public Institutions

When it comes to colleges and universities, the term *public* is generally synonymous with *state,* though there are some exceptions, like community colleges that are focused by region or county. Public higher educational institutions derive partial operational funding from federal, state, or local governments. State colleges and universities are legally seen as an "arm of the state" and typically afforded the privilege of sovereign immunity granted to state governments under the Eleventh Amendment (Holman 2020). And as described above, public institutions educate the vast majority of students or approximately 77% of all postsecondary students.

State universities are often exceedingly large, complex organizations that serve many students through flagship and satellite locations. Every state has at least one public university, and some have dozens. As discussed in the previous chapter, many state universities were formed as a result of the Morrill Land-Grants Acts of 1862, which gave states federal lands, often previously held by indigenous people, to fund and advance agricultural and mechanical education and to "open college doors to farmers' sons and others who lacked the means to attend the colleges then existing" (Morrill 1874, as cited in Duemer 2007, p. 136). The Second Morrill Act of 1890 provided further funding for those institutions. However, "money would not be distributed to states that considered race in admissions and had not established a separate college for colored students" (Wheatle 2019, p. 3), effectively establishing Black public institutions. The land-grant system also created the US Cooperative Extension Service, offering community-centered educational opportunities to agricultural producers and citizens throughout most of the counties and territories in the United States (Croft 2019). Because of the connection to agriculture and science, many of the public universities that offer veterinary medicine programs are land-grant universities.

Part 1: Public Higher Education Funding

Public higher education institutions have complex funding mechanisms to support their operations. Figure 20.1 depicts the interplay between students, state and local governments, institutions, the federal government, donors, and the economy (NCHEMS 2022).

Federal Funding

Federal funding for higher education programs in FY 2017 equated to 2% of the federal budget, or approximately US$ 75 billion (Pew Charitable Trusts 2019). Money comes into the system through two primary avenues: (i) student aid in the form of loans and grants and (ii) grants to the institution for research and other activities. Federal funding for Pell Grants and veterans' benefits grew significantly after the 2008 recession and still remain at levels greater than pre-2008. According to Pew (2019), 70% of Pell Grant funds are used at public universities, 61% of federal research dollars go to public universities, and just over one-third of veteran's benefits go to public universities. Federal funding accounts for approximately 13% of public college and university budgets.

State Funding

State governments have traditionally had a more direct role in funding public institutions, with a portion of state budget flowing directly to state institutions for operating costs. Historically, state residents are then given a discount on tuition, known as in-state tuition, as a recognition of the use of public funds to operate the higher education system. Over the last 40 years there has been a decline in the percentage of funds allocated to state universities. The shift of financing public higher education continues to move on to the student, who on average now carry 42% of the cost burden in 2021, up from 21% in 1980 (State Higher Education Executive Officers Association 2022). However, even with declining appropriations, higher education still averages the third-largest appropriation of funds across all states, only behind K-12 education and Medicaid, for a total of US$ 87.1 billion (Pew Charitable Trusts 2019).

Due to COVID-19 stimulus funding, many states were generally able to maintain prior appropriation levels during the pandemic, something that goes against the decades-long trend of decreasing state funding support for public institutions. Somewhat fortunately, while state appropriations have generally declined, federal funding has slightly increased on a per-student basis – though not enough to offset the declines in state funding. On average, state funding provides 21% of funds for public institutions. Meanwhile, the total tuition bill has continued to outpace funding by significant margins: over the last 20 years, out-of-state tuition at public universities has grown 141%, while in-state tuition has grown 175% (Kerr and Wood 2022a).

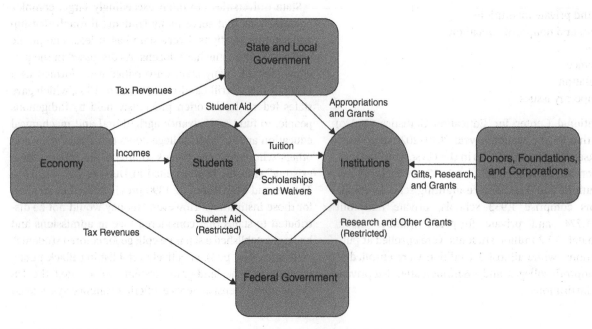

Figure 20.1 Public Higher Education Finance. *Source:* Created by Kimberly S. Cook.

Local Funding

Local funds allocated for higher education are typically used by community or two-year colleges. Often there are special taxing districts set up to support community colleges that pull from local property and sales taxes. In FY 2017, local funding for higher education was US$ 10.5 billion, or 4% of total institutional operating budgets (Pew Charitable Trusts 2019).

Endowments

Endowments are often large grants or donations that are given by private donors or foundations to an institution for a specific use. Due to subsidies from state governments, public universities traditionally did not seek endowments to offset costs. However, more recently, public universities have been pursuing endowed funds to help balance finances. The use of endowed funds can be restricted, for example, to pay for a faculty line such as an endowed chair, meaning that the funds can only be used to support that individual and their research efforts. Unrestricted endowed funds can be used to cover the cost of any purpose. However, the total amount that can be drawn per year is typically governed by the institution's board of directors and/or bylaws and averages around 5% (Lombardi et al. 2021).

According to the National Center for Education Statistics (2022b), the total market value of endowments at all colleges and universities, both public and private, in the United States at the end of the fiscal year 2020 was US$ 691 billion. Of the top 10 universities with the richest endowments, three were related to public universities or systems. These include the University of Texas at Austin, totaling US$ 13.8 billion, Texas A&M University – College Station at US$ 12.7 billion, and the University of Michigan – Ann Arbor valued at US$ 12.4 billion. Thus, it is obvious that in the face of rising student debt, rising operating costs, and diminishing state support, public institutions are seeking more private funds to help defray the impact of these forces.

Part 2: Governance and Operations Structure

Operations of higher education institutions are complex. Higher education as an industry has traditionally adopted an approach of shared governance, an idea based on the concept of faculty actively participating in institutional governance. The platform of shared governance was codified by the American Association of University Professors (AAUP) more than 100 years ago and remains the hallmark of the decision-making process within the academy (AAUP 2022a).

Shared governance embodies the idea of shared responsibility between governing boards, the administration, and the institution's faculty. However, there is building concern about the realities and sustainability of shared governance as a successful governing model moving forward (Crellin 2010). The functions and processes of shared governance within a loosely coupled organization such as the academy can increase the strain and tension on the system. Collaboration between faculty senates and administration has been decreasing as frustration has grown over the lack of transparency, protracted decision timelines by faculty, and a move to more corporate operating models, all while the influence of federal, state, and local politics has put pressure on the relationships between governing boards and institutions. Figure 20.2 depicts a simplified structure of oversight and governance of a state flagship university.

State Higher Education Coordinating Boards

Many states have a higher education coordinating board or commission. Often, these are statutory boards created to oversee the planning, coordination, and budgeting of state institutions. Coordinating board members are often appointed by a combination of procedures, including direct appointment by governors, lieutenant governors, and state congress officials, and by confirmation by the state congress. Coordinating boards vary in their purposes and regulatory oversight by state. The Education Commission of the States provides information on state education policy, including higher education. More information can be found at: https://www.ecs.org.

University Governing Boards

There can be multiple levels of governing boards within the state's higher education system. If the state has large university systems, there may be a system-wide board of regents or governors and then one for each campus as well. McKinsey and Company (Bevins et al. 2020), identify the core functions of university boards as being centered in the following areas:

- *Strategy*. Setting and monitoring institutional strategy and planning.
- *Governance*. Recruiting and assessing president's performance.
- *Financials*. Overseeing budgets, financial management, and fundraising and investment activity.
- *Performance*. Establishing and overseeing key performance indicators (KPIs).
- *Risk*. Monitoring compliance with legal obligations, reviewing audits and investigations, and developing crisis-response strategies.
- *External relations*. Promoting partnerships with stakeholders and representing the university in the community.

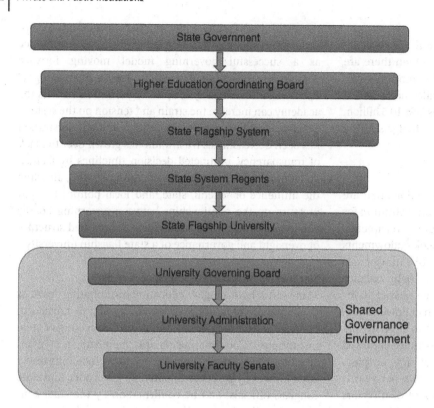

Figure 20.2 Simplified Public University Oversight.

A public institution's governing board members can be appointed by direct appointment by the governor or through a multistep political confirmation procedure. This process has given rise to the influence of politicians and their constituents. *The Chronicle of Higher Education* (Ellis et al. 2020), reported that of more than 400 board members appointed to public institutions, 70% were controlled by a single political party. Moreover, board members of the nation's flagship campuses or state systems contributed at least US$ 19.7 million in state-level political campaigns and partisan causes. A governing board has a fiduciary duty to elevate the concerns of the institution above the interests of the individual members, but currently, political interests pose threats to the ability of the members to carry out that duty independently.

University Administration

In a simplified form, the university administration often consists of three to four key leaders who govern the university under the purview of the college president. While position titles and responsibilities vary based on institution size and organization, these individuals make up the president's management team overseeing the key aspects of the university. These positions include:

- Vice-president of Administration and Finance, who oversees all administrative and day-to-day business functions of the university.

- Vice-president of Academic Affairs, sometimes known as the Provost, who oversees the academic operations and mission of the university.
- Vice-president of Student Affairs, who oversees the student support programs and services within the university.
- Many universities also include the Director of Athletics at the cabinet level due to the amount of revenue and expense that may flow through the athletic department. Other institutions may organize that division under administration or student services.

Faculty Organizations

In a shared governance environment, the faculty plays an active role in helping govern the institution. While the power of the faculty has diminished over time, it can still wield significant power through issuing statements and conducting votes of no confidence in institutional leaders. Since the faculty is independent and decentralized, to act as one body, a faculty organization such as a faculty senate or faculty union is usually established.

Faculty Senate While the faculty senate falls under the guidance of the provost, in a shared governance environment it can also be considered a stand-alone entity. Faculty senate is the body through which the teaching faculty participates in university governance (Johnston 2003). The faculty senate considers a broad range of topics including, but not limited to, curriculum and research, standards for academic and professional behavior, administrative concerns, general education requirements and assessment, and many other issues.

Because state funds are used to support institutions, institutions are seen as an arm of the government, which creates considerable scrutiny and political implications within both governing and operating decisions. Additionally, many documents and records of public institutions, including emails, are considered public information and may be requested under state open records acts. This can impact many faculty in terms of the confidentiality of research and other considerations.

Faculty Union

In addition to or in place of the faculty senate, institutions may have a faculty union. Faculty unions are primarily based at public institutions; they pursue collective bargaining and may address a wide variety of issues on campus, including the proportion of full-time faculty, required office hours, teaching loads, and course evaluations (Nelson 2011).

> Unionization in the public sector is based on state law, much of which expressly allows faculty to unionize. Formal unionization in the private sector is governed by federal law and the US Constitution, where the ability to unionize is much more uncertain. In 1980 the US Supreme Court, in *National Labor Relations Board (NLRB) v. Yeshiva University*, held that faculty at that institution were "managerial employees" and thus excluded from the coverage of the National Labor Relations Act. This has precluded the unionization of many private sector tenure-track faculty, though many nontenure-track faculty have been successful at unionizing. (AAUP 2022, n.p.)

Part 3: Accreditation

While not unique to higher education, the role accrediting bodies play is one of self-monitoring across the industry to help ensure institutions are meeting certain levels of quality as monitored by groups of their peers. "Accrediting agencies, which are private educational associations of regional or national scope, develop evaluation criteria and conduct peer evaluations to assess whether or not those criteria are met. Institutions and/or programs that request an agency's evaluation and that meet an agency's criteria are then 'accredited' by that agency" (US Department of Education 2022, n.p.). Accreditation is synonymous with credibility and respect in higher education. Thus, while accrediting bodies do not have traditional oversight within the system, their

influence in everything from mission and vision to online education and credits earned is significant. Accreditation is covered briefly here; for a more in-depth discussion of accreditation, please see Chapter 23.

Institutional Accreditation

In addition to the oversight in place for public institutions through governmental and internal structures, colleges are also required to be accredited by regional bodies in order to receive federal financial aid and any federal grants. The accrediting bodies are the same for both public and private institutions. The Council for Higher Education Accreditation lists the following information about regional accrediting agencies and their jurisdictions (CHEA 2022):

- Middle States Commission on Higher Education (MSCHE)
  - Degree-granting institutions which offer one or more postsecondary educational programs, including those offered via distance education, of at least one academic year in length at the Associate's or higher level in Delaware, the District of Columbia, Maryland, New Jersey, New York, Pennsylvania, Puerto Rico, the Virgin Islands, and any other geographic areas in which the Commission elects to conduct accrediting activities within and outside of the United States.
- New England Commission of Higher Education (NECHE)
  - The accreditation of institutions that award the bachelor's, master's and doctoral degrees and associate's degree-granting institutions that include in their offerings at least one program in liberal studies or another area of study widely available at the baccalaureate level of regionally accredited colleges and universities in Connecticut, Maine, Massachusetts, New Hampshire, Rhode Island, Vermont and internationally.
- Northwest Commission on Colleges and Universities (NWCCU)
  - The accreditation and pre-accreditation ("Candidacy status") of postsecondary degree-granting educational institutions in Alaska, Idaho, Montana, Nevada, Oregon, Utah, Washington, and internationally, and the accreditation of programs offered via distance education within these institutions.
- Southern Association of Colleges and Schools Commission on Colleges (SACSCOC)
  - Regional accrediting body for degree-granting institutions of higher education in Alabama, Florida, Georgia, Kentucky, Louisiana, Mississippi, North Carolina, South Carolina, Tennessee, Texas, Virginia, Latin America, and other Commission approved international sites, including the accreditation of programs offered via distance and correspondence education within these institutions.

- WASC Senior College and University Commission (WSCUC)
  - Institutions of higher education in the US and internationally that offer the baccalaureate degree or above at colleges in California, Hawaii, the Territories of Guam and American Samoa, the Commonwealth of the Northern Mariana Islands, the Republic of Palau, the Federated States of Micronesia and the Republic of the Marshall Islands.

Veterinary Programmatic Accreditation

In addition to institutional accreditation, many of the individual bodies within the university may be separately accredited. In veterinary medicine, the Council on Education (COE) is approved by the US Department of Education to accredit colleges and schools of veterinary medicine in the United States, Canada, and internationally (AAVMC 2022). The COE is supported by both the American Association of Veterinary Medical Colleges (AAVMC) and the American Veterinary Medical Association (AVMA).

> The AAVMC is responsible for appointing eight of the 20 members of the COE, and provides the funding to support these eight members. The AVMA appoints and funds eight members as well. The remaining four members are the three public members and the Canadian representative, who are selected by the COE and the Canadian Veterinary Medical Association, respectively.
>
> The COE has complete responsibility for the administration of the accreditation process. In addition to evaluating whether applicant institutions meet accreditation standards, council members also periodically review, suggest changes to, and evaluate feedback on the standards before revising them.
>
> The AAVMC appoints members representing preventive medicine and basic science, large animal clinical science, small animal clinical science, postgraduate education, veterinary medical research, another in basic science, and a representative from the AAVMC membership. Terms last six years and are filled as terms expire. (AAVMC 2022, n.p.)

Section 3: Private Institutions

Though many aspects of higher education are similar across public and private institutions, there are some variations. As noted at the top of the chapter, private higher education accounts for a considerably smaller proportion of students than public higher education. Serving about 23%

of higher education students, almost 3.4 million were enrolled at private nonprofit colleges, and 1.6 million attended private for-profit institutions (National Center for Education Statistics 2022a) in 2019–2020.

Part 1: For-Profit

Another area of difference across the spectrum of institutions, and within private education itself, is profit motivation. There is a subset of private schools which provide higher education for a profit. Many for-profit institutions are operated by corporations, including publicly traded ones, which are governed by a board of directors and managed to maximize profit and shareholder value. Overall, for-profit institutions have had a challenging history. Of degree-granting, postsecondary institutions, for-profits grew from 55 in 1977 to a maximum of 1,451 in 2013. In 2020, there were 704, or less than half the peak number (National Center for Education Statistics 2022a). The growth in for-profit education was spurred by a growing number of credential-seeking students, the accessibility of federal student aid, and the low cost of online education (Reigg Cellini and Turner 2019).

Overall, for-profit institutions enroll a greater number of underserved groups than public and private nonprofit institutions (Gilpin and Stoddard 2017). The growth in for-profit institutions has been linked to limitations in the public sector of higher education in terms of resources, response to market changes, and lack of services for nontraditional students. Thus, for-profit colleges have been providing access to higher education for students that have been historically marginalized. They have also been able to develop credentials and programs at a more agile pace than traditional institutions.

However, there has been considerable concern about the quality, value, and completion rates of for-profit education institutions. The six-year graduation rate for private for-profit institutions in 2020 was 29%, compared to 68% for private nonprofit institutions, and 63% for public institutions (National Center for Education Statistics 2022c). For-profit colleges also have higher tuition, debt burdens, and default rates than public institutions. Additionally, the perceived value of for-profit schools is considerably lower than all other institutions, with only 41% of Americans seeing the education at for-profit schools as worth the cost (New America 2022). Ultimately, for-profit colleges also have low rates of employment preparation for students (Reigg Cellini and Turner 2019). Since the peak of for-profit education in 2013, many institutions have filed bankruptcy or ceased operations, leaving many students with much debt, but little to no demonstrable evidence of courses completed toward a credential.

Part 2: Nonprofit

The most familiar type of private institution is private, non-profit institution, a designation under the US Internal Revenue Code qualifying organizations that meet its criteria as tax-exempt, charitable organizations. "To be tax-exempt under section 501(c)(3) of the Internal Revenue Code, an organization must be organized and operated exclusively for exempt purposes set forth in section 501(c)(3), and none of its earnings may inure to any private shareholder or individual" (Internal Revenue Service 2022, n.p.). The purposes allowed by the IRS include charitable, religious, educational, and scientific, among others. Further, the term charitable is defined to include the advancement of education or science, which institutions of higher education do. From here forward, use of the term *private* in this chapter refers to private, nonprofit institutions.

As described in the previous chapter, private colleges were the foundation of the US Higher Education system, and in many ways continue to lead the way. The Center for Measuring University Performance (Lombardi et al. 2021), lists only one public university, University of Michigan – Ann Arbor (#7) in their Top 10 American Research Universities. The other nine are private. They are: Columbia University (#1), Harvard University (#2), Massachusetts Institute of Technology (#3), Stanford University (#4), Duke University (#5), Johns Hopkins University (#6), University of Pennsylvania (#8), Yale University (#9), and Northwestern University (#10).

Part 3: Funding

The funding of private institutions is a bit more straightforward than public institutions, though it does not lack in complexity. Private colleges are known to be considerably more expensive than public colleges, due to the lack of government funding that goes directly to operating budgets in public schools. US News and World Report indicate that the average tuition and fees for ranked, private colleges for the 2022–2023 school year were US\$ 39,723 (Kerr and Wood 2022b). Meanwhile, out-of-state tuition at ranked public schools averaged US\$ 22,953 per year, while in-state tuition averaged US\$ 10,423 per year. As such, private universities and their students attempt to balance between tuition, financial aid, and student loans to meet tuition and budget demands. However, it is notable that tuition and fees at private universities have increased 134% in the past 20 years (Kerr and Wood 2022a).

Public Funding

Federal funding that is provided to private colleges, like public institutions, usually comes in two forms: research grants and funding or student aid. However, there is big difference in public funding between the allocation to public and private schools. According to the State Higher Education Executive Officers Association (Laderman 2020), in 2020, state governments provided US\$ 2.68 billion to private schools, which averages US\$ 563 per student. Almost 90% of state funds to private schools are in the form of financial aid to students. Conversely, states allocated US\$ 93.5 billion to public schools, or US\$ 8,436 per student, where less than 10% of state funds go to financial aid, instead going directly to operating budgets. Further, during the first two decades of the 2000s, enrollment at private institutions increased over 60%, while public schools grew by almost 30%. Concurrently, state funding and financial aid to private school students decreased while state financial aid to public school students increased.

> State operating appropriations declined on a per-FTE basis for both private and public institutions following the 2001 tech bust. After a few years of increases, appropriations to both institution types again declined during and following the Great Recession, but declines were far steeper for private institutions. In the last eight years, states have slowly reinvested in public operating appropriations, and there has been a partial recovery. On the other hand, state funding for private institutions remained near its all-time low until the last two years, when there was a slight increase (Laderman 2020, p. 4).

Fundraising

Additional ways that private institutions attempt to balance costs and expenditures is fundraising. From annual giving campaigns focused on alumni to capital campaigns to fund campus expansions, private schools rely on the philanthropy and generosity of others to offset tuition and expenses. The main groups that are targeted by university advancement and development offices are alumni, non-alumni with affinity or connections to the institution, corporations, and foundations. Their support can be donations, endowments with restrictions, loans, or even funds bequeathed in a will. According to the annual Voluntary Support of Education survey conducted by the Council for Advancement and Support of Education (Kaplan 2022), overall donations to higher education (both public and private) are on the rise, increasing by 4–6%. Some large donations from names like MacKenzie Scott and Michael Bloomberg have led the way (Moody 2022). However, due to concerns of current and future economic climates, there is some worry about giving in the near future.

Endowments and Annual Giving As discussed above in the public universities section, endowments have traditionally been more central to private institutions. According to the

Center for Measuring University Performance, the 2019 endowment asset values of the top 25 private research universities range from US$ 39.4 billion at Harvard to US$ 665 million at Yeshiva University. Meanwhile, Johns Hopkins doubled Harvard's annual giving number to lead this category with US$ 2.6 billion, whereas Yeshiva booked US$ 31 million from annual giving funds (Lombardi et al. 2021). All eight of the Ivy League schools have current assets valued in excess of US$ 5 billion, with Harvard (US$ 39.4b), Yale (US$ 30.3b), and Princeton (US$ 26.1b) all in excess of US$ 20 billion. Further, the areas of endowments are the most critical for the future of institutions. The study's authors anticipate that many small institutions with less than 2,000 students and lacking large endowments will struggle and ultimately close or be absorbed by others in the next decade, a trend which has already begun.

Discount Rates Much of the funds raised by private universities go to offset tuition costs via student aid. The discount rate is defined as "the total institutional grant aid awarded to undergraduates a percentage of the gross tuition and fee revenue the institution would collect if all students paid the full tuition and fee sticker price" (NACUBO 2017, n.p.). In an annual study by the National Association of College and University Business Officers (NACUBO 2022), the average institutional discount rate was 49% at private colleges, while the median discount rate was 58%. That means that schools are only collecting about half (or less) of the gross revenue that their sticker prices indicate while providing grants, fellowships, and scholarships for the other half. Many private schools rely on tuition discounting as a means to increase enrollment, as indicated by the fact that 83% of undergraduates at the schools surveyed received some aid. The median discount rate for highly selective institutions was lower than the average rate for all schools, meaning less aid to students and a higher tuition expense for students at highly selective institutions. However, that is not true for all highly selective, private institutions. Princeton, Harvard, and Stanford, among others, often meet students' full demonstrated needs through scholarships, fellowships, grants, and other approaches with no loans included (Kerr and Wood 2022c).

Part 4: Governance and Operations Structure

Because private institutions maintain their autonomy, there is no state oversight structure that mimics the role coordinating boards serve for public universities. Private universities must adhere to federal and state laws and maintain compliance with other regulations if they wish to continue to receive federal grants and accept federal student aid. However, to represent the collective voices of accredited, private nonprofit colleges, in 1976 the presidents of those institutions formed the National Association of Independent Colleges and Universities (NAICU 2022). NAICU serves as an industry lobby focused on issues related to student aid, tax policy, and government regulation. Additionally, as mentioned in the accreditation section, private institutions are subject to the same accreditation standards and bodies as public institutions.

As a nongovernmental entity, the governance structure for a private institution is much more streamlined. The institution, at the highest level, is directed by a board. While there may be a variance in the titles of the members, such as a board of trustees, governors, or directors, these individuals are tasked with setting the direction of the institution, approving budgets and tenure, determining strategy, and approving large changes or additions to the physical and programmatic aspects of the school, among other duties. The board also selects, evaluates, and sets compensation for the chief executive of the institution. This chief executive position maybe called the chancellor, the president, or other similar designation. Board members are often chosen for their ability to raise funds, their connections to the local or national community, alumni status, or because they have held important business and economic roles within the area.

Beyond the governance structures, general operations of private institutions are similar to public schools, varying by size, type, location, and classification. The variance across these elements provides a wide variety of institutions through which students have sought and continue to seek education after high school and beyond. However, all types of institutions now grapple with a range of challenges and opportunities that face the industry. These issues, some of which are highlighted below, will shape the future of higher education.

Section 4: Contemporary Issues

As we have shown, the landscape of higher education in the United States is complex. From size and funding to governance, the operations of institutions trudge along, most often *not* like a well-oiled machine. Then add to those challenges financial (in)stability, shared governance, promotion and tenure, student expectations, and a corporatization of the academy, and the complexity increases exponentially. When the operations are wrapped in a context of K-12 deficiencies; increasing demands for services, oversight, and compliance; increasing contingent faculty and decreasing tenured roles; decreasing public sentiment and support; and the explosion of educational technology, the higher education milieu is rife with change-inducing challenges that make the near and long-term future difficult to predict (Lombardi et al. 2020).

Part 1: Student Debt

The increasing rates of student debt have been a touchpoint for many. From discussions about student debt forgiveness programs to income-based repayment to increased questioning of the value of a degree and the increase in university costs, the concept of student debt colors much of the higher education environment. At private colleges, the share of first-time, full-time first-year students who received an institutional grant or scholarship in 2021–2022 was estimated to be 89.5% (NACUBO 2022). As we have established, private schools are typically more expensive than public, and scholarships and grants only offset part of the expenses. Undergraduate students at public four-year institutions borrow less than those at private schools, but the amount for both is still significant. Graduates in 2020 from a ranked private college borrowed an average of US$ 32,029, while public college graduates averaged US$ 26,627 of debt (Kerr and Wood 2022b).

Debt totals for all students grew sharply, by approximately 20% between 2009 and 2015, before stabilizing over the past few years. These amounts and the concern of borrowers about the worthiness of spending significant funds and incurring long-lasting debt is a topic that has lasting implications for the structure and sustainability of the current model of higher education. While the market for the traditional, residential college experience is likely to persist, there will no doubt be changes in the size of that market and the schools that have a tenuous financial situation are likely to struggle even more.

Part 2: Public Sentiment

As noted earlier, public funding and other means of public support have been declining for decades. According to New America's (2022) annual survey of sentiment on higher education, Americans' views on the positive impact of higher education have sharply decreased in the past few years – from 69% in 2020 to 55% in 2022. It is important to note that support for colleges and universities has become an inherently political issue, with nearly 75% of Democrats seeing institutions as having a positive effect, whereas only a third of Republicans view the effect favorably. However, public institutions remain an important investment, with support for use of tax dollars at public institutions remaining high: 79% support continual funding of community colleges, 68% support funding public four-year universities, and 63% are in favor of spending for minority-serving

institutions (MSIs). The continued fluctuation in sentiment, when coupled with the debt and funding challenges, creates uncertainty about the number of students who will continue to matriculate.

Part 3: Politics and Academic Freedom

One of the major areas of government and political influence, over and above funding, is the appointment of university governing board members. Board members may be appointed as political favors or in return for financial support of political candidates. "Every regional accreditor states that boards should be independent. Some accrediting agencies' standards explicitly require boards to be independent from political pressure, noting that this particular type of interference is problematic. If boards are unduly influenced by state lawmakers, the colleges they oversee could run afoul of these standards" (Ellis et al. 2020, n.p.).

Academic freedom is closely related to issues of free speech and institutional purpose. The AAUP adopted the following definition in its statement of principles in 1940.

> The purpose of this statement is to promote public understanding and support of academic freedom . . . Institutions of higher education are conducted for the common good and not to further the interest of either the individual teacher or the institution as a whole. The common good depends upon the free search for truth and its free exposition.
>
> Academic freedom is essential to these purposes and applies to both teaching and research. Freedom in research is fundamental to the advancement of truth. Academic freedom in its teaching aspect is fundamental for the protection of the rights of the teacher in teaching and of the student to freedom in learning. It carries with it duties correlative with rights. (AAUP 1940, n.p.)

Recently some state legislators have become involved in what should be taught in classrooms. While this appears to be limited to elementary and secondary schools, there is some concern it soon could be applied to higher education. In Idaho, a university general counsel has warned faculty to be very careful how issues related to reproductive freedom are discussed to avoid being in violation of state law. The Supreme Court weighed in on academic freedom in 1967 in the Keyishian v. Board of Regents case. In this case, the Court ruled that a professor could not be fired simply for being a member of the Communist Party. As Wermiel wrote, "Brennan's majority opinion is often credited with helping to boost the concept of academic freedom as a constitutionally protected value. 'Our Nation is deeply committed to safeguarding academic freedom, which is of transcendent value to all of us and not merely to the teachers concerned,' Brennan wrote" (Wermiel 2009, n.p.).

Speech related to contentious issues has been a source of controversy for years beginning in the 1960s. How should speech be regulated? Should any speech be regulated? Is offensive speech protected? Do institutions have an obligation to prevent students from disrupting a speaker with whom they disagree? If so, is that limiting the free speech rights of the disruptors? Who decides? These questions are being answered in the realm of public opinion but not definitively in courts. The Foundation for Individual Rights and Expression (FIRE) is dedicated to finding appropriate answers and policies for these questions. It is likely that speech will continue to be an issue, particularly as politicians become involved.

Part 4: Organizational Change

Over the last 50 years, higher education has moved away from the collaborative, collegial model of shared governance and a republic of scholars with academic freedom upon which the system was founded (Bleiklie and Kogan 2007). The changing tide has moved the academy toward a stakeholder organization with a corporate style of business management focused on productivity and revenue management (Taylor 2017). Concurrently, the size of the administration of higher education has drastically increased, when compared to the previous half century, raising both costs and bureaucracy, as roles traditionally overseen by faculty are offloaded onto professional staff. Nichols (1995), has termed this phenomenon the administrative lattice and noted that it has continued to grow and be rewarded with larger staff as higher education becomes more complex and layered with more regulations. Conversely, while the lattice has grown, the academic ratchet – a narrowing of faculty focus away from the broader institutional goals toward the interests of academic specialty – has been incentivized by reducing faculty teaching and advising in exchange for individual research and publications.

While the faculty-centered staffing model has shifted to an administrative-led approach, a shift in governance has also occurred. The collegial, shared governance model of a loosely coupled organization has given way to a more corporate style of management, with a top-down approach that emphasizes revenue and directs faculty instead of collaborating with them. Given some of the operating realities presented in this and the previous chapter, some elements of this shift may have been inevitable to help ensure the continuation of many schools. However, some scholars argue that this transition has minimized the university's

role as knowledge creator and disseminator for the betterment of society while increasing corporate activism and influence on campus (Taylor 2017).

Budgetary considerations and changing philosophies have impacted the core of higher education, the faculty. There has been a decrease in the number of tenured faculty over the last three decades, while there has been a considerable rise in the number of contingent or adjunct (part-time) faculty. While 57% of faculty in 1975 were full-time tenure track faculty, only one-third of professors hold that distinction today, with two-thirds being nontenured track positions (Taylor 2017; Chronicle of Higher Education 2020).

The contingent faculty roles are reliant on adequate enrollment and earn salaries that are much lower than those in tenure track positions. "Consequently, 25% of adjuncts across the US are receiving some form of public assistance, typically food stamps and Medicaid. This situation has prompted unionization efforts for faculty, staff, and graduate students, which tends to undermine the collegial climate that was highly valued" (Lombardi et al. 2020, p. 15).

Summary

The structure and operations of public and private higher education institutions are complex. The use of public funds in higher education, both public and private, increases the scrutiny under which institutions operate. Public institutions, as an arm of the government, have more complex funding and oversight models. Private institutions, while more streamlined, do share many of the same operating realities as their public counterparts. One of the more involved aspects of higher education administration as a whole are the funding models. Additionally, the governance and accreditation systems add levels of complexity. Finally, all of these contribute to or are impacted by the operating context of colleges and universities.

Some contemporary issues involved in the higher education environment covered in this chapter will have indelible impact on the future of many institutions. However, that is not to say that the future is bleak. The US higher education system continues to foster and develop innovations, research, knowledge, and advancements that move our understanding of our world forward. The value of that progress will continue to grow as the industry works to solve these and other issues in the future. A system such as ours will inherently have inefficiencies, but its decentralization is a strength as multiple missions create greater opportunities.

References

AAUP (1940). 1940 Statement of principles on academic freedom and tenure. https://www.aaup.org/report/1940-statement-principles-academic-freedom-and-tenure (accessed 30 September 2022).

AAUP (2022a). Collective bargaining. https://www.aaup.org/programs/collective-bargaining (accessed 30 September 2022).

AAUP (2022b). Shared governance. https://www.aaup.org/our-programs/shared-governance (accessed 30 September 2022).

AAVMC (2022). Accreditation. American Association of Veterinary Medical Colleges. https://www.aavmc.org/programs/accreditation (accessed 30 September 2022).

Bevins, F., Law, J., Sanghvi, S., and Valentino, R. (2020, November). Shaping university boards for 21st century higher education in the US. McKinsey: https://www.mckinsey.com/industries/education/our-insights/shaping-university-boards-for-21st-century-higher-education-in-the-us (accessed 30 September 2022).

Bleiklie, I. and Kogan, M. (2007). Organization and governance of universities. *Higher Education Policy* 20: 477–493. https://doi.org/10.1057/palgrave.hep.8300167.

CHEA (2022). Regional Accrediting Organizations. https://www.chea.org/regional-accrediting-organizations (accessed 30 September 2022).

Chronicle of Higher Education (2020, August 16). Tenure status of full-time and part-time faculty members, Fall 2018. https://www.chronicle.com/article/tenure-status-of-full-time-and-part-time-faculty-members-fall-2018 (accessed 30 September 2022).

Crellin, M.A. (2010). The future of shared governance. *New Directions for Higher Education* 151: 71–81. https://doi.org/10.1002/he.402.

Croft, G. H. (2019). The U.S. Land-Grant University System: An Overview. Congressional Research Service. https://crsreports.congress.gov/product/pdf/R/R45897 (accessed 30 September 2022).

Duemer, L.S. (2007). The agricultural education origins of the Morrill Land Grant Act of 1862. *American Educational History Journal* 34 (1): 135–146.

Ellis, L., Stripling, J., and Bauman, D. (2020, September 25). Public-College Boards and State Politics. The Chronicle of Higher Education: https://www.chronicle.com/article/public-college-boards-and-state-politics (accessed 30 September 2022).

Gilpin, G. and Stoddard, C. (2017). Does regulating for-profit colleges improve educational outcomes? *Journal of Policy Analysis and Management* 36 (4): 942–950.

Holman, C.M. (2020). State universities push the limits of eleventh amendment sovereign immunity at the Federal Circuit. *Biotechnology Law Report* 39 (5): http://doi.org/10.1089/blr.2020.29194.cmh.

Internal Revenue Service (2022). Exemption Requirements - 501(c)(3) Organizations. https://www.irs.gov/charities-non-profits/charitable-organizations/exemption-requirements-501c3-organizations (accessed 30 September 2022).

Johnston, S.W. (2003). Faculty governance and effective academic administrative leadership. *New Directions for Higher Education* 124: 57–63. https://doi.org/10.1002/he.130.

Kaplan, A. E. (2022). Voluntary Support. CASE. https://www.case.org/system/files/media/file/VSE%20Research%20Brief%20Key%20Findings%202020-21.pdf (accessed 30 September 2022).

Kerr, E. and Wood, S. (2022a, September 13). A Look at College Tuition Growth Over 20 Years. U.S. News and World Report. https://www.usnews.com/education/best-colleges/paying-for-college/articles/see-20-years-of-tuition-growth-at-national-universities (accessed 30 September 2022).

Kerr, E., & Wood, S. (2022b, September 12). U.S. News and World Report. See the Average College Tuition in 2022-2023: https://www.usnews.com/education/best-colleges/paying-for-college/articles/paying-for-college-infographic (accessed 30 September 2022).

Kerr, E. and Wood, S. (2022c). What you need to know about college tuition costs. U.S. News and World Report. https://www.usnews.com/education/best-colleges/paying-for-college/articles/what-you-need-to-know-about-college-tuition-costs (accessed 30 September 2022).

Laderman, S. (2020). State Higher Education Finance. SHEEO. https://shef.sheeo.org/wp-content/uploads/2021/05/SHEEO_SHEF_FY20_IB_Private_Funding.pdf (accessed 30 September 2022).

Lombardi, J., Abbey, C., and Craig, D. (2020). *The Top American Research Universities*. The Center for Measuring University Performance.

Lombardi, J., Abbey, C.W., Craig, D.D., and Collis, L.N. (2021). *The Top American Research Universities*. The Center for Measuring University Performance https://ir.aa.ufl.edu/topics/cmup (accessed 30 September 2022).

Moody, J. (2022, August 18). Colleges Report Strong Fundraising Year. Inside Higher Ed. https://www.insidehighered.com/news/2022/08/18/colleges-report-strong-fundraising-fiscal-year-2022 (accessed 30 September 2022).

NACUBO (2017, November 11). Tuition Discounting Study Glossary and Help Text. National Association of College and University Business Officers. https://www.nacubo.org/Research/2021/NACUBO-Tuition-Discounting-Study/

Tuition-Discounting-Study-Help-Text-and-Glossary (accessed 30 September 2022).

NACUBO (2022, May 19). Tuition discount rates at private colleges and universities hit all-time highs. NACUBO. https://www.nacubo.org/Press-Releases/2022/Tuition-Discount-Rates-at-Private-Colleges-and-Universities-Hit-All-Time-Highs#:~:text=In%20the%202021%20NACUBO%20Tuition,all%20undergraduates%E2%80%94both%20record%20highs (accessed 30 September 2022).

NAICU (2022). About NAICU. https://www.naicu.edu/about-naicu (accessed 30 September 2022).

National Center for Education Statistics (2022a). Degree-granting postsecondary institutions, by control and level of institution. Digest of Education Statistics: https://nces.ed.gov/programs/digest/d21/tables/dt21_317.10.asp (accessed 30 September 2022).

National Center for Education Statistics. (2022b). *Endowments. Fast Facts*: https://nces.ed.gov/fastfacts/display.asp?id=73 (accessed 30 September 2022).

National Center for Education Statistics (2022c). *Postsecondary Institutions*. 2022, from IES>NCES: https://nces.ed.gov/ipeds/TrendGenerator/app/answer/1/1 (accessed 30 September 2022).

National Center for Higher Education Management Systems (2022). NCHEMS. http://www.higheredinfo.org/catcontent/cat8.php (accessed 30 September 2022).

Nelson, C. (2011, March 9). What Faculty Unions Do. Martin Center for Academic Renewal: https://www.jamesgmartin.center/2011/03/what-faculty-unions-do (accessed 30 September 2022).

New America (2022). Varying Degrees. New America. https://www.newamerica.org/education-policy/reports/varying-degrees-2022 (accessed 30 September 2022).

Nichols, P. (1995). The ratchet and the lattice: understanding the complexity of the Modern University. *International Higher Education* 2: 4–6. https://doi.org/10.6017/ihe.1995.2.6177.

Pew Charitable Trusts (2019). Two decades of change in federal and State Higher Education Funding. https://www.pewtrusts.org/en/research-and-analysis/issue-briefs/2019/10/two-decades-of-change-in-federal-and-state-higher-education-funding (accessed 30 September 2022).

Reigg Cellini, S. and Turner, N. (2019). Gainfully employed? Assessing the employment and earnings of for-profit college students using administrative data. *Journal of Human Resources* 54 (2): 342–370.

State Higher Education Executive Officers Association (2022). State of Higher Education Funding: FY2021. Boulder. https://shef.sheeo.org/wp-content/uploads/2022/06/SHEEO_SHEF_FY21_Report.pdf (accessed 30 September 2022).

Taylor, A. (2017). Perspectives on the university as a business: the corporate management structure, neoliberalism and higher education. *Journal for Critical Education Policy Studies* 15 (1): 108–135.

U.S. Department of Education (2022). Database of Accredited Postsecondary Institutions and Programs. https://ope.ed.gov/dapip/#/home (accessed 30 September 2022).

Wermiel, S. (2009). Keyishian v. Board of Regents *(1967)*. The First Amendment Encyclopedia: https://mtsu.edu/first-amendment/article/15/keyishian-v-board-of-regents (accessed 30 September 2022).

Wheatle, K.I. (2019). Neither just nor equitable: race in the congressional debate of second Morrill Act of 1890. *American Educational History Journal* 46 (2): 1–20.

21

Higher Education Policies

Patricia Butterbrodt, PhD, MEd

Richard A. Gillespie College of Veterinary Medicine, Lincoln Memorial University, Harrogate, TN, USA

Section 1: Introduction

An institute of higher learning such as a college or university is a place where hundreds – or even thousands – of people come together daily to work, study, and socialize. Campuses include classrooms and laboratories, libraries and chapels, dormitories and fraternity and sorority houses, athletic fields and stadiums, and retail stores and eating establishments. Whenever such a complex physical facility accommodates such a myriad of individuals, rules and regulations must be in place to ensure the safety of all as well as the security of the physical environment. Policies are set to give guidance and parameters for anyone coming on the campus, physically and virtually. These policies are necessary to maintain the academic integrity of the curriculum and educational programs, the rights and privileges of the people involved, the safety and well-being of those same people, and the security and maintenance of the physical property and technology. When visiting a campus, enrolling as a student, or being hired as a faculty member or staff of the institution, it is important to be aware of these policies and those that apply to your situation as a visitor, student, or employee.

In many countries, there is a single government entity that is responsible for setting policies and procedures for educational institutions. In Great Britain, the Department for Education is overseen cooperatively by the Secretary of State for Education and the Minister of State for Higher and Further Education, who ensure that universities adhere to national policy (Office for Students 2022). In Japan, both public and private institutions of higher education are required to set internal policies and regulations that follow the 2014 National University Corporation Law, enacted in 2015 (Yamada 2018). In South Africa, the Department of Higher Education and Training oversees universities and other postsecondary education, with the Higher Education Policy Development and Research Directorate setting nationwide policies for colleges and universities (DHOT 2022). In Chile, the Division of the Undersecretary of Higher Education is responsible for developing and implementing policies and procedures that adhere to the laws of Chile, including Law No. 20,800, establishing regulations on administration of higher education (MINUDEC 2022).

In the United States, the educational system is incredibly complex. Each state is given power over its educational system, including the authority to set and uphold policies at its land-grant state universities. However, there are policies at the federal level that apply to all federally funded land-grant institutions, and to those private educational institutions that seek funding at the federal level. In 1965, the government passed the Higher Education Act (HEA) of 1965, or P.L. 89-329; Approved 8 November 1965. This act set provisions for institutions of higher learning to follow to receive any federal funding for their educational programs. Examples of the provisions addressed in the HEA include antidiscrimination (Sec. 111), protection of student speech and association rights (Sec. 112), institutional quality and integrity (Sec. 114), student representation (Sec. 115), binge drinking, drug, and alcohol abuse prevention (Secs. 119–120), diploma mills (Sec. 123), tuition for armed forces personnel and their dependents (Sec. 135), student financial aid procurement and delivery (Secs. 141–143), teacher quality and enhancement (Secs. 205–230), digital age learners (Secs. 231–234), STEM education, Historically Black Colleges and University financing, funding for Hispanic institutions, serving students with disabilities, several grants and scholarship programs, and much more (USDOE HEA 2022). This act is regularly reviewed and amended to address new issues that arise in society and on campuses and to delete provisions that no longer apply to current society.

Educational Principles and Practice in Veterinary Medicine, First Edition. Edited by Katherine Fogelberg.
© 2024 John Wiley & Sons, Inc. Published 2024 by John Wiley & Sons, Inc.

Each state has its own version of public university policies, based on the state-designated board that creates the policies and procedures. Whether the group is named a Board of Regents as in Colorado and Arizona, a Board of Trustees as in Ohio and California, a State Board of Higher Education as in Oregon, or an Executive Council of the Office of the Provost as in South Carolina, this group is responsible for reviewing and reaffirming, editing, or deleting current policies and procedures, as well as reviewing and adopting new policies. As McLendon and Perna (2014) explain, "state governments have long played the lead policy role for higher and postsecondary education. It is the actions taken or not taken by state policy-makers that primarily determine the future course of higher education attainment in the United States" (pp. 7–8). They go on to discuss the innovations of policy experimentation by several states and the numerous policies that have been created for funding, including merit scholarship programs, college savings plans, prepaid tuition programs, and policies permitting campuses to differentiate state tuition charges. States have also enacted structural changes in the government of performance funding, including funding based on graduation and completion rates. But McLendon and Perna (2014) point out that "despite the prevalence of these innovations and experiments, too little scholarship provides the empirical, theoretical, and applied policy insights that researchers and policy-makers need to be able to evaluate adequately the influence of state policies on higher education attainment" (p. 9). They encourage more research and knowledge on the part of the policy-makers to maximize the effectiveness of policies they implement.

For land-grant, state-based universities and colleges, there is a set of state policies that apply at every campus of the state educational system. Colleges and universities that are private, whether not-for-profit or for-profit, also have policies at the institutional level, and must also adhere to federal guidelines to receive any federal funding. Most colleges and universities desire full accreditation by their accrediting bodies, and as accreditation includes following these federal guidelines, their policies will in part look very similar to those of public institutions of higher learning. Private schools also usually have a Board of Trustees or equivalent group of decision-makers, but in these institutions, the President of the University could also have full power to adopt, edit, or veto policies based on the organizational design.

University policies are usually set by a Board of Trustees whose responsibility it is to address both national policy adherence and social and political issues of the day. Particularly, the state board is responsible for assuring that federal policies are followed, as detailed in the HEA in Section 495 (20 U.S.C. 1099a) – State Responsibilities (USDOE HOA 2022, p. 746). The state board enacts these policies, and each campus of the land-grant institution is responsible for adopting and upholding these policies. According to the state of Pennsylvania:

> University Policies are policies with broad application throughout the University system, designed to enhance the University's mission, promote operational efficiencies, and reduce institutional risk. Such policies help ensure compliance with applicable laws and regulations, promote ethical standards and integrity, and are approved in accordance with applicable procedures. (Pennsylvania State University 2015, n.p.).

The University of Tennessee explains that its policies provide guidance for employees to:

> Ensure compliance with state and federal laws and regulations; Maintain adequate internal controls to safeguard the university's assets; Provide consistent management of resources transactions across the system; and Understand the university's expectations for conducting university business and communicate these expectations to others as needed (University of Tennessee 2022, n.p.).

The University of Texas states that "University Policies are designed to communicate institutional rules for operation, organization, and programming of the university, including policy relating to students" (University of Texas 2022, n.p.), while Oregon State University says that "Through policies and standards, the university articulates the expectations of individuals, promotes efficiency, and supports compliance with laws and regulations" (Oregon State University 2022, n.p.). Similar phrasing is used in most university policy pages, indicating the purpose of the policies in place for the organization and running of the institution.

Institutions of higher learning are not all state-owned land-grant institutions. Many colleges and universities are privately owned, sometimes by a religious organization, such as the University of Notre Dame, which is owned by the Catholic church and governed by a President and Board of Trustees. Other private schools are independent entities, such as Cornell University in New York and Vanderbilt University in Tennessee. These not-for-profit private schools are often funded not only by tuition but by endowments from their founders and supporters. There are also for-profit independent institutions that are funded by tuition and investors, such as DeVry University, Grand Canyon University, and the University of Phoenix. While these institutions have their own policies and procedures addressing the same areas as state-owned and non-profit institutions, the educational survey results from these schools, such as degree completion and net cost to students, are much less favorable than their state and non-profit counterparts (NCES 2021, 2022). Nonetheless, all institutions of higher education have policies that dictate their business and educational endeavors.

Section 2: University Policy Areas

University policies cover all aspects of running the business of a university. The primary business of such an institution is, of course, education, and there are policies that cover the rights and responsibilities of the students. The faculty of a university are both teachers and employees, and the institutional policies cover faculty rights and responsibilities, as well as human and citizen rights in general for all people on campus. There are other employees, including administrators and staff of the central office and each department or college, and the policies also address the issues of employing faculty and staff in general.

The business of a university includes budget and fiscal responsibilities of the institution, dealing with tuition, funding, grants, donations, and other income, and with the expenses of property and facilities upkeep, utilities and equipment purchases and maintenance, employee salaries and benefits, marketing and recruiting, and other institutional expenses. Policies covering fiscal responsibility often address both how and what funding can come into the university and how and what expenses are allowed to go out. Policies also cover such situations as how students are selected for admission to the institution, the safety and security of the university, both in person and online, opportunities for travel and continuing education for faculty and staff, regulation of student organizations on campuses, corporations that do business on campus, and academic issues such as credits, degrees, and suspension and expulsion of students. At the University of Colorado, the Board of Regents divided the university policies into nine areas:

- CU System Administration
- Governance Policies
- Administration and Finance
- Education, Teaching, and Research
- Human Resources
- Information Technology
- Safety
- Student Life (University of Colorado 2022).

At the University of Florida, there are 12 categories of institutional policies:

- Academic Affairs
- Agriculture and Natural Resources
- Business Affairs
- Compliance
- Enrollment Management
- Finance
- Human Resources
- Inclusion, Diversity, Equity, and Access
- Information Technology
- Operations
- Research
- Strategic Communications and Marketing (University of Florida 2022).

Each of these areas of policy has subcategories that cover current and potential situations for administration, faculty, staff, and students at the institution. In contrast, the University of Connecticut has a web page listing all of its institutional policies in alphabetical order, with over 240 links on the list. Some links have a single policy with detailed explanation, such as the Space Management Policy. Other links lead to a web page that has a set of policies and procedures addressing a single issue, such as the page labeled "Minors" that discusses all the rules and regulations for students under the age of majority enrolled at the university (University of Connecticut 2022). While each college and university will have its own version of different categories, all institutions of higher education have sets of policies to address conditions and contexts in all aspects of the daily running of the business of higher learning.

Institutional policies are effective at all campuses of the institution. However, there are certain policies that can be implemented for individual departments or colleges within the greater institution. In those universities that include a College or School of Veterinary Medicine (CVM or SVM, from here forward referred to as a CVM), the CVM will have policies and procedures that apply only to the CVM and not necessarily to the college of education, the college of fine arts, or other colleges within the university. Also, undergraduate policies may or may not apply to postgraduate programs, and policies at one campus of a university might differ from policies at another campus of the same university. None of these college, department, or campus policies may override an institutional policy, but the colleges and departments may have policies that are different from each other.

As an example, consider the University of Illinois system. There are three main campuses of the University of Illinois – Urbana-Champaign (UIUC), Chicago (UIC), and Springfield (UIS). There is a set of system policies that are universally observed at all three campuses. In the Personnel section of their online policy page, one can find system policies that cover such categories as nondiscrimination, public affairs, contracts to be signed by the comptroller, the setting of fiscal year dates, legalities of intellectual property, and employment procedures. However, each campus also has policies and procedures specific to its own situations and programs. In the Student Policies section of the policy page, the Course Fee Guidelines are consistent across the system, while the Promotion and Tenure Guidelines and the Graduate Waiver Policy each have individual sections for each of the three campuses (UI 2022). In the student handbook for the Graduate College at the Urbana-Champaign campus, part I of the handbook preface states:

> All graduate students must follow Graduate College policies. Individual graduate programs may have additional policies specific to their students. Therefore, students should familiarize themselves with policies in their departmental handbook as well as those outlined here. Additionally, graduate students must also be aware of campus and university policies as well as state laws that could impact graduate students but are not under the jurisdiction or authority of the Graduate College (UIUC 2022, p. 4).

In a similar preface, the faculty handbook for the University of Illinois Springfield says:

> This handbook is intended as a general guide for faculty and academic staff. Some policies, procedures and information affect all three universities of the University of Illinois system while others are specific to UIS. In case of any discrepancy between the summaries or statements provided herein and the original University statue (*sic*), rule, regulation or policy upon which the Academic Staff Handbook is relying, the original is controlling (UIS 2022, n.p.).

Administrators in each college and department at a university must be familiar with the institutional policies and procedures. They are responsible for the adherence to those policies by all students, faculty, and staff at their own level within their own college. At the same time, those responsible for creating and upholding college-level policies and procedures must also ensure that they are not in conflict with those institutional policies.

Part 1: Individual Veterinary School Policies

While state and university policies have an effect on the faculty in every department, there are more specific policies decided at the department level that have a more direct impact on individual instructors. These are the policies that are important for every faculty member to become familiar with, as they set the standards at the college level. By learning and following the policies and questioning them when necessary, the faculty can make the learning environment less stressful both for themselves and students.

Policies at a veterinary school generally fall under several categories, including such areas as Admissions, Academic Affairs, Professional Behavior, Disciplinary, Facility, Research and Animal Use and Care, Student Organization functionality, and Student, Faculty, and Staff Code of Conduct. There are some policies that will be dependent upon outside influence, such as the AVMA or the AAVMC. Some policies will be dependent upon the influence of other schools at the university, such as medical, law, or other professional schools with similar regulations addressing similar issues. Still, other policies may be influenced by other colleges of veterinary medicine, in an effort to provide consistency within the profession. Finally, there could be policies that address unique situations that exist only on that campus or in that geographical or virtual environment. Most policies for a department or college, such as a CVM, are reviewed and revised annually and are published in a handbook format, both digitally and in hard copy.

Academic policies define the academic progression of students through the educational program. These policies affect the integrity of the curriculum and the educational program itself. Such policies may include how grades are calculated, class ranking, remediation, recession, and dismissal policies, elective options, and even the admissions procedure for the school. Many schools have prerequisites for their students, including a grade point average, passing certain prerequisite courses, hours of community service or professional experience, and more.

Policies addressing professional behavior are necessary to maintain a certain level of professionalism on and off campus for veterinary students. These policies could include a dress code, monitoring of off-campus acts such as intoxication or other illegal activities, rules for contacting and addressing faculty and administrators, proper interactions with other students, and other nonacademic expectations.

Disciplinary policies are those that follow up on students and employees who do not follow the professional or other policies. These will include the process of administration to dispense consequences for violating other policies, identification of the body responsible for such dispensation (e.g., student council, a faculty board, and the dean), and an appeals process.

Some policies are designed to protect the campus of the school and its facilities. While the university may have facility policies such as driving and parking policies, hours of building availability, and campus security policies, each college will have its own policies covering its own facilities.

In the case of a veterinary school, these policies could extend to a teaching hospital, a clinical skills laboratory or surgical suite, and even acreage owned by the college that houses large animals and their barns, stables, and equipment. Such facility policies could include who is allowed access to these facilities, who is and is not allowed to use the equipment, such as tractors and their implements, and use of the acreage or fields for community or organizations outside of the college.

As for the actual animals owned and housed at the college, there are policies addressing their use and care that start with federal mandates from the Public Health Service Policy on Humane Care and Use of Laboratory Animals, based on the Animal Welfare Act (7 U.S.C. 2131 et. seq.), and include state animal use regulations, followed by the policies of the Institutional Animal Care and Use Committee (IACUC) at the institution, whose responsibilities are outlined in the National Institutes of Health Office of Laboratory Animal Welfare publications (National Institute of Health 2021).

Accreditation requirements (covered fully in Chapter 23) for veterinary training include a minimum of one year of clinical experiences, and policies covering these situations are also unique to this type of medical training. Whether the college has its own teaching hospital on campus or the students are out in a distributive model of clinics, shelters, zoos, research facilities, and other independent entities, there are policies that guide the students, the faculty, the preceptors and employees, and the member sites as to the rules, regulations, expectations, and guidelines of supporting the students in their hands-on education. In the case of the distributive model of rotations. Each member site must agree to adhere to these policies to sponsor and host veterinary students at their clinic, lab, or place of business.

Policies particular to a college such as a CVM may also include committee information. Each college will have a structure of committees to handle individual situations. The Governance Document of the Iowa State University CVM has a section on standing committees. There are 17 standing committees at this CVM, including committees for Admissions, Computer Library and Information Management, a Budget Advisory Committee, Committees on Diversity and Inclusion, Promotion and Tenure, Research, and Safety. Each committee's procedural policies are published in the document, including the number of committee members and their qualifications, the responsibility of that committee, and identification of areas for which that committee is to develop and submit policies to be adopted by the college (Iowa State University 2022, pp. 7–8). Then each committee is responsible for developing and implementing policies addressing their specific area of governance.

Section 3: Faculty Responsibility to Policy

Among the most important policies to know as a faculty member are those academic policies that cover the instructional procedures for presenting content. The policies may decide how many lectures and labs are included in a course, and/or how the budget is allotted to the course for guest speakers, equipment, and supplies. Policies may cover research and publications and may address professional development requirements. All of these areas will have different policies at different schools. Each school has certain restrictions based on university policies and certain freedoms to set its own policies. Each school designs its instruction to meet the needs of the curricular design at that school, and no two schools present the content in the same manner. Often the curriculum content, if not the curricular design, will be organized in cooperation with other schools offering the same program. For a college of veterinary medicine, there are certain curricular areas required for accreditation, such as the theory and practice of medicine and surgery for a broad range of species, epidemiology, food safety, and the professional legal and ethical regulatory principles of veterinary medical services (AVMA COE 2022). Professional schools, such as colleges of veterinary medicine, often work together to create policies for consistency across the professional preparation institutions.

Another important policy for instructors is creating the syllabus of the course. The syllabus, covered fully in Chapter 8, is a published document outlining the expectations for the course and the rights and responsibilities of both the instructor(s) and the students. In most schools, the course director or instructor of record is responsible for the content in the syllabus, but also in most schools, there is either a template or a predesigned outline of what is required to be included at that university in a syllabus. The actual content, the list of lectures and labs, the testing and assessment design that will be used, the list of instructors and office hours, and other pertinent data may change from course to course. But there are usually legalities in every syllabus that outline university policies such as the Federal Educational Rights and Privacy Act (FERPA), Americans with Disabilities Act (ADA), security, and administration information. When writing the syllabus, it is imperative that the faculty not only include this university-based information but that each instructor is familiar with what it says and means. The faculty is responsible for assuring the published syllabus follows the policies of the university.

Once the course content and lecture and lab schedules are set, and the syllabus is written and published, the faculty proceeds with their instruction. However, the academic policies are in effect during the entire time the course is running and the faculty is employed. If the course is proceeding on schedule and the students are succeeding academically, the policies are generally followed by all involved as a matter of course. It is the unexpected situation or the student who is unsuccessful academically or behaviorally (professionalism) that causes the need to review and implement policies. The best case scenario for these situations is that the issue is already addressed in the published policies. If a student cheats on a written exam, if a student and a faculty have an inappropriate relationship, or if a student organization holds an unauthorized event or serves alcohol in an area where this is prohibited, the published policies should already be in place to address the procedure for handling the situation. A faculty member has the responsibility to follow the published policies in reporting the situation to the appropriate resource. If there is a policy in place, the administration then becomes responsible for carrying out the college or institutional policy addressing the issue.

There is the possibility that a situation may arise that is not addressed by any current policy. In that case, there is usually a general policy statement that would address these unique situations. This policy may indicate who would be responsible for working through such a situation or to whom such a situation should be referred for further information. Often when this occurs, a new policy is then created to address the unexpected situation, should it happen again in the future at that institution.

Part 1: Faculty Employment Policies

Just as academic policies cover the instructional design and presentation of content, there are employment policies that cover the benefits and responsibilities of faculty employed by the university. It is very important that faculty are familiar with these policies both for their own benefit and for legal protection. These policies are designed to protect the employees and to protect the university.

Employment policies cover such benefits as accumulation and use of leave time, faculty advancement and tenure, allowing guests on campus and in office areas, classrooms, labs, and areas where animals are housed, travel for business purposes, and even registration of vehicles and parking. For example, at one university, the policy may be that faculty have assigned parking sites while another university may not. Or at one university, faculty and staff may bring their children to work for one day if the local school system closes, while another university may say no children are allowed in the office area at all. Each university, college, or campus has rules and regulations that cover their policies and procedures concerning the faculty and staff, and it is the responsibility of those employees to know the policies and follow them.

Employment policies also cover legalities, with a written code of professional conduct and policies covering such topics as personal relationships between employees and adult students, conflicts of interest in scholarly endeavors, conducting personal business during work hours, and intellectual property. For example, a university may have a policy stating that photos and images of certain areas of the campus, such as a surgical lab or inside a storage area, are not to be shared publicly, including on social media. Another university may have a policy restricting use of the logo in any external publications, or requiring a copyright or trademark indication on any published works through the institution. There will be policies that address the use of technology and internet access on campus and during work hours, including time on social media or accessing banking or shopping sites through institutional internet. The consequences of violating these policies could include suspension without pay or termination of employment.

Changing Policies

Once a policy is approved and established, it is expected that students, faculty, and staff will adhere to the policy while enrolled or employed at the institution. However, the purpose behind a policy could change either with time or immediately.

Federal Level Policy Changes

At the federal level, changes to the HEA of 1965 have occurred several times over the past 50 years, according to the changing needs of society. For each change, a task force is established, a study is done on the current policy in question, the data are reviewed, and a recommendation to either make changes or reauthorize the policy as is made to the House Committee on Education and Labor. The committee may reject or approve the recommendation, which is then brought before Congress. Congress will review the recommendation, whether it be to reauthorize or to make changes; they then vote to approve or reject the recommendation for reauthorization or for each individual recommended change to the federal policy (USDOE 2022).

A recent task force, convened in 2018 by the Bipartisan Policy Center, spent a year and a half deliberating on the Higher Education Financing and Student Outcomes. The task force finally reached an agreement on a package of 45 recommendations presented to Congress in 2020 (Bitar 2020). When we say that it takes an act of Congress to change a policy, in this case, it is true. But as has been discussed, the federal government only handles a few major issues with education, and they are usually tied to funding. Most actual educational policies are set at the state level.

State Policy Level Changes

Each state has its own governance model as to how educational policies are reviewed and adopted. The states may have a state board of education, which may be elected or may be appointed by the governor. These boards may have a chief state education officer, who may be elected or may be appointed by the governor or by the board. There are two states – Minnesota and Wisconsin – that do not have state boards of education, and 30 states with some type of executive-level secretary role who makes major decisions. Oregon has the governor as the chief state school officer, and other states have educational officers, secretaries, or governance institutions. According to the Education Commission of the States blog page on policy, "State education governance can be complex and a bit of a mystery. . ." and "Many policy leaders work in separate branches of government or in different administrative agencies, so knowing how their relationships are structured helps us understand how different individuals and policy institutions are connected at the state level" (Railey 2017, n.p.). Therefore, the method by which policies are made and are changed is as varied as the states where they occur.

Sometimes a policy addresses an issue that changes with time and society. Sometimes these changes come gradually, such as uses of technology both as instructional tools and communication and social interaction. The policies addressing computer-based teaching have changed drastically in the past 30 years. In 1997, articles addressing the use of computers in teaching and taking exams found that computer-based education was a real possibility (Russell and Haney 1997; Stanika 1997; Herlehy 1997). In his article encouraging the use of technology in the higher education classroom, Herlehy (1997) stated "The only way an academic institution is going to be able to establish/enhance its reputation as a cutting-edge provider of technology education is to use those very technologies that are part of the curriculum and put them into practice in the administrative offices" (p. 11).

Twenty years later, the policies addressing technology were still in need of updating. When addressing policies for digital tools in administrative use, Saykili (2019) found that the same innovations that offer potential solutions to educational technologies also act as challenges, due to lack of proper policy and planning, resource allocation, and qualified staff. In this case, the policies previously in place were actually hindering the institution from keeping up with current technology. Saykili stated that "policymakers involved in education need to re-think the implications of digital connective technologies, the challenges and opportunities they bring to the educational scene while developing value-added policies regarding higher education" (p 4). In the 2020s, the use of computers both in instruction and

administration is an accepted, expected, common practice, with policies governing their use and restriction, thus fulfilling his prediction. As the technology changed, as the use of the technology changed, so the policies that covered technology changed. These were gradual changes that occurred naturally with time.

There are also changes in policy or creation of new policy that occur more immediately due to unexpected events, innovations in technology, or other unforeseen circumstances. In 2001, the United States experienced a horrific attack by international terrorists, resulting in an immediate change in security measures both in the United States and internationally. On university campuses, security policies reflected similar changes to protect the students and employees. In the mid-2000s, unmanned aerial vehicles (UAVs), or what are commonly called drones, became popular and accessible to the public. As drone use led to issues of controversy, policies were created to regulate the use of this technology to protect personal invasions of privacy as well as human and property damage. A study by Freeman and Freeland in 2019 on the UAV policy change states that "while some colleges and universities have responded to these risks by adopting stringent [policies] regarding UAV use . . . other higher-education institutions have done nothing, or enacted few rules." (p. 120). Policies differed widely on this issue.

In 2020, the COVID-19 pandemic brought changes to health policies, including policies regarding the wearing of face masks and staying certain distances apart, to public and private institutions across the globe. The COVID-19 pandemic also brought changes in policies addressing instruction and the college campus, encouraging more online teaching and assessment, expanding policies on working from home, and creating revisions in medical leave policy.

In cases, such as these that require immediate policy creation or changes, often those changes come directly from the president or the board of directors of the university, or the dean of the college. In other cases that are not as dire, policy changes have a procedure that could take weeks to months to make a final decision. Usually, when there is a request for a policy change, that request will be brought to the appropriate committee, who will review the recommendation and either reject or adopt the proposed change and then forward the recommendation to the institutional level committee or officer who will review and make the final decision on the rejection or approval of the change. If approved, the policy is then formally written, published, and distributed before being activated, a process that could take even more time. In their description of implementation of a new policy at a university, Whittaker and Anderson (2013) explain, "the most important and often most difficult aspect is likely to be in the mechanisms of implementation and dissemination, without which the existence of a policy is hardly worthwhile" (p. 40).

Changes in policy are not easily made. Often a policy has been in place for more years than the students or faculty have been at the institution, and is considered institutional tradition and history. When a policy is questioned or challenged, there must be justification for a change, and often that justification must be introduced, researched, documented, discussed, argued, and reintroduced before finally being brought to a vote and a decision made. In researching how changes to policy are successful, several studies have indicated the association with *actors* and networks as the driving factor to a policy change being made.

Actors are individuals who have interest in having the change occur or influence in making the decision on the change. Whether the individual is a student who is concerned about the rights of an underserved population, a faculty who feels the benefits currently offered are below standard or a community member who sees an opportunity to engage the university in an outreach opportunity, an actor could be someone who is passionate about a cause and feels a change in policy can help make the cause successful. An actor could also be a new dean, a vice president who is promoted to president of the university, or a new board member who has the political influence to make a change occur at the highest level. According to Saarinen and Ursin (2012), "effective policy entrepreneurs, as human actors, can be distinguished by the extent to which their identity and actions match the situation" (p. 148).

A *network* is a group of people who are either invested in the cause of an actor or who could be considered an actor in their own right. Sometimes a dynamic individual has political and social relationships that can be tapped to provide support for a change or support against making the change, thus creating a network. Other times, it is the network already in place, such as supporters of a political party's views or of a nonprofit organization's focus group, that initiates the actions for a change in policy. A study by Shearer et al. (2016) explored policy changes as being the result of institutions, interests, and ideas, called the "three Is," which are supported by networks of followers. Those networks then take those three Is and integrate them into changes in policy. Their study defines networks as "both empirically measurable sets of actors and their relationships, and as intentional governance or management structures with agency to act strategically" (Shearer et al. 2016, p. 1201). Often it is the influence of a network that brings about the introduction of a policy change, either from the outside into the institution, or from the inside of the decision-making group out to the populace.

In their literature review on higher education policy changes, Saarinen and Ursin (2012) found that the articles on agency approach to policy changes showed that "higher education policy change is an interactive process between various actors and domains within transient structures" (p. 149) and go on to point out that the actor-network theory of policy change shows the fluid nature of higher education policy, since actors and networks are interactive and transient. It is when an individual or group sees a need for a change and they take action to make that change happen that policy is updated to reflect the rules and regulations that best address the needs of the institution and the people involved in that institution.

Section 4: Summary

Policies are put in place to protect people, property, and the integrity of an institution. In the case of higher education, policies are designed to protect students, faculty and staff, the campuses, materials and equipment, and the curriculum and education provided. Higher education policies are designed to protect the rights of students and employees, to set rules and regulations for use of buildings, public areas, equipment, and supplies, and to ensure the integrity of the education that occurs and the resulting performance of graduates in their chosen fields.

These policies come from many levels and affect nearly all aspects of a university. In the United States, the national government sets policies that must be adhered to by state governments. States set policies that must be adhered to by colleges and universities. The accrediting bodies for higher education also set policies that universities must follow to maintain accreditation. Universities set policies that must be adhered to by each division or college. Colleges set policies that must be adhered to by each department or campus. Departments and campuses set policies that must be adhered to by the students, faculty, and staff who attend or work there. Each university, each college, each department or campus have policies that are similar to each other and policies that are distinct and unique to their own educational situations.

It is the responsibility of each level of policy-makers to disseminate information covering the requirements and expectations, as well as identify consequences for not following these policies. At the same time, it is the responsibility of each individual to know and understand the policies that apply to them in their own situations. Some policies can stand for years, even decades, and be understood almost innately. Other policies change often, and the individuals must keep abreast of changes and their implications to them as students, faculty, or staff.

The most common practice for universities to publish their policies is in a set of handbooks – a Student Handbook, an Employee Handbook, a Faculty Handbook – and some may have handbooks for each campus or each department. These handbooks are reviewed, updated, and published each year, some each semester, to be sure the information is disseminated as clearly and simply as possible. The handbooks are usually available both as hard copies on paper and in an online document. Every student, instructor, and staff member are made aware of the handbooks to assure adherence to policies and may be required to confirm receipt of this information, through a virtual or written signature. Thus the policies that have been created can be monitored and upheld to support the institution in their ongoing purpose of making the educational experience offered at their institution the best and most effective educational experience possible.

References

American Veterinary Medical Association Council on Education (AVMA COE) (2022). COE Accreditation Policies and Procedures. https://www.avma.org/education/accreditation/colleges/coe-accreditation-policies-and-procedures-principles (accessed 14 December 2022).

Bitar, J. (2020). The Higher Education Act: opportunities for bipartisan reform. *Liberal Education* 106 (1–2). https://eric.ed.gov/?id=EJ1261448.

Department of Higher Education and Training (DHOT) (2022). Higher Education Policy Development and Research. *Republic of South Africa*. https://www.dhet.gov.za/SitePages/Policy-Development-and-Research.aspx (accessed 14 December 2022).

Freeman, P. and Freeland, R. (2019). Red tape in higher education institutions: UAV policy. *ISPRS Annals of the Photogrammetry, Remote Sensing and Spatial Information Sciences* 4 (2/W5): 119–126. https://www.proquest.com/docview/2585371651?accountid=12101.

Herlehy, W. (1997). Education tailor-made for the times. *Journal of Aviation/Aerospace Education & Research* 7 (2): 9–14. https://www.proquest.com/docview/1689584337?OpenUrlRefId=info:xri/sid:wcdiscovery&accountid=12101.

Iowa State University (ISU) (2022). College Governance, Governance Document. https://vetmed.iastate.edu/sites/default/files/About/Faculty/GOVERNANCE-DOCUMENT-CVM-approved-2020.pdf (accessed 02 December 2022).

McLendon, M. and Perna, L. (2014). State policies and higher education attainment. *The Annals of the American Academy of Political and Social Science* 655: 6–15. https://www.jstor.org/stable/24541747#metadata_info_tab_contents.

Ministry of Education (MINEDUC), Division of the Undersecretariat (2022). About us. Ejecucion Subsecretaria de Educacion Superior. https://educacionsuperior.mineduc.cl/ (accessed 14 December 2022).

National Institutes of Health (NIH) (2021). The IACUC. https://olaw.nih.gov/resources/tutorial/iacuc.htm (accessed 06 December 2022).

Office for Students (2022). Guidance from Government. *Publications, Office for Students, United Kingdom*. https://www.officeforstudents.org.uk/publications/annual-review-2022/ (accessed 2 December 2022).

Oregon State University (2022). University Policies and Standards. https://policy.oregonstate.edu/ (accessed 02 December 2022).

Pennsylvania State University (2015). About Penn State Policies. https://policies.psu.edu/about (accessed 02 December 2022).

Railey, H. (2017). Who Makes Ed Policy in Your State? *EdNote: Your education policy blog, December 19, 2017. Education Commission of the States*. https://ednote.ecs.org/who-makes-ed-policy-in-your-state/ (accessed 15 December 2022).

Russell, M. and Haney, W. (1997). Testing writing on computers. *Education Policy Analysis Archives* 5 (3). https://doaj-org.lmunet.idm.oclc.org/article/4cafddc84c6f41029d61fb5600b1a04d.

Saarinen, T. and Ursin, J. (2012). Dominant and emerging approaches in the study of higher education policy change. *Studies in Higher Education* 37 (2): 143–156. https://web.s.ebscohost.com/ehost/pdfviewer/pdfviewer?vid=1&sid=12137afb-690e-4cff-a48b-2eca04f31890%40redis.

Saykili, A. (2019). Higher education in the digital age: the impact of digital connective technologies. *Journal of Educational Technology & Online Learning* 2 (1): 1–15. https://www.proquest.com/docview/2256216608?accountid=12101.

Shearer, J., Abelson, J., Kouyaté, B. et al. (2016). Why do policies change? Institutions, interests, ideas and networks in three cases of policy reform. *Health Policy and Planning* 31: 1200–1211. https://web.s.ebscohost.com/ehost/pdfviewer/pdfviewer?vid=2&sid=087c0c37-e6f0-4268-8de6-cdb3916227e5%40redis.

Stanika, D. (1997). The use of computers for teaching. *Journal of Special Education and Rehabilitation* 1 (3): 108–117. https://doaj-org.lmunet.idm.oclc.org/article/a6dffa24bfff4814bf6498d8d0d3d2bb.

United States Department of Education (USDOE) (2022). Office of Postsecondary Education – About OPE – Policy, *Planning, and Innovation*. https://www2.ed.gov/about/offices/list/ope/ppi.html (accessed 14 December 2022).

United States Department of Education – Higher Education Act (USDOE HEA) (2022). Higher Education Act of 1965 (HEA) As Amended Through P.L. 117-200, Enacted October 11, 2022. https://www.govinfo.gov/content/pkg/COMPS-765/pdf/COMPS-765.pdf (accessed 14 December 2022).

United States Department of Education, National Center for Education Statistics (NCES) (2021). IPEDS Data Explorer, Table 5. https://nces.ed.gov/ipeds/Search/ViewTable?tableId=32476&returnUrl=%2Fipeds%2FSearch (accessed 02 December 2022).

United States Department of Education, National Center for Education Statistics (NCES) (2022). Digest of Education Statistics. https://nces.ed.gov/programs/digest/d21/tables/dt21_326.15.asp (accessed 15 December 2022).

University of Colorado (2022). Campus Policies. https://www.colorado.edu/policies (accessed 2 December 2022).

University of Connecticut (2022). Policies & Procedures. https://policy.uconn.edu/posts-a-z/ (accessed 2 December 2022).

University of Florida (2022). UF Policy Hub. https://hub.policy.ufl.edu/s/ (accessed 2 December 2022).

University of Illinois (UI) (2022). University of Illinois System Resources Policies and Procedures. https://www.vpaa.uillinois.edu/cms/One.aspx?portalId=420456&pageId=423423 (accessed 2 December 2022).

University of Illinois Springfield (UIS) (2022). Academic Staff Handbook. https://www.uis.edu/academicstaffhandbook (accessed 2 December 2022).

University of Illinois Urbana-Champaign (UIUC) (2022). University of Illinois Urbana-Champaign Graduate College Handbook 2022–2023. https://grad.illinois.edu/sites/grad.illinois.edu/files/pdfs/handbook.pdf (accessed 2 December 2022).

University of Tennessee (2022). UT System Policy Website. https://policy.tennessee.edu/ (accessed 2 December 2022).

University of Texas (2022). University Policy Office. https://compliance.utexas.edu/university-policy-office (accessed 2 December 2022).

Whittaker, A. and Anderson, G. (2013). A policy at the University of Adelaide for student objections to the use of animals in teaching. *Journal of Veterinary Medical Education* 40 (1): 52–57.

Yamada, R. (2018). Impact of Higher Education Policy on Private Universities in Japan: analysis of governance and educational reform through survey responses. *Research Institute for Higher Education* 3 (15): 19–37. https://ir.lib.hiroshima-u.ac.jp/files/public/4/45645/2018042709391422207/HigherEducationForum_15_19.pdf.

22

Leadership in Higher Education

Erik H. Hofmeister, DVM, DACVAA, DECVAA, MA, MS

College of Veterinary Medicine, Auburn University, Auburn, AL, USA

Section 1: Introduction

Leadership in higher education (HE) is distinctly different from leadership in corporate or government environments (Lumby 2012). HE leaders are responsible for cultivating a creative environment with power distributed to faculty members who need relatively little direction, are beholden to a wide variety of constituents (not only shareholders, as with corporations, or their citizens, as with government entities), produce a widely disparate type of "products" (research, students, and services), and have outputs that are difficult to quantify (research impact, student preparedness, and service impact). Academic leaders often must confront basic questions that can never be resolved: Who are we? What are we here to do? How should we do it? (Gallos and Bolman 2021). With the COVID-19 pandemic, institutions have lost revenue, had increased expenses, fewer admissions, and an increased need for student support services (Gallos and Bolman 2021). All of these differences – and more – make it difficult to apply principles from other domains of leadership to HE. This necessitates an exploration of HE leadership as a separate style of leadership.

Beyond the difference between HE leadership and corporate and government leadership, leadership in veterinary academia is significantly distinct from leadership in HE. Consider the following: the number of applicants for faculty positions is dramatically different. Whereas many university units have dozens or hundreds of applicants for open faculty positions, clinical faculty positions in colleges of veterinary medicine (CVMs) rarely attract more than a handful of applicants and, often, zero applicants. This necessitates a different approach to faculty recruitment and retention. The explosion of adjunct faculty – up to 70% of teaching faculty in some institutions (Kezar et al. 2019) – has not occurred in veterinary medicine and

is unlikely to occur, as specialists with the expertise to teach in the veterinary curriculum are relatively rare. Many universities set salaries at a certain level of education, with no regard for market forces. In veterinary medicine, this leads to technical staff (who typically do not have advanced degrees) being grossly underpaid relative to their supply and demand.

Additionally, the clinical service responsibilities of veterinary faculty members are grossly misunderstood by upper administration in other programs (deans, provosts, vice presidents, and presidents). How does one calculate credit for a clinical rotation, where faculty spend 40–60 hours per week in instruction and service? If a week of clinics were considered a laboratory class, with three hours of lab over 15 weeks equaling one credit, a single week of clinics would be worth one credit. Multiplied by a typical faculty appointment of 50% clinic time means a clinical faculty member would be teaching 26 credits a year, not including lecture-based courses! How do veterinary leaders effectively communicate their needs to upper administration, given these massive disparities in roles, expectations, resources, and needs?

A model could be found in human medicine, but there are numerous differences in education between veterinary medicine and human medicine. Those differences include the amount of funding (lower in veterinary medicine), outcomes (training general practitioners in veterinary medicine as opposed to specialists in human medicine), debt-to-income ratio of graduates (lower income in veterinary medicine), learning comparative medicine in veterinary medicine, public health and zoonoses in veterinary medicine, financial issues (insurance and billing in human medicine versus communicating expenses to veterinary clients), euthanasia in veterinary medicine, communication (difficult in nonverbal veterinary patients), and regulation. Also, the interactions between academic health centers and the university versus the interaction between a college of veterinary medicine and the university are often dramatically different. For example, many academic health centers are their own separate entity, where faculty are compensated partly by the university and partly by the hospital. For these reasons, teaching leadership in veterinary medicine is distinctly different from teaching leadership in human medicine.

Beyond the academic leaders (department heads, directors, associate deans, and deans) in veterinary medicine, veterinary educators must also serve as leaders on a daily basis. They lead their classrooms, clinic teams, research laboratories (composed of students, staff, graduate students, and/or house officers), committees, services, sections, and professional associations. Moreover, as professionals, every veterinarian is expected to be a leader. Nearly every role a veterinarian occupies – from clinical practice to government work to research – involves managing and leading others. Preparing veterinary students, graduate students, and house officers to be leaders is an important task for veterinary educators. Serving as effective leaders, veterinary educators model leadership behaviors for their students, and applying principles of leadership can facilitate the veterinary educator in being successful across their wide variety of roles.

This chapter will introduce principles of leadership, including leadership theories that can be successfully applied to the unique context of veterinary HE; how leadership can be included in the curriculum (both formal and hidden); and provide suggestions for training veterinary students, graduate students, house officers, and faculty members to be effective leaders. It is expected that the reader will be prepared to present theories relevant to their context, discuss curriculum modifications to enhance leadership training and take active steps to enhance leadership skills in their students.

Section 2: Principles of Leadership

The distinction between management (controlling processes and making sure systems run smoothly so that things that need to get done are done) and leadership (creating vision, getting people on board with a direction, and inspiring others) has often been drawn, with management being derided as inferior to leadership. In reality, both management and leadership are required. In the literature, the line between the two is often blurred. Therefore, both management and leadership are addressed in this chapter.

Understanding the foundational principles and theories of leadership is important to develop a working understanding of leadership education. Just as there are educational theories (e.g., behaviorism, social learning theory, andragogy) that help educators focus their efforts in a directed, specific way, leadership theories exist that help to direct leaders' efforts. Most leadership theories have been created with a corporate or business context in mind. As mentioned in the Introduction, these theories may not be fully translatable to veterinary HE. Nonetheless, there are important concepts introduced in the theories that may be applicable to veterinary educators. Ultimately, a leadership theory of veterinary education does not exist, so these theories may serve as a foundation until such a theory is developed.

Theories have practical implications for veterinary leaders. For example, faculty satisfaction depends, in part, on the leadership style of administrators (Bateh and Heyliger 2014). Those administrators embracing passive/avoidant leadership styles had faculty with less job satisfaction (Bateh and Heyliger 2014). Theories also serve as a framework on which to build curricula and focus efforts directed at enhancing leadership competency. The theories presented here are not comprehensive, as the scholarship of leadership has produced hundreds of theories over the decades, but are chosen on the basis of the author's perception of their relevance to today's complex HE setting. The theories presented are transactional leadership, passive/avoidant leadership, transformational leadership, servant leadership, authentic leadership, self-determination theory (SDT), and HE culture. Furthermore, special considerations for women and underrepresented minorities (URM) in leadership positions are also presented.

Part 1: Transactional Leadership

Transactional leaders tend to focus on achieving specific behaviors in their followers by providing distinct rewards or punishments to motivate them. Leaders are often autocratic in their decision-making and provide a clear, singular direction. They set high goals for themselves and others and put emphasis on administrative issues with clear answers or outcomes (Bateh and Heyliger 2014). Transactional leaders tend to focus on the lower orders of Maslow's hierarchy of needs, such as the need for security (in the form of a salary) and belonging (in the form of gold stars, praise, or bonuses). Transactional leaders rarely seek to authentically develop their followers into independently acting entities.

Part 2: Passive/Avoidant Leadership

Passive leaders tend to maintain the status quo and not challenge conventions. Leaders tend to only act if a problem arises. Passive leadership is essentially an absence of leadership, and passive leaders tend to be primarily managerial.

Passive leaders avoid decisions and fail to model and reinforce appropriate behavior. Followers tend not to trust passive leaders, and this is generally acknowledged as a maladaptive leadership style (Holtz and Hu 2017).

Part 3: Transformational Leadership

Transformational leaders tend to focus on organizational objectives (Stone et al. 2004). Transformational leadership moves beyond self-interest or transactions (i.e., you do this and get rewarded) toward the good of the group and organization. This enhances follower performance and engagement. Transformational leaders focus on progress and development and foster an environment of trust where relationships can be easily formed. A shared vision, developed by a charismatic leader, is integral to this theory. Transformational leaders inspire followers, stimulate followers to be creative, and act as coaches for followers. Personal power, in the form of charisma, often determines the leader's overall effectiveness and may predispose the transformational leader to abuse of power. In HE, academic credibility (e.g., research and teaching) and experience in academia are also important competencies of effective transformational leaders (Spendlove 2007).

Part 4: Servant Leadership

Servant leaders tend to focus on the people who are their followers (Stone et al. 2004). The leadership focus is on fulfilling the needs of others. Servant leaders develop their followers, allowing them to flourish. Servant leaders derive their influence from servanthood and placing their trust in their followers. They value the people who comprise the organization, rather than the organization itself, and prioritize their follower's relationships and wellness. In so doing, the expectation is that the followers will invest in each other and the organization to succeed in the long term. The servant leader does not direct followers, but rather motivates and facilitates their activities. They use reciprocity to encourage followers, but this can have a negative effect where followers do not return the trust and freedom given to them, creating a breakdown in effective leadership. There may also be a risk of the servant leader "burning out" due to the outpouring of energy when engaging their followers, particularly in large academic units.

Part 5: Authentic Leadership

Authentic leaders tend to focus on their own internal awareness and lead a values-based mission (Gardner et al. 2011). Authentic leaders must lead in a way that honors their core values, beliefs, strengths, and weaknesses.

Authentic leaders are role models and focus on transcendent values like honesty, loyalty, and equality to motivate their followers. Leaders and followers gain self-awareness and have open, trusting relationships. Authentic leaders consider multiple sides and perspectives and make decisions in balanced ways. Authentic leaders embrace positive ethical and moral stances and create a values-based leadership style (Day et al. 2014). Authentic leadership requires followers who are also authentic and requires significant vulnerability on the part of the leader to be effective.

Part 6: Self-Determination Theory

Although not a theory of leadership, understanding SDT facilitates other leadership styles because it describes a theory to explain human motivation and behavior. SDT posits that people are motivated on a spectrum between amotivation (lacking any desire to act) to external regulation (acting to satisfy a simple desire or avoid harm) to internal motivation (acting out of interest and inherent satisfaction). External regulation can be equated to a transactional leadership approach – where followers only take actions to get something from the leader. Internal motivation may be achieved by transformational, servant, and/or authentic leadership styles, and in general results in people being happier and more satisfied (Bryman 2007).

Internal motivation is facilitated by providing followers with three elements: autonomy, competence, and relatedness. Autonomy is the ability to do as the individual desires, and academia is a place where autonomy abounds. Competence is the ability to improve in a skill, again a strength of academia. Relatedness is the ability to connect with others and form meaningful relationships. The classic model of motivation – where an individual does an action to get a reward or avoid a punishment – is not effective to motivate people in highly creative pursuits (Kohn 1993). Only when the three elements of SDT can be provided will people be internally motivated to excel in complex activities such as veterinary medicine.

Leaders can use SDT when they are considering an action and interacting with a follower. How can the leader assign an activity that gives the follower as much autonomy as possible? Perhaps by providing the follower the freedom to choose with whom to work, when to complete the task, or how to complete the task. How can the leader facilitate intrinsic motivation by providing opportunities to develop competence? Perhaps training sessions in teaching or research for faculty or continuing education (CE) for staff can be provided. Can the leader facilitate relatedness? Perhaps hosting social functions (within or outside the workplace), having meetings where individuals get to share and meet with each other, and highlighting the importance of the work for the community and society in general. Facilitating internal motivation by the followers will enhance their work experience and, ideally, the effectiveness of that work.

Part 7: Higher-Education Culture

Although not a leadership theory, the theory of HE culture has a meaningful impact on leaders. All leaders must understand the culture in which they work. HE culture and histories are often extensive and significantly influence the way leaders function. McNay's (1995) theory of organization is based on the degree of tightness on two characteristics: how policy is defined and how it is implemented (McCaffery 2010). The way these two levels of the two variables interact produces four cultures of HE.

The collegium culture has low levels of policy, low implementation, and emphasizes academic freedom led by senior professors as the dominant leaders. Students are regarded as apprentice academics and management is permissive, allowing faculty free reign. A bureaucratic culture has a loose policy but a tight implementation and focuses on rules and regulations and procedures. Leadership is formalized and students are evaluated as statistics. The corporate institution culture has tight control over both policy and implementation and focuses on loyalty to the institution and senior management. Leadership is political and decision-making is made largely by senior management rather than faculty, and students are considered customers. An enterprise culture has a tight policy but loose implementation and focuses on competence. Leadership is supportive of development and decision-making is focused on project teams, while students are regarded as valued customers.

Institutions tend to move from collegium to bureaucracy to corporate to enterprise throughout their existence, particularly in recent decades. However, some institutions may move directly from the collegium to an enterprise organization, and all institutions have some elements of each type of culture.

Part 8: Women and Underrepresented Minorities and Leadership

Individuals representing groups who traditionally have not held power in our society – such as women and URM – generally have more challenges in leadership roles (Eagly 2005). For the purposes of this material, URM includes racial and ethnic minorities, as well as any individual with characteristics that are not well represented in veterinary medicine, such as a different sexual orientation, religion, or disability. Their challenges in holding leadership roles are often

because followers automatically attribute characteristics to women and URM they may not actually have, solely based on these other characteristics (Devine et al. 2021).

Although women represent 80% of currently enrolled veterinary students (American Association of Veterinary Medical Colleges 2021) and 62% of the veterinary workforce, they represent only 49% of faculty members and 39% of veterinary HE leadership (Lloyd et al. 2008). Nonetheless, female faculty members expressed more interest in learning about leadership skills than male faculty members (Lloyd et al. 2008). However, societal incongruities between gender roles and leadership roles can present a challenge to women leaders in HE (Gardner et al. 2011). For example, classically masculine traits like risk-taking, confidence, and assertiveness are often associated with successful leadership (Muller-Kahle and Schiehll 2013). This creates a situation where women, who are equally effective as men at being leaders, face the challenge of legitimacy of their skills (Muller-Kahle and Shchiehll 2013). Ironically, companies with greater gender diversity show lower risk and deliver better performance (Perryman et al. 2016). This suggests the assumption that masculine leadership qualities are superior is false, and that HE settings embracing those masculine qualities may be at a disadvantage compared with their peer institutions.

In the United States, underrepresented racial and ethnic minorities represent ~22% of the veterinary student body and faculty members but only 13% of veterinary HE leadership (Lloyd et al. 2008). Unfortunately, the representation is so low that statistical analyses of URM are not performed (Lloyd et al. 2008). URM may not seek out leadership opportunities or may leave them due to inhospitable environments on campus, unrealistic role expectations, lack of mentoring, and tokenism (Wolfe and Dilworth 2015). Institutions may be able to improve conditions to facilitate recruiting and retaining URM leaders by embracing cultural pluralism and multiculturalism. In these paradigms, cultures are all embraced and viewed as neutral and dominant groups (e.g., white, straight, and able) are acknowledged while seeking unity and celebrating the enriched collective including all people (Wolfe and Dilworth 2015).

Section 3: Leadership Education

It is important to teach leadership in the veterinary curriculum. Leadership is about an interaction between the leader and the follower(s). In veterinary medicine, these interactions are obvious in the examples of a faculty member and a student, a veterinarian and a staff member, a club president and a member, a principal investigator and their team, and a practice owner and a veterinary employee.

Less obvious examples are when a patient suffers cardiac arrest and the first intern on the scene begins cardiopulmonary resuscitation (CPR) but then a resident appears on the scene, or when an associate professor is interacting with an assistant professor. Leadership dynamics can be separated into three descriptions of authority: positional authority, rank-based authority, and situational authority (Norton 2015).

Positional authority is the classic leader-follower pairing, where the leader has a professional position that explicitly puts them in a leadership role. Examples include practice owner, department chair, principal investigator, and club president. In business, this is often considered "direct reports" – the leader has ultimate control over the follower's activities and job-related rewards such as salary. As professionals with a substantial amount of education and expertise, veterinarians will naturally occupy roles of positional authority throughout their career. Therefore, veterinarians should be prepared and trained to occupy positional authority leadership roles.

Rank-based authority is encountered most commonly in hierarchical organizations, such as veterinary education (senior student, intern, resident, and faculty member), academia (assistant professor, associate professor, and professor), the military (lower enlisted, noncommissioned or petty officer, and commissioned officer), and business entities (assistant vice president, vice president, and president). In these circumstances, the interaction between the leader and follower is less pronounced than positional authority but still important. The leader rarely has direct control over the follower's job-related rewards, although they may have input into their job performance. Rank-based authority is valuable in emergency situations, where quick decisions must be made and followers have to act on the instructions given to them. Every veterinary student is faced with rank-based authority from the moment they start veterinary school, and many will pursue careers in highly hierarchical organizations, so learning to lead effectively in these circumstances is essential.

Situational authority is when an individual is faced with a specific situation where they have particular expertise and therefore can and should take a leadership role, which may be at odds with the typical position- or rank-based authority. For example, in a patient suffering cardiac arrest, a faculty member who rarely supervises CPR initially begins efforts, but then a senior resident in emergency and critical care appears. In this case, although the resident does not have positional authority and is below the faculty member in the academic hierarchy, they are clearly the most qualified to lead CPR efforts and should assume leadership in the situation. Situational authority may arise in nonemergency situations, too. For example, if, during a

department meeting, a faculty member indicates they have particular knowledge about a situation, they may take a leadership role. Veterinarians will encounter a variety of these situations where they are expected to be the leader and therefore must learn to lead effectively.

These simple categories of authority can be broken down even further, particularly in academic settings. At least nine types of authority have been identified in academic settings and explain why HE has developed elaborate systems of committees (Clark 1983). Committees and how they interact with leaders are important in HE settings. Leadership credibility depends on how, when, why, and where they hold meetings and with whom they hold them (McCaffery 2010). Critics of excessive committee work and meetings complain that such work is meaningless or is actively used to delay reaching a decision. Successfully managing committees and meetings are essential for leaders in HE, but is not generally explicitly taught.

Given these different situations and the role veterinarians fulfill as professionals who often occupy positions of authority, have a high rank in hierarchical organizations, and have expertise to provide them situational authority, it is essential that veterinarians are taught how to be effective leaders (Pearson et al. 2018). In human medicine, there is not a clear distinction in skills needed between those leaders in an official position (e.g., clinic director) versus those in everyday clinical leadership (e.g., daily clinical practice; Berghout et al. 2017). This emphasizes the importance of leadership for every clinical professional. Characteristics of effective leaders, leadership development, and the influence of the hidden curriculum must all be understood to effectively shape curriculum and produce veterinarians who are competent leaders.

Part 1: Characteristics of Effective Leaders

Research into individual characteristics of leaders is the longest-standing research topic in the science of leadership (Zaccaro et al. 2017). Part of the challenge of definitively defining leadership characteristics occurs because leadership is highly contextual. The skills a leader in a large corporation needs are different from the skills needed by a department chair (Bryman 2007). Leadership skills are also situational – skills that are helpful in some situations are detrimental in others. The specific contexts of leadership in a veterinary practice and in HE will be used as examples to highlight characteristics of effective leaders, realizing that even these represent a wide breadth of contexts and therefore generalities are difficult to apply.

Some characteristics associated with leadership cannot be changed, such as intelligence, height, and facial attractiveness (Zaccaro et al. 2017). Aesthetic attributes are used to form judgments of others, including leaders, because individuals use "thin-slice judgments," where impressions are made with scant amounts of information. Recognition of aesthetic attributes may be evolutionarily hard-wired to facilitate mate selection and assessment of healthiness (Devine et al. 2021). Social systems, such as racism and sexism, can bias individuals working with or selecting leaders. All of this leads to a bias toward tall, attractive, white men in leadership positions (Gündemir et al. 2014).

Aside from physical characteristics, which cannot be changed, some models have been devised with an exhaustive list of characteristics, such as the National Center for Healthcare Leadership's 26-item model (Calhoun et al. 2008). A handful of models have been developed that highlight the most important characteristics of medical practitioners and academic leaders, and form the foundation for the characteristics presented here.

In private practice veterinary medicine, characteristics of maintaining positive relationships, making decisions for the greater good of the business, a desire to make a difference, and good emotional intelligence have been described (Pearson et al. 2018). A model in human medicine has described personal integrity, effective communication, pursuing excellence, building and maintaining relationships, and thinking critically as important characteristics for leaders (Hargett et al. 2017). Another study in human medicine outlined the five most important competencies for physician leaders as communication skills, professional ethics, continuous learning, building coalitions, and clinical excellence (McKenna et al. 2004). A meta-analysis of leadership in human medicine reinforces the importance of clinical expertise in medical leaders (Berghout et al. 2017).

From this sample of the literature, it is evident that qualities for effective leadership in clinical veterinary medicine tend to focus on clinical excellence, integrity, communication, and interacting with others (i.e., emotional intelligence). Interestingly, this list is very similar to the qualities of a good clinical role model (Jochemsen-van der Leeuw et al. 2013). Clinical excellence is built into the curriculum of veterinary education, so it should come as a part of the veterinarian's routine training. Moral and ethical integrity does not accumulate passively during veterinary school, but actively teaching ethical behavior can result in improvements in moral judgment (Verrinder and Phillips 2015). Communication skills are now taught in the veterinary curriculum, and improvements in communication skills can be made by using the curriculum (Pun 2020). Similar to integrity, emotional intelligence does not accumulate passively through veterinary training (Adin et al. 2020), but can be learned (Crowley et al. 2019).

A systematic review of HE leadership produced a list of 13 characteristics that effective leaders display (Bryman 2007).

In addition to typical characteristics of leaders, such as providing vision, being a role model, and being respectful, effective academic leaders encourage participation in key decisions, create a collegial environment, advocate for their department, provide resources to stimulate scholarship, and enhance the department's reputation. Communication was the most important quality listed by Deans of CVMs (Haden et al. 2010). Communication, conflict resolution, diversity and inclusion, faculty work-life balance, operations of the university, and accreditation were the highest in importance according to a survey of 116 veterinary college administrations (Lloyd et al. 2019a). Successful leaders in academia find meaning in negative experiences and learn from trying and frustrating situations (Bennis and Thomas 2002).

Some of these characteristics of leaders, both in clinical practice and in HE, can be learned, nurtured, and developed. Experiential learning is an important element of leadership development, but leadership programs are equally essential.

Part 2: Leadership Development

Although some characteristics of leaders cannot be influenced, such as height or race, many characteristics of leadership can be developed and enhanced. Leadership development programs are ubiquitous in corporations, yet their addition to HE settings has only recently begun in earnest (Gallos and Bolman 2021). Leadership development is a dynamic process that occurs over time. Development also requires significant practice, and participation in workshops, programs, and seminars alone is insufficient to produce effective leaders (Day et al. 2014). Leaders who are better able to learn from their experiences tend to become better leaders (Day et al. 2014). As with any skill, leaders progress through novice, intermediate, and expert skill levels. Each level requires development of new knowledge and skills across broad realms. There is evidence that leadership skills can be enhanced with specific training, but there is an extremely wide variety of training programs in the literature, including duration (hours, days, months), method of delivery (workshop, seminar), and types of activities (coaching, role-playing; Martin et al. 2021). Therefore, a single leadership development strategy has yet to emerge as the model for future programs.

Development programs can be gauged in their efficacy on four outcomes: student response, student content knowledge, student application, and organization-wide results. The student response is how the student responds to the program: do they find it enjoyable, useful, etc. Student content knowledge is how much information about the topic (e.g., conflict resolution) the student acquires. Student application is how well the student can apply the principles to actual situations. Organization-wide results include outcomes like profits, turnover, etc.

Student responses are commonly very positive for leadership development programs (Reyes et al. 2019). Students in HE learning development programs tend to have good improvements on their content knowledge, but less improvement in their application of the knowledge (Reyes et al. 2019). The method of delivery and if the program was in-person or online did not significantly impact student outcomes, implying that any leadership development can be effective (Reyes et al. 2019).

In veterinary medicine, one description of a leadership program used a series of four one-day modules, workshops, lunchtime seminars, and a leadership library (Lloyd et al. 2008). Numerous leadership development programs have been used in veterinary medicine, including the AAVMC's Leadership Academy and PennVet Wharton (Lloyd et al. 2019b). The most common topics taught, according to participants, were general leadership training, conflict and mediation, personal assessment and self-reflection, financial topics, and hands-on experience with a leadership team. One publication that described teaching veterinary students leadership included developing skills in stress management, goal setting, conflict resolution, and giving and receiving feedback; participation in this program was associated with slightly lower stress scores and no difference in academic performance (Moore et al. 2007).

Part 3: Influence of the Hidden Curriculum

The hidden curriculum is what students learn from their experiences outside of the formal curriculum (e.g., classrooms and clinical rotations). The behavior of staff and faculty, assessment systems, institutional structure and rules, and student relationships all contribute to the hidden curriculum (Roder and May 2017). Although veterinary faculty tend to agree about the importance of teaching nontechnical competencies, including leadership, inclusion of leadership in the formal curriculum is often lacking (Lane and Bogue 2010). Faculty may assume that students will "pick it up," so do not need specific training in leadership skills. In fact, as has been mentioned, students do not passively improve as leaders without specific intervention (Verrinder and Phillips 2015; Crowley et al. 2019).

Relying on the hidden curriculum is not only ineffective, but it may be detrimental. Veterinary students have identified that the information they receive about professional skills is often a "do as I say not as I do," and observe that faculty and staff violate professional rules (Roder and May 2017). Without a specific leadership development curriculum, it is difficult to know what messages students receive about leadership. An explicit curriculum, with clearly articulated goals

and learning objectives, would minimize the influence of the hidden curriculum on veterinary leadership training.

Part 4: Incorporating Leadership into the Veterinary Curriculum

Making leadership training an explicit part of the veterinary curriculum requires faculty motivation and administration participation. The content must be selected and topics including communication, conflict resolution, self-reflection skills, developing and maintaining integrity, interpersonal relationships, and emotional intelligence are universally helpful for leaders in HE (Bryman 2007). Goals must be determined, ideally within the AAVMC's Competency-Based Veterinary Education (CBVE) framework. Many CBVE competencies draw on skills that should be a part of leadership development (Table 22.1). The content must be designed to achieve the stated goals and a variety of educational delivery methods are appropriate for teaching leadership. It can be tempting to put leadership along with professionalism and communication all in a single course, but that approach may lead to a lack of focus and to students viewing these topics as siloed, rather than connecting. Integrating leadership topics throughout the curriculum, intentionally and with faculty direction, ensures that students continue to improve their competency with leadership skills as they progress through the curriculum (Reyes et al. 2019).

The limitation in the veterinary school curriculum is often how to find the time to insert new content. Making sure that faculty believe in the importance of leadership is essential so that the time can be justified in the curriculum. Individual lectures, a series of lectures, a core course, and/or elective courses can be included in the curriculum to teach leadership topics.

Using effective leadership skills when seeking to modify the curriculum should result in improved outcomes. Faculty often express the desire for processes to be fair and legitimate (Gallos and Bolman 2021). To effect curriculum change, a leader should be open to feedback about the proposal, provide ample time for faculty to discuss, make changes in response to feedback, and repeat those steps as needed. Leaders seeking to make curricular changes should embrace the principles of patience, process, and persistence. Patience acknowledges that changes in academia often move at a very slow pace. Leaders use the process to ensure that the decision-making process is bolstered by the culture and history of the institution. Persistence is essential, as initiatives and programs come and go. The leader seeking actual change will need to demonstrate that this curricular change is important enough to persist in the face of challenges.

Table 22.1 Relationship between competency-based veterinary education competencies and opportunities for leadership development.

Competency number	Competency description	Leadership connection
1.1	Gathers and assimilates relevant information about animals	X
1.2	Synthesizes and prioritizes problems to arrive at differential diagnoses	
1.3	Creates and adjusts a diagnostic and/or treatment plan based on available evidence	
1.4	Incorporates animal welfare, client expectations, and economic considerations into the diagnostic or treatment plan	X
1.5	Prioritizes situational urgency and allocates resources	
1.6	Adapts knowledge to varied scenarios and contexts	X
1.7	Recognizes limitations of knowledge, skill and resources, and consults as needed	X
2.1	Performs veterinary procedures and postprocedural care	
2.2	Promotes comprehensive wellness and preventive care	
3.1	Applies population management principles in compliance with legal regulations and economic realities	X
3.2	Recommends and evaluates protocols for biosecurity	X
3.3	Advises stakeholders on practices that promote animal welfare	X
4.1	Recognizes zoonotic diseases and responds accordingly	
4.2	Promotes the health and safety of people and the environment	X
5.1	Listens attentively and communicates professionally	X
5.2	Adapts communication style to colleagues and clients	X
5.3	Prepares documentation appropriate for the intended audience	X
6.1	Solicits, respects, and integrates contributions from others	X
6.2	Functions as leader or team member based on experience, skills, and context	X
6.3	Maintains ongoing relationship to provide continuity of collaborative effort	X
6.4	Demonstrates inclusivity and cultural competence	X
7.1	Adopts an ethical approach to meeting professional obligations	X
7.2	Practices time management	X
7.3	Reflects on personal actions	X
7.4	Engages in self-directed learning and career planning	X
7.5	Attends to well-being of self and others	X
8.1	Weighs economic factors in personal and business decision-making	X
8.2	Delivers veterinary services compliant with legal and regulatory requirements	X
8.3	Advocates for the health and safety of patients, clients, and members of the team within the workplace	X
9.1	Evaluates health-related information	
9.2	Integrates, adapts, and applies knowledge and skills	X
9.3	Disseminates knowledge and practices to stakeholders	X

Part 5: Training Veterinarians to Be Leaders in the Profession

Leadership development for veterinary professionals can, and should, take place at multiple stages throughout their professional development. Programs launched for incoming students before they begin veterinary school, classes and programs throughout veterinary school, deliberate instruction for house officers (interns and residents), CE programs for practicing veterinarians, and faculty leadership development programs can all be employed to elevate the profession's leadership competency. The faculty presenting these topics must have a level of expertise, so faculty development may need to take place before leadership development can be extended to students. Some suggestions are provided below for learning activities aimed at veterinary professionals at different professional stages.

Part 6: Veterinary Students

A detailed description of a leadership program administered to students immediately before they begin their first year of veterinary school has been published by Moore and Klingborg (2001). Their program is five days long and looked to teach communication, openness, self-confidence, moving vision into action, courage, knowledge of issue complexity, and integrity. Lectures may provide foundational knowledge for students (e.g., basic concepts, definitions) but active learning, small group work, and role-playing exercise are preferable for students to practice skills and develop competency (Verrinder and Phillips 2015; Crowley et al. 2019).

Applying CBVE principles, in the first year, veterinary students may be introduced to leadership concepts, principles, and definitions. In the second and third years, they may engage in active learning exercises where they apply those principles to a variety of situations (e.g., conflict with a peer, solving a clinic system problem, and communicating a decision to employees). Based on the author's experience, in the clinical year, students are rarely evaluated on "leadership;" instead, it is often included under a broader topic of "professionalism." An important educational principle is that which is assessed is what students will focus on, so adding a separate assessment for leadership would encourage students to think about and practice improving their leadership skills (Roder and May 2017). Making expectations for leadership clear, including ethical behavior, self-reflection, and positive communication, will guide students in their development.

In addition to assessing leadership, simple activities can be added to the clinical year experience to expand leadership skills. Communication rounds, where students are encouraged to reflect on their communication and seek peer feedback, have been shown to be particularly effective for senior students (Meehan and Menniti 2014). When debriefing a case, the faculty can ask the student to reflect, and can also discuss nonmedical aspects of the case that may facilitate leadership development skills (e.g., managing conflict with a client).

A leadership project, which could be completed at the student's leisure, may be an effective way for students to reflect on their experiences in the context of leadership development (Jacobs et al. 2020). Opportunities to teach or reinforce leadership concepts also abound during clinical rotations if faculty are intentional in identifying those opportunities and making use of them.

Part 7: House Officers

Although some programs provide formal classes for house officers, training for interns and residents is expected to be primarily clinical in nature and dealing with direct patient care. However, there are opportunities to introduce leadership development of house officers beginning with orientation. It should be part of a required curriculum, but could also be presented as optional after-hours sessions and/or be incorporated into clinical training and teaching. Sessions presented during orientation should include foundational knowledge since the level of training in leadership among incoming house officers is inconsistent. Expectations for integrity and ethical behavior should be made explicit at the start of training. Too often, faculty rely on the hidden curriculum to teach these elements of leadership, which is ineffective (Roder and May 2017). Basic communication skills training, including how to handle conflict with their supervisors and clients, is also valuable.

Many house officer programs have weekly topics sessions, and leadership topics could be included throughout, such as on a quarterly basis. After-hours sessions, ideally where an incentive (e.g., a meal) is provided, would allow for delivery of leadership topics without crowding out other content. Overworked house officers may be disinclined to participate frequently in such activities, however, so incorporating leadership development into clinical training is likely to be the most effective and natural way to deliver such content. As with clinical veterinary students, clear expectations for leadership, making sure leadership is assessed, and including leadership topics in rounds and case discussions can all be used to develop house officers' leadership skills.

Part 8: Practicing Veterinarians

Most practicing veterinarians must participate in CE for license maintenance. Although most CE programs focus on lecture-based content delivery, some have workshops or laboratory opportunities where participants can have hands-on experience in developing leadership skills. The busy veterinarian must seek out those leadership CE experiences, potentially spending less time on medical topics. Unfortunately, veterinarians may not realize their important leadership roles, unless they are in a position of authority (Pearson et al. 2018). If leadership is emphasized in the veterinary curriculum, one would anticipate that more graduates will realize the importance of this skill. Intensive leadership development opportunities, such as the Veterinary Leadership Experience, are also available and have been shown to improve leadership skills up to one year after the program (Crowley et al. 2019).

Designing CE programs for leadership development must assume that the audience has a broad range of knowledge and experience with leadership, so foundational principles and definitions should be provided. Similar to teaching veterinary students, active learning and small group teaching should be used to practice leadership skills. Given the oft-limited time for CE content, limiting the content to a single aspect of leadership, such as conflict management, may be better than trying to cover a wide variety of leadership topics.

Part 9: Faculty Members

The foundation of all leadership development efforts must begin with the educators, who themselves must be trained in how to teach leadership (Lloyd et al. 2008). Veterinary faculty have expressed significant interest in leadership development (Lloyd et al. 2019b). The specific leadership topics of most interest were leading change, strategic thinking, leading teams, and leading without authority (Lloyd et al. 2019b). Faculty also indicated an interest in online development programs. One program in veterinary medicine described several key considerations for leadership development. Some of these included the ideas that leaders must be involved in the effort to develop leadership, that leaders have to serve as models for the type of leadership they want to develop, and that leadership development is an ongoing process, which requires a culture of learning.

External programs, such as the AAVMC Leadership Academy, are currently available to a select few individuals each year for faculty leadership development. Internal programs can be designed within each institution. Designing a leadership program should begin with a needs assessment, where faculty indicate what they believe their needs are for development and the faculty's preferred methods of content delivery (e.g., time of day, day of the week, and duration of sessions). Content should be delivered by individuals whom the faculty perceive as being competent and authoritative with the topics presented (McKenna et al. 2004). Faculty leadership development should be a continuous and iterative process, so new and existing faculty members can continue to enhance their skills.

Summary

Four-star Admiral William McRaven, after leaving his position as Chancellor of the University of Texas system after only three years, said, "The toughest job in the nation is the one of an academic- or health-institution president." Leadership in HE has numerous challenges that make it distinct from other domains of leadership. Leadership in veterinary medicine is further distinct because of the resources available in veterinary medicine, the number and nature of applicants for faculty and leadership positions, and the clinical responsibilities of faculty educators. Being an effective leader is challenging, but it is a skill that can be learned and practiced. Veterinary students, house officers, practicing clinicians, and faculty would all benefit from training in leadership skills.

References

Adin, D.B., Royal, K.D., and Adin, C.A. (2020). Cross-sectional assessment of the emotional intelligence of fourth-year veterinary students and veterinary house officers in a teaching hospital. *Journal of Veterinary Medical Educatuion* 47 (2): 193–201. https://doi.org/10.3138/jvme.0518-065r. Epub 2019 Jun 13. PMID: 31194633.

American Association of Veterinary Medical Colleges (2021). Annual data report 2020–2021 [internet]. Washington, DC. https://www.aavmc.org/about-aavmc/public-data (accessed 08 July 2022).

Bateh, J. and Heyliger, W. (2014). Academic administrator leadership styles and the impact on faculty job satisfaction. *Journal of Leadership Education* 13: 34–49. https://doi.org/10.12806/V13/I3/RF3.

Bennis, W.G. and Thomas, R.J. (2002). Crucibles of leadership. *Harvard Business Review* 80 (9): 39–45. PMID: 12227145.

Berghout, M.A., Fabbricotti, I.N., Buljac-Samardžić, M., and Hilders, C.G.J.M. (2017). Medical leaders or masters?-a systematic review of medical leadership in hospital settings. *PLoS One* 12 (9): e0184522. https://doi.org/10.1371/journal.pone.0184522. PMID: 28910335; PMCID: PMC5598981.

Bryman, A. (2007). Effective leadership in higher education: a literature review. *Studies in Higher Education* 32 (6): 693–710. https://doi.org/10.1080/03075070701685114.

Calhoun, J.G., Dollett, L., Sinioris, M.E. et al. (2008). Development of an interprofessional competency model for healthcare leadership. *Journal of Healthcare Management* 53 (6): 375–389; discussion 390–391. PMID: 19070333.

Clark, B.R. (1983). *The Higher Education System: Academic Organization in Cross-National Perspective*, 1e. Berkeley, CA: University of California Press.

Crowley, S.L., Homan, K.J., Rogers, K.S. et al. (2019). Measurement of leadership skills development among veterinary students and veterinary professionals participating in an experiential leadership program (the Veterinary Leadership Experience). *Journal of the American Veterinary Medical Association* 255 (10): 1167–1173. https://doi.org/10.2460/javma.255.10.1167. PMID: 31687900.

Day, D.V., Fleenor, J.W., Atwater, L.E. et al. (2014). Advances in leader and leadership development: a review of 25 years of research and theory. *The Leadership Quarterly* 25: 63–82.

Devine, R., Holmes, R.M., and Wang, G. (2021). Do executives' aesthetic attributes matter to career and organizational outcomes? A critical review and theoretical integration. *The Leadership Quarterly* 32 (1): 1–28.

Eagly, A.H. (2005). Achieving relational authenticity in leadership: does gender matter? *The Leadership Quarterly* 16 (3): 459–474.

Gallos, J.V. and Bolman, L.G. (2021). *Reframing Academic Leadership*, 2e. Hoboken , NJ: Jossey-Bass.

Gardner, W.L., Cogliser, C.C., Davis, K.M., and Dickens, M.P. (2011). Authentic leadership: a review of the literature and research agenda. *The Leadership Quarterly* 22 (6): 1120–1145.

Gündemir, S., Homan, A.C., de Dreu, C.K., and van Vugt, M. (2014). Think leader, think White? Capturing and weakening an implicit pro-White leadership bias. *PLoS One* 9 (1): e83915. https://doi.org/10.1371/journal.pone.0083915. PMID: 24416181; PMCID: PMC3885528.

Haden, N.K., Chaddock, M., Hoffsis, G.F. et al. (2010). Knowledge, skills, and attitudes of veterinary college deans: AAVMC survey of deans in 2010. *Journal of Veterinary Medical Education* 7 (3): 210–219. https://doi.org/10.3138/jvme.37.3.210. Erratum in: J Vet Med Educ. 2010 Winter;37(4):316. PMID: 20847329.

Hargett, C.W., Doty, J.P., Hauck, J.N. et al. (2017). Developing a model for effective leadership in healthcare: a concept mapping approach. *Journal of Healthcare Leadership* 28 (9): 69–78. https://doi.org/10.2147/JHL.S141664. PMID: 29355249; PMCID: PMC5774455.

Holtz, B.C. and Hu, B. (2017). Passive leadership: relationships with trust and justice perceptions. *Journal of Managerial Psychology* 32 (1): 119–130. https://doi.org/10.1108/JMP-02-2016-0029.

Jacobs, K.G., Kugler, J., Chi, J. et al. (2020). A mixed methods approach to understanding curricular impact of a capstone course on the self-efficacy of fourth-year medical students. *Cureus* 12 (8): e9537. https://doi.org/10.7759/cureus.9537. PMID: 32905172; PMCID: PMC7465827.

Jochemsen-van der Leeuw, H.G., van Dijk, N., van Etten-Jamaludin, F.S., and Wieringa-de Waard, M. (2013). The attributes of the clinical trainer as a role model: a

systematic review. *Academic Medicine* 88 (1): 26–34. https://doi.org/10.1097/ACM.0b013e318276d070. PMID:23165277.

Kezar, A., DePaola, T., and Scott, D.T. (2019). The gig academy: mapping labor in the neoliberal university. In: *Reforming Higher Education: Innovation and the Public Good*, 1e. Baltimore, MD: Johns Hopkins University Press.

Kohn, A. (1993). *Punished by Rewards. The Trouble with Gold Stars, Incentive Plans, as, Praise, and Other Bribes*, 1e. Boston, MA: Houghton Mifflin Company.

Lane, I.F. and Bogue, E.G. (2010). Faculty perspectives regarding the importance and place of nontechnical competencies in veterinary medical education at five North American colleges of veterinary medicine. *Journal of the American Veterinary Medical Association* 237 (1): 53–64. https://doi.org/10.2460/javma.237.1.53. . PMID: 20590495.

Lloyd, J.W., Stone, D.J., and King, L.J. (2008). Developing veterinary colleges and leaders: a whole-system approach. *Journal of Veterinary Medical Education* 35 (1): 138–144. https://doi.org/10.3138/jvme.35.1.138. PMID: 18339968.

Lloyd, J.W., Cantner, C.A., Mariani, V. et al. (2019a). *AAVMC Academic Administrator Leadership Development Needs Assessment – 2019*. American Association of Veterinary Medical Colleges.

Lloyd, J.W., Cantner, C.A., Mariani, V. et al. (2019b). *AAVMC Faculty Development Needs Assessment – 2019*. American Association of Veterinary Medical Colleges.

Lumby, J. (2012). *What Do we Know about Leadership in Higher Education? The Leadership Foundation for Higher Education's research*. Leadership Foundation for Higher Education.

Martin, R., Hughes, D.J., Epitropaki, O., and Thomas, G. (2021). In pursuit of causality in leadership training research: a review and pragmatic recommendations. *TheLeadership Quarterly* 32 (5): 101375.

McCaffery, P. (2010). *The Higher Education Manager's Handbook*, 2e. NY: Routledge.

McKenna, M.K., Gartland, M.P., and Pugno, P.A. (2004). Development of physician leadership competencies: perceptions of physician leaders, physician educators and medical students. *Journal of Health Administration Education* 21 (3): 343–354. PMID: 15379370.

McNay, I. (1995). From the collegial academy to corporate enterprise: the changing culture of universities. In: *TheChanging University?* (ed. T. Schuller), 105–115. Buckingham, UK: SRHE and OUP.

Meehan, M.P. and Menniti, M.F. (2014). Final-year veterinary students' perceptions of their communication competencies and a communication skills training program delivered in a primary care setting and based on Kolb's Experiential Learning Theory. *Journal of Veterinary Medical Education* 41 (4): 371–383. https://doi.org/10.3138/jvme.1213-162R1. PMID: 25148880.

Moore, D.A. and Klingborg, D.J. (2001). Development and evaluation of a leadership program for veterinary students. *Journal of Veterinary Medical Education* 28 (1): 10–15. https://doi.org/10.3138/jvme.28.1.10. PMID: 11548769.

Moore, D.A., Truscott, M.L., St. Clair, L., and Klingborg, D.J. (2007). Effects of a veterinary student leadership program on measures of stress and academic performance. *Journal of Veterinary Medical Education* 34 (2): 112–121. https://doi.org/10.3138/jvme.34.2.112. PMID: 17446636.

Muller-Kahle, M.I. and Schiehll, E. (2013). Gaining the ultimate power edge: women in the dual role of CEO and Chair. *The Leadership Quarterly* 24 (5): 666–679.

Norton, M.S. (2015). *The Changing Landscape of School Leadership: Recalibrating the School Principalship*, 1e. Lanham: Rowman & Littlefield Publishers.

Pearson, C.E., Butler, A.J., and Murray, Y.P. (2018). Understanding veterinary leadership in practice. *Veterinary Record* 182 (16): 460. https://doi.org/10.1136/vr.104485. Epub 2018 Feb 14. PMID: 29445011.

Perryman, A.A., Fernando, G.D., and Tripathy, A. (2016). Do gender differences persist? An examination of gender diversity on firm performance, risk, and executive compensation. *Journal of Business Research* 69 (2): 579–586. https://doi.org/10.1016/j.jbusres.2015.05.013.

Pun, J.K.H. (2020). An integrated review of the role of communication in veterinary clinical practice. *BMC Veterinary Research* 16 (1): 394. https://doi.org/10.1186/s12917-020-02558-2. PMID: 33076917; PMCID: PMC7569566.

Reyes, D.L., Dinh, J., Lacerenza, C.N. et al. (2019). The state of higher education leadership development program evaluation: a meta-analysis, critical review, and recommendations. *The Leadership Quarterly* 30: https://doi.org/10.1016/j.leaqua.2019.101311.

Roder, C.A. and May, S.A. (2017). The hidden curriculum of veterinary education: mediators and moderators of its effects. *Journal of Veterinary Medical Education* 44 (3): 542–551. https://doi.org/10.3138/jvme.0416-082. . PMID: 28876989.

Spendlove, M. (2007). Competencies for effective leadership in higher education. *International Journal of Educational Management* 21: 407–417. https://doi.org/10.1108/09513540710760183.

Stone, A.G., Russell, R.F., and Patterson, K. (2004). Transformational versus servant leadership: a difference in leader focus. *The Leadership & Organization Development Journal* 25 (4): 349–361.

Verrinder, J.M. and Phillips, C.J. (2015). Assessing veterinary and animal science students' moral judgment development on animal ethics issues. *Journal of Veterinary Medical Education* 42 (3): 206–216. https://doi.org/10.3138/jvme.0215-022R. Epub 2015 Jul 22. PMID: 26200702.

Wolfe, B. and Dilworth, P.P. (2015). Transitioning normalcy: organizational culture, African American administrators, and diversity leadership in higher education. *Review of Educational Research* 85 (4): 667–697. https://doi.org/10.3102/0034654314565667.

Zaccaro, S.J., Green, J.P., Dubrow, S., and Kolze, M. (2017). Leader individual differences, situational parameters, and leadership outcomes: a comprehensive review and integration. *The Leadership Quarterly* 29 (1): 2–43. https://doi.org/10.1016/j.leaqua.2017.10.003.

23

Accreditation: What It Is and Why It Is Important

Myrah Stockdale, MS (Educational Research Methods)
Campbell University College of Pharmacy and Health Sciences, Lillington, NC, USA

Malathi Raghavan, DVM, MS, PhD
Purdue University College of Veterinary Medicine, West Lafayette, IN, USA

Stacy L. Anderson, DVM, PhD, DACVS-LA
Lincoln Memorial University College of Veterinary Medicine, Harrogate, TN, USA

Section 1: Overview

Myrah Stockdale

Accreditation is a cyclical process of external review that institutions of higher education undergo to receive recognition (also known as accreditation) that their programs or curricula meet quality standards set by regional, national, or professional accrediting bodies (Keating 2015). Accreditation is also the status awarded following a successful accreditation process. Between external review cycles ongoing reporting and communication with accreditors is vital to maintaining an accreditation status. In the United States, colleges and universities seek institutional or national accreditation at the institutional level to establish value to consumers, validate quality standards, and qualify for federal financial aid. Professional programs such as Veterinary Medicine (AVMA-COE), Pharmacy (ACPE), and Nursing (CCNE) have specialized or professional (and sometimes called programmatic) accreditation bodies specific to their discipline. Specialized accreditation, which is voluntary, allows programs to demonstrate their academic quality, commitment to continuous quality improvement (CQI), and ability to meet rigorous discipline-specific standards necessary for entry-level competency.

For this reason, it is important for faculty, administrators, and program directors to understand their role in the accreditation process. In this section, readers will learn about the function and importance of accreditation and a brief history of accreditation within the United States.

Part 1: Definition of Terms

Accreditation – is both a status awarded for successfully completing an accreditation process (i.e., having accreditation or being accredited) and the evaluative process to determine if an institution or program meets acceptable criteria or standards as laid out by an accrediting body (i.e., undergoing an accreditation or accreditation review).

Standards of Accreditation/Accreditation Standards – a set of criteria for the evaluation and accreditation of an institution of program published by the accrediting body.

State Authorization – regulations established in 2010 but delayed until 2015 by the US Department of Education to enhance program integrity. The regulations apply to a university's compliance with individual statutes, regulations, and rules in each state in which it operates.

Gainful Employment – a metric established in 2014 by the US Department of Education to determine whether student debt is proportional to their relative earnings. Programs must demonstrate that the projected student loan payment will be less than 8% of total income. Programs sustaining a percentage of 12% or higher for two years are considered grounds for ineligibility for federal funds.

Part 2: What Is Accreditation?

Types of Accreditation

There are two primary types of accreditation for secondary or higher education – institutional and specialized (i.e., programmatic or professional). Institutional accreditation,

Educational Principles and Practice in Veterinary Medicine, First Edition. Edited by Katherine Fogelberg.
© 2024 John Wiley & Sons, Inc. Published 2024 by John Wiley & Sons, Inc.

as the name implies, encompasses the entire university or college. Institutional accreditors, in the United States, include both institutional and national accreditors (see Section 2 for more on this). A specialized accreditor accredits a particular program or school. To receive a specialized accreditation for a program, such as Veterinary Medicine, the institution must first be institutionally accredited. The process for institutional and specialized accreditors is parallel. Each establishes quality standards that are continually evaluated through accreditation cycles.

Part 3: Importance of Accreditation

Accreditation can impact an institution or programs' academic reputation, international rankings, research and innovation, funding, enrollment, quality of teaching, and graduate employability (Acevedo-De-los-Ríos and Rondinel-Oviedo 2022; Kumar et al. 2020). Federal loan and grant programs require that institutions meet institutional or national accreditation standards (more in Section 2) to receive federal funds. In the allied health sciences, professional accreditors, including Pharmacy, Nursing, and Social Work, indicate that successful program accreditation and professional licensure are strongly related (Dawn Apgar 2022). This should be unsurprising.

Professional programs are expected, by their specialized accreditors, to offer curricula and academic support that positively contributes to the necessary knowledge, skills, and attitudes (KSAs) needed to be professionally licensed. A veterinary medical student successfully completing an AVMA-COE accredited program should expect that they have been exposed to and assessed on the KSAs necessary to meet entry-level licensure expectations. The expectations from licensing boards are reciprocated. Most allied health science licensure boards, particularly in the United States, require that licensure candidates have educational credentials (e.g., degrees, certifications) from accredited institutions to sit for a licensure exam.

Further, specialized accreditors for allied health science programs have each accredited program annually update their websites with their first-time and/or overall pass rates for national licensure exams. Along with licensure pass rates, these accreditors require other important metrics (e.g., job placement at graduation, jurisprudence first-time pass rate, on-time graduation rate) to be updated and made publicly available. This provides transparency to program stakeholders (prospective students, current students, faculty, staff, etc.) on measures of quality that can be discerned between other accredited programs. Being accredited builds public trust, demonstrates commitment to CQI, and accountability to quality assurance.

Part 4: Accreditation Cycles

Academic or educational accreditation at its core is quality assurance. The term "accreditation" can be confusing as it describes both a process and a status. The process of accreditation is most often understood as the external review of a program or institution to determine if it meets predefined quality standards. While the accreditation process does include external review it also encompasses the self-study, official decision, and maintenance or ongoing monitoring. Section 3 of this chapter expands more on what to expect and how to prepare for self-study and the site visit. An accreditation status is the outcome of the accreditation process. Common accreditation statuses include: Intent to Apply, Accredited on Contingency, Probationary Accreditation, Full Accreditation, or Accredited (American Psychological Association n.d.; American Veterinary Medical Association 2022). All possible statuses are defined by an accrediting body. Accrediting bodies (or accreditors) are discussed extensively in Section 2 of this chapter.

Accreditation is not a one-time process or a fixed status, it is a cycle. The process is ongoing and iterative as programs and institutions are expected to demonstrate a commitment to CQI. An accreditation cycle (see Figure 23.1) typically has four sequential components: self-study, external review, status decision, and ongoing review.

Accreditation cycles are specified based on guidelines outlined by the accreditor in relation to accreditation status received. Full accreditations have the longest cycle (i.e., they require less frequent external reviews) while statuses less than full accreditation carry more frequent reporting or reviews to achieve full accreditation. For example, a program receiving a "probationary accreditation" status following an external review could be required to complete a focused self-study report and undergo a focused site visit within two years for the standard(s) that were deemed noncompliant. Following a successful focused review (i.e., all standards are deemed compliant), the program would receive a "full accreditation" status and would proceed with continual monitoring expectations (i.e., they would reenter the accreditation cycle). Once an institution or program receives an accreditation status, that status must be maintained via ongoing review or continued monitoring.

One noteworthy event sits outside of the accreditation cycle – the initial intention to seek accreditation. When an institution or program intends to seek initial accreditation, it submits an application to the accrediting body. The barriers to entry vary by accrediting body. Some accrediting bodies require formal training, completing a self-evaluation or readiness assessment, interviews, site visits, or other documentation to begin the formal process of seeking accreditation. The requirements to successfully apply for accreditation are outlined by each accreditor. This singular event sits adjacent to the cycle of accreditation as it is a one-time event that enters an institution or program into the cycle seen in Figure 23.1.

In the United States, academic accreditation is voluntary and conducted by nongovernmental accreditation bodies (see Section 2 for a more robust discussion) whereas internationally this varies. For example, Uganda has the Uganda National Council for Higher Education (UNCHE), a semi-autonomous government regulatory agency charged with licensing higher learning in the country (UNCHE 2022). Despite these differences, the steps in the accreditation cycles are similar.

Section 2: Abbreviated History of Accreditation in the United States

Myrah Stockdale

This section highlights events that shaped accreditation within the United States. This history is by no means exhaustive, nor is it complete. Accreditation in the United States continues to evolve and will no doubt look different in a decade's time.

Part 1: 1800s–1940s

While university accreditation processes are necessary to receive federal financial aid in the United States now, few know how accreditation began. Institutions of higher education developed voluntary accreditation membership associations in the late 1800s (Harcleroad 1980). These associations outlined peer-reviewed processes and standards for curricula, degrees, and transfer credits. Belonging to these associations allowed institutions to indicate they met quality standards. Until the 1940s, higher education accreditation in the United States remained unaffiliated with the federal government.

Part 2: 1940s–1960s

In 1944, following World War II, the United States passed the Servicemen's Readjustment Act (more commonly known as the G.I. Bill), which allocated federal funds to returning veterans for civilian education and training. Within five years of the G.I. Bill's passage, over 6000 for-profit schools emerged and applied for a portion of the billions allocated to service members' education and training (House Select Committee 1951). The often-predatory practices of those institutions prompted an investigation by the House Select Committee to Investigate Educational and

Table 23.1 Titles under the Higher Education Act (2020).

Title	Area covered
Title I	General Provisions
Title II	Teacher Quality Enhancement
Title III	Strengthening Institutions
Title IV	Student Assistance
Title V	Developing Institutions
Title VI	International Education Programs
Title VII	Graduate and Postsecondary Improvement Programs
Title VIII	Additional Programs

Training Program under GI Bill found that there were insufficient checks and balances to mitigate "bad actors" and to adequately protect students. Subsequently, the Veterans' Readjustment Assistance Act of 1952 was passed, which required schools receiving the GI Bill to be accredited (82nd Congress 1952). The Office of Education (now the US Department of Education) published a list of recognized accrediting agencies and outlined means for institutions that were not accredited to establish their legitimacy and successfully receive federal funds. Accreditation continued over the 1960s and 1970s to serve as the gatekeeper for federal funding.

Part 3: 1960s–1980s

The most notable expansions came in 1965 with the passage of the Higher Education Act (or HEA) and the National Vocational Student Loan Insurance Act (or NVSLIA). The HEA allowed all students seeking postsecondary education at accredited public and nonprofit institutions to access federal grants or loans. The HEA is organized under titles. As of 2020, the HEA is organized into the following eight titles (Table 23.1).

Similarly, the NVSLIA allowed students attending accredited trade schools and for-profit schools to access federal loans (but not grants). Both the HEA and NVSLIA were intended to increase the skilled workforce and create economic opportunity for Americans regardless of their familial wealth. The HEA was amended in 1972 to include Title IX (which prohibits discrimination based on sex in education programs and activities) and was reauthorized in 1980 and 1986 (Hannah 1996).

Part 4: 1980s–2000s

Leading up to the 1992 reauthorization of the HEA, concerns about high numbers of student loan defaults, illegitimate proprietary schools, and abuses of federal student loan programs made their way to Congress. Between 1983 and 1990, the total student loan volume doubled, and the number of loan defaults grew by more than 300% (Parsons 1997). These alarming statistics, along with wide-spread public scrutiny, led to the highly publicized "Nunn Hearings." The committee found that fraud and abuse were widespread throughout the for-profit college sector that contributed significantly to student loan inflation and student loan defaults (Permanent Subcommittee on Investigations of the Committee on Governmental Affairs 1991). The investigation laid out what later became amendments to the HEA that directly addressed loan and grant eligibility based on the length of program and quality indicators. Adding federal standards served to strengthen the role of accreditors. Accreditors were now required to evaluate the following common elements:

1) Program length, Degree/Credential offering, Tuition and fees, Credit hours to completion
2) Fiscal and Administrative Capacity/Scalability
3) Facilities and Equipment
4) Faculty and Staff
5) Curriculum
6) Recruiting, Advertising, and Admissions Practices
7) Student Support Services
8) Student Grievances
9) Grading, Policies, Catalogs
10) Measures of student success in relation to the mission, job placement, state licensing
11) Default rates on student loans.

Many of the 1992 amendments were reversed in 1998 as the House majority voted for less federal oversight in standards enforcement. Of note were the requirement for accreditors to review default rates (as well as to conduct their own investigations), and the requirement that accreditors check tuition and fees in relation to subject matter and program length were removed.

Continuing the trend of decreased oversight, HEA was amended further in 2008. During this period, the role of the federal government was reduced while the role of the institutional mission was increased. Accreditors were expected to measure institutions against quality standards with respect to the institutional mission. Alongside this amendment was another amendment that prohibited the Secretary of Education from establishing standards regarding the assessment of student achievement.

Part 5: 2010–2020s

Following the 2008 amendments, there was a notable shift in legislative tactics to protect access to federal student aid and decrease fraud. Rather than using accrediting bodies that were granted authority through the Department of Education, federal regulations were enacted. This created multiple accountability mechanisms.

The first was state authorization (State Authorization 2010). Authorization refers to the legal authority of an institution to operate within a state. This meant that institutions had to meet requirements of their state to be eligible for federal student aid. The second regulation was gainful employment. Under gainful employment, institutions must demonstrate that projected student loan payments will be less than 8% of a graduate's total income. Programs sustaining a percentage of 12% or higher for two years were considered grounds for ineligibility for federal funds. Keep in mind that these regulations did not remove accreditation requirements.

By 2012, a recurrent issue (seen in the 1950s, 1980s, and 1990s) emerged. Federal investigations exhibited drastically lower completion rates, higher student loan debt, and higher loan default rates in the for-profit sector. Due to concerns and language (or lack thereof) related to distance education, state authorization was delayed until 2015 and language related to distance education was not agreed upon until July 2020 (Student Assistance General Provisions 2022; Thompson et al. 2020).

In 2019, gainful employment was revoked. As of 2022, the regulation, as well as the verbiage related to the metric is being reconsidered. Issues of accountability, access, and equity are being discussed in relation to gainful employment.

Section 3: History of Accreditation in Veterinary Education

Malathi Raghavan

In 1863, around the time of establishment of an early version of the AVMA, then known as USVMA, veterinary medical practitioners were mostly uneducated or self-educated practitioners who called themselves farriers or veterinary surgeons (American Veterinary Medical Association n.d.). Therefore, a Committee on Intelligence and Education (CIE) was formed and in 1887 the association resolved to seek "uniform requirements for veterinary schooling and a standard graduation exam by a common examining board" (American Veterinary Medical Association n.d.). As early as 1913, membership in the AVMA required graduation from a three-year, accredited veterinary school. The Committee defined minimum educational standards known as the Essentials of an Approved Veterinary College, which the Association adopted in 1921. CIE was the early version of what we now know as the Council on Education and the Essentials of an Approved Veterinary College have, over the decades since, become the COE's Standards of Accreditation.

For AVMA-COE, the date of initial listing as a United States Department of Education (USDE) recognized accrediting agency was 1952 (AVMA 2022a). The COE was most recently reviewed for renewed recognition of the agency by AG staff and the National Advisory Committee on Institutional Quality and Integrity (NACIQI) in 2021. As it is on a five-year review cycle, 2026 is the date of the next scheduled review for renewal of recognition (USDE 2023a). USDE recognition (USDE 2023b) indicates that:

- The COE adopts policies and procedures that comply with the USDE-published guidelines of operation
- There are clearly documented standards of accreditation applied in a uniform, fair, and consistent manner to all veterinary programs seeking accreditation
- Students have access to reliable information
- Proper documentation of accreditation outcomes is overseen by the USDE in a timely manner.

All of this ensures buy-in from the public and peers in the veterinary and veterinary educational community.

In addition to being recognized by the USDE as a programmatic accreditor, the COE has also chosen voluntarily to be recognized by the Council for Higher Education Accreditor (CHEA 2023b), a nongovernmental organization that raises the bar on quality in the accreditation process (AVMA n.d.). While USDE's recognition of the COE offers students eligibility for receiving federal aid distributed under Title VII, CHEA's role can be described as additionally "accrediting the accreditor." Issues related to academic quality, best practices in accreditation, and continual improvement are the domains of CHEA's activity.

As the only accrediting body for programs leading to the DVM or VMD degree in the United States and Canada, accreditation by the COE is a requirement for veterinary students' eligibility to register for the North American Veterinary Licensing Examination (NAVLE). Successful NAVLE completion is a prerequisite for veterinary licensure and is required of an individual practitioner by all licensing bodies in the United States and Canada. For this reason, colleges of veterinary medicine in the United States and Canada voluntarily seek and maintain COE accreditation.

The college's accreditation status influences the college choice of prospective students' and their parents, who desire reasonable reassurance that a typical graduate of the accredited program will have the ability to register for the licensing exam, be in a position to be hired by employers, and be eligible to be recognized by state or provincial veterinary licensing boards. In addition, graduates of accredited schools are eligible to enter clinical training programs, such as residency programs, without further training toward educational equivalency (EE) qualifications. Accreditation by the COE also reassures employers that the quality of graduates will have entry-level competency in the practice of veterinary medicine in the United States and Canada. Last but not least, there is reasonable assurance that the public is protected from inadequately prepared graduates of an educational program.

Section 4: Accrediting Bodies

Part 1: Introduction

Myrah Stockdale

While accreditation is both a process and a status, accrediting bodies are the third-party organizations that outline accreditation processes, conduct evaluations, and award accreditation statuses. In the United States, the USDE does not directly accredit programs and institutions. Rather, the USDE has a process for approving and publishing reliable accrediting agencies. Only institutions that undergo accreditation with federally recognized accrediting bodies can receive federal funding. Accrediting bodies, just like institutions of higher education, undergo periodic reviews by the NACIQI, a joint committee. This section will expand on the varied role of accrediting bodies and discuss international accreditation. It will also expand Veterinary Medicine accreditation around the globe.

Part 2: Accrediting Agencies

Malathi Raghavan

Accrediting agencies carry out their authorized responsibility in two primary ways: (i) They develop meaningful evaluation criteria, and (ii) They conduct peer evaluations to assess whether those criteria are met by institutions that voluntarily seek accreditation. Additionally, the culture of accreditation promotes an environment of constant quality improvement. The authorized agencies belong to one of three types of accrediting agencies – regional, national, or programmatic (Council for Higher Education Accreditation 2023a). Currently, the labels "regional" and "national" accreditors are being phased out in favor of just institutional accreditors (Table 23.2).

Institutional accreditors are those who were previously known as regional and national accreditors.

Regional accrediting agencies: All regional accrediting commissions review and grant accreditation to academically oriented, nonprofit, or state-owned institutions of higher education. They review entire institutions and not just colleges or programs. There are seven in all and they historically tended to operate in specific regions inside the United States. For example, the Middle States Commission on Higher Education (MSCHE) accredits Carnegie Mellon University and Cornell University and University

Table 23.2 Institutional Accreditors in the United States.

Institutional Accreditation Agency
Middle States Commission on Higher Education (MSCHE)
New England Association of Schools and Colleges (NEASC)
Northwest Commission on Colleges and Universities (NWCCU)
Higher Learning Commission (HLC)
Southern Association of Colleges and Schools (SACSCOC)
Western Association of Schools and Colleges (WASC)
Accrediting Commission for Community and Junior Colleges (ACCJC) Western Association of Schools and Colleges

of Maryland, College Park, among others in a geographic region that includes Delaware, the District of Columbia, Maryland, New Jersey, New York, Pennsylvania, Puerto Rico, and the Virgin Islands. In 2020, however, the USDE removed the limitation on regional accreditors' geographic scope. And so, while we still refer to a type of accrediting agencies as "regional" they are more rightly thought of as institutional accrediting agencies with national scope. Geographic area of accrediting activities of MSCHE currently extends throughout the United States. Accreditation by these accrediting agencies is required to qualify for federal financial aid programs authorized under Title IV of the Higher Education Act (HEA).

National accrediting agencies: National accrediting agencies generally offer accreditation to schools or proprietary institutions that focus on vocational (career-based) or religious education. They operate across the entire country. One example of this type of agency is the Accrediting Commission of Career Schools and Colleges, which accredits the South Texas Vocational Technical Institute in Corpus Christi, TX, the Merryfield School of Pet Grooming in Ft. Lauderdale, FL, and the Aviation Institute of Maintenance in Teterboro, NJ.

Programmatic accrediting agencies or specialized accrediting agencies: These entities operate nationwide and review specific departments or programs in a particular field of study and demonstrate that the department or program meets established standards for that specific field of study. The AVMA-COE is an example of a programmatic accrediting agency, as is the Liaison Committee for Medical Education (LCME). The scope of the AVMA-COE is in the granting of accreditation and pre-accreditation ("Provisional Accreditation") of programs leading to professional degrees (DVM or VMD) in veterinary medicine in the United States. LCME is the accrediting body of educational programs leading to the MD and DO degrees.

Programmatic accrediting agencies use an accreditation procedure and standards that are created and streamlined

specifically for evaluating the quality of a program in a specific field of study, such as medicine (accrediting agency: LCME), dental (CODA), law (ABA), architecture (NAAB), pharmacy (ACPE), and veterinary medicine (COE). Most often by design, the institution that offers a specific program, like those leading to a veterinary degree, is accredited not only by the programmatic accrediting agency (COE) but also by an institutional accrediting agency (e.g., MSC). That is, more than one level of accreditation exists and is required for eligibility for USDE funds and loans for students. COE accreditation, although necessary for licensure eligibility, does not qualify the program to distribute federal financial assistance programs authorized under Title IV of the HEA. Accordingly, an accreditation standard of the AVMA-COE stipulates that the program is to be situated in and offered by a regionally accredited institution, such as a sponsoring university.

Part 3: Recognition of Accreditation Agencies

Recognition as a USDE-authorized accrediting agency is voluntarily sought by institutional accreditors, whether regional/institutional, national/vocational, or programmatic. To be recognized by the USDE as reliable authorities on the quality of education offered by individual institutions, all accrediting agencies must meet the criteria for recognition defined by the USDE (2023b). Key requirements to be met by accrediting agencies include:

Applying consistently and enforcing standards that ensure the education programs offered are of sufficient quality to meet the stated objective for which they are offered;

Using review standards that assess student achievement in relation to the institution's mission, including, as applicable, course completion, passing of state licensing examinations, and job placement rates;

Evaluating an institution's or program's curricula, faculty, facilities, and fiscal and administrative capacity; and

Meeting required operating and due process procedures with respect to the institutions and programs they accredit (Congressional Research Service 2022).

It is also a basic USDE requirement for an accrediting agency to demonstrate that its standards, policies, procedures, and decisions to grant or deny accreditation are widely accepted in the United States by educators and educational institutions (i.e., peers) as well as licensing bodies, practitioners, and employers in the field for which programs prepare their students.

Accrediting agencies undergo periodic reviews by the USDE Accreditation Group (AG) staff and the NACIQI. Public comments are sought by AG and NACIQI around the time of review of the accrediting agency. Once recommended by both AG staff and NACIQI, a senior

USDE official designated by the Secretary of Education makes the final decision regarding recognition or continued recognition of the accrediting agency (Congressional Research Service 2022).

Section 5: International Accreditation

Malathi Raghavan

With increasing globalization, accreditation also helps market an educational program to an international community of prospective students who are looking for reputable educational programs. An international college's accreditation status may influence a prospective student when determining which program they will attend, whether hailing from the United States, Canada, or elsewhere, because accreditation guarantees entry-level competency upon graduation in veterinary medicine as defined by the COE. Graduates of COE-accredited international schools also have the eligibility to enter postgraduate clinical training programs, (e.g., residency programs) without earning EE qualifications that graduates of non-COE accredited programs are required to earn. These are some reasons why COE accreditation is voluntarily sought by veterinary medical programs that are offered outside of the United States and Canada.

Take, for example, the Royal Veterinary College (RVC) in London, United Kingdom. It already holds accreditations from the Royal College of Veterinary Surgeons (RCVS) in the United Kingdom and from the European Association of Establishments for Veterinary Education (EAEVE), ensuring that RVC graduates are recognized as competent in the United Kingdom, Ireland, Australia, and New Zealand in addition to being recognized as meeting agreed upon and acceptable standards in Europe. In 1998, the college also received COE accreditation for the first time. It is not necessary for British and European students to graduate from a COE-accredited school if they expect to practice in the United Kingdom, Ireland, Australia, or New Zealand. However, since 1998, graduates of the RVC are also eligible to practice veterinary medicine in the United States or Canada as long as they comply with the state or provincial licensing requirements and immigration laws of either of these two destination countries. More importantly, graduates of COE-accredited schools in the United States and Canada are seen as having met the same educational standards as graduates of the AVMA-COE accredited school in the United Kingdom. Therefore, the United Kingdom must also apply the same licensing procedures and requirements to graduates of COE-accredited US and Canadian schools wishing to practice in the United Kingdom.

This mutually beneficial opportunity is underscored through a reciprocity agreement that exists between the AVMA and all foreign countries that have at least one AVMA-accredited veterinary school in that country, irrespective of the role of other local accrediting agencies or governmental oversight operating in that country (AVMA n.d.). This is one of the many benefits conferred by the COE on graduates of COE-accredited schools in the United States and Canada: the ability to work as a veterinarian in those countries where there is at least one COE-accredited veterinary program. In addition, prospective US and Canadian students have the option to study veterinary medicine in a COE-accredited program in another country and be eligible to register for the NAVLE and apply for licensure back home in the United States or Canada. As of 2022, 17 programs are accredited by the COE outside of the 33 programs in United States and five in Canada: four in Australia, three in the United Kingdom, two in Scotland, one in France, one in Ireland, one in Mexico, one in The Netherlands, one in New Zealand, one in Korea, and two in the West Indies (AVMA 2022b.)

The COE, sponsored by the AVMA, is an autonomous council of 20 voluntary members. Although it is situated within the AVMA, financed partially by the AVMA and partly supported by staff from the AVMA, there is a firewall between the COE and the Board of Directors of the AVMA. All COE decisions are independent and devoid of any potential conflicts of interest on the part of the AVMA (n.d.).

Membership in the COE consists of 17 veterinarians representing academia, research, private practice, large animal and small animal focus areas, public health professionals, non-private practice, nonacademic veterinarians (e.g., industry), and three members of the public. Eight of the 17 members are selected by the AVMA COE Selection Committee. Another eight members are selected by the AAVMC COE Selection Committee and one by the Canadian Veterinary Medical Association (CVMA). The COE itself appoints three public members to complete its roster of 20. One of the AAVMC-appointed members serves as an official representative of the AAVMC and the CVMA-appointed Canadian veterinarian officially represents the CVMA. The official AAVMC representative and the members selected by the AAVMC COE Selection Committee are funded by the AAVMC. The CVMA-appointed veterinarian is funded by the CVMA.

Only the CVMA is given a seat in the COE and, by extension, only Canada is invited to take part in the accreditation process of US (and Canadian) veterinary colleges. This is because the COE (as was its predecessor) is the authorized accrediting agency for veterinary medical education in Canada since 1921 (Banasiak 2012). The Canadian member represents the needs and interests of the CVMA and Canada, whose evolution of veterinary medical education and history of the profession are closely tied with that of the United States.

Although individual institutions in Mexico, Europe, Australia, and New Zealand voluntarily seek accreditation by the COE, unlike the situation in Canada, COE accreditation of veterinary programs is not required by the governments or licensing bodies of those countries, although it is recognized and accepted. In turn, from the American practitioner's point of view, there may be very little justification to invite to the table a representative from veterinary medical education systems and practice environments that are vastly different than those in the United States and Canada. The USDE or the US veterinary community may not see them as peer reviewers, as the COE accreditation process is built on a detailed peer-based assessment of compliance with standards for educational quality. These may be reasons why COE membership is not extended to those situated outside of the United States or Canada.

The COE is structured somewhat similar to the programmatic accreditor for programs conferring the Medical Doctor, or M.D., degree, the Liaison Committee for Medical Education (LCME; Liaison Committee on Medical Education 2023). Major similarities and differences are outlined in Table 23.3.

Table 23.3 History, Structure, Function of the Council on Education (COE) and the Liaison Committee for Medical Education (LCME): A Comparative Study.

	Council on Education	Liaison Committee for Medical Education
Accredits institutions granting:	DVM/VMD or equivalent degree	MD degree
Accreditation of distributive model schools:	Yes	Yes
Degree from accredited college gives student:	Prerequisite to register for NAVLE; degree recognized by state licensing authorities; eligibility for clinical residency programs	Prerequisite to register for USMLE step examinations; degree recognized by state licensing authorities; eligibility for clinical residency programs approved by ACGME
Year of establishment	1946	1942
Membership	20 volunteers (including 3 public members) No students	21 volunteers (including 2 public members) Two medical students
Members selected by	AVMA COE selection committee (8 professional members) AAVMC COE selection committee (8 professional members) CVMA (1 professional member) COE (3 public members)	AMA (8 professional members +1 student member) AAMC (8 professional members +1 student member) LCME (1 professional member +2 public members)
Information collection processes	Institutional self-study, site visit teams, site visit report, periodic reviews between site visits	Institutional self-study, site visit teams, site visit report, periodic reviews between site visits
Recognized as accrediting authority and oversight provided by	USDE and CHEA (voluntarily sought)	USDE
First recognized by the USDE in	1952	1952
CHEA recognition for the purpose of	Affirming that standards and processes of COE are consistent with quality, improvement, and CHEA-established accountability expectations	Not applicable
How often reviewed?	5-yr review cycle by USDE; 5 yr review cycle by CHEA	5-yr review cycle
USDE recognition for the purpose of	Federal student aid eligibility and quality assurance	Federal student aid eligibility and quality assurance
Recognition of accreditor by USDE gives students:	Eligibility to receive Health Professions Student Loans (HPSLs) under Title VII of the US Public Health Service Act	Eligibility for selected federal grants and programs, including Title VII funding administered by the US Public Health Service Act

Table 23.3 (Continued)

	Council on Education	Liaison Committee for Medical Education
Sponsoring organization(s)	AVMA. To a limited extent, the AAVMC and CVMA share responsibilities such as appointing members	AMA and AAMC
Funding	AVMA; AAVMC covers cost of members selected by AAVMC; fees from programs paying for accreditation reviews Differential fee structure between US/Canadian schools and international schools	50%–50% cost share between AMA and AAMC; fees from developing programs alone and not established schools
Staff support	AVMA staff and AAVMC to a limited extent	AMA and AAMC staff
Autonomy in decision-making	Enabled by firewall between sponsoring organizations and accreditor	Enabled by firewall between sponsoring organizations and accreditor
Geography of accrediting activities	United States, Canada, Mexico, United Kingdom France, Netherlands, Denmark, Australia, New Zealand	US and US passport-eligible geography such as PR; joint accreditation process together with Committee on Accreditation of Canadian Medical Schools (CACMS) since 1972. The LCME-CACMS partnership is set to end in 2025

Section 6: Accreditation of Veterinary Education Worldwide

Malathi Raghavan

Although degree-granting institutions seek accreditation voluntarily to demonstrate quality and competence of their graduates and enable students to secure financial aid, another important factor that drives the need for accredited status is the determination by the regional or national veterinary statutory board (VSB) regarding eligibility for licensure to practice. Graduation from a college accredited by an approved body is a prerequisite for licensure to practice. This is the case at least in the United States, Canada, Australia, New Zealand, and some countries such as the United Kingdom in Europe. However, the status of institutional accreditation may not necessarily be a prerequisite for veterinary practice in other countries and regions. In fact, the prevalence of accredited colleges and accrediting bodies varies widely across world regions, given that the prevalence of national medical education accrediting bodies is few in numbers and variable in their approaches in some regions of the world.

Part 1: Accreditation in the United Kingdom

Accreditation by the RCVS, the statutory regulator of the veterinary professions in the United Kingdom, is required by a veterinary college in the United Kingdom to graduate veterinarians who are eligible to register to practice veterinary medicine in the United Kingdom. Voluntarily-sought external review of the RCVS was recently carried out by the European Association for Quality Assurance in Higher Education (ENQA) so the RCVS could demonstrate that its accreditation processes are in line with best practices in Europe (Royal College of Veterinary Surgeons 2023). Therefore, accreditation activities of the RCVS are also in compliance with the European Standards and Guidelines in the European Higher Education Area (ESG). Accreditation by RCVS ensures graduates of accredited institutions are licensed to work in the United Kingdom (England, Scotland, Wales, and Northern Ireland), Ireland, Australia, New Zealand, and South Africa. The standards against which veterinary degree-granting programs are judged by the RCVS cover the following areas: organization, finances, physical facilities, equipment, faculty and teaching staff, admissions policies and procedures, curriculum (including extramural studies and externships), library and learning resources, Day One competencies for the new graduate, and performance in veterinary degree examinations.

Part 2: Accreditation in Europe

The European Association of Establishments for Veterinary Education (EAEVE), founded in 1988, is an association of veterinary medical colleges that has established minimum standards for veterinary medical education programs (European Association of Establishments for Veterinary Education 2023). EAEVE accredits colleges provided they are members of the association, although members are not all in Europe. The roster for membership includes, for example, the University of Sao Paulo, Brazil; Hebrew University of Jerusalem, Rohovot, Israel; Jordan University of Science and Technology; and several colleges from Japan.

The accreditation status conferred by EAEVE plays a slightly different role than that conferred by the COE or RCVS, in that approval or accreditation by EAEVE is not a prerequisite for licensure to practice or for registration as a veterinarian in Europe or elsewhere. In this respect, accreditation by EAEVE assures the meeting of standards set by participating member institutions. EAEVE accreditation is one way in which value is added over and above standards applied locally. For example, in some local standards, communication education may not yet be mentioned as a key component of veterinary education and training for professional success. But EAEVE includes specific recommendations for communication skills among the competencies listed as "Day One" skills, ensuring that communication skills are part of the curricula of veterinary colleges that are members of EAEVE. As is the case with COE accreditation, a benefit of accreditation by the EAEVE is the reciprocal recognition of veterinary graduates from countries that work together on setting accreditation standards, provided work visa regulations are met.

Part 3: Accreditation in Australia and New Zealand

The Australasian Veterinary Boards Council (AVBC) and its accrediting agency have statutory authority to accredit veterinary medical education programs in Australia and New Zealand. The accreditation system is managed by the Veterinary Schools Accreditation Advisory Committee (VSAAC), which reports to the AVBC. School site visits by VSAAC occur at least once every seven years. Compliance with 12 standards is reviewed annually (Australasian Veterinary Boards Council n.d.).

Part 4: Accreditation in Mexico

The Universidad Nacional Autónoma de México (UNAM) houses the oldest veterinary program on the American continent. Started in 1853, it is considered one of the most prestigious programs in the Americas and the world. Many founding faculty members of veterinary colleges in South American countries were educated at UNAM. The curriculum and standards at UNAM also influenced the programs in those countries. However, there was no formal system of assessing the quality of veterinary education in Mexico's 44 veterinary programs until 1995, when the National Council for Veterinary Medicine Education (CONEVET) was founded with the aim of promoting quality teaching and practice of veterinary medicine.

One of the factors influencing interest in the system of educational accreditation was Mexico's entry into the North American Free Trade Agreement (NAFTA) in 1994 (Taylor Preciado et al. 2005; Berruecos et al. 2004). CONEVET is in charge of both accreditation of colleges

and certification of individuals. While the accreditation process is carried out via college evaluations, the certification of individuals is carried out via national and specialist examinations.

Accreditation status is sought voluntarily by colleges. Accredited status makes colleges eligible to receive federal funds specifically allocated for accredited programs.

UNAM is the only institution in Mexico (and all of Latin America) that has sought COE accreditation and it has been accredited by the COE since 2011 (Larkin 2011).

Part 5: Accreditation in Asia

In East Asia, the Accreditation Board for Veterinary Education in Korea (ABOVE-K) was established in 2010 and recognized as an accreditation body of veterinary education in 2011 by the Ministry of Agriculture, Food, and Rural Affairs, which is in charge of issuing veterinary licensure for practicing veterinary medicine in Korea. ABOVE-K accredits and evaluates veterinary educational programs and has developed the National Licensing Examination since 2012 (Accreditation Board for Veterinary Education in Korea n.d.).

For Central Asia, the Veterinary Council of India (VCI) is the statutory body that regulates veterinary practice in India since 1984. The VCI establishes minimum standards of veterinary education and approves public and private colleges that grant recognized veterinary qualifications to practice veterinary medicine in India (Veterinary Council of India 2023). In Malaysia, veterinary educational programs are accredited by the Malaysian Veterinary Council (Malaysian Veterinary Council 2023).

Part 6: Oversight of Veterinary Education in South Africa

The South African Veterinary Council (SAVC) monitors the standards of veterinary training in South African educational institutions and also administers the registration examination that a new veterinarian is required to pass to practice veterinary medicine (South African Veterinary Council 2023).

Part 7: Oversight of Veterinary Education in Brazil

Owing to its vast geographic distribution, rich history, numerous political and administrative divisions, and diverse regional needs for veterinary services, Brazil has a complex system of oversight of veterinary education offered in over a hundred programs. The structures of these programs differ based on whether they are offered in state universities, faculties (equivalent to colleges in the US) or schools, or private universities or schools. The Ministry of National Education establishes curricular directives for the programs and administers the National Examination of Courses that all students must pass at the end of their educational programs. Another examination, the National Examination of Professional Certification, is administered by the Federal Council of Veterinary Medicine, which, along with its system of Regional Councils of Veterinary Medicine, establishes the guidelines for the practice of veterinary medicine in Brazil. Once the certification is earned, the new graduate can enroll in a Regional Veterinary Council as a requirement to practice veterinary medicine in Brazil (Branco Germiniani 2004).

Part 8: In the Absence of Accreditation

Not all countries have a concept of accreditation by a third party. One reason may be that some countries do not have an accrediting overseer, another may be that the cycle of accreditation is managed by a centralized authority, such as a Ministry for Education (or its equivalent) that singularly controls postsecondary educational institutions nationally. The Ministry or its equivalent stipulates the curriculum to be taught, the number and background of students to be admitted, the number of faculty to be employed, and the allocated budget for those colleges that are state-sponsored or state-financed. Graduation from state-approved colleges implies meeting the standards for Day One competency expected by the Ministry or its equivalent agency and the regional or national VSB (Gallant 2016.)

Part 9: Educational Equivalency Certifications: ECFVG and PAVE

Graduates of non-COE accredited veterinary schools who wish to practice in the United States or Canada for reasons of migration or other, as in the case of US citizens or Canadians who choose to study elsewhere, are required to earn an EE certification to be eligible to register for the NAVLE. Once the NAVLE is successfully completed, the graduate of a non-COE accredited veterinary program becomes eligible to register with a state or provincial licensing body.

The EE certification is a credential earned by graduates of non-COE accredited veterinary colleges as the necessary route to be eligible for professional licensure. The existence of the EE certification route not only offers a path to meaningful pursuit of the profession for the graduates of the non-COE accredited college, but it also protects the US and Canadian public and helps a prospective employer and the corresponding licensing body assess the individual qualifications of such graduates without attempting to determine the standards of education offered in the nonaccredited college. Equally important is the fact that by evaluating the individual's skills against the standards set by the COE, EE certification protects the value of veterinary degrees earned

from COE-accredited schools by maintaining the quality and standards of veterinary medicine practiced by all in the United States and Canada. Two such programs currently exist in the United States: the certification offered by the Educational Commission for Foreign Veterinary Graduates (ECFVG) and the certification by the Program for Assessment of Veterinary Education Equivalence (PAVE).

The ECFVG certification is a four-step, assessment-based process. Those seeking to obtain ECFVG certification must: provide proof of graduation from an educational institution that is either accredited or authorized as a D.V.M. or equivalent-degree granting institution by authorities in that country; provide proof of English language proficiency; demonstrate entry-level veterinary medical knowledge by passing a standardized, computer-based exam; and demonstrate entry-level (Day One) clinical skills expected of a graduate from a COE-accredited college. The concept of an assessment-based EE certification offered by the ECFVG is very much like that of a foreign medical graduate from a program not accredited by the LCME completing the ECFMG program (AVMA n.d.).

The PAVE certification is also a four-step process. However, the fourth step of the process is successful completion of a clinical year at a college of veterinary medicine. The clinical year is similar in structure and function to the clinical year rotations in a traditional US-based program, the vast majority of which occur during the fourth year of the curriculum (one in the United States, the University of Arizona's CVM, currently has a three-year program, which spans the entire calendar year rather than the more traditional academic year). Successful completion of PAVE establishes eligibility to register for NAVLE (American Association of Veterinary State Boards n.d.).

Thus, the major difference between the ECFVG and the PAVE certifications is that while PAVE offers an opportunity to train within the United States, the ECFVG is purely assessment based.

The ECFVG certification is recognized by Canada's National Examining Board (NEB) of the CVMA and the Canadian veterinary licensing authorities; it is also accepted by the AVBC for eligibility to practice veterinary medicine in Australia and New Zealand. The PAVE certification is accepted by a number of state licensing boards in the United States and by the AVBC, but not by the CVMA.

Part 10: Recognized Accreditation Policy

In human medicine, there has been a move toward promoting the concept of educational accreditation by regional or national entities worldwide since 2010. This has been the result of the Educational Commission for Foreign Medical Graduates (ECFMG) instituting a new requirement for ECFMG certification. In the future, foreign medical graduates registering to earn an ECFMG certification as a prerequisite to undergo further training or to practice medicine in the United States must graduate from a nationally or regionally accredited educational institution. While this requirement can be seen as a step toward protecting the American public who are served by internationally educated physicians, indirectly, this decision also promotes excellence in international medical education since accreditation enhances the quality of educational processes anywhere and therefore gradually worldwide (Shiffer et al. 2019).

Section 7: The Process of Accreditation

Part 1: Overview

Myrah Stockdale

This section serves as practical guide to successfully navigate the accreditation process and achieve successful outcomes. It delves into the intricacies of the accreditation preparation process and accreditation cycle mentioned in section one. It provides an overview of the steps necessary for a program or institution to be successful in achieving a full accreditation status. There is an outline of first-time accreditation needs followed by a discussion accreditation cycle and processes necessary for successful accreditation status – particularly the self-study process and site visit process. This section is unique, as it incorporates project management concepts, which may improve self-study processes. The section also explores the critical role of key stakeholders, such as faculty, staff, students, and administrators, in the accreditation process.

Part 2: Definition of Terms

Self-Study – documentation written and compiled by a program or institution to demonstrate compliance with accreditation standards. Includes both narrative and numeric data. This documentation is submitted to the accrediting body ahead of an external review and serves as the foundation of an accreditation review.

Site Visit – the on-site (although this can be hosted digitally in some cases) portion of the external review process. Following the review of the self-study documentation, the accrediting body will send a trained team of reviewers to assess factors that cannot be adequately described in writing. Often involves observation, interviews, and group discussions over a period of two to five days.

Mission – communicates the purpose of the organization, what is valued, and how it will serve stakeholders. In higher education accreditation, it is common for quality standards to be measured against how well they satisfy the mission statement.

Vision – communicates the organization's aspirations and what they wish to become.

Strategic Plan – The strategic plan utilizes the vision (where an organization wants to be), along with the mission (how the organization operates day-to-day), to inform a strategy to achieve the vision (Bart and Baetz 1998). Under the overarching strategy are goals and measures to gauge the success of the plan. Strategic plans typically have a 3–10-year timeframe.

Continuous Quality Improvement – the iterative and ongoing process to achieve measurable improvement in indicators of quality such as: efficiency, effectiveness, performance, accountability, or outcomes. CQI is more than a single project, it is a commitment to long-term data-driven improvement.

Distributive Clinical Teaching Model – the use of workplace-based placements outside of the institution to accomplish clinical training.

Traditional Clinical Teaching Model – the use of a dedicated teaching hospital that is operated by the institution to accomplish clinical training.

Part 3: First-Time Accreditation

Stacy L. Anderson

A new veterinary medical program begins the process of program accreditation by submission of a written request for accreditation to the COE. A Dean of a College or School of Veterinary Medicine must have, at minimum, a DVM, VMD, or an equivalent degree. Within the letter, a new program should request a date for a consultative site visit that is conducted by the COE site visit team using published policies and procedures. The consultative site visit is funded by the institution and provides an unofficial appraisal of the program as it relates to planned compliance with the Standards of Accreditation. Eight weeks prior to the consultative site visit, the proposed program will submit a self-study that outlines its plan to meet each accreditation standard. The COE will provide a report following the consultative site visit. The program must address all points within the report to the satisfaction of the COE prior to moving to the next step.

The desired outcome after the consultative site visit is to secure a letter of reasonable assurance from the COE, at which point the proposed program should feel comfortable admitting their first class under provisional accreditation. The first class must be admitted within three years of receiving the letter of reasonable assurance or the process will have to restart from the beginning. To be eligible to receive a letter of reasonable assurance, the veterinary college/school must be part of a parent institution that is accredited by an institutional or national institutional accrediting body recognized by the USDE that is legally authorized to confer a professional degree and employs a veterinarian as the dean or chief executive office of the veterinary college/school.

A program under provisional accreditation may function as a fully accredited program until a final comprehensive site visit is completed. Under provisional accreditation, the program must prepare and submit interim reports that address how the program is maintaining the 11 standards of accreditation as it develops. The final comprehensive site visit for provisionally accredited programs occurs when the first class is in its final year of the program and uses the same policies and procedures as fully accredited programs as the assessment standard. Any deficiencies identified during the comprehensive site visit must be addressed to the satisfaction of the COE prior to a program being awarded full accreditation. Once fully accredited, accreditation is reevaluated every seven years.

Summary of the process from AVMA COE site:

1) Receipt of written request for accreditation.
2) Receipt and review of appropriate reports submitted by the college.
3) A comprehensive site visit to the college.
4) Preparation of a report of evaluation by the site visit team.
5) Review of the evaluation report by the full Council on Education.
6) Assignment by the full Council of a classification of accreditation.
7) Interim reports including any changes to the application of Standards – annually for accredited schools, and every six months for those provisionally accredited, granted Reasonable Assurance, on probationary accreditation, or accredited with minor deficiencies.

8) Reevaluation (self-study and comprehensive site visit) at intervals of no more than seven years or after any major change. Focused site visits may be required at Council discretion.
9) Upon written notification, a college may postpone or cancel a scheduled accreditation site visit or may withdraw from the accreditation process at any time (Table 23.4).

Part 4: Expanding on the Accreditation Cycle

Myrah Stockdale

In section one we established that the accreditation cycle (refer to Figure 23.1) includes: self-study, external review, decision, and continued monitoring. Each event in the accreditation cycle is multipart. This subsequent section will discuss the components of the cycle (e.g., self-study) overall, provide guidance on timeline planning, and breakout key considerations.

Accreditation Cycle: Self-Study

The self-study process is a crucial component of the accreditation cycle, as it allows institutions and programs to demonstrate their compliance with accreditation standards through the provision of evidence and documentation. This process not only serves as proof of an organization's commitment to quality standards and CQI but also offers valuable insights for future development.

The self-study report is prepared by various stakeholders within the organization, including but not limited to faculty, staff, administration, and students. It is then submitted to the accrediting body for external review, usually six to eight weeks prior to a scheduled site visit. The length of the self-study document may vary depending on the accreditor and the institution or program, with some

Table 23.4 Side-by-side comparison of steps required for new DVM program.

Institutional or National Accreditor	Discipline Accreditor (AVMA COE)
	Hire Dean who is a DVM, VMD, or equivalent
	Program developed
Program approved by institution	Self-study submitted >8 weeks before consultative site visit
Substantive change request submitted	Consultative site visit
Substantive change request approved	Submit report to apply for Letter of Reasonable Assurance
	Letter of Reasonable Assurance granted for provisional accreditation
	First-class admitted
	Interim reports submitted every six months
	Comprehensive site visit when first class is in final year of program
	Full accreditation awarded

accreditors providing specific guidelines for writing and formatting the report. For example, the Accreditation Council for Pharmacy Education (ACPE) currently has 25 standards for Doctor of Pharmacy programs, and states that no standard should exceed six pages in length (maximum narrative length 150 pages) without appendices. In contrast, the American Veterinary Medical Association Council on Education (AVMA-COE), which accredits Doctor of Veterinary Medicine programs has 11 standards and requires that the final self-study document be no more than 50 pages in length. Accreditors may also provide additional resources, such as external review or site visit rubrics and accreditation guidance documentation, to support institutions and programs during the self-study process.

The self-study process is time-intensive, requiring careful analysis of strategic priorities, identification of mission or purpose-related areas of improvement, and adaptation to changing environments. The process also necessitates a thorough examination of strategic priorities, identification of areas requiring improvement in relation to the organization's mission or purpose, and adaptation to changing environments. A self-study requires data, analysis, and a contextualized narrative to describe the extent to which the institution or program meets each quality standard. In addition to writing a narrative, accreditors outline expected data and trends to be included for each standard (e.g., admissions, first-time graduation rate, first-time license pass rate, feedback from various stakeholders), as well as appendices to be included to supplant the narrative (e.g., syllabi, assessment plan, evaluation templates/rubrics, faculty credentials, organizational charts). Atop the expected data, trends, and appendices, institutions and programs are encouraged to include other pertinent data, trends, or appendices that add meaning to the narrative.

The self-study process is a significant undertaking that requires a large allocation of time and resources. A program should consider allocating 12–24 months to the self-study process to ensure a comprehensive and thorough examination of all accreditation standards. For institutions seeking institutional reaffirmation, the timeline for the self-study process may need to be extended, depending on the size and complexity of the organization.

Effective preparation and planning are essential to the development of a successful self-study. The self-study is a complex, time-limited project that requires a high degree of precision, making it an ideal opportunity to integrate principles of project management (Dominelli et al. 2007). By utilizing project management techniques, such as setting clear objectives, establishing timelines, and assigning roles and responsibilities, the self-study process can be streamlined and made more efficient.

Additionally, it is important to establish clear communication channels and regularly review the progress of the self-study process to ensure that all stakeholders are aware of the status of the project and any issues or concerns that may arise. Furthermore, it is essential to identify and address any potential roadblocks or obstacles early on to minimize the risk of delays or setbacks.

The following sections of this chapter will provide more detailed information on project management considerations and key events in the self-study process, providing guidance on how to effectively plan, execute, and evaluate the self-study process to achieve successful accreditation.

Self-Study Project Management Considerations

As higher education has become increasingly more complex, accreditation has also become more intricate to capture these complexities. Institutions of higher education are multifaceted organizations with layered hierarchies (e.g., programs nested under colleges that are nested under the institution). Student services provide education-adjacent support to the students that they serve (e.g., recreation intramural sports, involvement activities, career services, and counseling). While faculties are responsible for the development and delivery of curricula, nonacademic units are responsible for the aforementioned student services as well as managing the business aspects of the organization (e.g., finance, human resources, talent acquisition, research, contracts, legal). The self-study process requires input from both educators and administrators to provide a robust picture of both the academic (teaching, research, and scholarship) and nonacademic (management, allocation of resources, activities to increase organizational continuity) activities at the institution or program (Costa et al. 2014).

Given the complexity and the multifaceted nature of the self-study process, it is important for institutions to approach the process with a strategic and organized approach. One effective way of achieving this is by treating the self-study process as a project manager would treat a project. This approach involves managing the process as a time-bound, resource-intensive, and scoped endeavor. By applying project management techniques and tools, institutions can effectively plan, execute, and evaluate the self-study process to achieve successful accreditation.

Project management practices, such as developing project plans, anticipating and addressing challenges, and implementing strategies to execute the project to completion, can be adapted to benefit the self-study process (Project Management Institute 2022). Furthermore, by borrowing planning and organizational tools from the discipline of project management, faculty and administrators can make the self-study process less arduous. While not all project management practices may apply to higher education, the following practices have been demonstrated to have potential usefulness in the context of developing an accreditation self-study (Trilling and Ginevri 2017).

The effective management of people, processes, and products is essential for a successful accreditation self-study.

People:

- Select cochairs or leadership that can manage motivations, interactions, and facilitate teamwork among the self-study membership.
- Select membership that understands the organization, is committed to quality, and brings various perspectives and strengths to the team.
- Gain commitment from team members on goals.
- Communicate clearly and often with all stakeholders (faculty, administrators, students, preceptors, staff, etc.) the expectations, responsibilities, progress, and any changes.
- Engage creative and effective critical thinking when encountering challenges.

Process:

- Use effective project management strategies that support the nature of accreditation and the complexities of self-study.
- Consider outlining the project using project cycle phases such as Define, Plan, Do, and Review.
- Maintain flexibility in both thought processes and methodology are prerequisites for adeptly navigating any project cycle.
- Create a clear project definition with a detailed scope.
- Outline the chronological timeframe including key events (e.g., training of members, initial drafting, initial reviews, second drafting)
- Develop, work from, and regularly update a work plan.
- Hold meetings and communicate regularly with self-study membership.
- Document and evaluate the process fidelity to inform future self-study iterations.

Product(s):

- Develop high-quality deliverables (e.g., self-study documents and evidences).
- Develop high-quality self-study products or deliverables in accordance with project goals.
- Seek feedback on products or deliverables to provide quality and expectations that have been satisfied.

The effective management of people, processes, and products leads to higher collective performance as well as process improvement in future iterations. The practices above lead us to an expanded discussion on project management considerations, which have value in the accreditation self-study.

Leadership, Team, and Stakeholders

In the context of an accreditation self-study, the selection and management of leadership, team members, and stakeholders is a crucial aspect of project management. Effective leadership, in the form of one person or cochairs, is essential for the successful completion of the self-study process. These leaders should possess integrity, trustworthiness,

and a familiarity with the organization and accreditation standards. They do not need to be experts in all aspects of the organization or the standards. However, they should be resourceful, creative critical thinkers, and have a firm understanding of team dynamics and motivation. It is important to recognize that the self-study process can be a lengthy endeavor, often spanning 12–24 months or more. Therefore, the leadership team should be consistent throughout the duration of the project and consider factors such as faculty and administrator contract periods, which may affect the continuity of the self-study process.

The selection of committed and dedicated leadership, team members, and stakeholders is central to the successful completion of the accreditation self-study process. The leadership team, responsible for managing and guiding the self-study process, should possess integrity, trustworthiness, and a familiarity with various parts of the organization and accreditation standards. They should be resourceful, able to support team members in finding the necessary tools and resources, and possess strong critical thinking skills and an understanding of team dynamics. While there are infinite means to organize the self-study team, two of the major functions of the team will be to write and review. The team which will be writing should be composed of individuals who understand the organization and are committed to quality and bring various perspectives and strengths to the team. Be mindful that writing for a self-study is different than writing and producing academic paper. If those which are responsible for writing have not written on a self-study prior, they will need guidelines, resources, examples, and potentially training. Lack of writing support may produce inconsistent writing styles across the narratives. The team which reviews the writing should be robust, providing feedback and suggesting revisions to make sure the self-study document is thorough, accurate, and meets accreditation standards. Similar to the support for those writing (which may overlap with the reviewers), consider the experience in reviewing self-study documents. Outline where possible expectations given to those writing, rubrics that will be used by the site reviewers, and other guidance (e.g., how to refer to the program, first or third-person perspective, terms or acronyms used across the document). Guidance and training will allow leadership to proactively guide teams to developing documents which represent the program or institution well. Further, consider using multiple perspectives in the review process, where possible. This includes not only internal reviewers (e.g., faculty, students, staff) but also external stakeholders such as alumni and professional advisors, who can provide a unique perspective on the program. This added reviewership allows the program or institution to understand the degree to which the narratives and support documentation accurately articulate the state of the program or institution. Overall, having a well-rounded and dedicated team and stakeholders is essential for the successful completion of the self-study process and achieving accreditation.

Initially, leadership at the institution or program (e.g., Provost, Dean, VP of Academic Affairs) should identify:

- Essential leadership roles and responsibilities
  - Cochairs
  - Members
- Necessary expertise or perspectives, including:
  - Administrators, department chairs/program directors
  - Faculty and staff most familiar with areas of the standards
  - Finance
  - Assessment, CQI, Outcomes
  - Curriculum
  - Support Services (e.g., financial aid, recruiting, career services, student support)
  - Institutional Effectiveness.

Once cochairs have been selected, they should consider reviewers and other stakeholder voices to be included in the writing and review of self-study documents early. For example,

- Alumni with understanding of the program(s) components
  - Recent graduates can bring a unique perspective as a recent student, graduate, and a young professional
- Current students
  - If the leadership team considers student reviewers, it is recommended that students in various cohorts, majors, and with varied experiences be considered. A first-year student likely has different experiences than second year, and students primarily in classrooms or labs have different experiences than those on experiential rotation and/or clinical clerkships.

Incorporating students and alumni into the writing and review of the self-study can provide valuable feedback and unique perspectives. However, it is important to note that the primary responsibility for writing the self-study document should fall on the faculty, staff, and administration team. This is because they are most familiar with the organization and accreditation standards. It is recommended that students and alumni augment reviewing on standards and in areas where they are most knowledgeable (e.g., student services and curriculum). This feedback serves two key purposes. Firstly, it enables the program or institution to gain valuable insights into these critical aspects. Secondly, when discussing the process with site reviewers, it demonstrates that the documentation was developed comprehensively, taking into account the perspectives of all stakeholders.

While students and alumni can serve as reviewers and provide feedback on the self-study document, they can also ask questions that an external reviewer may also ask. However, it is important to consider their unique schedules and responsibilities, such as classes and work. To accommodate these schedules, meetings can be scheduled around them or they can be given the option to review drafts independently and submit feedback to a specified point person by a specific deadline.

As an additional consideration to garner greater student participation, self-study participation can be considered as part of community-service requirements for students. Demonstrating how to incorporate self-study participation into students' resumes not only meets their needs but can helps gather valuable feedback. Much like the support needed for faculty, staff, and administrative team members it is important to provide guidance and information to students and alumni about the self-study process, its importance, and the team's expectations for their participation. This can help ensure that they have a clear understanding of the process and their role in it. While the current group may not require training, it is advisable for leadership to explore methods of educating students and alumni on the process, rather than expecting them to review documents independently. For example, with students, having an in-person short education and editing session during times that work for their schedules can increase participation.

Internal Reviewers

- Consider individuals that can review and edit the team's drafts. These individuals can be from other programs at the institution or college (e.g., English, another health science department, institutional effectiveness office, etc.) or from the same program (i.e., individuals not working on the self-study draft).
- For some programs, writing teams may include the entire faculty and staff. These individuals can still serve as internal editors and reviewers in the process, despite being writers. It is recommended that the writing teams consider exchanging drafts, thereby editing documents that were not initially developed by them or their team.
  - Any program hoping to use this strategy should consider this when outlining its process.

External Reviewers

Incorporating external reviewers into the self-study process can provide valuable feedback and perspectives on the institution's or program's compliance with accreditation standards and areas for improvement. External reviewers can bring a fresh perspective and may have experience with similar institutions or programs, allowing them to provide insight and suggestions for improvement. They can also help identify any potential blind spots or areas that the internal team may have overlooked. Additionally, involving external reviewers can help increase the credibility and validity of the self-study document, as it demonstrates that the institution or program is open to outside review and willing to make improvements based on that feedback. Overall, incorporating external reviewers into the self-study process can provide valuable insights and help ensure that the self-study document is thorough, accurate, and meets accreditation standards.

- Consider external reviewers from peer organizations which can review for soundness, coherence, and understanding.
  - External reviewers can be cost prohibitive if there are no reciprocal relationships established between programs or institutions (e.g., deans or assessment staff agreeing to review one another's self-study), an option that can help offset costs.

In addition to having the right people in place, it is also important to have a clear and structured plan for managing the self-study process. This can be achieved by utilizing effective project management strategies that support the cyclical nature of accreditation and the complexities of the self-study process. By treating the self-study as a project with a project cycle, it can be more manageable as project management practices can assist in the development of an accreditation self-study.

Project Cycles

A project cycle is a framework for managing a project from start to finish. The cycle repeats for each project and supports the effective and efficient management of a project. There are several frameworks for project cycles and each is intended to help ensure the project is completed on time, within budget, and to the satisfaction of all stakeholders. While many project cycle frameworks exist, the two frameworks discussed in this section are the Define, Plan, Do, Review project cycle, and Planning, Execution, Monitoring, and Controlling (PEMC). Each will be outlined with its general benefits and shortcomings. An applied self-study-related example will follow the general discussions.

Define, Plan, Do, Review The Define, Plan, Do, Review cycle is a simple, four-step process that is easy to understand and follow.

The steps are:

1) Define – project goals.
2) Plan – how to achieve the project's goals.
3) Do – the work.
4) Review – results and process.

The primary benefit of using a Define, Plan, Do, Review cycle is that it provides a clear structure and direction for the self-study process. The primary limitation of this project cycle framework is that it is less comprehensive and may be less effective in managing larger or more complex projects.

A Define, Plan, Do, Review cycle overall for a self-study covers the following in each stage:

- *Define*. In the first phase, the scope of the self-study project is defined, including the accreditation standards that will be addressed, the goals and objectives of the self-study, and the key stakeholders who will be involved. The team establishes the overall project timeline and milestones and outlines the roles and responsibilities of team members.
- *Plan*. In this phase, the team develops a detailed project plan, which includes outlining the specific tasks and activities that need to be completed, identifying the resources (e.g., personnel, budget) required, and developing a schedule for completing the work.
- *Do*. The team executes the steps to the plan during this phase. This may include conducting research, collecting data, drafting the self-study document, and building appendices. The cochairs will monitor progress and adjust as needed.
- *Review*. In the fourth and final phase, the team reviews the completed self-study document, incorporating feedback. Once the document is finalized, it is submitted for review to the accrediting body. To complete this phase the team will evaluate the overall process and identify areas for improvement for future self-studies.

A comprehensive illustration of the Define, Plan, Do, Review cycle in a 24-month self-study process is provided below. This example outlines a clear timeline and delves into the finer details of the self-study process. Additionally, it offers helpful advice for cochairs and project managers who may be using this framework for their self-study endeavors.

Define (Month 1–3):

- Determine the scope and objectives of the accreditation self-study process.
  - Scope:
    - o The accreditation self-study will cover all aspects of the college's operations, including its academic programs, research activities, clinical services, and support functions.
    - o The self-study will involve a comprehensive review of the college's policies, procedures, and performance data to assess its compliance with accreditation standards.
  - Objectives:
    - o To evaluate the college's compliance with the most recently published AVMA accreditation standards and identify areas for improvement.
    - o To assess the quality and effectiveness of the college's academic programs, research activities, and clinical services.
    - o To determine the college's strengths and weaknesses and prioritize areas for improvement.
    - o To engage all stakeholders, including faculty, staff, students, and alumni, in the self-study process to ensure its comprehensive and objective nature.

- o To prepare a comprehensive self-study report to AVMA specifications and plan of action to present to the accrediting body.
- o To implement the plan of action and continuously monitor and evaluate the college's operations and processes to ensure ongoing compliance with accreditation standards.
- Identify the accrediting body and review its standards and requirements.
  - *Accreditor.* American Veterinary Medical Association (AVMA)
  - Current Standards to be included in self-study (https://www.avma.org/education/accreditation-policies-and-procedures-avma-council-education-coe/coe-accreditation-policies-and-procedures-self-study)
    - o Organization
    - o Finances
    - o Physical Facilities and Equipment
    - o Clinical Resources
    - o Information Resources
    - o Students
    - o Admission
    - o Faculty
    - o Curriculum
    - o Research Programs
    - o Outcomes Assessment
- Assemble a team of stakeholders, including administrators, faculty, staff, students, preceptors, and alumni, to participate in the self-study process.
  - More specifically, this is determining the approach to completing the self-study process.
  - Determining how each stakeholder will interact with the self-study process.
  - Could also be developing the space and organizational components needed to host documents, data, and guidelines.
    - o E.g., utilizing an online accessible file system to organize files by standard
  - This is a great time to plan logistics as well as consider any notes from prior self-study practices.

Plan (Month 4–6):

- Develop a detailed timeline and budget for the self-study process.
  - Begin the timeline planning in reverse, placing most important dates/events first (e.g., self-study submission deadline)
    - o Consider setting project completion deadline two to four weeks prior to hard deadline in case of unexpected delays.
    - o Keep in mind the flow of the College and University in determining deadlines (e.g., finals, midterms, student breaks, faculty contracts). Always build in

buffer time for unanticipated challenges that may arise in the process.
  - Budgets could include items such as:
    - o Personnel:
    - o The hiring of a self-study coordinator or additional staff (e.g., editor) as needed.
    - o This may also look like a stipend for faculty who take on additional responsibilities related to cochairing the self-study.
    - o Providing compensation and benefits for self-study team members.
    - o Equipment and Supplies:
    - o Purchasing or leasing equipment, software, and supplies needed for the self-study process (e.g., Statistical software, videoconferencing systems, office supplies, a dedicated copier or printer)
    - o Providing materials for data collection and analysis.
    - o Travel:
    - o Covering travel expenses for site visits and presentations.
    - o Many accreditors host a workshop or conference for programs that are preparing for a site visit. This can be digital or in person. The program will likely need to send the cochairs.
    - o Could be for travel or time associated with a mock site visit.
    - o Reimburse expenses incurred by self-study team members.
    - o This could include meals for meetings, supplies purchased by the team members, and travel expenses.
    - o Professional Services:
    - o Hire consultants or contractors to support the self-study process.
    - o It is recommended that a program utilize an external reviewer, consider a mock site visit, and discuss the self-study process with experts.
    - o Miscellaneous:
    - o Cover miscellaneous expenses, such as printing and mailing costs, advertising and outreach expenses, and legal fees.
- Assign tasks and responsibilities to the self-study team.
- Determine the methods and tools to be used to collect and analyze data.
  - This may be discussed in the Define phase but should be finalized in the Plan phase.

Do (Month 7–12):

- Conduct an internal review of the college, including its policies, procedures, and operations.
  - This includes:
    - o the review of procedural alignment between College and program policies and processes against accreditation standards and expectations.

o the evaluation of performance and efficiency of College or program operations including academic programs, research activities, clinical services, and support functions. There should be a discussion regarding action plans and CQI.

o the collection and analysis of performance data (e.g., faculty productivity, student achievement, clinical services) resulting in a discussion of strengths and weaknesses of the program or College.

o the extent to which stakeholders are engaged in the self-study process as well as in providing feedback for the program or College.

o the review of financial management and prioritization of the program from the University. A look at the effectiveness of financial management should be included.

o the internal review of program or College resources needed to achieve its goals and objectives.

- Collect and analyze data from various sources, including student and faculty surveys, focus groups, and performance data.
  - Often an accreditor has annual or regular surveys delivered to stakeholders such as faculty, graduating students, preceptors, and alumni. The accreditor will want to see that the data is being reviewed and utilized.
- Identify areas for improvement and prioritize them based on their impact and feasibility.
  - This could include using procedures such as Value Stream Mapping, Pareto Analyses, Statistical Process Control, Root Cause Analysis, or Define-Measure-Analyze-Improve-Control (DMAIC).

Review (Month 13–15):

- Synthesize the data collected and analyze it to determine the college's strengths and weaknesses.
  - More specifically, this would include:
    o Data collection and management,
    o Data cleaning and preparation,
    o Data synthesis,
    o Data analysis, and
    o Interpretation and presentation of results.
  - Additionally, the organization and access to the data should be managed to ensure all members of the team that need data for writing or editing can review relevant data.
- Write a comprehensive self-study report addressing the accrediting body's standards and requirements.
  - Leadership should outline a report format prior to team engagement in writing. Consider:
    o Writing Voice (i.e., 1st person, 3rd person)
    o Formatting (e.g., 12-pt, Times New Roman, Single Spaced)
    o Use of headers and sub-headers
    o Length of sections

o Content in each section (e.g., consider if all sections have relevant data).

- Writers will need to consider the standard-specific guidelines as they write and edit.

- Develop a quick reference guide for communicating with internal stakeholders and those directly interacting with the site visit team.
- Develop the appendices for the self-study.
- Prepare a plan of action to address any identified areas of improvement.
  - Should be included in each standard.
- Review and edit self-study documents.
  - Recommend that a smaller team of experts and editors work on the revision process to keep writing voice similar.
- Hold meeting with stakeholders to educate them on self-study process, documentation, and quick reference guide. Hold time for questions, and allow access to documents for edits and questions.
- Vote from faculty body endorsing the self-study and appendices.

Planning (Month 16–18):

- Submit the self-study report to the accrediting body.
  - This process has become digital however, some accrediting bodies still require a printed copy to be submitted as well.
- Prepare for a site visit from the accrediting body and provide necessary documentation and information.
  - Mock Site visit should happen during this time.
- Implement the plans of action to address any identified areas of improvement.
- Monitor and evaluate the college's operations and processes to ensure ongoing compliance with accreditation standards.

It is important to note that this timeline is just a general outline and may vary depending on individual needs and circumstances. The Define, Plan, Do, Review cycle helps ensure that key tasks are completed and that the self-study document and appendices represent the program/organization and meet the accreditation standards. The built-in review process allows for regular review and feedback on the progress of the project, which helps to identify and address issues early on.

Part 5: Planning, Execution, Monitoring, and Controlling

The PEMC cycle, on the other hand, is a more detailed project management framework. It includes four stages:

1) *Planning.* Establishing project goals and objectives, determining the resources required, and creating a plan for achieving the objectives.

2) *Execution*. Carrying out the project plan, including tasks and activities, using the resources allocated.

3) *Monitoring and Controlling*. Keeping track of progress, managing risks, and adjusting as needed to stay on track and achieve the project objectives.

4) *Closing*. Finalizing all project activities, ensuring that all project deliverables have been completed, and documenting lessons learned for future reference.

The benefits of this cycle include a more structured and organized approach to the self-study process, better tracking of progress and budget, and a more thorough and accurate self-study document. The shortcoming could be the high level of management and coordination required for the project, which could be resource intensive. Please note that the added complexity in this model can make it harder for team members to follow and implement.

A PEMC (Planning, Execution, Monitoring, and Controlling) cycle for a self-study process could include following under each stage:

- Planning
  - Define the project scope and objectives,
  - identify key stakeholders and team members, and
  - develop a project plan, budget, and risk management plan.
- Execution
  - Kick off the project,
  - establish governance,
  - set up meetings,
  - begin writing the self-study document, and
  - coordinate with stakeholders.
- Monitoring
  - Edit and revise documents
  - continuously track progress against the plan, budget, and resources, and
  - communicate progress to stakeholders.
- Controlling
  - Prepare the final report and
  - use project data to develop plan.

Like the Define-Plan-Do-Review framework, the PEMC framework is also illustrated in a 24-month self-study process below. Despite its touted complexity (which may be less obvious in the example below), it is crucial to keep in mind that the PEMC framework is more flexible and adjusts to changes in the timeline and deviations from the expected pattern. Much of the differentiation between the two frameworks will depend on how they are utilized by the cochairs or project managers.

Planning (Months 1–3):

- Form the self-study team and establish roles and responsibilities.

- The PEMC condenses the Define and Plan stages into the "Planning" stage. This is well seen in this first bullet point.
- Define the scope and objectives of the project.
  - The scope and objectives will be the same as from the above example.
- Develop a detailed project plan including timelines, budgets, and resource requirements.
  - This will look similar to the above example but will be done earlier in the project cycle.
- Identify any potential risks and develop contingency plans.
  - The PEMC model commonly includes risk planning in the earliest steps.
  - This could be included in either project cycle model.

Execution (Months 4–12):

- Conduct an internal review of the college and gather supporting documentation.
  - Refer back to the "Do" section in the prior example for an expansion on what this includes.
- Synthesize the data collected and analyze it to determine the college's strengths and weaknesses.
  - This still includes:
    - Data collection and management,
    - Data cleaning and preparation,
    - Data synthesis,
    - Data analysis, and
    - Interpretation and presentation of results.
- Write the self-study report, addressing the accrediting body's standards and requirements.
  - Notice that the PEMC gets into writing the self-study report sooner in the project cycle.
- Develop the appendices for the self-study.
- Identify areas for improvement and prioritize them based on their impact and feasibility.

Monitoring (Months 13–20):

- Have external reviewers review the self-study, appendices, and other documentation.
- Edit, revise, and update the self-study and appendices as needed.
- Implement prioritized improvements, documenting changes and effects.
  - The site visit team may ask about these initiatives while on site. Having documentation on their implementation and initial impact could be helpful evidence of continuous improvement.

Controlling (Months 21–22):

- Evaluate the outcomes of the self-study process and make any adjustments as needed.

This will inform the Review and Planning stage. By capturing the effectiveness of processes in achievement of outcomes there will be documentation and evidence for future self-studies.

- Review the self-study report to ensure accuracy and completeness.
- Submit the self-study report to the accrediting body for review.

Review and Planning (Months 23–24):

- Review the feedback from the accrediting body.
- Develop a plan for future improvements based on the feedback received.

Determining which project cycle framework to use depends on the specific needs of the project and team. The Define, Plan, Do, Review cycle is simple and flexible, while the PEMC cycle is more detailed and comprehensive. Both frameworks can be adapted or enhanced to suit specific needs if they are tailored to the project and team.

Part 6: Projects Versus Ongoing Operations

For those more familiar with project management concepts it can be important to differentiate between the terms "project" and "ongoing operation." In assessment, these may be discussed as projects versus CQI. However, these two concepts often get confused when discussed outside of project management circles. Projects are temporary (i.e., they have a distinct beginning and end), have a fixed budget, and produce something unique. Completing a strategic initiative such as "adopting products or services which significantly increase research capacity within the next three years" is an example of a project. It has a clear scope and endpoint (e.g., selection, purchase, and implementation of products or services which increase institutional research capacity within three years).

The example project might include the following breakdown:

- reviewing the current research capacity, needs, constraints (e.g., time), and vision,
- identifying challenges facing current research efforts and meeting vision, and
- establishing criteria for evaluating products and services
  - e.g., degree to which varied needs are met, price point or expected cost, integration capacity, quality of support, training availability, impact on institutional research.
- identifying products or services which can
  - be implemented in the given timeframe.
  - address challenges facing institutional research efforts.
- considering potential survey platforms against established criteria
- selecting a survey platform
  - gaining institutional support for choice
- purchasing and launching survey platform.

The project ends at the point where the scope is met. The selected platform's performance will likely be regularly evaluated as part of the institution's ongoing operations. The ongoing evaluation of the platform's ability to continue to meet the institutions continuing (or evolving) research needs could lead to one of the following outcomes:

1) *Evaluation outcome.* The platform continues to meet the majority of needs; no action is recommended
   a) *Action.* None taken
2) *Evaluation outcome.* The platform meets many but not all needs; recommendation for additional support products/services
   a) *Action.* Develop a project to select, purchase, and implement new supporting products/services
3) *Evaluation outcome.* The platform no longer meets the needs; recommendation to purchase a new platform
   a) *Action.* Develop a project to select, purchase, and implement a new survey platform purchase.

In this example, it is clear how timebound projects (purchasing a survey platform) can create ongoing operations (evaluation of survey platform for meeting continuing research needs) and the reciprocal (the evaluation of the platform triggering a new project). Accreditors expect that higher education assessment and accreditation practices are handled as ongoing operations despite often discussing their cycles like projects. Most higher education administrators have heard the phrase "closing the loop." The phrase refers to using data from a cycle to inform direction (e.g., improvements) or a future cycle. This is precisely how accreditation, CQI, and assessment processes serve as an example of what project management refers to as ongoing operations. There is an expectation that programs or institutions are continually evaluating data and practices to make improvements (or better alignment to standards), therefore making accreditation an ongoing operation. This delineation, while important for other project management concepts, is less important in project cycles.

Both projects and ongoing operations can utilize project cycles despite the naming convention. Ongoing operations treat individual cycles (e.g., accreditation cycle) as projects where the final step (e.g., review) is to take learning from the prior cycle to the new cycle. Think of it as an iterative project cycle. While the people involved, process undertaken, or products produced may change between iterations, the act of meeting and continually documenting accreditation standards iterate after an accreditation status is awarded. Similarly, when assessing curricular outcomes, it is expected that findings from the first iteration of curricular assessment will inform improvements for the next iteration. These ongoing operational processes assume that once a cycle completes then another cycle will begin.

Each project will encounter fluctuations during its life cycle. Project cycles are used to segment or outline a project's flow from its initial conception through to its final completion. Project cycles are often defined by their phases or iterations such as the "define-plan-do-review" framework from above. Iterations are specified segments of time meant to accomplish a portion of the overall project. Often iterations are seen as "mini-projects." Iteration names vary by project manager and context. In technology and software development, the discover-design-develop-test naming convention is often used for project cycles. The naming of iterations is less important than the concept of segmenting the project into smaller achievable portions to deliver the ultimate product. Inside the iterations effective project managers utilize "increments," which further break down the iteration into smaller chunks.

Both iterative and incremental approaches in project management involve breaking down a project into smaller, manageable parts and working on them one at a time. The iterative approach involves repeating the process of planning, execution, and evaluation until the project is completed. The incremental approach involves breaking down the project into smaller parts and completing them one at a time, with each part building on the previous one. Both approaches allow for flexibility and adaptability in the project, as progress can be evaluated, and adjustments can be made as needed.

As demonstrated above, an iterative and incremental approach can help break a complex project into a manageable series of iterations and increments. This approach is included in this chapter because it is advantageous for multifunctional or cross-functional teams like accreditation self-study writing teams. Projects employing the PEMC framework often use both iterative and incremental or blended approaches as it captures more complexity. However, this concept is not constrained or required for any project cycle framework.

Part 7: Timeline Development

Within project cycle frameworks, it's important to take into account considerations related to the development of timelines. A project's life cycle is finite. To optimize the available time, the timeline of the self-study should be outlined at the outset of the project and monitored throughout.

To build a timeline for a project, consider the following steps:

- Define the project goals and objectives.
  - Overall self-study goals
- Break down the project into smaller, manageable segments.
  - Iterations/phases
  - Increments/tasks (Figure 23.1)
- Assign a start and end date to each segment.
- Identify any dependencies between increments or tasks and ensure that they are scheduled in the correct order.
- Review and adjust the timelines as needed, considering potential roadblocks or delays.
- Communicate the timeline to all stakeholders.
- Continuously monitor progress and adjust the timeline as needed.

Tools such as Gantt charts, spreadsheets, or Project management software (if available) can be helpful in visualizing and managing the self-study timeline. For some accreditors, this timeline can be a helpful appendix to demonstrate the writing and reviewing process for the self-study.

Part 8: Timelines and Communication

The below timelines taken from a 2023 PharmD self-study demonstrate how this team communicated their overall timeline and further broke out more specific goals by semester. Each subcommittee had further refined timelines. These high-level (i.e., less detailed) communication

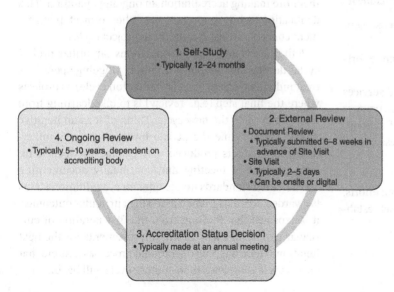

Figure 23.1 Common accreditation cycle.

pieces led to greater understanding of all team members and allowed the initial drafts to be completed by April 2022 (one month ahead of time). Feedback from the teams showed that timelines and guidance (e.g., 3rd person, 12 pt, Times New Roman, use introduction paragraphs) like those presented above drove overall process understanding while more detailed timelines developed by the writing teams gave the members structure as they wrote and refined their drafts.

The leadership team for this self-study laid out expectations early for their writing teams. During the first meeting of leadership (this school had seven faculty writing subcommittees, each with a faculty chair) of the cochairs and faculty chairs (collectively the leadership team), after discussing the self-study and site visit, timelines, team membership, and report expectations the following expectations were outlined,

a) Educate yourselves on the standards that your subcommittee is responsible for.
   i) You will be considered the expert for your team. While we are here to assist, you should understand the standards and be able to answer most questions raised by your team.
b) Review the existing data available for your standards, available in the Network drive (link provided).
   ii) Summarize data so that you can share it with your writing team when you meet.
c) Review the guidance document related to your standards (i.e., ACPE's Rubric 2.0). Develop a plan for your team to draft their standard narratives that addresses the guidance.
d) Setup a Meeting with your Team for January or February 2022.

   iii) Please invite co-chairs to initial meeting
   iv) Initial meeting needs to address the following:
       1) Education on standards, data, guidelines
       2) Timeline for accomplishing writing.
       3) Team Expectations

Following the expectations were the next meeting dates and agendas stating what should be discussed and was expected to be accomplished during these meetings. The subsequent meeting invites were sent directly following the close of the initial meeting. Meeting invites also had meeting agendas. The leadership team expressed that clear, concise, and timely communication was essential for their success as subcommittee chairs. They knew what they needed to accomplish, who to work with (their subcommittee of people) and who to contact if they had questions or concerns, how to approach their task, and when products were available (Figures 23.2 and 23.3).

Timelines are an important component of communication in the self-study process. This team continued to update the timeline as the process became clearer. The cochairs presented segments of the timeline with more details, as seen in the Spring 2022 timeline. These tools were helpful as the self-study leadership met with subcommittees and faculty.

Part 9: Tips for Success

- Frequently communicate goals, criteria, and progress toward the self-study document.
  - Communication can be emails, trainings, meetings, posters, or other modalities of interest.
  - Communicate with members of the team but also with the organization. It is important that all faculty and staff have an understanding of the process, the expectations, and the goals over the course of the accreditation cycle.
- Ask for continuous feedback throughout the process and be open to adapting as necessary.
  - Sometimes direction changes to fit the organization and that is okay. That is part of embracing CQI.
- Goals can be refined over time depending on the duration of the self-study (e.g., a 24-month timeline may have clear deadlines over the initial three to six months and approximate ones that develop more as time passes).

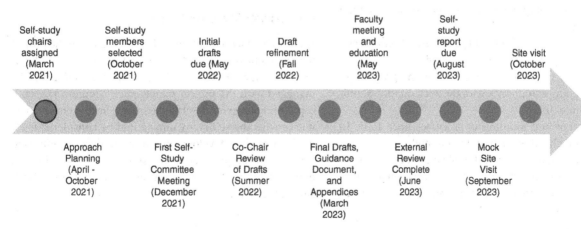

Figure 23.2 Example high-level timeline from a PharmD self-study.

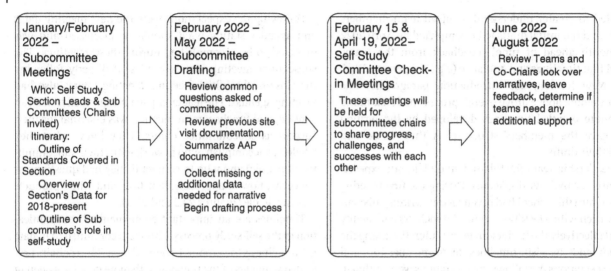

Figure 23.3 Example spring 2022 timeline from same PharmD self-study.

Part 10: Preparing for the Self-Study

Achieving success in a self-study calls for exceptional project management abilities, reliable data gathering, and thorough evaluation. The key to preparing for a self-study and on-site visit lies in using project cycles for planning, considering the complexities of your program or organization, and creating flexible timelines. It is also important to familiarize yourself with the specific expectations and requirements set forth by your accrediting body.

A program undergoing accreditation will need to consider the following:

- Adhering to the most recently published standards and guidelines set forth by the accrediting body.
  - This is particularly important with professional accreditation bodies as they often update standards.
- Gathering and providing evidence of compliance with the accreditation standards and guidelines.
  Many accreditation bodies outline the expected artifacts needed to satisfy standards compliance. However, your program/institution will want to consider its unique nature and the artifact(s) needed to demonstrate the way those unique components contribute to accreditation compliance.
- Involving key stakeholders in the accreditation process, such as faculty, staff, students, and graduates.
- Continuously monitoring and assessing the program to ensure ongoing compliance with the accreditation standards and guidelines.
  - Assessment and monitoring processes need to be in place well ahead of writing the self-study.
  - If a new program or institutional component is implemented prior to the self-study site visit, ensure that there are assessment and monitoring procedures

planned and outlined, which ensure this component meets expectations.
- Being prepared to address any issues or concerns that may arise during the accreditation process.
  - Every program has areas of improvement; during the self-study process work to identify the areas where issues or concerns may be raised.
  - Recognize that if a self-study writing process is initiated 12–24 months prior to the site visit, there is time to develop a means to address areas of improvement.
- Being open to feedback and willing to make changes to improve the program.
  - Review and feedback are crucial in the self-study process.
  - Plan to have reviewers and writers work in successions in order to produce an accurate narrative, appendices, and supporting documentation.
- Communicating effectively with the accrediting body to ensure a smooth and successful accreditation process.
  - Accrediting bodies often have a point of contact which can help with questions that may arise in the self-study process.

Part 11: Self-Study Key Events

A great deal has been discussed above related to the project management of self-study. This section serves as a high-level overview of the overall self-study events that will be managed with the project management frameworks, concepts, and processes described earlier. These events are key markers for the self-study and should be considered early in the timeline development. It is in these events that cochairs or project managers should consider effective practices for the effective and successful completion of self-study objectives.

Standards Review

Before embarking on the self-study process, it is important that the self-study team review the most current standards produced by the accreditor. If guidance documentation, site visit rubrics, or other information related to the standards is provided, it is recommended that the team review those as well. These documents will illuminate the expectations of the accrediting body when drafting a narrative and creating appendices to support the standards. Additional questions related to the expectations may be directed to the accrediting body if they are not found on the website or in the provided documentation.

Drafting, Data Collection, Analysis

Gathering data and analysis will coincide with drafting narratives and appendices. With proper assessment and monitoring cycles, many years of data will have been analyzed to inform the program or institution. However, there may be data, such as national or peer comparative data, which will need to be assembled, trended, and analyzed as a part of the self-study writing process. Determining the data needed should be done early in the process as the narrative will weave the processes, data, and actions taken as a result of data analysis together into a cohesive account.

Review and Finalization

Throughout the writing process, review should be done to ensure that standard expectations are met and narratives capture program/institutional realities. At the completion of writing, the entire self-study should be reviewed by a small team of editors. These editors will review narrative accuracy, voice, tone, and composition. It is recommended that following the final review, the faculty, staff, and stakeholders be given an opportunity to review and endorse (or vote) on the document. Once the faculty, staff, and stakeholders have had time to review the document it will be finalized.

Stakeholder Education and Communication

While communication should be consistent throughout the self-study process, it is recommended that the team develop a means of communicating the most salient points included in the self-study narrative and appendices to faculty, staff, and stakeholders. Remind stakeholders of the goal of the process, what has happened to date, and what is left to be done. If the overall document is 50+ pages, as is the case with accreditors such as ACPE, the team may want to consider providing short highlights per standard. This is especially true for those individuals that will be interacting with the site visit team.

Submission

Each accrediting body has a predetermined time before a site visit that they will request the self-study be submitted (e.g., 6–12 weeks). This submission may take place in a digital system or manually (although the manual option is falling out of favor). Plan to submit the self-study before the deadline as systems can falter.

Section 8: Additional Considerations

Part 1: Distributive Models

Stacy L. Anderson

Distributive models of clinical education are becoming increasingly common in the United States as new veterinary medical programs are developed. Distributive clinical education is commonly employed in human medical education, having evolved from the traditional teaching hospital model to meet the educational needs of the growing health profession and to address deficiencies in learning opportunities provided by teaching hospitals (Ellaway and Bates 2018; Cooke et al. 2010). Distributive models rely on workplace rotations for students to undergo clinical training rather than providing training in an institutionally operated teaching hospital.

For programs that choose to use a distributive model for clinical training, there are specific policies and procedures outlined by the COE for obtaining and maintaining accreditation. Due to the novelty of distributive clinical year teaching models, it is important to check regularly for updated policies and procedures as they have been evolving over the past few years with revisions occurring almost annually.

The primary consideration for distributive models during the accreditation process happens during the site visit. Rather than visit one teaching hospital, site visitors will visit all sites that deliver core clinical training. Due to the continued definitions of what is considered "core" training, the number of sites could vary among programs. Current distributive models used anywhere from 20 to 100 sites for clinical training. Given that a site visit is funded by the program, it can take considerable resources from a program with distributive clinical training to facilitate a site visit.

Mock Site Visit

Before a site visit, it is worth considering a mock site visit. A mock site visit is a simulated accreditation visit that is conducted by a program or institution before an actual accreditation visit by an accrediting body. It is designed to simulate the experience of an actual accreditation visit as closely as possible and is typically conducted by a team of external evaluators who are familiar with the accreditation process and the standards and guidelines of the accrediting body.

The purpose of a mock site visit is to give the program or institution an opportunity to practice and prepare for the actual accreditation visit. It allows the program or institution to identify and address any issues or concerns that may arise during the accreditation process, and to make any necessary improvements or revisions to the program or institution. It also allows the program or institution to test its readiness, the effectiveness of its self-study report, and the level of preparedness of the faculty and staff.

During the mock site visit, the evaluators will review the program or institution's self-study report, conduct interviews with faculty, staff, students, and other stakeholders, and visit classrooms and other facilities. They will also provide feedback and recommendations for improvement to the program or institution.

Mock site visits are a useful tool for programs and institutions to prepare for the actual accreditation visit and increase their chances of success. They can help to identify areas of weakness and provide an opportunity to fix them before the actual visit.

Part 2: Developing a Quick Reference Guide

Myrah Stockdale

Another optional addition to the self-study and site visit preparation is the development and distribution of a Quick Reference Guide related to the self-study. This document serves as a quick communication tool from the program or organization to stakeholders. While the self-study document will be available to stakeholders, there are many who will not find the time to read it in its entirety. A quick reference guide allows stakeholders to review the full self-study in a summated way. Keep the user in mind when building this guide.

Concepts to include or consider in developing a Quick Reference Guide:

- Purpose and Goals – include brief statements related to the goal of the self-study and site visit. Below is an excerpt from an internal document from the Campbell University College of Pharmacy and Health Sciences Doctor of Pharmacy 2023 Quick Reference Guide.

"it is important to remember that we want to showcase our strengths and achievements. The team members will come prepared with questions and will be seeking to gather information on how [. . .] program meets accreditation standards. Let's aim to make a positive impression and highlight our achievements during their visit" (from author's files).

- Self-Preparation – include common questions that faculty may need to consider in addition to understanding the portions of the self-study that most directly impact their position. Also, they need to be flexible as the team may shift plans.
  - What initiatives or programs are you implementing in your area to support student success?
  - How do you measure and evaluate the effectiveness of these efforts?
  - What changes or improvements have you made or are you currently planning to make in your area?
- What to do is a Site Visitor asks for Additional Documentation – give the email address of the cochairs (or other administrative support) and guidance on what to include, like the requestor's name.
- How to use the guide – while it may seem obvious to those who worked extensively on the self-study it may seem nebulous to others why this guide exists and how to use it.
  - To be well-prepared for the upcoming visit, it is essential that you familiarize yourself with the (Program or Organization) Self-Study. You can choose to do this by either using the quick guide provided, which highlights relevant examples from each standard as they pertain to the (Accrediting Body) standards, or by reading the entire self-study. We recommend focusing on the standards that are most closely related to your role and using the quick guide for the other standards.
- Include a summary of standards table, as demonstrated in Table 23.5.
- Include snapshots of each standard including
  - The name and language of the standard,
  - The high-level "what is it" with examples,
  - Identified areas of improvement, and
  - Any other pertinent information related to that standard (i.e., something everyone should know).

Each standard should be a page or less (unless it is a robust standard). The preparation of the Quick Reference Guide

Table 23.5 Sample FAQ layout.

Section	Standard	Best for
I Educational outcomes	1) Foundational Knowledge	Instructors, Curriculum Committee Members
	2) Essentials for Practice and Care	Instructors, Curriculum Committee Members
	3) Approach to Practice and Care	Instructors, Curriculum Committee, Preceptors
	4) Personal and Professional Development	Instructors, Curriculum Committee, Preceptors

can be done alongside the development of the self-study and appendices. The team could also include a sample schedule for the visit with the purpose of each meeting outlined.

Accreditation Cycle: External Review

Once the self-study is submitted to the accreditor, it is shared with a team of trained reviewers who will later visit the institution or program (i.e., the site visit team). The review team's number and composition will vary based on the accrediting body and the type of visit (consultative, comprehensive, focused). The team will review the documentation in preparation for the site visit, taking notes on areas of interest. The site visit is typically scheduled to last from 2 to 5 days.

The purpose of the site visit is to verify and clarify information provided in the self-study. To verify the self-study, the review team will conduct interviews with stakeholders (e.g., administrators, staff, faculty), group discussions (e.g., committees, admissions office, students), and review relevant facilities and equipment. The site visit team is there to ensure that quality standards are being met and that CQI is systematized (i.e., there are data-informed improvement cycles built into processes).

Traditionally, these visits were physically on-site. However, in the wake of the Coronavirus pandemic, many accreditors developed means to review sites virtually. While most accreditors are shifting back to the on-site review standard, some are continuing to explore the cost-savings (i.e., reduction in site visit-travel-related expenses) afforded with virtual site visits. Accrediting bodies employing virtual site visits have published guidelines and expectations (e.g., ACPE), which can be found in the resources section of this textbook. While the modality is different, virtual review teams are expected to complete analogous processes to on-site visits.

Preparation for Site Visit

Preparation for the site visit includes the activities of the self-study and activities following the submission of the self-study, such as a mock site visit and faculty meetings to discuss the self-study, appendices, quick reference guide, and improvements prioritized. While developing the documentation will take up the vast majority of the timeline (likely, months 1–20), the short period between the submission of the self-study and the site visit is critical for a successful accreditation site visit. Because the ultimate goal of the process is to successfully be accredited, not taking time to discuss the process and expectations could result in underprepared stakeholders who cannot speak as experts (or give conflicting accounts) on the program or organization during the site visit. This lack of expertise or conflict of information could raise concerns with the site visit team and impact the ultimate decision made by the accrediting body. While it is uncommon to have an accreditation fully revoked (only the most egregious failures result in this), there are statuses less than accredited that could be attained (e.g., probation, under monitoring). Failure to meet full accreditation following a self-study and site visit typically results in additional reporting requirements (e.g., annual reports on standards meeting less than expectation), a focused site visit, and a requirement to update websites and other recruiting materials regarding accreditation status (which could harm recruiting and retention). All this is to say, prepare for the site visit diligently as with the self-study.

Here are some steps a program or institution can take to prepare for an accreditation site visit, following the submission of the self-study:

- Identify key stakeholders and prepare them for interviews with the accreditation team, including students, faculty, staff, alumni, and community members.
- Prepare a schedule of activities, including site visits, meetings, and interviews, which will be conducted by the accreditation team.
  - See Appendix A for an outline of common Site Team activities and meetings as well as their purpose.
- Identify any areas of concern or weakness and develop an action plan to address them before the accreditation visit.
  - Educate your key stakeholders on what has been done to address these issues.
  - Identify and implement those identified as the highest priority.
    o There is more on this in the extended Define-Plan-Do-Review example.
- Consider conducting a mock site visit to simulate the actual accreditation visit and to test the program or institution's readiness.
  - While this is optional, it is highly recommended.
  - This can be accomplished with an external team or an internal team (e.g., cochairs, individuals from institutional effectiveness office, other health science programs, and new faculty who have done site visits at other schools), if external is cost prohibitive.
- Gather relevant documentation and evidence, such as student work samples, syllabi, and program evaluations, which demonstrate compliance with the standards and guidelines.
  - These may be included as appendices or may be in addition to the submitted documentation.
  - As new improvement projects are implemented, keep documentation that outlines what was done and any impacts made.
- Appoint a point person or team to coordinate the accreditation visit and ensure that all activities run smoothly.
  - This will likely be the cochairs of the self-study committee but does not have to be.

It is important to note that preparation for an accreditation visit should be a continuous process and not a last-minute activity. While this portion of the project cycle is short, it is vital for meeting the accreditation goals. Programs and institutions should be proactive in identifying areas for improvement and implementing changes to ensure compliance with accreditation standards.

During a Site Visit

During an accreditation site visit, an accreditation team, typically composed of peer evaluators, conducts an on-site evaluation of a program or institution to assess its compliance with the standards and guidelines of the accrediting body. The site visit is typically divided into two parts: a review of the program or institution's self-study report, and an on-site evaluation, known as the site visit.

- *Self-study review.* The accreditation team will review the program or institution's self-study report, appendices, and other relevant documents. They may ask for additional information, documentation, or clarification from any stakeholder.
- *On-site evaluation.* During the site visit, the team will visit the program or institution's facilities, observe classes, and conduct interviews with faculty, staff, students, and other stakeholders.
- *Meetings.* The accreditation team will conduct meetings with different groups of stakeholders, such as faculty, staff, students, preceptors, committees, and administrators. The meetings are typically focused on specific topics such as program outcomes, assessment, academic support and student services, facilities, and resources.
- *Feedback and recommendations.* At the end of the visit, the accreditation team will provide feedback and recommendations for improvement to the program or institution. They will also provide a written report outlining their findings and recommendations.

Schedules for the site visit team are negotiated several weeks before the team's arrival so both the institution/program and team understand the flow of the on-site evaluation. Once these are solidified, faculty, staff, students and others that will be meeting with accreditors need to be aware of the timeline and expectations.

It is important to note that the site visit is a collaborative and flexible process, and the program or institution should be prepared to provide evidence of compliance with the standards and guidelines of the accrediting body. The program or institution should also be prepared to answer questions and provide additional information as needed.

Appendix A outlines a typical site visit schedule. This table includes the purpose of these meetings and should assist stakeholders or first-time cochairs in communicating the importance of individual meetings held by the site visit team.

Accreditation Cycle: Action or Decision

While the site review team will discuss some of their findings with the chief academic officer at the conclusion of the site visit, the final decision will not be made until the accrediting body's board meets. Following the site visit, the site visit team drafts an evaluation team report (ETR) for the accreditor. The ETR along with the site visit documentation is reviewed by the board of the accrediting body (minus any members that attended the site visit) before an official decision is made. During the next scheduled board meeting (usually held 1–4 times annually), a decision regarding the accreditation status will be made. The institution or program will be alerted officially of its accreditation status following the meeting. If a decision of less than full accreditation is made (e.g., probationary accreditation), then an action plan for getting to full accreditation will be outlined.

Accreditation Cycle: Ongoing Review or Continued Monitoring

Continual monitoring procedures are outlined and published by individual accrediting bodies to establish measures of accountability. Institutions and programs must maintain compliance with accreditation standards between external reviews. Most often maintenance or continual monitoring involves annual as well as interim reporting related to the institution or program's critical functions and reporting of substantive changes (e.g., changes to mission or purpose, organizational structure, legal status, student contact hours, establishing satellite campuses, major enrollment changes) as they occur. Institutions or programs that fail to meet continual monitoring expectations may have their accreditation status revoked, withdrawn, or suspended.

Summary

This comprehensive chapter delves into the intricacies of the accreditation process in higher education institutions and veterinary medicine on a global scale. It covers the history and significance of accreditation in the United States, highlighting the common elements and accreditation cycles. The role of accrediting bodies, including the recent shift from regional to institutional accreditation, is thoroughly explored. Furthermore, the unique history and reach of veterinary medicine accreditation are detailed. This chapter also focuses on the practical side of the accreditation process, providing valuable advice and guidance for anyone seeking to achieve and maintain accreditation status. With a thorough examination of the self-study process and the integration of project management concepts, the chapter serves as an indispensable resource for ensuring a successful and seamless accreditation experience.

References

82nd Congress (1952, July 16). H.R. 7656 - 82nd Congress. An Act to provide vocational readjustment and to restore lost educational opportunities to certain persons who served in the Armed Forces on or after June 27, 1950. Washington, DC: U.S. Congress. www.congress.gov (accessed 02 February 2023).

Accreditation Board for Veterinary Education in Korea (ABOVE-K) (n.d.). http://www.abovek.or.kr/eng/file/Information_Leaflet.pdf (accessed 14 August 2023).

Acevedo-De-los-Ríos, A. and Rondinel-Oviedo, D.R. (2022). Impact, added value and relevance of an accreditation process on quality assurance in architectural higher education. *Quality in Higher Education* 28 (2): 186–204. https://doi.org/10.1080/13538322.2021.1977482.

American Association of Veterinary State Boards (n.d.). International pathway. https://www.aavsb.org/pave (accessed 14 August 2023).

American Psychological Association (n.d.). About APA accreditation. Other Accreditation Statuses. https://www.accreditation.apa.org/other-statuses (accessed 14 August 2023).

American Veterinary Medical Association (2022a). A comparison of accrediting bodies, 2015. https://www.avma.org/sites/default/files/resources/AccreditationComparison.6.26.2015.pdf (accessed 14August 2023).

American Veterinary Medical Association (2022b, October 30). AVMA Center for Veterinary Education Accreditation. Accredited Veterinary Colleges: Public Notice. https://www.avma.org/education/center-for-veterinary-accreditation/accredited-veterinary-colleges (accessed 14 August 2023).

American Veterinary Medical Association (n.d.). History of the AVMA. https://www.avma.org/about/history-avma (accessed 14 August 2023).

American Veterinary Medical Association. (n.d.). COE Recognition by the Council for Higher Education Accreditation. AVMA Council on Education https://www.avma.org/education/accreditation/colleges/coe-recognition-council-higher-education-accreditation (accessed 14 August 2023).

American Veterinary Medical Association (n.d.). What does the reciprocity agreement with foreign countries mean? https://www.avma.org/education/accreditation/colleges/what-does-reciprocity-agreement-foreign-countries-mean (accessed 14 August 2023).

American Veterinary Medical Association (n.d.). COE accreditation policies and procedures. https://www.avma.org/education/center-for-veterinary-accreditation/accreditation-policies-and-procedures-avma-council-education-coe/coe-accreditation-policies-and-procedures-accreditation (accessed 14 August 2023).

American Veterinary Medical Association (n.d.). Educational Commission for foreign veterinary graduates. https://www.avma.org/education/ecfvg (accessed 14 August 2023).

Dawn Apgar (2022). Linking social work licensure examination pass rates to accreditation: the merits, challenges, and implications for social work education. *Journal of Teaching in Social Work* 42 (4): 335–353. https://doi.org/10.1080/08841233.2022.2112809.

Australasian Veterinary Boards Council (n.d.). Program accreditation. https://avbc.asn.au/veterinary-education/program-accreditation (accessed 14 August 2023).

Banasiak, D. (2012). Rooted in knowledge. In: *The AVMA: 150 Years of Education, Science, and Service* (ed. K. Matushek), 161–178. Schaumburg, IL: American Veterinary Medical Association.

Bart, C.K. and Baetz, M.C. (1998). The relationship between mission statements and firm performance: an exploratory study. *Journal of Management Studies* 35: 823–853.

Berruecos, J.M., Trigo, F.J., and Zarco, L.A. (2004). The accreditation system for colleges of veterinary medicine in Mexico and a comparison with the AVMA system. *Journal of Veterinary Medical Education* 31 (2): 111–115.

Branco Germiniani, C. (2004). Veterinary education in Brazil: past, history, current issues. *Journal of Veterinary Medical Education* 31 (1): 28–31.

Congressional Research Service (2022, December 20). An overview of accreditation of higher education in the United States. https://sgp.fas.org/crs/misc/R43826.pdf (accessed 14 August 2023).

Cooke, M., Irby, D.M., and O'Brien, B.C. (2010). *Educating Physicians: A Call for Reform of Medical School and Residency*. Stanford, CA: Jossey-Bass.

Costa, Giovane, Maccari Emerson, Martins Cibele, Kniess Claudia. (2014). Project Management in Higher Education Institutions: Pro-Administration Case. https://www.researchgate.net/publication/275658788_Project_Management_in_Higher_Education_Institutions_Pro-Administration_Case (accessed 14 August 2023).

Council for Higher Education Accreditation (2023a, January 11). Regional accrediting Organizations. https://www.chea.org/regional-accrediting-organizations (accessed 14 August 2023).

Council for Higher Education Accreditation (2023b, January 11). Accreditation and recognition in the United States. https://www.chea.org/accreditation-recognition-united-states (accessed 14 August 2023).

Dominelli, A., Iwanowicz, S.L., Bailie, G.R. et al. (2007). A project management approach to an ACPE accreditation self-study. *American Journal of Pharmaceutical Education* 71 (2): 23. https://doi.org/10.5688/aj710223.

Ellaway, R. and Bates, J. (2018). Distributed medical education in Canada. *Canadian Medical Education Journal* 9 (1): e1–e5.

European Association of Establishments for Veterinary Education (2023). The association, foundation, mission, objectives. https://www.eaeve.org (accessed 14 August 2023).

Gallant, N. (2016). Why veterinary school accreditation matters. *Canadian Veterinary Journal* 57 (3): 227–229.

Hannah, S.B. (1996). The higher education act of 1992: skills, constraints, and the politics of higher education. *The Journal of Higher Education* 67 (5): 498–527. https://doi.org/10.2307/2943866.

Harcleroad, F. (1980). *Accreditation: History, Process, and Problems*. AAHE-ERIC.

House Select Committee (1951). *Investigation of GI Schools: Hearings before the House Select Committee to Investigate Educational and Training Program under GI Bill*. Washington, DC: Government Printing Office.

Keating, S.B. (2015). *Curriculum Development and Evaluation in Nursing*. New York, NY: Springer Publishing Company.

Kumar, P., Shukla, B., and Passey, D. (2020). Impact of accreditation on quality and excellence of higher education institutions. *Investigación Operacional* 41 (2): 151–167.

Larkin, M. (2011). Mexican school joins an elite group: Hemisphere's oldest veterinary school is COE-accredited. *Journal of the American Veterinary Medical Association* https://www.avma.org/javma-news/2011-04-15/mexican-school-joins-elite-group (accessed 14 August 2023).

Liaison Committee on Medical Education (2023). Scope and purpose of accreditation. https://lcme.org/about (accessed 14 August 2023).

Malaysian Veterinary Council (2023, January 11). About us. www.mvc.gov.my/about (accessed 14 August 2023).

Parsons, M. (1997). *Power and Politics: Federal Higher Education Policymaking in the 1990's*. Albany: Statue University of New York Press.

Permanent Subcommittee on Investigations of the Committee on Governmental Affairs (1991). *Abuses in Federal Student aid Programs*. Washington: U.S. Government Printing Office https://files.eric.ed.gov/fulltext/ED332631.pdf (accessed 14 August 2023).

Bernie Trilling, Walter Ginevri (2017). Project Management for Education: The Bridge to 21st Century Learning.

Project Management Institute (2022). *A Guide to the Project Management Body of Knowledge (PMBOK Guide)*, 7e. Project Management Institute.

Royal College of Veterinary Surgeons (2023 January 11). External review of the rCVS by the ENQA. www.rcvs.org.uk/setting-standards/accrediting-primary-qualifications/rcvs-enqa-review (accessed 14 August 2023).

Shiffer, C.D., Boulet, J.R., Cover, L.L., and Pinsky, W.W. (2019). Advancing the quality of medical education worldwide: ECFMG's 2023 medical school accreditation requirement. *Journal of Medical Regulation* 105 (4): 8–16.

South African Veterinary Council (2023, January 11). Evaluation of Veterinary Training: Standards and operating procedures. https://savc.org.za/wp-content/uploads/2021/09/SAVC_VET-SER-FRAMEWORK_2019_FINAL.pdf (accessed 14 August 2023).

State Authorization (2010). Federal Register. https://www.federalregister.gov/documents/2010/10/29/2010-26531/program-integrity-issues (accessed 14 August 2023).

Student Assistance General Provisions (2022). https://www.federalregister.gov/documents/2022/10/20/2022-22822/student-assistance-general-provisions-federal-family-education-loan-program-and-william-d-ford (accessed 14 August 2023).

Taylor Preciado, J.J., Galindo Garcia, J., and Villagomez Zavala, D.A.F. (2005). Plans and hopes for veterinary education in Mexico. *Journal of Veterinary Medical Education* 32 (4): 389–398.

Thompson, P.N., Gunter, K., Schuna, J.M., and Jr., Tomayko E. J. (2020). Are all four-day school weeks created equal? A national assessment of four-day school week policy adoption and implementation. *Education Finance and Policy* 1–50: https://doi.org/10.1162/edfp_a_00316.

U.S. Department of Education (2023a, January 11). Programmatic Accrediting Agencies. Accreditation in the United States https://www2.ed.gov/admins/finaid/accred/accreditation_pg4.html#National_Institutional (accessed 14 August 2023).

U.S. Department of Education (2023b, January 11). Overview of Accreditation in the United States. Accreditation in the United States. https://www2.ed.gov/admins/finaid/accred/accreditation.html#Overview (accessed 14 August 2023).

UNCHE (2022, October 30). Who We Are. National Council for Higher Education. https://unche.or.ug/who-we-are (accessed 14 August 2023).

Veterinary Council of India (2023, January 11). About VCI. http://vci.dadf.gov.in (accessed 14 August 2023).

Additional Resources

ACPE Guide and Policies for Virtual Site Visits Approved by ACPE Board July 2020 Version 2, minor updates January 2021.

Appendix A   A Typical Mock Site Visit Schedule

	First Day		
Approx. Time	**Activity**	**Attendees**	**Purpose –** *Overall the team looking to help, looking for noise, verifying*
1 hour	MEETING: Dean	Full Site Visit Team Dean	Provide an overview of the program and its current status, including any challenges faced by the program and its leadership, highlight significant accomplishments or events, assess the position of the program's leadership, and discuss the program's vision and future direction
1 hour	MEETING: Self-Study Committee	CoChairs of Self-Study Primary Internal Writers and Reviewers of Self Study Full Site Visit Team	Discuss the preparation of the self-study documentation to gain an understanding of the preparation
15 min	Break	Full Site Team	Even reviewers need a break
1 h	MEETING: Students	Selection of Students from Across Curriculum ($\sim n = 5$) Site Team Members[a]	Inquire about details related to the program, including the communication process, application and admission process, available resources, academic policies and how they are disseminated, and the overall student experience
1 h	LUNCH	Dean, Self-Study Leadership, selected faculty, staff, students Full Site Team	Informal discussion and questions that have not yet come up in the review
1 h	MEETING: Curriculum Committee	Curriculum Committee Site Team Members[a]	Examine recent developments and changes within the program, explore the composition and organization of the committee, determine the frequency of their meetings, understand the level of autonomy given, investigate the upcoming projects and initiatives, and investigate the process of decision-making and approval
1 hour	MEETING: Experiential Office	Members of Experiential Education Site Team Members[a]	Examine recent developments and changes within the program, explore the composition and organization of the committee, determine the frequency of their meetings, understand the level of autonomy given, investigate the upcoming projects and initiatives, and investigate the process of decision-making and approval. Team will likely inquire about the level of support provided
15 min	Break	Full Site Team	Even reviewers need a break
1 h	MEETING: Admissions Committee	Admissions Committee Site Team Members[a]	Examine recent developments and changes within the program, examine the composition and organization of the committee, determine the frequency of their meetings, understand the level of autonomy given, investigate the upcoming projects and initiatives, and investigate the process of decision-making and approval Inquire about the level of support for recruiting and the availability of resources, investigate the admissions process, examine the method of conducting interviews
30 min	MEETING: Dean and Self-Study Leadership	Dean Self-Study Cochairs Full Site Team	Debrief on day's activities, discuss needs, and expectations for following day

		Second Day	
Time	**Activity**	**Attendees**	**Purpose**
1 h	MEETING: Executive Leadership	Full Site Visit Team Dean Executive Leadership for Program	Examine the formation and role of the committee, describe the leadership style of the dean, explain the function and purpose of the committee and the dean's role within it, discuss the relationship between the committee and the dean (e.g., consensus or advisory), identify any challenges faced by the school/program, and discuss the actions being taken to address those challenges
1 h	MEETING: Provost and other Financial Officers	Site Team Members[a] Dean Provost Financial Officers at College and University	Examine the relationship with the program or college to the University. Explore the financial commitment to the program under review. Discuss budget or other financial concerns
1 hour	MEETING: Assessment Committee	Assessment Committee Site Team Members[a]	Examine recent developments and changes within the program, explore the composition and organization of the committee, determine the frequency of their meetings, understand the level of autonomy given, investigate the upcoming projects and initiatives, and investigate the process of decision-making and approval Inquire about the upcoming initiatives and projects, investigate the level of support and buy-in from the faculty, and explore strategies to increase it
15 min	Break	Full Site Team	Even reviewers need a break
1 h	MEETING: Meetings with individual faculty	Selection of faculty from program (~$n = 5$) Full Site Team	The Site Team will conduct individual meetings simultaneously to optimize the time and number of people met Provide an overview of the school's direction, explain the research, development, promotion and tenure process, describe the resources available, and discuss any challenges faced by the school It is during these interviews that "noise" often arises
1 h	LUNCH	Dean, Self-Study Leadership, selected faculty, staff, students Full Site Team	Informal discussion and questions that have not yet come up in the review
1 h	MEETING: Preceptors	Selection of preceptors from program (~$n = 5$) Site Team Members[a]	In a group setting, the team will discuss the readiness of the students precepted, the resources provided to preceptors, the opportunities for development, the communication channels with the program, the evaluation method used for students, and the access to university resources such as journals and interlibrary loan Emphasis will be placed on the aspects of Development, Communication, and Students
1 hour	MEETING: Student Affairs	Student Affairs Staff Student Affairs Leadership Site Team Members[a]	Discuss the available resources for students, evaluate the adequacy of staff to provide effective support, identify any challenges faced by the department/office, assess the level of administrative support, identify trends in student behavior, mental wellness, and study skills, and describe the development programs offered for both students and faculty
15 min	Break	Full Site Team	Even reviewers need a break
1 h	MEETING: Site Team	Full Site Team	Internal discussion to debrief on visit
1 h	MEETING: Dean and Self-Study Leadership	Dean Self-Study Cochairs Full Site Team	Debrief on visit. Preliminary decision will be discussed at this time

[a] May not be the full team, some may be viewing facilities, reviewing documents, or hosting interviews with individuals (faculty, staff, preceptors, etc.)

24

Leaving Thoughts and the Future of Veterinary Education

Katherine Fogelberg, DVM, PhD (Science Education), MA (Educational Leadership)
Virginia-Maryland College of Veterinary Medicine, Blacksburg, VA, USA

Section 1: Introduction

> Times and conditions change so rapidly that we must keep our aim constantly focused on the future.
> Walt Disney

This textbook provides a lot of information about education broadly and veterinary education specifically where it can – which is just what I envisioned when I proposed this book to Wiley over two years ago. I wanted to publish a textbook that laid a solid foundation in educational philosophy, theory, and psychology, as well as one that had some practical information that I had not seen in other textbooks aimed at education. I wanted to publish a book that would help veterinary educators and would also have parts that could help *any* educator at the university level – there seem to be rather few out there, and none quite as comprehensive as this one. Of course, the fact that it is, when possible, veterinary specific, makes it even better – not that I am biased. I never actually thought it would be accepted, and even as I read the letter from the publisher indicating that it was, in fact, going to be published, I think I was still in a bit of shock. It was an ambitious proposal; one that I could never have imagined I would engage with even five years ago. It has certainly been an experience – mostly good – and I am pleased to see it finally in print.

I have no idea, really, how many folks will want to buy this textbook, though everyone I have spoken to about it has expressed interest and gratitude that such a book is being published. There are not a lot of veterinary education-centric textbooks out there, and I truly hope that this one finds its place on the shelves of at least one person at every veterinary program – I firmly believe it is that good! But I also hope others will find it useful – those in higher education in general, or who teach in professional programs, or

are stressing because they are getting ready to go through their first accreditation (or 10th). There is a little something for everyone in higher education contained within this textbook, and I am thankful that I have so many colleagues who were willing and able to contribute their expertise.

In the end, however, my primary audience is veterinary educators. We are in higher education and professional programs instruction, so there are a number of overlaps between us and human medicine or nursing or law school in terms of what we can, should, and actually do in the classrooms, labs, and clinics we educate within. However, veterinary medical education (VME) presents some unique challenges that other professional programs do not – and while we are working hard to continue producing high-quality veterinarians, it is becoming increasingly challenging to do so. The challenges we face are not insurmountable, but they are beginning to feel as though they could become so quickly. Not all of them will be mitigated by educating our educators, of course, but a good many of them could be at least managed better by doing so. If you are reading this textbook, I want to thank you for wanting to learn more about education and all the complexities of doing it *well*.

As for the quote that opens this chapter, a little background. My husband and I have no kids, but we still love DisneyWorld: it is our opinion that it is more fun to visit Disney as adults and without kids for a variety of reasons. On one of our many trips to the most magical place on Earth, we were at Epcot and wandering through the maze of barriers they had built due to ongoing construction. Along the barriers they had a variety of quotes from Walt Disney, including the one that opens this chapter – and it resonated with me particularly because on that trip, I had just received notice that I was a finalist for a job I had applied for in veterinary education. I thought perhaps it would come in handy, and it most certainly did.

For those of you unfamiliar with the process of on-site interviews in academia, suffice it to say that it can be a long two or three days, depending on the institution. It's one of those rites of passage every aspiring academic must go through, it seems, and while it consists of lots of meetings with lots of people up and down the chain, it also usually requires the candidate to put together and deliver a presentation that is open to the entire college and often, nowadays, delivered in a hybrid manner. Sometimes the search committee asks you to come up with your own topic, sometimes they provide one for you. In my case, for this particular interview, a topic had been provided for me: What did I see as the challenges and opportunities in VME?

It was a meatball for me (to use a baseball term); it seemed like a topic that was right up my alley. I dove in and created a presentation that was – well, pretty awful! But after some reconsideration, I had a light bulb moment and was able to create a presentation of which I am, to this day, very proud. I did not get the job (in case you were wondering), although I did have a couple of other interviews for similar roles and was eventually successful. Sadly, I was never able to reuse this presentation for those other interviews, but I knew it would come in handy someday – and here we are. In a parallel fashion, I had written this chapter already and was ready to have someone read it over for editing, but something was holding me back. It just did not feel quite right. It was not awful, but it was not me; it had the content but did not feel like it had a compelling purpose. I asked myself, is anyone really going to want to read all these words? I felt pretty sure the answer was "no." Thus, on one of my (increasingly less frequent) morning runs, it popped into my head that perhaps this was the time to revisit that presentation I had created a couple of years ago of which I was so proud. So, let's jump into why I think about veterinary education as a *wicked problem*, and why I believe it is so pertinent now and will continue to be well into our future.

Section 2: The Power of Veterinary Medical Education

> With great power comes great responsibility. Voltaire
> With wicked problems come wicked opportunities
> K. Fogelberg

VME is the gatekeeper to entering the profession of veterinary medicine as a doctor. There are, of course, other ways to enter the profession – as a veterinary assistant, kennel keeper, receptionist, or credentialed veterinary technician. Some of these require schooling, others on-the-job training. But the only way to become a veterinarian is to go through a veterinary medical training program, most often known as a college or school of veterinary medicine. It doesn't matter in what continent or country you live; it doesn't matter if the program is accredited or not accredited. To become a veterinarian, a doctor of medicine who treats animals other than humans, you must go through a veterinary medical training program. That is power.

Contrary to popular belief, power is not always a bad thing. It can be leveraged for both good and evil; it can enable people to accomplish great and wonderful things, even as it can also corrupt and cause inequalities. The power we hold as veterinary educators change people's lives – for those who get accepted to veterinary school, it should be for the better. Because what we do in our classrooms, labs, and hospitals every day affects the lives of hundreds of thousands of animals and people – but before it can do that, it affects the lives of thousands of budding veterinarians. And it is our responsibility – and privilege – to ensure future veterinarians are informed, skilled, and thoughtful – aka, *competent* – once they graduate. But we must also ensure they are healthy enough to function as human beings, as sisters and brothers, aunts and uncles, mothers and fathers, friends and life partners.

This does not mean that we should cater to students' every whim. On the contrary, this means that we must make the hard decisions that come with being leaders – something every educator is, whether they want to be or not. It means balancing our high expectations of students with the realities of day-to-day life. It means managing our own lives in a way that can model what that looks like – bumps and all. And it means establishing a culture where those balanced expectations are the norm rather than the exception.

As educators, we have one of the hardest jobs in the world. And yes – I am biased – but I strongly believe veterinary educators have one of the hardest professional jobs in the world. I will make my argument for why in a bit. But here, let us first discuss why *education* is one of the hardest professions – this is where the idea of the *wicked problem* comes in.

Part 1: Wicked Problems: Defined and Examples

Horst Rittel and Melvin Webber, two professors at the University of California at Davis, first coined the phrase *wicked problem* in 1973: "We use the term wicked in a meaning akin to that of 'malignant' (in contrast to 'benign') or 'vicious' (like a circle) or *'tricky' (like a leprechaun)* or 'aggressive' (like a lion, in contrast to the docility of a lamb)" – the emphasis is mine, because "tricky" is how I perceive veterinary education most closely fitting into the wicked problem mold. They also identified 10 criteria that must be met for a problem to be classified as wicked:

1) There is no definitive formulation.
2) There is no stopping rule.
3) Solutions are not true or false, only good or bad.
4) There is no immediate or ultimate test of a solution.
5) Every solution is a one-shot operation.
6) There are an endless number of solutions/approaches.
7) Each solution is essentially unique.
8) All solutions are considered a symptom of another problem.
9) The problem's descriptions determine its possible solutions.
10) The planner has no right to be wrong.

A few prime examples of wicked problems include climate change, *educational policy*, hunger, poverty, public health, sustainability, and terrorism. That is a pretty heavy-duty list – and I did not put educational policy there myself (though I did emphasize it here). It does help you see, though, that education writ large is an issue – though perhaps it has not been applied to a specific sector of education as I do in this chapter.

In the following sections, I will address each of these criteria as it specifically relates to VME in an attempt to convince you that VME is a wicked problem and, as such, requires us to consider its place, role, and challenges. It is also important for us to view VME through this lens as educators because we are on the front lines of the profession – we are the (essentially) all-powerful gatekeepers, opening and closing the gates to those who wish to become veterinarians based on our processes. And for those who have the gate opened, we need to ensure it is not a floodgate (or a wide-open firehose), but rather a gate that allows our students to walk through, encounter challenges that are difficult but not impossible, and supports them appropriately as they navigate each challenge so they leave their programs as competent, healthy, and strong practitioners – no matter what that practice may look like.

Part 2: VME as a Wicked Problem

There Is No Definitive Formulation

At the time I write this chapter, there are 54 American Veterinary Medical Association Council on Education (AVMA-CoE) accredited veterinary programs globally and *every program is different,* yet all of them, of course, meet the accreditation requirements and standards that have been outlined by the AVMA-CoE. As such, at least by quantitative measures, each of these programs produce "successful" veterinarians (successful being defined

slightly differently, depending upon whom you ask). Thus, there is no identifiably "perfect" veterinary program – there is no definitive formulation.

There Is No Stopping Rule

Wicked problems lack an inherent logic that signals when they are solved. What does that mean for VME? What does "perfect" even mean in VME? How would we even know it if had actually created a "perfect" VME program or curriculum? Take a moment to consider what beacon(s) would indicate that our graduates are truly "day one ready"?

These questions indicate that VME is a constantly evolving problem that requires continuous attention. And to be fair, we will likely never reach a "perfect" veterinary education program – but we should certainly continue striving to do so. What we absolutely cannot do is continue what we currently are doing and lulling ourselves into thinking that it is "good enough." We ask our students to be lifelong, reflective practitioners – is it not important, then, for us to ask ourselves to do the same in education with regard to our current approaches and practices?

Solutions Are Not True or False, Only Good or Bad

If we consider the multiple areas of VME that are challenging us right now, an entire book could be written on this criterion alone. But one that tends to dominate the conversations right now (and has historically): the rising costs of education. Again, contrary to popular belief, there are both good and bad consequences of this cost increase. Let's start with the good: the rising costs of education improve facilities and potentially quality faculty/staff because it increases the income coming into the state (public universities) and program (private universities). The bad? Rising costs of tuition impact graduates' financial viability for those who rely on government and private loans to fund their education (it took me 29 years to pay off my student loans – not all of them from veterinary school, but a good chunk of them certainly were).

Another challenge we are dealing with on a large scale now, and one that has been growing significantly over the past couple of decades, is the poor state of mental health and well-being across our profession. While this elephant lurked in the shadows for far too long, it is now emerging and becoming a focus for those at all levels and across all industries in which veterinarians are employed. It would be pretty difficult to convince anyone that addressing the problem is a waste of time and resources – resources that have been increasingly allocated to these efforts, especially in the last 10 years or so. This is great because it is working to improve the quality of life for our veterinary students and faculty, which we hope will help them beyond graduation and retain them in university roles. Perhaps this will also help improve our internal views of the profession – one that, as of 2018, saw around 60% of veterinarians saying they would not recommend veterinary medicine to someone else as a profession to pursue (Lau 2018). So, what is the downside to this, you may be wondering? Well, increased resources require more funding, which can contribute to increasing the cost of the program overall – which, in turn, affects the quality of life for new graduates who are indebted because they now carry an even heavier student loan burden upon graduating.

Not only, then, are solutions to the many individual issues in VME challenging to address, but they are also often good chasing bad or bad chasing good. We can easily get stuck in this negative feedback loop without understanding how it started in the first place and how we can stop it.

There Is No Immediate or Ultimate Test of a Solution

There are multitude examples of issues in VME that aptly illustrate this criterion. One of the first that comes to my mind is the issue of diversity, equity, inclusion, and belonging (DEIB) policies and procedures. It is pretty clear that a small but growing cohort of people has been doing this intentional work for a long time; it is also clear that what we are doing is not acutely changing the face of VME or the profession. Change is being made, but it is creeping and incremental; spotty and variably accepted. Figuring out how to change culture – whether it is to increase DEIB or change a toxic one – is not going to happen overnight. And there is never going to be a definitive multiple choice (or other type) exam that we can collectively "pass" that demonstrates our solution is "right."

A couple of other examples that may hit close to home for you include changing curricula, how we increase recognition and rewards for good teaching, and deciding to implement different approaches to teaching. Let's consider each of these in relation to this idea that there is no immediate or ultimate test of a solution.

There is currently a sweeping movement toward outcomes-based veterinary education, which is – at least in my view – a response to the traditional "sit and get" curricula that have dominated the veterinary – and higher education – landscape for decades. On the surface and in theory, this is a good thing – the idea that we want our students to obtain mastery is not new and is, in fact, the goal of all veterinary programs – and has been for a while. Consider this: veterinary students become veterinarians overnight. It is a transition they have been working toward for years and years, of course, but the actual change itself is literally overnight – one day the student is a student, the next day, they walk across the stage, get called "doctor" officially for the first time, and walk off the stage and into practice. That practice may be an internship or a "real job"

out in a clinic. With this outcome in mind, our curriculum is having difficulty keeping up with its current form. And, of course, there is the AVMA's requirement that curriculum be thoughtfully revisited every so often.

Regardless of the causes for curricular review and revision, the fact remains that anyone going through this process realizes while we come up with solutions that we *think* will help us evolve, we do not actually *know* for years – and even after years, we learn quickly that there is no single assessment we can deliver and use to determine whether we have been successful in our change.

Every Solution Is a One-Shot Operation

We have all been faced with choices we had to make that we only had one chance to make. These decisions happen on small and large scales everyday, from what we eat (or do not) for breakfast to whether we should start a family, from what to major in during our studies to where we decide to earn our degree(s). With each of these decisions, there are varying levels of opportunities to change the choice the next time, but the decision in real-time is a one-shot operation: once you make the decision, you do not get to go back and change it.

How does this relate to VME? Well, when it comes to curricular changes, you get one shot when you implement it – you do it or you don't. And you have to wait for a while to determine if it worked, or sort-of worked, or did not work at all the way you hoped. In other words, you have no real opportunity to learn whether your solution is a good one through trial and error in the sense of a scientific experiment, nor do you have the luxury of using a control group and a treatment group. Can you imagine running different curricula simultaneously for the number of years you would have to do that to get decent enough data to support your ultimate decision? Logistics aside, the ethical aspects of this are just unacceptable.

Beyond that, when (potential) solutions are selected and implemented, you cannot go back and "fix" any flaws in the solution you have decided to deploy. With curricular changes, this is eminently true. You can, of course, go back to the "old" curriculum if you discover that the "new" curriculum just is not doing what you thought it would, but you cannot go back and change the curriculum for the students who went through the "new" one – they have already completed their studies and are out in the world, for better or for worse. Thus, curricular changes are one-shot operations whose implemented solutions are irreversible – so you better make that implemented solution (or single shot) count!

There are other examples within VME that illustrate this criterion, too; I am certain you can think of many on your own. The faculty shortage (clinical and teaching); DEI and the decision to either make it a priority or not; the lack of veterinary educational research (VER). I will leave it to you to figure out why these are "one-shot operations" and to think of others that fall under this criterion. I hope my curricular example has, at the very least, gotten your wheels turning with respect to how many different ways this could be applied in VME.

There Are an Endless Number of Solutions/Approaches

On the flip side of the one-shot operation, this criterion is equally confounding. While the implementation of your selected solution or approach is, indeed, a one-shot (or one-time) deal, arriving at the "best" path forward can be overwhelming. How many different ways can we construct a VME program? There are, in theory, an infinite number of models that could be successfully (or unsuccessfully) employed. There is some evidence to support this, in fact – all you need to do is look at the small subset of VME programs that are accredited through the AVMA-CoE. With 54 accredited veterinary schools around the world, if you study each one you would quickly find that there are 54 different approaches to curriculum and curriculum mapping, meeting societal demand, increasing DEI, improving mental health and wellness issues, improving views of the profession, research, creating and rewarding good educators, and on and on. In fact, even the number of years required for the programs differs somewhat from country to country – with some programs condensed into three years (as with University of Arizona) and others requiring six years (as with University of Utrecht in the Netherlands). Thus, there is no "well-described set of permissible operations that may be incorporated into the plan" (Rittel and Webber 1973, p. 164).

All Solutions are Considered a Symptom of Another Problem

The eighth criterion for a problem to be considered wicked is that every solution really arises from the need to address the symptom of another problem. What does this mean? Well, we have been unable to aptly balance supply and demand when it comes to producing veterinarians and counteracting the loss of existing veterinarians (whether due to attrition, retirement, or just not enough being trained). But this is a symptom of the issues being driven by personal, social, governmental, and economic issues.

Consider this: students graduating from veterinary school today have an average debt load of over US$ 160,000 in the United States (for those carrying debt). This debt is crippling personally for many both financially – as they try to figure out how to make student loan payments while still having a decent quality of life – and emotionally, as they often choose to go into an area of practice that does not align with their true passion because of the debt they have acquired. I certainly ended up practicing small animal medicine for 13 years because I had a

six-figure student debt load, and that was the only way I was going to be able to pay it back and live a life that was not a continuation of my life as a poor veterinary student! I certainly don't regret having that experience, but my first choice was NOT clinical practice, and my mental health certainly suffered during those years because of it. This is just as true for those wishing to go into equine practice, rural practice, or those considering additional specialty training. But one of the ongoing solutions to this issue is to maintain (at least in the United States) a four-year program, regardless of its increasing lack of tenability. The argument for this is that we do not want to increase the already overwhelming debt load of our new graduates, thus the current solutions are certainly symptoms of another problem.

The Problem's Descriptions Determine Its Possible Solutions

As veterinary educators, we perform many tasks throughout the days and years. The allocation of time and effort to each of the following tasks (which is not even close to an exhaustive list) varies from person to person and institution to institution, but in general, the vast majority of us work to generate new scientific knowledge, generate new educational knowledge and insights, improve animal, human, and ecosystem health, develop the next generations of veterinarians, and provide high-quality learning opportunities to veterinary students. Therefore, it is each of our individual ways of describing the problem that, when collected together, helps us determine the most viable possible solutions. In other words, how we perceive, analyze, and prioritize these duties, along with our many others, determines our approaches to creating solutions.

Each Wicked Problem Is Essentially Unique

Each wicked problem is different from other problems – wicked or otherwise. As a profession, we have long taken our lead from human medicine, and that has been incredibly helpful in many ways. But in others – in ways that are important – I believe that following that lead has held us back. Consider the ways that veterinary medicine is unique from human medicine – and feel free to add your thoughts to this list, as it is by no means exhaustive.

Veterinary medicine focuses on animal health but also encompasses human, environmental, and ecosystem health. It is comparative and broad, both in the species covered and the topics considered important. Human medicine focuses on a single species at a very detailed level, leaving many of the pieces of medicine that veterinarians learn about to other members of the human medical team (pharmacists, dentists, and optometrists, for example), and have a significant number of supporting team members who augment their roles (psychologists, social workers, nurses, for example).

In veterinary medicine, supply and demand rely largely on *disposable income* rather than a "right to health," which is the driving force behind human medicine. As a result, veterinarians are far more service oriented (as a whole) than human medicine is – we have more patients and clients than we can handle currently, but if those patients and clients decide to take their business elsewhere, it hurts our bottom line. There is no large-scale insurance industry (though it is growing) to ensure that pets receive the care they should get on a regular and emergency basis; as clinicians, veterinarians rely on people being willing to spend their real dollars in real time to keep us afloat.

Another unique aspect of VME is that the current VME model was built on the human education model, and the human medical education model changed rapidly (or as rapidly as an overly large institution can) in response to the Flexner Report, written by Abraham Flexner and published in 1910. Widely viewed in medical education as one of the most influential treatises on medical training, Flexner's influence is still widely seen today – in the way we move students through a fairly standard and time-based curriculum that lays the foundations of medicine in the preclinical years to prepare students for clinical rotations/clerkships in the final years of their program, for example. In human medicine this is a 2 + 2 version, with two years studying the "basic sciences" and two years applying that information during clinical rotations, often referred to as clerkships. (I will leave the negative effects of Flexner's report for another time, though there are plenty of published articles exploring the damage done by the changes Flexner wrought – you can get a brief summary at AAMC.org if you desire.)

Such clerkships vary in length from program to program and are designed to expose medical students to a wide variety of specialties – from psychology to radiology, surgery to internal medicine, neurology to obstetrics and gynecology, and so on and so forth. In human medicine, clerkships are primarily spent at off-site hospitals or clinics rather than at an attached teaching hospital. There are, however, a few programs with hospitals attached in the United States, and while I was unable to find a comprehensive list of those programs, the *New York Times* reports that about 26% of hospitals in the United States are designated as teaching hospitals (Frakt 2017).

Given that there are currently 192 medical schools in the United States (including allopathic and osteopathic), the vast majority of human medical programs use what is termed the "distributive model" of clinical education. This system appears to work reasonably well for human medicine; it has worked for a very long time and for very good reason: medical programs prepare students to become specialists – in essence, medical school is an intermediate degree-granting program, in that it produces MDs or DOs, but those physicians are *not yet ready to practice*

autonomously (this was lightly touched upon the section discussing how each wicked problem is essentially unique). Indeed, only those who continue on to, and complete, their required residencies in a specialty (usually) of their choosing and pass the requisite associated examinations can ultimately become licensed to practice as autonomously acting physicians. (This is why medical programs are referred to as undergraduate medical education in most countries; it is the residency that is considered graduate medical education, as this is the terminal training that serves as the basis of qualification to practice medicine without supervision). Thus, the purpose of a medical education program is not to produce a ready-to-practice physician; rather, it is to produce a physician with enough broad medical knowledge and experience to be able to take on an additional three to seven years of specialized training.

Returning our focus to VME and remembering that the veterinary education model was fashioned after the human medical education model, the idea that it serves veterinarians as well as it serves physicians is a bit absurd when you take the time to think about it. In a standard four-year (academic year based) or three-year (calendar year based) veterinary curriculum, students are expected to learn and effectively apply knowledge and skills spanning seven core species, practice management and business, communication and professional skills, and public health. Because veterinarians are truly expected to be competent across species, and across medical topics, this means that veterinary students are absorbing information covering not only those seven species and associated skills but also the specific specialty areas (broadly) that physicians receive little to no training in unless they pursue a residency in the area. Thus, while veterinary students are typically using three classroom-based years to gain the information needed to be licensed and medical students are doing this in only two, veterinary students are learning the anatomy, physiology, pharmacology, toxicology, neurology, microbiology, histology, pathology, nutrition, dentistry, dermatology, internal medicine, surgery, etc. of seven species in an attempt to be prepared for clerkships, lasting anywhere from 12 to 18 months. At the end of this journey, veterinary students are (ideally) licensed to practice autonomously the day after they walk across that stage and are called "doctor" for the first time.

If reading this exhausts you, it has achieved its aim: veterinarians understand this mountain, while I fear the vast majority of others in society have no idea the task laid upon the shoulders of veterinary educators, students, and practitioners. It takes a LOT to become a veterinarian. This is not to impugn the difficulties faced by other professional programs; it is merely highlighting the unique challenges veterinary educators face every day. Challenges that are, as of this writing, beginning to crush the veterinary profession as we grapple with how to continue producing "day one ready" veterinarians in the face of ever-rising volumes of medical advancements that continue to expand the information students must learn even as we refuse to consider changes to our current education model that are literally bursting at its ever-weakening seams.

The Planner Has No Right to Be Wrong

Finally, when it comes to wicked problems, whatever solution we come up with and decide to implement, we cannot get it wrong (no pressure, huh?). The aim of solving wicked problems is "not to find truth, but to improve some characteristics of the world where people live" (Rittel and Webber 1973, p.167). This means that those who provide solutions "are liable for the consequences of the solutions they generate; the effects can matter a great deal to the people who are touched by those actions" (Rittel and Webber 1973, p. 167).

It is a heavy lift, and it is one that our students – and our profession – rely on those of us in VME to get "right." Are we doing OK, right now? Yes, but just barely. Society is evolving rapidly and so is veterinary medicine; we are in significant danger of being left behind if we do not embrace the opportunity to evolve faster and become more agile. Our programs are becoming increasingly difficult to staff with qualified and interested clinicians and teachers, our students are demanding more evidence that what we are doing is preparing them for success in their careers, and the general public is becoming increasingly alarmed at the lack of access they have to veterinary professionals in all sectors of animal health. We are stretched too thin, and as everyone knows, when something is stretched thin enough, eventually it breaks.

Section 3: Moving Veterinary Education Forward

So what? Why did I spend so many words on explaining why VME is a wicked problem and ask you to read my thoughts? Because I hope I have convinced you that VME needs a makeover. I have felt this way since the first year I entered veterinary school almost 20 years ago, and I feel even more strongly that this is true today. In a lovely twist of irony, you spent a good bit of your time reading this textbook and learning about the history of education – how it started, why it started, the evolutions we went through to figure out how people learn, and now I am asking you to consider the future. It is a question I ask myself often – for those who know me, they may say I ask it too often (I can't help it, I'm a planner). It is a question I asked – rhetorically – during many job interviews with veterinary programs over the years and one that always raised eyebrows but never raised really solid answers. So I ask you, someone

who is clearly engaged in education at a depth that is not yet true of every veterinary instructor: *What is our vision for the profession in 50 years?*

I ask this question in reference to veterinary education specifically, for some obvious reasons and for some that may not be so obvious. My suspicion is that other professional programs should be asking the same question if they are not already. Indeed, I also suspect that universities in general need to take a close and critical look at their purposes and goals – in an era of ever-increasing student loan debt that affects undergraduate, graduate, and professional students alike; is consistently challenged by societal evolutions and political machinations (from both the right and the left); is increasingly viewed as a business rather than an institution of education; and threatens to become a dinosaur with the rapid growth in access through technology, higher education must look at itself and consider its future. And, as I have hopefully convinced you, education is generally a *wicked problem* on a larger scale; in this, at least, VME is not alone.

The obvious reasons I posed this question include those you have probably already figured out: I am a veterinarian and veterinary educator, and the author of a textbook about veterinary education with a slightly broader slant toward education as a whole. But the less obvious reasons (to some, at least) are those that involve where we currently stand in VME. It is those less obvious reasons that led me to outline for you why I view VME as a wicked problem: it is not because we should be throwing our hands up in despair, lamenting the fact that we will never "get it right." No – it is because I firmly believe that with wicked problems come wicked opportunities – opportunities that are staring us in the face right now, that should push us out of our comfort zone to consider new and creative ways to address the issues we face – the issues that make VME a wicked problem.

For me, the biggest issue we have is that we are a profession asking students to obtain competencies in a wide variety of fields (medicine, public health, communication, practice management, and the like) covering a minimum of seven species *in just four years*. With the increasing pace of medical discoveries that must be taught, the time for teaching shrinks each year because more is being packed into it. We are, as I put it somewhat succinctly the other day during a conversation with a colleague, trying really hard to pack 10-lb of poop into a 5-lb bag. And, as we can only reasonably expect, we are failing miserably. It is a well-supported idea that we can only lean into the future by understanding and learning about and from the past. To be better, we must know more so we can teach better and lead our students to better learning. But we must also be willing to candidly reflect upon that past. What have we done in a superior manner? What have we failed to do well? And what have we settled on doing well enough?

None of these questions is easy to answer. The last question is potentially the trickiest, at least in my opinion. No one wants to look at themselves and say, "Wow! We've really settled and still managed to get things done." Not exactly the thought we all want to have about a profession we have poured so much of ourselves – individually and collectively – into. But we must. Reflecting on what we have settled on doing well enough is not necessarily a bad thing; no one is great at everything, after all.

One prime example of where we are currently settling for "good enough" is the veterinary teaching hospital (VTH). Our VTH model is great in theory, and it has certainly provided thousands – no, tens of thousands – of veterinarians an education of which they can be proud. New graduates have been able to walk out of schools with this traditional teaching model knowing what to look for and how to treat the many zebras we know of across species. They have been taught the "gold standard" of care when it comes to those zebras, and that was good enough for a long while. Until we started doing surveys of employers and realizing that while our new graduates were great at recognizing things like liver shunts and cardiac anomalies, rare neoplasias, and unusual fungal infections, most were unable to diagnose ear mites, demodectic mange, strangles, bloat, or hardware disease – though I will nod to the large, equine, and food animal folks and say that, in general, they have done a better job of preparing a truly general practice (GP)-ready graduate than those in the field where I practiced longest – small animal (primarily dogs and cats).

Unfortunately, our current VTH model is simply unsustainable. Veterinary programs have stuck relentlessly to the teaching hospital paradigm: there are currently 54 accredited veterinary schools around the world, 32 of which are located in the United States (30 are fully accredited, 2 are provisionally accredited as they have not yet graduated their first class of students at the time of this writing). Of those 32 programs, the vast majority have a VTH attached to it, through which the students rotate to learn about and acquire the skills needed to become a "day one" ready veterinarian. Or at least, this is what proponents of the VTH model would like you to believe. One only needs to read the scathing commentary by Dr. Robert Marshak (2015), to see at least one veterinarian with experience across the profession who believes the VTH is the only way to produce high-quality, well-trained veterinary graduates. And while Dr. Marshak certainly makes some excellent points, there are definitely some holes in his argument; let us consider the following quote:

> . . .the argument that teaching hospitals are unaffordable, and therefore obsolete, is bogus and a disservice to those teaching hospitals that are advancing clinical medicine and financially helping their parent institutions.

> Teaching hospitals are powerful magnets attracting the most gifted clinicians, interns, residents, veterinary and graduate students, and veterinary scientists. Largely through referrals, teaching hospitals attract the most perplexing clinical cases that are essential to challenging students' ability to develop and work through a differential diagnosis, consult the literature, and judiciously use laboratory tests and technical resources. (Marshak 2015, n.p.)

It is certainly true that VTHs provide excellent opportunities for advancing both bench science and clinical medicine, and that they provide a service to their communities that are not always found elsewhere. However, VTHs are no longer the "powerful magnets" Marshak refers to – while academic institutions writ large do not seem to be experiencing a shortage of applicants for tenure and nontenure track educators at all levels, veterinary medical colleges are experiencing significant shortages of *qualified applicants* who desire to work in an academic institution. Part of the reason for this is salary, but the biggest driver behind this is *quality of life*. Why would any veterinarian, particularly one who is specialty trained, want to work in a VTH for far less pay but more stress and working hours that are equal to or longer than they would be in private or corporate practice? Why would any veterinarian, particularly one who is specialty trained, want to work at a VTH, where they have to juggle a fragmented medical system, other faculty, staff, students, patients, and clients, when they could work in private practice and see more cases with less headaches?

Do not misunderstand me; there are still a good number of folks who decide they want to try academia out. Some of them make the leap after years in practice, while others (a decreasing few) choose to go directly into academia after their many years of education and training. But the shortage of veterinarians we are experiencing as of this writing (that has only continued to worsen over the last decade) is hitting academia particularly hard: for those graduating from veterinary school with an average student loan debt of over US$ 160,000 (and some students leaving with US$ 250,000 or more in loans), it is difficult to convince them to do an internship and residency, only to come back to academia to make far less than they could in practice – sometimes as much as 50% less, in fact – sometimes even a greater percentage less than that. (I recently learned of a colleague who left a CVM and is now working 20 hours a week making twice the salary they made as a full professor.) It is *this* that is the primary issue with VTHs – and what makes them untenable for the foreseeable future in my view.

But I also take to task Marshak's sentiment that students need "the most perplexing clinical cases that are essential to challenging students' ability to develop and work through a differential diagnosis, consult the literature and judiciously use laboratory tests and technical resources." While I absolutely agree that students need to be able to develop clinical reasoning skills, understand the value of diagnostic tests, and be comfortable using high-quality literature, this can be accomplished with cases that are less complex and prepare them for the real world of GP – regardless of species. The truth is that the majority of our students who run into one of those "perplexing cases" are most likely to either not be able to diagnose it or they will diagnose it and *refer them to a specialist* whenever possible. Thus, our students need to learn how to diagnose and treat the "horses" – the cases that are going to come in on a daily basis. In other words, not the kinds of cases routinely seen in a VTH by specialty-trained, and usually board-certified, veterinarians (the "perplexing cases," aka, the "zebras").

It is easy to forget how few veterinary specialists there really are – when you are a student you are surrounded by them, so you assume that a good chunk of veterinarians go on to specialty training, certification, and practice. But the reality is that only about 12% of veterinarians are board-certified specialists according to the AVMA, which means that VTHs are teaching specialty – often tertiary care – knowledge and skills to a very small fraction of students who will go on to become specialists themselves (Cima 2018). This is supported by the fact that, according to the AVMA, GPs make up about 66% of veterinary professionals (Lester 2021). I am not great at math, but those numbers fail to make sense to me: why would we invest 70% of our efforts into the 12% of students who will ultimately end up in specialty training and/or practice (that 12% has held fairly steady over the years, in case you are wondering – for one documented reason, that being the lack of residencies available – and likely for several other reasons I do not have the information to support). My point is, of the approximately 80% of veterinarians who are clinicians (the other 20% are working in academia in nonclinical roles, industry, government, public health, and the like), we are educating them on cases the vast majority will never manage in practice.

Granted, seeing ear mites in cats and navicular disease in horses is not going to challenge students for very long, but the first few times they see them, those types of GP cases will challenge them and create opportunities for them to engage in critical thinking, clinical reasoning, and consulting the literature as needed (see Chapter 6 and its section on clinical teaching). Diagnosing ear mites in cats is relatively straightforward, in fact, speaking as someone who has 10+ years of small animal GP under my belt. But the first time anyone diagnosis anything, it is going to challenge them – and there are plenty of cases in GP that will challenge folks on a regular basis. My first year in practice I managed complex DKA, IMHA, pancreatitis, diabetes mellitus, Cushing's disease, Addison's disease, and other

medicine cases – all cases GPs see and treat on a regular basis that are not usually seen in a tertiary care facility (though they certainly do occasionally show up). These cases were not necessarily perplexing to me, but they were still challenging, and they still made me think about what diagnostics I needed versus what I wanted, how I would communicate my recommendations and findings to my clients, and how such cases were best managed. Why would they not do the same for veterinary students?

Beyond this discussion and regardless of which side of the fence you fall on, based on the statistics alone it makes little sense for us to be hanging on to an antiquated model of veterinary education. Throw in the financial challenges (though this can be overcome) and the lack of human resources available to staff this traditional model, and this clinging to an ideal just does not hold water anymore. *We must evolve if we are to survive and thrive* – if it is good enough for Darwin's finches, it should be good enough for us.

To those out there reading this and fuming, maybe doing an Elmer Fudd steam session (apologies to those of you too young to understand this reference), please know that I am NOT saying we should dump VTHs. There are many reasons to keep VTHs – not the least of which include those points made by Marshak (2015), regarding their value in public service, fundraising, and scientific contributions. I would add that the specialists in VTHs are also an irreplaceable resource for the small (but steady) number of students who think they would like to become specialists themselves. The opportunity to work alongside and learn from board-certified specialists and residency-trained clinicians in a VTH is indispensable for those students, and incredibly important for the interns and residents who have already started down the specialty path. We are certainly seeing a growth in the number of private and corporate specialty clinics, to be sure, but not all of those are interested in training the next generation of specialists; in a VTH, that is a core part of the clinician's job.

Thus, VTHs are not the veterinary education apocalypse-inducing behemoths that some proponents of the distributive model may argue they are, but they are also not the only way we can train students to be competent veterinarians the day they graduate. As a graduate of a program that followed the VTH education model, I can say with complete honesty that I had great technical and patient care skills, but I had much to learn about being a "doctor." And this had little to do with the clinicians who taught me – it had to do with the model within which those clinicians had to teach. On the ladder of learning in a VTH, it starts with the clinician, steps down to the 3rd-year resident, 2nd-year resident, 1st-year resident, intern, credentialed technician, and then clinical student for those clerkships that are also training specialists, which is most of them.

Not an ideal learning situation that provides the students an opportunity to work on those "zebras" that present themselves.

Having already established that fewer veterinarians are entering academia, our inability to adequately staff and maintain VTHs also means we are often unable to provide the caseload and learning opportunities during clerkships that students need to become proficient. And even when we do have good caseloads, VTH models selectively (at least currently in the United States) teach specialty medicine and procedures most of the time – particularly in small animals, but in equine, production, and small ruminant animals as well. It has only really been in the last two or three decades that we have seen VTHs nod to GP – particularly in small animal (large animal, at least on the food animal side, has more traditionally focused on production medicine and herd health, which tends toward GP as a rule) – so that our students are provided the opportunity to handle and learn from cases the majority of them will see during their clinical careers. In fact, about 66% of our students (as you read in Chapter 6) go into GP, regardless of species type, which means we are spending 70% of our time teaching them on referral cases that most of them will never manage during their careers. The exception, as of just a couple of years ago, is the Royal Veterinary College, which has updated its graduation requirements to include a minimum of 38 weeks of extramural studies (EMS), 26 of which must be clinical practice oriented, meaning that just over 70% of RVC's clinical rotations must be completed in real, working practices – most of which are GP (RVC n.d.). This is an important shift that others using the VTH model should take note of and one that probably should have happened many years ago.

While this may feel like a bit of a soapbox, the stark reality is that we have fewer veterinary specialists desiring to go into academia and an outdated educational model that is moving itself toward obsolescence because it is so caught up in what it used to do that it is clinging to the past rather than working to become the future. The current system does not serve faculty, staff, or students well – which we are seeing manifest itself through increasing mental health issues in those same populations. My current program has two dedicated counselors for preclinical students and one full-time social worker who supports clinical faculty, staff, students, and clients – and all three of them are some of the busiest people I know. We have an epidemic of suicides and students who are taking anxiety meds just to get through school; we have faculty who are constantly asked to do more and more with less and less. And this is not limited to those running programs with VTHs; this is a profession-wide issue that starts well before veterinary school begins and continues well past graduation.

Part 1: If Not a VTH, Then What?

Having graduated from a top-tier veterinary program that educated me in the VTH tradition, I distinctly remember graduating and feeling like I was really well-trained in patient care and a number of technical skills, but I certainly lacked confidence in "doctoring." I understood how to write a detailed medical note and perform treatments, but still needed work on creating those treatment plans and figuring out appropriate diagnostic plans, too. In a VTH, finances are far less of a concern than they are in GP, yet we were never taught how to prioritize our diagnostics; that I had to figure out on my own.

Being an older student and, therefore, an older graduate, I was simply not willing to continue taking extremely low pay to work extremely high hours for another year, nor did I have any interest in specialty practice – I had entered veterinary school after already having a 10-year career that required me to work my way up from the bottom, and at 35 I was unwilling to start at the bottom again; four years of professional school was long enough. Although I had little desire to go into clinical practice, the few faculty positions I applied for were not offered to me, but the two veterinary jobs I applied for were. Did I go into shelter medicine, where my heart was, or private practice, where the caseload would be high and the salary higher? I chose the latter, facing US$ 140,000 in student loan debt and wanting to live like an adult.

While my first job ended on a sour note, I do like to say that I was provided an internship experience without the internship pay and hours. Oh, I worked a lot of hours, but I was also appropriately remunerated. I was an eager new graduate, hungry to learn and take on challenging cases that the seven other doctors in my practice were less enthusiastic about. My clinic was both a day and emergency practice, so I had the chance to take on overnights and manage complicated cases of medicine and surgery on a regular basis: GDVs, HBCs, and hemangiosarcomas; dietary indiscretions resulting in foreign bodies needing removal on the surgery side, in addition to those challenging medical cases previously presented. I became competent and confident after a few months and with each success because I had the help of seasoned doctors who were willing to answer my numerous questions and assist when asked.

But I was, in my anecdotal experience, the exception rather than the rule. I stayed in touch with several good friends and classmates who had very different experiences and commiserated with many a year after graduation when we ran into each other at a popular conference as we all worked to earn our required CE. Many had already quit their first jobs and moved on to another; several were unhappy but could not leave for a variety of reasons, and others felt as though they were just then feeling like "real doctors." For those of us brave enough to start our practice careers without additional training, it felt like we were doing OK but certainly could have been better prepared. It felt, at least to me, that my program – representative of the majority of programs – was trying to be good but was still going at it the wrong way and, therefore, was still settling for doing it "well enough."

Fast forward 15 years, and there are a few programs coming online that have decided to try something "new" – or at least new to veterinary medicine. The distributive model of clinical education is our new answer to training veterinary students; it decreases the overall costs associated with opening and operating a new school (at least in theory), gives students "real world" experience before they graduate, and decreases the need for retaining specialty trained clinicians who are increasingly difficult to attract and retain in traditional VTH-model programs. But it is still extremely expensive for students, and the quality of their clinical experiences varies vastly from practice to practice. The caseload is generally one that most students will see, but depending upon the veterinarians responsible for training the students, the amount of actual case management and quality of learning are highly variable. This is true of both medical and surgical cases, and particularly from the surgery standpoint, a lack of practice during the clinical year can increase the anxiety a graduate may experience once they have graduated.

Because of the challenges faced in achieving good quality control of participating practices, in some ways, the distributive model has caused us to revisit a problem we had already solved in the VTH model: the lack of general surgical experience before graduation (ovariohysterectomy and castration in cats and dogs; castrations in piglets, horses, cattle, sheep, and goats; c-sections in all animals; etc.). And, this model also places the burden of coordinating travel, lodging, and additional budgeting squarely upon the student during their third year of classroom-based studies – a time, I might argue, that is one of the most pivotal to their success. In short, while the distributive model certainly addresses some concerns associated with the VTH model, in some ways it just swaps one set of problems for another. But perhaps distributive model schools will become the norm and we will get better at quality control. Maybe students who go through such training will be better organized and more capable in the end because of the scheduling and logistical challenges they faced during their schooling. Human medical programs have, after all, been successfully training physicians this way for decades.

We have additional struggles that we have been ignoring or denying for far too long that are now spilling over and demanding attention as well. High rates of depression, anxiety, and yes, suicide. Incredibly high debt to income ratio for our new graduates, VTHs struggling to staff appropriately and overworking the staff we do have, from veterinarians to credentialed veterinary technicians to front desk receptionists. Too few schools recognizing that there is more to being a veterinarian than clinical practice and a licensing process that is fraught with issues and decreasingly serves the profession as a whole. We are still the whitest of all the healthcare professions and have yet to solve the puzzle of how to invite in and include those populations of underserved and underrepresented minorities – whether they be racial/ethnic, gender, neurodiverse, physically and/or mentally disabled, religious, or anything that is not the "norm," which has traditionally been set by and measured next to the middle or upper-class white male. Thus, even while we are a female-dominated profession, we are still primarily white and, in a group of around 115,000 strong and growing (slowly, but growing), we still see limited female leadership in industry, academia, and practice (to say nothing of the lack of other types of diversity).

And our clients are also being left behind; in the practicing world, the costs of owning and taking care of a pet or pleasure animal are separating the haves from the have nots. It is rapidly becoming an elitist endeavor to own a pet in the United States. So yes, our profession is struggling in many ways. Perhaps you do not see the direct connection between these struggles and veterinary education specifically; perhaps you do. Regardless of which side you fall on, the connection is most certainly there.

Overall, there are certainly many pieces of our profession that need to change for us to remain viable. Some are issues that VME cannot directly impact but could certainly be affected if we are willing and able to apply our creativity and passion to change it. Others are issues that are clearly tied to VME, and while there are arguments for each of the two current types of VME clinical training programs, I believe strongly that the wicked problem of VME must be met with equally wicked changes. One of those wicked changes is, perhaps, being more intentional in the education of our veterinary educators. We have already started this process through the creation of the Academy of Veterinary Educators (AVE), an organization that is already 500+ members strong with participants from all walks of the profession and from around the world. The steady increase in distributive models of veterinary education indicates to me that the profession is willing to change – perhaps it just needs a stronger push. The conversations are opening up around accreditation and what it should really do, and I increasingly hear folks willing to entertain the idea of species-specific licensure. These are hard conversations, but imperative ones if we are to move the veterinary profession.

Part 2: A Vision for the Future?

Where do YOU see the veterinary profession in 50 years? What will it look like? Take a moment to think about that – maybe even jot down some of your ideas. Depending on where you are in your career, your thoughts may be very different than your mentors or teachers or friends or administrators or. . .well, you get the idea. But that's OK. Variety is the spice of life, right? Regardless of the differences, I do hope there is at least one similarity – that being that we are still around as a profession and continuing to advance animal, human, and environmental health in ways we might not be able to predict now. But to do that, to stick around and continue to make the impact we are making now (or a bigger one – let us face it, we have a lot to offer!) – we *must* change. And the start point of that change must be in the academy – where every veterinarian begins their professional career.

Remember that veterinary schools are powerful. They are the gatekeepers of the profession – only those allowed to pass through these gates can ever legally call themselves a doctor of veterinary medicine; there is absolutely no other accepted path. Unlike being an educator, you cannot decide one day that you are a veterinarian, apply for a job, and get hired. There are years of training and rigorous assessments involved; mechanical and technical skills that must be acquired and repeatedly demonstrated; and a final, grueling exam that must be passed before the title of veterinarian is earned. You cannot simply watch another veterinarian for years, practice the skills you have observed while occasionally asking for help, and rely on experience to call yourself a doctor. *Yet we allow others and ourselves to do this every day when it comes to the profession of education.*

So perhaps, instead of focusing on whether traditional VTH versus distributive models are the best ways to educate our students and produce enough veterinarians to meet the ever-growing and urgent demand, we should be focusing on the crux of the problem: why are we fitting ourselves into an educational model that is failing to fit our needs? Consider this: we are adding medical knowledge at an increasingly rapid pace and finding skills and information our graduates need but have not acquired during their programs based on employer and new graduate surveys. Our response has always been, where do we put this in the curriculum? Admirable, but unsustainable in the current models – regardless of traditional or distributive. The Mythbusters once did a show to determine whether you could, indeed, put 10-lb of poop into a 5-lb bag. Not surprisingly, the only way they could achieve this feat was to fully dehydrate the poop. So, this begs the question: did they really fit 10-lb of poop into that 5-lb bag? Most reasonable people would say no – they just took out a big chunk of it to

make it fit! This is the perfect analogy for our current veterinary education conundrum: do we continue to try to pack 10-lb of poop into a 5-lb bag by dehydrating it and calling it good? Or do we *change the size of the bag so it can store the amount of poop we have to put in it?*

If all this talk of poop and bags bothers you, my apologies. Veterinarians talk about poop more than any other professional I know of – including gastroenterologists. My point is, we have been boxed into a four-year veterinary curriculum for far too long. The only variation on this theme in the last 100 years or so has been to compress the curriculum further – into three years – and it remains to be seen whether this experiment is as successful as the current progenitors predicted it would be. I have no answer for why four years has become the norm in the United States; I suspect it is based on the overall undergraduate model (which has increasingly adapted, by the way), and later it became the bedrock for the argument many made regarding the financial concerns of students (adding more years would only increase the burden on the student). I am not aware of any studies demonstrating this is actually true, but it certainly seems to make sense. But our system is crumbling and we are scrambling; rather than patching the wall, though, maybe it's time to tear it down and build it up brand new – stronger, more flexible, and capable of serving our students even better. I believe this is possible – it will just take someone, or a group of someones, who are brave enough to do it.

Part 3: My Vision for the Future

To start, we must become more flexible with our curricula. There are many ways to do this – and currently, the defense of our time fence is more about finances than it is about anything else. Understandably so, given the amount of debt US students are increasingly graduating with. However, there are ways to fit the content we currently squeeze into three or four years into more years with, potentially, less stress, less money, and more flexibility. Many of you have probably thought about a 2+ or 3+ curriculum (similar to the British system); some have perhaps thought of a curriculum similar to many human medical programs abroad that start students right after high school, going through a five- or six-year curriculum (similar, but not exactly the same as, the British system). But what about a part-time curriculum? What about a flex curriculum? What about a hybrid (virtual + face-to-face [F2F]) program? Let us explore each of these below.

If COVID taught us anything, it taught us that we need to be a bit more flexible, or flexibility will be forced upon us. Medical schools have been giving students the option to attend lecture-based classes for decades and have seen their students continue to be successful. Instead of being in a large classroom with potentially disruptive classmates and/or trying to act as if they are paying attention when, in fact, they are texting their _____ (fill in the blank), students have the option of organizing their day around the required activities they must attend (clinical skills labs, wet labs, etc.) and viewing lectures when it best suits them. For those who are early birds, this might mean doing so at 6 in the morning, when they are brightest and most energetic. For night owls, this might be midnight or 1 a.m., after they have had time to engage in the amount of sleep they need and socializing they wish to enjoy. Students are, first and foremost, people with lives – lives that we should respect, even if we cannot always accommodate them.

That is not to say that students should not be encouraged to attend class. If you have learned anything from this text, I hope you have concluded that research is emphatic in its finding that students who attend classes in person tend to learn more, retain more, and achieve more in the long run. The ability to have questions answered in real time, to get clarity on topics that might be slightly – or very – muddy, and to interact with classmates is incredibly impactful. It also helps build those professional relationships and networks that will sustain them throughout their careers – an incredibly important but often ignored part of the learning process. Additionally, the idea that we can replace the need to interact with people with floating faces on screens goes against the grain of all that we are as a species. To be sure, the vast amount of our sensory input comes through our visual cortex (80%, based on the literature), but there are four other senses as well – three of which are deprived of their use when we go virtual for learning or deliver content asynchronously. Feel, smell, taste – all three are involved with learning. Doubt it? Take a moment to reflect on a memory you hold sharply. What triggers that memory to flood? My guess is that it has to do with a certain smell, perhaps a favorite food, or the comfort that comes from the touch of someone – whether that someone is human or some other kind of animal. It is all the senses that help us learn; it is all the senses that play a role in our understanding of the world and the creatures that inhabit it.

That said, however, we must not neglect the fact that not everyone can make it to the classroom from 8a or 9a until 5p every day. Our students are people first and foremost, remember? Many have children, spouses, and families. Many come from backgrounds that have provided them with few opportunities to succeed, yet they have found a way to do so. But our educational system – from the time they graduate high school – throws higher and higher barriers in front of them. From figuring out how to navigate the government financial aid system to understanding how to advocate for their rights, the system is set up to challenge them in ways that often lead them to failure rather than success. So, what are some ways we can increase access to our programs? Increasing access is one way to increase diversity; it's awfully hard to think of yourself as a veterinarian (or lawyer, or physician, or. . .) when you do not see others who look like you or came from a background similar to yours.

Technology – and more specifically computer and internet technology – is definitely one answer. It is not the perfect one, of course, as there are still many in this country who lack access to one or the other, but it is certainly one tool we can and should better leverage in the veterinary profession. If we provide opportunities for students to attend virtually for topics (such as the basic sciences) that are traditionally taught via lecture, why should not students be able to do so in their comfy clothes with a cup of coffee (or a Coke) in their hands? Yes, learning science tells us that attending classes in person is generally the best way for adults to learn, but sometimes it is nice to just sit and listen, knowing you can go back later to catch that word or phrase you could not quite make out during the lecture. It might not be the answer to all the ills of educational access, but it is certainly one worth exploiting.

Let's go back to those students who have family or other obligations that sometimes dictate whether they are able to go back to school full time. If we offered a part-time program of study (the only other professional program I could find that did this was law school), we could offer some flexibility in attendance, potentially decrease their debt loads (they would be able to continue working while in school, so may not need to take out the maximum amounts offered to them through government funding), and might even help address the mental health crisis. If you had been able to take courses part time as a veterinary student, how might that have helped you? For me, I would have been able to learn at a slightly slower pace – something that would have been welcome as a 31-year-old student – and had the time to really review and dig into the information being delivered. I would not have had to sacrifice my study time for my mental and physical health time, something I made a conscious effort to do during school that resulted in lower grades but someone who (barely) made it through school feeling decent about myself. I would have the opportunity to truly master the information I needed to master to feel ready to tackle clinical rotations – not knowing it all, of course, but knowing enough that when asked a question during rounds I wasn't frozen in fear because I recognized the words but couldn't quite put it all together.

What if we offered a hybrid program? One where students were able to take their courses online and do their labs in person? How much more accessible might that be? Or perhaps we do offer those 2- or 3-plus four-year programs, where the pre-veterinary track has undergraduates studying the basic sciences and moving into the clinical applications in their first year of the professional program. My point is, we need to get creative with our approaches to veterinary education – the *entirety* of veterinary education – rather than just focusing on the VTH versus distributive model debate. Veterinary education is currently a 5-lb bag, and we need a bigger bag if we are to really serve our students well.

Section 4: Conclusion and Leaving Thoughts

It is not all gray skies and rain clouds. Lest we leave this chapter on a sad note, let us remember there are plenty of things we are doing well. We have built a reputation as a profession that has lasted well over a century – we are more trusted than most and respected the same. Our students are the best and the brightest and they continue to shine well in all walks of the veterinary halls. We help millions of pets and come out of veterinary school with knowledge of and skills in a multitude of species and content – from companion animals to farm animals to exotic pocket pets. We have some grasp of how to act professionally and run a business, know a bit about public health, and at least are aware of the best ways to communicate with clients and with each other. As a whole, we have an incredibly vast capacity to adapt and problem-solve in creative and rapid ways. Our colleagues are constantly growing, learning, and

stretching themselves to do more – and we already do a *lot*. Exhibit A – you are reading a book about an entirely new discipline, because you have recognized a need and discovered a passion for not settling, for rectifying our failures, and for ensuring that moving forward we educate our students better than we ever have before. That is something to brag about; *this* is something to be proud of.

I am thrilled that you are reading this book and excited (I hope) to apply your new-found knowledge in your classrooms, labs, clinics, and hospitals (teaching or otherwise). I am so hopeful as I see our profession finally coming around to the idea that education is not just something we decide to do one day – it is something that requires learning about, training in, and practice. It is amazing that we have the AVE, which is in the process of establishing a credentialing process for those veterinary educators who desire to be recognized as experts in the field (some of you may already be recognized as such by the AVE). But I want you to do more! I want you to consider how knowing about education can help veterinary medical programs evolve and embrace the future; I want you to use your knowledge and begin applying it in a way that not only makes our profession better but also pushes our profession beyond its comfort zone and addresses the biggest elephant in the room: our current educational model is simply unsustainable. This is the thought I will leave you with; this is the challenge I put forth to you. In its simplest form, it comes down to this: What is your vision for the future of our profession 50 years from now, and how must we educators change and influence others to change so that we can get there?

References

Cima, G. (26 September 2018). Specialists in short supply: Universities, private practices struggle to find certain specialists, blame lack of residency training programs. https://www.avma.org/javma-news/2018-10-15/specialists-short-supply (accessed on 23 February 2023).

Frakt, A. (5 Jun 2017). Teaching hospitals cost more, but they could save your life. https://www.nytimes.com/2017/06/05/upshot/teaching-hospitals-cost-more-but-could-save-your-life.html#:~:text=About%2026%20percent%20of%20hospitals,over%20half%20of%20all%20admissions (accessed 2 March 2023).

Lau, E. (2018). Survey: majority of veterinarians don't recommend the profession. Study finds young practitioners struggling. *VIN News Service* https://news.vin.com/default.aspx?pid=210&Id=8421012&f5=1 (accessed 13 March 2023).

Lester, B. (2021). 'Just' a GP General practitioners are the heart and soul of veterinary medicine, so stop discounting their career choice. https://todaysveterinarybusiness.com/gp-veterinary-medicine (accessed 23 February 2023).

Marshak, R. (13 July 2015). Long live the veterinary teaching hospital: distributive model puts profession on path toward economic decline, mediocrity. https://news.vin.com/default.aspx?pid=210&catId=14426&id=6869519 (accessed 2 March 2023).

Rittel, H.W.J. and Webber, M.M. (1973). Dilemmas in a general theory of planning. *Policy Sciences* 4 (2): 155–169. http://www.jstor.org/stable/4531523.

Royal Veterinary College (n.d.). EMS Policy and accompanying guidance. www.rcvs.org.uk/lifelong-learning/students/veterinary-students/extra-mural-studies-ems/ems-policy-and-accompanying-guidance (accessed 23 February 2023).

Index

Note: Page numbers followed by *f* indicates figure and *t* indicates table.

Educational Principles and Practice in Veterinary Medicine, First Edition. Edited by Katherine Fogelberg.
© 2024 John Wiley & Sons, Inc. Published 2024 by John Wiley & Sons, Inc.